JUST SO[ME] [OF] [THE]
GROUNDBREAKING ALTERNATIVE USES
DESCRIBED IN THIS BOOK

WELLBUTRIN
A popular antidepressant also prescribed
to treat chronic lower back pain.

BOTOX
This popular cosmetic injection also can relieve
severe headaches and migraines.

XANAX
Can relieve irritable bowel syndrome
as well as anxiety disorders.

PROZAC and ZOLOFT
These two popular antidepressants can relieve
the symptoms of menopause.

FOSAMAX
This well-known osteoporosis medication
can also aid with spinal cord trauma.

CELEXA
This antidepressant can also help
the emotional symptoms associated
with Alzheimer's disease dementia.

NEURONTIN
A drug developed to treat seizures
that can relieve painful cluster headaches.

PRESCRIPTION DRUGS

Alternative Uses, Alternative Cures

Over 1,500 New Uses
for FDA-Approved Drugs

KEVIN LOUGHLIN, M.D.
Medical Editor-in-Chief
JOYCE GENERALI, M.S., R.Ph.
Pharmaceutical Editor-in-Chief

Amjad Almahameed, M.D., Alina Bridges, D.O., Kevin Brown, M.D., Diana Dell, M.D., Michael Dempsey, D.O., J.C. Garbutt, M.D., Daniel Hinthorn, M.D., Ahmet Höke, M.D., Ph.D., Frieda Hulka, M.D., Priya Jamidar, M.D., A. Lawrence Ossias, M.D., Ernesta Parisi, D.M.D., Omega Silva, M.D.

Produced by The Philip Lief Group, Inc.

PREVIOUSLY PUBLISHED AS
The Guide to Off-Label Prescription Drugs

POCKET BOOKS
New York London Toronto Sydney

Pocket Books
A Division of Simon & Schuster, Inc.
1230 Avenue of the Americas
New York, NY 10020

Produced by The Philip Lief Group, Inc.
130 Wall Street
Princeton, NJ 08450
www.TPLG.org

Cover design by Janet Perr
Cover photograph by Jupiter Images

Manufactured in the United States of America

10 9 8 7 6 5 4 3

ISBN-13: 978-0-7432-8671-8
ISBN-10:   0-7432-8671-5

Contents

PART II: Drug Profiles

PART III: Drug Information

Medical Contributors and Consultants

MEDICAL EDITOR-IN-CHIEF
Kevin Loughlin, M.D. is at Brigham and Women's Hospital, a teaching hospital of Harvard Medical School. He has been selected for "Best Doctors in America" and "Top Doctors" by The Center for the Study of Services in Washington, D.C. He currently serves as the Director of Urologic Research. Dr. Loughlin has published more than 200 articles, abstracts, and letters in publications such as *New England Journal of Medicine, Journal of Urology*, and *Laboratory Medicine*. He lives in Boston, MA, with his wife and three children.

PHARMACEUTICAL EDITOR-IN-CHIEF
Joyce Generali, M.S., R.Ph. is Director of the Drug Information Residency Program and of the Drug and Information Center at Kansas University Medical Center. The center's international mission is to provide information regarding accurate drug therapy that is current and unbiased. She is also a clinical professor at Kansas University and a member of *Woman's Day* Health Advisory Panel and *Medzine* Health Panel. She is the author of ten books for doctors and pharmacists including the *Technician's Pocket Drug Reference, Drug Reaction Alerts*, and *Pharmacy Examination Review Book*.

MEDICAL ADVISORY BOARD
Amjad Almahameed, M.D.
Division of Vascular Medicine in the Department of Cardiovascular Medicine, Cleveland Clinic Heart Center

Alina G. Bridges, D.O.
Division of Dermatology, Mayo Clinic, Rochester, MN

Kevin K. Brown, M.D.
Director, Clinical Interstitial Lung Disease Program, National Jewish Medical and Research Center

Diana Dell, M.D., FACOG
Assistant Professor, Department of Psychiatry and Behavioral

Health and Department of Obstetrics and Gynecology, Duke University Medical Center

Michael Dempsey, D.O.
Private Practice, Physical Medicine and Rehabilitation

James C. Garbutt, M.D.
Professor of Psychiatry, University of North Carolina at Chapel Hill

Daniel Hinthorn, M.D., FACP
Professor of Internal Medicine, Pediatrics, and Family Medicine; Director, Division for Infectious Diseases, University of Kansas Medical Center

Ahmet Höke, M.D., Ph.D.
Assistant Professor of Neurology, The Johns Hopkins University School of Medicine

Frieda Hulka, M.D.
Clinical Assistant Professor, University of Nevada School of Medicine; Private Practice General Surgery, Reno, Nevada

Priya A. Jamidar, M.D.
Assistant Professor of Medicine, Director of Interventional Endoscopy Section of Digestive Diseases, Department of Internal Medicine, Yale University School of Medicine

A. Lawrence Ossias, M.D.
Private Practice; Assistant Attending Physician, Mount Sinai Medical Center

Ernesta Parisi, D.M.D.
Assistant Professor, Division of Oral Medicine, UMDNJ-New Jersey Dental School

Omega Silva, M.D., FACP
Professor Emeritus of Medicine, George Washington University; Medical Review Officer, Employee Health Programs, Bethesda, MD

EDITORIAL STAFF

Senior Editor: Leslie Meredith

Managing Editor: Judy Capodanno

Project Editor: Albry Montalbano

Contributing Writers: Diana Benzaia, Karen Golebowski, Kristen Golebowski, Jan Green, Celeste May Krauss, Pauline Lerner, Jennifer LiMarzi, Deborah J. Shuman

Pharmaceutical Researchers: Jillian Ast, Clinton Boor, Kent Brand, Nicole Brand, Amy Braun, Lisa Buchholz, Maggie Carey, Lucy Carter, Lindsay Coombs, Josh Coppersmith, Scott Craig, Joseph Dellalo, Cori Dirickson, Ryan Doyle, Valerie Emming, Allison Fetter, Morissa Friesen, Lela Fung, Laura Gampper, Vernessa Griffin, Jenny Hu, Wisam Kandah, Tim Kerr, Jessica Koerner, Lindsey Leiker, Brandi McCullough, Susan Meadows, Phiyen Nguyen, Tuan Nguyen, Vinh Nguyen, Whitney Owecke, Jamie Patel, Amy Perry, Mandy Petz, Jennifer Ploetz, Sara Rangust, Catarina Rozman, Brandon Schminke, Kezia Schweiterman, Frank Tra, Hiue Tran, Joseph Truong, Brandy Williams

Medical Researchers: Priscilla Chung, Kimberly Lee, Patricia Volin, Joanne Yi, Jenn Yoo

Editorial Associate: Marybeth Fedele

Chief Copyeditor: Jon Bowen

Design and Production Director: Annie Jeon

Introduction

As consumers we make decisions every day. We check the ingredients before choosing a particular brand of cereal; we compare cars before buying a new one; and we check reviews before taking in a Friday night movie. So, if we go through such lengths to make the right decisions about our everyday indulgences, shouldn't we take the same care when making decisions about the prescription drugs we take? Now, fortunately, with *Prescription Drugs: Alternatives Uses, Alternative Cures*, we can.

Before a prescription drug hits the market, it must be studied in clinical trials and undergo rigorous evaluation by the Food and Drug Administration for a specified use. Once approved, this is called the "on-label" use. However, it is increasingly common for researchers and physicians to discover that some drugs also have benefits when used for "off-label" indications, *additional* uses beyond what the FDA first approved. For example, the popular drug Rogaine (generically known as *minoxidil*), was originally approved to treat high blood pressure. However, when it was used for this purpose, researchers and doctors discovered that the drug also spurred hair growth in bald men. Eventually, Rogaine became widely prescribed for this secondary use.

Prescribing drugs for off-label use is legal, and physicians are doing it more often each year. **Today, 1 out of every 4 prescriptions written is off-label** and most physicians agree that prescribing off-label drugs is a vital tool in their arsenal for managing patient care. *Prescription Drugs* is designed to be an equally vital tool for patients: the first guide of its kind to provide a comprehensive, up-to-date overview of the breakthrough off-label uses of prescription drugs, so you can know the facts about what your doctor is prescribing to you and be used as an important resource to initiate discussions with your doctor.

The information provided in this book is intended to help you make more informed decisions with your doctors about which prescription drugs you are putting into your body. So, if your doctor prescribes Effexor (generically known as *venlafaxine*), a popular antidepressant, to treat hot flashes associated with menopause or breast cancer—now you can find out why. With this book you can learn about the independent studies and clinical trials that have been performed to test Effexor for hot flashes. You can read about the results from published data, possible risks, and the success rate for the drug used for this purpose, and whether it has been widely studied. With this information in hand—information you would not otherwise have—you can work in tandem with your doctor and decide what course of treatment is best for you.

The book will also help you learn about different off-label options that may work for you. Suppose you suffer from migraines. Your physician has prescribed a number of different on-label prescriptions, but none has worked for you. One makes you so drowsy you cannot function. Another is effective but makes you very nauseated. A third alternative doesn't have any significant side effects, yet it does nothing to ease your pain. After many frustrating months of taking ineffective medication, you turn to *Prescription Drugs*, go to the "Brain and Nervous System" chapter, and peruse the "Migraine" section. Here, you find a variety of breakthrough off-label options: one of them is Botox (*botulinum toxin type A*). Botox is approved by the FDA for a popular use: "Temporary Improvement of Moderate to Severe Facial Lines." Yet along the way, doctors began to find that some of their patients who used Botox for cosmetic reasons also experienced fewer migraines. However, you might be hesitant about its effectiveness for migraines and have questions such as: Have independent studies been conducted for the use of this drug for migraines? What were the results? When tested for this off-label use, did it help one population more than another? Are there any particular risks, side effects, or contraindications? But with this resource guide that includes selected information about recent independent studies and results, you can initiate a discussion regarding the possibility of Botox with your doctor, and, ultimately, make an informed decision on whether it might be a viable possibility for you. By consulting *Prescrip-*

tion Drugs, you can be more proactive in becoming informed about your healthcare.

What Is the Definition of "Off-Label"?

The term "off-label" has a fairly broad definition. Technically, a drug is being prescribed off-label anytime it is used in a way that is different from what is indicated on the package insert, or as it is more officially known, the product labeling. Most often, that designation refers to instances where a medication is prescribed for a condition that is different from the one for which it received FDA approval. But sometimes, drugs are given in a different dosage, particularly when prescribed for a different segment of the population, such as children or pregnant women, and those instances are also considered off-label uses of the drug. Whenever the patient designation, condition, dosage, or type of administration is different from what is specifically indicated in FDA-approved labeling—this, too, is considered an "off-label" use.

Originally, the phrase "off-label" referred not only to "off-label" use of medications but also to "unlabeled," "unapproved," or "nonapproved" uses. Since these terms are misleading—creating the erroneous impression that the FDA evaluated these drugs and disapproved of their use—the expression "off-label" has become the preferred term for this type of drug therapy, and has made its way into the medical lexicon because it is far more accurate.

And what do doctors think of prescribing drugs off-label? In one recent survey, virtually all of the respondents regard this practice as a vital alternative in optimizing patient care in some cases. "There is a direct relationship between the physician and patient, and off-label options allow a more accurate choice of alternative medications to be used in the medical treatment," say Drs. Alexander Tabarrok and Daniel B. Klein. And doctors emphatically agree: in one national survey, over 500 were asked, "What would be your position on a proposal to change FDA law so that physicians could NOT prescribe drugs for off-label use?" An overwhelming 94% said they would be opposed to such a change. Researchers, doctors, and other medical professionals see several key advantages to allowing off-label applications for existing drugs. First, with careful evaluation of published data and a critical assessment of the benefit-risk ratio, it offers physicians more latitude and the ability to customize their approach to patients' needs. Secondly, off-label use may offer alternatives for patients who have not responded to conventional therapy.

In recent years, doctors have been prescribing off-label drugs with more and more frequency. For example, in 1998, health-care professionals wrote an estimated 58 million prescriptions off-label. Just five years later, in 2003, that number virtually doubled—reaching an unprecedented 115 million. In monetary terms, that is nearly 13 billion dollars spent on off-label drugs. If that number continues to grow (and every indication suggests it will), the need for patient knowledge and awareness of these expanded off-label drug options will be increasingly important.

In fact, it's likely that you have taken an off-label medication sometime—or many times—without even realizing it. Though the overall average for off-label use is about 25%, that figure is estimated to be as high as 50 to 90% for certain types of medications. Common disorders such as Lyme disease, insomnia, arthritis, osteoporosis, PMS, diabetes, fibromyalgia, high blood pressure, and allergies are all being successfully treated with off-label prescription drugs.

What You Will Find in This Book

Prescription Drugs is organized in a user-friendly format, with all data handily cross-referenced so you can find information either by ailment (Part One) or by drug (Part Two), and additional pertinent drug information in Part Three.

In Part One—the section organized by ailment—breakthrough off-label drug possibilities are listed for each disorder within a main chapter; this section includes a summary of selected medical research findings (from studies, trials, and other reputable sources) that explain the use of the drug, how the medication works for the particular illness, and results from studies. Part Two offers abbreviated profiles of the drugs mentioned in the book—including their FDA-approved indications, their off-label uses, food and drug interactions, side effects, and important warnings. Part Three provides several useful lists of additional drug information, including recently approved FDA drugs, sugar-free drug products, alcohol-free drug products, and more.

A medical advisory board comprised of highly qualified physicians and pharmaceutical experts—representing a wide variety of medical specialties—has reviewed the medical data and information provided. The medical advisory board chose drugs that had the most data on their off-label use including clinical trials and private and independent studies. Results for the included trials are reported, including how effective the drugs were and what side effects occurred. Not all the drugs included here are the best current therapy, but the advisory board wanted to include the most up-to-date information available. The information on the studies is from a vast array of medical journals, periodicals, and other published sources.

These findings reflect scientific data—they *are not* meant to be interpreted as an endorsement that a particular medication is superior to other available therapies or that it will be effective in your particular therapy. That decision must be made by a health professional who is familiar with your medical history and conditions and will gather more data before making a decision. The inclusion of a drug does not mean that it is necessarily recommended, nor does the exclusion of a drug mean that it is not recommended. It is important to note that not all risk and safety information may be addressed in the reviewed studies. Other information in this guide comes from some of the foremost health information organizations nationwide, such as the National Institutes of Health, the American Diabetes Association, the American Heart Association, and the American Urological Association.

What You Will Not Find in This Book—And Why

As you peruse the pages of *Prescription Drugs*, you will find that the entries are comprehensive but not complete—that is, they offer detailed profiles of off-label uses for certain medicines but not for every drug available for every imaginable malady. One of the most noteworthy exceptions is drugs related to the treatment of cancer. Cancer-related drugs are truly a subspecialty all their own, and it would require a separate volume to cover the topic adequately. In addition, cancer therapies are fast changing, and experimental treatment is widespread. Also, we have not provided dosages for any of the drugs in either Part I or Part II as, especially for off-label uses, doctors may try different dosages according to your medical history and needs.

How to Use This Book

You can find information either by the illness in question or by the medication.

Part I is organized into 20 chapters by the system of the body, with ailments associated with that main topic. Part II offers a compendium of corresponding drug profiles in alphabetical order by generic drug name.

Each ailment section in Part I includes a brief description of a particular disorder, organized alphabetically within the chapter, followed by individual entries of all the currently appropriate off-label drugs that might be used to treat that disorder. Under every ailment listed, you'll find, first, the "Commonly Prescribed (On-Label)" drugs approved to treat the ailment, then, the generic and brand names of each relevant "Off-Label Prescription Breakthrough Option" drug, its off-label use, complete with a concise explanation of how/why the drug may act in this particular off-label application and any special studies that discuss the drug's effectiveness in its off-label use.

Part Two includes a profile for drugs listed in Part One— over 400 medications. Each individual profile gives an up-to-date summary about the drug, including uses for approved indications, side effects, interactions with other drugs, herbs, or foods, and warnings. These data, although comprehensive, are not complete, and you should consult your doctor prior to making any changes in therapy.

How to Talk to Your Doctor

Of course, *Prescription Drugs* is not intended to be a self-diagnostic tool. Nor should this book be a substitute for the expertise of a physician. Your doctor is best equipped to assess symptoms and prescribe treatment based on your personal medical history, a physical examination, and diagnostic tests. Patients should always consult a physician before discontinuing a prescription drug or starting any drug treatment.

Prescription Drugs offers both the generic and brand name options for each drug. The inclusion of specific brand names does not imply that these specific products were used in the summarized trials nor that the products are equivalent, but are provided as a helpful guide for you to become familiar with the drug names. It is up to your doctor to decide which brand might work best for you. (This book also includes a user-friendly index of generic drug names, brand names, and drug class names.)

In today's health care environment, both patients and physicians know how important it is for every patient to become better informed about the treatments he or she receives. Patients must also become more active in determining their own treatment options. To do this, they need sound medical information. And a lot of patients do try to find that information. In a 2005 New York Times/CBS News poll of 1,111 adults, 44% of those who had received a diagnosis said they sought additional information about their condition from sources other than their doctor such as the Internet, TV broadcasts, pharmaceutical advertising, and sometimes absorbing frightening bits of incomplete or misleading information. But this way of gathering information can be overwhelming and confusing. *Prescription Drugs* is designed to help readers, patients, and all medical health consumers cut through the welter of health claims to the essential facts they need.

It's important for you to have a good relationship with your health care provider—a relationship that welcomes open, honest, and educated dialogue. With *Prescription Drugs*, you can start that dialogue and feel secure that you have the best information available to decide with your doctor the course that is right for you.

—Dr. Kevin Loughlin
Brigham and Women's Hospital
Harvard Medical School Teaching Hospital

PART I

AILMENTS AND DISORDERS

BRAIN AND NERVOUS SYSTEM DISORDERS

Alzheimer's Disease

Alzheimer's disease, a neurological condition that affects an estimated four million people nationwide, results in the death of nerve cells in the brain. Symptom onset begins gradually, often as mild forgetfulness, and may be falsely attributed to normal aging. As the disease progresses cognitive abilities decrease, people are unable to make decisions or perform everyday tasks, and some patients may undergo personality changes. In its later stages, Alzheimer's disease causes dementia and ultimately death.

Commonly Prescribed (On-Label) Drugs: *Donepezil, Galantamine, Memantine, Rivastigmine, Tacrine*

OFF-LABEL PRESCRIPTION DRUGS
BREAKTHROUGH OPTIONS

Generic: **Aripiprazole** *(ay-ri-PIP-ray-zole)*
Brand: **Abilify**

Aripiprazole belongs to the class of drugs known as antipsychotics and is used mainly for schizophrenia and schizoaffective disorder. It works to control psychotic symptoms by regulating two key brain chemicals associated with emotional health, serotonin and dopamine. By interacting with these brain chemicals, aripiprazole adjusts and restores balance to the levels of serotonin and dopamine in the brain.

There is evidence that aripiprazole may be useful in treating Alzheimer's patients who exhibit psychotic symptoms. A 10-week study of 208 patients with Alzheimer's disease–associated psychosis in *Journal of Clinical Psychopharmacology* compared the safety, effectiveness, and tolerability of aripiprazole versus placebo. The aripiprazole group showed significant reduction in psychosis symptoms, suggesting that this drug is safe and well tolerated.

For more information see page 1025.

Generic: *Atorvastatin* (a-TORE-va-stat-in)
Brand: *Lipitor*

Atorvastatin belongs to the class of drugs called HMG-CoA reductase inhibitors, more commonly known as statins. It is used to lower cholesterol, primarily LDL cholesterol or "bad" cholesterol, which is responsible for the development of arterial plaque leading to a heart attack or stroke. Unlike other statins, atorvastatin can also reduce fat levels, another risk factor for heart disease. Statins prevent the liver from producing cholesterol by blocking the cholesterol production enzyme.

Laboratory evidence shows that the cholesterol-induced production of a neurotoxin may precipitate Alzheimer's disease. Therefore, by reducing the production of cholesterol by using a cholesterol-lowering statin, the production of this neurotoxin may also decrease, potentially slowing the progression of Alzheimer's disease.

In a clinical trial, patients with mild to moderate Alzheimer's disease received atorvastatin calcium or placebo. The study found that reducing the circulation cholesterol levels improved measurements of Alzheimer's disease compared with placebo. However, these data, while encouraging, were not deemed statistically significant. Researchers believe the results of the study are promising, but additional clinical trials are needed to establish further the role of atorvastatin in treating Alzheimer's.

For more information see page 1030.

Generic: *Buspirone* (byoo-SPYE-rone)
Brand: *BuSpar*

Buspirone is an antianxiety medication used to treat anxiety disorders or short-term symptoms of anxiety. It works by stimulating nerve cells and altering neurochemically transmitted messaging. Unlike the more commonly prescribed antianxiety medications in the benzodiazepine class, you will not feel the effects of this therapy until after two or more weeks of treatment.

In Alzheimer's disease, buspirone is thought to alleviate depression and psychosis that complicate dementia. Studies of its use in Alzheimer's disease are very limited, but in an evaluation of studies, approximately 40% of patients had a positive response to buspirone.

For more information see page 1061.

Generic: **Carbamazepine** (kar-ba-MAZ-e-peen)
Brands: **Carbatrol, Epitol, Tegretol, Tegretol XR**

Carbamazepine is used to control seizures in epilepsy, to relieve pain due to trigeminal neuralgia, and in the treatment of mania and bipolar disorders. In Alzheimer's disease, this drug may modify brain chemical (neurotransmitter) activity.

Several small studies suggest that carbamazepine may reduce agitation in people with dementia including Alzheimer's patients. In a six-week study, 21 patients with Alzheimer's disease who had been previously and unsuccessfully treated with antipsychotics received either carbamazepine or placebo. Researchers followed up with patients at six weeks, evaluated them using a variety of psychiatric scales, and found significant improvements in symptoms of Alzheimer's disease, although the hallucination evaluation favored the placebo group. The study provided support for initial reports of the efficacy of carbamazepine in improving and stabilizing hostility in patients with Alzheimer's disease; however, additional long-term studies are needed to extend these findings.

For more information see page 1068.

Generic: **Citalopram** (sye-TAL-oh-pram)
Brand: **Celexa**

Citalopram, from the class of drugs known as selective serotonin reuptake inhibitors or SSRIs, is used to treat depression and acts to restore the brain's chemical balance by increasing the supply of the neurotransmitter serotonin. It acts as an emotional stabilizer and, theoretically, may be effective in treating many of the symptoms associated with Alzheimer's disease.

A study of 98 people in *British Journal of Psychiatry* evaluated the clinical efficacy of citalopram versus placebo in Alzheimer's patients. After four weeks, patients treated with citalopram showed a significant reduction in emotional bluntness, confusion, irritability, anxiety, fear/panic, depressed mood, and restlessness. Only very few, mild side effects were reported. Another study of citalopram in patients with Alzheimer's disease and dementia found similar results with the drug reducing emotional disturbance symptoms, but showing no improvement in psychomotor and cognitive behavior. Both studies were small, but indicate promise in the treatment of emotional symptoms associated with Alzheimer's disease dementia.

For more information see page 1096.

Generic: **Divalproex** *(DI-val-PROE-ix)*
Brands: **Depakote Delayed Release, Depakote ER, Depakote Sprinkle**

Divalproex is an anticonvulsant drug used in the treatment of manic episodes associated with bipolar disorder, complex partial seizures associated with epilepsy, and for the prevention of migraine headaches. Although how it works has not yet been established, its activity may be related to increased brain levels of gamma-aminobutyric acid (GABA).

In patients with Alzheimer's disease, divalproex seems to reduce behavioral agitation, a common manifestation of dementia. In a 10-patient study, patients were started on divalproex sodium and evaluated between two to five weeks. Of the ten patients enrolled, five patients showed improvement, which suggests that divalproex may be effective for behavioral agitation in elderly patients with dementia; however, larger studies are needed.

For more information see page 1147.

Generic: **Fluoxetine** *(floo-OKS-e-teen)*
Brands: **Prozac, Prozac Weekly, Sarafem**

Fluoxetine is an antidepressant from the selective serotonin reuptake inhibitor (SSRI) class, used to treat depression, obsessive-compulsive disorder (OCD), bulimia nervosa, premenstrual dysphoric disorder, and panic disorder. Compared to other SSRIs fluoxetine has a strong energizing effect, making it highly effective for treating depressed mood and lack of energy.

There have been several studies and case reports of fluoxetine treating Alzheimer's disease symptoms. One study reported success with fluoxetine for six months in the treatment of severe obsessive-compulsive symptoms in an Alzheimer's disease patient. Another researcher reported that fluoxetine also exhibited positive mental reasoning effects in treating depression in people with Alzheimer's.

For more information see page 1192.

Generic: **Gabapentin** *(GA-ba-pen-tin)*
Brand: **Neurontin**

Gabapentin is used to manage post-herpetic neuralgia in adults and partial seizures associated with epilepsy. It has also been used to control agitation and aggression in people with dementia based on the rationale that certain anticonvulsant medications have positive effects in reducing mania and aggressive behavior.

While no specific studies of gabapentin in the treatment of Alzheimer's disease patients have been conducted, several case reports and studies have reviewed gabapentin in treating elderly patients with dementia. In a 24-patient, two-year review published in *American Journal of Geriatric Psychiatry*, researchers analyzed gabapentin's effects on aggressive and agitated behaviors in nursing home patients diagnosed with dementia. Seventeen of 22 patients were deemed much or greatly improved, four were minimally improved, and only one was noted as unchanged. Two of the patients had to discontinue use of gabapentin due to excessive sedation, but no other significant side effects were reported. Further data are needed to support the findings of the study.

For more information see page 1206.

Generic: **Haloperidol** *(ha-loe-PER-i-dole)*
Brands: **Haldol, Haldol Decanoate**

Haloperidol is used to treat psychotic disorders and control tics and vocal utterances associated with Tourette's syndrome. It works by interfering with the effects of brain chemicals on the nerves. Haloperidol has had some success in treating Alzheimer's disease–related psychosis and delusions. One study showed that neuroleptic drugs such as haloperidol resolve delusions and psychotic behavior in about 20% more patients than placebo; however, there is limited evidence of one neuroleptic being superior than another. Another study compared high-dose haloperidol, low-dose haloperidol, and placebo in 71 people with Alzheimer's disease and psychosis or disruptive behavior. High-dose haloperidol produced a 30% greater improvement in symptoms than low-dose or placebo; however, 20% of patients receiving the high dose experienced tremors, restlessness, and muscle contractions.

For more information see page 1217.

*Generic: **Olanzapine** (oh-LAN-za-peen)*
*Brands: **Zyprexa, Zyprexa Zydis***

Olanzapine belongs to the class of drugs known as atypical antipsychotics. In tablet form, it is used in the treatment of schizophrenia, acute bipolar mania, and bipolar disorder. In injection form, olanzapine is used to treat agitation associated with schizophrenia and bipolar mania. The most common side effects associated with olanzapine are a feeling of being unable to sit still, constipation, dizziness, drowsiness, objectionable behavior, orthostatic hypotension, and weight gain.

In people with Alzheimer's disease, olanzapine has been shown to be an effective treatment for psychotic behavior. Low doses are more effective than higher doses. An eight-week trial published in *Journal of Neuropsychiatry & Clinical Neurosciences* study found that olanzapine may be beneficial for Alzheimer's disease patients experiencing neuropsychiatric symptoms.

For more information see page 1381.

*Generic: **Paroxetine** (pa-ROKS-e-teen)*
*Brands: **Paxil, Paxil CR***

Paroxetine, an antidepressant in the class of drugs called selective serotonin reuptake inhibitors (SSRIs), is used to manage depression, obsessive-compulsive disorder, panic disorder, and premenstrual dysphoric disorder. It blocks the reuptake of serotonin by the nerves that release it, an action that allows more serotonin to be available to be taken up by other nerves.

Data is limited about paroxetine in the treatment of people with Alzheimer's disease. Some reports say it is successful in reducing agitation in Alzheimer's disease patients. In a study of patients with coexisting depression and dementia, paroxetine reduced the severity of illness and showed global improvement at weeks two, four, eight and at the study's conclusion. The study found paroxetine to be effective and well tolerated.

For more information see page 1395.

Generic: **Quetiapine** *(kwe-TYE-a-peen)*
Brand: **Seroquel**

Quetiapine is in the class of drugs known as atypical antipsychotic and is used in treating schizophrenia and mania associated with bipolar disorder.

In a study, 333 patients with Alzheimer's disease, vascular dementia, or mixed dementia and severe clinical symptoms of agitation received quetiapine or placebo. A total of 219 patients completed the 10-week study, which found that quetiapine reduced agitation in elderly patients with Alzheimer's disease without leading to a decline in mental function. Fifty-seven percent of patients were noted as much improved or very much improved, compared to 32% in the placebo group. Quetiapine was generally well tolerated.

For more information see page 1440.

Generic: **Risperidone** *(ris-PEER-i-dohn)*
Brands: **Risperdal, Risperdal M-TAB**

Risperidone is an antipsychotic medication that works by interfering with several brain chemicals. Side effects with risperidone are usually mild and may include insomnia, hypotension, weight gain, and extrapyramidal symptoms.

Several studies have been conducted to evaluate the effects of risperidone in the treatment of aggression, agitation, and psychosis associated with dementia and Alzheimer's disease. In one clinical trial, 345 elderly patients received placebo or risperidone for a 12-week period. The study found that low-dose risperidone resulted in significant improvement in aggression, agitation, and psychosis associated with dementia. These results have been repeated in other smaller studies with good drug tolerability.

For more information see page 1456.

Generic: **Sertraline** *(SER-tra-leen)*
Brand: **Zoloft**

Sertraline belongs to the drug class known as selective serotonin reuptake inhibitors (SSRIs), which change the level of serotonin in the brain. It is used to treat depression, obsessive-compulsive disorder, panic disorder, and post-traumatic stress.

Several studies have evaluated sertraline in the treatment of Alzheimer's disease–related symptoms. One study of 44 people with Alzheimer's disease–related depression showed that, in the sertraline-treated group, 38% of patients responded positively, 46% partially responded, compared with 20% and 15% respectively in the placebo group. A similar study of 22 patients published in *International Journal of Geriatric Psychiatry* produced equivalent results. Like many other drugs in this class, however, additional studies are needed to fully assess their effect on Alzheimer's disease.

For more information see page 1468.

Generic: **Trazodone** *(TRAZ-oh-done)*
Brand: **Desyrel**

Trazodone, primarily used to treat depression, is in a class of medications called serotonin modulators. It works by increasing the amount of serotonin to help maintain mental balance. Studies conducted in patients with Alzheimer's disease and dementia have shown that trazodone improves diverse symptoms including sadness, emotional disorders, irritability, fear, psychomotor instability, and delirant ideas.

For more information see page 1521.

AUTOIMMUNE NEUROMUSCULAR DISEASES

Autoimmune neuromuscular diseases are caused by an overactive immune response by the body against substances and tissues normally present. In other words, the body attacks its own cells and tissues. There are more than 40 human diseases classified as either definite or probable autoimmune diseases. Almost all autoimmune diseases appear without warning or apparent cause, and most patients suffer from fatigue.

Chronic Inflammatory Demyelinating Polyneuropathy

Chronic inflammatory demyelinating polyneuropathy is a neurological disorder characterized by progressive weakness and impaired sensory function in the legs and arms. The disorder is caused by damage to the myelin (the layers around the nerve fibers) of the peripheral nerves. It is more common in young adults, and in men more than women. Symptoms often include tingling or numbness, weakness of the arms and legs, loss of deep tendon reflexes, fatigue, and abnormal sensations.

Commonly Prescribed (On-Label) Drugs: *Azathioprine, Immune Globulin*

OFF-LABEL PRESCRIPTION DRUGS
BREAKTHROUGH OPTIONS

Generic: ***Cyclophosphamide*** *(sye-kloe-FOS-fa-mide)*
Brands: ***Cytoxan, Neosar***

Cyclophosphamide belongs to the class of drugs known as alkylating drugs and is primarily a cancer treatment used to treat Hodgkin's disease, lymphomas, leukemias, and other tumors. It is a derivative of mustard gas and works by disrupting DNA and interfering with normal cell function to kill the cell. Cells that divide rapidly (and thus replicate their DNA rapidly like cancer cells) are especially targeted by cyclophosphamide.

Common first-line therapies in treating chronic inflammatory demyelinating polyneuropathy include corticosteroids, plasmapheresis, and IV immunoglobulin IgG. For people who do not respond to these treatments, limited research has shown that cyclophosphamide may be helpful. In one small study of patients who were unresponsive to common first-line therapies with high-dose cyclophosphamide, all patients improved in function and muscle strength. Nerve conduction improved in 75% of the patients. While data are limited, cyclophosphamide shows promise as a second-line treatment therapy for treating chronic inflammatory demyelinating polyneuropathy.

For more information see page 1123.

Generic: **Cyclosporine** *(si-klo-SPOR-een)*
Brands: **Gengraf, Neoral, Sandimmune**

Cyclosporine A is used primarily to prevent organ rejection in transplant recipients. While data is somewhat limited, studies have shown cyclosporine to be an important treatment of chronic inflammatory demyelinating polyneuropathy especially as a second-line treatment. In a review of 19 patients with chronic inflammatory demyelinating polyneuropathy, who had failed treatment with corticosteroids, plasmapheresis, IV immune globulin, patients were divided into two groups, one with progressive disease and one relapsing based on types and response to treatment they had received in the past. The study found cyclosporine A to be effective and safe for these patients.

For more information see pages 1125 and 1127.

Generic: **Mycophenolate Mofetil**
(mye-koe-FEN-oh-late MAH-feh-till)
Brands: **CellCept, Myfortic**

Mycophenolate mofetil is an immunosuppressive drug used to prevent organ rejections in transplant patients. Like other immunosuppressive therapies, it is primarily used in patients where first-line therapies such as corticosteroids and immunoglobulin have failed.

In a study of 21 patients with chronic inflammatory demyelinating polyneuropathy, treatment with mycophenolate mofetil improved three patients. No significant differences occurred in the strength or sensory scores before or after treatment, however, so researchers concluded that the drug induced a modest benefit in approximately 20% of their patients and stabilized patient condition, allowing reduction of steroid or IV immunoglobulin therapy.

For more information see page 1344.

Generic: **Rituximab** *(ri-TUK-si-mab)*
Brand: **Rituxan**

Rituximab works with the immune system against non-Hodgkin's lymphoma. It targets a type of B cell involved in non-Hodgkin's lymphoma and causes the immune system to destroy only those cells.

Preliminary data support the use of rituximab in chronic inflammatory demyelinating polyneuropathy. The results thus far suggest that patients resistant to intravenous immunoglobulin IgG administration may benefit from treatments that deplete B cells such as rituximab.

For more information see page 1457.

Guillain-Barre Syndrome

Guillain-Barre syndrome is a rare disorder in which the body's immune system attacks part of the peripheral nervous system. The first symptoms include varying degrees of weakness or tingling sensations in the legs that may spread to the arms and upper body. Symptoms can increase in intensity until the muscles are unusable and the patient is almost paralyzed. In these cases, the disorder is life threatening and considered a medical emergency. The precise cause is unknown.

Commonly Prescribed (On-Label) Drugs: *None*

OFF-LABEL PRESCRIPTION DRUG
BREAKTHROUGH OPTION

Generic: **Immune Globulin IgG, IV**
(EH-mune GLOB-ewe-lyn)
Brands: **Gamimune N, Gammar-P, Polygam**

Immunoglobulins are proteins found in human blood and are an important part of the body's defense against disease. Immunoglobulin therapy is administered when a person's body does not produce enough of its own or needs a temporary boost in immunoglobulin to help treat a specific disease. The therapy helps the body fight off infection and control the symptoms of many chronic diseases.

Clinical trials have shown that immunoglobulin is effective in reducing the time to functional recovery. Approximately 10% of patients with Guillain-Barre syndrome deteriorate after initial stabilization following intravenous immunoglobulin and often require repeated treatment.

For more information see pages 1234 and 1235.

Myasthenia Gravis

Myasthenia gravis is a chronic autoimmune neuromuscular disease distinguished by varying degrees of weakness of the skeletal muscles. Muscle weakness typically increases during periods of activity and improves after periods of rest. Certain muscles such as those that control eye and eyelid movement, facial expression, chewing, talking, and swallowing are often, but not always, involved in the disorder. The muscles that control breathing and neck and limb movements may also be affected.

Commonly Prescribed (On-Label) Drugs: *Ambenonium, Edrophonium, Neostigmine, Pyridostigmine, Tubocurarine*

OFF-LABEL PRESCRIPTION DRUGS
BREAKTHROUGH OPTIONS

Generic: **Azathioprine** *(ay-za-THYE-oh-preen)*
Brand: **Imuran**

Azathioprine is an immunosuppressant medication used to prevent rejection of transplanted kidneys. It is also used for treatment-resistant forms of severe, active rheumatoid arthritis.

Several studies have investigated azathioprine treatment of myasthenia gravis. One study analyzed the clinical records of 33 myasthenia gravis patients treated with anticholinesterase medications. Researchers concluded that azathioprine plus steroids improved outcome. Another study found that immune modulators addressed the underlying autoimmune process in myasthenia gravis but were associated with potential complications and side effects. Researchers proposed that patients with generalized myasthenia who have significant weakness beyond the eye muscles and who remain symptomatic, despite treatment with cholinesterase inhibitors, are candidates for immune modulation.

For more information see page 1033.

Generic: **Cyclophosphamide** *(sye-kloe-FOS-fa-mide)*
Brands: **Cytoxan, Neosar**

Cyclophosphamide belongs to the class of alkylating drugs, which are used to treat Hodgkin's disease, lymphomas, leukemias, and other tumors. It is a derivative of mustard gas and works by binding to DNA, interfering with normal cell function, and killing the cell. Cells that divide rapidly (and thus replicate their DNA rapidly) are especially targeted by cyclophosphamide.

In one clinical trial, 23 myasthenia gravis patients, who were either not responding to treatment or exhibiting steroid-related side effects, received treatment for 12 months with intravenous cyclophosphamide or placebo. Changes of muscle strength, steroid and pyridostigmine requirements, and development of ventilatory failure or swallowing impairment were evaluated at zero, three, six, and 12 months. At 12 months, five subjects on cyclophosphamide had tapered off their steroids whereas no patient on placebo achieved further reductions. Cyclophosphamide improved muscle strength at three and six months. This study suggests that intravenous cyclophosphamide allows reduction of steroid usage without muscle strength deterioration or cyclophosphamide-related side effects.

For more information see page 1123.

Generic: **Cyclosporine** *(si-klo-SPOR-een)*
Brands: **Gengraf, Neoral, Sandimmune**

Cyclosporine is used to prevent rejection of kidney, liver, and heart transplants. It is also used in psoriasis and severe cases of rheumatoid arthritis and related diseases by inhibiting a group of cells, known as T-lymphocytes, which are important to immune system function but contribute to the development of autoimmune diseases.

Researchers studied 57 patients with myasthenia gravis who took cyclosporine for an average of 3.5 years. Fifty-five (96%) had clinical improvement within approximately seven months. Corticosteroids were discontinued or decreased in 95% of 38 patients taking them. Five percent could not afford or tolerate the drug.

In another small study in *Journal of Neurology,* nine people with severe myasthenia gravis received cyclosporine A for two years. During cyclosporine A treatment seven of nine patients improved their muscle strength. In all the patients except one the corticosteroid dosage was reduced and in seven of the nine patients the dose reduction was over 50% with subsequent reduction of the corticosteroid side effects.

For more information see pages 1125 and 1127.

Generic: **Mycophenolate Mofetil** *(mye-koe-FEN-oh-late MAH-feh-till)*
Brands: **CellCept, Myfortic**

Mycophenolate mofetil is an immunosuppressive drug approved for use in certain organ transplant patients to prevent organ rejection by suppressing the immune system. Those with myasthenia gravis may benefit from therapy with mycophenolate mofetil when other immunosuppressive treatments have been ineffective or contraindicated. Patients with myasthenia gravis would take much smaller doses of mycophenolate mofetil than transplant patients, so common adverse effects are limited and mainly related to gastrointestinal problems including nausea and diarrhea, low white blood counts, anemia, and skin rash.

Mycophenolate mofetil has shown promising effects in myasthenia gravis patients in preliminary studies and is currently being studied in two trials to better establish its role in treatment. The results of one trial in the treatment of uncontrolled, stable myasthenia gravis were promising and suggested greater improvement in the patients who received mycophenolate mofetil compared to placebo. Additional research is needed.

For more information see page 1344.

Generic: **Prednisone** (pred-NIS-zone)
Brands: **Deltasone, Liqui-PRED, Meticorten, Orasone, Sterapred**

Prednisone is an oral, synthetic corticosteroid used for suppressing the immune system and inflammation. Synthetic corticosteroids work similarly to hydrocortisone, the naturally occurring corticosteroid produced in the body by the adrenal glands. Corticosteroids have many effects on the body, but are most often used for their anti-inflammatory effects, particularly in conditions where the immune system plays an important role, including arthritis, colitis, asthma, bronchitis, certain skin rashes, and allergic or inflammatory conditions of the nose and eyes.

A review article analyzed the results of several published studies of treatments of myasthenia gravis with corticosteroids, including prednisone. Two trials compared prednisone with placebo. In the first study of 13 patients, the prednisone group's improvement was found to be slightly greater at six months. In the second short-term study of 20 patients, the improvement was found to be significantly greater at two weeks. Another two trials compared glucocorticosteroids with azathioprine. In one trial, the rate of treatment failure was greater in the prednisone group. These limited trials suggest that corticosteroid treatment including prednisone offers significant short-term benefit in myasthenia gravis compared with placebo.

For more information see page 1429.

HEADACHE

Headaches can occur on one part of the head or involve the entire head. Pain associated with headache varies from person to person, and may be sudden and sharp or dull and constant. Other symptoms such as nausea can also occur. The main types of headaches include tension, migraine, menstrual migraine, and cluster. An estimated seven out of 10 people experience at least one headache each year; the majority of headaches endure for only a few hours, but some can persist for weeks. Several causes of headaches include but are not limited to scalp and neck muscle tension, allergies, and hormonal imbalance. For more information on headaches in children, see headaches in the Children's Health Disorders chapter on page 210.

Cluster Headache

Cluster headaches occur in groups or clusters and last for an extended time. Cluster headache pain is extremely severe, but the attack is short-lasting. Pain is centered around one eye, which may become inflamed and watery. Nasal congestion may accompany the cluster headache on the affected side of the face. Cluster headaches can occur in the middle of the night, and often happen at about the same time each day during the course of a cluster. Treatment includes inhalation of oxygen, triptans, ergotamines, and steroids, among others.

Commonly Prescribed (On-Label) Drugs:
Dihydroergotamine, Ergotamine, Sumatriptan

OFF-LABEL PRESCRIPTION DRUGS
BREAKTHROUGH OPTIONS

Generic: **Baclofen** *(BAK-low-fen)*
Brands: **Kemstro, Lioresal**

Baclofen belongs to a class of drugs known as muscle relaxants; it is used to relieve muscle spasms and contractions in conditions such as multiple sclerosis.

Researchers at the Meir General Hospital in Israel evaluated the use of baclofen in 16 patients treated during the cluster period and two weeks after. After a week, 12 patients' cluster headache attacks stopped. One patient was substantially better and became attack-free by the end of the following week. In the remaining three patients, the cluster headache attacks became worse and corticosteroid drugs were given. Three of the 16 patients had an additional cluster period, which resolved with a second course of baclofen. Researchers concluded that baclofen was effective and well tolerated for cluster headache. Furthermore, the drug retained its efficacy on repeated cluster attacks.

For more information see page 1037.

Generic: **Cortisone** *(KOR-ti-sone)*
Brand: **Cortisone Acetate**

Cortisone belongs to a class of drugs known as corticosteroids and is used to reduce swelling, redness, itching, allergic reactions, skin problems, asthma, and arthritis, among other conditions. Along with other drugs such as lithium and verapamil, cortisone is considered a first-line preventive drug for cluster headaches. Cortisone is very effective for cluster headache and works quickly. It is usually given for one or two weeks during the peak of the cluster series. Taking cortisone may increase your risk of infection. When you no longer need cortisone, you must gradually reduce the dose so the body can adjust.

Few clinical trials evaluate the use of cortisone for preventing cluster headache. In one article, German researchers noted that cortisone, along with several other drugs, is helpful for treating and preventing cluster headaches.

For more information see page 1118.

Generic: **Gabapentin** *(GA-ba-pen-tin)*
Brand: **Neurontin**

Gabapentin belongs to a class of drugs known as anticonvulsants and is used to help control some types of seizures in treating epilepsy. It is also used to control pain associated with shingles and has been evaluated for other pain conditions, including migraine. Anticonvulsant drugs, such as gabapentin, are becoming increasingly popular for migraine prevention. It is thought that gabapentin's effects on pain may be related to release of the brain chemical GABA, which regulates the perception of pain, but the precise way gabapentin works is not fully understood.

In clinical trials, gabapentin has been used for the treatment of cluster headache in fewer than 20 patients. In one trial, 12 adult patients with chronic or episodic cluster headache received gabapentin and, at four months, all reported no new attacks. Patients in the episodic group reported a decrease in mean headache duration from 35 days to 10 days. All patients had complete pain relief within the first eight days of gabapentin therapy and long-term effects had continued at the three-month follow-up examination. In trials, gabapentin has been well tolerated— drowsiness was the only reported side effect. Withdrawal symptoms have been reported with abrupt termination of use.

For more information see page 1206.

Generic: **Indomethacin** *(in-doe-METH-a-sin)*
Brands: **Indocin, Indocin I.V.; Indocin SR**

Indomethacin belongs to a class of drugs known as nonsteroidal anti-inflammatory drugs (NSAIDs), and is used to relieve inflammation and pain associated with rheumatoid arthritis and other inflammatory conditions.

Researchers in Japan documented the use of indomethacin in a 36-year-old man with cluster headache associated with hemicrania continua (a type of headache that involves the face). In this patient, continuous, dull or pressure-type headache appeared on the same side of the head during the third month of a prolonged cluster period, and varied in the severity of pain. The continuous headache lasted more than three months, and significantly responded to indomethacin. Researchers concluded that indomethacin may deserve consideration for the treatment of continuous headache.

For more information see page 1238.

Generic: **Topiramate** *(TOE-pie-rah-mate)*
Brand: **Topamax**

Topiramate is a member of a class of drugs known as anti-epileptics, used to control seizures (convulsions) in adults or children with various forms of epilepsy. It is also used to prevent migraine headaches and treat other conditions.

A number of studies and case reports use topiramate for cluster headache. German researchers recognize topiramate as the only drug that provided pain relief in acute cluster headache and noted the positive benefits of topiramate in people with cluster headache. In three patients, topiramate was effective but it produced intolerable side effects in two patients.

For more information see page 1516.

Cluster Headache Prevention

In most people, cluster headache prevention requires daily drugs since the headaches are severe and difficult to stop. Criteria for the use of preventive drugs for cluster headaches include the following: the cluster headaches are not easily stopped with drugs; the cluster headaches occur daily and last longer than 15 minutes; and the person is willing to take drugs and endure potential drug side effects. Preventive drugs for cluster headache include SSRIs, calcium channel blockers, anticonvulsants, steroids, ergotamines, and lithium, among others.

Commonly Prescribed (On-Label) Drugs: *Methylergonovine*

OFF-LABEL PRESCRIPTION DRUGS
BREAKTHROUGH OPTIONS

Generic: **Baclofen** *(BAK-low-fen)*
Brands: **Kemstro, Lioresal**

Baclofen belongs to a class of drugs known as muscle relaxants; it has antispasmic and pain-relieving properties and is used to relieve muscle spasms and contractions in conditions such as multiple sclerosis.

In an Israeli study, 16 patients with cluster headache were treated with daily baclofen in three divided doses for the cluster period and two weeks after. Within one week, 12 patients reported that cluster attacks stopped. One patient was substantially better and became attack-free by the end of the following week. In the remaining three patients, the attacks worsened and corticosteroid drugs were prescribed. Three of the 16 patients had an additional cluster period, which cleared with a second course of baclofen. Researchers concluded that baclofen was effective, safe, and well tolerated for cluster headache, and appeared to retain its efficacy on repeated clusters. In another report, these same researchers noted that baclofen was well tolerated for the prevention of cluster headache.

For more information see page 1037.

*Generic: **Gabapentin** (GA-ba-pen-tin)*
*Brand: **Neurontin***

Gabapentin belongs to a class of drugs known as anticonvulsants, and is used to help control some types of seizures in the treatment of epilepsy. It is also used to control pain associated with shingles and has been evaluated for pain conditions, including headache. Anticonvulsant drugs, such as gabapentin, are becoming increasingly popular for headache prevention. Gabapentin's pain-relief effects may be related to release of the brain chemical GABA, which regulates the perception of pain.

In a case in China, gabapentin was found to be effective in the treatment and prevention of cluster headache. A 38-year-old man with a history of cluster headaches was treated with gabapentin, which treated and prevented cluster headache. In an Italian study, patients with episodic or cluster headache took gabapentin and, after eight days of treatment, all were pain free. Additionally, the drug reduced cluster headache duration 16% to 40% of the previous average headache bouts (in patients with episodic cluster headache).

For more information see page 1206.

*Generic: **Lithium** (LITH-ee-um)*
*Brands: **Eskalith, Eskalith CR, Lithobid***

Lithium is used to control both mania and depression; it helps to control extreme mood swings in manic-depressive illness. Lithium can prevent or reduce manic-depressive episodes. In fact, according to doctors at the Robbins Headache Clinic in Northbrook, Illinois, lithium is very helpful for chronic cluster headaches and considered helpful for episodic cluster headaches.

Lithium may be combined with other cluster headache drugs such as verapamil and/or cortisone. In low doses, lithium is usually well tolerated.

The short- and long-term effects of lithium in cluster headache were evaluated in 90 patients. Sixty-eight had episodic cluster headache and 22 the chronic form of the disease. Eleven of the 22 patients with chronic cluster headache showed a definite, constant, short-term, and long-term improvement. In seven of the 22 patients, lithium treatment provided excellent results at first but was later followed by some transient worsening. In the remaining four patients, only partial benefits were observed upfront and treatment proved still less effective after a few months.

For more information see page 1286.

Generic: *Topiramate* (TOE-pie-rah-mate)
Brand: *Topamax*

Topiramate is a member of a class of drugs known as anti-epileptics, which are used to control seizures (convulsions) in adult or children with various forms of epilepsy. It is also used to prevent migraine headaches and treat other conditions. It may also help people with chronic pain syndromes.

In a case study, 10 patients with cluster headaches unresponsive to previous drugs were treated with topiramate. Cluster remission occurred within one to three weeks in nine patients. Cluster period duration was reduced in nine patients. Side effects of topiramate were mild and included drowsiness, numbness or a feeling of "pins and needles," and word-finding difficulty. Researchers concluded that the positive results seen with the use of topiramate require additional study.

In another study, 26 adults with episodic or chronic cluster headache were treated with topiramate at bedtime. Fifty-eight percent of patients achieved remission within 14 days; 27% achieved remission within the first week. Moreover, 23% of patients had greater than 50% reduction in the number of cluster headache attacks. Side effects of topiramate included numbness, altered taste, memory impairment, weight loss, and drowsiness. Researchers concluded that topiramate is effective for preventing episodic and chronic cluster headache.

For more information see page 1516.

Generic: **Verapamil** *(Vur-AP-ah-mill)*
Brands: **Calan, Calan SR, Covera-HS, Isoptin SR, Verelan, Verelan PM**

Verapamil belongs to a class of drugs known as calcium channel blockers, and is used to treat irregular heartbeats and high blood pressure. It relaxes blood vessels so the heart does not have to pump as hard. It also increases the supply of blood and oxygen to the heart to control chest pain. Research has shown that calcium channel blockers, such as verapamil, are effective in the prevention of migraine and cluster headache. This drug changes the way calcium ions move into muscle cells and blood vessels, thereby preventing blood vessel changes that may cause certain types of headache.

First-line prevention of episodic cluster headaches includes verapamil, lithium, and cortisone drugs. Among experts, verapamil is considered to be the main drug for cluster headache prevention. Overall, verapamil is well tolerated and effective in preventing both episodic and chronic cluster headache. Verapamil may be used along with cortisone (a steroid drug).

In a German study, nine patients with episodic and three patients with chronic cluster headache took verapamil. In episodic cluster headache, early treatment with verapamil stopped attacks within 20 days in 80% of patients; late treatment onset was successful within 10 days in 67% of patients. Early treatment shortened duration of headaches by four times. Researchers concluded that chronic cluster headache probably requires higher doses. In another study, 48 patients with cluster headache were treated with verapamil. Thirty-three patients (69%) improved more than 75%. No significant differences were seen between episodic and chronic cluster headache.

For more information see page 1544.

Lumbar Puncture-induced Headache

Lumbar puncture-induced headache is a recognized complication of lumbar punctures most commonly from an epidural, and is related to the loss of cerebrospinal fluid. If you are sitting or in an upright position, the pain is relieved once you lie down. Nausea, photophobia (unusual sensitivity to light), or other vision changes may accompany lumbar puncture-induced headache. Symptoms are managed with bed rest, remaining in a reclined position, and drug treatments.

Commonly Prescribed (On-Label) Drugs: None

OFF-LABEL PRESCRIPTION DRUG
BREAKTHROUGH OPTION

Generic: **Sumatriptan** *(soo-ma-TRIP-tan)*
Brand: **Imitrex**

Sumatriptan belongs to a class of anti-headache or anti-migraine drugs, and is used to treat severe migraine headaches. With sumatriptan, many people find that they are headache-free; others report that their headaches are much less painful and they are able to resume their normal activities even though they are not entirely headache-free. Sumatriptan may relieve other symptoms that occur together with a migraine headache such as nausea, vomiting, light sensitivity, and sound sensitivity.

There have been a few studies evaluating sumatriptan for lumbar puncture-induced headache. In a small study, 10 patients with lumbar puncture-induced headache were given a single injection of sumatriptan or placebo. Based on results from this study, researchers do not recommend sumatriptan for this type of headache in people who fail to respond to standard headache treatments.

In a study of six people with lumbar puncture-induced headache, four of the six achieved long-lasting headache relief with a single injection of sumatriptan and needed no other treatment.

For more information see page 1487.

Menstrual Migraine

Menstrual migraine is a type of headache that occurs in women two days before and up until the last day of menstruation. Factors that play a role in the development of menstrual migraine include hormone levels, blood platelet dysfunction, decreased levels of brain magnesium, decreased natural brain endorphins, and increased secretion of prostaglandins (a substance that causes inflammation in brain blood vessels). A variety of treatments are used to manage menstrual migraine, including hormone drugs and pain drugs.

Commonly Prescribed (On-Label) Drugs: *None*

OFF-LABEL PRESCRIPTION DRUGS
BREAKTHROUGH OPTIONS

Generic: **Danazol** *(DA-na-zole)*
Brand: **Danocrine**

Danazol is a synthetic steroid that slows the production of the female hormone estrogen and has similar activity to male sex hormones, or androgens. It is used to relieve the symptoms of endometriosis (a condition in which tissue that normally lines the uterus grows in abnormal locations such as the ovaries, fallopian tubes, and abdominal cavity) by shrinking abnormal tissue, which forms the lining of the womb. It is thought that danazol works on menstrual migraine by suppressing estrogen levels thereby preventing attacks.

In a study at the Headache Institute for Women, in Southfield, Michigan, 131 women between the ages of 20 years and 51 years with a primary diagnosis of migraine were enrolled. None of the subjects responded to placebo treatment, but after two months of danazol, 63% reported a greater than 75% improvement in their headaches. Nearly 83% of subjects continued with danazol for an additional year and remained almost migraine-free. In this study, danazol efficacy was continued throughout the treatment course, with only mild side effects. Danazol was found to be especially helpful in women who suffered from premenstrual migraine. In this group, 75% of subjects reported significant relief from migraine. It was concluded that a stable, low level of estrogen achieved with the use of danazol may be effective in controlling menstrual migraine.

For more information see page 1129.

Generic: **Leuprolide** *(loo-PROE-lide)*
Brands: **Eligard, Lupron, Lupron Depot, Lupron Depot-Ped, Viadur**

Leuprolide is a synthetic protein similar to a natural hormone produced in the body known as gonadotropin-releasing hormone (GnRH). Regular injections of leuprolide decrease the levels of testosterone in men and estrogen in women. Leuprolide may be used in diseases such as prostate cancer and endometriosis and may be useful for menstrual migraine by suppressing levels of estrogen.

At the Headache Institute for Women, 21 women with menstrual migraine were given leuprolide to suppress estrogen levels. Leuprolide effectively controlled migraines in 52% of the 21 participants in this two-year study. It was concluded that the low level of estrogen achieved by leuprolide is an effective treatment for menstrual migraine.

Experts at the Robbins Headache Clinic in Northbrook, Illinois, identified gonadotropin-releasing hormone agonists, such as leuprolide, as last-resort options for menstrual migraine and recommended that these drugs be reserved for women with menstrual migraines resistant to both hormonal therapy and treatments for nonmenstrual migraines.

For more information see page 1274.

Generic: **Mefenamic acid** *(me-fe-NAM-ik AS-id)*
Brand: **Ponstel**

Mefenamic acid belongs to a class of nonsteroidal anti-inflammatory drugs (NSAIDs). It relieves inflammation and pain associated with rheumatoid arthritis, osteoarthritis, menstrual cramps, and premenstrual discomfort.

A researcher at the Dubai Specialized Medical Center and Medical Research Laboratories in the United Arab Emirates treated 24 women with menstrual migraine for two consecutive menstrual periods; during one period they received mefenamic acid and during another period they were given placebo. Each treatment was given at the start of migraine symptoms and the dose was repeated every eight hours during menstruation. Results from this study showed that 79.16% of women had significant pain relief with mefenamic acid compared with 16.6% of women treated with placebo. Additionally, 83.3% of patients treated with mefenamic acid were able to function compared with 12.4% of those on placebo. The researcher concluded that mefenamic acid is significantly superior to placebo and is a safe, effective treatment for acute menstrual migraine.

For more information see page 1300.

Migraine

Migraines are recurrent, throbbing, or pulsating headaches that often run in families, and strike three times as many women as men. They often occur on one side of the head and can be accompanied by nausea, vomiting, sensitivity to light, sound, and smells, sleep disruption, and depression. They may be triggered by menstrual or altered sleep cycles, missed meals, sunlight, certain foods, excessive noise, stress, or underlying depression. Attacks tend to become less severe with age.

Commonly Prescribed (On-Label) Drugs: *Almotriptan, Aspirin, Dihydroergotamine, Eletriptan, Ergotamine, Frovatriptan, Isometheptene, Methysergide, Naratriptan, Propranolol, Rizatriptan, Sumatriptan, Timolol, Topiramate, Valproic Acid, Zolmitriptan*

OFF-LABEL PRESCRIPTION DRUGS
BREAKTHROUGH OPTIONS

Generic: **Botulinum Toxin Type A** *(BOT-yoo-lin-num TOKS-in type aye)*
Brands: **Botox, Botox cosmetic**

Botulinum toxin type A belongs to a class of drugs known as injectable neurotoxins. Neurotoxins block the nerves' ability to make muscles contract thereby paralyzing muscles. This drug prevents the release of a nerve chemical in the body known as acetylcholine and so it prevents muscle cells from contracting. This injectable neurotoxin is used to treat neck muscle spasms, and uncontrollable blinking, to control misaligned or "lazy eyes," and to reduce the appearance of forehead frown lines in adults 65 and younger.

Among headache experts, botulinum toxin type A is considered to be a novel, preventive treatment for migraine without major side effects. Studies have found this drug to be a potentially cost-effective treatment for migraine. In a three-year study involving 271 headache patients, including migraine, botulinum toxin type A significantly reduced the frequency of headache, regardless of headache type. The number of days with headache each month was reduced from 18.9 to 8.3 at last treatment, which translates into a 56% reduction. Moreover, headache severity decreased from 2.4 points at the beginning of the study to 1.8 points at the last treatment, and was highly significant in people with migraine and other types of headache. Finally, 95% of patients in this study reported no adverse reactions with botulinum toxin type A treatment. Patients with localized neck pain and headaches, and headaches that do not respond to conventional treatments, are likely candidates for botulinum toxin type A treatment for migraine.

For more information see page 1051.

Generic: **Lidocaine** (LYE-doe-kane)
Brands: **Anestacon, Xylocaine**

Lidocaine, when used as a topical analgesic and anesthetic, causes a loss of feeling in the skin and surrounding tissues. It is often used to relieve pain caused by sunburn, insect bites, poison ivy, and minor cuts and scratches. In studies, lidocaine has been given in single increments in one nostril during 30 seconds (or in both nostrils if headache affects both sides of the head). This is usually given again at two minutes if headache persists. Also, lidocaine has been given in four sprays, and two sprays are repeated, if necessary, in 15 minutes.

Lidocaine may work by targeting nerve centers in the body. In one trial with 81 patients, intranasal lidocaine acted rapidly, and was effective in 55% of adult patients with migraine within 15 minutes after one or two doses. Compared with placebo, headache relapse rates were significantly lower in the lidocaine group of patients. Relapses usually occurred within one hour; 42% of patients in the lidocaine group and 83% of patients in the placebo group had headache relapse. In this study, 58% of patients who responded to intranasal lidocaine for migraine had continuous symptom relief at 24-hour follow-up. Side effects of intranasal lidocaine in this study included local burning, nasal numbness, throat numbness, and unpleasant taste. This drug is not commercially available in intranasal formulation and requires special compounding by your pharmacist. In addition, to avoid toxicities and ensure proper administration, patients require special instructions for administration when using this drug intranasally. Using the topical commercial product in the nose is NOT recommended as this might result in an overdose of the drug.

The effects of intranasal lidocaine solution were evaluated in a study involving 23 people with migraine or migraine plus daily dull headache. Researchers administered lidocaine via eyedropper vial in the nostril. Findings from this study revealed that lidocaine stopped migraine attacks; 52.2% of patients had complete or near complete relief with the use of this drug.

For more information see page 1283.

Generic: **Magnesium Sulfate** *(mag-NEE-zhum SUL-fate)*
Brand: **Magnesium Sulfate**

Magnesium sulfate, a naturally occurring mineral, is also classified as an anticonvulsant, antiarrhythmic, and laxative drug. It is often used to prevent or correct low blood magnesium caused by malnutrition, to prevent or treat seizures during pregnancy, to prevent abnormal heart rate after a heart attack, and is administered orally as a laxative to relieve constipation. Magnesium sulfate is an important component in the body, particularly for normal nerve and muscle function. It is given by injection into a muscle or vein in a hospital or clinic.

Since researchers have found magnesium deficiency to be responsible for some migraines, using magnesium to treat migraine has been proposed. In a study of 30 patients with moderate or severe migraine in Turkey, 15 patients received intravenous (IV) magnesium sulfate during 15 minutes. The other 15 patients received saline IV. All patients who received magnesium sulfate responded to treatment. Migraine pain was completely gone in 13 patients (86.6%); diminished in two patients (13.4%); and in all 15 patients treated with magnesium sulfate, associated migraine symptoms disappeared. Those patients who initially received saline in this study were then given magnesium sulfate; and all patients responded to this drug. In 14 patients

(93.3%) in this group, the migraine attack stopped; in one patient (6.6%), the pain intensity decreased. In all 15 patients in this group, migraine-associated symptoms completely stopped. Therefore, IV magnesium sulfate may be an efficient, and well-tolerated drug for the treatment of migraine attacks. Another study in Brazil concluded that magnesium sulfate can be used for the treatment of all symptoms of migraine with aura (visual symptoms or vision loss), or as an add-on treatment for associated symptoms in people with migraine without aura.

For more information see page 1292.

Generic: **Metoclopramide** *(met-oh-kloe-PRA-mide)*
Brand: **Reglan**

Metoclopramide has a number of uses: it is a dopamine-receptor antagonist, an anti-emetic (drug that stops or prevents nausea and vomiting), and a stimulant of upper gastrointestinal (GI) activity. It is used in a wide variety of GI disorders, particularly gastroesophageal reflux disease (GERD), and to prevent chemotherapy-induced nausea and vomiting.

Metoclopramide has been successful in treating migraines. Experts have affirmed that metoclopramide injected directly into the muscle may be considered as an add-on treatment to control nausea in people with acute migraine attacks; the IV formulation may be used alone to relieve migraine pain. Across the medical literature, metoclopramide hydrochloride has been identified as a possible option to treat and prevent nausea and vomiting, and to speed up the absorption of anti-migraine drugs.

In a study at the Albert Einstein College of Medicine in New York City, patients received IV metoclopramide hydrochloride alone or in combination with magnesium sulfate in the emergency room. Researchers unexpectedly found that the addition of magnesium to metoclopramide may reduce the effectiveness of metoclopramide in relieving migraine.

For more information see page 1318.

Migraine Prevention

The goal of migraine prevention is to reduce the occurrence of migraine headache. Physicians will prescribe preventive treatment if migraines are frequent, disabling, or associated with neurologic features, or if acute treatment is ineffective or overused. It is recommended that the selected drug be tested in the absence of interfering or ineffective drugs, so your doctor needs to consider other diseases or conditions that you have. It is important to note that only a few drugs available for migraine prevention have proven effective. Also, some preventive drugs take weeks or months before they are completely effective.

Commonly Prescribed (On-Label) Drugs: *Topiramate, Valproic Acid*

OFF-LABEL PRESCRIPTION DRUGS
BREAKTHROUGH OPTIONS

Generic: **Amitriptyline** *(a-mee-TRIP-ti-leen)*
Brand: **Elavil**

Amitriptyline belongs to a group of drugs known as tricyclic antidepressants (TCAs) used to relieve depression. Tricyclic antidepressants, such as amitriptyline, are also considered effective in migraine prevention, especially for people with migraine who are prone to depression. In general, the doses used to treat migraine are lower than the doses used to treat depression, so side effects are less noticeable. Amitriptyline influences the body's use of a chemical known as serotonin; therefore, its use can result in improvements in migraine and depression.

In clinical guidelines set forth by the American College of Physicians-American Society of Internal Medicine, amitriptyline is considered the most frequently studied antidepressant and it is used to prevent migraine. In clinical studies, amitriptyline is recommended as a first-line drug for preventing migraine.

In an article on the off-label uses of antidepressants in *American Family Physician* journal, fluvoxamine, an antidepressant, was considered as effective as amitriptyline for migraine prevention. In this Hungarian study of 64 people with migraine, amitriptyline significantly reduced the number of migraine attacks, although its use resulted in severe drowsiness. Fluvoxamine also reduced the number of migraine attacks and produced slight side effects. The researcher concluded that fluvoxamine may be an alternative for preventing some types of migraines.

For more information see page 1009.

Generic: **Atenolol** *(a-TEN-oh-lole)*
Brand: **Tenormin**

Tenormin belongs to a class of drugs known as selective beta-blockers, and is typically used to reduce the workload of the heart and help it beat more regularly. It controls high blood pressure and relieves chest pain, and can be a useful medication after a heart attack. Atenolol is sometimes used to prevent migraine headaches.

Compared with another beta-blocker drug, propranolol, atenolol has fewer side effects. In general, beta-blockers are considered to be the most widely used drug class for migraine prevention. Atenolol is among a number of beta-blocker drugs that offer beneficial effects when compared with placebo or propanolol. Additionally, atenolol may offer two-fold benefits to patients with migraine and high blood pressure. According to researchers in France, beta-blockers, such as atenolol are considered first-choice drugs for preventing migraine.

For more information see page 1027.

Generic: **Baclofen** *(BAK-loe-fen)*
Brands: **Kemstro, Lioresal**

Baclofen belongs to a class of drugs known as muscle relaxants; it is used to relieve muscle spasms and contractions in people with conditions such as multiple sclerosis. It has anti-spasmic and pain-relieving properties.

In a study by researchers in Israel, 16 people with cluster headache were treated with daily baclofen, given during the cluster headache period and for two weeks after. After one week of treatment, 12 patients reported that their cluster headaches stopped. One patient was reported to be significantly better and became attack-free by the end of the following week. In the remaining patients, the cluster headache attacks worsened and corticosteroid-type drugs were given. Of the 16 patients, three had another cluster headache period, which was eventually controlled with the use of baclofen. Researchers concluded that baclofen appears effective and well tolerated for cluster headache.

In another 12-week trial with 54 patients with migraine in Israel, baclofen was effective in 86.2% of patients, with more than 50% headache reduction compared with before treatment. Three patients in this study could not tolerate the drug because of side effects. Researchers concluded that baclofen is effective for the prevention of migraine.

For more information see page 1037.

Generic: **Botulinum Toxin Type A** *(BOT-yoo-lin-num TOKS-in type aye)*
Brands: **Botox, Botox cosmetic**

Botulinum toxin type A is classified as an injectable neurotoxin. Neurotoxins block the nerves' ability to make muscles contract, thereby paralyzing muscles. This injectable neurotoxin is used to treat neck muscle spasms and uncontrollable blinking, to control misaligned or "lazy eyes," and to reduce the appearance of forehead frown lines in adults 65 and younger. The way the drug works in headache prevention is not completely understood.

In a study, the effects of botulinum toxin type A compared with placebo were evaluated in 123 people with migraine. Results showed that botulinum toxin type A improved migraines for up to three months, decreased the incidence of migraine, decreased migraine severity, and decreased the number of days that migraine drugs were needed. Researchers concluded that botulinum toxin type A was safe and effective, and reduced migraine frequency, severity, medication use, and associated vomiting.

In a study of 30 patients with migraine, botulinum toxin type A as a preventive migraine drug was evaluated. Single- and multiple-site injections were given. Botulinum toxin type A was found to provide improvement for up to three months, and reduced the frequency of migraine attacks, the duration of migraine, the use of migraine drugs, and nausea. Researchers concluded that botulinum toxin type A is effective for migraine prevention.

For more information see page 1051.

Generic: **Candesartan** *(kan-de-SAR-tan)*
Brand: **Atacand**

Candesartan belongs to a class of drugs known as angiotensin 2-receptor antagonists (ARBs), and is used to lower high blood pressure and prevent subsequent stroke, heart failure, and kidney damage. Heart drugs, such as candesartan, possibly because of their action on vascular tone, have been useful in preventing migraine attacks.

In a 12-week trial, 60 patients with two to six migraines per month received placebo or candesartan. Compared with placebo, candesartan significantly reduced migraine occurrence. Patients on candesartan also had significantly lower blood pressure compared with placebo. There were 32 adverse events in the candesartan group compared with 44 adverse events in the placebo group. Common side effects of candesartan included dizziness, fainting, upper respiratory tract infection, musculoskeletal symptoms, other infections, and gastrointestinal problems.

In a case report from Japan, candesartan successfully reduced the incidence and severity of headache in patients with high blood pressure. Migraine disability scores and high blood pressure were also reduced. Researchers concluded that in people who cannot tolerate other migraine drugs and have high blood pressure, candesartan is a unique, attractive drug for the prevention of migraine.

For more information see page 1065.

Generic: **Diltiazem** *(dil-TYE-a-zem)*
Brands: **Cardizem, Cartia XT, Dilacor XR, Diltia XT, Taztia XT, Tiazac**

Diltiazem belongs to a class of drugs known as calcium channel blockers, used to treat cardiovascular disorders. Diltiazem relaxes the blood vessels so the heart does not have to pump as hard. It changes the movement of calcium ions into muscle cells of blood vessels, which can sometimes prevent the blood vessel changes that contribute to migraine, thereby preventing headaches by improving blood flow.

According to the American College of Physicians-American Society of Internal Medicine, diltiazem is a recommended preventive migraine drug based on expert consensus and clinical use. However, evidence from clinical studies on the use of this drug for migraine prevention is variable.

For more information see page 1146.

Generic: **Doxepin** *(DOKS-e-pin)*
Brands: **Prudoxin, Sinequan**

Doxepin belongs to a class of drugs known as tricyclic antidepressants, used to treat depression and anxiety, and may be particularly useful in people with depression and migraine. Antidepressants may reduce migraine frequency by regulating a chemical in the brain known as serotonin. In general, doxepin doses for migraine are lower than that for depression; therefore side effects may be less noticeable. Side effects associated with doxepin include upset stomach, drowsiness, weakness or tiredness, excitement or anxiety, insomnia, nightmares, dry mouth, skin sensitivity to sunlight, and appetite or weight changes.

According to the American College of Physicians-American Society of Internal Medicine, doxepin is a recommended preventive migraine drug based on expert consensus and clinical use. Doxepin is among the most frequently used tricyclic antidepressants for migraine depression, as noted in a medical journal article. This article recommended that the drug be given as a small dose because of doxepin-associated drowsiness.

For more information see page 1154.

Generic: **Fluoxetine** *(floo-OKS-e-teen)*
Brands: **Prozac, Prozac Weekly, Sarafem**

Fluoxetine belongs to a class of antidepressant drugs known as selective serotonin reuptake inhibitors (SSRIs) used to treat mental depression. It is also used to treat obsessive-compulsive disorder (OCD), bulimia nervosa, and premenstrual dysphoric disorder (PMDD). How fluoxetine and other antidepressants work to prevent migraine is uncertain, but this type of drug has been shown to be useful in a variety of painful states including headache. Fluoxetine acts only on the neurotransmitter serotonin and may reduce the frequency of migraine by regulating serotonin levels in the brain.

According to migraine treatment guidelines established by the U.S. Headache Consortium, fluoxetine was significantly better than placebo for preventing migraines. The American Council for Headache Education reported that SSRI-type drugs, such as fluoxetine, have fewer side effects than TCA-type antidepressants and are a reasonable option for persons with mood disorders and migraine. In fact, if you cannot tolerate or fail to respond to other standard migraine prevention drugs, you can try fluoxetine.

For more information see page 1192.

*Generic: **Fluvoxamine** (floo-VOKS-a-meen)*
*Brand: **Luvox***

Fluvoxamine belongs to a class of antidepressant drugs known as SSRIs, and is used to treat obsessive-compulsive disorder (OCD). The way fluvoxamine and other antidepressants work to prevent migraine is uncertain, but this type of drug is useful in a variety of painful states including headache. Fluvoxamine acts only on the neurotransmitter chemical serotonin and may reduce the frequency of migraine by regulating serotonin levels in the brain.

According to the U.S. Headache Consortium recommendations, fluvoxamine may be used to prevent migraine, based on expert consensus and clinical experience. However, evidence is lacking from clinical trials for the use of fluvoxamine for this condition. SSRI-type drugs, such as fluoxetine, have fewer side effects than TCA-type antidepressants and may be an option for people with mood disorders and migraine.

In a study in Hungary, amitriptyline (an antidepressant) and fluvoxamine were tested in 64 people with migraine. Amitriptyline significantly reduced the number of headache attacks, but caused severe drowsiness in many patients. Fluvoxamine also reduced the number of headache attacks but caused only slight side effects. These findings suggest that fluvoxamine may be a viable treatment alternative for migraine prevention.

For more information see page 1199.

Generic: **Gabapentin** *(GA-ba-pen-tin)*
Brand: **Neurontin**

Gabapentin belongs to a class of drugs known as anticonvulsants, used to help control seizures in the treatment of epilepsy. It is also used to control pain associated with shingles and has been evaluated for pain conditions, including migraine, as its pain-modulating properties may regulate the perception of pain. Anticonvulsant drugs, such as gabapentin, are becoming increasingly popular for migraine prevention.

International and domestic studies that have evaluated gabapentin for migraine prevention suggest that it is effective. In a study of 63 patients with migraine (with or without aura), gabapentin significantly reduced migraine frequency and intensity among 30 patients who received it. In this study, adverse events were mild to moderate in severity.

Similarly, in a large study, 143 people with migraine received daily doses of gabapentin or placebo for 12 weeks. At the end of 12 weeks, the migraine rate had declined from 4.2 migraines before treatment to 2.7 migraines after treatment in those who received gabapentin. This decrease was significantly greater than the decrease from 4.1 migraines to 3.5 migraines among those who received placebo. Of the 56 gabapentin recipients, 46% had at least a 50% reduction in the four-week migraine rate. Drug-related adverse events (sleepiness and dizziness) led to drug withdrawal in 13% of patients in the gabapentin group compared with 7% in the placebo group. The researchers concluded that gabapentin is an effective and well-tolerated preventive for migraine.

For more information see page 1206.

Generic: **Imipramine** *(im-IP-ra-meen)*
Brands: **Tofranil, Tofranil-PM**

Imipramine belongs to a class of antidepressant drugs known as TCAs used to treat depression. According to the American Council for Headache Education, TCA-type antidepressants are thought to be effective, especially for people who have both migraine and depression. In general, the doses of TCA antidepressants, such as imipramine, tend to be lower than those needed to treat depression. Therefore, the side effects associated with this drug may be less noticeable, including upset stomach, drowsiness, weakness or tiredness, excitement, anxiety, difficulty sleeping, nightmares, dry mouth, skin sensitivity to sunlight, and changes in appetite or weight.

The TCA-type antidepressants seem to vary in the way they are absorbed, distributed, and excreted in the body. In a review article published in *Current Medical Research and Opinion*, imipramine was occasionally used for migraine prevention. The U.S. Headache Consortium recommends imipramine for migraine prevention in their practice guidelines.

With the exception of amitriptyline, the TCAs have not been thoroughly studied for migraine prevention; a search of the medical literature produced very little evidence of its use for migraine prevention. In one article, researchers with the Adelman Headache Center in Greensboro, North Carolina, noted that imipramine is very inexpensive for migraine prevention, and recommended that it replace another drug as a second-line drug for treating this condition.

For more information see page 1230.

Generic: **Lisinopril** *(lyse-IN-oh-pril)*
Brands: **Prinivil, Zestril**

Lisinopril belongs to a class of drugs known as angiotensin-converting enzyme (ACE) inhibitors, and is used alone or in combination with other drugs to treat high blood pressure. Lisinopril works by decreasing chemicals in the body that tighten blood vessels, thereby smoothing the flow of blood and allowing the heart to pump more efficiently.

In migraine prevention, lisinopril and other drugs of this class may be effective because they improve on blood vessel tone. In a trial, 60 adults with two to six migraines per month were given placebo or lisinopril for 12 weeks. Compared with placebo, lisinopril use resulted in a decrease in hours with headache (20%) and frequency of headache (17%). Despite the beneficial headache reductions lisinopril provided, however, there was no difference in quality of life between the treatment groups. The researchers concluded that lisinopril offers important preventive effects in migraine. Other studies also consider it a useful, well-tolerated preventive drug for migraine.

For more information see page 1284.

Generic: **Metoprolol** *(me-toe-PROE-lole)*
Brands: **Lopressor, Toprol-XL**

Metoprolol belongs to a class of drugs known as selective beta-blockers. It is often used alone or in combination with other drugs to treat high blood pressure, to prevent chest pain, and to treat heart attacks by slowing the heart rate and relaxing blood vessels so the heart does not have to pump as hard. Sometimes metoprolol is used to prevent migraine headaches.

An article in *Current Medical Research and Opinion* noted that beta-blockers are the most widely used drug class in migraine prevention. They are thought to prevent migraine by improving blood flow. The long-acting formulation of this drug may be given once daily. For some patients, the beneficial effects of metoprolol may be two-fold, as it may treat both high blood pressure and prevent migraine.

For more information see page 1321.

Generic: **Mirtazapine** *(mir-TAZ-a-peen)*
Brands: **Remeron, Remeron SolTab**

Mirtazapine belongs to a class of drugs known as antidepressants, used to treat depression by increasing certain types of activity in the brain.

According to the U.S. Headache Consortium practice guidelines, mirtazapine is recommended for migraine prevention based on expert consensus and clinical experience. In one patient study at Louisiana State University School of Medicine, mirtazapine was given to a 60-year-old man with depressive symptoms who found that it also prevented migraine headaches. He reported that if he felt migraine symptoms early on, he would take an extra mirtazapine tablet to prevent its onset. According to the patient, taking the extra tablet resulted in a decrease of four or five migraines per month to one per month. Researchers concluded that mirtazapine may be useful in preventing migraine, although more clinical studies are needed.

For more information see page 1332.

Generic: **Nadolol** *(nay-DOE-lole)*
Brand: **Cogard**

Nadolol, a beta-blocker, treats high blood pressure and prevents chest pain by slowing the heart rate and relaxing the blood vessels so the heart does not have to pump as hard. It is often used to prevent migraine headaches, since beta-blockers may prevent headaches by improving blood flow; therefore, they are the most widely used drug class in the prevention of migraines.

Nadolol may be particularly helpful in people who have high blood pressure and suffer from migraine. There is limited data on the efficacy of nadolol for migraine prevention, but this drug is recognized to have some utility for prevention. The medical literature contains a few brief reports of the use of nadolol for migraine prevention. In an article by French researchers, nadolol, along with a number of other beta-blocker drugs, was a first choice for preventing this debilitating condition. In a study by researchers in Spain, combination therapy with a beta-blocker (nadolol) and sodium valproate appears to be "good migraine prevention" in people who are resistant to these drugs when used alone.

For more information see page 1347.

Generic: **Nortriptyline** *(nor-TRIP-ti-leen)*
Brands: **Aventyl, Pamelor**

Nortriptyline belongs to a class of antidepressant drugs known as sedating TCAs, and is used to treat depression. In general, antidepressants may be helpful in preventing migraine by regulating serotonin levels in the brain.

TCA-type antidepressants may be particularly useful for patients with depression who also suffer from migraine. TCAs vary widely in the way they are absorbed, distributed, and excreted in the body. Nortriptyline is among the most commonly used TCA-type drugs for migraine prevention. The U.S. Headache Consortium recommends the use of nortriptyline for migraine prevention based on expert consensus and clinical experience. Researchers at the School of Pharmacy at West Virginia University noted that the prevention of chronic, recurrent tension headaches is best achieved with nighttime TCAs, particularly nortriptyline.

For more information see page 1378.

Generic: **Phenelzine** *(FEN-el-zeen)*
Brand: **Nardil**

Phenelzine belongs to a class of antidepressant drugs known as nonspecific monoamine oxidase (MAO) inhibitors, and is used to treat depression. It is occasionally used to treat headaches and other conditions. Phenyelzine may help prevent migraine by regulating the levels of the brain chemical, serotonin.

Current Medical Research and Opinion notes that phenelzine has been used to prevent migraines when other treatments fail. If you take this drug, though, you must adhere to a restricted diet to prevent high blood pressure.

For more information see page 1408.

Generic: **Tiagabine** *(tie-GA-been)*
Brand: **Gabitril**

Tiagabine belongs to a class of drugs known as anticonvulsants, and is used to treat partial seizures by increasing the amount of GABA available in the brain. This action may also reduce the incidence of migraine.

Researchers at the New England Center for Headache, in Stamford, Connecticut, noted that tiagabine has not been extensively studied for migraine prevention. Overall, the use of anticonvulsants for migraine prevention is increasing, based on the idea that migraine and epilepsy share several features and respond to many of the same drugs. In a study of 41 patients taking tiagabine, five patients were free from migraine and 33 of 41 patients had at least a 50% reduction in migraine attacks. The U.S. Headache Consortium recommends tiagabine for migraine prevention, based on expert consensus and clinical experience.

For more information see page 1510.

Generic: **Tizanidine** *(tye-ZAN-i-dine)*
Brand: **Zanaflex**

Tizanidine belongs to a class of drugs known as muscle relaxants, and is used to alleviate spasms caused by multiple sclerosis and other conditions that reduce muscle tone.

Studies of tizanidine have shown it to be useful in chronic headache. In one study, tizanidine had a statistically significant benefit compared with placebo. At the Michigan Head-Pain and Neurological Institute in Ann Arbor, Michigan, the efficacy and safety of tizanidine was evaluated in 39 patients with more than 15 headaches (including migraine) per month. Patients in this study received 2 mg of tizanidine at bedtime to start; this dose was then increased to a median daily dose of 14 mg by week four of the study. With the use of tizanidine, overall headache frequency declined, headache intensity decreased, and duration of headache was reduced. Researchers concluded that this drug is effective for headache prevention.

For more information see page 1515.

Generic: *Trazodone* (TRAZ-oh-done)
Brand: *Desyrel*

Trazodone, a serotonin modulator, belongs to a class of drugs known as antidepressants. It treats depression by increasing the levels of the brain chemical serotonin. Side effects associated with trazodone include headache, upset stomach, vomiting, bad taste in the mouth, stomach pain, diarrhea, constipation, changes in appetite, weight changes, weakness or tiredness, nervousness, and confusion, among others. Although trazodone is recommended by the U. S. Headache Consortium for preventing of migraine, based on expert consensus and clinical experience, there is very little clinical data in the medical literature on its efficacy and safety in patients.

In an eight-month trial, researchers in Italy examined the efficacy of trazodone in 40 children with migraine (without aura) ranging in age from seven years to 18 years. Patients in Group A received oral trazodone for 12 weeks, while patients in Group B received placebo. After a four-week washout period, Group A was then given placebo and Group B was treated with trazodone for another 12 weeks. During the first treatment period, both the frequency and the duration of the migraine episodes were significantly reduced in both groups. During the second, a significant, additional improvement in both parameters was seen only in Group B. In this study, no side effects were observed at any time. Results from this study showed that, similar to other antidepressants, trazodone is a valid treatment option for children with migraine.

For more information see page 1521.

Generic: *Venlafaxine* (ven-la-FAX-een)
Brands: *Effexor, Effexor XR*

Venlafaxine belongs to a class of antidepressant drugs known as SSRIs, and is used to treat depression. It is also used to treat general anxiety disorder (GAD) and seasonal affective disorder (SAD). Venlafaxine works by increasing certain kinds of activity in the brain. Side effects associated with venlafaxine include upset stomach, drowsiness, weakness, tiredness, excitement, anxiety, difficulty sleeping, nightmares, dry mouth, skin sensitivity to sunlight, changes in appetite or weight, and headache.

Venlafaxine is recommended as a migraine prevention drug according to the U.S. Headache Consortium guidelines, based on expert consensus and clinical experience. However, it is important to note that there is little to no evidence from clinical trials with this drug. In general, SSRIs may be especially useful in people with mood disorders and migraine. Moreover, SSRIs produce fewer side effects compared with TCA-type drugs.

In a study in *Headache*, 60 patients with migraine (without aura) received venlafaxine dosed at 75 mg or 150 mg, or placebo. In this study, a significant difference in the number of headache attacks was seen between the venlafaxine 150-mg group and placebo. Additionally, 80% of patients in the 75-mg group and 88.2% of patients in the 150-mg group reported their treatment to be "good" or "very good." Researchers concluded that venlafaxine was more effective than placebo, and is safe and well tolerated for migraine prevention. In a review study evaluating 170 patients with migraine or other type of headache, venlafaxine was given in doses ranging from 37.5 mg/day to 75 mg/day. Results from this study showed that venlafaxine significantly reduced the frequency of moderate-to-severe headaches.

For more information see page 1542.

Generic: **Verapamil** *(vur-AP-ah-mill)*
Brands: **Calan, Calan SR, Covera-HS, Isoptin SR,
Verelan, Verelan PM**

Verapamil belongs to a class of drugs known as calcium channel
blockers, and is used to treat irregular heartbeats and high blood
pressure. It relaxes blood vessels so the heart does not have to
pump as hard. It also increases the supply of blood and oxygen to
the heart to control chest pain. Verapamil may be used to treat migraine headaches; it may prevent migraine by improving blood
flow by changing the movement of calcium ions into muscle cells
of blood vessels. Side effects associated with verapamil include
constipation, dizziness, lightheadedness, upset stomach, heartburn, excessive tiredness, feeling of warmth, slow heartbeat, and
vivid dreams.

In general, it takes about two weeks for this drug to work. There is
limited evidence for the use of verapamil for migraine prevention.
In three trials, significant differences were found with this drug, but
the relevance of the findings were uncertain because of high patient
dropout rates in two of the studies. Among the calcium channel
blockers used for migraine prevention, verapamil happens to be the
most widely studied and is considered the first-line choice within its
class. Some researchers believe that calcium channel drugs, such as
verapamil, may be more effective than beta-blockers in patients
with migraine (with aura) or those with complicated migraine. Verapamil may be particularly useful in those patients with high
blood pressure and migraine.

In three studies, 10 of 12 patients, eight of 14 patients, and 20 of
23 patients showed improvement with verapamil. All studies
demonstrated verapamil to be significantly more effective than
placebo in migraine prevention.

For more information see page 1544.

Tension Headache

The International Headache Society (IHS) classifies episodic tension headache as 10 previous headache episodes lasting from 30
minutes to seven days and happening less than 180 times per year.
Pain symptoms of tension headache include at least two of the following: pressing/tightening located on both sides of the head; mild

to moderate intensity; not triggered by physical activity; not accompanied by nausea or vomiting; and possible sensitivity to light, sound, or both. Treatment of tension headache includes over-the-counter (aspirin, acetaminophen) or prescription drugs.

Commonly Prescribed (On-Label) Drugs: None

OFF-LABEL PRESCRIPTION DRUGS
BREAKTHROUGH OPTIONS
---

*Generic: **Botulinum Toxin Type A** (BOT-yoo-lin-num TOKS-in type aye)*
*Brands: **Botox, Botox cosmetic***

Botulinum toxin type A belongs to a class of drugs known as injectable neurotoxins. Neurotoxins block the nerves' ability to make muscles contract thereby paralyzing muscles. Botulinum toxin type A works by preventing the release of a nerve chemical in the body known as acetylcholine, thus preventing muscle cells from contracting. This injectable neurotoxin is used to treat neck muscle spasms and uncontrollable blinking, to control misaligned or "lazy eyes," and to reduce the appearance of forehead frown lines in adults age 65 and younger. Side effects associated with botulinum toxin type A include allergic reactions, temporary muscle weakness or discomfort at injection site, skin rash, sensitivity to light, and headache.

In people with tension headache, botulinum toxin type A may direct muscular relaxation and reduce feeling thereby alleviating tender and trigger points associated with tension-type headaches. Improvements in tension-type headache were first realized in patients receiving botulinum toxin type A injections for cosmetic treatment of wrinkles. A number of clinical studies evaluated botulinum toxin type A for tension headache treatment. In these studies, doses of botulinum toxin type A have ranged from five units per site to 20 units per site to 30 units to 50 units divided (three to five sites). It has been suggested that this drug be injected at the site of pain or trigger points and not on a standardized or predetermined basis for affected patients.

In a study, 60 adult patients with chronic tension-type headache were selected to receive 150 units of botulinum toxin diluted in normal saline solution. Of the treated patients, 63% reported a 50% improvement in facial pain. Moreover, all 46 patients with chronic tension headache reported a 50% improvement in headache pain. In this study, no adverse drug reactions were seen. Researchers concluded that botulinum toxin type A was effective in improving facial and headache pain associated with tension headaches. Side effects of botulinum toxin type A seen in clinical trials include headache worsening and a weak feeling in the neck muscles.

For more information see page 1051.

Generic: **Lorazepam** *(lore-AZ-ee-pam)*
Brands: **Ativan, Lorazepam Intensol**

Lorazepam belongs to the benzodiazepines class of drugs, which slow down the central nervous system and help relieve anxiety and nervousness. A doctor may prescribe lorazepam for tension-type headache. Side effects include constipation, diarrhea, difficulty sleeping, nightmares, dizziness, drowsiness, clumsiness, headache, memory loss, nausea, and vomiting.

In general, benzodiazepines cause sedation and are habit forming; therefore, their use requires close monitoring by doctors. They are considered a last resort and not a first choice for the management of tension-type headache. An article in a medical journal noted that two trials found insufficient evidence regarding the effects of benzodiazepine-type drugs compared with placebo and other treatments for tension-type headache. The researcher also emphasized that regular use of benzodiazepine drugs has adverse effects and concluded that they are ineffective or harmful for chronic tension headache. Even though benzodiazepines, such as lorazepam, have been used to treat tension-type headache, controlled trials are quite limited in the medical literature.

For more information see page 1287.

Generic: **Tizanidine** *(tye-ZAN-i-deen)*
Brand: **Zanaflex**

Tizanidine is classified as a muscle relaxant drug, and can relieve but not cure muscle spasms caused by medical conditions such as multiple sclerosis and brain and spinal injuries. A number of studies evaluated the use of tizanidine for tension-type headache and other types of headache. Researchers in Finland compared tizanidine with placebo in 185 adults with chronic tension-type headache. The treatment period was six weeks and patients received either 6 mg or 12 mg of tizanidine or placebo (all given orally once per day). Of the 185 patients, 160 completed the study and headache severity decreased similarly across both active drug treatment groups and placebo. It was concluded that tizanidine, in doses up to 12 mg, was not superior to placebo for the treatment of chronic tension-type headache.

In another trial, researchers in Finland examined the efficacy of tizanidine compared with placebo in 37 women with chronic tension-type headache. Treatment in this study consisted of 6 mg/day of tizanidine divided into three doses; the daily dose could be increased up to 18 mg/day depending on response to the drug. Compared with placebo, tizanidine was found to be statistically more effective than placebo for pain control, number of days free of headache, the number of headache drugs needed, and the dose of study medication needed. Side effects associated with tizanidine in this study were drowsiness and dry mouth. Researchers concluded that tizanidine is effective in the treatment of chronic tension-type headache in women. Side effects include blurred vision, constipation, drowsiness, dry mouth, tiredness, and weakness.

For more information see page 1515.

Tension Headache Prevention

Approximately 69% of men and 88% of women develop tension headache during their life. Tension headaches can be episodic or chronic; pain may affect both sides of the head, or it can be localized to the forehead, temples, or back of head. Prevention includes use of drugs in the following classes: antidepressants, beta-blockers, and anticonvulsants. Doctors will usually start tension headache treatment with newer types of antidepressants, and will increase the dose until you get a therapeutic effect.

Commonly Prescribed (On-Label) Drugs: *None*

OFF-LABEL PRESCRIPTION DRUGS
BREAKTHROUGH OPTIONS

Generic: **Baclofen** *(BAK-low-fen)*
Brands: **Kemstro, Lioresal**

Baclofen belongs to a class of drugs known as muscle relaxants, and is used to relieve spasms and cramping of muscles in conditions such as multiple sclerosis. It affects a major inhibitory neurotransmitter (known as gamma-aminobutyric acid or GABA) in the brain and has anti-spasmic and analgesic properties. A few studies support baclofen's use as a migraine and cluster headache prevention drug. Side effects associated with baclofen include changes in taste, confusion, constipation, diarrhea, difficulty sleeping, dizziness, drowsiness, dry mouth, headache, increased passing of urine, muscle weakness, nausea, vomiting, weakness, and tiredness.

Most of the studies involving baclofen involve other headache types. In a study in Israel, nine patients with cluster headache were given baclofen 15 mg to 30 mg in three divided doses. Within one week, six of the nine patients reported that their headache attacks stopped. One patient was substantially better and became free of headache attacks by the end of the following week. The remaining two patients' headache attacks worsened and corticosteroid drugs were prescribed. Researchers concluded that baclofen appeared to be effective and well tolerated for the prevention of cluster headache.

In another study, also in Israel, 54 patients with migraine (with and without aura) were given baclofen (15 mg to 40 mg) in three divided doses for 12 weeks. It was effective in 86.2% of the patients with greater than 50% reduction in headache from the start of the study. Three patients could not tolerate the drug because of adverse reactions. Researchers concluded that baclofen was effective for preventing migraine.

For more information see page 1037.

Generic: **Botulinum Toxin Type A** *(BOT-yoo-lin-num TOKS-in type aye)*
Brands: **Botox, Botox Cosmetics**

Botulinum toxin type A belongs to a class of drugs known as injectable neurotoxins, which block the nerves' ability to make muscles contract, thereby paralyzing them. Botulinum toxin type A prevents the release of a nerve chemical known as acetylcholine and so prevents muscle cells from contracting. It is used to treat neck muscle spasms and uncontrollable blinking, to control misaligned or "lazy eyes," and to reduce the appearance of forehead frown lines. The way it works to prevent headache is not completely understood. Side effects associated with the drug include allergic reactions, temporary muscle weakness or discomfort at injection site, skin rash, sensitivity to light, and headache.

Botulinum toxin type A has been widely studied for the treatment and prevention of a variety of headache types. In a 2000 study in *Neurology* journal, patients with chronic tension-type headache resistant to standard treatment were given multiple injections (in a variety of sites) with botulinum toxin type A (40 units to 95 units). Patients had decreased headache severity, decreased tenderness, and headache-free days. Adverse reactions were rarely seen and researchers concluded that botulinum toxin type A may effectively prevent chronic tension-type headache.

In general, patient case reports and clinical trials suggest that migraine and tension-type headaches may respond well to botulinum toxin type A. The effect of a single treatment can last for up to three months. Overall, it reduces the frequency and severity of headaches, reduces the headache disability that it causes, improves quality of life, and reduces the need for headache drugs. It is recommended that botulinum toxin type A be used in the difficult-to-treat cases of chronic migraine and chronic tension-type headache.

For more information see page 1051.

Generic: **Candesartan** *(kan-de-SAR-tan)*
Brand: **Atacand**

Candesartan belongs to a class of drugs known as angiotensin 2-receptor antagonists (ARBs), and is used to lower high blood pressure and prevent stroke, heart failure, and kidney damage. Heart drugs, such as candesartan, are useful in preventing headaches, possibly because they act on blood vessels. Side effects include back pain, cough, dizziness, headache, sore throat, nasal congestion, and runny nose.

The medical literature has little information on the use of candesartan for the prevention of tension-type headache, although its efficacy and safety for migraine headache were studied by researchers in Tokyo, Japan. Eight patients with migraine and hypertension who could not tolerate other headache drugs were successfully treated with candesartan; their migraine severity and blood pressure reduced. Researchers concluded that candesartan is a unique, desirable migraine prevention drug in patients with concomitant hypertension. In a 2004 study in *Headache*, researchers evaluated the use of off-label prescription drugs used in a specialty headache practice. Candesartan accounted for 4% of off-label headache prescription drugs. Researchers concluded that it is reasonable to use off-label drugs, such as candesartan, in treating some headache conditions.

For more information see page 1065.

Generic: **Fluoxetine** *(floo-OKS-e-teen)*
Brands: **Prozac, Prozac Weekly, Sarafem**

Fluoxetine belongs to a class of antidepressant drugs known as selective serotonin reuptake inhibitors (SSRIs), and is used to treat mental depression, obsessive-compulsive disorder (OCD), bulimia nervosa, and premenstrual dysphoric disorder (PMDD). How fluoxetine and other antidepressants prevent tension-type headache is uncertain, but this type of drug has helped a variety of painful states including headache. Fluoxetine acts only on the neurotransmitter chemical, serotonin, and so may reduce the frequency of migraine by regulating serotonin levels in the brain. Side effects include anxiety, nervousness, decreased appetite, decreased sexual ability or drive, skin rash, diarrhea, drowsiness, increased sweating, nausea, tiredness, weakness, trembling, shaking, and difficulty sleeping, among others.

Researchers at the University College London Medical School in England compared the use of fluoxetine and desipramine (an antidepressant drug) in the treatment of chronic tension headache and depression. Patients received either fluoxetine or desipramine for 12 weeks. Of the 25 patients who completed the study, 12 received fluoxetine and 13 desipramine. Neither group showed a significant difference at the start of the study or in change of pain, reduction in the use of pain drugs, or changes in depression scores. However, 72% of patients who completed the study improved.

In a study published in *Headache*, prescriptions of newer antidepressants (venlafaxine) accounted for 15% of off-label drugs used for headaches. Researchers concluded that off-label drugs are reasonable for treating headache disorders.

For more information see page 1192.

Generic: **Levetiracetam** *(lee-va-tye-RA-se-tam)*
Brand: **Keppra**

Levetiracetam belongs to a class of anti-epileptic drugs, and is used to control partial seizures (convulsions); it may be prescribed with other drugs to help control convulsions. Side effects associated with its use include dizziness and drowsiness. Since 1970, anti-epileptic drugs have been used to prevent headache; the advent of newer drugs in this class has spurred research on their effects on pain.

Valproic acid and topiramate are among the commonly used anti-epileptic drugs for preventing tension-type headache. In a study published in *Headache*, levetiracetam accounted for 2% of the off-label drugs used for headaches. Researchers evaluated the use of off-label drugs in a specialty headache practice and concluded that off-label drugs are reasonable to use to treat headache disorders.

In a review article in Italy, levetiracetam was among anti-epileptic drugs mentioned for the prevention of migraine headache. The authors noted that anti-epileptic drugs may be useful in preventing migraine headaches as some have reduced the monthly frequency and severity of attacks. Other researchers in Brazil noted that levetiracetam may be useful to prevent migraine headaches, but more clinical trials are needed to confirm its safety and efficacy.

For more information see page 1276.

Generic: **Tizanidine** *(tye-ZAN-i-deen)*
Brand: **Zanaflex**

Tizanidine, an alpha2-adrenergic agonist, belongs to a class of drugs known as muscle relaxants, and is used to alleviate spasms in multiple sclerosis and other conditions, and increase muscle tone. Tizanidine may help prevent tension-type headache.

In a 12-week study conducted at the Michigan Head-Pain and Neurological Institute, tizanidine was associated with a decline in headache frequency and headache intensity, and improvements in mood, sleep, and quality of life. During weeks nine through 12, 67% of patients had improved more than 50% since the start of the study. Overall headache frequency decreased from 22.83 days/month to 15.83 days/month.

In a 2004 study published in *Headache*, tizanidine accounted for 3% of the off-label drugs used in headache disorders. In a review article by a researcher at the University of Health Sciences/ Chicago Medical School, tizanidine was used to prevent tension-type headaches. The researcher noted that tizanidine has been useful in chronic headache. Additionally, in one trial, tizanidine had a statistically significant benefit versus placebo. This researcher concluded that tizanidine is effective in primary headache disorders.

For more information see page 1515.

Generic: **Venlafaxine** *(ven-la-FAX-een)*
Brands: **Effexor, Effexor XR**

Venlafaxine belongs to a class of antidepressant drugs known as SSRIs, and is used to treat depression, general anxiety disorder (GAD), and seasonal affective disorder (SAD). Venlafaxine works by increasing certain kinds of activity in the brain. In animals, venlafaxine has been shown to be an effective pain reliever. Studies evaluating venlafaxine for pain have shown that this drug may alter pain tolerance thresholds thereby providing a pain-relieving effect in headache or other conditions. Side effects include upset stomach, drowsiness, weakness, tiredness, excitement, anxiety, difficulty sleeping, nightmares, dry mouth, skin sensitivity to sunlight, changes in appetite or weight, and headache.

In a study, 170 adults with migraine or chronic tension-type headache were treated with venlafaxine for six months. Results showed that the mean frequency of tension headaches decreased from 24/month to 15.2/month. Thirty percent of patients with tension-type headache had 50% reduction in headaches and 41% of patients with moderate to severe tension-type headaches had greater than 50% reduction in headaches with the use of venlafaxine. Adverse drug reactions seen in this study, which led to discontinuing venlafaxine, included nausea, difficulty sleeping, and excessive tiredness and weakness. Researchers concluded that venlafaxine has potential as a headache prevention drug.

For more information see page 1542.

MISCELLANEOUS DISORDERS

When the brain is damaged, it can malfunction and lead to complete loss of consciousness (coma), disorientation, or an inability to pay attention (delirium). The type and severity of brain dysfunction depend on how extensive brain damage is, where the damage is, and how quickly the disorder causing it is progressing. The nervous system is also vulnerable to damage and malfunction (from diseases and injuries), for example from nerve degeneration that causes Alzheimer's or Parkinson's disease. Bacteria or viruses can infect the brain or spinal cord, causing encephalitis or meningitis.

Charles Bonnet Syndrome

Charles Bonnet Syndrome (or CBS) is named after a Swiss philosopher who first described this condition in 1760 when he noticed that his grandfather, who was blinded by cataracts, described seeing birds and buildings that did not exist. CBS is a condition in which people with sight problems start to see things that they know are not real (visual hallucinations). CBS affects people with sight difficulties and normally only people who have lost their sight later in life. However, it can affect people of any age.

Commonly Prescribed (On-Label) Drugs: None

OFF-LABEL PRESCRIPTION DRUGS
BREAKTHROUGH OPTIONS

Generic: **Donepezil** *(doh-NEP-e-zil)*
Brand: **Aricept**

Donepezil is used to treat Alzheimer's disease. It works by increasing the amount of certain brain chemicals. Side effects associated with donepezil include upset stomach, diarrhea, difficulty falling asleep or staying asleep, vomiting, muscle cramps, excessive tiredness, appetite loss, pain, headache, and dizziness, among others.

There is no established treatment for CBS, although a number of drugs have been used, including donepezil. Since cholinergic drugs have been successful in treating patients with visual hallucinations associated with Alzheimer's disease, researchers in Japan reported the use of this drug in a 73-year-old woman with CBS who had glaucoma in both eyes since her 30s. During her lifetime, she had progressive bilateral visual impairment. At age 68, she underwent cataract surgery in both eyes. About four months after her surgery, her vision worsened and visual hallucination quickly appeared. She described these visions as black and round flying objects, but knew they were not real. After one month, the hallucinations became colorful and in shapes of flowers and lattice; the frequency and duration of the hallucinations increased as well. She was treated with a number of drugs for five months, and then tried donepezil. The dose was increased two weeks later and hallucinations decreased in both eyes, so she was maintained on this dose without any adverse effects.

For more information see page 1150.

Generic: **Mirtazapine** *(mir-TAZ-a-peen)*
Brands: **Remeron, Remeron SolTab**

Mirtazapine is a mood elevator used to treat depression. It works by increasing certain types of activity in the brain. Some side effects include drowsiness, dizziness, anxiousness, confusion, weight gain, dry mouth, and upset stomach.

There is no established treatment for CBS; however, a number of drugs have been used, including mirtazapine. Two researchers from Omaha, Nebraska, reported the use of mirtazapine in a

59-year-old African American man who was hospitalized for pneumonia. On the fifth day of his hospitalization, he had visual hallucinations, which had been occurring for three years, included people and farm animals, most often occurring in the evening. After he was diagnosed with CBS, he was given mirtazapine at bedtime. Within three days, his visual hallucinations were reduced, and he had no recurrence of hallucinations at his one-month follow-up. Doctors chose mirtazapine because of the drug's properties and favorable safety record in elderly patients and concluded that it is an effective, safe, and well-tolerated drug for CBS.

For more information see page 1332.

Multiple Sclerosis

Multiple sclerosis (MS) is an unpredictable disease of the central nervous system (CNS) that predominantly strikes young women. Generally believed to be an autoimmune disease (the body's immune system attacks itself), it involves damage to the myelin sheath of nerve tissue. Symptoms include fatigue, mobility impairment, pain, depression, sensory disorders (vision, hearing, and touch), poor balance, and muscle weakness and spasms, with the first symptoms usually occurring between the ages of 20 and 40. Presently there is no cure for MS. The diagnosis may be delayed due to nonspecific and uncertain symptoms. MS has the tendency to move into remission and spontaneously exacerbate. Researchers are now investigating many different therapies for slowing disease progression and minimizing recurrences; some of these therapies have been approved by U. S. FDA to reduce frequency of exacerbations.

Commonly Prescribed (On-Label) Drugs: *Corticotropin, Gadopentetate Dimeglumine, Glatiramer, Interferon Beta-1A, Interferon Beta-1B, Methylprednisolone, Mitoxantrone, Natalizumab, Prednisone, Triamcinolone*

OFF-LABEL PRESCRIPTION DRUGS
BREAKTHROUGH OPTIONS

Generic: **Alemtuzumab** *(ay-lem-TU-zoo-mab)*
Brand: **Campath**

Alemtuzumab is a biologic (made from living cells) drug that is derived from DNA. It belongs to a new class of drugs called humanized monoclonal antibodies. Alemtuzumab is used to treat certain types of leukemia in patients whose previous therapies failed. This drug is only administered intravenously (IV) under the supervision of a doctor experienced in cancer therapies. Side effects include blood count disorders, increased risk of infections, and infusion reactions.

According to researchers in the United Kingdom, alemtuzumab has shown clinical benefit in patients receiving treatment during the early phase of MS, when disease activity is attributed to inflammation within the body. In a study, 58 patients with secondary progressive multiple sclerosis (SPMS) and relapsing-remitting multiple sclerosis (RRMS) were treated with alemtuzumab. The RRMS group had MS for a mean of 2.7 years, and the SPMS group had the disease for a mean of 12 years. Of the two groups, the patients with SPMS had fewer relapse rates during a mean of seven years, yet had progressive disability and an initial profound T-cell (a type of lymphocyte) count depletion. Of the treated patients with RRMS, only one patient relapsed. The study determined that alemtuzumab was associated with a reduction in the annual relapse rates in patients with RRMS. Other medical literature associates alemtuzumab treatment in MS to nerve cell growth, which fosters healing and prevents further deterioration. This evidence suggests new research is needed to study damage caused by MS and possibilities of nerve fiber survival.

For more information see page 992.

Generic: **Amantadine** *(a-MAN-to-deen)*
Brand: **Symmetrel**

Amantadine belongs to a class of drugs known as antivirals, used to prevent or treat influenza (flu) infections. This antiviral drug has also shown activity against viruses that belong to the *Flaviviridae* family of viruses, to which hepatitis C virus belongs. It has been used for many years as a drug of choice in combating fatigue and has been used to treat fatigue in patients with MS. It works by facilitating the release of dopamine (i.e., a nervous system hormone) from nerve cells. Amantadine is also used in Parkinson's disease.

Since this drug has an antiviral action, and MS exacerbations are triggered by infections, experts suggest that the use of amantadine can reduce the amount of flare-ups by preventing viral infections. In a two-year study, fewer exacerbations resulted in those treated with amantadine versus placebo. Intermittent therapy is suggested due to the diminished effects of the drug after a few months. Caution should be taken by patients with kidney disease to prevent toxicity. It is usually well tolerated, but side effects of amantadine include insomnia, mood disturbances, allergic reactions, confusion, and hallucinations.

Other opposing literature suggests the studies involving amantadine in MS for fatigue are poorly documented and new research needs to be conducted.

For more information see page 1001.

*Generic: **Amitriptyline** (a-mee-TRIP-ti-leen)*
*Brand: **Elavil***

Amitriptyline belongs to a class of drugs called tricyclic antidepressants (TCAs), used in the treatment of symptoms of mental depression, including anxiety. Amitriptyline is thought to improve mood by raising the level of neurotransmitters (the brain messenger chemicals norepinephrine and serotonin) thereby improving anxiety with its sedative effects.

Side effects of amitriptyline include dry mouth, mild drowsiness, photosensitivity, urinary retention, tinnitus (ringing in the ears), and confusion. It should be taken at night due to its sedative effects. It may take up to two to three weeks to take effect.

MS patients may suffer neuropathic pain—pain that arises from nerve dysfunction, not a result of direct injury. Painful paresthesias (burning sensations, pins and needles, and stabbing pains) are caused by damage to the regulating pathways of the brain and spinal cord. This type of pain has also been treated with amitriptyline. Other off-label uses of this drug include migraine prevention, tension headache prevention, chronic pain, fibromyalgia, neuropathy, and trigeminal neuralgia (a facial nerve disorder). TCAs should not be used in combination with another type of antidepressant called MAO inhibitors.

For more information see page 1009.

*Generic: **Azathioprine** (ay-za-THYE-oh-preen)*
*Brand: **Imuran***

Azathioprine belongs to a class of drugs known as immunosuppressives (decrease immune activity) usually prescribed to prevent rejection of transplanted organs and in rheumatoid arthritis. The use of azathioprine may decrease proliferation of immune cells, thus reducing autoimmune activity (body's attack of its own tissues). Side effects include increased chances of infections, hair loss, loss of appetite, nausea, vomiting, skin rash, discolored urine and stool, fever, chills, sore throat, low back pain, and joint pain.

Since MS is believed to be an autoimmune disease, azathioprine has been used to treat it. A survey conducted among 2,000 practitioners to inquire about the types of immunosuppressants given for the treatment of MS, and from 702 MS centers in France, found that azathioprine was used most frequently. Other immunosuppressive treatments included cyclophosphamide, methotrexate, and mitoxantrone.

In a study of 23 patients with relapse-remitting MS (RRMS) combination therapy with azathioprine and interferon beta (1a) had promising results. Although trials involving the investigation of azathioprine in the treatment of MS are small in sample size and have various limitations, most suggest that it reduces the relapse rate of the disease. The drug's effect on progression of disability has not been studied.

For more information see page 1033.

*Generic: **Carbamazepine** (kar-ba-MAZ-e-peen)*
*Brands: **Carbatrol, Epitol, Tegretol, Tegretol XR***

Carbamazepine is an anticonvulsant approved for the treatment of seizures in epilepsy, pain in trigeminal neuralgia, and in patients with bipolar disorder (manic-depressive illness). It has been associated with rash and neurologic (nervous system function) side effects, particularly when administered in higher doses. Other side effects include drowsiness, headache, fatigue, dry mouth, and blood disorders, to guard against which patients require regular monitoring of blood counts and liver function.

Dystonic (abnormal movement) spasms associated with MS may be treated with carbamazepine, which medical literature has noted to be beneficial. This drug and other anticonvulsants/muscle relaxants have helped in painful muscle spasms that occur with MS.

In other medical literature, however, carbamazepine has been known to exacerbate ataxia (muscular weakness and dysfunction). Ataxia is a common symptom in MS as well as in other disorders including diabetic polyneuropathy (a complication of diabetes involving the nerves). One study involved the combination of low-dose gabapentin combined with either carbamazepine or lamotrigine in the treatment of trigeminal neuralgia (a facial nerve disorder) in MS. Of the 11 patients with MS and trigeminal neuralgia, six were not able to tolerate carbamazepine due to side effects and were started on combination therapy of gabapentin and carbamazepine, but the decreased dose did not yield any pain relief. The same was found in the group treated with lamotrigine.

For more information see page 1068.

Generic: **Clonazepam** (kloe-NA-ze-pam)
Brand: **Klonopin**

Clonazepam is a benzodiazepine that has anxiolytic (suppresses anxiety), sedative, and anticonvulsant properties and belongs to a class of drugs called central nervous system (CNS) depressants. It is used in the treatment of panic and seizure disorders. Side effects include drowsiness, clumsiness, ataxia, behavior problems, rash, back pain, blood disorders, increased salivation, and withdrawal symptoms. It also tends to become addictive. Clonazepam adds to the effect of alcohol and other CNS depressants (sleep aids, muscle relaxants, antihistamines, and pain drugs) and may lose efficacy with cigarette smoking.

Clonazepam has shown benefit in the treatment of tremor, pain, and ataxia (uncoordinated movement), eye movement disorders, muscle spasms, stiffness, postural tremor, and walking difficulties associated with MS. Although limited scientific data are available on this drug and MS, as a sedative/anticonvulsant it has helped control symptoms by depressing CNS activity. It may be difficult to distinguish between common symptoms of MS and certain side effects of clonazepam; therefore patients should communicate any reactions they notice. Clonazepam has also been used in the treatment of Parkinson's disease.

For more information see page 1107.

Generic: **Cyclophosphamide** *(sye-kloe-FOS-fa-mide)*
Brands: **Cytoxan, Neosar**

Cyclophosphamide belongs to a class of drugs called antineoplastic (drugs used to treat cancer) alkylating drugs, which decrease or inhibit the growth of cancerous cells. The most commonly reported side effect of cyclophosphamide is decreased blood cell counts. Other side effects include thinning hair, skin discolorations, loss of appetite, unusual bleeding/bruising, cough, congestion, fever, dizziness, chills, shortness of breath, sore throat, nausea and vomiting, and rash.

Chemotherapeutic drugs, such as cyclophosphamide, can help treat symptoms of MS, particularly in secondary progressive MS (SPMS) and worsening relapsing-remitting MS (RRMS). Since MS has autoimmune tendencies, and cyclophosphamide has shown selective immune effects in patients suffering from MS, off-label use of this drug has been ongoing for years. Other medical literature only suggests treatment with cyclophosphamide when patients have failed therapy with other common treatments.

In an Italian study, 10 patients with rapidly transitional MS received a combination treatment with cyclophosphamide and interferon-beta. The patients had been treated previously with interferon-beta alone with no benefit. When cyclophosphamide was added to treatment regimens, they had a decreased number of relapses and an improvement in tissue analysis.

For more information see page 1123.

Generic: **Diazepam** *(dye-AZ-e-pam)*
Brands: **Diastat, Diazepam Intensol, Valium**

Diazepam, which is a benzodiazepine-type drug, induces a calming effect of the central nervous system (CNS). It possesses anti-anxiety, anticonvulsant, sedative, and skeletal muscle relaxant properties. It is closely related to clonazepam, as mentioned above. Diazepam is prescribed for anxiety-related disorders and alcohol withdrawal. Common side effects of diazepam include drowsiness and fatigue; dependence and withdrawal symptoms upon abrupt discontinuation are possible. Any unusual side effects such as behavior problems, convulsions, hallucinations, anger, confusion, mental depression, and difficulty concentrating should be discussed with a doctor. Diazepam has the potential to magnify effects of alcohol and other CNS depressants (antihistamines, sleep aids, pain drugs, muscle relaxants, and anticonvulsants).

In MS, diazepam is used primarily for the relief of muscle spasm, stiffness, difficulty walking, and muscle spasticity. Along with other drugs, it can contribute to sexual dysfunctions including decreased libido, erectile problems, and abnormal ejaculation. Although scientific data are limited on the use of benzodiazepines in MS, diazepam is also used for tremors. Patients with MS may experience spasticity (uncontrolled contraction or squeezing) of the bladder, which involves discomfort and pain. Diazepam also has been used to treat these contractions due to its sedating properties. It may be difficult to distinguish between symptoms associated with MS and some side effects of diazepam; therefore, patients have regular appointments with their doctor to communicate any concerns.

For more information see page 1139.

Generic: **Dronabinol** *(droe-NAB-i-nol)*
Brand: **Marinol**

Dronabinol is a derivative of cannabinoid (primary ingredient in marijuana) and is used to treat anxiety, nausea, and pain in cancer, rheumatoid arthritis (RA), and acquired immunodeficiency syndrome (AIDS). Patients who previously failed traditional therapies, or have numerous allergies and sensitivities, have found relief with cannabinoid derivatives. Cannabinoid research has recently become a field of study in science and medicine, and is influencing the development of cannabinoid-based products for RA and MS. Data derived from research in this area suggest that cannabinoids have a role in pain control, memory, anxiety reduction, euphoria, and nausea. The most powerful effects include diminished psychomotor activity, impaired judgment, and the potential for abuse.

Many MS symptoms include musculoskeletal pain, spasm pain, and central pain. Central pain is the most common (33%) and affects nervous system pathways from the sclerosing (hardening) of the plaques (damaged areas of tissue). Cannabinoids have positive effects on central pain. In a study in Denmark, 24 patients received treatment for three weeks with either dronabinol or placebo to evaluate the effect on spontaneous pain in patients with definitive MS. Those treated with dronabinol had superior results over placebo on spontaneous pain in the last week of therapy. A relative reduction in pain intensity of 20.5% was found among the dronabinol group, and quality of life improved, as well. Adverse events included dizziness, fatigue, myalgia (muscle pain), and muscle weakness. Use of dronabinol has been recommended in patients who previously failed or were insufficiently treated with anticonvulsants, antidepressants, or opioids.

For more information see page 1159.

Generic: **Fluoxetine** *(floo-OKS-e-teen)*
Brands: **Prozac, Prozac Weekly, Sarafem**

Fluoxetine belongs to a class of drugs known as selective serotonin reuptake inhibitors (SSRIs), also referred to as antidepressants, which can alter levels of brain chemicals and are used for mental depression and panic disorder. Depression often accompanies other symptoms in MS and antidepressants may be included in treatment regimens. Before depression is diagnosed, doctors should rule out poor sleep patterns, medical conditions, and any other possible drug side effects. Patients should be encouraged to exercise regularly along with taking antidepressant drugs.

Fluoxetine is among many antidepressants prescribed for depression as well as fatigue in MS. It is generally well tolerated, yet should be taken in the morning to avoid sleep disturbances. Other common side effects include dry mouth and dizziness.

In one case study from Canada, a 41-year-old woman with MS and a 12-month history of severe depression (non-suicidal) had been treated previously with doxepin hydrochloride with limited effects. Doxepin hydrochloride was discontinued and exchanged for fluoxetine. Six weeks after beginning fluoxetine, she reported mood improvements, less hostility, less emotional lability, and improved concentration at work. One side effect was fatigue, which resolved when she switched to nighttime administration. Her sensory problems, including numbness, also improved.

In a clinical trial of fluoxetine and amitriptyline in MS patients, fluoxetine had a greater effect on cognitive disturbances (another symptom of MS) than amitriptyline.

For more information see page 1192.

Generic: **Gabapentin** *(GA-ba-pen-tin)*
Brand: **Neurontin**

Gabapentin belongs to a class of drugs known as anticonvulsants, used to help control seizures in the treatment of epilepsy. It is also used to control pain associated with shingles and has been evaluated for a number of other pain conditions and neurologic and psychiatric disorders. Gabapentin's pain-modulating properties may be related to release of the neurotransmitter GABA in the spinal cord neural pathways that regulate the perception of pain. Gabapentin has also shown promising results in the treating of diabetes-related neurologic pain.

Gabapentin has been used in MS to treat neuropathic pain (which arises from nerve dysfunction, not a result of injury), trigeminal neuralgia (a type of neuropathic pain and facial nerve disorder), intractable pain, ocular ataxia (abnormal movement of eye muscles), tremors, and muscle spasticity. In some medical literature, many of these symptoms combined are named "paroxysmal symptoms" (includes trigeminal neuralgia, painful tonic spasms, dysesthetic or paresthetic symptoms). The most common side effects are dizziness and somnolence.

In Italy, a small clinical study evaluated the effect of gabapentin on paroxysmal symptoms in 10 patients with MS by testing a nerve reflex of the eyes. It was concluded that gabapentin may help paroxysmal symptoms in MS when other therapies are intolerable or ineffective.

One study of low-dose gabapentin combined with either carbamazepine or lamotrigine (other anticonvulsants) in the treatment of trigeminal neuralgia (a facial nerve disorder) in MS, however, did not help relieve pain. In the 11 patients with MS and trigeminal neuralgia, six were unable to tolerate carbamazepine due to unwanted side effects, and were started on combination therapy of low-dose gabapentin and carbamazepine, but the decreased dose of drug did not help, either. The same effects were found in the group treated with lamotrigine.

At the University of Colorado, a study evaluated the effects of gabapentin on spasticity and found that gabapentin reduced the impairment of spasticity when compared with placebo.

For more information see page 1206.

Generic: **Imipramine** (im-IP-ra-meen)
Brands: **Tofranil, Tofranil-PM**

Imipramine is a TCA and is indicated for depression. The way this antidepressant works is not well understood, but it seems to act on brain chemicals. Side effects include sensitivity to the sun, drowsiness, blurry vision, urinary retention, dry mouth, and constipation.

Imipramine has also been used off-label for different types of urinary incontinence (loss of control in bladder functions). Some patients with MS have urinary problems including urgency, frequency, and urge incontinence—usually referred to as "neurogenic bladder." Some literature suggests that 65% of patients with MS suffer from the problem, which are due to detrusor hyperreflexia (involuntary contractions of the bladder muscle).

In a study from Israel involving 16 patients with MS who were suffering with detrusor hyperreflexia, imipramine was combined with propantheline (anti-spasmotic). Although no change was noted in bladder capacity, 14 of 16 patients showed significant improvement in urinary symptoms. This combination therapy seems to decrease parasympathetic (nervous system) activity while increasing sympathetic (nervous system) activity. Imipramine may relieve other symptoms such as bowel spasms and sensory symptoms, including numbness and tingling.

For more information see page 1230.

Generic: **Immune Globulin** *(EH-mune GLOB-ewe-lyn)*
Brand: **BayGam**

Immune globulin (IgG) is a concentrated antibody (immune cell) preparation that can provide immediate short-term immune protection for those at risk of certain diseases, including viral or bacterial infections. Typically, it is used to treat exposure to measles, varicella (chicken pox), rubella, IgG deficiency, and viral hepatitis A prevention.

The damage to the myelin sheath in MS is thought to be an immune-related reaction, similar to damage in other diseases that have responded well to IgG therapy, including Guillain-Barre syndrome (autoimmune disorder that attacks the peripheral nervous system) and certain polyneuropathies (nerve damage involving pain).

In clinical studies, IgG therapy in patients with acute severe MS has produced favorable responses. In relapsing-remitting MS (RRMS), however, IgG therapy in high doses failed to help.

During pregnancy, MS relapse rates tend to decrease; however, after delivery, relapse rates increase. In one study in Italy of pregnant patients, high doses of IgG showed a slight increase in relapse rates six months after delivery, yet remained lower than those women who were untreated.

A systematic literature review analyzed 10 clinical trials involving IgG therapy in MS. In one clinical trial, some evidence to support the preventive treatment of RRMS was suggested.

For more information see pages 1234 and 1235.

Generic: **Isoniazid** *(eye-soe-NYE-a-zid)*
Brand: **Nydrazid**

Isoniazid is used as first-line treatment and prevention of tuberculosis (TB) in combination with other drugs. It belongs to a large class of drugs, commonly called anti-infectives. TB is a highly contagious bacterial disease of the lung that is difficult to treat because the bacteria have become drug-resistant. Therefore, isoniazid treatment must be continued for six to 12 months, and some TB drugs may be taken up to two years. Isoniazid is available in pill form, syrup, and injection. Patients with liver dysfunction and chronic alcoholism may not be able to take isoniazid as it can cause severe liver damage. Side effects include peripheral neuropathy, upset stomach, and hepatitis. Vitamin B-6 may be taken to decrease incidence of peripheral neuropathy (painful nerve damage), and to prevent gastrointestinal irritation.

Isoniazid treatment can help patients with MS, typically the related eye muscle disorders. In three case studies performed at a neurology clinic in Italy, three patients with MS with pendular nystagmus (involuntary rhythmic movement of the eyes) were treated. Two of the three patients experienced abolished and relieved oscillopsia (swinging vision). The third patient's eye recordings failed to show any effects on nystagmus, but visual acuity improved significantly. Isoniazid also helped cerebellar tremors found in patients with MS. Other treatments found effective in pendular nystagmus include valproic acid, trihexyphenidyl, and clonazepam. In other medical literature, isoniazid has been recommended in the treatment of vertigo and tremors in MS.

For more information see page 1246.

Generic: *Lamotrigine* (la-MOE-tri-jeen)
Brand: *Lamictal*

Lamotrigine belongs to a class of drugs known as anticonvulsants, also called antiepileptics, approved for the treatment of seizures and bipolar disorder. Lamotrigine can cause severe rash, which may be fatal or cause permanent disability. One serious reaction associated with this drug (1% of pediatric patients; 0.3% of adults) is Stevens Johnson syndrome, a fatal skin reaction. Patients must let their doctors and pharmacists know all drugs they are taking to prevent dangerous interactions. Some of the many side effects include loss of balance, blurry vision, difficult concentration, drowsiness, dizziness, and irritability. Serious side effects, which require immediate attention, include chest pain, depression, worsened or more frequent seizures, and swelling of the extremities.

In one clinical study, 21 patients with relapse-remitting and secondary progressive MS were studied to evaluate add-on treatment of lamotrigine in burning paresthesias (numbness and tingling), pain, and painful tonic spasms (PTS). Fifteen patients with pain and burning paresthesias, and eight patients with PTS received lamotrigine. Previous and concomitant treatment included other anticonvulsants, steroids, or muscle relaxants. Results suggested improvements in limb pain, paresthesias, and PTS symptoms. Benefits lasted at least four months, and in one patient they lasted one year.

For more information see page 1268.

Generic: **Methotrexate** *(meth-oh-TREKS-ate)*
Brands: **Rheumatrex, Trexall**

Methotrexate, a chemotherapy drug, belongs to a class of drugs known as immunosuppressants. Methotrexate is used to treat certain types of cancer and inflammatory diseases such as rheumatoid arthritis, lupus, and a number of dermatologic disorders.

Low-dose oral methotrexate has been used in the treatment of patients with chronic progressive MS. In clinical studies, treatment with methotrexate weekly for up to two years can reduce active disease and the progression of disability. Patients who benefit most from methotrexate have secondary progressive MS (SPMS). Long-term treatment with methotrexate must be carefully monitored due to risk of liver toxicity.

In one study in Italy, 20 patients with chronic progressive MS received low dose methotrexate. After one year of therapy, 15 were still receiving treatment, 10 were stable; and 12 sustained 18 months of therapy with eight stable patients. Side effects included elevated liver enzymes and local herpes zoster. Although no changes were noted on magnetic resonance image (MRI) scans, the study determined that methotrexate is useful as an add-on treatment in patients who had no response to interferon-beta.

For more information see page 1312.

Generic: **Methylphenidate** *(meth-il-FEN-i-date)*
Brands: **Concerta, Metadate CD, Metadate ER, Methylin, Methylin ER, Ritalin, Ritalin LA, Ritalin-SR**

Methylphenidate is a mild central nervous system (CNS) stimulant used to treat attention-deficit hyperactivity disorder (ADHD) and narcolepsy (sudden and uncontrollable attacks of drowsiness and sleep). In the medical literature, methylphenidate has treated symptoms of fatigue in MS. It alleviates the fatigue, but may also interfere with sleep. An expert opinion paper from the National Multiple Sclerosis Society recommends methylphenidate in managing fatigue in MS patients. About 50% to 60% of those with MS report fatigue as one of the most troublesome symptoms, apart from disease course or level of disability. The paper also suggested treating other MS symptoms contributing to fatigue, drug adjustments (for drugs that induce drowsiness), and energy conservation strategies. Methylphenidate has also been used in the treatment of fatigue found in patients infected with the human immunodeficiency virus (HIV).

This drug should not be used in severe depression, alcohol or drug dependence, hypertension, psychosis, or seizure disorders. Side effects of this drug may include restlessness, abnormal behavior, slurred speech, and appetite disturbances. Serious side effects include tachycardia (rapid heart rate), hallucinations, and hypertension.

For more information see page 1315.

Generic: **Modafinil** (moe-DAF-i-nil)
Brand: **Provigil**

Modafinil is a central nervous system (CNS) stimulant prescribed for narcolepsy (sudden and uncontrollable attacks of drowsiness and sleep), obstructive sleep apnea (periodic cessation of breathing at night), and shift work sleep-related disorders. It is used to promote wakefulness and alertness. It works by changing the amount of certain natural substances in the area of the brain that control sleep and wake cycles. Modafinil has also been used in the treatment of fatigue in MS. Side effects include jitteriness, anxiety, headache, mood swings, insomnia, and palpitations.

An expert opinion paper from the National Multiple Sclerosis Society recommended modafinil to manage MS-related fatigue. The paper also suggested treating other MS symptoms contributing to fatigue, drug adjustments (for drugs that induce drowsiness), and energy conservation strategies.

In a clinical trial at Ohio State University, 72 patients with MS were treated with modafinil or placebo over nine weeks. No serious adverse events were found in either group, and common side effects included nausea and headache. Sixty-five patients completed the trial, and the study concluded that treatment with modafinil significantly improved fatigue and was also tolerated well.

For more information see page 1338.

*Generic: **Nortriptyline** (nor-TRIP-ti-leen)*
*Brands: **Aventyl, Pamelor***

Nortriptyline belongs to a class of drugs called tricyclic antidepressants (TCAs), and is used to treat mental depression. TCAs work with certain chemicals in the brain to adjust mood. Nortriptyline is available in pill and liquid form, and may take a few weeks to reach its full effect. Other uses of nortriptyline include panic disorders, chronic pain, certain skin conditions, and premenstrual depression.

Nortriptyline may intensify effects of alcohol and central nervous system (CNS) depressants (sleep aids, muscle relaxants, antihistamines, and pain drugs). Side effects include dry mouth, constipation, weight gain, drowsiness, excitement or anxiety, photosensitivity (light sensitivity), changes in sex drive, and irregular heartbeats. Studies of this drug have not been performed to evaluate its effect in pregnancy. TCAs should not be used in combination with another type of antidepressants called MAO inhibitors. Although limited scientific evidence is available, nortriptyline, like other TCAs, have been used in the management of MS.

Patients with MS often are diagnosed with endogenous (from within the body) mental depression, which nortriptyline has helped. Nortriptyline may also help relieve neuropathic pain associated with progressive MS, which involves paresthesias (numbness, tingling, and pain) of the extremities, a result of the damage to the nerves.

For more information see page 1378.

Generic: **Ondansetron** *(on-DAN-se-tron)*
Brands: **Zofran, Zofran ODT**

Ondansetron is an anti-emetic, which prevents nausea and vomiting induced by anesthesia, chemotherapy, and radiation therapy. It may be administered by injection or taken in a tablet form. Side effects include diarrhea, headache, constipation, rash, lightheadedness, dry mouth, and drowsiness. Serious side effects include allergic reactions, muscle cramps or uncontrollable movements, and irregular heartbeats, all of which require immediate medical attention.

In a New Zealand study in *Journal of Pain and Symptom Management*, two patients with debilitating, chronic nausea associated with MS were evaluated for symptom management. One patient, a 43-year-old woman with a clinical presentation of MS, began to experience persistent nausea without vomiting with intractable vertigo within a few months of disease onset. Her nausea worsened with positional changes, became constant, and resulted in anorexia, and a weight loss of 25%. Combination drugs including prochlorperazine, metoclopramide, cyclizine, haloperidol, and lorazepam were used to treat the nausea and vertigo but were ineffective. After ondansetron was administered, however, the patient's nausea improved within one day. She had continued treatment for five years and gained total control of nausea and experienced fewer bouts of vertigo.

The second patient, a 35-year-old woman with MS, also experienced acute vertigo and nausea. Successful treatment with high dose oral ondansetron resulted in a 50% improvement in control of nausea. Based on this limited data, ondansetron may control nausea and vertigo in patients with MS, thereby improving quality of life by minimizing discomfort.

For more information see page 1387.

Generic: **Phenytoin** *(FEN-i-toyn)*
Brand: **Dilantin**

Dilantin belongs to a class of drugs known as anticonvulsants or antiepileptics, primarily used to treat epilepsy. It targets chemicals in the brain that maintain balance. Usually, it is taken on a full stomach to avoid gastric upset. Common side effects may include drowsiness, constipation, irritated gums, headache, and insomnia.

MS patients who have sensory symptoms, including numbness and tingling (neuropathic pain), may find relief with phenytoin, which improves balance and prevents some common sensory disturbances.

Phenytoin is effective when used in combination with carbamazepine, when either therapy alone has been ineffective. In some pre-clinical (testing on mice and rat animal models) studies, phenytoin has demonstrated neuroprotection (nerve protection) by decreasing inflammatory reactions associated with MS and other inflammatory nerve disorders.

Phenytoin has also been recommended for patients with MS who have tonic seizures (seizures that last 15 seconds to 60 seconds with no change in consciousness). Although tonic seizures are not very common in MS, anticonvulsants can control them.

For more information see page 1413.

Generic: **Simvastatin** *(SIM-va-stat-in)*
Brand: **Zocor**

Simvastatin is a cholesterol-lowering drug of the group called "statins" to lower cholesterol used when diet and exercise are not enough. In patients with coronary heart disease and elevated cholesterol, simvastatin is used to reduce the risk of death, stroke, and heart attack. It reduces the amount of cholesterol produced and increases the rate it is removed from the body. Patients with liver or kidney disease should not be given simvastatin because it can cause further damage. Side effects of this drug include gastrointestinal upset, headache, insomnia, dizziness, and fatigue.

Some unexpected effects of this drug on the immune system prompted simvastatin to be tested in the treatment of MS. Statins have complex immunomodulation effects within the body. In comparison to available therapies for MS, which are costly and may require injections, simvastatin is relatively inexpensive and is taken by mouth. In a study of 30 patients with relapse-remitting MS, oral simvastatin for six months reduced lesions seen by magnetic resonant image (MRI) scanning by 44%, and the drug was tolerated well. According to this study, the inflammatory pathology in MS may be ameliorated by simvastatin. Additional research is presently ongoing to evaluate the safety and effectiveness of simvastatin and other statins in treating MS.

For more information see page 1474.

Generic: *Tiagabine* (tie-GA-been)
Brand: *Gabitril*

Tiagabine belongs to a class of drugs known as anticonvulsants, and is used to treat partial seizures (a type of epilepsy). Side effects associated with tiagabine include dizziness, drowsiness, lack of energy, weakness, unsteadiness, depression, hostility, anger, irritability, confusion, abnormal thinking, increased appetite, upset stomach, and nervousness, among others. Some of the off-label uses for this drug are spasticity, migraine headaches, and mood disorders.

In a study conducted in Italy, seven patients with painful spasms in MS who got no relief from other drugs (gabapentin, baclofen, diazepam, or clonazepam) were enrolled in a trial of therapy with tiagabine. The mean patient age was 45 years, and the mean disease duration 7.1 years. No other drugs with similar action were taken during the study. Four of seven patients experienced relief of the painful tonic spasms after therapy with tiagabine. The recovery from spasms was sustained within one month of treatment, while efficacy had been maintained for three months. However, the spasticity level did not change during the study as with other drugs, such as tizanidine. Two patients dropped out of the study due to side effects. Tiagabine may be a new therapy for painful spasms in MS, but larger trials are needed to determine safety and efficacy.

For more information see page 1510.

Generic: *Topiramate* (TOE-pie-rah-mate)
Brand: *Topamax*

Topiramate is a new drug, belonging to a class called anticonvulsants. It is used in the treatment of epileptic seizures and in the prevention of migraine headaches.

Although how topiramate works is not fully understood, it modulates the neurotransmitter GABA in the brain. Side effects include dizziness, shakiness, rapid heartbeat, sweating, confusion, blurry vision, headache, and weakness. Serious side effects may include worsening of seizures, bleeding or bruising, chest pain, and trouble breathing.

Recent studies of topiramate suggest that it protects nerve cells against damage and so it has been studied in the treatment of MS in patients who experience paroxysmal symptoms (includes: trigeminal neuralgia, painful spasms, dysesthetic or paresthetic symptoms).

In one clinical trial involving 13 patients diagnosed with MS and paroxysmal symptoms, patients received an increasing dose of topiramate each week until they responsed optimally. Three patients did not complete the study due to severe and persistent dizziness and nausea. Neurophysiological (involving nerve stimulation) tests were performed prior to therapy onset and at 12 weeks to evaluate the effect of the drug on paroxysmal symptoms. All who completed the study responded to treatment, but none achieved regression. There was no distinct connection between the drug responses and increased doses. From the study, the evidence suggests that topiramate may be effective in those suffering from paroxysmal symptoms related to MS, and have tried other conventional therapies, but further studies are needed.

For more information see page 1516.

SLEEP DISORDERS

Sleep disorders prevent you from getting restful sleep and, as a result, can cause daytime sleepiness and dysfunction. There are about 80 different kinds of sleep disorders, and about 70 million Americans suffer from them. The most common sleep disorders include insomnia, sleep apnea, restless legs syndrome (RLS), and narcolepsy. A doctor diagnoses sleep disorders based on physical exams, sleep diaries, and a variety of diagnostic tests.

Insomnia

Insomnia is a sleep disorder in which you have difficulty falling asleep or staying sleep. People with insomnia may have one or more of the following symptoms: difficulty falling asleep; waking up often during the night and having trouble going back to sleep; waking up too early in the morning; and having unrefreshing sleep. Insomnia varies in how long it lasts and how often it occurs; it can be short-term (acute insomnia) or can last for a long time (chronic insomnia).

Commonly Prescribed (On-Label) Drugs: *Acetophenazine, Chloral Hydrate, Diphenhydramine, Doxylamine, Estazolam, Eszopiclone, Ethchlorvynol, Ethinamate, Flurazepam, Glutethimide, Methyprylon, Paraldehyde, Pentobarbital, Quazepam, Secobarbital, Temazepam, Triazolam, Zaleplon, Zolpidem*

OFF-LABEL PRESCRIPTION DRUGS
BREAKTHROUGH OPTIONS

Generic: ***Mirtazapine*** *(mir-TAZ-a-peen)*
Brands: ***Remeron, Remeron SolTab***

Mirtazapine is a mood elevator used to treat depression. Your doctor may prescribe an antidepressant drug, such as mirtazapine, to treat insomnia. Clinical trials with antidepressants have shown a wide range of effects on one's ability in addition to effects on daytime sleepiness. Some side effects associated with mirtazapine include drowsiness, dizziness, anxiousness, confusion, weight gain, dry mouth, and upset stomach.

Mirtazapine improved sleep in patients with depression. Alternatively, 8% to 48% of patients with depression who were treated with mirtazapine reported daytime sleepiness compared with 18% of patients who received placebo. In a small study of six patients with major depression and insomnia, mirtazapine decreased in sleep latency significantly and significantly increased total sleep time and sleep efficiency during the first two weeks of treatment.

Researchers at the University of Connecticut Health Center in Farmington compared mirtazapine with another antidepressant, fluoxetine, in patients with major depression and insomnia. Nineteen patients in this study received mirtazapine or fluoxetine for eight weeks. The mirtazapine group significantly improved in sleep latency and sleep efficiency after only two weeks of treatment.

For more information see page 1332.

Generic: **Trazodone** *(TRAZ-oh-done)*
Brand: **Desyrel**

Trazodone is used to treat depression by increasing the levels of the brain chemical serotonin. It is also used to treat schizophrenia, anxiety, alcohol abuse, and abnormal uncontrollable movements that may be caused by certain drugs. Side effects include headache, upset stomach, vomiting, bad taste in the mouth, stomach pain, diarrhea, constipation, changes in appetite, weight changes, weakness or tiredness, nervousness, and confusion, among others.

Although trazodone is mainly used to treat depression and anxiety disorders, it has been effective for insomnia. Compared with zolpidem (a drug used for insomnia), trazodone was less effective but was found to be more effective than placebo. Trazodone also helps patients with both insomnia and depression.

For more information see page 1521.

Narcolepsy

Narcolepsy is a neurological disorder of sleep regulation. Persons with narcolepsy have excessive daytime sleepiness and intermittent, uncontrollable episodes of falling asleep during the daytime. These sudden sleep attacks may occur during any type of activity at any time of the day. Narcolepsy usually begins between the ages of 15 and 25, although it can happen at any age. Symptoms include hallucinations, cataplexy, and paralysis. In many cases, narcolepsy is undiagnosed and, therefore, goes untreated.

Commonly Prescribed (On-Label) Drugs: *Amphetamine, Dextroamphetamine, Methylphenidate, Modafinil, Sodium Oxybate*

OFF-LABEL PRESCRIPTION DRUGS
BREAKTHROUGH OPTIONS

Generic: **Clomipramine** *(kloe-MI-pra-meen)*
Brand: **Anafranil**

Clomipramine belongs to a class of drugs known as tricyclic antidepressants (TCAs), used to treat depression and obsessive-compulsive disorder (OCD). Additionally, clomipramine reduces the frequency of cataplexy (abrupt attacks of muscular weakness or decreased muscle tone often associated with narcolepsy) and other narcolepsy symptoms. Side effects include drowsiness, dry mouth, upset stomach, vomiting, diarrhea, constipation, nervousness, decreased sexual ability, and headache, among others.

Clomipramine is widely known to block a type of sleep known as rapid eye movement (REM) sleep. A researcher with St. George's Hospital Medical School in London reported the use of clomipramine in a 57-year-old man with narcolepsy, which began around the age of 18 years and had worsening symptoms. He was taking a number of medications for his sleep disorder. He was evaluated in a sleep laboratory, and subsequently treated with clomipramine. At a follow-up visit, the patient's REM sleep decreased, total sleep time increased, and the time spent awake was slightly decreased. He also had longer intervals of wakefulness. Despite the fact that there were no changes in sleep attacks, the patient was pleased that his narcoleptic symptoms (hallucinations, cataplexy, a feature of narcolepsy where the person experiences a sudden loss of muscle tone and falls to the floor, and paralysis) were gone. Overall, in this case study, clomipramine increased the time spent asleep and resulted in clearer intervals of wakefulness.

For more information see page 1105.

Generic: **Fluoxetine** *(floo-OKS-e-teen)*
Brands: **Prozac, Prozac Weekly, Sarafem**

Fluoxetine belongs to a class of antidepressant drugs known as selective serotonin reuptake inhibitors (SSRIs). It is used to treat mental depression, obsessive-compulsive disorder (OCD), bulimia nervosa, and premenstrual dysphoric disorder (PMDD). Side effects include anxiety, nervousness, decreased appetite, decreased sexual ability or drive, skin rash, diarrhea, drowsiness, increased sweating, nausea, tiredness, weakness, trembling, shaking, and difficulty sleeping, among others.

Fluoxetine is effective in treating cataplexy. Researchers at the VA Greater Los Angeles Healthcare System and UCLA School of Medicine in Sepulveda, California, noted in *Sleep* that a number of drugs including fluoxetine are effective for narcolepsy, although the quality of published clinical evidence supporting them varies. Scheduled naps can help combat sleepiness although this is not a first-line treatment.

In a study by researchers at the Barrow Neurological Institute, in Phoenix, Arizona, six patients with poorly controlled cataplexy were given a single dose without any change in their current drugs. Once benefit occurred, their other drugs were discontinued or reduced. Patients experienced a reduction of 92% of cataplexy episodes/week. Based on these results, fluoxetine appeared to effectively suppress cataplexy and reduced the need for other, less desirable, anticataplectic drugs.

For more information see page 1192.

SPASM DISORDERS

Spasm disorders encompass a number of conditions such as restless legs syndrome, periodic limb movement disorder, and tardive dyskinesia, among others. Muscle twitches are the result of spontaneous local muscle contractions that are involuntary. These contractions usually affect individual groups of muscles connected to a particular motor neuron in the body. Some muscle twitches are normal whereas others indicate a neurological disorder. Muscle spasms can cause cramps, and may be induced by certain drugs. Serious causes of spasms, such as motor neuron disease, muscle diseases, or denervation, may be accompanied by weakness, muscle wasting, and other symptoms. For more information on these disorders in children see Seizures and Spasms Disorders in the Children's Health Disorders chapter on page 245.

Epilepsy Seizures

Epilepsy is a brain disorder in which clusters of nerve cells in the brain have abnormal signaling, which causes strange sensations, emotions, and behavior, and sometimes seizures, muscle spasms, and loss of consciousness. Epilepsy can be caused by other disorders or injury. Doctors have identified more than 30 different types of seizures. About 60% of people with epilepsy have focal (also known as partial) seizures.

Commonly Prescribed (On-Label) Drugs: *Acetazolamide, Carbamazepine, Ethotoin, Fludeoxyglucose F 18, Levetiracetam, Mephenytoin, Methsuximide, Oxcarbazepine, Phenacemide, Phenobarbital, Primidone, Secobarbital, Zonisamide*

OFF-LABEL PRESCRIPTION DRUG
BREAKTHROUGH OPTION

Generic: **Pregabalin** *(pre-GAB-a-lin)*
Brand: **Lyrica**

Pregabalin belongs to a class of drugs known as antiepileptics, used to treat pain and seizure disorders, often combined with other drugs. It is also used to manage post-herpetic neuralgia, or shingles, a type of nerve pain caused by the herpes virus. Pregabalin affects chemicals and nerves that are involved in the cause of seizures and some type of pain. Side effects include dizziness, poor coordination, drowsiness, blurred vision, weight gain, swelling of the hands and feet, unexplained muscle problems, dry mouth, and tremor.

Researchers affiliated with U.S. institutions evaluated pregabalin as an add-on treatment in patients with partial seizure not responsive to other drugs. In this multicenter, 12-week study, patients received placebo or pregabalin 150 mg or 600 mg. Both pregabalin 150 mg and 600 mg were significantly more effective than placebo in reducing seizure frequency. Seizure frequency was reduced 20.6% for patients taking the smaller dose and 47.8% for those taking the larger. Treatment-related adverse events in this study included somnolence, dizziness, and weight gain. Overall, both doses of pregabalin were effective and well tolerated as an add-on treatment in patients with partial seizure.

For more information see page 1431.

Gilles de la Tourette Syndrome

Gilles de la Tourette Syndrome, or Tourette's Syndrome (TS), is a neurological disorder characterized by tics (involuntary, rapid, sudden movements or vocalizations that occur repeatedly in the same way). The most common first symptom is a facial tic such as rapidly blinking eyes or mouth twitches. Involuntary sounds such as throat clearing and sniffing, or tics of the limbs may be first signs of TS. The cause of TS is not clear although the disorder may stem from abnormal activity of the brain chemical (neurotransmitter) dopamine. Other neurotransmitters and receptors may be involved.

Commonly Prescribed (On-Label) Drugs: Haloperidol

OFF-LABEL PRESCRIPTION DRUGS
BREAKTHROUGH OPTIONS

*Generic: **Baclofen** (BAK-low-fen)*
*Brands: **Kemstro, Lioresal***

Baclofen belongs to a class of drugs known as muscle relaxants; it is used to relieve muscle spasms and contractions in conditions such as multiple sclerosis. Baclofen may be effective in treating Tourette's Syndrome (TS). Side effects include changes in taste, confusion, constipation, diarrhea, difficulty sleeping, dizziness or drowsiness, dry mouth, headache, increased urination, muscle weakness, nausea, vomiting, and weakness or tiredness.

According to researchers at The Johns Hopkins Hospital in Baltimore, Maryland, baclofen is one of the first-line drugs for tic suppression. A study of baclofen in 264 patients showed a 95% reduction in tic severity. Researchers from the Department of Neurology and Pediatrics investigated the effectiveness of baclofen for the treatment of tics in children with TS. The children received random four-week medication cycles of baclofen and placebo. All showed some reduction in total tics with baclofen treatment and no major side effects. Children with TS may benefit from treatment with baclofen, although improvements may be related to factors other than tics. Larger studies that compare baclofen with other tic-suppressing drugs are recommended.

For more information see page 1037.

Generic: **Clonazepam** *(kloe-NA-ze-pam)*
Brand: **Klonopin**

Clonazepam belongs to a class of drugs known as benzodiazepines. It is used to control seizures and relieve anxiety. Clonazepam may be used to treat symptoms of Parkinson's disease, twitching, schizophrenia, and to manage pain. It has been used to treat movement disorders such as TS. Side effects include drowsiness, dizziness, tiredness, weakness, dry mouth, diarrhea, upset stomach, and appetite changes. This drug may be habit-forming, and with long-term use, some persons may become tolerant to the drug's effects.

According to researchers at The Johns Hopkins Hospital in Baltimore, Maryland, clonazepam is one of the first-line drugs for tic suppression. The use of clonazepam was documented in a patient case study at Texas Tech University Health Sciences Center in El Paso, Texas, of a 16-year-old boy with a history of infrequent tics that had become more severe over time. He had very frequent tics in the face, shoulders, and to a lesser extent hands. With decreased activity, the tics decreased slightly. Additionally, his tics were accompanied with grunting sounds and short whistles. Doctors treated him with clonazepam and, at follow-up, his tics were minimized. The daily clonazepam dose was increased and, at the next follow-up, the patient was improved with few tics. After additional improvement, this patient's dose was reduced.

For more information see page 1107.

Generic: **Clonidine** *(KLON-i-deen)*
Brands: **Catapres, Catapres-TTS, Duraclon**

Clonidine is classified as an antihypertensive drug, and is used to treat high blood pressure. It works by stimulating certain brain receptors, which relax blood vessels in other parts of the body, causing them to widen. Side effects include dizziness, lightheadedness, drowsiness, dry mouth, and constipation.

According to researchers at The Johns Hopkins Hospital in Baltimore, Maryland, clonidine is one of the first-line drugs for tic suppression, and benefits persons with TS. It may take up to six weeks to exhibit effects in TS, however.

Researchers at Yale University School of Medicine conducted a 12-week study comparing clonidine and placebo in the treatment of 47 persons with TS. Tic severity declined for both groups, but the magnitude of response was greater in the group receiving clonidine. Clinician-rated measures of motor tic severity, the degree to which the tics are "noticeable to others," motor tic counts from videotaped interviews and parent-rated measures of impulsivity and hyperactivity were the most responsive to clonidine treatment. The most common side effects were fatigue, dry mouth, dizziness, and irritability. These findings show that clonidine is more effective than placebo in reducing some of the tic and other behavioral symptoms associated with TS.

For more information see page 1108.

*Generic: **Guanfacine** (GWAHN-fa-seen)*
*Brand: **Tenex***

Guanfacine belongs to a group of drugs known as antihypertensives, which relax blood vessels and relieve high blood pressure. Side effects associated with guanfacine include blurred vision, constipation, depression, difficulty sleeping, drowsiness, dry mouth, headache, minor sexual problems, skin rash, sweating, and weakness.

According to researchers at The Johns Hopkins Hospital in Baltimore, Maryland, guanfacine is one of the first-line drugs for tic suppression, and has been shown to benefit persons with TS. In fact, guanfacine can treat both TS and ADHD (attention-deficit hyperactivity disorder), two conditions that often occur together.

Researchers at Yale University School of Medicine in New Haven, Connecticut, studied guanfacine in 10 children (ranging in age from eight to 16 years) with TS and ADHD. Duration of follow-up was four to 20 weeks. Results of the study showed that guanfacine was associated with significant decreases in severity of motor and phonic tics. The most common side effects in this study were transient sedation and headaches. Researchers concluded that guanfacine may be a safe, alternative therapy for children with ADHD in the presence of tics.

For more information see page 1216.

Generic: *Risperidone* (RIS-peer-i-dohn)
Brands: *Risperdal, Risperdal M-TAB*

Risperidone belongs to a class of drugs known as antipsychotics, used to treat schizophrenia. It is also prescribed to treat other mood disorders. Risperidone reduces mental problems and helps the person stay in touch with reality. According to researchers at The Johns Hopkins Hospital in Baltimore, Maryland, risperidone is considered to be a second-line drug for TS symptoms. Side effects include constipation, decreased sexual ability, difficulty sleeping, drowsiness, dizziness, headache, increased or decreased saliva, menstrual irregularities, nausea and/or vomiting, and stomach pain, among others.

Risperidone has been useful in other conditions with tic symptoms and studies have evaluated it for TS symptoms. In one study of risperidone, there was a 36% to 56% reduction in vocal and motor tics in nine of 11 patients (ranging in age from 19 years to 52 years). In another study, there was a 26% to 66% reduction in tic scores in seven children (ranging in age from 11 years and 16 years). In a study of 58 patients with TS (ranging in age from eight to 53 years), risperidone provided 58% improvement; however, 21% of patients dropped out of the study because of side effects.

For more information see page 1456.

Generic: *Ziprasidone* (ze-PRAZ-eh-don)
Brand: *Geodon*

Ziprasidone treats the symptoms of schizophrenia, such as auditory or visual hallucinations, suspiciousness of others, mistaken beliefs and delusions, or withdrawal from normal activities. Side effects include constipation, mild dizziness, drowsiness, headache, nausea, vomiting, and upset stomach.

Ziprasidone for the treatment of TS has been evaluated in one clinical trial where many of the patients (ranging in age from seven years to 17 years) also had other conditions (ADHD, OCD). All 28 patients had to be free of other psychotropic drugs for at least four weeks before starting the study. Ziprasidone reduced total tic score and global severity score significantly when compared with placebo. The most commonly reported side effect was mild sedation. Researchers acknowledged the benefits of ziprasidone in the treatment of TS, although more research is needed.

For more information see page 1551.

Hiccups

Hiccups are repeated spasmodic involuntary contractions of the diaphragm that occur when you inhale. Practically everyone has hiccups at some point, but they usually go away. Chronic episodes lasting longer than 48 hours are called intractable hiccups and can be invasive, causing sleep difficulties, inability to eat, and depression. This spasm disorder may be triggered by certain foods, drinks, drugs, or behavior; treatments include drugs and other non-drug interventions.

Commonly Prescribed (On-Label) Drugs: *Chlorpromazine*

OFF-LABEL PRESCRIPTION DRUGS
BREAKTHROUGH OPTIONS

Generic: ***Baclofen*** *(BAK-low-fen)*
Brands: ***Kemstro, Lioresal***

Baclofen belongs to a class of drugs known as muscle relaxants; it is used to relieve muscle spasms and contractions in conditions such as multiple sclerosis. Side effects associated with baclofen include changes in taste, confusion, constipation, diarrhea, difficulty sleeping, dizziness or drowsiness, dry mouth, headache, increased urination, muscle weakness, nausea, vomiting, and weakness or tiredness.

Baclofen is among the many drugs used to treat hiccups. In one small trial, two weeks of baclofen treatment was more effective than placebo in increasing hiccup-free periods, although it did not change the frequency of hiccups. Across patient case studies, hiccup improvement or complete resolution of hiccups with baclofen was seen in almost all instances. Onset of hiccup relief was seen in as early as 24 hours, although in some patients, reducing the dose or stopping the drug resulted in hiccup relapse. After relapse, patients responded to baclofen once again. In general, baclofen appears to be well tolerated. Researchers concluded that this drug is a useful option for patients with hiccups of various causes that are unresponsive to other therapies.

For more information see page 1037.

*Generic: **Carbamazepine** (kar-ba-MAZ-e-peen)*
*Brands: **Carbatrol, Epitol, Tegretol, Tegretol XR***

Carbamazepine belongs to a class of drugs known as mood stabilizers. Depending on its use, this drug also may be classified as an antineuralgic, antidiuretic, or an anticonvulsant. Carbamazepine is used to control some types of epileptic seizures; also it may be used to relieve neurogenic pain, prevent bipolar disorder symptoms, and treat a certain type of diabetes, alcohol withdrawal, and some mental illnesses. Side effects include, but are not limited to clumsiness, unsteadiness, dizziness, drowsiness, lightheadedness, and nausea and vomiting.

A number of case study reports document the use of carbamazepine for hiccups. Researchers at Washington University School of Medicine in St. Louis, Missouri, reported successful hiccup resolution in one of three patients with stroke and hiccups of at least 48 hours. Carbamazepine, in general, has been effective in treating intractable hiccups caused by central lesions (brain and spinal cord). In one patient with multiple sclerosis and intractable hiccups, carbamazepine stopped the hiccups within 24 hours. When the patient stopped the drug, hiccups reccurred, but when he began taking carbamazepine again, the hiccups resolved within 24 hours. Carbamazepine is effective in spasm disorders involving lesions of the brainstem and cervical cord.

For more information see page 1068.

*Generic: **Gabapentin** (GA-ba-pen-tin)*
*Brand: **Neurontin***

Gabapentin belongs to a class of drugs known as anticonvulsants, and is used to help control some types of epileptic seizures. It is also used to control pain associated with shingles and may be prescribed for other nervous system disorders. In the treatment of hiccups, gabapentin may help to regulate the diaphragm and inspiratory muscle excitability.

Gabapentin has been combined with baclofen and other drugs for hiccup treatment. Side effects include blurred or double vision; cold or flu-like symptoms; delusions; dementia; drowsiness; hoarseness; lack or loss of strength; lower back or side pain; swelling of the hands, feet, or lower legs; and trembling and shaking; among others.

In most cases documenting the use of gabapentin, patients responded to treatment on the first day, usually after the second dose of gabapentin. Those patients requiring a six-day regimen of treatment required extra gabapentin doses for hiccup recurrences. Across these case studies, gabapentin is well tolerated, and no patients stopped treatment because of side effects. Overall, gabapentin may be a useful alternative in patients with intractable hiccups from various causes that have been unresponsive to other treatments.

For more information see page 1206.

*Generic: **Haloperidol** (ha-loe-PER-i-dole)*
*Brands: **Haldol, Haldol Decanoate***

Haloperidol is used to treat schizophrenia; it reduces mental symptoms and helps keep patients in touch with reality. This drug may be used to control tics and vocal outbursts in patients with Tourette's Syndrome, and treat behavioral problems in children with severe conduct disorders (mood swings, aggressive behavior). Side effects include anxiety, blurred vision, breast pain, constipation, decreased sexual ability, drowsiness, dry mouth, menstrual changes, and weight gain, among others.

In an article in *American Journal of Psychiatry*, two patients with intractable hiccups were treated with intramuscular (IM) haloperidol. Hiccup remission occurred within one hour. Although haloperidol has few adverse cardiovascular effects, it has been associated with extrapyramidal reactions (movement disorders such as restlessness, muscular spasms of the neck, muscle stiffness). Thus, its use for hiccups is limited by these significant side effects.

In another case report, researchers at Washington University School of Medicine in St. Louis, Missouri, reported successful treatment of hiccups in patients participating in stroke rehabilitation with haloperidol, baclofen, or carbamazepine.

For more information see page 1217.

Huntington's Disease

Huntington's disease is a progressive, degenerative, and inherited disease that causes certain nerve cells in the brain to waste away. Signs and symptoms of Huntington's chorea (incessant, quick, and jerky movements seen with this disorder) usually develop during middle age. The earliest signs and symptoms of Huntington's disease often include personality changes and decreased cognitive abilities. A person with early disease may be irritable, angry, paranoid, or depressed. As the disease progresses, a person may develop sudden, jerky, involuntary movements throughout the body and other symptoms.

Commonly Prescribed (On-Label) Drugs: *None*

OFF-LABEL PRESCRIPTION DRUGS
BREAKTHROUGH OPTIONS

Generic: ***Clozapine*** *(KLOE-za-peen)*
Brand: ***Clozaril***

Clozapine belongs to a class of drugs known as antipsychotics, used to treat schizophrenia in patients who have not been helped by or are unable to take other drugs. Side effects include constipation, dizziness, lightheadedness, drowsiness, mild headache, increased watering of mouth, nausea, vomiting, and weight gain.

Researchers at the National Institute of Mental Health Laboratory in Bethesda, Maryland, evaluated clozapine in 12 patients with abnormal involuntary movement associated with Huntington's disease or Tourette's Syndrome in a trial. Two patients were dropped from the study because of complications, but two patients showed a marked, beneficial decrease in movements. The remaining patients did not have a significant therapeutic benefit with treatment. Seven out of 10 patients in this study experienced moderate or marked side effects.

Researchers concluded that clozapine proved clinically ineffective in treating patients with Tourette's Syndrome and two patients with atypical drug-induced dyskinesias. Two patients with Huntington's disease in this study showed significant reductions in abnormal movements although not without side effects.

For more information see page 1111.

Generic: Olanzapine (oh-LAN-za-peen)
Brands: Zyprexa, Zyprexa Zydis

Olanzapine belongs to a group of drugs known as atypical antipsychotics. This drug is used to treat psychotic mental disorders such as schizophrenia, bipolar disorder, and agitation that occur with schizophrenia and bipolar mania. Side effects include sour stomach, belching, change in walking and balance, constipation, difficulty speaking, dizziness, drowsiness, dry mouth, headache, heartburn, runny nose, and sleepiness, among others.

Olanzapine lacks the dangerous side effects of other antipsychotic drugs (clozapine); therefore, researchers have studied the effects of this drug in persons with Huntington's disease. Researchers in Israel used olanzapine for 11 patients (five of whom were men) with Huntington's disease. Nine patients were treated for 9.8 months. Disease symptoms improved in five patients; two patients dropped out because of drug eruption and lack of efficacy. It was concluded that olanzapine is a good alternative treatment in Huntington's disease, primarily for the psychiatric symptoms. Researchers in Spain described two patients with a predominantly "chorea-typed" Huntington's disease whose abnormal movements lessened after treatment with olanzapine. In these two patients, the drug was well tolerated.

For more information see page 1381.

*Generic: **Riluzole** (RIL-yoo-zole)*
*Brand: **Rilutek***

Riluzole is classified as an amyotrophic lateral sclerosis (ALS) therapy drug, used to treat ALS, commonly referred to as Lou Gehrig's disease. This drug is not a cure for the disease but it can extend survival in the early stages and possibly extend the time until windpipe surgery is needed. Riluzole may cause abdominal pain, gas, dizziness, drowsiness, appetite loss, numbness or tingling around the mouth, and liver problems.

Researchers in Austria studied riluzole in nine patients with Huntington's disease to evaluate its effects on motor impairment, functional disability, cognitive impairment, and behavioral abnormalities. In this study, riluzole was well tolerated, and did not lead to liver toxicity. At three months, movements improved, chorea decreased, and total functional capacity significantly improved compared with riluzole. At twelve months, however, this beneficial effect was not maintained. Researchers concluded that olanzapine exhibits anti-choreatic effects and more sustained effects on psychomotor speed and behavior in patients with Huntington's disease, although more research is needed.

For more information see page 1453.

*Generic: **Ziprasidone** (ze-PRAZ-eh-don)*
*Brand: **Geodon***

Ziprasidone belongs to a class of drugs known as atypical antipsychotic drugs, used to treat the symptoms of schizophrenia, such as auditory or visual hallucinations, suspiciousness of others, mistaken beliefs (delusions), or withdrawal from normal activities. Side effects include constipation, mild dizziness, drowsiness, headache, nausea, vomiting, and upset stomach.

Researchers in Austria demonstrated that ziprasidone is useful in different stages of Huntington's disease. In one of these case studies, a 34-year-old woman with Huntington's disease was unable to eat or dress without assistance. She was given ziprasidone and her chorea symptoms visibly decreased and her gait and fine motor tasks also improved over a few days.

In the second case study, a 61-year-old man with Huntington's disease was successfully treated with ziprasidone. Improvement was seen as early as the next day after start of treatment. In the third case study, a 42-year-old woman with Huntington's disease was treated with ziprasidone and a clear improvement began two days after the start of treatment.

These studies show that this drug may be helpful in the treatment of chorea symptoms, since it does not impair fine motor tasks or gait as some typical antipsychotics do.

For more information see page 1551.

Periodic Limb Movement Disorder

Periodic limb movement disorder (PLMD) is one of the most common neurological disorders. It affects people only during sleep, and is characterized by behavior ranging from shallow, continual movement of the ankle or toes, to wild and strenuous kicking and flailing of the legs and arms. Movement of the legs is more common than arm movement. Abdominal, oral, and nasal movement may accompany PLMD. Movements generally occur for 0.5 to 10 seconds, in intervals separated by five to 90 seconds. Arousals or awakening may be associated with the movements. The incidence of PLMD increases with age.

Commonly Prescribed (On-Label) Drugs: None

OFF-LABEL PRESCRIPTION DRUGS
BREAKTHROUGH OPTIONS

Generic: **Bromocriptine** *(broe-moe-KRIP-teen)*
Brand: **Parlodel**

Bromocriptine is used as a growth hormone suppressant, lactation blocker, and an antidyskinetic drug (among others) depending on the syndrome it is used to treat. Bromocriptine is also used to treat Parkinson's disease; it works by stimulating certain parts of the brain and nervous system that are involved in this disease. Side effects associated with its use include dizziness, lightheadedness, and nausea.

Dopaminergic drugs, such as bromocriptine, are considered to be the treatment of choice for PLMD. Researchers in Canada evaluated six narcoleptic (a sleep disorder) patients and found no change in nocturnal sleep organization, daytime somnolence, or psychomotor performance during bromocriptine use. However, periodic limb movements in sleep (PLMS) were significantly reduced with the use of bromocriptine.

Researchers in the Sleep/Wake Disorders Center at Presbyterian Hospital of Dallas, Texas, conducted a retrospective review of 49 patients with restless legs syndrome (RLS) or PLMS treated with the dopamine agonists L-dopa/carbidopa, bromocriptine mesylate, or both. Researchers found that in the extended follow-up group of 47 patients, four failed to respond to L-dopa or bromocriptine, five discontinued treatment because of side effects, and two reported loss of therapeutic effect within the first month.

For more information see page 1054.

*Generic: **Carbidopa-Levodopa** (kar-bi-DOE-pa lee-voe-DOE-pa)*
*Brands: **Sinemet, Sinemet CR***

Carbidopa-levodopa are classified as anti-Parkinsonian drugs. The combination of carbidopa and levodopa treat the symptoms of Parkinson's disease, including tremors, stiffness, and slowness of movement. Side effects are common and include dizziness, upset stomach, vomiting, appetite loss, difficulty speaking, taste changes, decreased attention span, memory loss, nervousness, nightmares, difficulty sleeping, and headaches, among others.

Dopaminergic drugs, such as carbidopa-levodopa, are considered the treatment of choice for PLMD. A single small dose is usually given one hour before sleep. In two clinical trials comparing carbidopa-levodopa to propoxyphene (an opiate drug), carbidopa-levodopa was much more effective than the opiate in reducing leg movements before and during sleep. Researchers at the Stanford University Sleep Disorders Clinic and Research Center in Stanford, California, reported that a 51-year-old man with Machado-Joseph disease and PLMD was successfully treated with carbidopa-levodopa and temazepam (a benzodiazepine drug).

Researchers at Johns Hopkins University Sleep Disorders Center in Baltimore, Maryland, found that RLS symptoms occur in the afternoon and evening prior to taking the next nightly dose of carbidopa-levodopa. These symptoms occurred in 31% of PLMS patients and 82% of RLS patients treated with this drug combination. The symptoms were greater in patients with more severe RLS symptoms and for patients taking higher doses. It was concluded that symptoms could be minimized by keeping the dose low.

For more information see page 1070.

Generic: **Clonazepam** *(kloe-NA-ze-pam)*
Brand: **Klonopin**

Clonazepam belongs to a class of drugs known as benzodiazepines, used to control seizures and relieve anxiety. Clonazepam may be used to treat symptoms of Parkinson's disease, twitching, schizophrenia, and to manage pain. Side effects associated with clonazepam include drowsiness, dizziness, tiredness, weakness, dry mouth, diarrhea, upset stomach, and appetite changes. This drug may be habit forming, and with long-term use, some persons may become tolerant to its effects. Clonazepam may have a direct effect on PLM rather than a vague sedative effect.

Researchers at the University of Vienna and Sleep Laboratory in Austria evaluated the effects of clonazepam on sleep and awakening quality in 10 patients with RLS and 16 with PLMD. Clonazepam significantly improved sleep efficiency and sleep quality in both patient groups. In PLMD, clonazepam improved leg movements during time in bed, rapid eye movement (REM) sleep, and wakefulness; and showed more significant changes in various sleep and awakening measures than in RLS patients, although there were no significant intergroup differences. Researchers concluded that clonazepam, in both PLMD and RLS, greatly helped insomnia.

For more information see page 1107.

Generic: **Pergolide** *(PER-go-lide)*
Brand: **Permax**

Pergolide is an anti-Parkinsonian drug, used with the drugs levodopa or carbidopa to treat Parkinson's disease. Pergolide works by stimulating certain parts of the central nervous system (CNS) involved in this disease. It has also been prescribed for persons with RLS. Common side effects of pergolide include chest congestion, constipation, dizziness, lightheadedness, drowsiness, heartburn, lower back pain, muscle pain, nausea, runny or stuffy nose, trouble sleeping, and weakness, among others.

Dopaminergic agonists, such as pergolide, are considered the treatment of choice for PLMD. In fact, according to the Standards of Practice Committee of the American Academy of Sleep Medicine, pergolide is deemed effective in the treatment of PLMD and RLS. This recommendation is based on the largest clinical study involving this drug, in which 78.6% of patients continued with pergolide long-term, despite adverse effects (i.e., nausea, congestion, and mild augmentation). In most cases, these adverse events were minor or adequately controlled.

In 51 patients with RLS or PLMS, pergolide was found to be more effective than levodopa/carbidopa in patients with RLS. Levodopa/carbidopa was more effective in those patients with periodic limb movements.

For more information see page 1406.

Generic: **Selegiline** *(se-LE-ji-leen)*
Brand: **Eldepryl**

Selegiline helps to increase or extend the effects of drugs used to treat Parkinson's disease (levodopa or carbidopa), and slow the progression of the disease. Side effects associated with selegiline include anxiety, nervousness, blurred vision, changes in taste, constipation, diarrhea, difficulty sleeping, drowsiness, dizziness, dry mouth, appetite loss, weight loss, and nausea and/or vomiting, among others.

Selegiline is recognized as a potential drug for the treatment of PLMD by the Standards of Practice Committee of the American Academy of Sleep Medicine, since its effectiveness has not been established in clinical studies. Researchers at the University Health Network in Canada evaluated 31 patients with PLMD undergoing treatment with selegiline. Pre- and post-treatment overnight polysomnographs revealed a highly significant decrease in the number of PLMS/hour of total sleep time. The alerting effect associated with selegiline did not have a significant effect on patients' sleep efficiency or sleep-onset latency. Researchers concluded that selegiline is an alternative drug that doctors should consider for PLMD.

For more information see page 1466.

Restless Legs Syndrome

Restless legs syndrome (RLS) is a sensory-motor disorder that affects up to 10% of the population. Features of RLS include a desire to move the limbs; abnormal, uncomfortable, and/or painful sensations in the lower extremities; motor restlessness; a partial and temporary relief of these symptoms with activity; and worsening of symptoms in the evening or night. RLS can occur at any age, although it is usually seen in adults and tends to worsen with age. Motor symptoms of RLS include periodic leg movements (PLMs) that can occur during wakefulness or sleep.

Commonly Prescribed (On-Label) Drugs: None

OFF-LABEL PRESCRIPTION DRUGS
BREAKTHROUGH OPTIONS

Generic: ***Aripiprazole*** *(ay-ri-PIP-ray-zole)*
Brand: ***Abilify***

Aripiprazole belongs to a class of drugs known as antipsychotics. It is used to treat schizophrenia, by decreasing abnormal excitement in the brain. Side effects associated with aripiprazole include headache, nervousness, difficulty sleeping, drowsiness, lightheadedness, restlessness, constipation, weight gain, coughing, and runny nose, among others.

According to a professor at the UND School of Medicine and Health Sciences in Fargo, North Dakota, drugs such as aripiprazole may be useful in patients with restless legs syndrome (RLS) and psychotic symptoms or addiction issues who cannot take standard treatments (clonazepam, opiates, or dopamine-receptor agonists). A 42-year-old man with a long history of RLS, who had a history of substance abuse and dependence, major depressive disorder with psychotic features, and anxiety disorder could not use stimulants because they worsened his RLS. Other drugs helped his target symptoms, but his RLS continued. After treatment with aripiprazole, however, the patient reported that his RLS was gone. He continued with aripiprazole, and his RLS did not return. Further research of aripiprazole in this subpopulation of patients is needed, based on the findings from this patient case study.

For more information see page 1025.

Generic: **Clonazepam** *(kloe-NA-ze-pam)*
Brand: **Klonopin**

Clonazepam belongs to a class of drugs known as benzodiazepines, used to control seizures and relieve anxiety. Clonazepam may be used to treat symptoms of Parkinson's disease, twitching, schizophrenia, and to manage pain. Side effects include drowsiness, dizziness, tiredness, weakness, dry mouth, diarrhea, upset stomach, and appetite changes. This drug may be habit-forming, and with long-term use, some persons may become tolerant to its effects.

Benzodiazepines, particularly clonazepam, were the first drugs to be studied for the treatment of RLS. In one study, clonazepam reduced the total number of leg movements by about 50%, and the number of periodic limb movements associated with arousals to one third. Clonazepam practically suppressed periodic limb movements occurring within the first 10 minutes after the sleep onset.

Researchers at the University of Vienna and Sleep Laboratory in Austria measured the effects of clonazepam on sleep and awakening quality in ten patients with RLS and 16 patients with periodic limb movement disorder (PLMD). Compared with placebo, clonazepam significantly improved sleep efficiency and sleep quality in both patient groups, but failed to reduce periodic leg movements during hours of sleep. In PLMD, clonazepam improved periodic leg movements during time in bed, rapid eye movement sleep, and wakefulness and showed more significant changes in various sleep and awakening measures than in RLS patients, although there were no significant intergroup differences. Researchers concluded that in both PLMD and RLS, clonazepam helped insomnia.

For more information see page 1107.

Generic: **Gabapentin** *(GA-ba-pen-tin)*
Brand: **Neurontin**

Gabapentin belongs to a class of drugs known as anticonvulsants, and is used to help control some types of epileptic seizures. In clinical studies, gabapentin decreased essential tremor. Side effects of gabapentin include blurred or double vision; cold or flu-like symptoms; delusions; dementia; drowsiness; hoarseness; lack or loss of strength; lower back or side pain; swelling of the hands, feet, or lower legs; and trembling and shaking. The most commonly reported side effects in clinical trials with gabapentin include dizziness, nausea, and drowsiness.

The Mayo Clinic in Scottsdale, Arizona, evaluated gabapentin for the treatment of eight patients with RLS. Of the eight patients, four had a beneficial response, and three had almost complete resolution of RLS symptoms for up to six months. These findings are promising and more research is needed.

Researchers in Spain evaluated 24 patients with RLS treated with gabapentin or placebo. Compared with placebo, gabapentin reduced symptoms for RLS. Periodic leg movements during sleep (PLMS) were also significantly reduced, and sleep was improved with gabapentin. Patients with RLS symptoms and pain benefited most from treatment with gabapentin. Based on this study, gabapentin improves the sensory and motor symptoms of RLS and improves sleep and PLMS.

For more information see page 1206.

Generic: **Pergolide** *(PER-go-lide)*
Brand: **Permax**

Pergolide, a dopamine agonist, belongs to a class of drugs known as ergot alkaloids. It is used with the drugs levodopa or carbidopa to treat persons with Parkinson's disease. Pergolide stimulates certain parts of the central nervous system (CNS) that are involved in this disease. Pergolide may also help persons with RLS. Common side effects of pergolide include chest congestion, constipation, dizziness, lightheadedness, drowsiness, heartburn, lower back pain, muscle pain, nausea, runny or stuffy nose, trouble sleeping, and weakness, among others.

Pergolide has been proven to be a successful RLS treatment in clinical trials. In one trial, pergolide was found to be more effective than levodopa in reducing sleep time with jerking movements and increasing total time asleep or in bed.

In other studies, pergolide significantly lessened RLS severity and improved quality of life compared to placebo. In a consecutive series of 51 patients with RLS or PLMS, pergolide was more effective than levodopa/carbidopa in patients with RLS. Levodopa/

carbidopa was more effective in those patients with periodic limb movements.

For more information see page 1406.

Generic: **Pramipexole** (pram-eh-PEX-oll)
Brand: **Mirapex**

Pramipexole belongs to a class of drug known as anti-Parkinsonian drug. It is used to treat the symptoms of Parkinson's disease, including tremors, stiffness, and slowness of movement. Pramipexole has also been shown to reduce sensory and motor symptoms associated with RLS. In fact, it may be an alternative treatment in those patients with insufficient response to standard RLS drugs. Side effects of pramipexole include involuntary movements and motions, dizziness, drowsiness, upset stomach, heartburn, constipation, excessive tiredness, frequent urination, dry mouth, and decreased sexual desire.

In a European study, pramipexole was compared with placebo in 345 patients with RLS across 37 treatment centers. Patients received placebo or pramipexole for four weeks in a flexible dose-increasing fashion, followed by two weeks of treatment at a maintenance dose. Researchers found that the RLS rating score improvement was 12.3 points for the pramipexole group compared with 5.7 points for the placebo group. Nighttime symptomatic improvement was 32.3% for pramipexole versus 12.4% for placebo; daytime symptoms were also significantly improved with the drug (12.1% versus 1.5%, respectively). Researchers also noted that there were greater sleep improvements in the pramipexole group than the placebo group (29.9% versus 13.8%). Finally, 79% of patients in the pramipexole group versus 31% of patients in the placebo group reported no or mild mood disturbances after six weeks of treatment.

For more information see page 1422.

Generic: **Tramadol** (TRAM-a-dole)
Brand: **Ultram**

Tramadol belongs to a class of drugs known as analgesics, used to relieve moderate to moderately severe pain caused by surgery and chronic conditions such as cancer or joint pain. Side effects of tramadol include dizziness, weakness, headache, nervousness, agitation, mood changes, drowsiness, blurred vision, upset stomach, sweating, diarrhea, and vomiting. This drug can be habit-forming and abrupt cessation of the drug can cause withdrawal symptoms (nervousness, panic, sweating, etc.).

Tramadol has been evaluated in fewer than 15 adult patients with RLS. In a small clinical trial, tramadol improved in patient ratings of RLS symptoms. Eighty-three percent of patients rated tramadol therapy as more successful than their previous treatments. After three to six months of tramadol treatment, some patients experienced RLS symptoms again. Increasing the dose of tramadol, restarting the drug after a short break, or switching to another drug (i.e., levodopa) controlled these RLS reccurring symptoms. The most common side effects were abdominal pain, dizziness in the morning, tremor sensation, and itching. Researchers recommend tramadol over other opiate analgesics for the treatment of RLS, with sporadic treatment and careful monitoring.

For more information see page 1518.

Stuttering

Stuttering is a disruption of the normal pattern, rhythm, or timing of speech. Stuttering may present itself by repetition and prolongation of words, phrases, and sounds; it can also include hesitations or pauses that interrupt speech flow. Stuttering may be caused by developmental factors (occurring in childhood) or stroke or head injury. Mild stuttering is rarely treated, but persons with more severe forms of stuttering may need speech therapy or drug treatment.

Commonly Prescribed (On-Label) Drugs: *None*

OFF-LABEL PRESCRIPTION DRUG
BREAKTHROUGH OPTION

Generic: ***Paroxetine*** *(pa-ROKS-e-teen)*
Brands: ***Paxil, Paxil CR***

Paroxetine belongs to a class of drugs known as selective serotonin reuptake inhibitor (SSRI) antidepressants and is used to treat mental depression, obsessive-compulsive disorder (OCD), panic disorder, generalized anxiety disorder (GAD), social anxiety disorder (also known as social phobia), premenstrual dysphoric disorder (PMDD), and post-traumatic stress disorder (PTSD). SSRI-type drugs, such as paroxetine, may work by increasing the activity of the chemical serotonin in the brain. Side effects associated with the use of paroxetine include acid or sour stomach, belching, decreased appetite, decreased sexual desire, gas, heartburn, nervousness, pain or tenderness around the eyes and cheekbones, and sleepiness, among others.

There are three patient reports documenting the use of paroxetine for stuttering. Stuttering symptoms were characterized by repetitions of words/phrases and sounds/syllables in all sentence positions. After a few days of paroxetine treatment, improvement was seen. Some patients completely stopped stuttering after one month. No adverse drug reactions were reported. Paroxetine may be helpful in patients who stutter and who have depression or other mood disorders.

For more information see page 1395.

Tardive Dyskinesia (Drug-induced)

Tardive dyskinesia is a neurological syndrome caused by the long-term use of neuroleptic drugs (drug prescribed for psychiatric, GI, and some neurological disorders). It is characterized by repetitive, involuntary, purposeless movements (e.g., grimacing, lip smacking, rapid eye blinking, rapid movement of the arms and legs). Persons with tardive dyskinesia are treated on an individualized basis. The first step of treatment is to stop or minimize the neuroleptic drug, although symptoms of tardive dyskinesia can continue long after the drug is discontinued.

Commonly Prescribed (On-Label) Drugs: *None*

OFF-LABEL PRESCRIPTION DRUG
BREAKTHROUGH OPTION

Generic: **Ondansetron** *(on-DAN-se-tron)*
Brands: **Zofran, Zofran ODT**

Ondansetron belongs to a class of drugs known as anti-emetics, used to prevent nausea and vomiting after treatment with chemotherapy, radiation, or surgery. Side effects of ondansetron include constipation, diarrhea, fever, headache, abdominal pain, dizziness, drowsiness, dry mouth, and weakness, among others.

Since serotonin plays a role in tardive dyskinesia, which improves with the use of selective-serotonin antagonists, ondansetron has been prescribed for this drug-induced spasm disorder. In two major clinical studies of ondansetron, it significantly reduced the severity and symptoms of tardive dyskinesia, and improved the patients' psychotic symptoms. In a four-week trial, 10 adult patients with mild tardive dyskinesia and schizophrenia had significant reductions in tardive dyskinesia and psychiatric symptoms. Four patients had greater than 50% decrease of their dyskinesia symptoms.

In a 12-week trial of 20 adult schizophrenic patients with drug-induced tardive dyskinesia, ondansetron significantly reduced the severity and symptoms of tardive dyskinesia and improved psychotic symptoms.

For more information see page 1387.

TRAUMA

Trauma is defined as a wound, hurt, or injury to the body. Trauma can also be mental such as when a person feels great stress. Each year, about 1.5 million Americans sustain a traumatic brain injury, of which 75% are mild concussions. Mild brain trauma can cause temporary confusion and headache; a serious injury can cause death. A traumatic spinal cord injury can occur from a sudden blow to the spine that harms one or more of the vertebrae. Common causes of spinal cord injury in the U.S. include motor vehicle accidents, acts of violence, falls, sports or recreation injuries, and diseases.

Brain Trauma

Traumatic brain injury (TBI) is the result of a sudden, violent blow to the head. Causes of brain trauma include motor vehicle accidents, gunshots, falls, and other injuries. Most of the symptoms of brain injury appear right after or shortly after a blow to the head. Symptoms of mild brain trauma include a brief period of unconsciousness, headache, confusion, dizziness, sensory problems, mood changes, and memory or concentration problems. If the brain injury is moderate to severe, the symptoms include persistent headache, repeated vomiting or nausea, convulsions, inability to awaken from sleep, and slurred speech, among others.

Commonly Prescribed (On-Label) Drugs: None

OFF-LABEL PRESCRIPTION DRUGS
BREAKTHROUGH OPTIONS

Generic: **Donepezil** *(doe-NEP-e-zil)*
Brand: **Aricept**

Donepezil is used to treat Alzheimer's disease by increasing the amount of certain natural substances in the brain. Side effects associated with donepezil include upset stomach, diarrhea, difficulty falling asleep or staying asleep, vomiting, muscle cramps, excessive tiredness, appetite loss, pain, headache, and dizziness, among others.

Based on the efficacy seen with donepezil in Alzheimer's disease, it has also been investigated for TBIs and has been shown to improve cognitive function, particularly memory. Researchers at the University of Texas Health Science Center in San Antonio examined the effects of donepezil on short-term memory and sustained attention in patients with traumatic brain injury (TBI) in a 24-week trial. Eighteen post-acute patients with TBI and cognitive impairment were randomly assigned to group A (patients in this group were given donepezil for the first 10 weeks and then a placebo for another 10 weeks) or group B (patients in group B received the preparations in the opposite order). Researchers found that donepezil significantly increased auditory and visual testing scores from the beginning of the study. In group B, there was no significant change in the testing scores between the baseline and end of the placebo phase. An intergroup comparison at the 10-week assessment showed significantly improved testing scores in group A with donepezil over group B with the placebo. Results from this study showed that donepezil increased neuropsychologic testing scores in short-term memory and sustained attention in patients with post-acute TBI.

For more information see page 1150.

*Generic: **Gabapentin** (GA-ba-pen-tin)*
*Brand: **Neurontin***

Gabapentin is used to help control some types of epileptic seizures. It is also used to control pain associated with shingles. Side effects of gabapentin include blurred or double vision; cold or flu-like symptoms; delusions; dementia; drowsiness; hoarseness; lack or loss of strength; lower back or side pain; swelling of the hands, feet, or lower legs; and trembling and shaking, among others.

Researchers at Walter Reed Army Institute of Research, Silver Spring, Maryland, developed a rat model of brain trauma-induced nonconvulsive seizures to evaluate potential drug treatments. Rats were treated with an antiepileptic drug from one of seven different drug classes. Based on the results, researchers found that ethosuximide and gabapentin worked best.

For more information see page 1206.

*Generic: **Methylphenidate** (meth-il-FEN-i-date)*
*Brands: **Concerta, Metadate CD, Metadate ER, Methylin, Methylin ER, Ritalin, Ritalin LA, Ritalin-SR***

Methylphenidate belongs to a group of medicines called central nervous system (CNS) stimulants. It is used to treat attention-deficit hyperactivity disorder (ADHD), narcolepsy, and other conditions such as depressive disorders, particularly in persons who cannot take antidepressant drugs. Side effects of methylphenidate include appetite loss, nervousness, trouble sleeping, anger, dizziness, fear, headache, irritability, nausea, and nervousness, among others.

Psychostimulant drugs, such as methylphenidate, may be used to improve cognitive impairment in persons with TBIs and have been used to try to improve poor attention, distractibility, hyperactivity, impulsiveness, arousal problems, mood disorders, aggression, and memory problems. Psychostimulant drugs are thought to correct problems with neurotransmission in affected persons. Use of these drugs may improve brain dopamine levels and promote the brain recovery process.

Researchers affiliated with several U.S. academic institutions showed the use of methylphenidate in 30 patients with active seizure disorders corresponded with a decreased incidence of seizures. They concluded that this drug can be safely used in patients with TBIs, especially those at high risk for seizures.

For more information see page 1315.

Generic: *Modafinil* (moe-DAF-i-nil)
Brand: *Provigil*

Modafinil is a central nervous system (CNS) stimulant that is prescribed for narcolepsy, obstructive sleep apnea (i.e., periodic cessation of breathing at night), and shift work sleep-related disorders used to promote wakefulness and alertness. Side effects include headache, nervousness, anxiety, restlessness, dizziness, difficulty falling asleep, drowsiness, depression, mood swings, upset stomach, diarrhea, and constipation, among others.

Fatigue is a common symptom in a person with TBI, and results in major cognitive and behavioral dysfunction. Since modafinil is effective in narcolepsy, scientists and doctors used it to treat fatigue in TBIs. Ten patients with brain injury and fatigue or sleepiness caused by drugs, modafinil dramatically reduced daytime sleepiness in nine patients. It also moderately improved daytime sleepiness in three patients. The drug showed activity within one to two hours after the first dose, and lasted all day allowing for normal nighttime sleep. The most common adverse effect was GI upset. Modafinil has been shown to increase cognition, improve rehabilitation, and improve quality of life for patients with TBI.

For more information see page 1338.

*Generic: **Rivastigmine** (ri-va-STIG-meen)*
*Brand: **Exelon***

Rivastigmine belongs to a class of drugs known as cholinesterase inhibitors, and is used for the treatment of Alzheimer's disease. It improves mental function by increasing the amount of certain natural substances in the brain. Side effects of rivastigmine include upset stomach, vomiting, appetite loss, stomach pain, weight loss, diarrhea, weakness, dizziness, headache, and extreme tiredness, among others.

As a drug class, acetylcholinesterase inhibitors such as rivastigmine alleviate some of the main symptoms of chronic TBI. In Finland 111 patients with chronic stable TBI (with at least one of the following symptoms: fatigue, poor memory, diminished attention, or diminished initiation) randomly received donepezil, galantamine, or rivastigmine. Twenty-seven patients received donepezil, 30 received galantamine, and 54 received rivastigmine. Results showed that 61% of patients had a marked positive response and 39% of patients had a modest or no response to drug treatment. The main improvements involved attention and general function. Fifty-five percent of patients in this study wanted to continue therapy with one of these drugs. The therapeutic response came very quickly and at low doses. There were no significant differences in effect or tolerability among the three drugs. Researchers concluded that this class of drugs has potential benefits in treating chronic TBI.

For more information see page 1459.

Acute Spinal Cord Injury

The spinal cord and brain comprise the central nervous system (CNS), which controls most of the body's functions. The most common causes of spinal cord injury in the United States are motor vehicle accidents, acts of violence, falls, sports or recreation injuries, and diseases. The signs and symptoms of acute spinal cord injury depend upon the location and severity of the injury. Signs and symptoms include pain or intense stinging sensation caused by damage to the nerve fibers in the spinal cord, loss of movement, loss of sensation, loss of bowel or bladder control, and difficulty breathing, among others.

Commonly Prescribed (On-Label) Drugs: *None*

OFF-LABEL PRESCRIPTION DRUGS
BREAKTHROUGH OPTIONS

Generic: **Heparin** *(HEP-a-rin)*
Brand: **Heparin**

Heparin is used to decrease the clotting ability of the blood and help prevent harmful clots from forming in the blood vessels. Heparin does not dissolve blood clots that have already formed, but it may prevent the clots from becoming larger and causing more serious problems. A doctor will prescribe heparin as a treatment for certain blood vessel, heart, and lung conditions; it is also used to prevent blood clotting during open-heart surgery, bypass surgery, and dialysis.

Heparin is recommended by the American College of Chest Physicians in patients with acute spinal cord injury because of their high risk of deep vein thrombosis (blood clots) and pulmonary embolism (a mass that obstructs or occludes a blood vessel). Specifically, this drug is recommended to prevent thromboembolism in patients with acute spinal cord injury in rehabilitation programs.

Researchers in the United Kingdom compared heparin combined with another drug, warfarin, with enoxaparin in the prevention of thromboembolism in patients with spinal cord injury. Researchers found that four of the 101 patients given heparin/warfarin developed symptoms of venous thromboembolism compared with 13 of the 72 who were treated with enoxaparin.

There is no drug profile for this drug as data are pending.

Generic: **Methylprednisolone** *(meth-il-pred-NIS-oh-lone)*
Brands: **Medrol, Solu-Medrol, Depo-Medrol**

Methylprednisolone, a man-made corticosteroid developed to mimic a natural hormone produced by the adrenal glands, is used in inflammatory disorders, such as arthritis, asthma, and severe allergies, to block symptoms of inflammation. It is also used to treat certain cancers. Methylprednisolone may be used in persons with acute spinal cord injury to reduce inflammation and promote recovery. Side effects of methylprednisolone include upset stomach, stomach irritation, vomiting, headache, dizziness, insomnia, restlessness, depression, anxiety, acne, and increased hair growth, among others.

The Second National Acute Spinal Cord Injury Study (NASCIS) II showed that methylprednisolone in high doses provided neurologic improvements in persons with spinal cord injury, but high doses of methylprednisolone have become controversial based on the drug's serious side effects. Yet this drug may help to reduce inflammatory processes that occur in the first days following the trauma, a secondary injury process which causes deterioration in spinal cord function.

Methylprednisolone has been studied in rats with spinal cord injury by researchers in Korea who found that this drug may improve functional recovery. At the University of Miami School of Medicine, researchers found that methylprednisolone may be effective in reducing inflammation in persons with spinal cord injury, also based on studies involving rats.

For more information see page 1316.

*Generic: **Phenytoin** (FEN-i-toyn)*
*Brand: **Dilantin***

Phenytoin, a sodium channel blocker, belongs to a class of drugs known as anticonvulsants or antiepileptics. Primarily used for the treatment of epilepsy, it targets chemicals in the brain to treat convulsions and seizures by maintaining balance. In persons with acute spinal cord injury, phenytoin may protect spinal cord axons, preserve the action of nerve impulse conduction, and reduce neurologic deficits. Common side effects include drowsiness, upset stomach, vomiting, constipation, stomach pain, loss of taste, weight loss, difficulty swallowing, mental confusion, blurred vision, and insomnia, among others.

In spinal cord injury, a series of events occur on multiple levels within the body. Abnormal sodium movements within the body have been cited as one of the major problems in spinal cord injury. Blocking sodium channels in the body with certain drugs has been shown to reduce further injury and promote recovery from spinal cord trauma. Researchers in Turkey evaluated the neuroprotective effect of phenytoin, a sodium channel blocker, on experimental spinal cord injury in rats, and found that phenytoin appears to protect the spinal cord against injury by decreasing certain lipid reactions and by lessening neuronal damage.

For more information see page 1413.

Bone Loss Reduction in Spinal Cord Injury

Immobilization of the spinal cord after injury can result in bone changes, including decreases in bone mass and osteoporosis (thinning of the bones). Bone loss is greatest in the first three to four months after the initial injury, and usually stabilizes by 16 months. Loss of bone initially affects the entire body, but is then isolated to the paralyzed areas. The mechanisms by which bone loss occurs are not fully understood. A group of drugs known as bisphosphonates may be used to reduce bone loss.

Commonly Prescribed (On-Label) Drugs: *None*

OFF-LABEL PRESCRIPTION DRUGS
BREAKTHROUGH OPTIONS

Generic: **Alendronate** *(a-LEN-droe-nate)*
Brand: **Fosamax**

Alendronate is used to prevent or treat osteoporosis in women after menopause and to treat osteoporosis in men. It may be used to treat Paget's disease of the bone and osteoporosis caused by steroid drugs. Side effects include abdominal pain, difficulty swallowing, heartburn, irritation or pain of the esophagus, and muscle pain.

Bisphosphonate drugs, such as alendronate, act primarily by inhibiting normal and abnormal bone resorption. These drugs may help those with spinal cord injuries by reducing bone loss. In a case study, alendronate was used for two years in the treatment of bone loss associated with spinal cord injury and improved bone density in a 47-year-old patient with spinal cord injury.

In a six-month study in Brazil, 19 patients with chronic spinal cord injury were divided into a control group, which received calcium daily, and an experimental group of patients, which received calcium plus alendronate daily. The alendronate had a positive effect on bone mineral density in patients with spinal cord injury, so alendronate is a potential drug for the prevention and treatment of osteoporosis in this patient population.

For more information see page 994.

Generic: **Etidronate** *(e-ti-DROE-nate)*
Brand: **Didronel**

Etidronate is used to treat Paget's disease of the bone and to treat and prevent certain bone problems that may occur after hip replacement or spinal cord injury. Etidronate prevents bone breakdown and increases bone density (thickness). It also interferes with bone mineralization. Sometimes this drug is used to treat and prevent osteoporosis caused by steroid drugs. Side effects can include upset stomach, diarrhea, and bone pain.

Bisphosphonate drugs, such as etidronate, act primarily by inhibiting normal and abnormal bone resorption and may be helpful in reducing bone loss in patients with spinal cord injuries. Researchers evaluated the effects of etidronate on bone density in 13 patients with acute spinal cord injury. Rate of bone loss was significantly greater in the wheelchair group versus the patients that could walk (or ambulatory), although bone density was preserved in the etidronate ambulatory group. The researchers found that etidronate may prevent bone density loss in a select group of ambulatory patients with spinal cord injury.

Across the literature, bisphosphonate drugs, such as etidronate, have helped reduce bone loss, although further studies are needed to determine which drug is most effective.

For more information see page 1177.

Generic: **Pamidronate** *(pa-mi-DROE-nate)*
Brand: **Aredia**

Pamidronate is used to treat hypercalcemia, a condition characterized by an over-abundance of calcium in the blood, that can occur with some types of cancer. It is also used to treat Paget's disease of the bone, the spread of cancer to the bone, and a condition known as osteogenesis imperfecta. Side effects include abdominal pain, acid or sour stomach, belching, bladder pain, bloody or cloudy urine, body aches or pain, bone pain, constipation, degenerative disease of the joint, and diarrhea, among others.

Bisphosphonate drugs, such as pamidronate, act primarily to inhibit normal and abnormal bone resorption. Researchers at the University of Manitoba compared the effects of a six-month treatment with IV pamidronate with conventional rehabilitation without pamidronate on bone density of the spine and leg bones in 24 patients with acute spinal cord injury. They found that patients treated with IV pamidronate after acute spinal cord injury had significantly less bone density loss compared with those who did not receive pamidronate. Additionally, ambulatory subjects had significantly less bone density loss during the study than nonambulatory subjects. Side effects included fever, nausea, and injection site reactions, among others. Overall, this study concluded that IV pamidronate treatment and ambulatory ability in the first six months after an acute spinal cord injury prevents bone density loss.

For more information see page 1391.

*Generic: **Tiludronate** (tye-LOO-droe-nate)*
*Brand: **Skelid***

Tiludronate is used to treat Paget's disease. This drug slows the weakening of bone by decreasing the breakdown of bone. Side effects of tiludronate include upset stomach, diarrhea, stomach irritation or pain, gas, constipation, vomiting, decreased appetite, swelling of the feet or legs, headache, dizziness, and nasal congestion, among others.

Bisphosphonate drugs, such as tiludronate, act primarily on the bone by inhibiting normal and abnormal bone resorption. These drugs may be helpful in patients with spinal cord injuries by reducing bone loss. In a study of 33 paraplegic patients, two doses of tiludronate for three months were compared with placebo. Twenty patients completed this study. Nonsignificant bone volume decreases occurred in the lesser-dosage tiludronate group and the placebo group, and slight increases were seen in the larger-dosage tiludronate group. Researchers concluded that tiludronate seems effective in reducing bone resorption without impairments in bone formation.

As a drug class bisphosphonates act on the bone tissue and have minimal side effects. Across the literature, bisphosphonate drugs, such as tiludronate, have reduced bone loss, although further studies are needed to determine which specific drug is most effective.

For more information see page 1514.

TREMOR DISORDERS

Tremor involves a rhythmic, involuntary, oscillatory movement of body parts. A diagnosis of tremor disorders is made on careful evaluation of the patient's history and diagnostic tests. Tremors are classified as rest or action tremors. Rest tremors occur when the affected body part is completely supported against gravity. Examples of rest tremor include Parkinson's disease or drug-induced tremors. Action tremors are the result of voluntary muscle contraction and include drug or alcohol withdrawal tremors. Tremor disorders include essential tremor and Parkinson's disease.

Essential Tremor

Essential tremor is the most common movement disorder in the world, ranging from 4.1 to 39.2 cases per 1,000 persons younger than 60 years. The incidence and prevalence of essential tremor increases with age. In essential tremor the upper limbs, the head, lower limbs, voice, tongue, face, and trunk may be affected. Although essential tremor does not affect your survival, it can cause significant physical and psychosocial disability. People with essential tremor may have difficulty writing, drinking, eating, dressing, speaking, and completing other basic activities.

Commonly Prescribed (On-Label) Drugs: Propranolol

OFF-LABEL PRESCRIPTION DRUGS
BREAKTHROUGH OPTIONS

Generic: Botulinum Toxin Type A (BOT-yoo-lin-num TOKS-in type aye)
Brands: Botox, Botox cosmetic

Botulinum toxin type A is classified as an injectable neurotoxin, which blocks the nerves' ability to make muscles contract, thereby paralyzing muscles. This injectable neurotoxin is used to treat neck muscle spasms and uncontrollable blinking, control misaligned or "lazy eyes," and reduce the appearance of forehead frown lines in adults age 65 and younger. Side effects include allergic reactions, temporary muscle weakness or discomfort at injection site, skin rash, sensitivity to light, and headache.

In a study, 25 patients with moderate to severe essential hand tremor were injected with botulinum toxin type A into wrist muscles. Researchers found that 75% of patients treated with botulinum toxin type A had mild to moderate improvement four weeks after treatment compared with those patients treated with placebo.

In another trial of 133 patients with essential tremor, botulinum toxin type A was injected into wrist muscles for 16 weeks. Improvements in motor task performance and functional disability were inconsistent and appeared to be offset by adverse side effects. Nowadays, clinicians give reduced doses of botulinum toxin type A.

For more information see page 1051.

Generic: Clonazepam (kloe-NA-ze-pam)
Brand: Klonopin

Clonazepam belongs to a class of drugs known as benzodiazepines. This drug is used to control seizures, and to relieve anxiety. Clonazepam may be used to treat symptoms of Parkinson's disease, twitching, schizophrenia, and to manage pain. It has an inhibitory effect on the central nervous system (CNS) and facilitates the activity of the neurotransmitter GABA, and has been used to treat movement disorders such as Tourette's Syndrome

(TS). Side effects associated with clonazepam include drowsiness, dizziness, tiredness, weakness, dry mouth, diarrhea, upset stomach, and appetite changes. This drug may be habit-forming, and with long-term use, some people may become tolerant to the drug's effects.

There are limited data on the use of clonazepam, which has been reported to be of some value in the treatment of benign essential tremor. Researchers found that this drug was not effective for essential tremor. Conversely, in a patient case study involving a family with essential tremor of the arms, clonazepam offered therapeutic benefits. Some family members also had tremor of the trunk and legs on standing, but not on walking, sitting, or reclining. Other drugs (beta-blockers) had no effect on trunk or leg tremor, but clonazepam was effective. In a study of 20 patients with tongue tremor (associated with essential tremor), therapy with a number of drugs including clonazepam reduced this type of tremor.

For more information see page 1107.

Generic: **Gabapentin** *(GA-ba-pen-tin)*
Brand: **Neurontin**

Gabapentin belongs to a class of drugs known as anticonvulsants, used to help control some epileptic seizures. It is also used to control pain associated with shingles. Gabapentin may also be prescribed for other nervous system disorders. Side effects include blurred or double vision; cold or flu-like symptoms; delusions; dementia; drowsiness; hoarseness; lack or loss of strength; lower back or side pain; swelling of the hands, feet, or lower legs; and trembling and shaking; among others.

Gabapentin has been used to treat essential tremor as a second-line treatment. It is well tolerated by the elderly. One study demonstrated that gabapentin is as effective as propranolol (a beta-blocker drug) for essential tremor. In contrast, in a study of 20 patients with essential tremor, gabapentin added to other treatments for two weeks showed only a modest benefit. In a report by the American Academy of Neurology, gabapentin alone offered up to a 77% improvement in tremor, for 16 treated patients.

For more information see page 1206.

Generic: **Metoprolol** *(me-TOE-proe-lole)*
Brands: **Lopressor, Toprol XL**

Metoprolol belongs to a class of drugs known as selective beta-blockers. It is often used alone or in combination with other drugs to treat high blood pressure, prevent chest pain, and treat heart attacks. Metoprolol slows the heart rate and relaxes blood vessels so the heart does not have to pump as hard. Sometimes metoprolol is used to prevent migraine headaches, and may be used to treat movement disorders caused by drugs or illness. Side effects of metoprolol include dizziness, lightheadedness, tiredness, depression, upset stomach, dry mouth, stomach pain, gas or bloating, heartburn, constipation, skin rash or itching, and cold hands and feet.

Beta-blocker drugs, such as metoprolol, are usually used first in the treatment of essential tremor and may be effective. Overall, this drug is considered a substitute to propranolol, another beta-blocker drug that is often used to treat essential tremor.

According to the American Academy of Neurology, data on metoprolol for essential tremor are conflicting. In one study it improved tremor, but in another, it was ineffective.

For more information see page 1321.

Generic: **Nicardipine** *(nye-KAR-de-peen)*
Brands: **Cardene, Cardene IV, Cardene SR**

Nicardipine is a calcium channel blocker used to used to treat high blood pressure; it relaxes blood vessels so the heart does not have to pump as hard and increases the supply of blood and oxygen to the heart to control chest pain. If taken regularly, nicardipine controls chest pain, but it does not stop chest pain once it starts. It may be used to treat congestive heart failure. Side effects include headache, upset stomach, dizziness, tiredness, flushing, numbness, fast heartbeat, muscle cramps, and constipation, among others.

Researchers in Spain examined the effects of nicardipine in 11 patients with essential tremor. Each patient was given placebo, and on a separate occasion, a single oral dose of nicardipine followed by one month of sustained daily treatment. A single oral dose of nicardipine reduced the tremor amplitude compared to placebo, but after one month of persistent treatment, nicardipine failed to sustain the initial statistical improvement although it still reduced the tremor amplitude. Researchers concluded that a single oral dose of nicardipine can reduce essential tremor, but chronic treatment may not maintain improvement.

For more information see page 1358.

Generic: *Nimodipine* (nye-MOE-di-peen)
Brand: *Nimotop*

Nimodipine belongs to a class of drugs known as calcium-channel blockers, used to treat symptoms resulting from ruptured blood vessels in the brain (hemorrhages) by increasing blood flow to injured brain tissue. It may be used to treat or prevent migraine headaches since it changes the movement of calcium ions into muscle cells of blood vessels thereby improving blood flow. Side effects of nimodipine include headache, dizziness, lightheadedness, feeling of warmth, heartburn, fast or slow heartbeat, upset stomach, stomach pain, constipation, depression, and unusual bruising or bleeding.

Nimodipine is also used for essential tremor and may reduce tremor amplitude by 53%. According to a report issued by the American Academy of Neurology, nimodipine can possibly reduce limb tremor associated with essential tremor disorder and it is recommended for treating limb tremors.

Researchers from Saudi Arabia evaluated nimodipine in 16 patients with essential tremor. Patients in this study were treated with placebo or nimodipine. Eight patients improved and one patient was withdrawn because of adverse effects. Researchers concluded that nimodipine is effective in some patients with essential tremor.

For more information see page 1361.

Generic: *Primidone* (PRI-mi-done)
Brand: *Mysoline*

Primidone is an anti-seizure drug. It was found to have anti-tremor activity when it was given to a patient with epilepsy and essential tremor. Side effects are common and include drowsiness, lack of coordination, irritability, excitement, upset stomach, tiredness, headache, and appetite changes.

The efficacy of primidone for essential tremor has been shown in a number of studies. Primidone has similar or even more efficacy than propranolol (a beta-blocker drug), with complete tremor suppression in a greater proportion of patients. It is most effective for hand tremor, and its efficacy for head and voice tremor are variable. After one year of treatment, about 10% to 15% of responders develop tolerance to the drug's effects.

In a short-term study, primidone was less tolerated than beta-blockers. Nearly one third of patients had short-term side effects (nausea, dizziness, etc.) with the drug that occurred in the morning and after the first nighttime dose and lasted up to four days. Only 12% of those patients experiencing side effects stopped treatment.

For more information see page 1432.

Generic: **Topiramate** *(TOE-pie-rah-mate)*
Brand: **Topamax**

Topiramate is used to prevent epileptic seizures, and may be used to prevent migraine headaches. Side effects include headache, nausea, tremor, fatigue, gastrointestinal upset, visual disturbances, sleepiness, and weight loss, among others.

The use of topiramate for essential tremor is limited to one trial and two studies. In the trial of 24 adults with essential tremor, topiramate provided significant reductions compared with placebo; improvements were recorded in tremor location, severity, specific motor tasks, and disabilities. In the smaller studies, topiramate improved tremors from 25% to 80%. The most common side effects seen with the use of topiramate in these studies included fatigue, abnormal and uncomfortable sensations, and drowsiness.

Overall, data suggest a beneficial but not curative effect of topiramate for essential tremor. According to the American Academy of Neurology, topiramate should be considered for the treatment of limb tremor associated with essential tremor.

For more information see page 1516.

Parkinson's Disease

Parkinson's disease (PD) is a chronic, progressive neurodegenerative disorder characterized by tremors, rigidity, slow movement, poor balance, and difficulty walking. In the U.S., PD affects one to 1.5 million people, and is more prevalent in whites. It is caused by the degeneration of dopamine-producing nerve cells in the brain. Once dopamine production is depleted, the motor system nerves are unable to control movement and coordination. Secondary symptoms of PD include constipation, difficulty swallowing, loss of bladder control, and loss of intellectual capacity, among others.

Commonly Prescribed (On-Label) Drugs: *Apomorphine, Bromocriptine, Entacapone, Ethopropazine, Levodopa, Levodopa/Carbidopa, Levodopa/Carbidopa/Entacapone, Pramipexole, Ropinirole, Selegiline, Tolcapone, Trihexyphenidyl*

OFF-LABEL PRESCRIPTION DRUGS
BREAKTHROUGH OPTIONS

Generic: **Clozapine** *(KLOE-za-peen)*
Brand: **Clozaril**

Clozapine belongs to a class of drugs known as antipsychotics, used to treat schizophrenia in patients who have not been helped by or are unable to take other medicines. It should not be used to treat behavioral problems in older adult patients who have dementia. Side effects of clozapine include constipation, dizziness, lightheadedness, drowsiness, mild headache, increased watering of mouth, nausea, vomiting, and weight gain.

Low doses of clozapine are used to treat drug-induced psychosis in PD even though there is a risk of agranulocytosis—a disease marked by high fever and a sharp drop in white blood cells. Studies have shown that clozapine, in small doses, can reduce the severity of levodopa (a Parkinsonian drug)-induced involuntary movements (known as dyskinesias) by about 50% in people with PD. Researchers in France evaluated clozapine in a study in 50 patients with drug-induced movements and PD. Results from this 10-week trial showed a reduction in the duration of "on" periods with levodopa-induced movements in favor of the clozapine group. It was concluded that clozapine is effective in the treatment of levodopa-induced dyskinesias in patients with severe PD. In another study, clozapine and quetiapine were equally effective for the treatment of PD psychosis.

For more information see page 1111.

Generic: **Gabapentin** (GA-ba-pen-tin)
Brand: **Neurontin**

Gabapentin belongs to a class of drugs known as anticonvulsants, and is used to help control some epileptic seizures. It is also used to control pain associated with shingles. Gabapentin may be prescribed for other nervous system disorders. Side effects of gabapentin include blurred or double vision; cold or flu-like symptoms; delusions; dementia; drowsiness; hoarseness; lack or loss of strength; lower back or side pain; swelling of the hands, feet, or lower legs; and trembling and shaking; among others.

Based on anecdotal reports that gabapentin was effective in relieving patients with leg cramps, tremor, rigidity, and PD, researchers at the University of Louisville in Kentucky further evaluated the drug for PD. Nineteen patients received gabapentin and improved with gabapentin compared with placebo. Additionally, their daily activities improved with gabapentin compared with placebo, but did not achieve statistical significance. Tremor improved with gabapentin. Overall, based on these results, gabapentin improved rigidity, bradykinesia, and PD tremor.

For more information see page 1206.

Generic: **Modafinil** (moe-DAF-i-nil)
Brand: **Provigil**

Modafinil is a central nervous system (CNS) stimulant prescribed for narcolepsy (sudden and uncontrollable attacks of drowsiness and sleep), obstructive sleep apnea (periodic cessation of breathing at night), and shift work sleep-related disorders. It is used to promote wakefulness and alertness. Side effects include headache, nervousness, anxiety, restlessness, dizziness, difficulty falling asleep, drowsiness, depression, mood swings, upset stomach, diarrhea, and constipation, among others.

Daytime sleepiness and fatigue is a common symptom in PD affecting nearly 40% of patients. Certain drugs used to treat PD are associated with excessive sleepiness and therefore are hazardous to patients who take them and attempt to perform certain basic activities. Compared with other PD drugs, modafinil appears to be useful for the treatment of excessive sleepiness.

In clinical studies of modafinil for PD-associated fatigue, there have been variable results. Fifteen adult patients with PD and excessive daytime sleepiness were chosen to receive modafinil or placebo for two weeks. Twelve patients completed this study. Modafinil significantly reduced sleepiness compared with placebo, although there were no differences with regard to estimated sleep time.

In another small study, modafinil made no difference in fatigue compared with placebo. Overall, the role of modafinil for PD is not completely known, and more studies are needed.

For more information see page 1338.

Generic: *Quetiapine* (kwe-TYE-a-peen)
Brand: *Seroquel*

Quetiapine is used to treat psychotic symptoms such as hallucinations, delusions, and hostility. About 50% of persons with advanced PD exhibit psychotic symptoms which quetiapine can treat. Side effects of quetiapine include dizziness, lightheadedness, constipation, stomach pain, headache, excessive weight gain, runny nose, rash, and ear pain, among others.

In clinical studies, quetiapine has shown promise as an effective drug for psychosis in PD and improves psychosis in PD without triggering movement disorders. Researchers at Emory University School of Medicine in Atlanta, Georgia, evaluated the effects of quetiapine for psychosis in 29 patients with PD who failed to respond to treatment with clozapine, risperidone, or olanzapine. In this 24-week trial, researchers found significant improvements in psychosis and no decline in motor functions. Furthermore, there were significant improvements in recall scores on cognitive tests. Researchers concluded that small doses of quetiapine may treat psychotic symptoms and improve cognition without worsening motor function in patients with PD.

For more information see page 1440.

*Generic: **Zolpidem*** *(zole-PE-dem)*
*Brand: **Ambien***

Zolpidem, a hypnotic drug, is used to treat insomnia. It helps affected persons get to sleep faster and sleep through the night. When sleep medicines are used every night for a long time, they may lose their effectiveness; therefore, they should be used only for short periods of time, such as one or two days, and should not be used for longer than one or two weeks. Side effects of zolpidem include stomach pain, daytime drowsiness, diarrhea, double vision, drugged feelings, dry mouth, general feeling of illness, headache, memory problems, and nausea, among others.

Isolated, positive trials on the use of zolpidem by patients with PD report improvement in motor symptoms and abnormal movements. The drug effects occur as fast as 15 minutes and are optimal within two hours of administration. Persistent use of zolpidem may lead to a reduced effect in some patients.

Among three patients, zolpidem provided 31% to 100% improvement in dystonia (prolonged, repetitive muscle contractions that may cause twisting or jerking movements of the body or a body part) and up to 40% improvement in Parkinsonism.

For more information see page 1556.

VESTIBULAR DISORDERS

Vestibular disorders occur often and affect people of all ages and all walks of life. According to studies from the National Institute of Health, 90 million Americans will complain to their doctors of dizziness at least once in their lifetime. Causes of vestibular disorders include injury, ear infections, and use of certain drugs such as antibiotics. The most common symptoms of vestibular disorders include dizziness, unsteadiness or imbalance when walking, vertigo, and nausea. These symptoms may be quite mild, lasting minutes, or quite severe and result in total disability.

Tinnitus

More than 50 million Americans have tinnitus to some degree. Tinnitus is the medical term for the perception of sound in one or both ears or in the head when no external sound is present. Tinnitus is often referred to as "ringing in the ears." Some people with tinnitus hear hissing, roaring, whistling, chirping, or clicking sounds. This disorder can be intermittent or constant with single or multiple tones; perceived volume can range from subtle to shattering. Some causes of tinnitus include ear wax build-up, environmental factors, the use of certain medications, and some types of trauma.

Commonly Prescribed (On-Label) Drugs: Nylidrin

OFF-LABEL PRESCRIPTION DRUG
BREAKTHROUGH OPTION

Generic: **Clonazepam** (kloe-NA-ze-pam)
Brand: **Klonopin**

Clonazepam is used to control seizures and relieve anxiety. It may be used to treat symptoms of Parkinson's disease, twitching, schizophrenia, and to manage pain. Side effects include drowsiness, dizziness, tiredness, weakness, dry mouth, diarrhea, upset stomach, and appetite changes. This drug may be habit-forming, and with long-term use, some people may become tolerant to its effects.

Since 1976, clonazepam, even in low doses, has been shown to be safe and effective for vestibular disorders. Researchers in Brazil surveyed 25 years of clinical experience with 3,357 outpatients treated with clonazepam for tinnitus (caused by different factors) during 60 days to 180 days. Researchers reviewed the medical records pertaining to a 0.5 or 1.0 mg/day of oral clonazepam. Tinnitus was improved in 32% of the affected patients. Side effects included light or mild drowsiness, depression, nightmares, or lowering of libido, which were reported by 16.9% of the patients as adverse, but which tended to subside with continued therapy. It was concluded that clonazepam is very useful and safe for the symptomatic treatment of patients suffering from tinnitus.

For more information see page 1107.

Vertigo

Vertigo is a false sensation of motion or spinning that leads to dizziness or discomfort. Persons with vertigo feel as though they are actually spinning or moving, or that their surroundings are in motion. There are two types of vertigo: peripheral and central. Peripheral vertigo occurs if there is a problem with the portion of the inner ear that controls balance or with the vestibular nerve. Central vertigo occurs if there is an abnormality in the brain. Associated symptoms include double vision, difficulty swallowing, facial paralysis, and slurred speech.

Commonly Prescribed (On-Label) Drugs: Diphenidol, Meclizine, Perphenazine

---

OFF-LABEL PRESCRIPTION DRUG
BREAKTHROUGH OPTION

Generic: **Clonazepam** (kloe-NA-ze-pam)
Brand: **Klonopin**

Clonazepam is used to control seizures and relieve anxiety. It may be used to treat symptoms of Parkinson's disease, twitching, schizophrenia, and to manage pain. Side effects associated with clonazepam include drowsiness, dizziness, tiredness, weakness, dry mouth, diarrhea, upset stomach, and appetite changes. This drug may be habit forming, and with long-term use, some people may become tolerant to its effects.

Since 1976, clonazepam, even in low doses, has been shown to be safe and effective for vestibular disorders. Researchers in Brazil conducted a retrospective survey of 25 years of clinical experience with 3,357 outpatients treated with clonazepam during 60 days to 180 days as a vestibular disorder treatment. Complete or substantial control of vertigo or nonvertigo-related dizziness was achieved in 77.4% of the vertigo patients. Light or mild drowsiness, depression, nightmares, or lowering of libido were reported by 16.9% of the patients as adverse side effects, which tended to subside with continued therapy. It was concluded that clonazepam is very useful and safe for the symptomatic treatment of patients suffering from vestibular disorders, such as vertigo.

For more information see page 1107.

CARDIOVASCULAR DISORDERS

ARRHYTHMIAS

Ataxia Cordis

See Atrial Fibrillation

Atrial Fibrillation

Atrial fibrillation (AF) is diagnosed as an abnormal rhythm of the heart. A heart without atrial fibrillation contracts and pumps blood at a regular rhythm such as at a rate of 60 beats per minute. While the heart may beat faster or slower with a shorter or longer interval between beats it maintains a constant interval at any one rate through regular electrical discharges, or currents, that travel through the heart and cause the muscle of the heart to contract. In people with AF, the electrical discharges are irregular and rapid and, as a result, the heart beats irregularly and, usually, rapidly. This is a common disorder that affects over half a million people yearly in the United States.

Commonly Prescribed (On-Label) Drugs: *Digitoxin, Dofetilide, Flecinide, Heparin, Verapamil, Warfarin*

OFF-LABEL PRESCRIPTION DRUG
BREAKTHROUGH OPTION

Generic: ***Amiodarone*** *(a-MEE-oh-da-rone)*
Brand: ***Cordarone, Pacerone***

Amiodarone is a medication used to treat life-threatening irregular heart rhythms (arrhythmias) and to maintain a normal heart rate in people who have not responded to other medications.

Amiodarone has been used orally and intravenously (IV) in the management of atrial fibrillation or flutter. According to physicians, IV amiodarone is the preferred or one of several preferred antiarrhythmic agents for the control of ventricular rates in patients with atrial fibrillation or flutter. However, most clinicians recommend that the drug be reserved for use within the first 48 hours of arrhythmia or in those in whom other rate-control measures are ineffective or contraindicated.

Long-term therapy with oral amiodarone alone or in combination with other antiarrhythmic agents has been effective for suppression and prevention of therapy-resistant atrial fibrillation. Limited data indicate that long-term amiodarone therapy may be effective in about 70% of patients with atrial fibrillation, including those whose arrhythmia is resistant to conventional therapy.

For more information see page 1007.

Crista Supraventricularis

See Supraventricular (Atrial) Arrhythmia

Paroxysmal Atrial Tachycardia

See Supraventricular Tachycardia

PSVT

See Supraventricular Tachycardia

Supraventricular (Atrial) Arrhythmia

Supraventricular arrhythmias happen in the upper chambers of the heart. Generally, supraventricular or "atrial arrhythmias" are not as serious as ventricular arrhythmias. Sometimes, they do not even require treatment. Atrial arrhythmias can happen in response to a number of things, including tobacco, alcohol, caffeine, and cough or cold medicines. The disorder also may result from rheumatic heart disease or an overactive thyroid (hyperthyroidism).

Commonly Prescribed (On-Label) Drugs: *Propafenone*

OFF-LABEL PRESCRIPTION DRUG
BREAKTHROUGH OPTION

Generic: **Atenolol** *(a-TEN-oh-lole)*
Brand: **Tenormin**

Atenolol is a beta-blocker medication used to treat chest pain (angina) and high blood pressure. It is also used after an acute heart attack to improve survival. This drug works by blocking the action of certain natural chemicals in the body such as epinephrine on the heart and blood vessels. The effect is a lowering of the heart rate, blood pressure, and strain on the heart.

Intravenous (IV) beta-blocking drugs, including atenolol, have been used in the treatment of various supraventricular tachyarrhythmias. IV beta-blocking agents also have been used to slow rapid ventricular response in patients with acute atrial fibrillation associated with a heart attack or other heart disorders. Use of a beta-blocker is one of the most effective means of slowing ventricular rate in atrial fibrillation. If a beta-blocker is used to control ventricular response in patients with acute atrial tachyarrhythmias (following acute heart attack), heart rate, blood pressure, and electrocardiogram (ECG) should be monitored. Also, the therapy should be discontinued when symptoms resolve or when blood pressure declines to less than 100 mm Hg or heart rate slows to less than 50 beats per minute.

For more information see page 1027.

Supraventricular Tachycardia

Supraventricular tachycardia (SVT) is a general term describing any rapid heart rate originating above the ventricles or lower chambers of the heart. SVT is an arrhythmia or abnormal heart rhythm. Specific types of SVT include: atrial fibrillation, AV nodal re-entrant tachycardia, and Wolff-Parkinson-White syndrome.

SVT generally begins and ends quickly. You may experience short periods of SVT and have no symptoms. However, SVT becomes a problem when it occurs frequently or lasts for long periods of time and produces symptoms. Common symptoms associated with SVT include palpitations, light-headedness, and chest pain. SVT may also cause confusion or loss of consciousness.

Commonly Prescribed (On-Label) Drugs: *Adenosine, Flecainide, Methoxamine*

OFF-LABEL PRESCRIPTION DRUG
BREAKTHROUGH OPTION

Generic: **Atenolol** *(a-TEN-oh-lole)*
Brand: **Tenormin**

Atenolol is a beta-blocker medication used to treat chest pain (angina) and high blood pressure used after a heart attack to improve survival. Intravenous (IV) beta-blocking agents, including atenolol, have been used in the treatment of various supraventricular tachyarrhythmias. According to researchers, the effectiveness of atenolol treatment for superventricular tachycardia is well known.

A study conducted at the Walsgrave Hospital in the United Kingdom of 60 patients undergoing coronary artery bypass surgery investigated the effect of a beta-blocker on supraventricular arrhythmias that occurred post operatively. Patients with good left ventricular function were divided into two groups: 30 patients treated with atenolol and 30 patients acted as controls. Eleven patients in the control group experienced arrhythmias while atenolol significantly reduced this incidence to one patient. Researchers concluded that the use of atenolol (started 72 hours before operation) is effective in reducing supraventricular arrhythmias following elective coronary artery bypass operations in patients with good left ventricular function.

For more information see page 1027.

SVT

See Supraventricular Tachycardia

Torsades de Pointes

Torsades de Pointes is a cardiac arrhythmia that may cause blackouts or even sudden death. The phrase "Torsades de Pointes" is French and literally means "twisting of the points," referring to the characteristic appearance of the electrocardiogram (ECG) during the rhythm abnormality. Torsades de Pointes occurs in individuals with genetic mutations in their genes that control sodium or potassium channels and is a frequent cause of sudden death in these individuals. It also occurs as a complication of drugs that prolong the QT interval (the interval that represents the time for electrical activation and inactivation of the heart's ventricles) by blockade of potassium channels. Doctors measure the time it takes for the QT interval to occur (in fractions of a second). By measuring the QT interval, they can determine it occurs in a normal amount of time, or it takes longer, which is then called a prolonged QT.

Commonly Prescribed (On-Label) Drugs: None

OFF-LABEL PRESCRIPTION DRUG
BREAKTHROUGH OPTION

Generic: **Magnesium Sulfate**
(mag-NEE-zhum SUL-fate)
Brand: **Magnesium Sulfate**

Magnesium sulfate is a medication most commonly used to control seizures in pregnancy and to treat low magnesium levels and problems related to kidney conditions (nephritis) in children. It is also used for preventing premature contractions in pregnancy and to treat heart attack and asthma patients.

In a review article, investigators in Israel concluded that treatment for Torsades de Pointes should focus on shortening the QT interval, noting that intravenous magnesium should be the first-line treatment choice for this condition, as it has proven effective in other trials and studies. Additionally, investigators at the Saitama Children's Medical Center in Japan conducted a study on six children diagnosed with Torsades de Points with long QT syndrome. An injection of magnesium sulfate was given to the patients over a 1- to 2-minute period, which was then followed by continuous administration for the next 2 to 7 days. Five of the children responded significantly to the initial administration; while one child required a higher dosage until Torsades de Pointes was eliminated. Researchers concluded that intravenous magnesium sulfate effectively treated children with Torsades de Pointes.

For more information see page 1292.

VT

See Ventricular Tachycardia

V Tach

See Ventricular Tachycardia

Ventricular Tachycardia

Ventricular tachycardia is a rapid heartbeat initiated within the ventricles (chambers that collect blood and then pump it out of the heart), characterized by three or more consecutive premature ventricular beats. Ventricular tachycardia is a potentially lethal disruption of normal heartbeat (arrhythmia) that may cause the heart to become unable to pump adequate blood through the body. The heart rate may be 160 to 240 (normal is 60 to 100 beats per minute). Ventricular tachycardia occurs in approximately two out of 10,000 people.

For more information on this disorder in children see Tachycardia on page 235 Children's Health Disorders.

Commonly Prescribed (On-Label) Drugs: *None*

OFF-LABEL PRESCRIPTION DRUGS
BREAKTHROUGH OPTIONS

Generic: **Atenolol** *(a-TEN-oh-lole)*
Brand: **Tenormin**

Atenolol is a medication known as a beta-blocker. It is used to treat chest pain (angina) and high blood pressure, and also used after a heart attack to improve survival. The drug works by blocking the action of certain natural chemicals in the body such as epinephrine on the heart and blood vessels. The result is a lowering of your heart rate, blood pressure, and strain on the heart.

Beta-blocking medications, including atenolol, have been shown to reduce the incidence of ventricular fibrillation associated with heart attacks and are considered among several preferred agents for the treatment of ventricular tachycardias. The efficacy of atenolol was studied by researchers in Thailand to determine the treatment for VA compared with placebo. The study involved 52 patients with VA. Researchers assessed the severity of symptoms and quality of life (QOL) at the start of the study and one month after atenolol. Exercise testing was also performed. According to researchers, results of this study showed that atenolol significantly decreased symptom frequency.

For more information see page 1027.

Generic: ***Magnesium Sulfate*** *(mag-NEE-zhum SUL-fate)*
Brand: ***Magnesium Sulfate***

Magnesium sulfate is a medication used to control seizures in pregnancy, to treat low magnesium levels and problems related to kidney conditions (nephritis) in children. It is also used for preventing premature contractions in pregnancy and to treat heart attacks and asthma. Use of magnesium sulfate is not recommended for the treatment of cardiac arrest except as an alternative therapy when the arrhythmias are suspected to be caused by low levels of magnesium in the blood. According to researchers, evidence suggests that magnesium sulfate also may be an effective treatment in antiarrhythmic drug-induced Torsades de Pointes even in the absence of magnesium deficiency.

For more information see page 1292.

Generic: ***Metoprolol*** *(me-toe-PROE-lole)*
Brands: ***Lopressor, Toprol-XL***

Metoprolol, a beta-blocker, slows the heart rate and reduces high blood pressure. It is used to treat angina (chest pain), high blood pressure, or irregular heartbeats. Beta-blocker medications, including metoprolol, have been shown to reduce the incidence of ventricular fibrillation associated with heart attack and is considered one of several preferred agents for the treatment of ventricular tachycardias.

Researchers suggest that the incidence of primary ventricular fibrillation (which is highest during the first four hours after a heart attack and then declines markedly) may be decreasing under current practices for acute heart attack management, possibly because of aggressive attempts at correction of electrolyte deficits and increased use of beta blocking drugs.

Routine use of intravenous (IV) beta blockers, including metoprolol, in patients without blood circulation problems is associated with a reduction in the incidence of early ventricular fibrillation. Therefore, it currently is recommended that IV followed by oral beta-blocker therapy be given (unless contraindicated) to all people following an acute heart attack.

For more information see page 1321.

Generic: **Phenytoin** *(FEN-i-toyn)*
Brand: **Dilantin**

Phenytoin is most commonly used to prevent and control seizures. This drug may also be used to treat certain types of irregular heartbeats and painful nerve conditions such as trigeminal neuralgia. A study conducted at the University of Pittsburgh School of Medicine examined the effectiveness of phenytoin in 69 of 87 patients undergoing a test that studies the heart's electrical system. In general, during the initial session lidocaine and procainamide were tested immediately after the start of the test, followed by phenytoin and quinidine during the next two sessions and then by additional drugs as needed. Nine of the 69 phenytoin trials were successful (13.0%), compared to eight of 57 trials (14.0%) with procainamide, four of 37 trials (10.8%) with quinidine and 0 of 41 trials (0%) with lidocaine. Researchers concluded that phenytoin is a well-tolerated drug.

For more information see page 1413.

Generic: **Verapamil** *(vur-AP-ah-mill)*
Brands: **Calan, Calan SR, Covera-HS, Isoptin SR, Verelan, Verelan PM**

Verapamil is a calcium channel blocker used to treat irregular heartbeats. Calcium is involved in blood vessel contraction and in controlling the electrical impulses within the heart. By blocking calcium, verapamil relaxes and widens blood vessels and can normalize heart rates.

Researchers in Japan investigated the efficacy of verapamil to terminate ventricular tachyarrhythmias. The study involved 390 patients with a diagnosis of acute heart attack. All patients received a procedure to relieve severe chest pain within six hours of onset of symptoms and 109 patients then experienced tachyarrhythmias induced by the restoration of blood flow (called reperfusion induced). Thirty-one patients (28%) were treated with verapamil for the immediate termination of reperfusion-induced ventricular tachyarrhythmias. The drug was effective in rapidly terminating all reperfusion-induced arrhythmias except for ventricular fibrillations. The side effects of treatment included temporary low blood pressure and slow heart beat, although all patients recovered. Based on these results, researchers concluded that verapamil can safely terminate reperfusion-induced ventricular tachyarrhythmias in a rapid manner.

For more information see page 1544.

Ventricular Tachycardia, Prevention of Recurrence and Sudden Death

Ventricular tachycardia (VT), usually defined as more than three consecutive electrocardiographic (ECG) complexes of ventricular origin at a rate of more than 100 beats/min, varies widely in severity. The vast majority of people with tachycardia and heart disease have VT.

Commonly Prescribed (On-Label) Drugs: *None*

OFF-LABEL PRESCRIPTION DRUGS
BREAKTHROUGH OPTIONS

*Generic: **Atenolol** (a-TEN-oh-lole)*
*Brand: **Tenormin***

Atenolol is a beta-blocker medication that is used to treat chest pain (angina) and high blood pressure. It is also used after an acute heart attack to improve survival. This drug works by lowering your heart rate, blood pressure, and strain on the heart.

Beta-blockers may be particularly useful early in the management of sustained polymorphic ventricular tachycardia (electrical storm) following acute heart attack, which often is unresponsive to conventional antiarrhythmic therapy. Members of a family were investigated by researchers at the Nicosia General Hospital in Cyprus because of three sudden deaths among them. Two young sisters, aged 12 and 16, died suddenly while swimming and running, while their 19-year-old brother died suddenly during emotional stress. In no case did autopsies reveal any structural abnormalities. Their 39-year-old mother and her 19-year-old daughter showed a history of syncopes (loss of consciousness due to decreased cerebral blood flow), while having a normal physical examination and normal ECGs. During a treadmill test, multiple premature contractions of the ventricle of the heart and bursts of ventricular tachycardia were observed. Members of this family have undergone several tests to determine the cause of their VT. The patients were given atenolol and were followed up for 18 months. Researchers concluded that this therapy was successful in reducing arrhythmias as assessed by serial treadmill tests.

For more information see page 1027.

*Generic: Beta-blockers such as **Bisoprolol** (bis-OH-proe-lol), **Carvedilol** (KAR-ve-dil-ole) and **Metoprolol** (me-toe-PROE-lole)*
*Brands: **Coreg (carvedilol), Lopressor, Toprol-XL (metoprolol), Zebeta (bisoprolol)***

Metoprolol, bisoprolol, and carvedilol are beta-blocker medications used to treat chest pain (angina), heart failure, and high blood pressure. These drugs work by lowering heart rate, blood pressure, and strain on the heart.

Beta-blockers may be particularly useful early in the management of sustained polymorphic ventricular tachycardia ("electrical storm") following acute heart attack, which often is unresponsive to conventional antiarrhythmic therapy. Despite routine use of angiotensin-converting enzyme (ACE) inhibitors, beta-blockers and spironolactone in patients with heart failure due to dilated cardiomyopathy (DCM), these patients still have a considerable death rate of five to 10%. Sudden unexpected death accounts for up to 50% of all deaths and is most often due to rapid ventricular tachycardia or ventricular fibrillation. Researchers note that the use of beta-blockers in patients with heart failure has been shown to reduce deaths considerably. This survival benefit has been demonstrated for bisoprolol, metoprolol, and carvedilol. Therefore, investigators conclude that one of these three beta-blocking agents should be administered routinely starting with low doses in all patients unless there is a contraindication to beta-blocker use.

For more information see pages 1047, 1073, and 1321.

*Generic: **Phenytoin** (FEN-I-toyn)*
*Brand: **Dilantin***

Phenytoin is used to prevent and control seizures. This drug may also be used to treat certain types of irregular heartbeats and painful nerve conditions like trigeminal neuralgia. Intravenous (IV) phenytoin sodium may be useful in the treatment of ventricular tachycardia and paroxysmal atrial tachycardia (bouts of rapid, regular heartbeats that begin and end suddenly), particularly in those patients who do not respond to conventional antiarrhythmic agents. Oral phenytoin and phenytoin sodium have been used for maintenance therapy in the management of cardiac arrhythmias.

Current treatments are used for significant arrhythmias. The degree of significance of ventricular tachycardia (VT) mostly depends on the type and degree of structural heart disease and the condition of the heart. In patients with low risk for sudden death no treatment is needed or antiarrhythmics administration. Conversely, in high-risk patients, implantation of a defibrillator may be necessary. In the prevention of recurrent arrhythmia and sudden death: amiodarone, sotalol, mexiletin, phenytoin, beta-blockers, radiofrequency ablation, implantablecardioverter-defibrillator and, in specific patients, verapamil, pacemaker or left ganglion stellatum denervation, may be used for treatment.

For more information see page 1413.

Generic: **Verapamil** *(vur-AP-ah-mill)*
Brands: **Calan, Calan SR, Covera-HS, Isoptin SR, Verelan, Verelan PM**

Verapamil is a calcium channel blocker medication used to treat irregular heartbeats. Calcium is involved in blood vessel contraction and in controlling the electrical impulses within the heart. By blocking calcium, verapamil relaxes and widens blood vessels and can normalize heart rates.

The majority of people who are diagnosed with ventricular tachycardia have underlying structural heart disease. However, there has been increasing evidence of multiple forms of ventricular tachycardia with distinct features and unique mechanisms. The most common form of ventricular tachycardia originates from the right ventricular outflow tract and is characterized by sensitivity to adenosine (a chemical in the body that has a role in energy transfer). Other forms of ventricular tachycardia include left ventricular tachycardia, due to reentry, which is sensitive to verapamil and automatic, propranolol-sensitive ventricular tachycardia.

For more information see page 1544.

Cardiac Arrest

Cardiac arrest is the sudden, abrupt loss of heart function. It is a medical emergency that, unless quickly corrected, is rapidly fatal. Cardiac arrest primarily results from cardiac causes, including electrical dysfunction (heart rhythms) in 80% of people and mechanical failure (pump functions) in 20%. Additional causes may include circulatory shock or abnormalities in ventilation leading to significant cardiopulmonary arrest. Although either the heart or lungs may fail first, both events usually are closely related.

Commonly Prescribed (On-Label) Drugs: *Norepinephrine*

OFF-LABEL PRESCRIPTION DRUGS
BREAKTHROUGH OPTIONS

*Generic: **Amiodarone** (a-MEE-oh-da-rone)*
*Brands: **Cordarone, Pacerone***

Amiodarone is a medication used to treat irregular heart rhythms (arrhythmias) and to maintain a normal heart rate. Data from most clinical studies indicate that the drug is effective in approximately 50–80% of patients with life-threatening ventricular arrhythmias, including those resistant to other antiarrhythmic agents. Previously, the potential severity of the drug's adverse effects generally had precluded amiodarone from being considered a first-line drug in treating life-threatening ventricular arrhythmias. The use of the drug generally was reserved for those in whom other antiarrhythmic agents were ineffective or not tolerated. Currently, however, amiodarone is considered a preferred or alternative drug for the management of various life-threatening ventricular arrhythmias, in part because of its apparent reduced risk of inducing arrhythmia activity. In addition, amiodarone is one of the few antiarrhythmics for ventricular tachyarrhythmias considered acceptable for geriatric patients and for patients with a progressive decline in cardiac function. Recently, the FDA required pharmacists to dispense a patient medication guide with each prescription, describing potential serious side effects of this medication.

For more information see page 1007.

*Generic: **Sodium Bicarbonate***
(SOW-dee-um bye-KAR-bun-ate)
*Brand: **Sodium Bicarbonate (IV)***

Sodium bicarbonate is used as a treatment of metabolic acidosis (characterized as an increase in total body acid). Sodium bicarbonate may also be used in advanced cardiovascular life support (ACLS) during cardiopulmonary resuscitation. In a study conducted at the Safar Center for Resuscitation Research at the University of Pittsburgh, the effects of sodium bicarbonate use on CPR outcome was analyzed. Analysis included only patients who had a cardiac arrest outside of the hospital and whose time from collapse to initiation was no longer than 30 minutes. Earlier and more frequent use of sodium bicarbonate was associated with higher early resuscitability rates and with better long-term outcome. Researchers concluded that sodium bicarbonate may be beneficial during CPR.

For more information see page 1477.

Generic: **Dobutamine** *(doe-BYOO-ta-meen)*
Brand: **Dobutrex**

Dobutamine is a medication that is used to treat heart conditions. The medication provides additional pumping strength by stimulating the heart muscle. Use of the drug in combination with dopamine for the management of heart failure and other heart problems is recommended by the American College of Cardiology (ACC) and American Heart Association (AHA).

When used to increase blood flow following a heart attack, dobutamine may be helpful as an addition to vasodilators such as sodium nitroprusside in people with left ventricular failure. Dobutamine also may be useful in people with low blood pressure cardiogenic shock following a heart attack once blood pressure has been stabilized. Dobutamine may be particularly helpful in the management of cardiogenic shock in patients with normal diastolic blood pressure and systolic pressures exceeding 100 mm Hg, since the drug provides the best support. Dobutamine should not be used alone if you are a severely hypotensive patient (when systolic blood pressure is less than 100 mm Hg).

For more information see page 1149.

Generic: **Magnesium Sulfate** *(mag-NEE-zhum SUL-fate)*
Brand: **Magnesium Sulfate**

Magnesium sulfate is used most commonly to control seizures in pregnancy, to treat low magnesium levels and problems related to kidney conditions (nephritis) in children. Magnesium sulfate has been administered intravenously (IV) as additional therapy to reduce cardiovascular morbidity and mortality associated with a heart attack. However, contradictory evidence of such beneficial effects has been reported and the precise role of the IV magnesium in the management of acute myocardial infarction needs to be more clearly explained.

Several studies have indicated a reduction in ventricular arrhythmias and/or mortality with early intravenous (IV) magnesium administration in patients with acute heart attack. In more than 2,000 patients with suspected heart attack and magnesium concentrations in the normal range, therapy with magnesium sulfate administered as a single IV injection (2 g) within 24 hours of onset of symptoms, followed by continuous IV infusion of the drug (16 g) over the next 24 hours. This treatment was associated with a reduction in death compared with that in placebo recipients.

Additionally, patients receiving IV magnesium had a 25% lower rate of congestive heart failure during hospitalization and a 21% reduction in heart disease-related mortality during long-term follow-up of at least 4.5 years.

For more information see page 1292.

*Generic: **Milrinone** (MIL-ri-none)*
*Brand: **Primacor***

Milrinone is used for the short-term treatment of congestive heart failure (CHF). Because researchers feel that clinical experience with milrinone is lacking, the manufacturers state that the drug is not recommended for use during the acute phase following a heart attack, and milrinone is not included in the current recommendations of the American College of Cardiology (ACC) and American Heart Association (AHA) for the management of a heart attack.

Phosphodiesterase (PDE) inhibitor drugs such as milrinone and inamrinone were developed with the hope that the different mechanism of action of these drugs would lead to improved cardiac output without the risk of arrhythmia associated with other treatments such as catecholamine drugs. However, excessive mortality observed with long-term milrinone therapy and unacceptable toxicity with long-term inamrinone therapy has limited the current use of these drugs. In addition, elimination of the drug from the body is problematic in critically ill patients. However, milrinone currently is recommended as an alternative drug that may be useful in advanced cardiovascular life support (ACLS) in adult and pediatric patients for improving cardiac output when other preferred drugs cannot be used or are ineffective in patients with severe heart failure or cardiogenic shock.

For more information see page 1330.

Cardiac Shock

See Cardiogenic Shock

Cardiogenic Shock

Cardiogenic shock is a disease state where the heart is damaged to the degree that it is unable to supply sufficient blood to the body. The most common cause is an acute heart attack, with left ventricular failure, but it can also be caused by mechanical complications. Cardiogenic shock complicates approximately 6 to 7% of heart attacks.

Commonly Prescribed (On-Label) Drugs: *Dopamine*

OFF-LABEL PRESCRIPTION DRUGS
BREAKTHROUGH OPTIONS

Generic: ***Milrinone*** *(MIL-ri-none)*
Brand: ***Primacor***

Milrinone is a drug that helps to dilate blood vessels. It increases the force with which the heart pumps and opens up blood vessels to facilitate blood flow. In a report published by investigators at the Saitama Medical School in Japan, they documented a case of a 19-year-old man with dilated cardiomyopathy (a condition where the heart is weakened and cannot pump blood efficiently) who developed cardiogenic shock. According to researchers, in this case, milrinone was lifesaving. A HeartMate left ventricular assist device was inserted as an emergency procedure, but removed after 189 days due to infection related to the device. Intravenous milrinone was administered because of recurrence of heart failure and, as a result, the symptoms disappeared. Subsequently, the patient successfully underwent heart transplantation. Researchers concluded that milrinone was effective as a therapeutic treatment of critical heart failure after removal of a heart assist device.

Another report by researchers at the Mayo Medical Center in Rochester, Minnesota, documented the case of a 55-year-old woman with delayed cardiogenic shock emerging within hours after a bursting of a blood vessel. Researchers documented that the patient had both cardiac and pulmonary injury. They administered dobutamine and milrinone, which resolved the complication.

For more information see page 1330.

*Generic: **Nitroprusside** (nye-tro-PRUS-ide)*
*Brand: **Nitropress***

Nitroprusside is a medication used for the immediate control of very high blood pressure. It is also used to treat certain heart problems such as congestive heart failure or to control bleeding during surgery. Heart function is determined by how much blood the heart can pump and at what rate it can pump. Changes of these variables may result in decrease of blood pressure, acute heart failure, or cardiogenic shock. Severe systemic low blood pressure often requires therapy with catecholamine (a chemical derived from amino acids) to restore circulation and to avoid organ damage. As the use of catecholamines is not aimed at the causes of problems, administration should be limited to an initial measure until correction of the underlying abnormalities can be achieved.

First-line intervention consists of restoring fluid as appropriate and use of dopamine to increase contractility and blood pressure. In acute left heart failure support with dobutamine or epinephrine may be necessary, frequently combined with a vasodilator such as sodium nitroprusside or nitroglycerine or phosphodiesterase-III-inhibitor.

For more information see page 1367.

Dilated Cardiomyopathy

Dilated cardiomyopathy (DCM) is a disease of the heart muscle that causes the heart to become enlarged and to reduce the ability of the heart to pump blood throughout the body. There are many possible causes including infection, injury, and genetics. Frequently the cause is unknown. The deterioration of heart function is usually slow and symptoms are commonly observed when the disease is quite advanced. Fluid can build up in the lungs and this congestion may cause you to experience a feeling of breathlessness.

Commonly Prescribed (On-Label) Drugs: *None*

OFF-LABEL PRESCRIPTION DRUGS
BREAKTHROUGH OPTIONS

*Generic: **Captopril** (KAP-toe-pril)*
*Brand: **Capoten***

Captopril belongs to a group of medications called ACE inhibitors (angiotensin-converting enzyme inhibitor). It is used to treat high blood pressure (hypertension). Captopril works by relaxing blood vessels, causing them to widen. Lowering high blood pressure helps prevent strokes, heart attacks, and kidney problems. This medication is also used to improve survival after an acute heart attack, help protect the kidneys from damage due to diabetes, and to treat congestive heart failure with other drugs such as diuretics.

A study reported in *Clinical Cardiology* looked at the effects of treatment with captopril or metoprolol on heart rate variability in 38 patients with mild to moderate symptoms of heart failure due to dilated cardiomyopathy (DCM). The study investigated and compared the effects of the ACE inhibitor captopril with those of the selective beta-blocker metoprolol on heart rate variability in patients with idiopathic DCM.

Captopril treatment increased heart rate. In the metoprolol group, there was an increase in both time and frequency of heart rate variability. Researchers observed that treatment with captopril and metoprolol increases heart rate variability in patients with DCM. This effect seems to be maintained for at least one month after therapy is stopped. The increase in heart rate variability seems to be more significant with metoprolol, and the two different treatment approaches may have effects that are of importance in patients with heart failure.

For more information see page 1066.

*Generic: **Enalapril** (e-NAL-a-pril)*
*Brand: **Vasotec, Vasotec I.V.***

Enalapril belongs to a group of medications called ACE inhibitors (angiotensin-converting enzyme inhibitor). It is used to treat high blood pressure (hypertension) in adults and children. It works by relaxing blood vessels, causing them to widen. A study examined the effect of treatment with ACE inhibitors on the long-term prognosis in 119 patients with dilated cardiomyopathy (DCM). Conventional therapy was used in 29 patients and 90 patients were treated with ACE inhibitors: 50 were taking captopril and 40 were taking enalapril. Patients treated with ACE inhibitors had a significantly better survival during the first to third year but the difference was not significant between the high- and low-dose groups. According to investigators, these results indicate that ACE inhibitors have a beneficial effect on prolonging the short- and long-term survival in DCM patients. It is strongly recommended by the investigators that all patients with DCM should be treated with ACE inhibitors unless contraindicated. Therefore, lower doses of ACE inhibitors appear to be equivalent to higher doses, and enalapril is preferable to captopril in the treatment of severe congestive heart failure.

For more information see page 1166.

Generic: *Metoprolol* (me-toe-PROE-lole)
Brands: *Lopressor, Toprol-XL*

Metoprolol is a beta-blocker medication used to treat chest pain (angina), heart failure, and high blood pressure. Lowering high blood pressure helps prevent strokes, heart attacks, and kidney problems. This drug works by blocking the action of certain natural chemicals in the body (such as epinephrine) that affect the heart and blood vessels. As a result, lowering of heart rate, blood pressure, and strain on the heart is accomplished.

In a study conducted at the Albert Einstein College of Medicine, researchers analyzed echocardiograms (ECG) of 72 patients with cardiomyopathy while receiving carvedilol or metoprolol for at least 24 months. Twelve months after beta-blocker initiation, the amount of blood pumped increased by greater than or equal to five percent in 75% of patients. Thus, the benefits of carvedilol or metoprolol on left ventricle function are long lasting in patients with cardiomyopathy.

For more information see page 1321.

Generic: **Propranolol** *(proe-PRAN-oh-lole)*
Brands: **Inderal, Inderal LA, InnoPran XL, Propranolol Intensol**

Propranolol is a beta-blocker used to treat chest pain (angina), high blood pressure, irregular heartbeats, migraine headaches, tremors, and other conditions. It is also used after an acute heart attack to improve survival. Lowering high blood pressure helps prevent strokes, heart attacks, and kidney problems. This drug works by blocking the action of certain natural chemicals in the body that affect the heart and blood vessels by lowering heart rate, blood pressure, and strain on the heart. A study conducted at the University of Illinois College of Medicine examined thirty patients with dilated cardiomyopathy. They were divided into three groups to receive intravenous injections of placebo, propranolol, or pindolol. The mean number of doses given was similar for both groups: 3.3 doses for the propranolol group and 3.4 for the pindolol group. Researchers concluded that compared to propranolol, pindolol was more effective in the treatment of dilated cardiomyopathy.

For more information see page 1438.

Cardiomyopathy, Hypertrophic

Hypertrophic cardiomyopathy (HCM) is a rare disorder and affects only one or two people out of 1,000. HCM is a form of cardiomyopathy (disease of the heart muscle) involving thickening of the heart muscle, which interferes with the heart's function. The thickening is often not symmetrical, affecting one part of the heart more than others and it may interfere with the heart's functioning by reducing the size of the ventricular chamber. It may also reduce the ability of the valves to work properly. The thickening of the heart muscle may, in some circumstances, obstruct the flow of blood out of the heart.

Commonly Prescribed (On-Label) Drugs: *None*

OFF-LABEL PRESCRIPTION DRUG
BREAKTHROUGH OPTION

Generic: **Verapamil** *(vur-AP-ah-mill)*
Brands: **Calan, Calan SR, Covera-HS, Isoptin SR, Verelan, Verelan PM**

Verapamil is a calcium channel blocker. Calcium is involved in blood vessel contraction and in controlling the electrical impulses within the heart. By blocking calcium, verapamil relaxes and widens blood vessels and can normalize heartbeats. Verapamil is used to treat chest pain (angina), high blood pressure, or irregular heartbeats.

Cardiac changes induced by verapamil can result in improvement and increased exercise tolerance. According to researchers, while the role of drug therapy in those with hypertrophic cardiomyopathy remains controversial, verapamil has improved defects and increased exercise capacity in such people. Some clinicians suggest that this therapy can be considered for relatively young patients with a family history of premature sudden death.

For more information see page 1544.

Cardiopulmonary Arrest

See Myocardial Infarction

Chronic Cardiac Insufficiency

Chronic cardiac insufficiency is mostly caused by the alteration of the heart's ability to contract. This defect causes an increase in the tension within the heart.

Commonly Prescribed (On-Label) Drugs: *None*

OFF-LABEL PRESCRIPTION DRUG
BREAKTHROUGH OPTION

Generic: **Betaxolol** *(be-TAKS-oh-lol)*
Brands: **Betoptic S, Kerlone**

Betaxolol is a medication used for chest pain (angina), high blood pressure, and irregular heartbeats. Effects were studied by investigators in Russia of a beta blocker in patients with chronic cardiac insufficiency (ChCI). A total of 47 patients with ChCI and an abnormality of the left ventricle were examined. Investigators stated that the use of betaxolol in the therapy of ChCI has been shown to be of significant benefit to people with this condition.

For more information see page 1045.

Congestive Heart Failure

Congestive heart failure (CHF), or heart failure, is a condition defined by a weakened heart that cannot pump enough blood. This can result from: narrowed arteries that supply blood to the heart muscle, coronary artery disease, or heart attack. The scar tissue that may form as a result of this condition can interfere with the heart muscle's normal work. Other potential causes include high blood pressure and heart valve disease due to past rheumatic fever. Primary disease of the heart muscle itself, called cardiomyopathy, or heart defects present at birth, congenital heart defects, as well as infection of the heart valves and/or heart muscle itself, endocarditis and/or myocarditis, can play a role in congestive heart failure.

Commonly Prescribed (On-Label) Drugs: *Amiloride, Bumetanide, Candesartan, Carvedilol, Deslanoside, Digitoxin, Dobutamine, Dopamine, Enalapril, Ethacrynic acid, Fosinopril, Furosemide, Hydrochlorothiazide, Inamrinone, Indapamide, Lisinopril, Metolazone, Metoprolol, Milrinone, Nitroprusside, Quinapril, Ramipril, Spironolactone, Torsemide, Trandolapril, Valsartan*

OFF-LABEL PRESCRIPTION DRUGS
BREAKTHROUGH OPTIONS

Generic: **Amiodarone** *(a-MEE-oh-da-rone)*
Brands: **Cordarone, Pacerone**

Amiodarone is a medication used to treat life-threatening irregular heart rhythms (arrhythmias) and to maintain a normal heart rate in patients who have not responded to other medications. In a study published in the *International Journal of Cardiology*, 21 patients who were diagnosed with CHF placed on a regimen of oral amiodarone. Researchers observed that patients with CHF had a greater benefit from combination dobutamine infusions and oral amiodarone. It is noted that recently the FDA required pharmacists to dispense a patient medication guide with each prescription, describing potential serious side effects.

For more information see page 1007.

Generic: **Atenolol** *(a-TEN-oh-lole)*
Brand: **Tenormin**

Atenolol is a beta-blocker medication used to treat chest pain (angina) and high blood pressure. It is also used after an acute heart attack to improve survival. This drug works by blocking the action of certain natural chemicals in the body, such as epinephrine, on the heart and blood vessels. This results in a lowering of the heart rate, blood pressure, and strain on the heart.

Chronic congestive heart failure is associated with abnormal heart rate turbulence (HRT). In a study conducted by researchers at the National Taiwan University College of Medicine and National Taiwan University Hospital, a 24-hour electrocardiogram (ECG) recording was obtained before and one and three months after giving atenolol therapy to 10 patients with advanced congestive heart failure. According to researchers, the study showed that abnormal heart rate turbulence caused by chronic congestive heart failure can be restored by beta-blocker therapy.

For more information see page 1027.

*Generic: **Bisoprolol*** *(bis-OH-proe-lol)*
*Brand: **Zebeta***

Bisoprolol is a beta-blocker used for chest pain (angina), high blood pressure, and irregular heartbeats. According to researchers, collective experience indicates that long-term therapy with beta-blockers can reduce heart failure symptoms and improve symptoms in patients with chronic heart failure and also can decrease the risk of death.

For more information see page 1047.

*Generic: **Felodipine*** *(fe-LOE-di-peen)*
*Brand: **Plendil***

Felodipine is used to treat high blood pressure (hypertension). Lowering high blood pressure helps prevent strokes, heart attacks, and kidney problems. Felodipine is known as a calcium channel blocker. By blocking calcium, this medication relaxes and widens blood vessels so blood can flow more easily. Echocardiographic (ECG) data were collected from 260 men with heart failure who were divided into two groups: one group receiving felodipine and the other group receiving a placebo. Researchers compared the differences at three months and at 12. At three months, no changes occurred in either group. At 12 months, felodipine patients achieved greater increases in heart function. Researchers concluded that felodipine was successfully added to heart failure therapy.

For more information see page 1182.

*Generic: **Hydralazine*** *(hye-DRAL-a-zeen)*
*Brand: **None***

Hydralazine is a medication that relaxes and expands blood vessels and is used to treat high blood pressure (hypertension). Hydralazine has been used effectively for the short-term treatment of severe congestive heart failure, often producing improvements in cardiac function and exercise tolerance. A few studies evaluating the long-term effects of hydralazine have suggested that beneficial effects may be sustained. However, conflicting results have been reported and tolerance to the drug can occur. In a study in patients with chronic congestive heart failure who were receiving conventional therapy, addition of hydralazine hydrochloride given at the same time as isosorbide dinitrate resulted in a 25–30% decrease in overall mortality rates.

For more information see page 1219.

Generic: **Isosorbide Dinitrate**
(eye-soe-SOR-bide dye-NYE-trate)
Brands: **Dilatrate-SR, Isochron, Isordil, Sorbitrate**

Isosorbide dinitrate is a medication that relaxes blood vessels allowing more blood to flow through. This improves blood flow to the heart. Oral dose forms are used to prevent angina (chest pain). The addition of isosorbide dinitrate plus hydralazine to standard therapy improved survival in heart failure patients who were African American, according to the African American Heart Failure Trial study. Researchers suggest that isosorbide dinitrate plus hydralazine should be added if heart failure persists.

For more information see page 1249.

Generic: **Isosorbide Mononitrate** *(eye-soe-SOR-bide mon-oh-NYE-trate)*
Brands: **Imdur, ISMO, Monoket**

Isosorbide Mononitrate is used to prevent chest pain (angina) and reduce strain on the heart in patients with heart disease (coronary artery disease). Isosorbide mononitrate relaxes and widens blood vessels so blood can flow more easily. In a study, oral isosorbide mononitrate or placebo was administered to 136 patients who were treated for heart failure. No adverse effects such as low blood pressure were observed with isosorbide mononitrate, although headache was reported in 19% of the people. Therefore, researchers observed that isosorbide mononitrate added to captopril increased exercise time in patients with heart failure.

For more information see page 1251.

Generic: **Nitroglycerin IV** *(nye-troe-GLI-ser-in)*
Brands: **Nitro-Bid-IV**

Nitroglycerin relaxes blood vessels, allowing more blood to flow through. Intravenous nitroglycerin is widely used in the treatment of this condition. In a study conducted at Keck School of Medicine in Los Angeles, investigators evaluated the effects of nitroglycerin in patients with heart failure. They concluded that the results were disappointing and failed to show a significant status of the blood system or improvement of symptoms compared with placebo. The initial beneficial effect achieved with the appropriate dose of nitroglycerin is limited by a development of nitrate tolerance. Researchers suggest that more information needs to be obtained in large-scale studies to evaluate the effect of variable doses of nitroglycerin on short- and long-term cardiovascular outcome before intravenous nitroglycerin can be recommended as a standard therapy for heart failure.

For more information see page 1364.

Generic: **Nitroprusside** *(nye-tro-PRUS-ide)*
Brand: **Nitropress**

Nitroprusside is a medication used for the immediate control of very high blood pressure. It is also used to treat certain heart problems such as congestive heart failure or to control bleeding during surgery. Nitroprusside is a valuable treatment, but its use is usually restricted to patients in the intensive care unit who are undergoing monitoring. Although recovery is the rule, the in-hospital mortality for acute heart failure is high and the readmission rate is very high. Researchers suggest that prevention of acute heart failure by avoiding factors known to cause this condition remains the most cost-effective strategy.

For more information see page 1367.

Generic: **Prazosin** *(PRA-zoe-sin)*
Brand: **Minipress**

Prazosin relaxes and expands blood vessels. It is used to treat high blood pressure (hypertension). Although partial or complete tolerance to the effects of prazosin has reportedly developed rapidly in some patients, the response may be temporary and/or corrected by dosage adjustment. Most studies evaluating the long-term effects of prazosin have suggested that beneficial clinical and blood system effects are sustained; however, conflicting results have been reported. According to investigators, further studies are needed to determine the efficacy and role of prazosin for the long-term treatment of severe congestive heart failure.

For more information see page 1426.

*Generic: **Spironolactone** (speer-on-oh-LAK-tone)*
*Brand: **Aldactone***

Spironolactone is used to treat high blood pressure. Lowering high blood pressure helps prevent strokes, heart attacks, and kidney problems. It is also used to treat swelling caused by certain conditions such as heart failure. Low-dose spironolactone therapy has been used in conjunction with angiotensin-converting enzyme (ACE) inhibitors, diuretics, and occasionally cardiac glycosides in patients with severe congestive heart failure (CHF) whose condition has not improved with an ACE inhibitor and a diuretic alone. The related use of spironolactone with an ACE inhibitor had been considered relatively contraindicated because of the potential for developing severe hyperkalemia (a life-threatening illness caused by higher than normal levels of potassium in the blood).

A study was conducted on 1,663 patients with moderate or severe CHF and other complications. Researchers concluded that spironolactone in addition to standard therapy such as an ACE inhibitor and a loop diuretic with or without a cardiac glycoside was associated with decreases in overall mortality and hospitalization rates compared with standard therapy and placebo.

For more information see page 1478.

Heart Arrest

See Cardiac Arrest

Heart Failure

See Congestive Heart Failure

Left Ventricular Dysfunction

Left ventricular dysfunction is a cardiac disorder that impairs, either structurally or functionally, the ability of your left ventricle of the heart to fill with or eject blood. This type of disorder is characterized by shortness of breath, fatigue, and fluid retention. Coronary artery disease is the underlying cause of heart failure in roughly two-thirds of patients with left ventricular dysfunction.

Commonly Prescribed (On-Label) Drugs: None

OFF-LABEL PRESCRIPTION DRUG
BREAKTHROUGH OPTION

Generic: **Nitroglycerin** *(nye-troe-GLI-ser-in)*
Brands: **Nitro-Time, Nitrogard, NitroQuick, Nitrostat, Nitro-Tab**

Nitroglycerin is a medication that relaxes blood vessels, allowing more blood to flow through. This improves blood flow to the heart. Oral dose forms are used to prevent angina (chest pain). This medication is not appropriate for treating an attack of chest pain that is already in progress.

It has been shown by investigators that 30-minute infusions of intravenous nitroglycerin in patients with a heart attack are able to lower left ventricular filling pressure and improve left ventricular function. In a study published in the *British Heart Journal* 30 patients with acute heart attack received one- to three-hour infusions of intravenous nitroglycerin. An improvement in ventricular function was noted in patients with the most severe left ventricular dysfunction. According to researchers, all patients heart attacks, irrespective of the presence or absence of left ventricular failure, showed improvement during nitroglycerin infusion.

For more information see pages 1363–1366.

Acute Myocardial Infarction

Acute myocardial infarction (also known as a heart attack) is the death of heart muscle from the sudden blockage of a coronary artery by a blood clot. Coronary arteries are blood vessels that supply the heart muscle with blood and oxygen. Blockage of a coronary artery deprives the heart muscle of blood and oxygen, causing injury to the heart muscle. Injury to the heart muscle causes chest pain and pressure. If blood flow is not restored within 20 to 40 minutes, irreversible death of the heart muscle will begin to occur. Muscle continues to die for six to eight hours, at which time the heart attack usually is "complete." The dead heart muscle is replaced by scar tissue. Approximately one million Americans suffer a heart attack each year. Four hundred thousand of them die as a result of their heart attack.

Commonly Prescribed (On-Label) Drugs: *Alteplase, Anistreplase, Aspirin, Dalteparin, Enoxaparin, Lisinopril, Ramipril, Reteplase, Streptokinase, Technetium Tenecteplase, Trandolapril, Warfarin*

OFF-LABEL PRESCRIPTION DRUGS
BREAKTHROUGH OPTIONS

Generic: **Dobutamine** *(doe-BYOO-ta-meen)*
Brand: **Dobutrex**

Dobutamine is a medication used to treat heart conditions. This medication provides additional pumping strength by stimulating the heart muscle. Dobutamine is used to increase cardiac output in the short-term treatment of patients with heart disease, cardiac surgical procedures, cardiac arrest, or acute heart attack. Researchers state that the safety of dobutamine hydrochloride following a heart attack has not been established. The use of the drug in combination with dopamine for the management of heart failure syndromes associated with left ventricular dysfunction is included in current recommendations of the American College of Cardiology (ACC) and American Heart Association (AHA) for acute myocardial infarction management.

For more information see page 1149.

*Generic: **Esmolol** (ES-moe-lol)*
*Brand: **Brevibloc***

Esmolol is a beta-blocker used for temporary control of heart rate and blood pressure. According to researchers, esmolol has effectively reduced heart rate, arterial blood pressure, and angina in patients with acute myocardial ischemia (oxygen deprivation to the heart muscle), including those with a heart attack or unstable angina. The efficacy and safety of esmolol have been shown in clinical settings involving patients with unstable angina, heart attack, atrial fibrillation or flutter, and supraventricular tachycardia. Researchers concluded that esmolol is relatively safe in the management of high blood pressure or tachyarrhythmias associated with congestive heart failure or chronic obstructive lung disease where beta-blockers are otherwise contraindicated.

For more information see page 1174.

*Generic: **Low Molecular Weight Heparin** (HEP-a-rin)*
*Brand: **Hep-Lock***

Heparin is an anticoagulant medication used to prevent the blood from clotting. It is used to prevent and treat conditions of blood clotting. Some evidence, principally from studies conducted prior to the widespread use of aspirin for acute heart attack, suggests that treatment with full-dose heparin followed by short-term therapy with oral anticoagulants may reduce the risk of early recurrence in selected patients. According to researchers, heparin treatment initiated during hospitalization and followed by oral anticoagulant therapy for approximately one month may reduce recurrence of acute heart attack. Many clinicians recommend full-dose intravenous (IV) heparin therapy followed by short-term therapy with low molecular weight heparin or warfarin in patients with acute heart attack who are at high risk of artery blockage.

There is no drug profile for this drug as data are pending.

Generic: **Lepirudin** *(leh-puh-ROO-din)*
Brand: **Refludan**

Lepirudin is a "blood thinner" (anticoagulant) used to treat patients who have developed a reaction to another type of anticoagulant such as patients with heparin-induced conditions. It is also used along with aspirin to treat worsening chest pain and certain types of heart attacks.

Efficacy and safety of lepirudin are based principally on the results of two studies in patients with a heparin-induced condition. Clinical efficacy was evaluated beginning at initiation of lepirudin therapy. Researchers concluded that lepirudin is effective in preventing cardiovascular death in patients with unstable angina.

For more information see page 1272.

Generic: **Nitroglycerin** *(nye-troe-GLI-ser-in)*
Brand: **Nitro-Bid IV**

Nitroglycerin is a medication used to relax blood vessels allowing more blood to flow through. Oral dose forms are used to prevent angina (chest pain). The use of nitroglycerin is one of the principal initial therapies in the management of patients with acute heart attack. The drug has been used to reduce myocardial ischemia (oxygen deprivation to the heart muscle) and improve survival after acute myocardial infarction. According to researchers, intravenous (IV) therapy with the drug allows for more precise minute-to-minute control during early management of acute heart attack.

During a heart attack, intravenous nitroglycerine therapy has demonstrated favorable properties, and some studies have shown that nitrates reduce the size of the attack. However, researchers are unsure if this could improve prognosis. A study, cited by researchers in Norway, showed reduced mortality (35%) of early intravenous nitrate therapy. However, researchers state that newer and larger studies have not documented a positive effect. Nitroglycerine administered intravenously is, according to present knowledge of researchers, recommended during the first 24 hours after a heart attack.

For more information see pages 1363–1366.

Myocardial Infarction, Post-incident

The outcome for a person who has had a heart attack depends on the following factors: time to treatment; strength of heart contraction; presence of rhythm disturbances; extent of coronary artery disease and number of coronary arteries involved; presence of congestive heart failure or dangerously low blood pressure; complications such as valve leakage; previous heart attacks, angioplasty, or bypass surgery; and whether the artery causing the heart attack has been successfully dilated so blood can flow through it to the heart muscle.

Commonly Prescribed (On-Label) Drugs: *Alteplase, Anistreplase, Aspirin, Dalteparin, Enoxaparin, Lisinopril, Ramipril, Reteplase, Streptokinase, Technetium Tenecteplase, Trandolapril, Warfarin*

OFF-LABEL PRESCRIPTION DRUG
BREAKTHROUGH OPTION

Generic: **Acebutolol** *(a-se-BYOO-toe-lole)*
Brand: **Sectral**

Acebutolol is a medication used for chest pain (angina), high blood pressure, and irregular heartbeats. A study published in the *American Journal of Cardiology* was conducted to assess the efficacy of one year of treatment by acebutolol in high-risk patients who had survived a heart attack. At one year there was a statistically significant (48%) reduction in total mortality in favor of acebutolol. Additionally, a long-term survey was undertaken to document the survival rate of patients who had acute heart attack. The study involved 586 patients who were followed up for at least five years. During follow-up, 74 deaths (24.8%) occurred in the acebutolol group and 96 (31.1%) in the placebo group. Thus, investigators concluded that the initial benefit obtained in one year of treatment by acebutolol lasts for an expected five years.

For more information see page 983.

Pericarditis

Pericarditis is a disorder caused by inflammation of the pericardium, which is the sac-like covering of the heart. The pericardium has an inner and outer layer with a small amount of lubricating fluid between them. When the pericardium becomes inflamed, the amount of fluid between the two layers increases. This squeezes the heart and restricts its action.

Commonly Prescribed (On-Label) Drugs: Penicillin G

OFF-LABEL PRESCRIPTION DRUGS
BREAKTHROUGH OPTIONS

Generic: **Azathioprine** *(ay-za-THYE-oh-preen)*
Brand: **Imuran**

Azathioprine is used to prevent rejection of transplanted organs and for cases of severe arthritis that do not respond to other therapies. In a report published in *Circulation* patients over the age of 40 underwent a cardiac study because of progressive heart failure. Two patients with active inflammation received prednisone and azathioprine in addition to conventional drug therapy for heart failure. Researchers determined at the eight-month follow-up, cardiac function improved considerably in azathioprine patients but remained unchanged in conventionally treated patients, of whom one died.

For more information see page 1033.

Generic: **Colchicine** *(KOL-chi-seen)*
Brand: **None**

Colchicine is a medication used to treat and prevent gout and has also been studied in various trials for its effectiveness in treating patients who have experienced acute pericarditis and who have not responded to traditional treatments. In a study done in Spain, nine patients who suffered at least three relapses of pericarditis despite being treated with acetylsalicylic acid, indomethacin, prednisone, or a combination were given colchicine. All patients treated with colchicine responded well and did not suffer a recurrence of pericarditis. After two years, follow up examinations were conducted and researchers found no relapses of pericarditis. They also observed marked differences between symptom-free periods before and after treatment with colchicine. Researchers concluded that colchicine may be an effective treatment of recurrent pericarditis.

For more information see page 1115.

*Generic: **Indomethacin** (in-doe-METH-a-sin)*
*Brands: **Indocin, Indocin I.V., Indocin SR***

Indomethacin treats the pain, swelling, and stiffness associated with arthritis, gout, bursitis or tendonitis. Indomethacin can also be used to reduce the pain, fever, and inflammation of pericarditis. One of the most common cardiac causes of recurrent chest pain following a heart attack is acute pericarditis. A study found that pericarditis occurred in about 20% of patients following a heart attack.

Some evidence indicates that the effects of indomethacin daily in relieving post-heart attack pericarditis are comparable to those of aspirin daily. However, while indomethacin can provide effective relief, researchers state that evidence suggests that the drug may cause increased coronary vascular resistance. Additionally, there is evidence that indomethacin may cause thinning of developing scar tissue. Researchers believe that indomethacin's usefulness and efficacy in the management of pericarditis associated with heart attack are less well established by evidence and opinion than those of aspirin and therefore aspirin should be considered the treatment of choice for post-heart attack pericarditis.

For more information see page 1238.

Post-MI Pericarditis

See Pericarditis

Post Myocardial Infarction Pericarditis

See Pericarditis

MISCELLANEOUS
HEART DISORDERS

Cocaine-Induced Coronary Syndrome

Cocaine causes constriction of the coronary arteries, with a decrease in the blood flow. There can be a variety of problems in normal heart function including: arrhythmia, chest pain, or myocardial infarction. The majority of cocaine users are younger than 40, have no cardiac risk factors, and have no history of previous cardiopulmonary disorders.

Commonly Prescribed (On-Label) Drugs: *None*

OFF-LABEL PRESCRIPTION DRUG
BREAKTHROUGH OPTION

Generic: **Nitroglycerin IV** *(nye-troe-GLI-ser-in)*
Brand: **Nitro-Bid IV**

Nitroglycerin is a medication that relaxes blood vessels, allowing more blood to flow through. This improves blood flow to the heart. Oral dose forms are used to prevent angina (chest pain).

A study was undertaken at the University of Florida Health Science Center to compare the use of lorazepam plus nitroglycerine versus nitroglycerine alone in the reduction of cocaine-induced chest pain in the emergency department. Patients were given nitroglycerine or nitroglycerine plus lorazepam intravenously every five minutes for a total of two doses.

Chest pain was recorded on a scale of 0 to 10 at start of treatment and then at five minutes after each dose. The nitroglycerine-only group consisted of 15 patients and the nitroglycerine-plus-lorazepam group consisted of 12 patients. Five minutes after initial treatment, scores for the two groups were 5.2 and 3.9, respectively. Five minutes after the second treatment, the scores were 4.6 and 1.5, respectively. Researchers concluded that the early use of lorazepam with nitroglycerine was more efficacious than nitroglycerine alone, and appeared to be safe in relieving cocaine-associated chest pain.

For more information see page 1364.

Heparin-Induced Thrombocytopenia

One third of hospitalized patients in the United States, or about 12 million a year, receive heparin. Heparin-induced thrombocytopenia (HIT) occurs in three percent of patients who receive intravenous heparin for treatment of deep vein thrombosis or pulmonary embolism. Thrombocytopenia is a condition characterized by low platelet count. It occurs when platelets are lost from the circulation faster than they can be replaced from the bone marrow where they are made. This may result in you experiencing spontaneous bleeding. Low-molecular-weight heparin causes HIT less often (incidence, about 0.5%) than unfractionated heparin.

Commonly Prescribed (On-Label) Drugs: *Argatroban, Lepirudin*

OFF-LABEL PRESCRIPTION DRUGS
BREAKTHROUGH OPTIONS

Generic: **Bivalirudin** *(bye-VAL-I-roo-din)*
Brand: **Angiomax**

Bivalirudin is a "blood thinner" used in patients with certain heart problems such as unstable angina during a type of heart procedure like coronary angioplasty. This medication helps prevent blood clots from forming during and after this type of procedure and is usually used along with aspirin.

The use of heparin in patients with heparin-induced thrombocytopenia (HIT) may result in severe complications or death. Researchers at Gaston Memorial Hospital examined four patients with severe thrombocytopenia after heparin exposure. These people with suspected HIT underwent coronary bypass surgery with bivalirudin. A continuous bivalirudin infusion was used during surgery. Researchers stated that anticoagulation with bivalirudin during bypass surgery was effective and uncomplicated. The duration of the operation was not prolonged and perioperative blood loss and transfusion rates were acceptable. According to researchers, these results provide further evidence of the efficacy of bivalirudin for anticoagulation in HIT patients.

For more information see page 1049.

*Generic: **Fondaparinux** (fon-da-PARE-i-nuks)*
*Brand: **Arixtra***

Fondaparinux is a type of "blood thinner" medication used to help prevent the formation of blood clots following hip or knee surgery. A report by physicians at the General Hospital of Karditsa in Greece documented a case of a man with a history of coronary artery disease and recent stent implantation and who developed severe heparin-induced thrombocytopenia. This occurred two months after stent implantation. The patient was treated with fondaparinux sodium. Researchers observed that there were no complications and platelet counts were restored to normal levels.

They concluded that this evidence suggests that fondaparinux eventually may prove to be valuable for preventing and treating thrombosis in patients with HIT.

For more information see page 1201.

Idiopathic Edema

Idiopathic edema refers to a disorder occurring in young, menstruating women in the absence of cardiac, hepatic, or renal disease. Fluid retention may initially occur premenstrually but often becomes persistent. Obesity and emotional problems (including depression and neurotic symptoms) are commonly part of this syndrome.

***Commonly Prescribed (On-Label) Drugs:** None*

OFF-LABEL PRESCRIPTION DRUG
BREAKTHROUGH OPTION

Generic: **Captopril** *(KAP-toe-pril)*
Brand: **Capoten**

Captopril is a drug that belongs to a group of medications called ACE inhibitors. It is used to treat high blood pressure (hypertension). It works by relaxing blood vessels, causing them to widen. Lowering high blood pressure helps prevent strokes, heart attacks and kidney problems.

Women resistant to dietary weight loss may have a type of idiopathic edema. In a study published in *Endocrine Practice* of 200 women, four drugs used previously for treating idiopathic edema were compared to determine their efficacy in causing weight reduction. After six months of treatment, the percentage of treated groups losing at least 10% of starting weight was 6% for hydrochlorothiazide, 8% for spironolactone, 68% for dextroamphetamine sulfate, and 4% for captopril. The percentage losing greater than 20% of starting weight in the same treatment groups was 28% for dextroamphetamine therapy but 0% for the other three groups.

Based on these results, researchers concluded that some women who are resistant to dietary weight loss may have a mild type of water retention that is not affected by diuretics or ACE inhibitors like captopril but responsive to dextroamphetamine.

For more information see page 1066.

VALVE DISORDERS

Aortic Valve Regurgitation

In aortic valve regurgitation, the aortic valve does not close properly. With each heartbeat, some of the blood pumped into the aorta leaks back (regurgitates) through the faulty valve into the left ventricle. The body doesn't receive enough blood, so the heart must work harder to make up for it. Typically, symptoms do not develop for decades because the heart compensates by enlarging so that it can pump out more blood.

Commonly Prescribed (On-Label) Drugs: None

OFF-LABEL PRESCRIPTION DRUG
BREAKTHROUGH OPTION

---

*Generic: **Hydralazine** (hye-DRAL-a-zeen)*
*Brand: **None***

Hydralazine is a medication that relaxes and expands blood vessels and is used to treat high blood pressure (hypertension). In studies of long-term therapy in patients with chronic aortic regurgitation, a reduction in regurgitation has been observed by investigators during treatment with hydralazine, nifedipine and ACE inhibitors.

For more information see page 1219.

Mitral Valve Regurgitation

Mitral valve regurgitation, or mitral regurgitation, is a condition in which the mitral valve doesn't close tightly, allowing blood to flow backward in the heart. When the mitral valve does not function properly, blood cannot move through the heart or to the rest of your body as efficiently. Mitral valve regurgitation is also called mitral insufficiency or incompetence. The condition frequently causes fatigue and shortness of breath.

Commonly Prescribed (On-Label) Drugs: None

OFF-LABEL PRESCRIPTION DRUG
BREAKTHROUGH OPTION

---

*Generic: **Nitroprusside** (nye-tro-PRUS-ide)*
*Brand: **Nitropress***

Nitroprusside intravenous is used for the immediate control of very high blood pressure. Nitroprusside is also used to treat certain heart problems (congestive heart failure) or to control bleeding during surgery. A review conducted at Tufts University School of Medicine examined the results of vasodilator therapy in patients with chronic regurgitant lesions of the aortic and mitral valves. In patients with chronic aortic or mitral regurgitation, the short-term administration of nitroprusside, hydralazine, nifedipine or an angiotensin-converting enzyme (ACE) inhibitor produced significant effects.

For patients with chronic mitral regurgitation, knowing the cause of the lesion is a prerequisite for choosing appropriate therapy. Researchers suggest that the preferred long-term therapy for chronic mitral regurgitation is an ACE inhibitor. However, researchers concluded that there are no long-term studies that support the use of this therapy.

For more information see page 1367.

Sibson Aortic Vestibule

See Aortic Valve Regurgitation

Vestibulum Aortae

See Aortic Valve Regurgitation

VASCULAR SYSTEM DISORDERS

Angina Pectoris

See Stable Angina

Aortic Aneurysm

An aneurysm is a bulge in a blood vessel, much like a bulge on an over-inflated inner tube. Aneurysms are dangerous because they may burst. The aorta, the main artery leading away from the heart, can sometimes develop an aneurysm. Aortic aneurysms usually occur in the abdomen below the kidneys (abdominal aneurysm), but may occur in the chest cavity. This can happen if the wall of the aorta becomes weakened by build-ups of fatty deposits called plaque. This is called atherosclerosis. Aneurysms may also be due to an inherited disease such as Marfan syndrome.

Commonly Prescribed (On-Label) Drugs: None

OFF-LABEL PRESCRIPTION DRUGS
BREAKTHROUGH OPTIONS

Generic: **Esmolol** *(ES-moe-lol)*
Brand: **Brevibloc**

Esmolol is a beta-blocker used for temporary control of heart rate and blood pressure. Researchers state that adverse effects of long-acting beta-blockers may include bradycardia (slow heart rate), heart failure, and bronchospasm (acute narrowing and obstruction of the respiratory airway). These effects may limit their usefulness because these conditions persist for a long time after discontinuation of treatment. Researchers feel that this may be detrimental, especially in patients with compromised cardiac function.

For more information see page 1174.

Generic: **Nitroprusside** *(nye-tro-PRUS-ide)*
Brand: **Nitropress**

Nitroprusside sodium is a medication used for the immediate control of very high blood pressure. Nitroprusside is also used to treat certain heart problems (congestive heart failure) or to control bleeding during surgery.

In a study conducted at Duke University Medical Center, 20 patients undergoing abdominal aortic aneurysm (AAA) surgery received either nitroprusside sodium or amrinone. Researchers concluded that amrinone provides equivalent blood system control to nitroprusside sodium during abdominal aortic aneurysm surgery because it allows moderate reductions in blood pressure without affecting other measurements.

For more information see page 1367.

*Generic: **Propranolol** (proe-PRAN-oh-lole)*
*Brands: **Inderal, Inderal LA, InnoPran XL, Propranolol Intensol***

Propranolol is a medication used to treat high blood pressure. Intravenous or injection is used for life threatening heart arrhythmias and to temporarily replace oral dosage forms of this drug when undergoing surgery. An abdominal aortic aneurysm (AAA) is defined as a localized dilation of the artery that is 1.5 times the diameter of the normal segment.

According to researchers, beta-blockers such as propranolol have not been shown to modify aneurysm growth rates, but drop-out rates in the studies have been high. Antibiotics do show a modest benefit.

For more information see page 1438.

Brain Attack

See Stroke

Cerebrovascular Accident

See Stroke

Chronic Peripheral Arterial Occlusive Disease

See Peripheral Artery Disease

CVA

See Stroke

Dissecting Aneurysm

See Aortic Aneurysm

Hyperpiesis

See Hypertension

Hyperpiesia

See Hypertension

Hypertension

Hypertension is another name for high blood pressure. This generally means that systolic blood pressure is consistently over 140 (systolic is the "top" number of your blood pressure measurement, which represents the pressure generated when the heart beats) diastolic blood pressure is consistently over 90 (diastolic is the "bottom" number of your blood pressure measurement, which represents the pressure in the vessels when the heart is at rest). Either or both of these numbers may be too high.

Commonly Prescribed (On-Label) Drugs: *Acebutolol, Amiloride, Amlodipine, Amlodipine/Atorvastatin, Amlodipine/Benazepril, Apraclonidine, Atenolol, Atenolol/Chlorthalidone, Benazepril, Bendroflumethiazide, Benzthiazide, Betaxolol, Bisoprolol, Bisoprolol/Hydrochlorothiazide, Bosentan, Candesartan, Candesartan/Hydrochlorothiazide, Captopril/ Hydrochlorothiazide, Carteolol, Carvedilol, Chlorothiazide, Chlorthalidone, Cyclothiazide, Delapril, Deserpidine, Diazoxide, Doxazosin, Enalapril, Enalapril/Hydrochloro- thiazide, Eplerenone, Epoprostenol, Eprosartan, Eprosartan/Hydrochlorothiazide, Fenoldopam, Fosinopril, Furosemide, Guanabenz, Guanadrel, Guanethidine, Guanfacine, Hydralazine, Hydrochlorothiazide, Hydroflumethiazide, Iloprost, Indapamide, Irbesartan, Irbesartan/Hydrochlorothiazide, Isradipine, Labetalol, Latanoprost, Lisinopril, Lisinopril/Hydrochlorothiazide, Losartan, Losartan/Hydrochlorothiazide, Mannitol, Meca- mylamine, Methyclothiazide, Methyldopa, Metolazone, Metoprolol, Mibefradil, Minoxidil, Moexipril, Nadolol, Nitric Oxide, Nitroprusside, Olmesartan, Olmesartan/ Hydrochlorothiazide, Penbutolol, Phentolamine, Pindolol, Polythiazide, Prazosin, Propranolol, Quinapril, Quinethazone, Ramipril, Rescinnamine, Reserpine, Saralasin, Spironolactone, Telmisartan, Telmisartan/Hydrochlorothiazide, Terazosin, Thiopental, Timolol, Tolazoline, Torsemide, Trandolapril, Trandolapril/Verapamil, Treprostinil, Triamterene/*

Hydrochlorothiazide, Trichlormethiazide, Trimethaphan,
Valsartan, Valsartan/Hydrochlorothiazide, Verapamil

OFF-LABEL PRESCRIPTION DRUG
BREAKTHROUGH OPTION

---

*Generic: **Ethacrynic Acid** (eth-a-KRIN-ik AS-id)*
*Brand: **Edecrin***

Ethacrynic acid is a diuretic that is used to decrease the amount of water in the body by increasing urination. It is used to decrease body fluid and swelling of the hands or feet (edema) and for high blood pressure. Ethacrynic acid has been used orally in the management of hypertension, either alone or in combination with other antihypertensive drugs. Although some clinicians have reported good results with ethacrynic acid daily, they noted high incidences of adverse gastrointestinal effects and heart rate increased substantially in some people. Ethacrynic acid or other diuretics such as bumetanide, furosemide, or metolazone may be preferred to thiazides if you suffer from renal insufficiency or congestive heart failure. Because sodium excretion may be impaired (resulting in sodium retention and increased blood pressure) in those with renal insufficiency, relatively large dosages of diuretics such as ethacrynic acid rather than thiazide diuretics may be necessary for blood pressure control.

For more information see page 1175.

Hypertensive Crisis

Hypertensive crisis is a severe increase in blood pressure that can lead to a stroke. Extremely high blood pressure, greater than 180/110 millimeters of mercury, can damage blood vessels. Blood vessels become inflamed and may leak fluid or blood. As a result, the heart may not be able to pump blood efficiently. Hypertensive crisis, both "emergency" and "urgent," requires immediate medical attention. A crisis requires immediate hospitalization in an intensive care unit with immediate treatment.

***Commonly Prescribed (On-Label) Drugs:** None*

OFF-LABEL PRESCRIPTION DRUGS
BREAKTHROUGH OPTIONS

*Generic: **Captopril** (KAP-toe-pril)*
*Brand: **Capoten***

Captopril is a drug that belongs to a group of medications called ACE inhibitors. It is typically used to treat high blood pressure (hypertension). It works by relaxing blood vessels, causing them to widen. This medication is also used to improve survival after a heart attack, to help protect the kidneys from damage due to diabetes, and with other drugs to treat congestive heart failure.

Most hypertensive emergencies require hospitalization and are treated initially with appropriate therapy such as nitroprusside sodium, nitroglycerin, and labetalol. Oral therapy with captopril also can effectively reduce blood pressure rapidly in such emergencies. When oral therapy is considered preferable to IV or injection, captopril has been regarded by physicians as a drug of choice for rapidly reducing blood pressure in patients with hypertensive crises. Because even oral therapy for hypertensive crises can result in profound hypotension (low blood pressure) and adverse heart effects such as heart attack or stroke, you should weigh the benefits versus risk of captopril with your physician.

For more information see page 1066.

*Generic: **Nitroglycerin IV** (nye-troe-GLI-ser-rin)*
*Brand: **Nitro-bid IV***

Nitroglycerin intravenous (IV) is a medication used to control high blood pressure, congestive heart failure, lung congestion, and chest pain, especially in heart attack patients. It decreases the workload on the heart by enlarging blood vessels. Hypertensive emergencies are those situations requiring immediate blood pressure reduction, although not necessarily to normal ranges, in order to prevent or limit target organ damage.

If IV nitroglycerin is used in the management of a hypertensive emergency, the initial goal of this therapy is to reduce arterial blood pressure by no more than 25% within minutes to one hour, followed by further reduction if stable toward 160/100 to 110 mm

Hg within the next two to six hours, avoiding excessive declines in pressure that could cause renal, cerebral, or coronary conditions. If this blood pressure is well tolerated and you are clinically stable, further gradual reductions toward normal can be implemented in the next 24–48 hours.

For more information see page 1364.

Lung Embolism

See Pulmonary Embolism

Ministroke

See Transient Ischemic Attack

Orthostatic Hypopiesis

See Orthostatic Hypotension

Orthostatic Hypotension

Orthostatic hypotension is a sudden fall in blood pressure that occurs when a person assumes a standing position. It may be caused by hypovolemia (a decreased amount of blood in the body), resulting from the excessive use of diuretics, vasodilators or other types of drugs, dehydration, or prolonged bed rest. The disorder may be associated with a variety of medical disorders. Symptoms, which generally occur after sudden standing, include dizziness, lightheadedness, blurred vision, and syncope (temporary loss of consciousness).

Commonly Prescribed (On-Label) Drugs: *None*

OFF-LABEL PRESCRIPTION DRUG
BREAKTHROUGH OPTION

*Generic: **Fludrocortisone** (floo-droe-KOR-ti-sone)*
*Brand: **Florinef***

Fludrocortisone is used to treat low levels of corticosteroid hormones such as Addison's disease. Fludrocortisone has been used with some success to increase systolic and diastolic blood pressure in patients with severe hypotension (low blood pressure) that does not respond adequately to other treatments. Most patients can be treated successfully with blood volume expansion or fludrocortisone or both in combination with another drug. Additionally, researchers note that desmopressin acetate and erythropoietin are useful supplementary drugs in patients with symptoms that are more resistant to treatment. It should be noted that a small group of patients remain resistant to all therapeutic modalities.

For more information see page 1189.

Peripheral Artery Disease

Peripheral arterial disease (also called PAD) refers to a problem with blood flow in the arteries. Your arteries carry blood to the muscles and organs in the body. When the arteries are affected, they become narrow or blocked. The most common cause of narrow or blocked arteries is the buildup of fatty deposits. This is called atherosclerosis. The most common complaint of people who have PAD is claudication (a pain in the calf or thigh muscle that occurs after walking a certain distance, perhaps a block or two. The pain stops after rest).

Commonly Prescribed (On-Label) Drugs: *None*

OFF-LABEL PRESCRIPTION DRUGS
BREAKTHROUGH OPTIONS

Generic: **Lovastatin** *(LOE-va-sta-tin)*
Brands: **Altocor, Altoprev, Mevacor**

Lovastatin is an enzyme blocker also known as a "statin." It is used along with a proper diet to help lower cholesterol and fats (triglycerides) in the blood. In general, physicians prescribe this drug after non-drug treatment options such as diet change, increase in exercise, weight loss. Reducing cholesterol and triglycerides help prevent strokes and heart attacks.

Researchers state that using statins in people with coronary artery disease (CAD) and high cholesterol reduces the risk of cardiovascular mortality, coronary events, stroke, intermittent claudication, and congestive heart failure. Statins are also effective in reducing cardiovascular events in the elderly who have high cholesterol without cardiovascular disease. Data from the Heart Protection Study favor treating patients at high risk for vascular events with statins regardless of age.

For more information see page 1290.

Generic: **Pravastatin** *(PRA-va-stat-in)*
Brand: **Pravachol**

Pravastatin is an enzyme blocker also known as a "statin." It is used along with a proper diet, to help lower cholesterol and fats (triglycerides) in the blood. Reducing cholesterol and triglycerides help prevent strokes and heart attacks. A study including 885 men with coronary artery disease (CAD) investigated pravastatin treatment's effects on the coronary cavity. Researchers observed that pravastatin treatment positively affects carotid and femoral artery walls.

For more information see page 1424.

Generic: **Simvastatin** *(SIM-va-stat-in)*
Brand: **Zocor**

Simvastatin is an enzyme blocker, also known as a "statin." When used along with a proper diet, it can help lower cholesterol and fats (triglycerides) in the blood. This can reduce cholesterol and triglycerides, preventing strokes and heart attacks.

A study was conducted in Brazil to assess the effect of simvastatin in 25 patients with stable angina and dyslipidemia (which describes a range of disorders that involve abnormally high and low lipoprotein levels) undergoing clinical treatment. The patients were divided into two groups: the simvastatin group and the placebo group. After a four- to six-month follow-up period, they underwent new laboratory and exercise tests. A significant reduction in the variation of total cholesterol and LDL-C levels was observed in the simvastatin group, compared to the placebo group. Patients receiving simvastatin also improved their functional capacity, subjectively assessed by the angina pectoris classification of the Canadian Cardiovascular Society. According to researchers these results suggest that the association of simvastatin and conventional treatment in patients with stable angina reduces the lack of blood flow and oxygen to the heart and can be used with this group of patients, particularly those considered ineligible for invasive therapeutic intervention.

For more information see page 1474.

Generic: **Warfarin** *(WAR-far-in)*
Brands: **Coumadin, Jantoven**

Warfarin is used to prevent and treat harmful blood clots. This medication helps to keep blood flowing smoothly in the body by decreasing the amount of clotting proteins in the blood. Preventing harmful blood clots helps to reduce the risk of a stroke or heart attack.

Patients with peripheral artery disease suffer from a high incidence of reduced blood flow and oxygen to the heart. The role of oral anticoagulants such as warfarin in patients with symptomatic peripheral artery disease is limited. Researchers are unsure whether the use of oral anticoagulants reduces morbidity and mortality.

For more information see page 1547.

Peripheral Atherosclerosis

See Peripheral Artery Disease

Peripheral Vascular Disease (PVD)

See Peripheral Artery Disease

Postural Hypotension

See Orthostatic Hypotension

Pulmonary Embolism

A pulmonary embolism is a blood clot that travels to the lungs. Often, the clot forms in another part of the body, usually in the veins of the legs. Large clots can be fatal. Pulmonary embolism is estimated to occur in one to two people per 1,000 each year in the United States.

Commonly Prescribed (On-Label) Drugs: *Alteplase, Dextran, Fondaparinux, Heparin, Streptokinase, Urokinase*

OFF-LABEL PRESCRIPTION DRUG
BREAKTHROUGH OPTION

Generic: ***Isoproterenol*** *(eye-soe-proe-TER-e-nole)*
Brand: ***Isuprel***

Isoproterenol is a drug that relaxes the smooth muscle in the lungs and dilates airways to improve breathing. It is used in the treatment of asthma, chronic bronchitis, and emphysema. Isoproterenol has also been used by intravenous (IV) infusion to treat pulmonary embolism. Patients with acute pulmonary embolism are at risk for early death. Researchers feel that norepinephrine, isoproterenol hydrochloride, and epinephrine may be effective treatments.

For more information see page 1248.

Pulmonary Hypertension

High blood pressure in the arteries that supply the lungs is called pulmonary hypertension (PHT). The blood pressure measured by cuff on the arm is not directly related to the pressure in the lungs. The blood vessels that supply the lungs constrict and their walls thicken, so they are unable to carry as much blood as needed. As in a kinked garden hose, pressure builds up and backs up. The heart works harder, trying to force the blood through. If the pressure is high enough, eventually the heart will not be able to keep up and the amount of blood circulating through the lungs is reduced resulting in reduced oxygen. You may then become tired, dizzy, and short of breath.

Commonly Prescribed (On-Label) Drugs: Bosentan, Epoprostenol, Iloprost, Nitric oxide, Tolazoline, Treprostinil

---

OFF-LABEL PRESCRIPTION DRUGS
BREAKTHROUGH OPTIONS

Generic: **Hydralazine** (hye-DRAL-a-zeen)
Brand: **None**

Hydralazine is a medication that relaxes and dilates blood vessels, resulting in lowered blood pressure. It is used to treat hypertension (high blood pressure). A study published in *The New England Journal of Medicine* evaluated the effects of hydralazine in four patients with pulmonary hypertension, before and 48 hours after starting therapy with oral hydralazine. Data were obtained at rest in four patients and also during exercise in three. After hydralazine, total pulmonary resistance at rest fell and pulmonary arteriolar resistance was reduced. Researchers concluded that hydralazine can reduce pulmonary resistance in some patients with pulmonary hypertension.

For more information see page 1219.

Generic: **Sildenafil** *(sil-DEN-a-fil)*
Brand: **Viagra**

Sildenafil is used to treat male sexual function problems (impotence or erectile dysfunction) by blocking a certain enzyme in the body.

A study reported in *Thorax* explored a strategy for treating high altitude pulmonary arterial hypertension (HAPH). In the study, 689 patients living at high altitudes were screened for HAPH by medical examination and electrocardiography (ECG). At three months, patients on sildenafil for every eight hours had a significantly lower pulmonary artery pressure at the end of the dosing interval than those on placebo. It also improved six minute walk distance by 45.4 m. Sildenafil was well tolerated. Therefore, researchers feel that sildenafil is an attractive drug for the treatment of HAPH. It should be noted that this drug has the potential for significant drug interactions, and you should not use it if you are maintained on nitrates.

For more information see page 1472.

Generic: **Tadalafil** *(tah-DA-la-fil)*
Brand: **Cialis**

Tadalafil is used to treat impotence or erectile dysfunction. Sildenafil, vardenafil, and tadalafil are a new class of drugs that have been developed for treatment of erectile dysfunction in patients. According to researchers, a growing number of studies in recent years suggest that tadalafil may be used for treatment of pulmonary hypertension. Investigators believe that future studies of tadalafil could have an enormous impact in treating this disorder. They note that this drug has the potential for significant drug interactions, and you should not use it if you are maintained on nitrates.

For more information see page 1491.

Generic: **Vardenafil** *(var-DEN-a-fil)*
Brand: **Levitra**

Vardenafil is used to treat male sexual function problems. A study conducted in Germany examined its effect on pulmonary and systemic blood systems and gas exchange parameters in patients with pulmonary arterial hypertension (PAH). Sixty PAH patients who underwent right heart catheterization (procedure to insert a thin plastic tube into an artery or vein in the arm or leg) received short-term nitric oxide inhalation and were subsequently given either sildenafil, vardenafil, or tadalafil. All three drugs caused significant pulmonary vasorelaxation, with maximum effects being obtained after 40 to 45 minutes (vardenafil), 60 minutes (sildenafil), and 75 to 90 minutes (tadalafil). Significant improvement in arterial oxygenation was only noted with sildenafil. Researchers assert that careful evaluation of each new drug, when being considered for PAH treatment, has to be undertaken. Additionally, these drugs have the potential for significant drug interactions and should not be used if you are maintained on nitrates.

For more information see page 1538.

Raynaud's Disease

See Raynaud's Syndrome

Raynaud's Syndrome

Up to one fifth of the adult population has Raynaud's syndrome. In response to cold or stress, the fingers of patients with Raynaud's syndrome undergo characteristic circulatory changes. The fingers typically become white, caused by vasoconstriction, then blue, caused by capillary stagnation and, finally, red. Women are more commonly affected than men and the condition may be familial or associated with connective tissue diseases such as scleroderma or lupus. Raynaud's syndrome can be classified as primary or secondary. Primary Raynaud's syndrome is characterized in patients that have no other underlying disease or causes such as connective tissue disease. Secondary Raynaud's syndrome, although less common but more complex and serious, occurs in patients who have an underlying disease that causes this syndrome.

Commonly Prescribed (On-Label) Drugs: Isoxsuprine

OFF-LABEL PRESCRIPTION DRUGS
BREAKTHROUGH OPTIONS

Generic: Calcium Channel Blockers such as ***Amlodipine*** *(am-LOE-di-peen)*, ***Captopril*** *(KAP-toe-pril)*, ***Diltiazem*** *(dil-TYE-a-zem)*, and ***Felodipine*** *(fe-LOE-di-peen)*
Brands: *Norvasc (amlodipine); Capoten (captopril); Cardizem, Cartia XT, Dilacor XR, Diltia XT, Taztia XT, Tiazac (diltiazem); Plendil (felodipine)*

Amlodipine, captopril, diltiazem, and felodipine are used to treat high blood pressure or chest pain (angina). These medications are known as a calcium channel blockers. By blocking calcium, amlodipine, captopril, diltiazem, and felodipine relaxes and widens blood vessels so blood can flow more easily. Lowering high blood pressure helps prevent strokes, heart attacks, and kidney problems.

Treatment of Raynaud's syndrome in patients with severe disease includes drugs that promote circulation. The calcium-channel antagonists, particularly nifedipine, are the most thoroughly studied drug class for the treatment of Raynaud's syndrome. Approximately two thirds of patients respond favorably, with significant reductions in the frequency and severity of attacks. Nifedipine use is often limited by the appearance of adverse circulation effects such as headache or peripheral edema (abnormal build-up of fluids in ankle and leg tissues). Calcium channel blockers such as amlodipine, captopril, diltiazem, felodipine also appear to be effective in patients with Raynaud's syndrome and may be associated with fewer adverse effects.

Additionally, a trial published in *Angiology* examined the therapeutic effects of diltiazem on occupational Raynaud's syndrome. Seventeen men were studied, and no patient had cardiovascular disease. Diltiazem was given to the patients orally for six weeks, three times daily. Before and after this treatment period, evaluation of the symptoms was reviewed as well as laboratory blood tests. The overall effectiveness of diltiazem therapy was assessed by evaluating the changes in symptoms, peripheral function and the occurrence of side effects. No side effects occurred during the treatment period. The collective effectiveness of diltiazem was reported as 64.7%. Researchers concluded that diltiazem can be effective in long-term treatment of patients with Raynaud's syndrome.

For more information see pages 1011, 1066, 1146, and 1182.

Generic: *Clonidine* (KLON-i-deen)
Brands: *Catapres, Catapres-TTS, Duraclon*

Clonidine is a medication typically used to treat high blood pressure. It works by stimulating certain brain receptors (alpha adrenergic type), which results in the relaxing of blood vessels in other parts of the body, causing them to widen. At the Department of Psychiatry and Behavioral Neurosciences at Wayne State University School of Medicine, investigators examined the involvement of skin and hormone reactions in patients with Raynaud's syndrome and scleroderma. Ten patients with Raynaud's syndrome and scleroderma and 10 healthy volunteers were studied. Methacholine, nitroprusside sodium, and clonidine were administered while finger blood flow was measured using a procedure to measure changes in limb circumference.

Compared to the controls, the patients showed diminished responses to methacholine and to clonidine. However, both groups showed similar responses to nitroprusside sodium. Researchers concluded that the findings were consistent with previous evidence of skin cell damage in scleroderma blood vessels. They believe that failure to release nitric oxide may play a role in Raynaud's syndrome in patients with scleroderma.

For more information see page 1108.

Generic: *Fluoxetine* (floo-OKS-e-teen)
Brands: *Prozac, Prozac Weekly, Sarafem*

Fluoxetine is a selective serotonin reuptake inhibitor (SSRI) that is typically used to treat depression, obsessive-compulsive disorder, panic attacks, certain eating disorders (bulimia), and a severe form of premenstrual syndrome (premenstrual dysphoric disorder or PMDD). A study conducted at the University College School of Medicine in London compared fluoxetine with nifedipine as treatment for primary or secondary Raynaud's syndrome. Twenty-six patients with primary and 27 patients with secondary Raynaud's syndrome were assigned to receive six weeks of treatment with fluoxetine or nifedipine. There was a reduction in attack frequency and severity of Raynaud's syndrome in patients treated with either fluoxetine or nifedipine but the effect was statistically significant only in the fluoxetine-treated group.

Analysis conducted by the researchers showed that the greatest response was seen in females and in patients with primary Raynaud's phenomenon. A significant improvement in the response to cold was also seen in female patients with primary Raynaud's syndrome treated with fluoxetine but not in those treated with nifedipine. No significant adverse effects occurred in the fluoxetine-treated group. Researchers concluded that the study confirmed the tolerability of fluoxetine and suggested that it would be effective as a treatment for Raynaud's syndrome. They believe that more trials are warranted to assess fluoxetine's therapeutic potential further in this condition.

For more information see page 1192.

Generic: **Losartan** *(loe-SAR-tan)*
Brand: **Cozaar**

Losartan is typically used to treat high blood pressure (hypertension) and to help protect the kidneys from damage due to diabetes. It is also used to lower the risk of strokes in patients with high blood pressure and an enlarged heart. This drug works by blocking the hormone angiotensin thereby relaxing blood vessels, causing them to widen.

At the Royal Free Hospital in London, a study compared the efficacy and tolerability of losartan with nifedipine for the treatment of primary and secondary Raynaud's syndrome. In the trial, patients with primary Raynaud's syndrome or Raynaud's syndrome secondary to systemic sclerosis received 12 weeks' treatment with either losartan or nifedipine.

Researchers evaluated the severity and frequency of Raynaud's syndrome episodes and measurements including changes in the skins temperature and blood flow through the body's tissues. There was a reduction in the severity of Raynaud's syndrome episodes following treatment with losartan and with nifedipine but this effect was greater in the losartan aspect of the study: episode frequency was reduced only in the losartan group. According to investigators, this study confirmed the tolerability of short-term treatment of Raynaud's syndrome with losartan and the data suggest its clinical benefit. They also concluded that further evaluation of this drug as a long-term treatment for systemic sclerosis-associated Raynaud's syndrome should be considered, since it may have additional disease-modifying potential.

For more information see page 1289.

Generic: **Nicardipine** *(nye-KAR-de-peen)*
Brands: **Cardene, Cardene IV; Cardene SR**

Nicardipine is a calcium channel blocker medication. Calcium channel blockers have been used in the treatment of primary and secondary Raynaud's syndrome. Researchers have observed a beneficial effect of this drug on Raynaud's syndrome. The efficacy of slow-releasing nicardipine was assessed in a clinical trial conducted in Italy. After a three-week period, slow-releasing nicardipine was significantly more useful than placebo. Researchers observed that the number of Raynaud's syndrome episodes per week decreased and severity of discomfort and hand disability scores improved. According to investigators, these results show that slow-releasing nicardipine is generally well tolerated and can provide effective improvement in Raynaud's syndrome patients without underlying diseases.

For more information see page 1358.

Generic: **Nifedipine** *(nye-FED-i-peen)*
Brands: **Adalat CC, Apo-Nifed (PA), Novo-Nifedin, Nu-Nifed, Procardia**

Nifedipine is a calcium channel blocker medication. Calcium is involved in blood vessel contraction. By blocking calcium, nifedipine relaxes and widens the blood vessels. It is typically used to treat chest pain (angina). Nifedipine has been used effectively in the management of Raynaud's phenomenon and is considered by investigators as a drug of choice for the management of this condition.

The drug has reduced the frequency, duration, and severity of attacks in patients with Raynaud's syndrome. However, not all patients with this condition respond to nifedipine and intolerable adverse effects such as headache and flushing may limit the usefulness of the drug in some other patients. Although most experience with nifedipine in the management of Raynaud's phenomenon had been with short-acting formulations of the drug, recent concerns such as risks of serious hypotension (low blood pressure) and associated cardiovascular consequences about the safety of short-acting nifedipine have prompted the manufacturers to warn against use of this preparation in conditions for which safety and efficacy have not been fully established. Therefore, while not studied as extensively as short-acting nifedipine, researchers suggest that extended-release nifedipine preferably should be used when the drug is indicated for the management of Raynaud's syndrome. The extended-release preparation of nifedipine appears to be better tolerated than the short-acting preparation in patients with this condition.

For more information see page 1360.

Generic: **Nitroglycerin (topical)** *(nye-troe-GLI-ser-in)*
Brands: **Minitran, Nitrek, Nitro-Bid, Nitro-Dur, Transderm-Nitro**

Nitroglycerine is a medication that relaxes blood vessels, allowing more blood to flow through and improving blood flow to the heart. Oral dose forms are used to prevent angina (chest pain). To investigate responses in fingers to topical nitroglycerine in patients with primary Raynaud's syndrome, systemic sclerosis, and healthy control subjects, a study was done at the University of Manchester Rheumatic Diseases Centre using a non-invasive technique to measure blood flow through the body's tissues.

Ten patients with primary Raynaud's syndrome, 13 with sclerosis, and 10 control subjects were studied. After the initial test, 2% nitroglycerine ointment was rubbed on the finger for 1 minute; placebo ointment was rubbed on the second finger for 1 minute, and the third finger remained untreated. Further testing of these three fingers was conducted immediately, 10, and 20 minutes after ointment application. There was increased blood flow response to nitroglycerine compared with placebo. The change in blood flow over time differed significantly between placebo and nitroglycerine but not between placebo and no ointment application: blood flow increased with nitroglycerine and decreased with placebo/no treatment at 10 and 20 minutes. As well as demonstrating the effectiveness of topical nitroglycerine in patients with Raynaud's syndrome and sclerosis, researchers believe that this study illustrates the ability of testing to identify local circulatory effects.

For more information see page 1363.

Generic: **Prazosin** *(PRA-zoe-sin)*
Brand: **Minipress**

Prazosin is a medication that relaxes and expands blood vessels. It is used to treat high blood pressure (hypertension). A review of studies conducted at the University of Western Ontario looked at the effects and toxicity of prazosin versus placebo for the treatment of Raynaud's syndrome in scleroderma. Researchers concluded that prazosin had been found to be more effective than placebo in the treatment of Raynaud's secondary to scleroderma. However, the positive response is modest and side effects are not rare in those taking prazosin. According to researchers, prazosin is modestly effective in the treatment of Raynaud's phenomenon secondary to scleroderma.

For more information see page 1426.

Generic: **Verapamil** *(vur-AP-ah-mill)*
Brands: **Calan, Calan SR, Covera-HS, Isoptin SR, Verelan, Verelan PM**

Verapamil is a medication that acts as a calcium channel blocker to treat chest pain (angina), high blood pressure, or irregular heartbeats. Calcium is involved in blood vessel contraction and in controlling the electrical impulses within the heart. By blocking calcium, verapamil relaxes and widens blood vessels and can normalize heartbeats.

A study conducted in Bulgaria looked at the short and prolonged treatment of Raynaud's syndrome with calcium channel blockers. The efficacy of nifedipine, verapamil, and felodipine was evaluated in a 14-day treatment of 61 patients with Raynaud's syndrome. Researchers observed that nifedipine and felodipine were better tolerated, but felodipine led to more reactions. Verapamil was least efficient and exerted a weak circulatory action. Twenty patients with systemic scleroderma were given nifedipine daily in the course of one year and the frequency, duration, and expression of the attacks of Raynaud's syndrome decreased. According to researchers, the study allows the recommendation of nifedipine as the drug of choice for the treatment of Raynaud's syndrome in the systemic connective tissue diseases.

For more information see page 1544.

Reversible Ischemic Neurologic Disease (RIND)

See Transient Ischemic Attack

Severe Hypertension

Severe hypertension is elevated blood pressure not yet leading to significant organ damage. In these patients, the hypertension does not necessarily require treatment during an emergency department visit but does require close follow-up with a primary care physician for long-term blood pressure control. In these cases, beginning antihypertensive therapy in the emergency department may be appropriate and should be done in consultation with your primary care physician, who will be caring for you after the visit. Severe hypertension is also referred to as Stage 3 hypertension and the blood pressure range is: systolic 180 to 209 mm Hg (top number), and diastolic 110 to 119 mm Hg (bottom number).

Commonly Prescribed (On-Label) Drugs: *Fenoldopam*

OFF-LABEL PRESCRIPTION DRUG
BREAKTHROUGH OPTION

Generic: **Nitroglycerin IV** *(nye-troe-GLI-ser-in)*
Brand: **Nitro-bid IV**

Nitroglycerin IV is a medication used to control high blood pressure, congestive heart failure, lung congestion, and chest pain, especially in heart attack patients. IV nitroglycerin is used to control blood pressure in hypertension associated with cardiovascular procedures. It is also used to control blood pressure in patients with severe hypertension or in hypertensive crises and for the immediate reduction of blood pressure in patients in whom such reduction is considered an emergency (hypertensive emergencies). The medication is also used for the treatment of congestive heart failure or pulmonary edema associated with heart attacks and for the treatment of angina pectoris if you have not responded to recommended dosages of nitrates and/or a beta-blocking drug.

For more information see page 1364.

Stable Angina

Angina is a pain or discomfort in the chest and is caused by insufficient blood flow to the heart. Symptoms include tightness, heavy pressure, squeezing, pain, or crushing chest pain. Angina affects 3 to 5% of the population and can be alleviated through rest or medication within a short period of time, usually within fifteen minutes.

Commonly Prescribed (On-Label) Drugs: *Bepridil*

OFF-LABEL PRESCRIPTION DRUG
BREAKTHROUGH OPTION

Generic: ***Acebutolol*** *(a-se-BYOO-toe-lole)*
Brand: ***Sectral***

Acebutolol is a medication used for chest pain (angina), high blood pressure, and irregular heartbeats. Acebutolol has been used in the management of chronic stable angina pectoris. Like other beta-blockers, use of acebutolol in chronic stable angina may reduce the frequency of angina attacks, allow a reduction in nitroglycerin dosage, and increase the patient's exercise tolerance.

In people who do not respond to maximal dosages of a beta-blocker or nitroglycerin alone, use of the two drugs in combination may be beneficial. Researchers suggest that combination therapy with a beta-blocker and a nitrate appears to be more effective than either drug alone. Beta-blockers weaken effects of an abnormally rapid heartbeat associated with nitrate therapy; while nitroglycerin counteracts the potential increase in left-ventricular blood volume and diastolic pressure associated with a decrease in heart rate.

For more information see page 983.

Stroke

A stroke occurs when there is insufficient blood supply to the brain, causing brain tissue to be deprived of nutrients. Strokes are the third-leading cause of death in the United States, affecting nearly 700,000 Americans annually. Symptoms include sudden numbness, weakness, loss of speech, blurred vision, and confusion. Medical treatment should be sought immediately for anyone experiencing a stroke.

Commonly Prescribed (On-Label) Drugs: None

OFF-LABEL PRESCRIPTION DRUG
BREAKTHROUGH OPTION

*Generic: **Fluoxetine** (floo-OKS-e-teen)*
*Brands: **Prozac, Prozac Weekly, Sarafem***

Fluoxetine is a selective serotonin reuptake inhibitor (SSRI) used to treat depression, obsessive-compulsive disorder, panic attacks, certain eating disorders (bulimia), and a severe form of premenstrual syndrome (premenstrual dysphoric disorder or PMDD). This medication works by restoring the balance of natural substances (neurotransmitters) in the brain, thereby improving mood and feelings of well being.

Fluoxetine may be given to treat post stroke depression, which is a common psychiatric condition after stroke and can have negative effects on rehabilitation therapy and functional recovery. In a study conducted by the Vienna University Medical School, researchers administered fluoxetine to 54 patients experiencing post-stroke depression while undergoing rehabilitation therapy. They found that patients treated with fluoxetine were significantly less depressed in follow-up visits 18 months after inclusion, and no side effects were detected. Researchers concluded that fluoxetine was a well-tolerated and safe treatment for patients who suffered a stroke.

For more information see page 1192.

Stroke Risk Reduction

The brain is an extremely complex organ that controls various body functions. If a stroke occurs, blood flow may not be able to reach the region that controls a particular body function. Knowing the risk and controlling what is possible (weight and diet for example) is your best defense against having a stroke. Both coronary heart disease and stroke share many of the same risk factors such as cholesterol disorders, high blood pressure, smoking, diabetes, physical inactivity, and being overweight or obese.

Commonly Prescribed (On-Label) Drugs: *Aspirin, Aspirin/Dipyridamole, Dipyridamole, Losartan, Pravastatin, Ramipril*

OFF-LABEL PRESCRIPTION DRUGS
BREAKTHROUGH OPTIONS

Generic: ***Captopril*** *(KAP-toe-pril)*
Brand: ***Capoten***

Captopril is a drug that belongs to a group of medications called ACE inhibitors. It is used to treat high blood pressure (hypertension). It works by relaxing blood vessels, causing them to widen. Lowering high blood pressure helps prevent strokes, heart attacks, and kidney problems. Although the risks and benefits of aggressive antihypertensive therapy in those with acute stroke are not fully understood, control of blood pressure at intermediate levels (systolic/diastolic blood pressures of about 160/100 mm Hg) is considered appropriate by physicians until the patient's condition has improved or stabilized. Administration of an ACE inhibitor in combination with a thiazide diuretic has been shown to lower recurrent stroke rates.

According to researchers in the Department of Medicine at New York Medical College, data clearly indicates that treatment with antihypertensive drugs reduces the incidence of all strokes in men (by 34%), women (by 38%), elderly persons (by 36%), including those older than 80 years (by 34%), younger persons, those with systolic and diastolic hypertension, persons with isolated systolic hypertension, and in those with a history of stroke. Blood pressure should be reduced to less than 140/90 mm Hg. Researchers also suggest that the overall data also shows that reduction of stroke in persons with hypertension is related more to a reduction in blood pressure than to the type of antihypertensive drugs used.

For more information see page 1066.

Generic: *Low Molecular Weight Heparin* (HEP-a-rin)
Brand: *Hep-Lock*

Heparin is an anticoagulant medication that prevents the blood from clotting. Full-dose heparin therapy has also been used preventively in progressive stroke or to prevent blockage of a blood vessel by a blood clot in paralyzed or immobile patients. Researchers feel that because conclusive data are not available, the decision to use anticoagulant therapy in progressive stroke must be individualized. Heparin therapy for the prevention of cerebral thrombosis (a stroke caused by a clot in an artery leading to the brain) in evolving stroke is now generally regarded as not useful by physicians. It is generally agreed by researchers that anticoagulants are of no value and should not be used in completed stroke and that the drugs may actually increase the risk of fatal cerebral hemorrhage in these patients. High blood pressure and atherosclerosis (hardening of blood vessels) are major factors in cerebrovascular disease and control of strokes is more dependent on the control of these factors than on anticoagulation.

There is no drug prfile associated with this drug, as more data are pending.

Generic: *Warfarin* (WAR-far-in)
Brands: *Coumadin, Jantoven*

Warfarin is used to prevent and treat harmful blood clots. This medication helps to keep blood flowing smoothly in the body by decreasing the amount of clotting proteins in the blood. Warfarin is sometimes commonly referred to as a "blood thinner." Conditions that increase risk of developing blood clots include a certain type of irregular heart rhythm (atrial fibrillation), heart valve replacement, or a recent heart attack. Preventing harmful blood clots helps to reduce the risk of a stroke or heart attack.

Some experts approve the consideration of early anticoagulation for the treatment of large-artery strokes and for progressing stroke when the suspected mechanism is ongoing thromboembolism (a blood clot that forms inside a blood vessel). Early anticoagulation is most likely to benefit patients who are at high-risk for early recurrent embolism such as in patients with mechanical heart valves or severe congestive heart failure. Researchers suggest that a brain imaging study should be performed prior to initiation of anticoagulant therapy in order to exclude hemorrhage and estimate the size of the clot. Anticoagulation is not recommended if you have large clots, uncontrolled hypertension, other bleeding conditions, or other potential contraindications to such anticoagulation.

For more information see page 1547.

Stroke Volume

See Stroke

Thrombectomy in Peripheral Artery Disease

Thrombolysis is the treatment to break up abnormal blood clots that are restricting blood flow. Thrombolytic therapy dissolves these blood clots using various medications administered directly into the clot through a catheter. Thrombectomy is the disruption of a blood clot using one of several mechanical devices. One or both of these methods can be used to dissolve and remove blood clots. Thrombolysis can greatly improve blood flow and reduce or eliminate the related symptoms and effects without the need for more invasive surgery.

Commonly Prescribed (On-Label) Drugs: *None*

OFF-LABEL PRESCRIPTION DRUG
BREAKTHROUGH OPTION

Generic: **Warfarin** *(WAR-far-in)*
Brands: **Coumadin, Jantoven**

Warfarin sodium is used for the prevention and treatment of venous thrombosis (a blood clot that forms within a vein) and complications associated with atrial fibrillation and/or cardiac valve replacement. The drug also is used to reduce the risk of death and thromboembolic events such as stroke or embolism following a heart attack. Because the effects of warfarin are delayed, heparin is the anticoagulant of choice when an immediate effect is required. Warfarin generally is used for follow-up anticoagulant therapy after the effects of full-dose heparin therapy have been established and when long-term anticoagulant therapy is indicated.

Warfarin has been used in patients with peripheral arterial occlusive disease (a condition where the artery is narrowed). In patients undergoing thrombolectomy (a procedure done to remove clots from a blood vessel), it is recommended to use heparin followed by oral anticoagulation to prevent recurrent embolism. Long-term oral anticoagulation with warfarin, with or without aspirin, is recommended by physicians in selected patients.

For more information see page 1547.

Transient Ischemic Attack

Transient ischemic attack is a brief episode in which the brain gets insufficient blood supply. The symptoms vary depending on the area where the blockage occurs but can include sudden numbness or weakness in the face, arm or leg, confusion or trouble speaking, severe headaches, and dizziness. Transient ischemic attack is a critical sign of impending stroke. Failure to quickly recognize and evaluate this warning sign could mean you are missing an opportunity to prevent permanent disability or death. The 90-day risk of stroke after a transient ischemic attack has been estimated to be approximately 10 percent, with one half of strokes occurring within the first two days of the attack. The 90-day stroke risk is even higher when a transient ischemic attack results from a narrowing of the carotid artery.

Commonly Prescribed (On-Label) Drugs: None

OFF-LABEL PRESCRIPTION DRUG
BREAKTHROUGH OPTION

Generic: **Warfarin** (WAR-far-in)
Brands: **Coumadin, Jantoven**

Warfarin is used to prevent and treat harmful blood clots. This medication helps to keep blood flowing smoothly in the body by decreasing the amount of clotting proteins in the blood. Preventing harmful blood clots helps to reduce the risk of a stroke or heart attack.

Researchers state that the value of anticoagulant therapy in patients with transient ischemic attacks (TIAs) has not been definitely established and routine use of such therapy in these patients generally is not recommended. According to researchers, there is some evidence that full-dose heparin therapy followed by warfarin-derivative therapy may decrease the frequency of TIAs and subsequent stroke, especially during the first few months of anticoagulant therapy. However, they caution there is no evidence that anticoagulant therapy reduces mortality associated with TIAs. When warfarin is contraindicated for prevention of stroke, aspirin is an alternative therapy.

For more information see page 1547.

Unstable Angina

Chest pain that persists for a long period of time or that occurs with a lower level of effort, even at rest, is classified as unstable angina. This is a serious form of angina, and anyone experiencing it should seek emergency care immediately.

Commonly Prescribed (On-Label) Drugs: Dalteparin, Enoxaparin

OFF-LABEL PRESCRIPTION DRUGS
BREAKTHROUGH OPTIONS

Generic: **Esmolol** *(ES-moe-lol)*
Brand: **Brevibloc**

Esmolol is a medication used for temporary control of heart rate and blood pressure.

Physicians use beta-blocker medication as part of the standard therapeutic measures for managing unstable angina. These measures also include therapy with aspirin and/or clopidogrel, low-molecular weight heparin and nitroglycerin. The American College of Cardiology (ACC) and the American Heart Association (AHA) recommend administration of an IV beta-blocker followed by oral beta-blocker therapy if you have unstable angina and are at high risk of death or nonfatal heart attack. They also recommend oral beta-blocker therapy for lower-risk patients.

For more information see page 1174.

Generic: *Low Molecular Weight Heparin* (HEP-a-rin)
Brand: *Hep-Lock*

Heparin is an anticoagulant medication used to prevent blood clotting. It is used to prevent and treat venous thrombosis (a blood clot in the vein), pulmonary embolism and other conditions of blood clotting. Low molecular weight heparin is used as part of standard therapeutic measures for managing unstable angina.

Researchers believe that early initiation of IV heparin therapy appears to be necessary for beneficial effects in patients with unstable angina since initiation of the drug more than 24 hours following onset of symptoms has failed to reduce angina and heart attack. In clinical studies in patients with acute unstable angina, researchers suggest that continuous IV infusion of the drug is effective. The optimal duration of IV heparin therapy in acute unstable angina has not been defined, but reactivation of the disease as recurrent unstable angina and/or heart attack has occurred following discontinuance of the drug. According to investigators, some evidence suggests that therapy with aspirin may prevent or substantially reduce the incidence of these recurrent adverse events.

There is no drug profile associated with this drug, as more data are pending.

Generic: *Lepirudin* (leh-puh-ROO-din)
Brand: *Refludan*

Lepirudin is a "blood thinner" (anticoagulant) used to treat patients who have developed a reaction to another type of anticoagulant (patients with heparin-induced thrombocytopenia). Lepirudin is used for prevention of further blood clots in patients with heparin-induced thrombocytopenia (HIT, a condition where platelets are lost from circulation faster than they can be made from the bone marrows) accompanied by thromboembolic complications. Efficacy and safety of lepirudin for this indication are based principally on the results of two studies in patients with HIT. Patients included in these studies had a reduction in platelet count of at least 30–50%. Efficacy was evaluated on the basis of the limb amputation, or new complications between the lepirudin and control groups.

For more information see page 1272.

Unstable Angina Pectoris

See Unstable Angina

Vasodepressor Syncope

See Vasovagal Syncope

Vasovagal Syncope

A simple faint (vasovagal syncope) occurs due to an exaggerated response by the nervous system. As a result, heart rate and blood pressure drop, which reduces blood flow to the brain and leads to fainting. In some cases, the cause of a simple faint cannot be determined. But common triggers include: standing for long periods, dehydration, coughing, urination, having a bowel movement, and emotional distress.

Commonly Prescribed (On-Label) Drugs: *None*

OFF-LABEL PRESCRIPTION DRUGS
BREAKTHROUGH OPTIONS

Generic: ***Fluoxetine*** *(floo-OKS-e-teen)*
Brands: ***Prozac, Prozac Weekly, Sarafem***

Fluoxetine is a selective serotonin reuptake inhibitor (SSRI) that is typically used to treat depression, obsessive-compulsive disorder, panic attacks, certain eating disorders (bulimia) and a severe form of premenstrual syndrome (premenstrual dysphoric disorder or PMDD).

In a report by physicians at the Onassis Cardiac Surgery Center in Greece, a man was admitted to the center who had a history of syncope. His symptoms were not alleviated with treatment using isoprenaline. The patient was then given fluoxetine, which successfully treated the condition. Researchers suggest that the use of fluoxetine may be of benefit to patients with vasovagal syncope.

For more information see page 1192.

Generic: **Paroxetine** *(pa-ROKS-e-teen)*
Brands: **Paxil, Paxil CR**

Paroxetine is a selective serotonin reuptake inhibitor (SSRI) that is typically used to treat depression, panic attacks, obsessive-compulsive disorder (OCD), social anxiety disorder (social phobia), post-traumatic stress disorder (PTSD) and generalized anxiety disorders (GAD). Orthostatic hypotension, characterized by symptoms of dizziness, faintness or lightheadedness upon standing, is caused by low blood pressure. It may be caused by syncope. According to a researcher in Italy, paroxetine showed efficacy in treating orthostatic hypotension in one trial that included a small number of patients. However in another study paroxetine failed to show a significant effect on regulating blood pressure or nerve activity. According to researchers, until more data from studies become available, the use of paroxetine for this indication cannot be confirmed.

For more information see page 1395.

CHILDREN'S HEALTH DISORDERS

CHILDHOOD DISEASES

Cerebral Palsy

Cerebral palsy (CP) is an umbrella-like term used to describe a group of chronic disorders that impair control of movement. These disorders appear in the first few years of life and generally do not worsen over time. The term cerebral refers to the brain's two halves, or hemispheres, and palsy describes any disorder that impairs control of body movement. Faulty development or damage to motor areas in the brain disrupts the brain's ability to adequately control movement and posture.

Commonly Prescribed (On-Label) Drugs: *None*

OFF-LABEL PRESCRIPTION DRUGS
BREAKTHROUGH OPTIONS

Generic: ***Botulinum Toxin Type A***
(BOT-yoo-lin-num TOKS-in type-aye)
Brands: ***Botox, Botox cosmetic***

Botulinum toxin type A is a medication that blocks the action of muscles. It is used in the treatment of certain eye disorders such as cross eyes and eye twitches. It is also used to treat severe underarm sweating, certain spasms, movement disorders, tremors, and cosmetic skin treatment.

Botulinum toxin type A injection is a well-recognized treatment for children with spastic cerebral palsy (CP); however, no study has compared the long-term effectiveness of this approach. A study in *The Journal of Neurosurgery* reported on 62 children with spastic paralysis CP in the same rehabilitation program, along with 19 healthy volunteers. The walking ability was assessed in the three groups of children at one week before treatment, and three, six, 12 and 20 months after treatment. Based on the analysis of walking velocity, cadence, and step length, the botulinum toxin type A group demonstrated rapid improvement post treatment but the improvement became insignificant after 12 months, even with repeated botulinum toxin type A injections at four-month intervals. The healthy volunteers did not display a significant change in gait. Researchers suggest that the effectiveness of botulinum toxin type A injection may be short-lived.

For more information see page 1057.

Generic: *Glycopyrrolate* (glye-koe-PYE-roe-late)
Brand: *Robinul, Robinul Forte*

Glycopyrrolate is a medication that slows the activity of the stomach and intestines and reduces acid secretion. It is used with anesthesia medications before surgery and in the treatment of peptic ulcers. This drug is also used to decrease saliva and phlegm in the mouth and throat.

Sialorrhea or drooling or excessive salivation is a common problem in neurologically impaired children especially in those with cerebral palsy. It is most commonly caused by poor oral and facial muscle control. Contributing factors may include hypersecretion of saliva, misaligned teeth, and an inability to recognize salivary spill. Sialorrhea causes a range of physical and psychosocial complications, including chapping, dehydration, odor, and social stigmatization.

A Norwegian team of researchers found that glycopyrrolate was effective in patients with cerebral palsy who had sialorrhea. Researchers administered glycopyrrolate three to four times daily to the patients and concluded that glycopyrrolate effectively reduced drooling. Glycopyrrolate is best used for shorter periods of time in controlled dosages.

Treatment options range from conservative ones such as observation, to more aggressive measures such as medication, radiation, and surgical therapy. Researchers have found that anticholinergic medications, such as glycopyrrolate are effective in reducing drooling, but their use may be limited by side effects.

For more information see page 1214.

Clarke-Hadfield Syndrome

See Cystic Fibrosis

Cystic Fibrosis

Cystic fibrosis (CF) is an inherited condition affecting the cells that produce mucus, sweat, saliva, and digestive juices. Normally, these secretions are thin and slippery, but in CF, a defective gene causes the secretions to become thick and sticky. Respiratory failure is the most dangerous consequence of CF. Each year approximately 3,200 Caucasian babies are born in the United States with CF. The disease is much less common among African-American and Asian-American children. Most babies born with CF are diagnosed by age three, although mild forms of the disease may not be detected until the third, fourth or fifth decade of life.

Commonly Prescribed (On-Label) Drugs: *Acetylcysteine, Aztreonam, Ceftazidime, Chloramphenicol, Dornase alfa, Fusidic Acid, Medium Chain Triglycerides, Pancrelipase, Ticarcillin/Clavulanic Acid, Tobramycin, Ursodiol*

OFF-LABEL PRESCRIPTION DRUGS
BREAKTHROUGH OPTIONS

Generic: ***Dexamethasone*** *(deks-a-METH-a-sone)*
Brands: ***Decadron, Dexameth, Dexone, Hexadrol***

Dexamethasone reduces swelling and inflammation and is used in a variety of disorders such as skin diseases (psoriasis, hives), allergic conditions, breathing problems, cancer, blood disorders (anemia), digestive problems, eye disorders and for arthritis/bursitis.

A study conducted by Italian researchers was undertaken to evaluate the safety and efficacy of glucocorticoids, hormones that raise blood sugar levels, in patients with CF. Nine CF patients received increasing amounts of dexamethasone to obtain a slow delivery of this drug in their blood circulation. Subsequently, eight additional patients received dexamethasone at one-month intervals to evaluate the efficacy of continuous release in circulation of low doses of this drug. Repeated administrations at four-week intervals for 15 months showed that very low doses of this drug provide significant improvement in some breathing measures and significantly reduced relapses due to bacteria. Researchers have found that the administration of very low doses of glucocorticoids using dexamethasone is possible without side effects.

For more information see page 1138.

Generic: **Fluticasone** *(floo-TIK-a-sone)*
Brands: **Cutivate, Flonase, Flovent, Flovent HFA, Flovent Diskus, Flovent Rotadisk**

Fluticasone works directly in the lungs to make breathing easier by reducing the swelling and inflammation of the airways. This medication must be used regularly to prevent the wheezing and shortness of breath caused by asthma, bronchitis, or some types of emphysema.

Inhaled fluticasone propionate is widely used to reduce lung inflammation in chronic obstructive pulmonary disease, but the potential effects of fluticasone propionate on airway cells from patients with CF are unknown. In CF, an inflammatory lung response occurs through a defective protein that makes the body susceptible to the bacteria *Pseudomonas aeruginosa*, which causes the airway to become filled with a thick mucus. The presence of these bacteria in the body leads to a chronic inflammation that further damages the lung cell surface.

Corticosteroids such as fluticasone have long-term benefits in suppressing the potentially damaging inflammatory response within the airways of patients with CF. Fluticasone proprionate is especially helpful in children with CF who are wheezy and have associated asthma. A study conducted in France found that fluticasone propionate exerts an anti-inflammatory effect by blocking a signal leading to a reduced level in lung cells.

For more information see page 1197.

*Generic: **Prednisolone** (pred-NISS-oh-lone)*
*Brands: **Prednisolone, Prelone***

Prednisolone is a corticosteroid medication that reduces swelling. It is used for many conditions, including skin diseases and breathing problems as well as certain cancers, blood disorders, eye problems, arthritis, digestive problems and hormone replacement.

In cystic fibrosis, airway obstruction and respiratory infection leads to inflammation and eventually long-term lung damage, respiratory failure, and death. Inflammation occurs early in the disease process. Anti-inflammatory agents, such as oral steroids, are used to reduce inflammation. A study assessed the effectiveness of oral steroids in cystic fibrosis with particular regard to lung function. Short-term use of oral steroids was studied for respiratory infections separately (up to 30 days) compared to long-term anti-inflammatory use (greater than 30 days). The Cochrane Cystic Fibrosis and Genetic Disorders Group specialist trials register was reviewed for information. Researchers concluded that oral prednisolone appeared to slow the progression of lung disease in cystic fibrosis but this benefit must to be weighed against the occurrence of adverse events associated with corticosteroids.

For more information see page 1428.

*Generic: **Prednisone** (pred-NIS-zone)*
*Brands: **Deltasone, Liquid Pred, Meticorten, Orasone, Sterapred***

Prednisone decreases your immune system's response to various diseases to reduce symptoms such as swelling and allergic-type reactions. It is used to treat conditions such as arthritis, blood disorders, breathing problems, certain cancers, eye problems, immune system diseases, and skin diseases.

Inflammation has been increasingly recognized as a major factor in the development of CF lung disease. The use of anti-inflammatory medications to slow lung deterioration has been the focus of much research over the past two decades. Oral corticosteroids are effective but are associated with significant adverse effects when used long-term. However, a study conducted at Baylor College of Medicine evaluated the effectiveness of prednisone for improving lung health in CF patients. This investigation found that the patients who received prednisone had more growth, lower hospitalization rate, and better pulmonary function than those who received a placebo.

For more information see page 1429.

Generic: **Theophylline** *(theo-FILL-in)*
Brands: **Bronkodyl, Quibron-T, Theo-24, Theolair, Theochron**

Theophylline, a derivative of caffeine, is a bronchodilator drug, meaning that it is a type of medication used to improve breathing by opening air passages in the lungs. It is commonly used in the treatment of asthma, chronic bronchitis, and emphysema. Theophylline is a systemic medication that is carried in the blood stream throughout the body.

Canadian researchers from the Children's Hospital in Winnipeg reported that in a recent survey of 9,500 cystic fibrosis patients, 75% used an inhaled bronchodilator. While the use of bronchodilators remains controversial in the treatment of cystic fibrosis, other studies on oral and intravenous treatments are being conducted. Researchers have had some success in treating lung function with the use of intravenous theophylline. Additionally, some researchers believe that theophylline may be able to reverse steroid resistance in chronic obstructive pulmonary disease and other inflammatory diseases.

For more information see page 1507.

Fibrocystic Disease of the Pancreas

See Cystic Fibrosis

Juvenile Chronic Arthritis

See Juvenile Rheumatoid Arthritis

Juvenile Rheumatoid Arthritis

Juvenile rheumatoid arthritis (JRA) is arthritis that causes joint inflammation and stiffness for more than six weeks in a child of 16 years of age or less. Inflammation causes redness, swelling, warmth, and soreness in the joints, although many children with JRA do not complain of joint pain. Any joint can be affected and inflammation may limit the mobility of affected joints. One type of JRA can also affect the internal organs. Doctors classify JRA into three types by the number of joints involved, the symptoms, and the presence or absence of certain antibodies found by a blood test.

Commonly Prescribed (On-Label) Drugs: Aurothioglucose, Choline Salicylate, Rofecoxib

---

OFF-LABEL PRESCRIPTION DRUGS
BREAKTHROUGH OPTIONS

Generic: **Anakinra** *(an-a-KIN-ra)*
Brand: **Kineret**

Anakinra is a protein medication used either alone or in combination with other medications to treat the symptoms of rheumatoid arthritis such as pain or swelling in adults. Anakinra is not a cure for rheumatoid arthritis. However, anakinra has been studied in children with polyarticular juvenile rheumatoid arthritis (JRA) (a disorder that affects five or more joints). Approximately 65% of patients developed injection-site reactions and 68% demonstrated a response to the medication. Anakinra may have increased efficacy in systemic JRA (which is a type of arthritis that affects the entire body).

This effective medication is an important addition to available therapies. Although originally developed for rheumatoid arthritis and Crohn's disease in adults, it has been found to be effective in the treatment of juvenile rheumatoid arthritis. Its role is currently being defined in other autoimmune disorders such as uveitis, sarcoidosis, interstitial lung disease, vasculitis, inflammatory myopathies, and Sjogren syndrome.

Research has examined the use of the anakinra in two patients with therapy resistant systemic juvenile rheumatoid arthritis. Both patients experienced immediate and sustained resolution of symptoms, in one case after years of treatment with other immunosuppressive therapies.

For more information see page 1018.

*Generic: **Auranofin*** *(au-RANE-oh-fin)*
*Brand: **Ridaura***

Auranofin is a medication used to treat pain, swelling, and stiffness associated with arthritis that is not controlled by other therapies. Auranofin is used in the management of rheumatoid arthritis in adults whose symptoms progress despite an adequate regimen of nonsteroidal anti-inflammatory drugs (NSAIDs).

Results of clinical studies in adults with active rheumatoid arthritis receiving auranofin suggest that the drug is generally effective in decreasing the number of painful and/or tender and swollen joints, the duration of morning stiffness, improving rheumatoid activity index and increasing grip strength. In studies, auranofin has generally been more effective than placebo in relieving symptoms. Auranofin does not possess direct treatment for juvenile rheumatoid arthritis, but as a result of its anti-inflammatory and antiarthritic effects, therapy with the drug generally results in a reduction of disease-associated pain.

Researchers believe further well-designed studies are needed to conclusively determine whether the drug can reduce the severity or rate of progression of joint space narrowing and bone erosion associated with rheumatoid arthritis.

For more information see page 1032.

*Generic: **Diclofenac*** *(di-KLOE-fen-ak)*
*Brands: **Voltaren Ophthalmic***

Diclofenac is a nonsteroidal anti-inflammatory drug that relieves pain and reduces inflammation. It is typically used to treat headaches, muscle aches, dental pain, menstrual cramps, and athletic injuries. It is also used to treat pain, swelling, and stiffness associated with arthritis. Diclofenac has been used with good results in a number of children for the management of JRA. Results of these studies suggest that usual dosages of the drug are more effective than placebo in decreasing the number of painful, swollen, and tender joints. Researchers believe further studies are needed to evaluate the efficacy and safety of diclofenac in the management of juvenile rheumatoid arthritis.

Researchers in Italy evaluated the clinical efficacy of diclofenac sodium in the treatment of polyarticular juvenile chronic arthritis which is a type of arthritis that affects five or more joints, usually the same joints on both sides of the body. Treatment of 26 patients aged two to 16 years was studied. Treatment was started only if previous anti-inflammatory drugs had been considered ineffective after a prolonged use (three to 12 months). Diclofenac sodium was given by tablets and/or suppositories, which (may require special compounding prescription). Diclofenac sodium was particularly effective on joint pain and morning stiffness but also on joint swelling and functional capacity. Researchers noticed a tendency of JRA to improve during the trial period. The drug was well tolerated.

For more information see pages 1142 and 1143.

*Generic: **Infliximab** (in-FLIKS-e-mab)*
*Brand: **Remicade***

Infliximab inhibits a protein called tumor necrosis factor (TNF). This results in decreased swelling and decreased immune system function. Infliximab is effective in treating rheumatoid arthritis and certain bowel diseases such as Crohn's disease in adults, since swelling and an overactive immune system likely play a role in these diseases. Biological drugs that are currently available for the treatment of inflammatory disorders include infliximab, adalimumab, etanercept, and anakinra, with many more in development.

Italian researchers evaluated the efficacy and safety of infliximab with methotrexate in juvenile idiopathic arthritis (JIA). Twenty-four young adults with long-lasting, therapy-resistant JIA were enrolled in a two-year study. Patients received intravenous infliximab at weeks 0, 2, and 6, and every 8 weeks thereafter plus methotrexate. Significant improvements were observed in the number of joints with active disease. Pain discomfort as well as patients' and physicians' global assessments of disease status were assessed. There were significant improvements in pain scores, patients' global assessment of disease status, and physicians' global assessment of disease status. Researchers concluded that infliximab plus methotrexate showed high effectiveness and safety in short- and medium-term treatment of long-lasting therapy-resistant JIA.

For more information see page 1239.

Generic: **Methylprednisolone** *(METH-il-pred-NIS-oh-lone)*
Brands: **Depo-Medrol, Medrol, Solu-Medrol,**

Methylprednisolone is used to treat various conditions such as allergic disorders; arthritis; blood diseases; breathing problems; certain cancers; eye diseases; intestinal disorders; collagen and skin diseases. It decreases the body's immune response to these diseases and reduces symptoms such as swelling and redness. Methylprednisolone is a corticosteroid hormone.

A study published in the *British Journal of Rheumatology* documented the use of intravenous methylprednisolone in children with juvenile chronic arthritis (JCA). Eighteen children were treated. Ten patients (55%) had a loss of all symptoms one month after the intravenous administration and eight (45%) had a reduction in the active joint count. At this time, five of the patients on oral prednisolone had achieved a reduction in dosage. Altogether, patients had a good response, with several going into remission. Physicians concluded that intravenous methylprednisolone provides good short-term benefit in patients with JCA.

For more information see page 1316.

Generic: **Nabumetone** *(na-BYOO-me-tone)*
Brand: **Relafen**

Nabumetone is a medication used to reduce pain, swelling, and joint stiffness from arthritis. This medication is known as a nonsteroidal anti-inflammatory drug (NSAID).

Once-a-day dosing with nabumetone has been shown to be effective in adults with rheumatoid arthritis. Dosing recommendations for nabumetone in children and adolescents with juvenile rheumatoid arthritis (JRA) was studied by Arthritis Associates of South Florida, which examined children with JRA aged two to 16 years who required NSAIDs for control of symptoms. NSAIDs were discontinued one day prior to study initiation to minimize disease flare. Patients received nabumetone once daily for 12 weeks. An overall assessment of efficacy was determined based on the percentage of patients who did not experience a flare. Routine safety assessments were completed for all patients. In total, 99 patients with JRA were enrolled and 89 completed the study.

Nabumetone demonstrated a safe profile with no loss of efficacy compared to alternative treatment in children with JRA.

For more information see page 1346.

Kawasaki Syndrome

Kawasaki disease is a rare condition in children (usually between the ages of 2 and 5) that involves inflammation of the blood vessels. The condition is usually accompanied by a fever that lasts at least five days. Other classic symptoms may include: red eyes, lips and mouth; a rash; swollen red hands and feet; and swollen lymph nodes.

Commonly Prescribed (On-Label) Drugs: Immune Globulin IV

OFF-LABEL PRESCRIPTION DRUGS
BREAKTHROUGH OPTION

Generic: **Infliximab** *(in-FLIKS-e-mab)*
Brand: **Remicade**

Infliximab inhibits a protein called tumor necrosis factor (TNF). This results in decreased swelling (inflammation) and decreased immune system function (immunosuppression). A study was undertaken at the Children's Hospital of San Diego to evaluate the use of infliximab for treatment of patients with Kawasaki syndrome who fail to have a fever or who experience persistent arthritis after treatment with intravenous immuno globulin (IVIG) and high-dose aspirin. Cases were collected from clinicians throughout the United States who had used infliximab for patients with Kawasaki syndrome who had either persistent arthritis or persistent or recurrent fever at equal to or greater than 48 hours following infusion of IVIG. Response to therapy with cessation of fever occurred in 13 of 16 patients. C-reactive protein (CRP), a test that measures concentrations of a protein that indicates acute inflammation, determined that the CRP level was elevated in all but one patient before infliximab infusion and the level was lower following infusion in all 10 patients in whom it was re-measured within 48 hours of treatment. There were no infusion reactions to infliximab and no complications attributed to infliximab administration in any of the patients.

For more information see page 1239.

GROWTH DISORDERS

Growth disorders may be caused by diseases of the kidneys, heart, gastrointestinal tract, lungs, bones, or other body systems. Other symptoms or physical signs in children with these illnesses usually give clues as to the disease causing the growth delay. However, poor growth may be the first sign of a problem in some of these conditions.

McCune-Albright Syndrome

The predominant features of the McCune-Albright syndrome occur in three areas: the bony skeleton, the skin, and the endocrine system. In all three systems, the extent of the abnormality and, in the case of the endocrine system, the nature of the abnormality, are highly variable from case to case, depending on the specific tissues involved and the extent of involvement. Although changes in ovary, bone, and skin tissue are most common, other endocrine and non-endocrine tissues also may be affected, including the adrenal, thyroid, pituitary, liver, and heart.

Commonly Prescribed (On-Label) Drugs: *None*

OFF-LABEL PRESCRIPTION DRUGS
BREAKTHROUGH OPTIONS

Generic: ***Anastrozole*** *(an-AS-troe-zole)*
Brand: ***Arimidex***

Anastrozole is most commonly used as an antineoplastic medication, meaning that it inhibits the maturation of abnormal cell growth. Usually, testolactone is used to treat conditions with excessive estrogen synthesis, such as precocious puberty in McCune-Albright syndrome (MAS). Unfortunately, daily treatment with testolactone requires three to four doses, 10-20 tablets, and even at these doses it is sometimes ineffective. A study reported in the *Journal of Pediatric Endocrinology & Metabolism* examined patients with MAS with the highly selective aromatase inhibitor anastrozole. Additionally, tamoxifen was added for one year but was discontinued when an ovarian cyst developed with markedly elevated estradiol levels. Estradiol levels returned to normal after resuming anastrozole-only treatment. Researchers found that the potent estrogen suppressive action and simple dosage regimen of anastrozole suggest it may be advantageous compared to other aromatase inhibitors such as testolactone or anti-estrogens.

For more information see page 1020.

Generic: **Flutamide** (FLOO-ta-mide)
Brand: **Eulexin**

Flutamide is a drug that inhibits the maturation of abnormal cell growth. During puberty, estrogen causes breast maturation and growth of the uterine lining in girls and accelerates linear growth and bone maturation in both boys and girls. Decreasing the biosynthesis of estrogen can slow these processes.

Researchers at National Institutes of Health conducted a study of 12 children with growth disorders. They found testolactone, in combination with flutamide, improved the control of growth and bone maturation compared with conventional therapy. In a six-year study of 10 boys with familial male precocious puberty, testolactone, in combination with spironolactone, decreased rates of growth and bone maturation and increased predicted adult height. Testolactone had no important adverse effects in any group of patients, although the need for a four-times-daily dosing schedule made compliance difficult for many families. Researchers concluded that suppressing of estrogen with testolactone was effective therapy and that more potent and specific inhibitors of aromatase could further improve the treatment of these disorders.

For more information see page 1196.

Generic: **Medroxyprogesterone Acetate**
(me-DROKS-ee-proe-JES-te-rone AS-eh-tate)
Brand: **Provera**

Medroxyprogesterone acetate is a female hormone used most commonly to treat amenorrhea (lack of menstrual flow), abnormal bleeding from the uterus, or endometriosis. It is also used to treat certain types of cancer and menopausal symptoms. Progestins such as medroxyprogesterone lower the risk of estrogen-related cancer of the uterus during hormone replacement therapy.

Researchers in India evaluated seven children presenting with Cafe-au-lait spots (skin markings that range in color from black to bluish-gray), bony abnormalities and/or sexual precocity. All seven children had large Cafe-au-lait spots, while bony abnormalities were seen in five. Six girls had precocious puberty with large ovarian follicles and elevated estradiol levels. Medroxyprogesterone acetate was used for all of the children. Five girls on follow up for six months showed termination of menstrual episodes and regression of ovarian follicles in three, regression in breast size in one and three girls continued to grow at a height velocity within the 95th percentile for their age.

For more information see page 1297.

Generic: **Pamidronate** *(pa-mi-DROE-nate)*
Brand: **Aredia**

Pamidronate acts on bone to help regulate blood calcium levels. Bone abnormalities are one of the main features of McCune-Albright syndrome. Encouraging therapeutic results have been achieved, mainly in adults, with pamidronate. In a study by the Department of Internal Medicine at the University of Turin, researchers examined newer bone growth in 11 children and adolescents with McCune-Albright syndrome who were treated with pamidronate. After treatment, significant decreases in bone alkaline phosphatase (an enzyme found in all tissues) were found. Bone mineral density significantly increased during treatment. There were signs of healing as thickening of the cortical bone was found in some cases.

For more information see page 1391.

Generic: **Tamoxifen** *(ta-MOKS-I-fen)*
Brand: **Nolvadex**

Tamoxifen is a drug that blocks the action of the hormone estrogen. It is most commonly used in the treatment and prevention of breast cancer in women. A one-year trial conducted at the James Whitcomb Riley Hospital for Children examined tamoxifen treatment for precocious puberty in 28 girls with MAS. Patients received tamoxifen daily. Compared with before the study, vaginal bleeding episodes decreased, growth velocity slowed, and rate of bone maturation decreased. No adverse events occurred. Researchers concluded that tamoxifen treatment of precocious puberty in MAS results in a reduction of vaginal bleeding and significant improvements in growth and of skeletal maturation.

For more information see page 1493.

Generic: **Testolactone** *(tes-toe-LAK-tone)*
Brand: **Teslac**

Testolactone is an antineoplastic agent, meaning that it prevents the growth of abnormal cell growths. McCune-Albright syndrome was diagnosed at 2.5 years in a boy, with a lower limb fracture and cafe-au-lait markings (skin markings that range in color from black to bluish-gray). At the age of 7.5, the child's bone age was that of a nine-year-old. Between the age of 8 to 8.5 years, the child's growth increased further, with bone age advancing from 9 to 12 years in one year. The child was treated with octreotide, flutamide and testolactone. Testolactone resulted in control of precocious puberty, slowing of growth demonstrated by the return to normal jaw size and tooth spacing, sweating, acne, and facial appearance.

For more information see page 1500.

Puberty Disorders

Puberty is the period of physiological and anatomical development when the organs of sexual reproduction mature and become functional. This is not to be confused with adolescence, which is a socially defined period of psychological development that is sociocultural. In girls, the onset of menstruation and the development of the breasts mark this maturation. In boys, the biological markers of puberty are the enlargement of the external genitalia and the production of semen.

Two common puberty disorders are precocious and delayed puberty, which can develop in either boys or girls; however, treatment various depending on the sex. Precocious puberty or "early puberty" is a condition in which the changes that normally accompany puberty, such as breast or genital development and growth of pubic hair, occur at an unexpectedly early age. Delayed puberty is defined as a condition in which a boy or girl has passed the usual age of the onset of puberty without develeoping any physical or hormonal signs that it is beginning. Delayed puberty may occur due to undernutrition as a symptom of a systemic disease, or to abnormalities of the reproductive system (hypogonadism) or a response to sex hormones.

Commonly Prescribed (On-Label) Drugs: Histrelin, *Leuprolide, Nafarelin, Testosterone*

OFF-LABEL PRESCRIPTION DRUGS
BREAKTHROUGH OPTIONS

---

*Generic: **Letrozole*** *(LET-roe-zole)*
*Brand: **Femara***

For delayed puberty in boys, letrozole may be prescribed. Letrozole is most commonly used as an antineoplastic agent, which is a drug that prevents the maturation of abnormal cell growths. In a study published in the *Journal of Endocrinology & Metabolism*, six boys were followed up without treatment (control group) and eight boys received low-dose testosterone with letrozole once a day for 0-12 months (treatment group). In the control group, bioactivity increased during the course of puberty. During 0-12 months of the study, the boys in the treatment group had faster rate of pubic hair growth than the control boys. Overall, the average bioactivity during 12 months of follow-up correlated strongly with the associated changes in genital and pubic hair stages. Researchers concluded that these results suggest that the combination of testosterone and letrozole given to boys with constitutional delay of puberty accelerates puberty.

For more information see page 1273.

Generic: **Medroxyprogesterone acetate**
(me-DROKS-ee-proe-JES-te-rone AS-eh-tate)
Brand: **Provera**

Medroxyprogesterone acetate is a female hormone. It is most commonly used to treat amenorrhea (lack of menstrual flow), abnormal bleeding from the uterus, or endometriosis. It may be used to treat girls with precocious puberty.

Precocious puberty is defined as the onset of pubertal development before the age of eight years in girls or nine years in boys. Central precocious puberty (CPP) has similar physical and hormonal characteristics to normal puberty. Precocious puberty is characterized by rapid growth and advancement of skeletal age. The skeletal advancement is greater than the growth increase, so that final adult height is compromised. Long-acting hormone drugs such as medroxyprogesterone acetate are the current therapy of choice for central precocious puberty, having demonstrated effectiveness in halting the precocious development associated with this condition with minimal side effects.

For more information see page 1297.

Generic: **Methylphenidate** *(meth-il-FEN-i-date).*
Brands: **Concerta, Metadate CD, Metadate ER, Methylin, Methylin ER, Ritalin, Ritalin LA, Ritalin-SR**

Methylphenidate is a mild stimulant that works by affecting the levels of chemicals in the nervous system. This medication is used most commonly in the treatment of attention deficit disorder and may be prescribed for familial male precocious puberty.

Familial male precocious puberty is a form of precocious puberty resulting from a mutation of a hormone receptor. Behavior problems are associated with the early onset of puberty. Sexual hyperactivity can be treated with psychostimulants such as methylphenidate. Researchers have found that the effectiveness of methylphenidate in reducing sexual hyperactivity with and without male precocious puberty needs further evaluation.

For more information see page 1315.

Generic: **Spironolactone** *(speer-row-no-LACK-tone)* and
Testolactone *(tes-toe-LAK-tone)* in combination therapy
Brands: **Aldactone** *(spironolactone)*, **Teslac** *(testolactone)*

Spironolactone can be used in combination with testolactone in the management of precocious puberty. Such therapy has effectively controlled acne, spontaneous erections, and aggressive behavior, and slows accelerated growth and skeletal maturation, at least in the short term, in boys with familial precocious puberty. Neither drug alone effectively controls pubertal characteristics nor the rate of growth and skeletal maturation in boys with this condition, although some benefit such as height velocity with testolactone alone may be apparent. Testolactone generally prevents the gynecomastia (a benign enlargement of the male breast) that may be associated with spironolactone. While spironolactone currently is the most widely used drug in familial male precocious puberty, alternative drugs that avoid some of the potentially serious adverse effects of spironolactone therapy are being studied for this condition and congenital adrenal hyperplasia.

Researchers believe that additional study and experience are needed to further determine the best regimens for the management of these forms of precocious puberty and the long-term effects of such therapy, and such patients should be managed in consultation with experts in the diagnosis and treatment of these conditions. Combinations of testolactone with flutamide or with spironolactone also have been studied in the complex regimen of therapy for boys and girls with congenital adrenal hyperplasia caused by a steroid deficiency; the rationale for the addition of such therapy to the therapeutic regimen was similar to that for familial male precocious puberty, which is to control hormone effects and accelerated growth and skeletal maturation.

For more information see page 1478.

HEADACHES

Migraine

Migraine headaches seem to be caused in part by changes in the level of a body chemical called serotonin. Serotonin plays many roles in the body, and it can have an effect on the blood vessels. When serotonin levels are high, blood vessels constrict. When serotonin levels fall, the blood vessels dilate. This swelling can cause pain or other problems. Many things can affect the level of serotonin in the body, including level of blood sugar, certain foods, and changes in the estrogen level of women. There are two main types of migraines: migraines with aura and migraines without aura. The aura that accompanies some migraines may be in the form of lines or spots before the eyes, total darkness, or speech impairment, and the aura usually occurs 10 to 30 minutes before the onset of the migraine.

Migraines can occur in children and adults; however, there are no labeled uses for drugs in the prevention or treatment of migraines in children. In order to determine the appropriate therapy for migraines in children, physicians use results of trials conducted on adult migraine sufferers. Many of the drugs used to treat migraines are approved only for adults, making them off-label when prescribed to children.

Commonly Prescribed (On-Label) Drugs: None

OFF-LABEL PRESCRIPTION DRUGS
BREAKTHROUGH OPTIONS

Generic: **Rizatriptan** *(rye-za-TRIP-tan)*
Brands: **Maxalt, Maxalt-MLT**

Rizatriptan is a medication used to treat acute migraine attacks in adults. This drug does not, however, prevent future migraine attacks. The current guideline for using rizatriptan is based principally on the results of four studies conducted on adults who were administered rizatriptan tablets and two studies of rizatriptan orally disintegrating tablets in adults with moderate to severe headaches. In these studies, substantially more patients receiving single doses of rizatriptan achieved a response (mild or no headache pain) two hours after treatment compared with patients receiving placebo. Rizatriptan also relieved symptoms of migraine other than headache (including nausea, photophobia and phonophobia), reduced the need for supplemental migraine therapy, and improved functional ability. Limited data from studies of up to one year in duration suggest that rizatriptan has remained effective throughout subsequent migraine attacks. Researchers have found that data from several comparative studies indicate that rizatriptan is at least as effective as oral sumatriptan in alleviating the pain associated with migraine two hours after treatment. Based on these results, physicians have prescribed rizatriptan to children with migraines.

For more information see page 1460.

Generic: **Sumatriptan** (soo-ma-TRIP-tan)
Brand: **Imitrex**

Sumatriptan treats migraine attacks in adults once they occur. It is not effective in preventing migraines. This medication is not to be used for other types of headaches. In clinical studies involving adults, approximately 70–88% of patients receiving sumatriptan attained relief of migraines within one to two hours compared with 18–39% of placebo recipients; at two hours, 48–65% of sumatriptan-treated patients were pain-free. Relief of migraine headache generally begins as early as 10 minutes following subcutaneous (underneath the skin) administration of sumatriptan and lasts for a maximum of two hours.

Relief of migraine symptoms with oral sumatriptan therapy is slower than that with subcutaneous (underneath the skin) administration of the drug, generally occurring 0.5–3 hours after single oral doses; maximum pain relief is attained within three to six hours. In clinical trials, 50–73% of patients receiving sumatriptan in single oral doses obtained relief of headache pain (defined as no pain or only mild pain) within two hours compared with 10–33% of patients receiving placebo. Sixty five to 78% of patients receiving sumatriptan reported relief of pain at four hours. These results suggest that sumatriptan may be an effective treatment for migraines in children; however, researchers note that you must first consult your doctor.

For more information see page 1487.

Generic: **Zolmitriptan** *(zohl-mi-TRIP-tan)*
Brands: **Zomig, Zomig ZMT**

Zolmitriptan is used to treat migraine headache attacks in adults. It does not prevent migraine headaches from occurring and should not be used for other types of headaches such as cluster headaches. Efficacy of zolmitriptan has been evaluated for the acute treatment of migraine attacks in several studies in adults with moderate to severe headaches. In these studies, substantially more patients receiving zolmitriptan achieved a response (mild or no headache pain) two hours after treatment than those receiving placebo. The drug also relieved symptoms of migraine other than headache (including nausea) and reduced the need for supplemental migraine therapy. In long-term studies, zolmitriptan remained effective during subsequent migraine attacks. Researchers feel that this drug may be an effective treatment for children who suffer from migraines.

For more information see page 1554.

Migraine Prevention

To minimize the onset and the effects of migraines, most individuals can use alternative, non-drug measures. However, it may be necessary to incorporate drugs into prevention options to minimize the frequency and severity of migraines and, in some causes, to treat the symptoms or terminate the attack altogether.

Commonly Prescribed (On-Label) Drugs: *None*

OFF-LABEL PRESCRIPTION DRUGS
BREAKTHROUGH OPTIONS

Generic: **Carbamazepine** *(kar-ba-MAZ-e-peen)*
Brands: **Carbatrol, Epitol, Tegretol, Tegretol XR**

Carbamazepine is typically used to prevent and control seizures. This medication is known as an anticonvulsant or anti-epileptic drug. It is also used to relieve trigeminal neuralgia, a type of nerve pain. This medication works by reducing excessive nerve signals in the brain and restoring the normal balance of nerve activity.

Researchers at the University of Hawaii at Manoa reviewed fourteen trials conducted on adult migraine sufferers to compare anticonvulsants with placebo. One trial showed that anticonvulsants, considered as a class, including carbamazepine, reduced migraine frequency by 50% or more, relative to placebo. They concluded that anticonvulsants appear to be both effective in reducing migraine frequency and reasonably well tolerated. Based on these results, carbamezapine may prevent migraines in children.

For more information see page 1068.

Generic: *Cyproheptadine* (si-proe-HEP-ta-deen)
Brand: *Periactin*

Cyproheptadine is an antihistamine medication that provides relief of seasonal and nonseasonal allergy symptoms such as watery and itchy eyes, runny nose and sneezing. It is also used to relieve itching and hives due to some skin conditions. Cyproheptadine reportedly has been effective in some patients for the management of migraines. It is more commonly prescribed to children, as it has been shown to be only slightly effective in adults.

Cyproheptadine is known as a sedating antihistamine, as it enters the brain in significant quantities and induces drowsiness. Researchers are unclear as to how cyproheptadine works to prevent migraines. It is believed that since cyproheptadine also blocks serotonin, a chemical in the brain, that this has an effect in the prevention of migraines. The chemical, serotonin, is a factor in the cause of migraines.

For more information see page 1128.

Generic: *Metoprolol* (me-toe-PROE-lole)
Brands: *Lopressor, Toprol-XL*

Metoprolol is a beta-blocker medication typically used to treat chest pain (angina) and high blood pressure. It is also used after an acute heart attack to improve survival. This drug works by blocking the action of certain natural chemicals in the body such as epinephrine on the heart and blood vessels. The effects of the medication are the lowering of heart rate, blood pressure, and strain on the heart.

Metoprolol has been used for the prevention of migraine headache. When used preventively, metoprolol can prevent migraine or reduce the number of attacks in some patients. Results of comparative studies suggest that metoprolol may be comparable to propranolol for this indication. However, the U.S. Headache Consortium states that the quality of evidence for metoprolol is not as compelling as it is for propranolol for this indication. Metoprolol is not recommended for the treatment of a migraine attack that has already started.

For more information see page 1321.

Generic: **Propranolol** *(proe-PRAN-oh-lole)*
Brands: **Inderal, Inderal LA, InnoPran XL, Propranolol Intensol**

Propranolol is a beta-blocker medication typically used to treat chest pain (angina), high blood pressure, irregular heartbeats, migraine headaches, tremors, and other conditions. It is also used after an acute heart attack to improve survival. This drug works by blocking the action of certain natural chemicals in the body (such as epinephrine) that affect the heart and blood vessels. This results in a lowering of heart rate, blood pressure, and strain on the heart.

Propranolol may be used for the prevention of common migraine headache. When used preventively, the drug can prevent common migraine or reduce the number of attacks in some patients. The U.S. Headache Consortium states that there is good evidence from multiple well-designed clinical trials that propranolol has medium to high efficacy for the prevention of migraine headache. Propranolol is not recommended for the treatment of a migraine attack that has already started nor for the prevention or treatment of cluster headaches.

For more information see page 1438.

Generic: **Topiramate** *(TOE-pie-rah-mate)*
Brand: **Topamax**

Topiramate is typically used to treat a seizure disorder (epilepsy). This medication is also used to prevent migraine headaches. Several well-documented studies have shown that topiramate is a well-tolerated, effective treatment for migraine prevention.

A study published in *Headache* reported on the use of topiramate as a preventive treatment for migraines in adults. Researchers were interested in assessing the efficacy of topiramate on health-related quality of life in migraine sufferers. The 26-week trial studied the preventive effects of topiramate on patients' performance of daily activities, emotional function, and restriction of daily activities due to migraines. Researchers found topiramate positively effective in all three of these areas, concluding that this prevents migraines and improves daily lives. They believe that this drug may be effective in the prevention of migraines in children.

For more information see page 1516.

Generic: **Valproic Acid** *(val-PRO-ick acid),*
(SOE-dee-um val-PROE-ate)
Brands: **Depacon, Depakene, Depakote Delayed Release, Depakote ER, Depakote Sprinkle**

Valproic acid is a medication typically used to treat seizure disorders. It works by restoring the balance of certain natural substances (neurotransmitters) in the brain. Migraine is a cause of recurrent headache in childhood. The efficacy of valproic acid is well known in the preventive treatment of adult migraine, but there are few studies involving the drug's effect in childhood migraine. To determine the efficacy of valproic acid in the preventive treatment of childhood migraine, 15 children with migraine were included in a study conducted by researchers in Turkey.

Headache severity was measured and assessed. All of the subjects were asked to keep a headache diary for eight weeks. Valproic acid was initiated in 10 subjects, and therapy continued for at least 12 weeks. The observed side effects were dizziness, drowsiness, and increase in appetite; none required drug withdrawal. In two cases, headache attacks recurred after the cessation of valproate, and therapy was restarted. Valproic acid appears to be effective and safe in selected patients with childhood migraine.

For more information see page 1534.

MENTAL HEALTH DISORDERS

The term mental illness describes various mental and emotional conditions. When mental illness interferes with life activities such as learning, reasoning, communication, and sleeping, it is called a psychiatric disability. The intensity, type, and duration of mental illness symptoms vary between people. Many times, mental health disorders can be effectively controlled through medication.

Attention Deficit Hyperactivity Disorder

Attention Deficit Hyperactivity Disorder (ADHD) is a condition that becomes apparent in some children in the preschool and early school years. It is hard for children with ADHD to control their behavior and/or focus their attention. It is estimated that between three and five percent of children have ADHD, or approximately two million children in the United States. This means that in a classroom of 25 to 30 children, it is likely that at least one will have ADHD.

Researchers believe that in selecting the appropriate drug treatment, consideration should be given to the child's daily school and after-school schedule, the presence of aggressive symptoms, and the risk of diversion. Careful selection of an appropriate medication regimen and active engagement of the child, parents, and teacher in daily management may help to ensure long-term adherence.

Commonly Prescribed (On-Label) Drugs: *Atomoxetine, Dexmethylphenidate, Methylphenidate*

OFF-LABEL PRESCRIPTION DRUGS
BREAKTHROUGH OPTIONS

Generic: ***Bupropion*** *(byoo-PROE-pee-on)*
Brands: ***Wellbutrin, Wellbutrin SR, Wellbutrin XL, Zyban***

Bupropion is an antidepressant medication typically used to treat depression and also used to treat smoking cessation. In a study conducted by researchers at the Massachusetts General Hospital, they examined the effects of bupropion on adults with ADHD in a 6-week trial. They found that sustained-release bupropion was effective in adult patients with ADHD. Given the success of this drug on ADHD adult sufferers, researchers suggest that it may be effective in treating children with ADHD. Bupropion and most tricyclic antidepressants are sound options for managing core behavioral symptoms and, to some extent, cognitive symptoms.

For more information see page 1058.

Generic: *Clonidine* (KLON-i-deen)
Brand: *Catapres, Catapres-TTS, Duraclon*

Clonidine is a medication used to treat high blood pressure. It works by stimulating certain brain receptors (alpha adrenergic type), which results in the relaxing of blood vessels in other parts of the body, causing them to widen. Clonidine has been used for the treatment of ADHD. Although pooled data from an analysis of studies in children with ADHD indicate that the drug has produced a moderate reduction in symptoms of ADHD, stimulants such as methylphenidate and amphetamines remain the drugs of choice for the management of ADHD because of their greater efficacy compared with that of other drugs.

Clonidine generally has been shown to be more effective than placebo in the treatment of core symptoms of ADHD. However, because clonidine may improve motor tics in patients with Tourette's syndrome, some experts recommend its use as an add-on therapy in pediatric patients with ADHD whose related tic disorder is not controlled with a stimulant alone. In pediatric patients without such related psychiatric disorders, use of clonidine for the treatment of ADHD usually is not recommended, because of the current lack of evidence establishing safety and efficacy.

For more information see page 1108.

Generic: *Desipramine* (des-IP-ra-meen)
Brand: *Norpramin*

Desipramine is a tricyclic antidepressant used to treat depression, obsessive-compulsive disorders, and bed-wetting in children over six years of age. The advantages of a tricyclic antidepressant for ADHD are they can be given at home, do not have the same abuse potentials as some other types of drugs, and symptom recurrence and insomnia are less likely. Desipramine is the most studied of the tricyclic antidepressants for the treatment of ADHD. Researchers concluded that this drug improves behavior and reduces motor activity, making it an effective drug for the treatment of ADHD in children.

For more information see page 1132.

Generic: **Fluoxetine** *(floo-OKS-e-teen)*
Brand: **Prozac, Prozac Weekly, Sarafem**

Fluoxetine is a drug known as a selective serotonin reuptake inhibitor (SSRI). It is used to treat depression, obsessive-compulsive disorder, panic attacks, certain eating disorders (bulimia), and a severe form of premenstrual syndrome. This medication works by restoring the balance of natural substances (neurotransmitters) in the brain, thereby improving mood and feelings of well being.

A study conducted for six weeks on 19 children with ADHD found that 60% of the patients experienced moderately improved symptoms of ADHD. Additionally, another team of researchers found that fluoxetine used in combination with methylphenidate improved symptoms of ADHD and depression.

For more information see page 1192.

Generic: **Gabapentin** *(GA-ba-pen-tin)*
Brand: **Neurontin**

Gabapentin is used with other medications to help control seizures in adults and children three years of age and older. It is also used to relieve nerve pain associated with shingles infection in adults.

Gabapentin is an anticonvulsant drug used as add-on therapy in therapy-resistant partial epilepsy. The mechanism of gabapentin is unknown, but the drug has a good safety profile, which allows its use in high-risk patients. Several reports have described the successful use of gabapentin for bipolar disorders in adults, but there are few studies in the use of gabapentin in children and adolescents. A study conducted at Yale University examined a 12-year-old boy with a history of ADHD, reading disorder, mixed receptive and expressive language disorder, encopresis (fecal incontinence) and bipolar disorder II. He was treated with gabapentin added to methylphenidate. Within three weeks, the improvement and stabilization of mood symptoms was remarkable, as noted by mother, teacher, and clinician, and remained so for six months of follow-up.

For more information see page 1206.

Generic: *Guanfacine* (GWAHN-fa-seen)
Brand: *Tenex*

Guanfacine is a medication typically used to treat high blood pressure. Stimulants are a highly efficacious and safe treatment for attention-deficit/hyperactivity disorder (ADHD), with 75%–90% of patients responding well if two different stimulants such as amphetamine and methylphenidate are used.

Stimulants may be prescribed if a child's academic performance is below average, based on his or her learning abilities, and at the occurrence of behavioral problems that arise when it appears that ADHD is a contributing factor. There are longer and shorter acting stimulant drugs that may be used in combination in order to prevent rebounding. Researchers warn that when administering stimulants, doctors need to pay close attention needs to be paid to the side effects of weight loss and slow growth due a suppression of appetite. Guanfacine is a slow-acting drug that may be given to the child in the evening. It is useful for treating tics, sleep disorders, impulsiveness, and hyperactivity. Researchers concluded that it is not suitable for distractibility or shortened attention span. It may take 4 to 5 weeks for this drug to have noticeable results.

For more information see page 1216.

Generic: *Imipramine* (im-IP-ra-meen)
Brands: *Tofranil, Tofranil-PM*

Imipramine is used to treat depression, obsessive-compulsive disorders, and bed-wetting in children over six years of age. This drug is a second-line treatment option for patients with ADHD. It may be prescribed when the patient does not respond to first-line treatment medications. However, if the child suffers from ADHD and bedwetting, imipramine may be prescribed as it has a proven record of success in treating patients with bedwetting disorders. It should be noted that imipramine may induce night terrors and should be discontinued if this happens.

For more information see page 1230.

Generic: **Modafinil** *(moe-DAF-i-nil)*
Brand: **Provigil**

Modafinil is typically used to treat excessive daytime sleepiness associated with narcolepsy, problems breathing while asleep, or shift work sleep disorder. Previous clinical evidence suggested that modafinil may improve clinical features of children with ADHD. This hypothesis was tested in a study of 24 children by researchers at Marshall University. The average ADHD scores improved for the modafinil group compared with a decline for control patients. Total scores for the modafinil group improved from 76.6 to 68.2 compared with improvement from 77.7 to 76.0 for control subjects. Ten of 11 treatment patients were reported as "significantly" improved, whereas eight of 11 children were reported as manifesting "no" or "slight" improvement. Researchers concluded that modafinil may be a useful treatment for children with ADHD, particularly in those who also have anorexia, which may limit the use of stimulants.

For more information see page 1338.

Generic: **Paroxetine** *(pa-ROKS-e-teen)*
Brand: **Paxil, Paxil CR**

Paroxetine is a selective serotonin reuptake inhibitor (SSRI) used to treat depression, panic attacks, obsessive-compulsive disorder, social anxiety disorder, post-traumatic stress disorder, and generalized anxiety disorders. Paroxetine does not treat the core symptoms of ADHD but may be effective for irritability, anxiety, or depression that can accompany ADHD. This drug has fewer side effects than tricyclic antidepressants and does not require as much medical monitoring, but does make some children jittery. However, the drug does interact with other medications so it is very important, as always, to let your doctor know what other medications your child is taking before starting a regimen of paroxetine.

For more information see page 1395.

Generic: **Sertraline** *(SER-tra-leen)*
Brand: **Zoloft**

Sertraline is a selective serotonin reuptake inhibitor (SSRI) used to treat depression, panic attacks, obsessive compulsive disorders, post-traumatic stress disorder, social anxiety disorder, and a severe form of premenstrual syndrome and other related disorders.

ADHD and major depression are common ailments throughout life, and these two disorders may occur at the same time. In a study conducted at Case Western Reserve University, seven pediatric patients with ADHD and major depression were examined. For all 11 patients, symptoms of major depression appeared to respond well to either fluoxetine or sertraline. Using fluoxetine or sertraline daily, there was no adverse behavioral effects. However, no improvement in ADHD symptoms was observed in any patient during the administration of fluoxetine or sertraline when used alone. Combination treatment with a psychostimulant seemed necessary for chronic ADHD symptoms to be effectively addressed. No patient developed suicide impulses, increased aggressiveness, mania, or other problematic side effects.

Researchers concluded that this combination therapy was well tolerated and appeared to be effective in treating both ADHD and depressive symptoms. According to the study, the results suggest that add-on treatment with psychostimulants might be a safe and effective intervention for children treated with fluoxetine or sertraline who have persistent ADHD symptoms.

For more information see page 1468.

Generic: **Venlafaxine** *(ven-la-FAX-een)*
Brand: **Effexor, Effexor XR**

Venlafaxine is an antidepressant used in the treatment of depression. It works by restoring the balance of natural chemicals (neurotransmitters) in the brain, thereby improving mood and feelings of well being.

A study conducted by Turkish researchers was undertaken to determine effectiveness of venlafaxine in the treatment of children and adolescents with ADHD. A six-week trial of venlafaxine was conducted in 13 children and adolescents with ADHD and without depression. The researchers concluded that venlafaxine was significantly effective in reducing the severity of symptoms in ADHD. Side effects such as stomachache and headache disappeared after the second week of treatment. These preliminary data suggest that venlafaxine may be an effective medication in the treatment of some children and adolescents with ADHD.

For more information see page 1542.

Autism

Autism is a complex developmental disability that typically appears during the first three years of life. The result of a neurological disorder that affects the functioning of the brain, autism affects the normal development of the brain and impedes social interaction and communication skills. Children and adults with autism typically have difficulties in verbal and non-verbal communication, social interactions, and leisure or play activities. Autism is a spectrum disorder that affects each individual differently and to varying degrees of severity. As many as 1.5 million Americans, children and adults, are thought to have autism today.

Commonly Prescribed (On-Label) Drugs: None

OFF-LABEL PRESCRIPTION DRUGS
BREAKTHROUGH OPTIONS

*Generic: **Clonidine** (KLON-i-deen)*
*Brands: **Catapres, Catapres-TTS, Duraclon***

Clonidine is used to treat high blood pressure. It works by stimulating certain brain receptors, which results in the relaxing of blood vessels in other parts of the body, causing them to widen. Lowering high blood pressure helps prevent strokes, heart attacks, and kidney problems.

A study undertaken by the College of Pharmacy at the University of Arizona evaluated the effects of clonidine on patients with autism. The trial lasted four weeks and involved male autistic patients between the ages of 5 to 33. Researchers observed the patients in seven, 20 to 30 minute intervals and rated the patients in five categories of social relationships, sensory responses, effectual reactions, language ability, and sensory motor behavior. At the end of the trial, researchers noted improvement in the categories of social relationships, sensory responses, and effectual reactions due to the administration of clonidine. The drug was also effective in reducing the severity of the illness. It has a calming effect on patients, enabling them to carry out social interactions, and minimizes inattention and repetitive behaviors. However, clonidine causes substantial fatigue and sedation.

For more information see page 1108.

Generic: *Cyproheptadine* (si-proe-HEP-ta-deen)
Brand: *Periactin*

Cyproheptadine is an antihistamine that provides relief of seasonal and nonseasonal allergy symptoms such as watery and itchy eyes, runny nose, and sneezing. It is also used to relieve itching and hives due to some skin conditions.

In an eight-week trial at Tehran University of Medical Sciences, assessment of the effects of cyproheptadine plus haloperidol in the treatment of autism was undertaken. Children between the ages three and 11 years with a clinical diagnosis of autism and severely disruptive symptoms related to autistic disorder received either cyproheptadine/haloperidol (Group A) or haloperidol/placebo (Group B). Patients were assessed by a third-year resident of psychiatry at the start of the study and after two, four, six, and eight weeks of starting medication. The primary measure of the outcome was the Aberrant Behavior Checklist-Community (ABC-C) and the secondary measure of the outcome was the Childhood Autism Rating Scale (relating to people and verbal communication).

The ABC-C and the Childhood Autism Rating Scale scores improved with cyproheptadine. No significant difference in neurological side effects was observed between the two groups. The results suggest that the combination of cyproheptadine with a conventional antipsychotic may be superior to conventional antipsychotic alone for children with autistic disorder.

For more information see page 1128.

*Generic: **Haloperidol** (ha-loe-PER-i-dole)*
*Brands: **Haldol, Haldol Deconoate***

Haloperidol is used to treat symptoms of certain types of mental health conditions such as schizophrenia to control movements or effects of Tourette's syndrome, or to control severe behavioral problems in children.

For autistic patients who have excess motor activity associated with autism, haloperidol is a helpful treatment. It is a dopamine antagonist (meaning that it affects the part of the brain that controls motor behaviors). A study by the Department of Psychiatry at New York University Medical Center evaluated learning and behavioral symptoms in patients with autism who were treated with haloperidol. The study consisted of 40 autistic children. Researchers found that haloperidol significantly decreased negative behavior and reduced hyperactivity and fidgetiness, which in turn affected the children's learning. Thirty-six parents of the patients requested that their child remain on haloperidol after the conclusion of the study.

In a follow-up study conducted five years later to assess whether the findings from the original trial would be replicated, a total of 45 autistic children were studied. Researchers examined the effects of haloperidol and concluded that the patients exhibited calmness without sedation and had decreases in hyperactivity, temper tantrums, and withdrawal. Overall, researchers concluded that chronic administration of haloperidol is therapeutically effective for up to 4.5 years, allowing autistic children to remain with their families and in educational programs. However, an adverse effect of long-term use of haloperidol may be the inducing of tardive dyskinesia (uncontrolled facial tics). For this reason, this drug must be monitored by your physician.

For more information see page 1217.

*Generic: **Methylphenidate** (meth-il-FEN-i-date)*
*Brands: **Concerta, Metadate CD, Metadate ER, Methylin, Methylin ER, Ritalin, Ritalin LA, Ritalin-SR***

Methylphenidate is used to treat attention disorders (attention deficit hyperactivity disorder, or ADHD) as part of a total treatment plan including psychological, educational, and social measures. This medication is a mild stimulant that works by affecting the levels of chemicals (neurotransmitters) in the nervous system.

Thirteen children with autism and symptoms of attention-deficit hyperactivity disorder (ADHD) participated in a study by the University of Pittsburgh School of Medicine to evaluate the effects of methylphenidate. Eight subjects responded positively, based upon a minimum 50% decrease on a scale that measures symptoms. Ratings of stereotypy (repetitive behavior that does not appear to be a function of social consequence) and inappropriate speech, which are often associated with autistic core features, also decreased. However, no changes were found on the Child Autism Rating Scale, another global assessment scale of autistic symptomatology. Significant adverse side effects occurred in some children, including social withdrawal and irritability. Results suggest that methylphenidate can be effective for children with autism and ADHD symptoms, but this group of children seems particularly susceptible to adverse side effects.

For more information see page 1315.

Generic: *Olanzapine* (oh-LAN-za-peen)
Brand: **Zyprexa, Zyprexa Zydis**

Olanzapine is a medication used to treat certain mental/mood conditions (schizophrenia, bipolar mania). It works by helping to restore the balance of certain natural chemicals in the brain (neurotransmitters).

Conventional neuroleptic drugs alleviate symptoms in children with autistic disorder; however, they are known to cause dyskinesias (uncontrolled facial tics). Olanzapine may have less risk for dyskinesia, but its efficacy in autistic disorder has not been established. A study at MCP Hahnemann University in Philadelphia was designed to investigate the safety and effectiveness of olanzapine as a treatment for children with autistic disorder by using haloperidol as a comparison treatment. In a parallel groups design, 12 children with autistic disorder received six weeks of treatment with either olanzapine or haloperidol. Outcomes were measured on the Clinical Global Impressions (CGI) scale and the Children's Psychiatric Rating Scale (CPRS). Both groups' symptoms were reduced. Five of six in the olanzapine group and three of six in the haloperidol group were rated as responders according to the CGI scale. Subjects showed improvement on the CPRS Autism Factor. Side effects included drowsiness and weight gain. Researchers concluded that these findings suggest that olanzapine is a promising treatment for children with autistic disorder.

For more information see page 1381.

Generic: **Pimozide** *(PI-moe-zide)*
Generic: **Orap**

Pimozide works in the nervous system to help control involuntary or unconscious movements (tics) both physical and verbal. It is used to reduce tics in persons with Tourette's Disorder.

A study was conducted at New York University School of Medicine to explore the efficacy and safety of pimozide, over a three-week period, in 8 hospitalized autistic children. Intellectual functioning ranged from moderate to profound mental retardation. Symptoms included severe withdrawal, stereotypes, hyperactivity and/or hypoactivity, aggressiveness, and temper tantrums. Decreases of behavioral symptoms appeared on all measures including the Children's Psychiatric Rating Scale, Clinical Global Impressions, and Global Clinical Judgments Scale. Of the five hypoactive children, four showed a decrease in hypoactivity, whereas one child worsened. Researchers concluded that these findings are promising and indicate the need for further study.

For more information see page 1416.

Generic: **Risperidone** *(RIS-peer-i-dohn)*
Brands: **Risperdal, Risperdal M-TAB**

Risperidone is typically used to treat schizophrenia and bipolar disorder (manic phase). It works by helping to restore the balance of certain natural substances in the brain (neurotransmitters).

Risperidone has been used for the management of severe behavioral problems associated with autistic disorders. Results of studies indicate that risperidone is an effective treatment for decreasing some of the more disruptive behavioral problems such as aggression, anger, uncooperativeness, hyperactivity, self-injurious behavior, and tantrums in children and adolescents (5–17 years of age) with autistic disorder. Although not curative, medicines such as risperidone generally are used to facilitate the child's adjustment and engagement in intensive, targeted educational programs. Risperidone has not been shown to improve the core symptoms of autism such as language deficits and social withdrawal and some clinicians state the drug should be reserved for treating moderate to severe behavioral problems associated with autistic disorders. The possible risks of weight gain, involuntary movements, and other reactions associated with the drug should be considered.

For more information see page 1456.

Generic: **Ziprasidone** *(ze-PRAZ-eh-don)*
Brand: **Geodon**

Ziprasidone is used to treat schizophrenia. A preliminary evaluation of the safety and effectiveness of ziprasidone in children, adolescents and young adults with autism was conducted at the Indiana University School of Medicine. Twelve patients with autism or received treatment with ziprasidone for at least six weeks. Six of the 12 patients were considered responders based on a Clinical Global Impression Scale rating of "much improved" or "very much improved." Temporary sedation was the most common side effect. No cardiovascular side effects, including chest pain were reported. Five patients lost weight, five had no change, one gained weight, and one had no follow-up weight measured. Significant weight gain was not observed in this short-term trial.

Researchers concluded that ziprasidone appears to have the potential for improving symptoms of aggression, agitation, and irritability in children, adolescents and young adults with autism.

For more information see page 1551.

Childhood Anxiety

All children experience anxiety, which is expected and normal at specific developmental stages. For example, from approximately age eight months through the preschool years, healthy youngsters may show intense distress when separated from their parents or other persons with whom they are close. Young children may have short-lived fears such as fear of the dark, storms, animals, or strangers. If anxieties become severe and begin to interfere with the daily activities of childhood, such as separating from parents, attending school and making friends, evaluation and advice from a child or adolescent psychiatrist may be needed. Drug treatment in children and adolescents must take into account the child's environmental influences and be part of an overall treatment plan where individual, familial, and cultural issues are addressed.

Commonly Prescribed (On-Label) Drugs: None

OFF-LABEL PRESCRIPTION DRUGS
BREAKTHROUGH OPTIONS

Generic: **Clomipramine** *(kloe-MI-pra-meen)*
Brand: **Anafranil**

Clomipramine is an antidepressant with antidepressant and antiobsessional properties used in the treatment of obsessive compulsive disorders (OCD). It may take two to three weeks before the full effects of this medication are noticed. Although it is not known how clomipramine affects OCD or other anxiety-related illness, it does have a mild sedative effect, which researchers think may be helpful in alleviating the anxiety component often accompanying depression. Increasing evidence supports the use of tricyclic antidepressants such as clomipramine in conjunction with therapy to treat childhood anxiety disorders. Generally, clomipramine is well tolerated by children and adolescents.

For more information see page 1105.

Generic: **Fluoxetine** *(floo-OKS-e-teen)*
Brands: **Prozac, Prozac Weekly, Sarafem**

Fluoxetine is a selective serotonin reuptake inhibitor (SSRI) used to treat depression, obsessive-compulsive disorder, panic attacks, certain eating disorders (bulimia), and a severe form of premenstrual syndrome.

Researchers have found that effective treatment of childhood anxiety disorders with medications may improve functioning and stress management. There are many reviews, but few studies, that examine the effect of psychotropic medication on anxiety disorders in children and adolescents. Most of the understanding comes from literature on adult medication trials. Available data indicate relative effectiveness of serotonin selective reuptake inhibitors in many childhood anxiety disorders, along with minimal side effects and good tolerability. Many other psychotropic medications have been considered and used to manage anxiety.

The SSRIs are considered a first-line therapeutic treatment for anxiety disorders in children and adolescents. Numerous other psychotropic medications may be considered, alone or in combination. However, this treatment must be used under the guidance of your physician as there are reports of SSRIs, most notably fluoxetine, causing suicide, hallucinations, and other serious adverse effects.

For more information see page 1192.

Generic: **Fluvoxamine** *(floo-VOKS-a-meen)*
Brand: **Luvox**

Social anxiety is the third largest psychological problem in the United States. It is believed that social anxiety, or social phobia, affects 15 million Americans a year, many of them teenagers. Fluvoxamine is used to treat obsessive-compulsive disorders (OCD). There has been a great deal of excitement about the publication of the RUPP Anxiety Study, demonstrating efficacy for fluvoxamine in socially phobic (SP) youth. Given that SP starts in childhood and adolescence, researchers believe more data are needed to support the use of drug treatment in this age group. Additional research needed includes: more investigation into what is required for social phobic individuals who respond well to medication and move into full remission; comparing the effectiveness of different drugs; research to help doctors predict how people will respond to a particular type of treatment; research of treatment resistance; and research on combining two types of effective treatments together.

For more information see page 1199.

Generic: **Sertraline** *(SER-tra-leen)*
Brand: **Zoloft**

Sertraline is a selective serotonin reuptake inhibitor (SSRI) used to treat depression, panic attacks, and other disorders.

A study at Duke University Medical Center was undertaken to assess the therapeutic benefits, response pattern, and safety of sertraline in children with social anxiety disorder. Fourteen children with a diagnosis of social anxiety disorder were treated in an eight-week trial of sertraline. Diagnostic and primary outcome measures included the Anxiety Disorders Interview Schedule for Children, Clinical Global Impressions scale (CGI), Social Phobia and Anxiety Inventory for Children, and a standardized behavioral avoidance test.

As measured by the CGI (Improvement subscale), 36% (5/14) of subjects were classified as treatment responders and 29% (4/14) as partial responders by the end of the eight-week trial. Self-report and behavioral measures showed significant clinical improvement into normal range across all domains measured. Sertraline was generally well tolerated. In this study researchers concluded that sertraline resulted in significant improvement in symptoms of childhood social anxiety disorder.

For more information see page 1468.

MISCELLANEOUS DISORDERS

Bone Cysts

Simple bone cysts are fluid-filled cavities in the bone. They occur most often in children and in the long bones of the arms or legs. The cause is not known, but the cysts are not related to cancer. A bone cyst may weaken the affected bone, increasing the risk of fracture. Bone cysts usually do not cause symptoms and are often discovered only after a fracture of the affected bone. They may also be detected incidentally on an x-ray done for some other reason.

Commonly Prescribed (On-Label) Drugs: *None*

OFF-LABEL PRESCRIPTION DRUG
BREAKTHROUGH OPTION

Generic: **Calcitonin** *(kal-si-TOE-nin)*
Brands: **Miacalcin, Miacalcin Spray**

Calcitonin is a medication used to treat brittle bone disease (osteoporosis) in women who are at least five years past menopause. Calcitonin works by slowing bone loss to help maintain strong bones and reduce risk of fractures.

A case report published in the *American Journal of Neuroradiology* by physicians at West Virginia University, documented a case of an 11-year-old girl presenting with neck pain and diagnosed as having a bone cyst. Minimally invasive treatment was performed with injections of calcitonin and methylprednisolone, two injections separated in time by two months. The cyst completely resolved over a period of six months, indicating injections should be tried first or as an add-on therapy to surgery for treating these benign tumors, especially those in the spine where treatment can involve complex, risky surgery.

For more information see page 1063.

Croup

Croup is an infection that causes the trachea (windpipe) and larynx (voice box) to swell. Usually part of a cold, croup causes fever, hoarseness, and a barking, hacking cough. It also may cause a crowing noise (called stridor) when the child breathes in through the narrowed windpipe. Croup usually lasts five to six days and symptoms most commonly occur in children one to three years old. Symptoms may be worse at night.

Commonly Prescribed (On-Label) Drugs: *None*

OFF-LABEL PRESCRIPTION DRUG
BREAKTHROUGH OPTION

Generic: **Dexamethasone** *(deks-a-METH-a-sone)*
Brands: **Decadron, Dexameth, Dexone, Hexadrol**

Dexamethasone reduces swelling and inflammation and is used for skin diseases, allergic conditions, breathing problems, cancer, blood disorders, digestive problems, eye disorders, and arthritis/bursitis.

Viral croup is the most common cause of upper airway obstruction in children six months to six years of age. Parainfluenza virus accounts for the majority of cases. The disease is characterized by varying degrees of inspiratory stridor, barking cough, and hoarseness because of laryngeal and/or tracheal obstruction. Treatment has altered dramatically in the past decade. Good evidence supports the routine use of a corticosteroid such as dexamethasone in all children with croup. Intervention at an earlier phase of the illness reduces the severity of the symptoms and returns to a health care practitioner for additional medical attention, visits to the emergency department, and admission to the hospital. Most children respond to a single, oral dose of dexamethasone. For those who do not tolerate the oral preparation, nebulized budesonide or intramuscular dexamethasone are reasonable alternatives.

For more information see page 1138.

Hemangioma

Hemangiomas are tufts of extra blood vessels that commonly occur in children, usually on the surface of the skin (strawberry hemangiomas). Those that are deeper in the skin are sometimes called cavernous hemangiomas. Some are mixed strawberry and cavernous hemangiomas. Most children with hemangiomas have only one. Many have a few. Rarely, children have many, both on the skin and in the internal organs. Some have enough extra vascular tissue to cause anemia or platelet problems.

Commonly Perscribed (On-Label) Drugs: *None*

OFF-LABEL PRESCRIPTION DRUGS
BREAKTHROUGH OPTIONS

Generic: **Imiquimod** *(i-mi-KWI-mod)*
Brand: **Aldara**

Imiquimod is a medication used to treat precancerous and cancerous skin conditions. It is also used to treat external genital and anal warts (or condyloma). It is not recommended for use to remove human papilloma virus (HPV) growths.

A case report published by physicians at Case Western Reserve University School of Medicine treated a four-month-old girl with infantile hemangioma affecting the chest wall. The lesion had appeared one week after birth, and was rapidly enlarging. It had also become painful. Treatment with topical 5% imiquimod cream three times a week after 10 days, and it completely disappeared after 10 weeks of therapy. The treatment was well tolerated.

In another study, ten patients with superficial infantile hemangiomas were treated with imiquimod 5% cream for up to 16 weeks. Four patients achieved complete clinical resolution, three had excellent improvement, one showed moderate improvement, and one patient did not respond to therapy. Researchers concluded that imiquimod may be an effective alternative for the treatment of superficial hemangiomas.

For more information see page 1233.

Generic: **Interferon alpha-2A**
(in-ter-FEER-on AL-fa-too-aye)
Brand: **Roferon-A**

Interferon alfa is used in the treatment of malignant melanoma, hairy cell leukemia, chronic hepatitis B, chronic hepatitis C, non-Hodgkin's lymphoma, and AIDS related Kaposi's sarcoma. Interferons are natural proteins produced by the body's cells in response to viral infections.

Many studies have shown the efficacy of interferon alpha 2A in the treatment of hemangiomas. It is believed to inhibit migrant endothelial cells, the cells that compose the inside of blood vessels. Interferon alpha 2A has been prescribed to treat lesions that are unresponsive to steroids. Adverse side effects of using interferon alpha 2A include potential irreversible spastic diplegia, a stiffness in the limbs categorized by weak, stiff, or clumsy legs.

For more information see page 1241.

Nocturnal Enuresis (Bedwetting)

See Kidney and Urinary Tract Disorders

Pediculosis Capitis (Head Lice)

There are three common types of lice: head lice, body lice, and pubic lice (also called crabs). Head lice infect the scalp hair and are easiest to see at the nape of the neck and over the ears. Tiny eggs can be seen on the hair, appearing much like flakes of dandruff, but stuck firmly to the hair shaft instead of flaking off of the scalp. Lice can also live on clothing, carpets, or bedding. Head lice are spread very easily and cause intense itching, but they do not lead to a serious medical problem. More common in close, overcrowded living conditions, lice also spread readily among school children.

Commonly Prescribed (On-Label) Drugs: *Lindane, Malathion, Permethrin, Undecylenic Acid*

OFF-LABEL PRESCRIPTION DRUG
BREAKTHROUGH OPTION

Generic: ***Ivermectin*** *(eye-ver-MEK-tin)*
Brand: ***Stromectol***

Ivermectin is used to treat infections due to certain parasites. Pediculosis and scabies are caused by ectoparasites; patients usually seek help with itching. Head and pubic lice infestations are diagnosed by the appearance of insects or eggs. Primary treatment is topically administered 1% permethrin. However ivermectin may be prescribed in a single dose for treatment of head lice that are resistant to conventional forms of treatment. It is absorbed into the blood and kills the lice but has no effect on the eggs, which must be physically removed with a nit comb.

For more information see page 1258.

Tachycardia

Tachycardia is an abnormally rapid beating of the heart, defined as a resting heart rate of over 100 beats per minute. It can have harmful effects in two ways. First, when the heart beats too rapidly, it performs inefficiently (since there is not enough time for the ventricles to fill completely), causing blood flow and blood pressure to diminish. Second, it increases the work of the heart, causing it to require more oxygen while also reducing the blood flow to the cardiac muscle tissue, increasing the risk of ischemia and resultantly infarction.

Commonly Prescribed (On-Label) Drugs: *None*

OFF-LABEL PRESCRIPTION DRUG
BREAKTHROUGH OPTION

Generic: ***Magnesium Sulfate*** *(mag-NEE-zhum SUL-fate)*
Brand: ***Magnesium Sulfate***

Magnesium sulfate is most commonly used to control seizures in pregnancy, to treat low magnesium levels and problems related to kidney conditions in children. It is also used for preventing premature contractions in pregnancy and to treat heart attack and asthma patients.

Intravenous administration of magnesium sulfate is a very effective, safe treatment for Torsades de Pointes, a type of tachycardia associated with acquired long Q-T syndrome, a hereditary disorder that affects the heart's electrical rhythm. The optimal magnesium sulphate dosage and serum magnesium were determined in six children with Torsades de Pointes; four had congenital long Q-T syndrome and two had acquired long Q-T syndrome. They received an injection of magnesium sulfate over one to two minutes followed by continuous infusion for the next two to seven days. Of the six patients, five responded completely to the initial injections. One required a higher dose of the drug until Torsades de Pointes completely stopped. Therefore, intravenous magnesium sulfate infusion effectively treated Torsades de Pointes in children with long Q-T syndrome.

For more information see page 1292.

NEONATAL AND INFANT DISORDERS

Bronchopulmonary Dysplasia

Bronchopulmonary dysplasia (BPD) is a chronic lung disease of babies, which develops most commonly in the first four weeks after birth. It mostly occurs in babies who are born more than four weeks before their due dates, though sometimes the babies are full term. In BPD, the lungs do not work properly and the babies have trouble breathing. They need extra oxygen and may even need help from a breathing machine. Doctors think babies get BPD because their lungs are sensitive to something damaging in the environment, such as oxygen, a breathing machine, or an infection.

Commonly Prescribed (On-Label) Drugs: *None*

OFF-LABEL PRESCRIPTION DRUGS
BREAKTHROUGH OPTIONS

Generic: **Albuterol** *(al-BYOO-ter-ole)*
Brand: **Proventil, Ventolin, Volmax**

Albuterol relaxes the smooth muscle in the lungs and dilates airways to improve breathing. It is used in the treatment of asthma, chronic bronchitis, and emphysema. The inhaler enables the drug to reach deep into the lungs for maximum benefit.

Bronchodilators are frequently used as part of the therapeutic regimen of ventilated preterm infants. There is conflicting evidence about the efficacy of bronchodilators such as albuterol. However, doctors usually administer the bronchodilators to children on a trial basis to assess response, which should be evaluated every 5 to 10 minutes. If improvement occurs, aerosol treatment may be continued. A study at Albert Einstein Medical Center identified the most efficient, cost-effective nebulizer device for delivery of albuterol aerosol as a bronchodilator in ventilated preterm infants. Fifty-three premature infants being ventilated for respiratory distress syndrome (RDS) were studied. Twenty-four received standard doses of albuterol aerosol via jet nebulizer and 29 via a metered dose inhaler. Heart rate, respiratory rate, oxygen saturation, lung compliance, and airway resistance were monitored prior and 15 minutes after albuterol delivery. There were significant changes in health between pre- and postnebulizer treatment. Both groups significantly improved lung function with a 13-24% reduction in airway resistance and three to seven percent increase in lung compliance. Oxygen saturations also increased. These findings suggest that both MDI-spacer and jet nebulizer are equally effective in delivering the albuterol aerosol to the lower respiratory tract.

For more information see page 991.

Generic: **Dexamethasone** *(deks-a-METH-a-sone)*
Brands: **Decadron, Dexameth, Dexone, Hexadrol**

Dexamethasone is a corticosteroid that reduces swelling and inflammation in a variety of disorders such as skin diseases, allergic conditions, breathing problems, cancer, blood disorders, digestive problems, eye disorders, and for arthritis/bursitis.

Bronchopulmonary dysplasia (BPD) is a common cause of death in preterm babies and at present its treatment is unclear. Over the past three decades there has been a growing use of corticosteroids in the postnatal period; first for the treatment and then, more recently, for the prevention of BPD. Dexamethasone has been the most frequently used corticosteroid in neonatal units, although others, including hydrocortisone, prednisolone and methylprednisolone, have been studied, as have inhaled corticosteroids. Research indicates that corticosteroids improve respiratory function in the short term. However, there is a high risk of hypertension, hyperglycemia, and gastrointestinal complications in corticosteroid-treated babies. If administered in the first four days of life, the drug is associated with long-term neurodevelopmental delay. Corticosteroid use should be limited to exceptional clinical circumstances, such as a ventilator-dependent infant after the second week of life who cannot be weaned from ventilation and whose condition is worsening. If used, they should be prescribed at the lowest effective dose for the shortest possible time.

For more information see page 1138.

Generic: **Furosemide** *(fyoor-OH-se-mide)*
Brand: **Lasix**

Furosemide is a "water pill" (diuretic) that increases the amount of urine made, which causes the body to get rid of excess water and is used to treat high blood pressure. A study by researchers at Albert Einstein College of Medicine and Montefiore Medical Center reviewed the risks and benefits of diuretics in pre-term infants with or developing chronic lung disease (CLD). In pre-term infants greater than three weeks of age with CLD, a four-week treatment with thiazide and spironolactone improved lung compliance and reduced the need for furosemide. The drugs decreased the risk of death and tended to decrease the risk for lack of extubation after eight weeks in intubated infants who did not have access to corticosteroids, bronchodilators, or aminophylline. However, there is little or no evidence to support any benefit of diuretic administration on need for ventilatory support, length of hospital stay, or long-term outcome in patients receiving current therapy. No evidence supports adding spironolactone to thiazide, or adding metolazone to furosemide to improve the health of preterm infants with CLD. Therefore, in preterm infants greater than three weeks of age with CLD, acute and chronic administration of diuretics improve pulmonary mechanics.

For more information see page 1204.

Generic: **Ipratropium** *(i-pra-TROE-pee-um)*
Brand: **Atrovent, Atrovent HFA**

Ipratropium is used to treat lung diseases such as chronic bronchitis and emphysema. It relaxes the muscles around the airways so that they open up for easier breathing.

Chronic lung disease (CLD) occurs frequently in preterm infants. Bronchodilators have the potential to dilate small airways with muscle hypertrophy and might have a role in the prevention and treatment of CLD. A review of the medical literature by British researchers was conducted to evaluate the effect of bronchodilators, given preventively or as treatment for chronic lung disease, on mortality and other complications of preterm births. Initiation of bronchodilator therapy such as ipratropium had to occur within two weeks of birth for it to be effective. Researchers concluded that ipratropium could be a promising treatment for prevention of CLD.

For more information see page 1245.

Congenital Adrenal Hyperplasia

Congenital adrenal hyperplasia is a group of recessive disorders resulting from the deficiency of one of the five enzymes required for the synthesis of the hormone cortisol in the adrenal cortex. The most frequent is steroid 21-hydroxylase deficiency, accounting for more than 90% of cases. A severe form may have symptoms that include alterations in sexual maturation.

Commonly Prescribed (On-Label) Drugs: *Betamethasone, Cortisone, Dexamethasone, Fludrocortisone, Methylprednisolone, Prednisolone, Prednisone, Triamcinolone*

OFF-LABEL PRESCRIPTION DRUGS
BREAKTHROUGH OPTIONS

Generic: ***Flutamide*** *(FLOO-ta-mide)*
Brand: ***Eulexin***

Flutamide is a nonsteroidal antiandrogen. For the treatment of congenital adrenal hyperplasia, a new four-drug treatment regimen of flutamide, testolactone, reduced hydrocortisone dose and fludrocortisone has been shown to achieve normal growth and development after two years of therapy and may, therefore, represent a potential alternative approach to the treatment of children with this disease.

An investigation published in the *Journal of Endocrinology and Metabolism* reported on the effect of flutamide and testolactone versus flutamide alone on cortisol clearance in 13 children with classic 21-hydroxylase deficiency. The results showed that total body cortisol clearance was significantly lower during treatment with the four-drug regimen than during treatment with hydrocortisone and fludrocortisone.

For more information see page 1196.

*Generic: **Hydrocortisone** (HI-dro-KOR-ti-sone)*
*Brand: **Cortef***

Hydrocortisone is a medication called a corticosteroid. It reduces swelling. It is used for many conditions, including skin diseases and breathing problems.

Children with classic 21-hydroxylase deficiency require long-term glucocorticoid treatment to inhibit factors stimulated by the lack of missing steroids. The therapeutic goal is to use the lowest dose of glucocorticoid that adequately suppresses adrenal androgens and maintains normal growth and weight gain.

During the past 50 years since the discovery of cortisone therapy as an effective treatment for congenital adrenal hyperplasia (CAH), many advances have been made in the management of 21-hydroxylase deficiency. Despite these advances, the clinical management of patients with CAH is often complicated by other problems. New treatment approaches to classic CAH attempt to address these unresolved issues. At the National Institutes of Health, a clinical trial is investigating a new treatment regimen: a reduced hydrocortisone dose, an antiandrogen and an aromatase inhibitor. Peripheral blockade of androgens may also be helpful in the adult woman with CAH. Other promising new treatment approaches are also under investigation.

For more information see page 1222.

*Generic: **Testolactone** (tes-toe-LAK-tone)*
*Brand: **Teslac***

Treatment of congenital adrenal hyperplasia is not always completely successful due to a condition known as hyperandrogenism, which is caused by elevated levels of male sexual hormones in females. A study of a new four-drug treatment regimen containing flutamide, testolactone, reduced hydrocortisone dose and fludrocortisone showed better control of linear growth, weight gain, and bone maturation compared to the effects of a control regimen of hydrocortisone and fludrocortisone. Twenty-eight children have completed a two-year follow-up in a subsequent study comparing these two treatments. During two years of therapy, children receiving flutamide, testolactone, reduced hydrocortisone dose and fludrocortisone had significantly higher hormone levels. However, children receiving the new treatment regimen had normal growth rate and bone maturation and showed no significant adverse effects. Researchers concluded that the regimen of flutamide, testolactone, reduced hydrocortisone dose and fludrocortisone provides effective control of congenital adrenal hyperplasia with reduced risk of increasing levels of glucocorticoid, a steroid hormone.

For more information see page 1500.

Hyaline Membrane Disease of the Newborn

See Respiratory Distress Syndrome

Intraventricular Hemorrhage

Intraventricular hemorrhage (IVH) is bleeding inside or around the ventricles, the spaces in the brain containing cerebral spinal fluid. Intraventricular means within the ventricles, and hemorrhage means excessive bleeding. Intraventricular hemorrhage is most common in premature babies, especially very low birthweight babies weighing less than 1,500 grams (three pounds, four ounces).

Commonly Prescribed (On-Label) Drugs: None

OFF-LABEL PRESCRIPTION DRUG
BREAKTHROUGH OPTION

---

*Generic: **Indomethacin** (in-doe-METH-a-sin)*
*Brands: **Indocin, Indocin I.V., Indocin SR***

Indomethacin treats the pain, swelling and stiffness associated with arthritis, gout, bursitis, or tendonitis. Preventive treatment with indomethacin has been shown to effectively reduce the rate of intraventricular hemorrhage in pre-term babies, but there is the potential for unwanted side effects. A review of the medical literature between 1966 and 2002 was undertaken by researchers in Scotland to examine the effect of preventive indomethacin on death rates of preterm infants. Of nineteen trials, four reported long-term effects of indomethacin, including a reduction in the rate of severe intraventricular hemorrhage; no short-term gastrointestinal or renal adverse effects were detected. There was no significant difference between indomethacin and control groups in the important long-term outcome of death. Therefore, preventive indomethacin has a number of short-term benefits for the pre-term infant, but there is no evidence that it results in an improvement in the rate of survival free of disability.

For more information see page 1238.

Neonatal Apnea

The standard definition of apnea is cessation of inspiratory gas flow for 20 seconds, or for a shorter period of time if accompanied by bradycardia (heart rate less than 100 beats per minute), cyanosis, or pallor. Apnea has been classified into three types depending on whether there is activity of the muscles that act during inspiration, also known as inspiratory muscle activity. If inspiratory muscle activity fails following an exhalation, it is termed Central Apnea. If inspiratory muscle activity is present without airflow, this is termed Obstructive Apnea. If both central and obstructive apnea occurs during the same episode, this is termed Mixed Apnea.

Before a diagnosis of apnea of prematurity (AOP) is made, and treatment initiated, all causes of secondary apnea must be ruled out. Treatment will depend on the cause as well as effectiveness and tolerability of the treatment by the child. The primary goal of any treatment of AOP is to prevent the frequency of apnea lasting greater than 20 seconds and/or those that are shorter, but associated with cyanosis and bradycardia.

Commonly Prescribed (On-Label) Drugs: None

OFF-LABEL PRESCRIPTION DRUGS
BREAKTHROUGH OPTION

Generic: **Theophylline** *(theo-FILL-in)*
Brands: **Bronkodyl, Quibron-T, Theo-24, Theochron, Theolair**

Theophylline relaxes smooth muscle of the respiratory tract, producing relief of bronchospasm and increasing flow rates and vital capacity. This medication improves breathing by opening air passages in the lungs. It is typically used in the treatment of asthma, chronic bronchitis, and emphysema. Methylxanthines such as theophylline are the most widely used drugs to manage AOP. Due to the wider therapeutic use of caffeine and ease of once-daily administration, it should be the preferred drug.

For more information see page 1507.

Patent Ductus Arteriosus

The ductus arteriosus is a normal fetal structure, allowing blood to bypass circulation to the lungs. Since the fetus does not use his/her lungs (oxygen is provided through the mother's placenta), flow from the right ventricle needs an outlet. The ductus provides this, shunting flow from the left pulmonary artery to the aorta just beyond the origin of the artery to the left subclavian artery. The high levels of oxygen it is exposed to after birth causes it to close in most cases within 24 hours. When it does not close, it is termed a patent ductus arteriosus.

Commonly Prescribed (On-Label) Drugs: Indomethacin

OFF-LABEL PRESCRIPTION DRUG
BREAKTHROUGH OPTION

Generic: **Ibuprofen** *(eye-byoo-PROE-fen)*
Brands: **Motrin, Ultraprin**

Ibuprofen is a nonsteroidal anti-inflammatory drug (NSAID), which relieves pain and swelling. It is used to treat headaches, muscle aches, backaches, dental pain, menstrual cramps, arthritis, or athletic injuries, and to reduce fever and minor aches due to the common cold or flu.

Indomethacin is commonly used for the treatment of PDA but has renal failure as a main side effect. Ibuprofen seems to be efficient in closing the ductus with fewer side effects, but few studies are available in literature regarding its use in preterm infants. A study analyzed data to compare the efficacy and tolerability of ibuprofen and indomethacin for the treatment of PDA administered to preterm infants. Ibuprofen was found to be as efficient as indomethacin and could be an alternative treatment. NSAID treatment was found to affect, at least transiently, renal function. Further studies are needed to assess whether ibuprofen is really less nephrotoxic than indomethacin. It should be noted that intravenously administered ibuprofen is not commercially available in the United States.

For more information see page 1228.

Respiratory Distress Syndrome

Respiratory distress syndrome (RDS) is a life-threatening lung disorder that commonly affects premature infants. RDS results from insufficient levels of surfactant, a foamy fluid substance produced by the body between the 34 and 37 week of pregnancy. Surfactant is essential for the expansion of the alveoli or air sacs of the lungs. When an infant is born prematurely, his or her lungs have not produced the necessary amount of surfactant. Without surfactant, the lungs cannot inflate, resulting in RDS.

Commonly Prescribed (On-Label) Drugs: Beractant, Calfactant, Colfosceril, Poractant alfa

---

OFF-LABEL PRESCRIPTION DRUG
BREAKTHROUGH OPTION

Generic: **Methylprednisolone** *(meth-il-pred-NIS-oh-lone)*
Brands: **Depo-Medrol, Medrol, Solu-Medrol**

Methylprednisolone is typically used to treat a number of conditions such as allergic disorders, arthritis, blood diseases, breathing problems, certain cancers, eye diseases, intestinal disorders, and skin diseases. It decreases the body's immune response to these diseases and reduces symptoms such as swelling and redness.

Corticosteroids such as methylprednisolone are powerful drugs increasingly used in the perinatal and neonatal period. A single course of antenatal corticosteroids in women at risk of premature delivery is highly effective in reducing respiratory distress syndrome (RDS), intraventricular hemorrhage, and neonatal mortality, and also neurodevelopmental problems including cerebral palsy. However, there is less evidence to support the practice of multiple courses of corticosteroids, with some animal and human studies suggesting an association with neurological impairment and reduction in birth weight as well as lung weight. Systemic corticosteroids may have a role in infants who had repeated and required prolonged intubations and those with low blood pressure requiring medications for support. Alternative strategies for prevention of chronic lung disease, such as inhaled steroids, methylprednisolone and hydrocortisone, may need further studies.

For more information see page 1316.

SEIZURES AND SPASM DISORDERS

Epilepsy

See Seizure

Convulsion

See Seizure

Convulsions with fever

See Febrile Seizure, Prevention

Fit

See Seizure

Febrile Convulsion

See Febrile Seizure, Prevention

Febrile Seizure, Prevention

Febrile seizures are relatively common in children younger than five years old. Febrile seizures can occur when a child develops a high fever, usually with the temperature rising rapidly to 102 degrees Fahrenheit or more. While terrifying to parents, these seizures are usually brief and rarely cause any problems, unless the fever is associated with a serious infection, such as meningitis. A child who has a febrile seizure is *not* more likely to develop epilepsy.

Commonly Prescribed (On-Label) Drugs: None

OFF-LABEL PRESCRIPTION DRUG
BREAKTHROUGH OPTION

Generic: **Primidone** *(PRI-mi-done)*
Brand: **Mysoline**

Primidone is used to treat a seizure disorder. Researchers in Japan conducted a study of 196 children with febrile convulsions. Sixty nine were placed on phenobarbital, twice per day and 32 on primidone twice a day. The remaining 95 children were given sodium valproate. Recurrence of febrile convulsions during one year was not different among these five groups.

For more information see page 1432.

Seizures

Seizures are caused by abnormal electrical discharges in the brain. Symptoms may vary depending on the part of the brain that is stimulated, but seizures may be associated with unusual sensations, uncontrollable muscle spasms and loss of consciousness. Some seizures may be the result of a medical problem. Low blood sugar, infection, a head injury, accidental poisoning, or drug overdose may cause a seizure. A seizure may also be due to a brain tumor or other neurological abnormality. In addition, anything that results in a sudden lack of oxygen to the brain can cause a seizure. In some cases, the cause of the seizure may not be discovered. When seizures recur, it may indicate the chronic condition known as epilepsy.

Commonly Prescribed (On-Label) Drugs: None

OFF-LABEL PRESCRIPTION DRUG
BREAKTHROUGH OPTION

Generic: **Midazolam** *(MID-aye-zoe-lam)*
Brand: **Versed**

Midazolam is used to relax and calm patients (generally children) before certain medical procedures or before anesthesia for surgery. It also helps decrease memory of the event. A study conducted by British researchers and published in *The Lancet* reported on rectal diazepam and buccal midazolam being used for emergency treatment of epileptic seizures in children with or without fever. The study compared the safety and efficacy of these drugs for emergency-room treatment of children aged six months and older arriving at the hospital with active seizures and without intravenous access. The dose varied according to age. Two hundred nineteen separate episodes involved 177 patients. Therapeutic success was 56% for buccal midazolam and 27% for rectal diazepam. Researchers concluded that buccal midazolam was more effective than rectal diazepam for children presenting to hospital with acute seizures and was not associated with an increased incidence of respiratory depression. Buccal midazolam is not available in the United States.

For more information see page 1325.

West Syndrome

Infantile spasm (IS) is a specific type of seizure seen in an epilepsy syndrome of infancy and early childhood known as West Syndrome. The onset is predominantly in the first year of life, typically between three to six months. The typical pattern of infantile spasm is a sudden bending forward and stiffening of the body, arms, and legs, although there can also be arching of the torso. Spasms tend to begin soon after arousal from sleep. Individual spasms typically last for one to five seconds and occur in clusters, ranging from two to 100 spasms at a time. Infants may have dozens of clusters and several hundred spasms per day. Infantile spasms usually stop by age five, but are often replaced by other seizure types. West Syndrome is characterized by infantile spasms, hypsarrhythmia (abnormal, chaotic brain wave patterns) and mental retardation. Other neurological disorders, such as cerebral palsy, may be seen in 30-50% of those with West Syndrome.

Commonly Prescribed (On-Label) Drugs: None

OFF-LABEL PRESCRIPTION DRUGS
BREAKTHROUGH OPTIONS

Generic: **Clonazepam** *(kloe-NA-ze-pam)*
Brand: **Klonopin**

Clonazepam is used to treat seizure disorders and panic attacks. It belongs to a class of medications called benzodiazepines, which act on the central nervous system to produce a calming effect.

West Syndrome is resistant to treatment to most conventional antiepileptic drugs and only valproic acid, benzodiazepines, adrenocorticotropic hormone (ACTH), corticosteroids and vigabatrin have been effective. Benzodiazepines, notably nitrazepam and clonazepam have been effective in bringing spasms under control but emerging tolerance and significant side effects (decreased tone of selected muscles and drowsiness) precluded its wider use.

For more information see page 1107.

Generic: **Corticotropin** *(cor-ti-COE-troe-pin)*
Brand: **HP Acthar Gel**

Corticotropin is used for the treatment of adrenal gland insufficiency as well as in patients with normal adrenocortical function for its anti-inflammatory and immunosuppressant properties.

A study published in the *Journal of Child Neurology* examined corticotropin in the treatment of infantile spasms to evaluate several questions about: (1) the efficacy of doses of corticotropin in comparison with other drugs, especially with vigabatrin, and the efficacy in patients with tuberous sclerosis (condition where benign tumors affect the central nervous system with symptoms of seizures and mental retardation); (2) tolerability; and (3) long-term outcome. In two reports, high doses were not more effective than low doses but were more effective in another study. In the follow-up of the studies, there was no difference. In another study, the efficacy and relapse rates of corticotropin and vigabatrin treatment did not differ significantly. The high response rates in tuberous sclerosis complex were similar. Both drugs had severe side effects. In the long-term follow-up of 20 to 35 years, one third of the patients died, the intellectual outcome of the remaining patients was normal or slightly subnormal, and one quarter and one third of the patients were seizure-free. Corticotropin should be the first choice for treatment of infantile spasms. The side effects of corticotropin, unlike those of vigabatrin, are well known, treatable, and reversible.

For more information see page 1117.

Generic: **Lamotrigine** and **Topiramate** *(la-MOE-tri-jeen)* and *(TOE-pie-rah-mate)*
Brands: **Lamictal** *(lamotrigine)* **and Topamax** *(topiramate)*

Lamotrigine and topiramate help control seizure disorders. Treatment of catastrophic epilepsies such as infantile spasms remains a challenge to clinicians. For infantile spasms, adrenocorticotropic hormone has traditionally been the drug of choice in the United States but may be associated with serious side effects in some patients. Newer antiepilepsy drugs, such as topiramate, and lamotrigine may be useful in children with infantile spasms.

A study conducted at the American University of Beirut in New York City evaluated the efficacy and tolerability of lamotrigine in children diagnosed with infantile spasms who were within their first year of life. Seven children with infantile spasms received lamotrigine for 3 months. Researchers observed that the rate of spasms decreased from 8.71 per day to 3.61. The researchers concluded that lamotrigine is effective in treating infants less than a year old who suffer from infantile spasms.

A study conducted at King Hussein Medical Center in Amman, Jordan assessed the efficacy and safety of topiramate in therapy-resistant epilepsies in infants and young children. A trial performed in three hospitals on 47 children aged six-60 months with therapy-resistant epilepsy rated the efficacy of the drug according to seizure type, frequency, and duration. Topiramate was introduced as add-on therapy in a daily dose for two weeks, followed by increments at two-week intervals.

After a minimum treatment period of six months, 28 (60%) of the children had a satisfactory response (completely seizure-free or more than a 50% seizure reduction). The remaining 19 children (40%) had an unsatisfactory response (50% or less reduction in seizure frequency, no change or increased seizure frequency). Topiramate appeared to be equally effective in infantile spasms, Lennox-Gastaut syndrome, and children with other types of epilepsy, with no significant difference between those with a satisfactory and an unsatisfactory response. Mild to moderate adverse effects, mainly somnolence, anorexia, and nervousness were present in 25 (53%) of children. One of the children developed hypothyroidism.

Although the long-term safety and possible adverse effects of topiramate have not been fully established in infants and young children, this study shows that it is a useful option for children with frequent seizures unresponsive to standard anti-epileptic drugs.

For more information see pages 1268 and 1516.

Generic: **Prednisone** *(pred-NIS-zone)*
Brands: **Deltasone, Liquid Pred, Meticorten, Orasone, Sterapred**

Prednisone decreases the immune system's response to various diseases to reduce symptoms such as swelling and allergic-type reactions. It is used to treat conditions such as arthritis, blood disorders, breathing problems, certain cancers, eye problems, immune system diseases, and skin diseases.

Steroids are often an effective treatment for West Syndrome, but there have been few reports of steroid use in children with epilepsy outside the first year of life. Twenty-eight children aged 18 months to 10 years with intractable epilepsy were studied at the University of Alberta in Canada. Prednisone (six weeks daily and six weeks alternate therapy) was prescribed in addition to their regular antiepileptic medications. The parents kept seizure diaries and the children were regularly assessed for seizure frequency and side effects.

The follow-up period was for one to five years. Thirteen patients (46%) became seizure-free on prednisone and another 18 (40%) had a significant decrease in seizure frequency. Five patients (19%) had no change in seizure frequency. The best outcomes were seen in the absence group in which six out of seven patients became seizure free and in the Lennox-Gastaut syndrome group, in which seven out of 10 became seizure-free.

Side effects were uncommon and included weight gain in five patients and aggression in four patients. Prednisone therapy is a safe and effective adjunctive treatment for epilepsy. It should be considered as an alternative treatment for older children with intractable generalized epilepsy who have failed conventional antiepileptic therapy.

For more information see page 1429.

DIGESTIVE DISORDERS

BLEEDING DISORDERS

The gastrointestinal system is lined with delicate mucous membranes. Any damage to that lining, whether from ulcers, malignancies, or other disorders, can cause acute or chronic bleeding which needs to be treated and its recurrence prevented.

Acute Upper Gastrointestinal Bleeding

Acute upper gastrointestinal bleeding is a medical emergency. If the bleeding is not stopped with medication, surgery will be required. If the bleeding is not stopped by medical or surgical means, you are at serious risk of death.

Commonly Prescribed (On-Label) Drugs: *None*

OFF-LABEL PRESCRIPTION DRUGS
BREAKTHROUGH OPTIONS

Generic: **Octreotide** *(ok-TREE-oh-tide)*
Brands: **Sandostatin, Sandostatin LAR**

Octreotide, which has similar effects to a natural hormone called somatostatin, is typically given by injection to suppress growth hormone. Octreotide is used to treat the flushing and diarrhea associated with certain intestinal tumors. It does not cure these tumors but helps you live a more normal life. It is also used to treat acromegaly, a hormonal disorder.

An article in the *Journal of Gastroenterology and Hepatology* from a hospital in China reported on a study comparing octreotide, vasopressin, and omeprazole in the treatment of acute bleeding in patients with acute bleeding of the stomach due to congestive charge in the gastric mucus, known as portal hypertensive gastropathy. They divided 66 patients to one of the three therapies. Four hours after the drugs were infused by a nasogastric tube (a plastic tube inserted through the nose, down the back of the throat, through the esophagus and into the stomach), bleeding was controlled in 100% of those receiving octreotide, 64% of those receiving vasopressin, and 59% of those receiving omeprazole. Those receiving octreotide also required fewer blood transfusions to control bleeding and had fewer side effects. Follow-up endoscopy (which involves inserting a flexible tube down the throat into the stomach so the doctor can see the inside of the stomach with a special camera) showed dramatic improvement in redness and ulceration. The investigators concluded that octreotide appeared to be more effective in controlling acute bleeding in patients with hypertensive gastropathy.

For more information see page 1380.

Generic: *Omeprazole* (oh-ME-pray-zol)
Brands: *Prilosec, Zegerid*

Omeprazole belongs to a class of drugs called proton pump inhibitors approved for treating ulcers, gastroesophageal reflux, and other conditions caused by excessive acid in the stomach. They completely block the production of stomach acid by shutting down a system in the stomach known as the proton pump.

An article in the *International Journal of Clinical Practice* from Hahnemann University in Philadelphia, reported on a study to assess the benefits of omeprazole versus ranitidine in the treatment of acute upper gastrointestinal bleeding. The diagnosis had been confirmed by endoscopy (a flexible tube inserted down the throat into the stomach so the doctor can see the inside of the stomach with a special camera). They divided 92 patients to take one of the two drugs. The patients all had ulcers of the stomach or the duodenum or erosive gastritis. Based on recurrence of bleeding, stabilization of the lesion by repeat endoscopy, and patients' length of stay in the intermediate medical care unit, the investigators concluded that omeprazole was more effective than ranitidine in the medical treatment of acute upper GI bleeding.

For more information see page 1386.

*Generic: **Vasopressin** (veh-SO-prez-in)*
*Brand: **Pitressin***

Vasopressin is a peptide hormone also known as antidiuretic hormone (ADH) because its single most important effect is to conserve body water by reducing the output of urine. Its only FDA-approved use is for the treatment of diabetes insipidus. However, it also causes severe constriction of blood vessels, which leads to its usefulness in acute GI bleeding.

An article in from Corning Hospital & Robert Packer Hospital reports that vasoconstrictive agents, such as vasopressin, can be used prior to surgery in cases of GI bleeding. Vasopressin reduces the blood flow and facilitates formation healing over of the bleeding vessel. Twenty-four patients were included in the study. In 22 of the patients, bleeding was controlled. Of these, 12 received no further therapy and were discharged. Three patients developed recurrent bleeding within two to 12 months of discharge. Vasopressin infusion was used as the sole treatment and stopped the bleeding in 36 to 100% of the cases. Because the recurrence rates fluctuated between 27 and 71%, vasopressin infusion was used to stabilize people prior to surgery. The results are less than satisfactory in people with severe atherosclerosis and bleeding problems. The researcher noted that patients with cardiac problems sometimes have complications that may be overcome with use of nitroglycerine paste or drip.

An article in the *Journal of Hepatology* from the University of Milan addressed this problem by comparing vasopressin plus transdermal nitroglycerin (a skin patch) versus terlipressin (which is only available in the United States as an orphan drug, a drug used in the treatment of rare diseases) in the treatment of digestive bleeding in patients with cirrhosis of the liver. Terlipressin is a prodrug, that is one that is not active itself but breaks down into an active drug, in this case into vasopressin. By slow release, it provides three to four hours of biological activity, as opposed to only a few minutes with vasopressin. The investigators found that the terlipressin group had fewer side effects but with equal benefits to the vasopressin group in a 24-hour evaluation of treatment of acute bleeding.

For more information see page 1540.

Anal Columns

See Rectal Bleeding

Gastrointestinal Bleeding

GI bleeding is a symptom not a disorder. It may be caused by a wide range of problems including ulcers, varices (like varicose veins), cancer, benign tumors, injuries, infections, inflammation, colitis, or other causes. It is a particular problem in the intestines when the site of the bleeding cannot be located.

Commonly Prescribed (On-Label) Drugs: None

OFF-LABEL PRESCRIPTION DRUG
BREAKTHROUGH OPTION

---

*Generic: **Thalidomide** (tha-LI-doe-mide)*
*Brand: **Thalomid***

Thalidomide was created as a drug to treat morning sickness in pregnant women, but it was found to cause terrible birth defects and then banned around the world. According to the National Institutes of Health (NIH), studies are also being conducted to determine the effectiveness of thalidomide in treating symptoms associated with AIDS, some cancers, Crohn's Disease, and a number of rheumatic diseases. Its benefits in cancer appear to be related to its ability to inhibit the growth of new blood vessels. It is that ability of thalidomide that is harnessed when it is used for the treatment of severe intestinal bleeding.

An article in *Gut* reported on a series of six elderly people treated at Charite University Hospital in Berlin, Germany, who had severe intestinal bleeding. All had not responded to conventional treatments. Extensive diagnostic procedures had been unable to identify the site of bleeding. Three of the patients had Crohn's disease. For all six patients, bleeding subsided within two weeks of initiation of thalidomide. Discontinuation after some months of therapy led to recurrence of bleeding, which stopped after re-initiation of therapy. The investigators concluded that thalidomide may be a valuable therapeutic option in those with severe gastrointestinal bleeding, and further therapeutic evaluation of thalidomide in this type of use is warranted.

For more information see page 1505.

Prevention of Recurrence of Upper GI Bleeding

After upper gastrointestinal bleeding has been brought under control, your physician must assess whether this is a condition that is likely to occur again. If it is concluded that recurrence is likely, medical or surgical steps must be taken to prevent recurrence to help prevent another crisis.

Commonly Prescribed (On-Label) Drugs: None

OFF-LABEL PRESCRIPTION DRUGS
BREAKTHROUGH OPTIONS

*Generic: **Famotidine** (fa-MOE-ti-deen)*
*Brand: **Pepcid***

Famotidine belongs to a class of drugs called H2 blockers because it inhibits the action of histamine on cells that block acid secretion in the stomach. It is approved for the treatment of duodenal and gastric ulcers, dyspepsia and heartburn and their prevention, and other conditions related to stomach acid secretion. Studies have found that it is also effective in the prevention of recurrent upper gastrointestinal bleeding.

An article in *Alimentary Pharmacological Therapy* from the Kawasaki Medical School in Japan reported on a study of famotidine versus omeprazole in the treatment of bleeding peptic ulcer. They divided 400 people to take one of the two therapies, given by intravenous infusion, and monitored the duration of fasting, hospital stay, volume of transfused blood, recurrences of bleeding, and death. While bleeding recurrences were not significantly different, the average hospital stay was significantly shorter in the omeprazole group (18.4 days) than in the famotidine group (21.5 days). However there was no significant difference in the other symptoms. Researchers conclude that the two drugs are equivalent for prevention of recurrent bleeding.

For more information see page 1181.

Generics: Proton Pump Inhibitors such as **Omeprazole** *(oh-ME-pray-zol)* and **Pantoprazole** *(pant-oh-PRAY-zol)* *Brands:* **Prilosec, Zegerid (omeprazole), Protonix, Protonix IV (pantoprazole)**

Omeprazole and pantoprazole belong to a class of drugs called proton pump inhibitors. They are approved for treating ulcers, gastroesophageal reflux and other conditions caused by excessive acid in the stomach. They work by completely blocking the production of stomach acid. They do this by shutting down a system in the stomach known as the proton pump.

In an article on the prevention of upper GI bleeding in the *Scandinavian Journal of Gastroenterology* from Leyenburg Hospital in The Hague, Netherlands, the researchers point out that two trials show that patients who receive omeprazole run a significantly lower risk of bleeding than patients receiving ranitidine.

An article in the *World Journal of Gastroenterology* from the Kaohsiung Veterans General Hospital in Taiwan reported on a study to determine whether intravenous pantoprazole could improve the efficacy of ranitidine as an add-on treatment to prevent recurrence of bleeding after endoscopy therapy. They divided 102 patients to receive one of the two therapies. Bleeding occurred in 4% of the pantoprazole group compared to 16% of the ranitidine group. The investigators concluded that pantoprazole was the superior therapy.

For more information see pages 1386 and 1393.

Generic: **Ranitidine** *(rah-NIT-a-deen)* *BrandS:* **Zantac, Zantac EFFERdose**

Ranitidine is one of a group of drugs known as H2 agonists. It blocks the action of histamine on cells that inhibit stomach acid secretion. Ranitidine is approved for the treatment of gastric and duodenal ulcers, as well as maintenance of healed ulcers, dyspepsia, erosive esophagitis, gastroesophageal reflux, and other acid-related problems. It has also been used off-label for the prevention of upper gastrointestinal bleeding.

In an article in the *Scandinavian Journal of Gastroenterology* from Leyenburg Hospital in The Hague, Netherlands, the researchers state that two studies show that treatment with ranitidine is more effective than such treatment with sucralfate in the prevention of upper GI bleeding.

Another study, published in the *New England Journal of Medicine*, was based on a clinical trial involving 1,200 patients requiring mechanical ventilation. Half of the people were given ranitidine and half were given sucralfate. All were critically ill patients on mechanical ventilation, which placed them at increased risk for gastrointestinal bleeding from stress ulcers. Gastrointestinal (GI) bleeding developed in 1.7% of those who received ranitidine, compared to 3.8 % of those who received sucralfate. There was no significant difference in deaths or duration of stay in the intensive care unit between the two groups.

For more information see page 1443.

BOWEL DISORDERS

The large intestine is the last section of the gastrointestinal system. By the time digestive products reach it, almost all of the nutritionally useful products have been removed. The large intestine removes water from the remainder, passing semi-solid feces into the rectum to be expelled from the body.

Anal Fissure

An anal fissure is a small tear or cut in the skin lining the anus. The typical symptoms are extreme pain during bowel movements and red blood streaking the stool. A hard, dry bowel movement can cause a tear in the anal lining, resulting in a fissure. Or it may be caused by diarrhea and inflammation of the anorectal area, overly tight or spastic anal sphincter muscles, scarring, or an underlying medical problem.

Commonly Prescribed (On-Label) Drugs: Docusate

OFF-LABEL PRESCRIPTION DRUGS
BREAKTHROUGH OPTIONS

Generic: **Botulinum Toxin Type B**
(BOT-yoo-lin-num TOKS-in type-bee)
Brand: **Myobloc**

Botulinum toxin produces a protein that blocks the release of acetylcholine and relaxes muscles. Type B is just one of seven different types of botulinum toxin, and each has different properties and actions. Botulinum toxin type B is now approved to decrease the severity of abnormal head position and neck pain associated with cervical dystonia.

Conventional treatment of anal fissure has focused on relieving spasms of the internal sphincter (a band of muscle just inside the anus) and reducing anal sphincter pressure or drug induced anal dilation, according to *Off-Label Drug Facts.* According to researchers, botulinum toxin essentially paralyzes the muscles. Injection of the toxin into the sphincter muscle relaxes it and promotes healing.

A position statement by the American Gastroenterological Association stated that initial conservative care may be appropriate in the treatment of fissures, especially acute fissures—that is, those that are recent. Their list of suggested treatments included locally injected botulinum toxin.

However, an article in *The Lancet* reported on 10 patients with chronic anal fissure who had symptoms on average for more than a year. Each received three injections of botulinum toxin during a five-minute procedure. Pain after bowel movement disappeared in five patients and was reduced in four patients one week after the injections. After one month, pain after bowel movement was gone in seven patients and reduced in another. At two months, one more patient had reduced pain. Seven patients had healed-over fissure scars. Further follow-up showed no relapse in five patients; three required re-treatment with botulinum toxin. One patient dropped out and had surgical treatment. One patient who had a relapse reported that symptoms were much milder. No overall complications were reported during injection or followup. One patient had transient mild incontinence for about one day a month after treatment. No other side effects occurred. Chemical denervation produced by the toxin is not permanent but lasts for two to three months, which, in anal fissure, roughly corresponds to the time required for healing.

An article in *The New England Journal of Medicine* reported on a trial conducted at the Catholic University of Rome of botulinum toxin versus saline injections for chronic anal fissure in 30 patients, with 15 divided to each therapy. After two months, 11 patients in the botulinum group and 2 in the control group had healed fissures, and 13 in the treated group and four in the control group had relief. Subsequently 10 patients in the control group received botulinum injections and had their fissures healed after two months. No relapses occurred during an average of 16 months of follow-up. The investigators concluded that local botulinum toxin is an effective treatment.

For more information see page 1053.

Generic: **Diltiazem** (dil-TYE-a-zem)
Brands: **Cardizem, Cartia XT, Dilacor XR, Diltia XT, Taztia XT, Tiazac**

Diltiazem is in a class of medications called calcium-channel blockers. They work by dilating blood vessels so blood flows through more easily and the heart does not have to pump as hard. This also increases the supply of blood and oxygen to the heart. Diltiazem is approved to treat high blood pressure and angina (chest pain).

According to *Off-Label Drug Facts*, conventional treatment has focused on relieving spasms of the internal sphincter (a band of muscle just inside the anus) and reducing anal sphincter pressure or drug-induced anal dilation. The latter approach avoids the risk of permanent incontinence. Recently calcium channel blockers have been considered by physicians when laboratory testing demonstrated that the smooth muscle of the sphincter depends on extracellular calcium entering the cells for contraction, according to a study reported in *Diseases of the Colon and Rectum*.

In four eight- to 12-week trials, topical diltiazem gel or cream (not available commercially in the United States) applied to the anus was effective in reducing anal pain and bleeding. Researchers noted that it promoted healing in chronic anal fissures at rates ranging from 48 to 73%. In one study reported in the *British Journal of Surgery*, of 71 patients with fissures who had not healed after using stool softeners and local anesthetic creams, 73% healed using diltiazem. Of the remaining patients, eight healed after re-treatment with diltiazem, two required nitroglycerin, four were given botulinum toxin injections, and one needed surgery.

For more information see page 1146.

Generic: *Lidocaine Topical* (LYE-doe-kane)
Brands: *Anestacon, Xylocaine*

Lidocaine is an anesthetic. In its topical form it is approved for burns, contact dermatitis, skin wounds, and post-herpetic neuralgia. It is related to the medication dentists inject to relieve pain during dental procedures.

An article in the *American Family Physician* reported a study in which two topical combination preparations were compared. One contained topical nifedipine (which dilates blood vessels and relaxes the anal sphincter) and lidocaine ointment, while the other contained hydrocortisone acetate ointment (an anti-inflammatory) and lidocaine ointment. Both were given every 12 hours. At the end of six weeks, healing of anal fissures occurred in 94.5% of those in the nifedipine combo group and 16.4% of those in the hydrocortisone group. No significant side effects were reported. The investigators concluded that topical nifedipine with lidocaine gel is effective and well tolerated.

For more information see page 1283.

Generic: *Nifedipine* (nye-FED-i-peen)
Brands: *Adalat, Procardia*

Nifedipine belongs to a class of drugs called calcium channel blockers. Nifedipine is approved for the treatment of hypertension, although it is not clear how the drug dilates blood vessels to lower blood pressure. Calcium channel blockers came to be considered for fissures when laboratory testing demonstrated that the smooth muscle of the anal sphincters depends on extracellular calcium entering the cells for contraction, as reported in a study in *Diseases of the Colon and Rectum,* which also reported a study that divided 110 people with anal fissures to take either topical gel of nifedipine/lidocaine (not available commercially in the United States) or a hydrocortisone/lidocaine combination, applied every 12 hours. After six weeks, researchers observed that healing was significantly higher in the nifedipine group – 94.5% versus 16.4%.

The same journal also reported a study that divided 283 adults with anal fissures to receive either a topical gel of nifedipine only or a lidocaine/hydrocortisone combination, again applied every 12 hours. After only three weeks, 95% of the nifedipine group was healed versus 50% of the control group.

For more information see page 1360.

Generic: **Nitroglycerin** *(nye-troe²-GLIH-suh-rin)*
Brands: **Nitro-Bid Ointment, Nitrol**

Nitroglycerin is a vasodilator—a drug that dilates blood vessels—often prescribed to help manage angina (chest pain). Nitroglycerin is available in capsules, transdermal capsules, pills that dissolve under the tongue, a spray that dissolves in the mouth, and an ointment that is applied to the skin. It is under consideration for treatment of people with anal fissures.

The goal of conventional therapy is to relieve spasms of the internal sphincter (a band of muscle just inside the anus) and reducing anal sphincter pressure or drug-induced anal dilation, according to *Off-Label Drug Facts.* The latter approach, achieved with medication, avoids the risk of permanent incontinence. Drugs used to achieve this goal have included topical nitroglycerin. It dilates the blood vessels and thereby relaxes the muscles of the anal sphincter. Researchers believe it may promote healing by improving the supply of blood to the anal region, just as it improves blood supply to the heart.

The American Gastroenterological Association stated that initial conservative care may be appropriate in the treatment of fissures, especially acute fissures—that is, those that are recent—and suggested treatments included nitroglycerin.

For more information see pages 1363 and 1366.

Generic: **Sildenafil** *(sil-DEN-a-fil)*
Brand: **Viagra**

Sildenafil is normally prescribed for the treatment of impotence, but does not cause sexual stimulation. Rather, it solves an underlying problem that causes impotence. It enhances nitric oxide-induced relaxation of smooth muscles. This mechanism might be useful in reducing tight anal sphincters in people with anal fissures. Topical gel versions of sildenafil have already been available because they have been used with some success in clinical trials for post-menopausal women with sexual difficulties, as reported in the *British Journal of Obstetrics, Gynecology,* and *The Journal of Reproductive Medicine.*

An article in *Diseases of the Colon and Rectum* reported on a small trial conducted in Marbella, Spain, and the Southeast Georgia Regional Medical Center, Brunswick, Georgia. Researchers treated 19 people with chronic anal fissures with a topical sildenafil cream (which is not available in the United States). The data reported maximum resting anal sphincter pressures dropped approximately 18% in all patients. Only one did not achieve a reduction of more than 10%. These declines occurred within three minutes of applying sildenafil. The most common side effect was transient anal itching or burning, reported in 26%. Although this drug significantly reduces anal sphincter pressure in this small group, researchers believe that trials of larger groups are needed.

For more information see page 1472.

Anal Ulcer

See Anal Fissure

Chronic Constipation

Constipation is defined as having only hard, dry bowel movements, straining or difficulty moving your bowels, and passing your bowels infrequently, usually fewer than three times a week. People who are constipated may find it painful to have a bowel movement and feel as if they have not evacuated completely.

Commonly Prescribed (On-Label) Drugs: Tegaserod

OFF-LABEL PRESCRIPTION DRUG
BREAKTHROUGH OPTION

Generic: **Misoprostol** *(mye-soe-PROST-ole)*
Brand: **Cytotec**

Misoprostol inhibits the secretion of acid in the stomach and protects the delicate mucosal lining of the stomach. It does this by increasing bicarbonate and mucus production and is used to help prevent gastric ulcers in people who are taking nonsteroidal anti-inflammatory drugs. It can also cause uterine contractions and is also approved for use with mifepristone to help induce abortion in early pregnancy. According to *Off-Label Drug Facts*, misoprostel may also induce abdominal cramping and diarrhea in some people. This secondary effect may result from multiple factors, including changes in bicarbonate balance. As a result, misoprostol has been tried as a treatment for chronic constipation.

Digestive Disease Science reported on a trial in nine patients who had bowel movements only every four days. They were divided to receive misoprostol or a placebo three times a day for one week, then no drug for one week, then the opposite therapy for one week. Movement of food through the colon was normalized in 78% of patients after misoprostol treatment and significantly decreased compared to placebo (66 vs. 109.4 hours). Researchers observed that frequency of bowel movements significantly increased from 2.5 to 6.5 in those receiving misoprostol.

For more information see page 1334.

Chronic Diarrhea

When bowel movements consist of loose, watery stools that pass more than three times in one day, it is called diarrhea. When the condition lasts for more than two weeks, it is considered chronic. In an otherwise healthy person, chronic diarrhea may be a nuisance, but for someone with a weak immune system, it is a life-threatening illness. In general, diarrhea may be caused by an infection or by other diseases, or the cause may be unknown.

Commonly Prescribed (On-Label) Drugs: *Loperamide*

OFF-LABEL PRESCRIPTION DRUGS
BREAKTHROUGH OPTIONS

Generic: **Clonidine** *(KLON-i-deen)*
Brands: **Catapres, Catapres-TTS, Duraclon**

Clonidine belongs to a class called antihypertensive drugs. Different antihypertensive drugs act in different ways. Clonidine is an alpha-adrenergic stimulating agent that works by controlling nerve impulses along certain nerve pathways. This relaxes and dilates blood vessels so that blood passes through them more easily and blood pressure is lowered.

Studies in animals have shown that stimulation of alpha-adrenergic receptors promotes fluid and electrolyte absorption in the intestines, which could help alleviate diarrhea, according to an article in the *Annals of Internal Medicine* from the University of Chicago Hospitals and Clinics. Therefore the researchers conducted a study in three people with insulin-dependent diabetes who had persistent and severe chronic diarrhea seven to 12 times per day for two to three years. All infectious and other possible disease causes had been ruled out. Clonidine was given to each for periods averaging one month, then withdrawn for 10 to 14 days, and then restarted. All had a significant decrease in the volume of their diarrhea during clonidine treatment. While the frequency of movements did not change significantly, there was a clustering of movements into one or two periods during the day. An increase in stool consistency also occurred. Symptoms resumed when the drug was withdrawn and improved again when clonidine was re-initiated.

Subsequently, reports in the *American Family Physician and Gastroenterology* have supported the treatment of chronic diarrhea with clonidine, noting its beneficial effects on intestinal absorption and motility.

For more information see page 1108.

Generic: **Codeine** *(KOE-deen)*
Brand: **Codeine**

Codeine is an opiate derived from the opium poppy. Its primary approved use is as a narcotic pain reliever and is also a valuable ingredient in some cough suppressants. Constipation is a side effect of opioids that can be useful in treating severe diarrhea.

The *Journal of Clinical Investigation* from the Baylor University Medical Center, Dallas, Texas, reported on studies to explore the mechanism of this antidiarrheal effect of codeine. In people, codeine markedly reduced stool volume, but there was no evidence that the rate of intestinal absorption was stimulated. Codeine also caused a marked slowing of fluid movement through the jejunum (that part of the small intestine that is half-way down between its duodenum and ileum sections), but no effect on the movement of fluid through the ileum (the lower three-fifths of the small intestine) or colon (the large intestine from the ileum to the rectum).

Thus, while codeine may alleviate pain in diarrhea sufferers, the researchers concluded that codeine's benefits in diarrhea alleviation derives from increasing net intestinal absorption. It thereby reduces stool volume simply by increasing *contact time* of fluid with mucosal cells in a critical part of the small intestine, not by increasing the rate of absorption by the mucosal cells. According to investigators, these benefits may be especially important after a meal. Codeine will be less likely to be of benefit in people with very severe diarrhea when all parts of the intestine are continuously exposed to large volumes of fluid.

For more information see page 1113.

*Generic: **Octreotide** (ok-TREE-oh-tide)*
*Brands: **Sandostatin, Sandostatin LAR***

Octreotide has similar effects to a natural hormone called somatostatin. It is given by injection and suppresses the body's own growth hormone. It is used to reduce an oversupply of growth hormone that leads to a bone overgrowth disease called acromegaly, as well as flushing and diarrhea associated with certain tumors. It does not cure the tumor but eases the symptoms.

An article in *Current Treatment Options in Gastroenterology* from Baylor University Medical Center in Dallas, Texas, reports that octreotide is of great value in treating diarrhea due to endocrine tumors and dumping syndrome, but its efficacy in other conditions or in nonspecific chronic diarrhea is less well established.

An article in *Digestion* from the University Hospital in Zurich, Switzerland, reviewed the history of octreotide in the treatment of chronic diarrhea that had not responded to other treatments. Octreotide was considered for treating chronic diarrhea because it also inhibits gastrointestinal secretion, intestinal absorption, and pancreatic secretion. Studies had included patients with problems such as: chemotherapy-induced diarrhea; short-bowel syndrome; AIDS-associated diarrhea; graft vs. host disease; diabetes; enteric infections; and other conditions associated with chronic diarrhea not responding to standard treatment. According to researchers, most of these studies were not conclusive as they yielded negative or controversial results. The investigators concluded that octreotide may be tried in the treatment of therapy-resistant diarrhea, especially in AIDS-associated diarrhea, if other therapies fail, but large trials are needed to define the role of octreotide in chronic diarrhea treatment.

For more information see page 1380.

Crohn's Disease

Crohn's disease is an inflammatory bowel disease that generally causes inflammation in the lower part of the small intestine, although it can affect any part of the digestive tract, from the mouth to the anus. The main symptoms are pain and frequent diarrhea. Bleeding from the rectum may be serious and persistent, leading to anemia. Fever and weight loss also may occur. The cause of Crohn's disease remains unknown.

Commonly Prescribed (On-Label) Drugs: *Mesalamine, Sulfasalazine*

OFF-LABEL PRESCRIPTION DRUGS
BREAKTHROUGH OPTIONS

Generics: Purine Analogues such as ***Azathioprine***
(ay-za-THYE-oh-preen) and ***Mercaptopurine,***
(mer-kap-toe-PYOOR-een)
Brands: ***Imuran (azathioprine), Purinethol***
(mercaptopurine)

Azathioprine and mercaptopurine are related to uric acid. Azathioprine is a prodrug of mercaptopurine (a prodrug is a compound that breaks down into the active agent). Both are immune system modifiers. Azathioprine is approved for the treatment of rheumatoid arthritis and for the prevention of organ transplant rejection. Mercaptopurine is approved to treat certain types of leukemia.

These drugs are also known as antimetabolites because they prevent cells (including those in the immune system) from dividing. One theory of the cause of Crohn's disease is that it is an immune system disorder. According to an article from Gastroenterology Associates, when Crohn's cannot be maintained in remission with aminosalicylates such as mesalamine, balasalazide, and sulfasalazine, immune modifiers such as these purine analogues are used. They also help reduce the dose of corticosteroids needed. They are also used for patients who cannot tolerate aminosalicylates.

An article in *Gastroenterology* reported on a trial in which 131 patients were assigned to receive mercaptopurine, mesalamine, or placebo as postoperative therapy for Crohn's disease remission. After two years, mercaptopurine proved to be most effective in preventing recurrence, and the investigators concluded that it should be considered as a maintenance therapy after resection surgery.

For more information see pages 1033 and 1305.

Generic: ***Balsalazide*** *(bal–SAL–a–zide)*
Brand: ***Colazal***

Balsalazide belongs to a family of drugs called aminosalicylates. According to an article on *eMedicine* from Gastroenterology Associates, aminosalicylates are the first line of drugs used in the treatment of Crohn's disease. Although they are approved for the treatment of ulcerative colitis, they are used off-label for Crohn's disease. However, even when used for Crohn's disease, the primary benefit of balsalazide is for colonic disease. Some studies suggest balsalazide is better at maintaining remission than sulfasalazine, although it is also used for treating acute episodes.

Balsalazide is essentially a distant but more powerful cousin of aspirin. It is a potent anti-inflammatory medication. When balslazide reaches the large intestine, colonic bacteria breaks it down and releases the active ingredient called 5-ASA. Then the drug may decrease inflammation by blocking production of the metabolites of acid in the mucosa of the colon.

An article in *Advanced Drug Delivery Review* from the Dr. Margarete Fischer-Bosche-Institute of Clinical Pharmacology notes that 5-ASA can be delivered to the colon either by balasalazide orally or by direct rectal administration in the form of enemas, foam, or suppositories. However, researchers state that the oral forms provide greater benefit for disease in the small bowel.

For more information see page 1038.

Generics: Antibiotics such as **Ciprofloxacin**
(sip-roe-FLOX-a-sin) and **Metronidazole**
(me-troe-NI-da-zole)
Brands: **Ciloxan, Cipro, Cipro XR (ciprofloxacin), Flagyl, Flagyl ER, MetroCream, MetroGel, MetroLotion, MetroGel Vaginal (metronidazole)**

Ciprofloxacin and metronidazole are antibiotics that are effective against a broad range of bacteria. According to an article on *eMedicine* from Gastroenterology Associates, they are the most commonly used antibiotics prescribed for treating people with inflammatory bowel disease and are prescribed for Crohn's disease, most often for disease around the anus, for fistulas (abnormal connections between the intestines and other organs), or for inflammatory masses in the abdomen such as abscesses (infections). Antibiotics also may be of some use when treating ileitis. These antibiotics may be prescribed separately or together.

However, according to an Italian study reported in the *American Journal of Gastroenterology* metronidazole and ciprofloxacin were not clearly more effective than steroids at inducing remission in a trial of 41 patients with active Crohn's disease, nor did they clearly cause fewer side effects. But particularly in view of the number of patients who withdrew from the study, an editorial commentary called the study too small to show any difference between steroids and antibiotics in the active treatment of active Crohn's disease.

For more information see pages 1093 and 1322.

Generic: **Thalidomide** *(tha-LI-doe-mide)*
Brand: **Thalomid**

Thalidomide was created as a drug to treat morning sickness in pregnant women, but it was found to cause terrible birth defects and then banned around the world. It was later discovered to be a superb therapy for leprosy, quickly improving the skin lesions. This launched years of research on the immunomodulatory effects of thalidomide, eventually leading to its FDA approval for treating leprosy symptoms. According to the National Institutes of Health (NIH), studies have been done to assess thalidomide in AIDS, various cancers, and numerous rheumatic and connective tissue diseases. When thalidomide affects the immune system, it suppresses inflammation.

An article in *Alimentary Pharmacological Therapy* from the Hospital Saint Louis in Paris, France reported a study using thalidomide as a maintenance therapy in 15 patients with Crohn's disease. The average follow-up was 238 days. After 12 months, 83% remained in remission, although four (two still in remission) had dropped out due to suspected adverse effects. The investigators concluded that thalidomide appeared to be effective and relatively safe except in the case of women of childbearing age who may be pregnant.

An article in *Off-Label Drug Facts* reviewed several other case reports of children and adults with Crohn's disease. Investigators concluded that thalidomide has been effective in reversing oral and colonic ulcerations, with symptomatic improvement within two to four weeks, and reduced recurrences with continued therapy.

For more information see page 1505.

Diarrhea

Diarrhea is the occurrence of loose, watery stools more than three times in one day. While uncomfortable, it is a common problem that usually lasts a day or two and then disappears without any treatment. The typical adult has diarrhea about four times a year. However, prolonged diarrhea can be a serious concern because fluid loss can cause dehydration. Diarrhea may be caused by an infection, or a chronic problem, like an intestinal disease.

Commonly Prescribed (On-Label) Drugs: Bismuth Subsalicylate, Diphenoxylate, Furazolidone, Kaolin/Pectin, Sodium Bicarbonate

OFF-LABEL PRESCRIPTION DRUGS
BREAKTHROUGH OPTIONS

*Generic: **Azithromycin** (az-ith-roe-MYE-sin)*
*Brands: **Tri-Pak, Zithromax, Zithromax Z-Pak***

Azithromycin belongs to a class of medications called macrolide antibiotics. It is used to treat a wide range of infections caused by bacteria, including streptococcal infections of the ear, lungs, skin, and sinuses, and gonococcal and chlamydial infections. It works by stopping bacterial growth.

Campylobacter is a group of bacteria that causes disease in humans and animals. It is one of the most common bacterial causes of diarrhea illness in the United States, and is very common throughout the world. People diagnosed with *campylobacter* are often given prescriptions for the antibiotic ciprofloxacin, but the bacteria has become resistant to it in some areas. According to *Canadian Family Physician*, azithromycin is effective in treatment of ciprofloxacin-resistant *Campylobacter*.

Clinics of Infectious Diseases reported on a study from the Walter Reed Army Institute of Research, Washington, D.C., that evaluated azithromycin or ciprofloxacin daily for three days for the treatment of acute diarrhea among U.S. military personnel in Thailand, where ciprofloxacin resistance is prevalent. Researchers found that azithromycin was superior to ciprofloxacin in decreasing the excretion of *Campylobacter* and as effective as ciprofloxacin in shortening the duration of illness.

For more information see page 1034.

Generic: **Erythromycin** *(er-ith-roe-MYE-sin)*
Brands: **Akne-Mycin, E.E.S., Eryc, Ery-Tab, Erythrocin**

Erythromycin is an antibiotic approved to treat a wide range of infections caused by bacteria, such as streptococcal infections of the skin, ears, and sinuses, pneumococcal pneumonia, chlamydia, bronchitis; diphtheria; Legionnaires' disease; whooping cough; pneumonia; rheumatic fever; certain venereal diseases, and other infections. It is also approved for use before some surgery or dental work to prevent infection in certain people at risk for complications.

Erythromycin is also used off-label to treat a group of bacteria called *Campylobacter*, one of the most common bacterial causes of diarrhea disease in the United States and worldwide. Although ciprofloxacin is often prescribed for those diagnosed with *Campylobacter*, it has become resistant to it in some areas, and erythromycin has become the antibiotic of choice, according to an article in *eMedicine* from the State University of New York at Stony Brook. Researchers believe that erythromycin resistance remains low, and it can be used in children or women who are pregnant, in contrast to problems presented by ciprofloxacin in those patients.

A Norwegian study examined in the laboratory the susceptibility to erythromycin and ciprofloxacin of 296 *Campylobacter jejuni* strains isolated during the 1998-1999 period. They found that nearly one in four of the isolates likely from Norway was resistant to ciprofloxacin; all resistant isolates were acquired outside Norway. In contrast, researchers state that resistance to erythromycin was very rare, indicating that it should still be the drug of choice for campylobacteriosis.

For more information see page 1170.

Diverticulitis

Diverticula are little pouches in the colon (which comprises most of the large intestine) that bulge outward. They are weak spots in the "tubing" of the intestine. Simply having such diverticula is a condition called diverticulosis. The condition is more common as you age, afflicting about 10% of those over age 40 and about half of those over age 60. If the diverticula become infected or inflamed, it is called diverticulitis.

Commonly Prescribed (On-Label) Drugs: *None*

OFF-LABEL PRESCRIPTION DRUGS
BREAKTHROUGH OPTIONS

Generics: Combination Antibiotics, such as ***Amoxicillin-Clavulanate*** *(a-moks-i-SIL-in klav-yoo-LAN-ate),* ***Piperacillin-Tazobactam*** *(tye-kar-SIL-in ta-zoe-BAK-tam),* and ***Ticarcillin-Clavulanate*** *(tye-kar-SIL-in klav-yoo-LAN-ate)*
Brands: ***Augmentin, Augmentin ES-600, Augmentin XR (amoxicillin-clavulanate), Zosyn (piperacillin-tazobactam), Timentin (ticarcillin-clavulanate)***

Each of these is a combination antibacterial drug that puts together two different drugs that work in two different ways to offer a wider range of attack on multiple microbes that could be causing illness. In each instance, the first drug is a member of the penicillin family. The second drug is a beta-lactamase inhibitor that can kill most bacteria. The combination of these sets of drugs has been found to be effective for treating diverticulitis.

Such combination drugs are essential in the treatment of diverticular disease, according to an article from the University of California at Irvine Medical Center, in order to kill all organisms that are likely to be active in causing disease in the intestines. In particular, it is necessary to the two major classes. Therefore, the investigators urge treatment with combination therapy including regimens such as amoxicillin-clavulanate, piperacillin-tazobactam and ticarcillin-clavulanate.

Additionally, amoxicillin-clavulanate was mentioned by 14% of colon and rectal surgeon respondents in a survey as the oral antibiotic given post-surgically to acute diverticulitis patients at discharge. The survey was conducted by Brown University of Providence, Rhode Island and reported in an article in *Diseases of the Colon and Rectum*.

For more information see pages 1013, 1421, and 1511.

Generic: **Ampicillin-sulbactam**
(am-pi-SILL-in SUL-bak-tam)
Brand: **Unasyn**

This is a combination antibacterial drug. It brings together the antibiotic ampicillen with sulbactam sodium. According to an article on *eMedicine* from the University of California at Irvine Medical Center, treatment for diverticulitis must be able to kill all organisms likely to be causing disease. To accomplish this goal in complicated diverticulitis commonly requires treatment with combination therapy including sulbactam sodium.

Diseases of the Colon and Rectum reported on a survey conducted by Brown University of Providence, Rhode Island, of current medical treatment of patients with uncomplicated acute diverticulitis. Of fellows of the American Society of Colon and Rectal Surgeons, one-half used a single intravenous antibiotic, with second generation cephalosporins (27%) and ampicillin/sulbactam (16%) being the most common.

For more information see page 1016.

Generic: **Cefoxitin** *(se-FOX-i-tin)*
Brand: **Mefoxin**

Cefoxitin belongs to a group of antibiotics called the cephalosporins, which kill bacteria by interfering with their ability to form cell walls, so they break up and die. Cefoxitin is approved for a range of very severe infections, such as staphylococcal and streptococcal infections, and is given by injection or infusion. It is sometimes given before an operation to prevent infection after surgery.

According to an article on *eMedicine* from the University of California at Irvine Medical Center, cefoxitin may be effective in killing bacteria that are resistant to earlier cephalosporins and penicillins.

An article in *Clinical Therapeutics* reported on a study conducted by the Medical College of Virginia in Richmond, Virginia, comparing cefoxitin to combination therapy with gentamicin and clindamycin in the treatment of acute colonic diverticulitis. They divided 51 hospitalized patients, located at five different medical centers, to receive one or the other therapy. Cure rates of 90% and 85.7% were seen for cefoxitin versus the combination therapy, respectively. However, antibiotic-related toxicity was higher in the combination therapy group, as was the cost of treatment. Therefore, the investigators concluded that cefoxitin may be preferred in view of its narrower antimicrobial spectrum and lower cost.

For more information see page 1075.

Generic: Antibiotics such as ***Cephalexin*** (*sef-a-LEXS-in*), ***Ciprofloxacin*** (*sip-roe-FLOX-a-sin*), ***Clindamycin*** (*klin-da-MYE-sin*), ***Gentamicin*** (*jen-ta-MYE-sin*), ***Metronidazole*** (*me-troe-NI-da-zole*), and ***Rifampin*** (*ri-FAM-pin*)
Brands: Biocef, Keflex (cephalexin), Ciloxan, Cipro, Cipro XR (ciprofloxacin), Cleocin T, Clindagel, ClindaMax, Clindets (clindamycin), Garamycin, Genoptic, Gentacidin, Gentak (gentamicin), Flagyl, Flagyl ER, MetroCream, MetroGel, MetroLotion, MetroGel Vaginal (metronidazole), Rifadin (rifampin)

These are all broad-spectrum antibiotics, each belonging to a different "family" of antibiotics. For example, cephalexin is a cephalosporin, ciprofloxacin is a fluoroquinolone, gentamicin is an aminoglycoside, and metronidazole is an antiprotazoal. All are approved to treat various infections. Rifampin is an isoniazid approved for the treatment of tuberculosis. These antibiotics are usually prescribed together.

Because diverticular disease often involves infection with multiple organisms in the intestines, physicians suggest treatment with medicines that are able to kill a wide range of pathogens, according to an article on *eMedicine* from the University of California at Irvine Medical Center. Because some drugs, for example, kill anaerobes (such as *bacterids*), while others kill gram-negative organisms (such as *enterococci*), multiple drugs are needed. Therefore, as the investigators discuss, complicated diverticulitis is commonly treated with a combination of metronidazole or clindamycin with an aminoglycoside such as gentamicin or a third-generation cephalosporin such as cephalosporin. Milder cases are treated on an outpatient bases with a regimen that includes ciprofloxacin and metronidazole. Recently, rifampin has been used to treat milder cases of acute diverticulitis, either alone or in combination with other antibiotics.

In a case review on acute diverticulitis in the *New England Journal of Medicine*, the researchers urged the use of broad-spectrum antibiotic coverage. They referred to the use of ampicillin, gentamicin, and metronidazole as the "standard triple therapy."

For more information see pages 1077, 1093, 1101, 1212, 1322, and 1450.

Generic: *Imipenem-cilastatin*
(i-mi-PEN-em and sye-la-STAT-in)
Brand: *Primaxin*

This is a broad-spectrum antibiotic that combines two antibacterial drugs. It puts together imipenem, which is a thienamycin antibiotic, with cilastatin sodium, which is an inhibitor of a kidney enzyme. Imipenem-cilastatin is given by injection. Because it is so potent, it is used in a limited number of situations. It is approved for a number of bacterial infections, such as bone and blood infections, lower respiratory infections, and bacterial infections of the urinary tract and lungs.

According to an article on *eMedicine* from the University of California at Irvine Medical Center, treatment for diverticulitis must be able to cover all pathogens likely to be causing disease in the gut, including those known as anaerobes (such as *bacterids*) and gram-negative organisms (such as *enterobacteria* and *enterococci*). This typically requires therapy with combination drugs, such as ampicillin/sulbactam. However, as the article notes, in more severe cases, imipenem may be used.

An article in *Pharmacotherapy* compared the efficacy of imipenem-cilastin to a combination of clindamycin and gentamicin in the treatment of infections in 20 patients. The conditions treated included acute diverticulitis, extremity ulcers, peritonitis, perirectal abscess, soft-tissue abscess, and abdominal abscess. Similar rates of cure or improvement were achieved with the two therapies. The researchers concluded that imipenem-cilastin appears to be an effective antibiotic in treating infections due to multiple microbes.

For more information see page 1229.

Generic: **Rifaximin** *(rif-AX-i-min)*
Brand: *Xifaxan*

Rifaximin is a gastrointestinal-selective antibiotic that was specifically designed for the treatment of traveler's diarrhea due to *E. coli* infections. Unlike antibiotics that are absorbed throughout the body, rifaximin's beneficial effects are achieved with minimal systemic absorption (about 0.4%), thus reducing the potential for development of antibiotic resistance in the body and other systemic concerns such as drug interactions.

International Journal of Colorectal Diseases reported on a study from the University of L'Aquila in Italy that examined the efficacy of administration of rifaximin in patients with uncomplicated diverticular disease to assess its benefits in reducing episodes of diverticulitis compared to those receiving fiber supplementation only. In a trial, 968 patients were divided to receive rifaximin for seven days every month plus fiber or fiber alone. After 12 months, 56.5% of those on rifaximin versus 29.2% of those on fiber alone had no symptoms. The investigators concluded that the drug was effective in reducing episodes of diverticulitis.

European Review of Medical Pharmacology Science reported on another study from the University of L'Aquila in which patients with symptomatic or complicated diverticular disease were treated with rifaximin for 10 to 12 days during the acute phase in addition to the appropriate systemic antibiotics, followed by a preventive rifaximin regimen for seven days every month. Researchers suggest a possible role of rifaximin in the prevention of diverticular disease complications.

For more information see page 1452.

Granulomatous Colitis

See Ulcerative Colitis

Hemorrhagic Colitis

See Traveler's Diarrhea

IBS

See Irritable Bowel Syndrome

Irritable Bowel Syndrome

Irritable bowel syndrome (IBS) is a disorder that interferes with the normal functions of the large intestine (colon). It causes symptoms such as crampy abdominal pain, bloating, constipation, and diarrhea, although it does not permanently harm the intestines nor lead to bleeding. Usually symptoms can be controlled with diet, stress management, and prescription medication.

Commonly Prescribed (On-Label) Drugs: *Alosetron, Atropine, Dicyclomine, Loperamide, Tegaserod, Tridihexethyl Chloride*

OFF-LABEL PRESCRIPTION DRUGS
BREAKTHROUGH OPTIONS

Generic: ***Alprazolam*** *(al-PRAY-zoe-lam)*
Brands: ***Alprazolam Intensol, Xanax, Xanax XR***

Alprazolam is a triazolobenzodiazepine tranquilizer approved for the treatment of anxiety, general anxiety disorder, and panic disorder. More recently, it has been used off-label in combination with other medications in the treatment of IBS. A significant proportion of patients with generalized anxiety disorder have IBS.

The *Journal of Clinical Psychiatry* reported on a study of alprazolam in the treatment of IBS. The goal was to investigate whether treatment of generalized anxiety disorder would influence the course of IBS symptom severity. Investigators gave alprazolam to

32 patients for six weeks, and 94% of patients had full or partial alleviation of anxiety. Eighty-nine percent experienced a concomitant reduction in the severity of their IBS. For the majority, benefits continued to be felt as the drug was tapered over four weeks and for four weeks after its discontinuation. The researchers concluded that alprazolam treatment was safe, effective, and beneficial for IBS, with only limited post-treatment rebound of symptoms.

For more information see page 997.

Generic: **Amitriptyline** *(a-mee-TRIP-ti-leen)*
Brand: **Elavil**

Amitriptyline belongs to a class of drugs called tricyclic antidepressants, one of the older types of antidepressants. While depression may also affect people with irritable bowel syndrome, this drug's primary effects on the illness appears not to be psychological but are related to its ability to interfere with certain chemical messengers in the brain and thereby change the way the brain perceives pain messages.

Gut reported on a study from Vanderbilt University in Nashville of 19 women with painful IBS who received amitriptyline or placebo for one month and crossed over to the alternate treatment after a washout period with no therapy. Brain activation during rectal distension was compared when on and off the active drug. Results showed that amitriptyline reduced brain activation during pain in critical areas of the brain. The investigators concluded that it is likely to work in the central nervous system rather than peripherally to blunt pain and other symptoms exacerbated by stress in IBS.

For more information see page 1009.

Generic: **Clonidine** *(KLON-i-deen)*
Brands: **Catapres, Catapres-TTS, Duraclon**

Clonidine belongs to a class of antihypertensive drugs called alpha-adrenergic stimulating agents. Various antihypertensive drugs act in different ways. Clonidine works by controlling nerve impulses along certain nerve pathways. This dilates blood vessels, enabling blood to pass through more easily, thus lowering the pressure.

Clinics of Gastroenterology and Hepatology reported on a study from the Mayo Clinic evaluating clonidine in people with IBS and diarrhea as their main symptom. Investigators divided 44 patients to receive one of three doses of the drug or placebo. Response was measured by questioning patients every week and asking them to keep a diary of their stools for four weeks. According to the investigators, the intermediate dose of clonidine proved to be the most satisfactory to patients—both of the higher dose patients dropped out as did two of 12 in the lower dose group. It yielded firmer stools and easier stool passage. These benefits were not associated with any significant changes in the transit time of stool through the intestines.

For more information see page 1108.

Generic: **Imipramine** *(im-IP-ra-meen)*
Brands: **Tofranil, Tofranil-PM**

Imipramine belongs to a group of medications called tricyclic antidepressants, one of the older types of antidepressants. While it is common for depression to affect people with chronic diseases like irritable bowel syndrome, this drug's primary effect on the illness seems not to be psychological but related to its ability to affect intestinal motility.

Digestive Disease Science reported on a study from St. Bartholomew's Hospital in West Smithfield, London, on the actions of imipramine on small intestinal motor function in eight healthy adults and six people with IBS in which diarrhea was the main symptom. According to investigators, after five days taking imipramine, the velocity of food moving through the intestines was modified in both groups, supporting the theory that the drug can have therapeutic benefit unrelated to improvement in mood.

For more information see page 1230.

Generic: **Octreotide** *(ok-TREE-oh-tide)*
Brands: **Sandostatin, Sandostatin LAR**

Octreotide is a drug that has similar effects to a natural hormone called somatostatin. It suppresses growth hormone and is given by injection. It is approved to treat the symptoms associated with certain intestinal tumors, such as diarrhea and flushing, although it does not cure these tumors. It is also approved to treat a hormonal disorder called acromegaly.

An article in *Alimentary Pharmacological Therapy* from the Center for Neurovisceral Sciences and Women's Health in Los Angeles, California, reported on a study to assess the effects of octreotide in IBS. The drug has been reported to be beneficial in chronic pain but the underlying mechanisms are unknown. In one study, discomfort was assessed in seven IBS patients and eight healthy controls on three separate days using a computer-controlled device. Subjects received either placebo or low- or high dose octreotide. In a second study, such responses were measured in nine IBS patients before and after repetitive high-pressure mechanical signoid stimulation, a very uncomfortable procedure. Octreotide increased discomfort thresholds in IBS patients but not in controls, without changing rectal compliance. However, repetitive signoid stimulation resulted in decreased rectal discomfort thresholds in the patient group only, thus preventing the sensitizing effect of such stimulation on rectal discomfort. The investigators concluded that octreotide has an anti-hyperalgesic effect. Hyperalgesia is a condition of altered perception; for example, for some experiencing hyperalgesia, stimuli that would normally induce a trivial discomfort cause significant pain.

For more information see page 1380.

Nonspecific Ulcerative Colitis

See Ulcerative Colitis

Reginal Enteritis

See Crohn's Disease

Spastic Colon

See Irritable Bowel Syndrome

Traveler's Diarrhea

People get traveler's diarrhea by eating food and drinking water that contain germs to which their bodies are not accustomed. Other people who live in these areas often drink tap water that contains these same germs, but they do not get diarrhea because their bodies are used to the germs. The most common pathogens in traveler's diarrhea are *Escherichia coli, Campylobacter, Shigella, Salmonella,* and *Yersinia.* However, viruses and protozoa can also be the cause. Traveler's diarrhea can usually be avoided by carefully selecting foods and beverages.

According to the *American Family Physician,* approximately one-third of travelers to less developed areas of the world become ill from ingesting food or water contaminated with feces, and up to 20% of them develop bloody diarrhea and fever. Such illness requires medical treatment with an antibiotic to kill the bacteria. Unfortunately, many of the bacteria that cause such illness have become resistant to the standard antibiotics usually prescribed.

Commonly Prescribed (On-Label) Drugs: Loperamide

OFF-LABEL PRESCRIPTION DRUGS
BREAKTHROUGH OPTION

Generic: **Norfloxacin** (nor-FLOKS-a-sin)
Brand: **Noroxin**

Norfloxacin belongs to the quinolone family of antibiotics. It is approved for the treatment of acute gonococcal cervicitis and urethritis, prostatitis due to *E. coli,* certain urinary tract infections, and acute lower genitourinary gonorrhea.

Clinical Infectious Diseases reported on a study from the Helsinki University Hospital in Finland of the clinical efficacy of norfloxacin for treatment of traveler's diarrhea in 106 Finnish tourists vacationing in Morocco. The travelers were divided to receive either norfloxacin or a placebo twice daily for three days. All symptoms disappeared sooner in those taking norfloxacin. Most notably, the diarrhea subsided in 1.2 days in the norfloxacin group versus 3.3 days in the placebo group. Its disappearance occurred most quickly in those infected with *E. coli* (1 day) and *Salmonella*

(1.1 day) and was slightly slower in those infected with *Campylobacter jejuni* (1.8 days). The rates in those on placebo were 3.1, 4.1, and 5.0, respectively. No significant adverse effects occurred. The investigators concluded that norfloxacin was safe and effective in therapy for traveler's diarrhea.

For more information see page 1373.

Traveler's Diarrhea, Prevention of

People get traveler's diarrhea by eating food and drinking water that contain germs to which their bodies are not accustomed. They lack protective antibodies (infection-fighting agents in the blood) that attack these germs. Local people do not get sick from these germs, just as cooks and food handlers may have the germs that cause traveler's diarrhea on their hands, but they may not get sick themselves. In some cases, traveler's diarrhea can be avoided by careful food and beverage selection; in others, premedication may be appropriate.

Commonly Prescribed (On-Label) Drugs: None

OFF-LABEL PRESCRIPTION DRUG
BREAKTHROUGH OPTION

Generic: **Doxycycline** *(doks-i-SYE-kleen)*
Brands: **Adoxa, Doryx, Doxy-100, Monodox, Periostat, Vibramycin, Vibra-Tabs**

Doxycycline is an antibiotic that belongs to a class of drugs called tetracyclines. It is typically used to treat bacterial infections in many different parts of the body, including gonococcal, staphylococcal, cholera, chlamydial, typhus, syphilis, and other infections. It has also received a lot of attention because it is one of the few drugs that can treat anthrax.

Gastroenterology from the Baltimore City Hospitals and The Johns Hopkins University School of Medicine in Maryland, reported on a study to determine the efficacy of doxycycline for the prevention of traveler's diarrhea among 50 Peace Corps Volunteers during their first 10 weeks in Morocco. The volunteers were divided to receive either doxycycline or placebo for three weeks and were observed by investigators for an additional seven weeks. Eleven of 24 on placebo and two of the 26 on doxycycline developed diarrhea during treatment. One week after drug cessation, diarrhea frequency increased among those who had been taking doxycycline; by three weeks later there were no differences in the two groups.

According to the *American Family Physician*, preventive treatment with doxycycline for up to three weeks has been found to provide better results than bismuth subsalicylate. Increasingly, however, resistance to these antibiotics has become such a problem that their routine use is not recommended. Antibiotic prevention for traveler's diarrhea is now recommended by physicians only in specific situations, such as in the seriously immune-compromised person or the seriously ill person who would not be able to withstand a diarrhea illness.

For more information see page 1158.

Ulcerative Colitis

Inflammatory Bowel Disease (IBD) generally has two components: ulcerative colitis, which affects primarily the colon, and Crohn's disease, which primarily affects the lower part of the small intestine. Ulcerative colitis can be difficult to diagnose because its symptoms are similar to other intestinal disorders. It involves immune system abnormalities in which immune cells in the gut that should be protecting the body from infection are instead attacking healthy tissue and causing inflammation.

Commonly Prescribed (On-Label) Drugs: *Balsalazide, Mesalamine, Methylprednisolone, Olsalazine, Sulfasalazine*

OFF-LABEL PRESCRIPTION DRUGS
BREAKTHROUGH OPTIONS

Generic: **Azathioprine** *(ay-za-THYE-oh-preen)*
Brand: **Imuran**

Azathioprine is related to uric acid. It is a prodrug (a prodrug is a compound that breaks down into the active agent) of mercaptopurine. Azathioprine is classified as an immunosuppressant medication for the prevention of organ transplant rejection and treatment of rheumatoid arthritis. Although its exact mechanism of action in rheumatoid arthritis is not known, its effect in suppressing the immune system appears to decrease the activity of the disease. It prevents cells (including those in the immune system) from dividing.

Because ulcerative colitis is also believed to be an immune-mediated disease, azathioprine is believed to play a similar role and reduces the lymphocyte count—white blood cells that play an important role in the immune system. Because of this action, they take a long time to act—up to two to three months.

An article from Gastroenterology Associates reports that immune-modifying agents such as azathioprine should be used in ulcerative colitis if corticosteroids fail or are required for prolonged periods. They are used to prevent infection in people with fistulas (abnormal connections between the intestines and other organs).

For more information see page 1033.

Generic: *Cyclosporine* (si-klo-SPOR-een)
Brands: *Gengraf, Neoral, Sandimmune*

Cyclosporine is a very powerful immunosuppressant medication approved to prevent the rejection of transplanted kidneys, hearts, and livers. It has also been tried in other immune-mediated conditions such as ulcerative colitis.

Cochrane Database System Review reported that the introduction of cyclosporine has provided an alternative to surgery for severe ulcerative colitis. In two trials, cyclosporine was given intravenously. In one, two of 11 patients on cyclosporine failed to respond to therapy compared to all nine on placebo. However, three of the 11 patients who responded eventually went on to surgery, as did four of the placebo group. In the second trial, 30 patients received either cyclosporine or methylprednisolone. Five of the cyclosporine and seven of the methylprednisolone patients did not respond to therapy. After one year, seven of the nine in the cyclosporine group were still in remission, compared to four of eight in the steroid group, and the surgery rate was similar in both groups.

For more information see page 1127.

Generic: **Thalidomide** *(tha-LI-doe-mide)*
Brand: **Thalomid**

Thalidomide was developed to treat morning sickness in pregnant women, but was found to cause tragic birth defects and quickly banned worldwide. In an accidental discovery, an Israeli physician who knew that the drug also promoted sleep, prescribed it to one of his leprosy patients who had terrible insomnia and found that thalidomide was an excellent treatment for leprosy symptoms. In-depth research on its immunomodulatory effects led to FDA approval of thalidomide for treating leprosy. Since ulcerative colitis is also an immune-mediated disease, physicians have also explored the benefits of thalidomide for these patients.

According to *eMedicine*, experimental treatments such as thalidomide should be used only after all other therapies have failed and then should be used only by physicians familiar with their use.

British Medical Journal reported that a staff member with ulcerative colitis in a facility that treated leprosy patients, having observed the excellent results thalidomide provided for her patients, asked if she might undergo a trial of the drug. Within eight weeks, instead of three or four rounds of bloody bowel movements daily, she was down to one bowel movement a day and by 10 weeks, macroscopic blood had disappeared. Almost two years later, she considered her bowel to have been normal for about a year.

For more information see page 1505.

ULCERS

Ulcers are small erosions, most likely caused by a bacterial infection such as *H. pylori*. Stomach ulcer disease is common, affecting millions of Americans yearly. The size of a stomach ulcer can range between 1/8 of an inch to 3/4 of an inch.

Duodenal Ulcer

See Gastric Ulcer

Gastric Ulcers

Gastric ulcers are erosions or sores that form in the mucosal lining of the stomach. They are usually caused by an infection with *H. pylori* or an imbalance between the secretion of stomach acid plus an enzyme called pepsin and the stomach's mucosal lining, which leads to inflammation, or inflammation caused by nonsteroidal anti-inflammatory medications (NSAIDs), such as ibuprofen, which worsen acid problems.

Commonly Prescribed (On-Label) Drugs: *Cimetidine, Esomeprazole, Famotidine, Lansoprazole, Misoprostol, Nizatidine, Omeprazole, Ranitidine*

OFF-LABEL PRESCRIPTION DRUG
BREAKTHROUGH OPTION

Generic: **Sucralfate** *(soo-KRAL-fate)*
Brand: **Carafate**

Sucralfate acts by providing a barrier over the area to protect the mucosa from acid attack, inhibit activity of the digestive enzyme pepsin in gastric juices, and absorb bile acids. *Journal of Physiological Pharmacology* reported on laboratory studies supporting this treatment and further documented immune-mediated activity that suppressed the death of mucosal cells. According to investigators, this suggests that sucralfate might also be helpful in the stomach.

In an article on gastric and duodenal ulcers during pregnancy in *Gastrointestinal Clinics of North America* reported that physicians often have to treat dyspepsia (pain or an uncomfortable feeling in the upper middle part of your stomach) or heartburn (stomach contents coming back up into your throat). It is initially treated with dietary or lifestyle modifications. If symptoms do not remit, your physician may recommend sucralfate or antacids.

Journal of Gastroenterology and Hepatology reported that sucralfate has been effective in healing both duodenal and gastric ulcers together with mild esophagitis (inflammation of the esophagus), and it is safe for both short-term use and maintenance. Investigators believe that its potential advantages lie in the better quality of ulcer healing associated with longer duration of remission.

For more information see page 1482.

Gastric Ulcer, Prevention of

If stomach ulcers have been caused by *H. pylori*, they are cured by antibiotics, and that should end the problem. If caused by an imbalance of stomach acid and the stomach lining's mucosal protection or inflammation caused by NSAIDs, medication is used, but there is a high risk of recurrence and preventive efforts are needed.

Commonly Prescribed (On-Label) Drugs:
Lansoprazole/Naproxen

OFF-LABEL PRESCRIPTION DRUG
BREAKTHROUGH OPTION

Generic: **Sucralfate** *(soo-KRAL-fate)*
Brand: **Carafate**

Sucralfate appears to inhibit the activity of the enzyme pepsin, which interacts with stomach acids, and absorbs bile acids, thus providing further protection. These actions all suggest that sucralfate might also be helpful for preventing the recurrence of gastric ulcers after they have healed.

The American Journal of Medicine reported on a maintenance regimen of sucralfate to help reduce the relapse rate for duodenal ulcer disease. They divided patients with recently healed duodenal ulcers to receive sucralfate, cimetidine or placebo. After one year, 96 patients were examined by endoscopy (a small camera that is inserted through the mouth so a physician can see the esophagus, stomach, and duodenum). According to researchers, ulcers had recurred in 17 of 31 sucralfate patients, 19 of 32 cimetidine patients, and 28 of the placebo patients. The investigators concluded that sucralfate was at least as effective as cimetidine in preventing duodenal ulcer relapse. Further, referring to the prior remission study, the investigators noted that patients initially treated with cimetidine alone had a greater early relapse rate than those treated with sucralfate alone, a combination of sucralfate and cimetidine, or an antacid alone.

For more information see page 1482.

Mucosal Disease, Stress Related

Stress-related mucosal disease (SRMD) refers to a condition that may develop in the lining (mucosa) of the stomach and small intestine of critically ill patients in the intensive care unit (ICU). The physical or medical stresses on the body may cause erosions to develop in this lining leading to bleeding. Because upper gastrointestinal bleeding is often an indicator of poor prognosis, including death, care is focused on preventing such mucosal bleeding.

Commonly Prescribed (On-Label) Drugs: None

OFF-LABEL PRESCRIPTION DRUGS
BREAKTHROUGH OPTIONS

Generics: Proton pump inhibitors such as ***Lansoprazole (lan-SOE-pra-zole)*** and ***Pantoprazole (pant-oh-pray-zoll)***
Brands: ***Prevacid, Prevacid IV, Prevacid Solutabs (lansoprazole), Protonix, Protonix IV (pantoprazole)***

Lansoprazole and pantoprazole belong to a class of drugs called proton pump inhibitors (PPIs). They suppress more than 90% of stomach acid production and thereby treat a variety of disorders caused or worsened by such acid. These two drugs are variously approved for the treatment of problems such as duodenal and gastric ulcer treatment, NSAID-induced gastric ulcer, and prevention of recurrence of such ulcers, maintenance of ulcer healing, erosive esophagitis, and gastroesophageal reflux.

According to *Clinical Therapeutics*, PPIs significantly raise the pH of gastric fluid, reducing acid levels, for up to 24 hours after a single dose. For stress-related mucosal disease, investigators suggest using pantoprazole as an intravenous formulation, particularly for patients receiving mechanical ventilation in the ICU. Further, pantoprazole may have properties leading to longer duration of its antisecretory efficacy. While lansoprazole has few known drug interactions, pantoprazole has none.

Lansoprazole and pantoprazole are the only PPIs approved for intravenous administration in the United States. This gives physicians a special option if they wish to provide the medication by IV rather than orally. *Current Medical Research and Opinions* compared intravenous pantoprazole to intravenous cimetidine in 202 critically ill patients, the duration of targeted pH levels increased with all the pantoprazole dosing regimens, while tolerance developed on cimetidine.

For more information see pages 1269 and 1393.

*Generic: **Sucralfate** (soo-KRAL-fate)*
*Brand: **Carafate***

Sucralfate is approved for the treatment of regular duodenal ulcers—those in the first part of the small intestine. It does this by first creating a coating covering the hole in the mucosa, then blocking the pepsin enzyme that interacts with digestive acids, and finally blocking bile acids. Because the creation of a film barrier over the mucosa at risk in ICU patients would be valuable—as would blocking pepsin and bile acids—these mechanisms suggest that sucralfate might also be useful in treating patients with stress-related mucosal disease.

Clinical Therapeutics noted that sucralfate will not interfere with other drugs in the bloodstream because it only acts directly in the stomach and intestines. However, investigators feel that this can also be a drawback, because it creates a film over part of the gut, and so can decrease absorption of other oral drugs administered at the same time. Therefore, other drugs must be given at least two hours before sucralfate.

Nonetheless, *Critical Care Medicine* reported that 12.2% of providers choose sucralfate as their first-line agent for stress ulcer care.

For more information see page 1482.

NSAID-induced Ulcer

Ulcers are sores or erosions that form in the mucosal lining of the stomach. Among the several ways they can develop are through the frequent use of nonsteroidal anti-inflammatory medications (NSAIDs), such as ibuprofen. Some people do not realize that aspirin is also an NSAID. These drugs interfere with the metabolism of hormone-like substances in the body and upset the acid balance in the stomach.

Commonly Prescribed (On-Label) Drugs: *Misoprostol*

OFF-LABEL PRESCRIPTION DRUG
BREAKTHROUGH OPTION

Generic: **Sucralfate** *(soo-KRAL-fate)*
Brand: **Carafate**

Sucralfate is approved for treating ulcers that form in the duodenum, the initial part of the small intestine. The drug works by first creating a gooey "Band-Aid" over the erosive hole—an emergency first aid. Then it works on surrounding problems: blocking activity of the pepsin enzyme that interacts with stomach acids and adsorbing bile acids. Because ulcers caused by NSAIDs involve the same type of damage as those due to other causes in the duodenum, these actions suggest that sucralfate might also be useful in NSAID-caused ulcers. However, researchers feel that studies have been conflicting.

Drug Safety reported that sucralfate was ineffective in preventing gastric ulcers when compared to misoprostol. Among patients taking NSAIDs, only two of 122 taking misoprostol developed ulcers compared with 21 of 131 using sucralfate.

However, *Clinics in Gastroenterology and Hepatology* reported on a study of sucralfate in people with bleeding gastric ulcers caused by long-term treatment with NSAIDs. Patients received either sucralfate or placebo twice daily for six weeks in addition to their NSAIDs. At the end of the study, 68% of the sucralfate patients had no lesions, compared with 35% of the controls. The investigators concluded that sucralfate significantly reduced the gastric erosions.

For more information see page 1482.

PUD

See Gastric Ulcer

Stomach Ulcer

See Gastric Ulcer

UPPER GASTROINTESTINAL DISORDERS

The upper gastrointestinal system includes the mouth, the stomach, the esophagus (the long pipe that connects the mouth to the stomach), and the inferior esophageal sphincter (the muscle at the base of the esophagus that helps keep food and stomach acid in the stomach once it gets there). A variety of disorders in this system can cause discomfort, pain, nausea, and vomiting.

Dyspepsia

Dyspepsia is pain or an uncomfortable feeling in the upper middle part of your stomach. (The stomach is actually well above the belly button, not below it.) The feeling can include a sense of bloating or fullness, burping, gnawing or burning pain, nausea, heartburn (with small amounts of your stomach contents coming back up into your throat), and major vomiting.

Commonly Prescribed (On-Label) Drugs: *None*

OFF-LABEL PRESCRIPTION DRUGS
BREAKTHROUGH OPTIONS

Generic: ***Amitriptyline*** *(a-mee-TRIP-ti-leen)*
Brand: ***Elavil***

Amitriptyline belongs to a large class of drugs called tricyclic antidepressants or TCAs. Its effect in dyspepsia has nothing to do with depression but may involve its ability to interfere with certain chemical messengers in the brain. It inhibits the reuptake of two chemical messengers—called norepinephrine and serotonin—by brain cells and changes the way the brain perceives pain messages.

American Journal of Gastroenterology explored the wide use of TCAs in the treatment of patients with functional abdominal pain syndromes and studies that have shown that their benefit is not due to any antidepressant or sedating effect. To explore further potential effects, the researchers divided seven patients with dyspepsia to receive four weeks of amitriptyline versus placebo.

After three weeks of washout, each patient received the alternate treatment. At the end of the trial, all patients reported significantly less severe symptoms after four weeks of amitriptyline compared to placebo. The researchers concluded that the patients seemed to have developed an increased tolerance to aversive body sensations, suggesting that the improvement is related to an alternation in central nervous system chemistry.

For more information see page 1009.

Generic: **Cimetidine** *(sye-MET-i-deen)*
Brand: **Tagamet**

Cimetidine belongs to a class of drugs known as histamine H 2-receptor antagonists, also known as H 2-blockers. It helps reduce the release of acid in the stomach. Cimetidine is approved to treat duodenal ulcers and gastric ulcers and gastroesophageal reflux disease, to help maintain the healing of duodenal ulcer, and for some other conditions, such as Zollinger-Ellison disease, in which the stomach produces too much acid.

Scandinavian Journal of Gastroenterology reported on a Swiss study of cisapride and cimetidine in the treatment of dyspepsia. One hundred thirty-seven patients received one of the two drugs. After four weeks of treatment, a small but significant difference in favor of cisapride was found. No significant differences could be detected between drugs in the other four dyspepsia subtypes: nausea and vomiting; reflux-like; ulcer-like; and non-specific. The study confirmed the importance of classifying people into dyspepsia subtypes in selecting the most appropriate drug therapy.

For more information see page 1091.

Esophageal Motility Disorders

The esophagus is a muscular tube. When you swallow, coordinated muscular contractions of the esophagus propel the food or fluid from the throat to the stomach. If those contractions become discoordinated or weak, interfering with movement of food down the esophagus, this condition is called a motility disorder. Motility disorders cause difficulty in swallowing (dysphagia), regurgitation of food, and, in some people, a spasm-type pain.

Commonly Prescribed (On-Label) Drugs: None

OFF-LABEL PRESCRIPTION DRUGS
BREAKTHROUGH OPTIONS

Generic: **Diltiazem** (*dil-TYE-a-zem*)
Brands: **Cardizem, Cartia XT, Dilacor XR, Diltia XT, Taztia XT, Tiazac**

Diltiazem belongs to a class of medications called calcium-channel blockers or antagonists that are approved to treat high blood pressure and to control chest pain (angina). By affecting the movement of calcium into the cells of the heart and blood vessels, they relax blood vessels and increase the supply of blood and oxygen to the heart while reducing its workload.

An article in the *American Journal of Medicine* from the University of Florida Health Science Center in Jacksonville reports that the two most common esophageal disorders in patients with angina-like chest pain are esophageal motility disorders and gastroesophageal reflux. According to physicians, despite the variety of drugs available for treating esophageal chest pain, none has become the drug of choice. The investigators reviewed the various treatments, including calcium channel antagonists, noting that as reported in *Gastroenterology*, an extra benefit of these drugs is that some increase esophageal contractions.

Another article in the *American Journal of Medicine* from the National Naval Medical Center and Uniformed Services University of the Health Sciences at Bethesda, Maryland, described another esophageal motility disorder, nutcracker esophagus, as a condition in which swallowing contractions are too powerful. In up to half of patients, it is caused by gastroesophageal reflux. Researchers studied 22 patients of whom 14 completed the study. Diltiazem was compared with placebo, with each administered for eight weeks. Diltiazem resulted in considerably less powerful swallowing contractions. Researchers observed that after therapy, only nine of the 14 still met the criteria for the disorder.

For more information see page 1146.

Generic: **Sildenafil** *(sil-DEN-a-fil)*
Brand: **Viagra**

Sildenafil is approved for the treatment of male impotence. It achieves this by relaxing the smooth muscle cells of the corpus cavernosum in the penis, which leads to penile erection.

An article in *Off-Label Drug Facts* explored the esophageal motility disorder called achalasia in which there is a relative lack of contractions in the esophagus, so food does not move toward the stomach well. But more importantly, the valve at the base of the esophagus leading to the stomach does not relax as much as it needs to in order to allow food to pass from the esophagus to the stomach. On the theory that relaxation of this muscle would be useful as it is in erectile dysfunction, researchers have tried sildenafil in three very small trials.

European Journal of Clinical Investigation reported on a trial in which 14 patients received sildenafil or placebo. Sphincter tone and amplitude were significantly decreased in those on the active drug. *Gut* reported on a study in which 11 patients with various esophageal motility disorders, including achalasia, nutcracker esophagus, and esophageal spasm, received sildenafil orally. Measurements taken an hour later demonstrated improvements in the sphincter pressure in 82 percent of the patients. Nine patients then took sildenafil as needed to control symptoms; two discontinued therapy because of side effects (chest tightness or sleep disturbance).

Gastroenterology reported a study of 14 patients with achalasia in which a single dose of sildenafil reduced sphincter tone with benefits noted at 15 minutes and lasting less than one hour.

For more information see page 1472.

Esophagitis

Esophagitis is inflammation of the muscular tube that connects the throat to the stomach. Esophagitis can make it painful to swallow or may make it feel as if you have angina. It may be caused by gastroesophageal reflux disease, not swallowing pills properly, or many other disorders.

Commonly Prescribed (On-Label) Drugs: *Esomeprazole, Famotidine, Lansoprazole, Omeprazole, Rabeprazole, Ranitidine*

OFF-LABEL PRESCRIPTION DRUG
BREAKTHROUGH OPTION

Generic: **Sucralfate** *(soo-KRAL-fate)*
Brand: **Carafate**

Sucralfate was originally designed to treat the most common type of ulcers that occur in the duodenum—the first part of the small intestine. While sucralfate only has approval for duodenal ulcers, physicians have tried it on esophagitis because all of the acids involved can leak into the esophagus and cause inflammation there.

Endoscopy reported on 29 patients with acute necrotizing esophagitis over a year. The first symptom of their esophagitis had been upper gastrointestinal bleeding. Their treatment had included sucralfate, an acid-suppressive drug (omeprazole), and an antibiotic. While 10 of the men died of other diseases over the course of the five years, the other 19 recovered from their esophagitis. The investigators concluded that esophagitis is more common than previously recognized.

Another way in which esophagitis may occur is by taking pills improperly, without adequate fluid or with other medications, or not taking them with meals. The pills repeatedly dissolve in the esophagus, and the contents cause irritation and inflammation. *Current Treatment Options in Gastroenterology* notes that pill esophagitis is a preventable cause of illness when people receive appropriate advice on how and when to take their medications. Further, physicians can usually avoid prescribing drugs that are most likely to cause pill esophagitis.

For more information see page 1482.

Gastroesophageal Reflux Disease

At the bottom of the esophagus is a muscular ring called the lower esophageal sphincter (LES), which is supposed to open to let food down into the stomach and then immediately close to keep digesting food and stomach acids from going into the esophagus. If it fails and reflux touches the esophagus, it causes a burning sensation; when this occurs more than once or twice a week, it causes inflammation called reflux esophagitis or gastroesophageal reflux disease, or GERD.

Commonly Prescribed (On-Label) Drugs: *Cimetidine, Famotidine, Lansoprazole, Metoclopramide, Nizatidine, Omeprazole, Pantoprazole*

OFF-LABEL PRESCRIPTION DRUG
BREAKTHROUGH OPTION

Generic: **Tegaserod** *(teg-a-SER-od)*
Brand: **Zelnorm**

Tegaserod is an unusual drug: it is approved only for the treatment of women, but for a disease that affects both men and women. It is approved for short-term treatment in women who have irritable bowel syndrome (IBS) with constipation. It is also used to treat women younger than 65 years of age who have chronic constipation with an unknown cause. It acts by speeding the movement of stools through the bowels so that too much fluid is not absorbed out of them, thus leaving more fluid in the stool and allowing a softer bowel movement. Tegaserod does not cure irritable bowel syndrome, and its benefits last only while the drug is being taken. During that time, tegaserod decreases not only constipation but also pain, discomfort, and bloating in the abdominal area. Symptoms recur within a week or two after you stop taking the drug.

One of the ways in which tegaserod speeds stool through the bowel is by causing increased contractions in the intestines so that the stools cannot lag along their route. Physicians believe that such intensifying of muscular contraction can benefit gastroesophageal reflux disease by tightening the response of the LES. Nineteen patients received tegaserod or placebo for two weeks, after which each was given no therapy for a week and then switched to the alternate therapy for two weeks. They found that tegaserod caused a more than 50% decrease in reflux after meals in these people. The benefit seemed to result from enhanced esophageal acid clearance, improved gastric acid emptying, and reduced transient lower esophageal sphincter relaxations.

For more information see page 1496.

GERD

See Gastroesophageal Reflux Disease

Heartburn

See Gastroesophageal Reflux Disease

Nausea and Vomiting, Cisplatin-Induced

Cisplatin is used in cancer chemotherapy, given by intravenous infusion. The agonies of treatment for cancer are widely known, and nausea and vomiting after each bout of chemotherapy is perhaps one of the most feared. Nausea and vomiting may begin a few hours after the treatment is given and last for a few days. Indeed, the fear of such a side effect may become so severe that nausea can begin on the way to the hospital for treatment.

Commonly Prescribed (On-Label) Drugs: Ondansetron

OFF-LABEL PRESCRIPTION DRUGS
BREAKTHROUGH OPTIONS

Generic: **Dexamethasone** *(deks-a-METH-a-sone)*
Brands: **Decadron, Dexameth, Dexone, Hexadrol**

Dexamethasone belongs to a class of drugs called corticosteroids. It is related to the hormone cortisol made by the adrenal glands. Dexamethasone is approved to treat a wide range of autoimmune, inflammatory, and allergic diseases, as well as certain malignancies. Depending on the dose, it can suppress inflammation or even tamp down the immune system. Off-label, dexamethasone is often used in combination with other drugs to help prevent nausea and vomiting when cisplatin is given.

Journal of the Medical Association of Thailand reported on a comparison of two combinations to control cisplatin-induced vomiting. One was ondansetron, dexamethasone, and lorazepam, and the other was metoclopramide and dexamethasone. These physicians chose to rely on dexamethasone in both regimens.

Indian Journal of Cancer discussed the effective control of cisplatin-induced vomiting reported on 32 cycles of chemotherapy given to 16 patients. They were given metoclopramide alone in the first cycle and a combination of metoclopramide, dexamethasone, and lorazepam in the second. Vomiting was controlled in only 19% of cases who received the single drug, compared to 81% of those who received the combination therapy, reported physicians from the University College of Medical Sciences in Delhi, India, again supporting the benefits of dexamethasone.

For more information see page 1138.

Generic: **Lorazepam** *(lore-AZ-ee-pam)*
Brands: **Ativan, Lorazepam Intensol**

Lorazepam is approved to treat anxiety, anxiety with depression, and insomnia. Interestingly, according to the website of the National Institutes of Health, some doctors also prescribe it to people with irritable bowel syndrome, although it is unknown whether the physicians prescribe it to help alleviate their anxiety about their illness or because it will help calm their bowels.

Journal of the Medical Association of Thailand reported on a comparison of two combinations to control cisplatin-induced vomiting. One was ondansetron, dexamethasone, and lorazepam, and the other metoclopramide and dexamethasone. Patients received either the ondansetron or metoclopramide in their first cycle of chemotherapy but an alternative combination in the second cycle. The ondansetron, dexamethasone, and lorazepam combination provided significantly better control of vomiting and with fewer side effects than the alternative approach.

Indian Journal of Cancer reported on a comparison of a single versus a combination approach to control cisplatin-induced vomiting. Sixteen patients each received two cycles of chemotherapy. In the first round, they were given metoclopramide alone; in the second, a combination of metoclopramide, dexamethasone, and lorazepam. Vomiting was controlled in only 19% of cases who received the single drug, compared to 81% of those who received the combination therapy. This study supports the use of lorazepam in the treatment of cisplatin-induced vomiting.

For more information see page 1287.

Nausea and Vomiting, Chronic

Nausea and vomiting—the regurgitation of stomach contents—are common gastrointestinal complaints. When they persist in a person who has no other diagnosable disorder, it is called functional chronic nausea and vomiting. If the problem comes and goes, it is called cyclic.

Commonly Prescribed (On-Label) Drugs: None

OFF-LABEL PRESCRIPTION DRUGS
BREAKTHROUGH OPTIONS

Generic: Tricyclic antidepressants, such as ***Amitriptyline*** *(a-mee-TRIP-ti-leen)*, ***Desipramine*** *(des-IP-ra-meen)*, ***Doxepin*** *(DOKS-e-pin)*, ***Imipramine*** *(im-IP-ra-meen)*, and ***Nortriptyline*** *(nor-TRIP-ti-leen)*
Brands: ***Elavil (amitriptyline), Norpramin (desipramine), Prudoxin, Sinequan (doxepin), Tofranil, Tofranil-PM (imipramine), Aventyl, Pamelor (nortriptyline)***

Amitriptyline, desipramine, doxepin, imipramine, and nortriptyline all belong to a large class of drugs called tricyclic antidepressants or TCAs. Their effect in chronic nausea and vomiting has nothing to do with depression, although how they act is unclear. They inhibit the reuptake of two brain chemical messengers—called norepinephrine and serotonin. In so doing, they change the way the brain perceives pain messages. So they may be interfering with messages that say "throw up."

Because tricyclic antidepressants have been used successfully in the treatment of irritable bowel syndrome and unexplained chest pain, physicians at the Washington University School of Medicine in St. Louis, Missouri, decided to assess their benefits in functional nausea and vomiting. They reviewed the charts of 37 outpatients of whom 57% had chronic persistent symptoms and 43% had intermittent relapsing symptoms. In addition, 35% also had pain as a dominant complaint. All had been treated with tricyclic antidepressants, and 84% had at least moderate improvement, with complete disappearance of symptoms in 51%. According to researchers, doxepin appeared to be most effective, banishing symptoms in 100 of those who received it, although that represented a total of only 10 patients, and amitriptyline was effective in 75% of those who received it, representing 15 patients. Less effective were nortriptyline and desipramine.

For more information see pages 1009, 1132, 1154, 1230, and 1378.

Nausea and Vomiting, Prevention of Postoperative

One out of three people who has had surgery with general anesthesia will remember the experience because of the most troubling side effects of that anesthesia: nausea and vomiting. Despite decades of advances in surgical technique and improved anesthetic agents, postoperative nausea and vomiting continues to be a problem that prolongs patient recovery, lengthens hospital stays, and can even have a negative effect on the surgery itself.

Commonly Prescribed (On-Label) Drugs: *Cyclizine, Dolasetron, Metoclopramide, Scopolamine*

OFF-LABEL PRESCRIPTION DRUGS
BREAKTHROUGH OPTIONS

Generic: **Dexamethasone** *(deks-a-METH-a-sone)*
Brands: **Decadron, Dexameth, Dexone, Hexadrol**

Dexamethasone is approved to treat a wide range of autoimmune, inflammatory, and allergic diseases, as well as certain cancers. Before surgery, dexamethasone is often used in combination with other medications to help prevent nausea and vomiting.

American Journal of Health—Systems Pharmacology points out that people at high risk for postoperative nausea and vomiting should be given a preventive antiemetic drug to block receptors in the body that can cause nausea and vomiting and include dexamethasone.

Anesthesiology and Intensive Medicine reported on the use of a combination of metoclopramide and dexamethasone in the prevention of postoperative bleeding. Dexamethasone was added to another medication because the antiemetic effects of metoclopramide alone are low. Of 42 patients with a history of postoperative nausea and vomiting, 71% had no symptoms after their surgery. The researchers concluded that this combination proved to be effective and inexpensive. On the basis of this study, it is now used preventively at their hospital if only one risk factor for the problem exists.

For more information see page 1138.

Generic: **Haloperidol** *(ha-loe-PER-i-dole)*
Brands: *Haldol, Haldol Deconoate*

Haloperidol is a psychoactive drug approved for the treatment of schizophrenia. However, it also possesses antiemetic properties. Nonetheless, surgeons and anesthesiologists are cautious about using it because it may potentiate the action of drugs to kill pain (such as barbiturates), general anesthetics, and other drugs that depress the central nervous system.

In a study reported in *Anesthesiology*, physicians studied the anti-vomiting effect of haloperidol using information from 15 studies published between 1962 and 1988 and eight unpublished randomized trials. This research involved 1,397 adults who received haloperidol and 1,071 controls, of whom 1,994 involved postoperative nausea or vomiting. They concluded that in doses of 0.4 to 4 mg, haloperidol provided a 1.26 to 1.51 benefit improvement over placebo. The lower dose was as beneficial as the higher dose, but a lower dose of 0.25 was not useful. There were no reports of cardiac side effects at these doses, but some sedation and cardiac side effects occurred above these doses. The investigators concluded that within these guidelines, haloperidol is useful to prevent postoperative nausea and vomiting.

Anesthesia and Analgesia reported on a study from physicians at Queen's University in Ontario, Canada of single dose haloperidol to prevent postoperative nausea and vomiting after intrathecal morphine. (Intrathecal involves delivering a drug directly into the spinal cord.) This type of spinal anesthesia prevents pain in the lower part of the body and legs but it also frequently causes postoperative nausea and vomiting. One hundred eight patients having lower limb orthopedic surgery or endoscopic urologic procedures received haloperidol or placebo after an intrathecal morphine injection. In the first 12 hours, 76% of those on placebo but only 56% of those on 1 mg haloperidol and 50% of those on 2 mg haloperidol experienced postoperative nausea and vomiting. There were no side effects of the drug, and the investigators concluded that a single small dose was safe and effective.

For more information see page 1217.

Obesity

More than half of the U.S. population is overweight. But being obese is different from being overweight. An individual is considered obese when weight is 20% (25% in women) or more over the maximum desirable for his or her height. An adult who is more than 100 pounds overweight is considered morbidly obese. Obesity is also defined as a body mass index (BMI) over 30. Patients with a BMI between 25 and 29.9 are considered overweight, but not obese.

Commonly Prescribed (On-Label) Drugs: *None*

OFF-LABEL PRESCRIPTION DRUGS
BREAKTHROUGH OPTIONS

Generic: **Topiramate** *(TOE-pie-rah-mate)*
Brand: **Topamax**

Topiramate is used to treat epilepsy and prevent migraine headaches. Three clinical trials examined the use of topiramate for weight reduction in obese subjects. They included a six-month study, a two-year study of weight loss, and a 44-week study in subjects who had previously lost weight on a low-calorie diet. According to investigators, all three studies found topiramate to be significantly more effective than placebo. Notably, weight loss continued for one year and, perhaps, could have continued for a longer period. Topiramate was generally well tolerated, with adverse events being mild to moderate and mostly related to the central nervous system. Paresthesia (burning, itching or tingling of the skin) was a frequent occurrence, but did not lead to withdrawal of greater than five percent of the people in any study.

For more information see page 1516.

Generic: **Zonisamide** *(zoe-NIS-a-mide)*
Brand: **Zonegran**

Zonisamide is an anti-epileptic drug. Weight loss was a side effect associated with zonisamide treatment in epilepsy clinical trials. A 16-week trial was undertaken at Duke University Medical Center to evaluate the efficacy of zonisamide for weight loss in obese adults with an optional extension of the same treatment for another 16 weeks. Fifty-five (92%) women and five (8%) men participated. Patients received zonisamide or placebo. All were prescribed a balanced hypocaloric diet and compliance was monitored in patients' food diaries. Zonisamide therapy was started orally, with gradual increase to and further increase for patients losing less than five percent of body weight at the end of 12 weeks. Placebo dosing was identical. Of 60 patients, 51 completed the 16-week phase. According to researchers, the zonisamide group lost more body weight than the placebo group during the 16-week period. Seventeen (57%) of 30 in the zonisamide group and three (10%) of 30 in the placebo group lost at least five percent of body weight by week 16. Of the 37 participants who entered the extension phase, 36 completed week 32. Zonisamide was tolerated well, with few adverse effects. Researchers concluded that zonisamide and hypocaloric diet resulted in more weight loss than placebo and hypocaloric diet in the treatment of obesity.

For more information see page 1557

EAR, NOSE, AND THROAT DISORDERS

EAR DISORDERS

Ear disorders can affect anyone at any age. While many of the common ear disorders involve infections, others include structural or sensory damage. Common ear disorders include barotitis media, Ménière's disease, labyrinthitis, otitis externa, acute otitis media, and chronic otitis media, among others. Hearing loss, vertigo (a sense of spinning and/or dizziness), earache, and discharge from the ear are some of the common symptoms. When ear problems arise, other areas may be affected such as the nose, sinuses, teeth, tongue, tonsils, pharynx (throat), larynx (voice box), salivary glands, and facial joints.

See Acute Otitis Media

Acute Otitis Media

Acute otitis media (AOM), or middle ear infection, is a bacterial or viral, usually secondary to a respiratory infection. Although this infection can occur at any age, it is most common in young children, particularly in infants and toddlers. Microorganisms may migrate from the throat to the middle ear through passages that connect to the ear. Secondhand smoke has been designated a risk factor in AOM. Symptoms include persistent severe earache, hearing loss, fever (up to 105°F), nausea, vomiting, and diarrhea. Fluid with blood or pus may also drain from the ear, and the eardrum can appear red and swollen.

Commonly Prescribed (On-Label) Drugs: *Cefdinir, Cefprozil, Erythromycin/Sulfisoxazole, Loracarbef, Trimethoprim*

OFF-LABEL PRESCRIPTION DRUGS
BREAKTHROUGH OPTIONS

Generic: **Ampicillin-sulbactam**
(am-pi-SIL-in–SUL-bak-tam)
Brand: **Unasyn**

Ampicillin-sulbactam is a penicillin-derivative antibiotic used to treat many different bacterial organisms that cause abdominal, skin, gynecologic, and urinary infections. Rash is a common adverse event associated with this antibiotic. Caution should be exercised with ampicillin-sulbactam, as some persons are allergic to penicillin. Ampicillin-sulbactam can be given as an intravenous infusion or injection.

Forty-one children with AOM were studied by the Pediatric Department at University of Pittsburgh in Pennsylvania. Researchers evaluated the treatment of antibiotic therapy with ampicillin-sulbactam. At six weeks of treatment, 66.7% of children treated with the drug were free from infection. However, four children experienced a recurrence of AOM after treatment, and a high incidence of diarrhea was noted. In another study at the University of Pittsburgh, ampicillin-sulbactam was compared with amoxicillin-clavulanate (a commonly used antibiotic drug for AOM). This study determined that ampicillin-sulbactam provides beneficial results in persons with AOM. More gastrointestinal effects were noted with ampicillin-sulbactam compared with patients treated with amoxicillin-clavulanate.

For more information see page 1016.

Generic: **Clindamycin** *(klin-da-MYE-sin)*
Brands: **Cleocin, Clindamycin**

Clindamycin belongs to a class of drugs known as antibiotics, and is usually reserved for use in more serious infections because it is associated with colitis (inflammation of the large intestine). Clindamycin works by blocking bacterial protein production and stopping bacterial growth. This antibiotic can be taken by mouth and injection.

In a six-year study at Baylor College in Houston, Texas, antibiotics were studied to learn more about antibiotic resistance (unresponsiveness to treatment) in AOM. Based on study findings, a certain type of bacteria associated with AOM was found to be susceptible to clindamycin. Other medical literature favors clindamycin in those who have received and failed initial treatments after three days. In case study analysis of an outbreak of AOM due to penicillin-resistant pneumococci in Kentucky, clindamycin (among other nonpenicillin-type drugs) provided relief to 70% of treated patients because of bacterial susceptibility to this antibiotic.

For more information see page 1099.

Generic: **Gatifloxacin** *(ga-ti-FLOKS-a-sin)*
Brand: **Tequin**

Gatifloxacin belongs to a class of drugs known as quinolone antibiotics and is used to treat acute sinus, lung, or urinary tract infections and sexually transmitted bacterial infection. This drug may be taken orally, in tablet form, or by injection. Common side effects associated with gatifloxacin include nausea, vaginitis (irritation or inflammation of the vagina), diarrhea, headache, dizziness, and irregular heart beats. In general, gatifloxacin is used in people who are unresponsive to other AOM therapies.

In one study, gatifloxacin was compared with amoxicillin/clavulanate in the treatment of recurrent otitis media (OM) and AOM in treatment failures in children. Three hundred fifty-four infants and children with recurrent OM or AOM failure received gatifloxacin or amoxicillin/clavulanate. Results showed that both drugs were well tolerated; the most common side effect was diarrhea. Researchers concluded that treatment with gatifloxacin once daily was as effective as amoxicillin/clavulanate twice daily. In other medical literature, gatifloxacin has been noted as a third-line treatment option in AOM.

For more information see page 1208.

Chronic Otitis Media

Chronic otitis media (COM) is recurrent or persistent otitis media, a bacterial or viral infection in the middle ear, usually secondary to a respiratory infection. A chronic ear infection may be more destructive than an acute ear infection because its effects are prolonged or repeated, and it may cause permanent damage to the ear. A chronic, long-term ear infection may show less severe symptoms; therefore, the infection may remain unnoticed and untreated for a long time. COM symptoms include ear ache or fullness in the ear, hearing loss, fever, nausea, vomiting, and diarrhea. Fluid with blood or pus may also drain from the ear, and the eardrum can appear red and swollen.

Commonly Prescribed (On-Label) Drugs: None

OFF-LABEL PRESCRIPTION DRUGS
BREAKTHROUGH OPTIONS

Generic: **Ampicillin-sulbactam**
(am-pi-SIL-in–SUL-bak-tam)
Brand: **Unasyn**

Ampicillin-sulbactam is a penicillin-derivative antibiotic used to treat many different bacterial organisms that cause abdominal, skin, gynecologic, and urinary infections. Rash is a common adverse event associated with this antibiotic. Caution should be exercised with ampicillin-sulbactam, as some persons are allergic to penicillin. Ampicillin-sulbactam can be taken through IV or as an injection.

In COM, ampicillin-sulbactam provides similar clinical benefits as seen in AOM. A study conducted in Italy evaluated the treatment of COM and chronic sinusitis (infection and inflammation of the sinuses). According to investigators, results from this study showed that ampicillin-sulbactam is an effective treatment; in patients with COM, the isolated bacteria analysis revealed a 100% susceptibility to ampicillin-sulbactam. Additionally, use of this antibiotic produced a 63% recovery and 26% improvement in treated patients. In other medical literature, ampicillin-sulbactam is considered effective for acute and COM because of its affinity for bacterial strains that produce beta-lactamases, the most common types that cause otitis media. In other clinical studies, ampicillin-sulbactam has been combined with steroids and shown positive benefits in patients affected with this ear disorder.

For more information see page 1016.

*Generic: **Budesonide Nasal** (byoo-DES-oh-nide)*
*Brands: **Entocort EC, Pulmicort Respules, Pulmicort Turbohaler, Rhinocort Aqua***

Budesonide belongs to a class of drugs known as corticosteroids, which are similar to natural steroids found in the body. In general, steroids host a number of functions within the body, including the maintenance of minerals and fluids, fat storage, glucose metabolism, cell growth, and inflammation. Corticosteroids are used in a number of diseases including endocrine disorders, cancer, arthritis, and in autoimmune disorders. Corticosteroids can be taken by mouth, injection, inhalation, and in the nose.

Intranasal budesonide is used in the treatment of inflammatory conditions of the respiratory system, and is considered safe in children. Budesonide nasal has shown clinical benefits in the treatment of COM infections with abnormal collection of fluid in the ear or without symptoms when used with other antibiotic drugs. In a study conducted in Turkey, 62 patients in three treatment groups were given: intranasal budesonide plus an antibiotic, or antibiotic alone, or no treatment. The budesonide-treated group had higher rates of infection cure.

Physicians recommend that intranasal steroids be taken cautiously to reduce the risk of side effects. In children, the most serious adverse effect is a diminished rate of growth. In clinical studies, researchers feel that budesonide has shown evidence of growth suppression; other intranasal corticosteroids have shown higher rates of suppression in comparison with budesonide.

For more information see page 1055.

*Generic: **Ciprofloxacin-hydrocortisone otic***
(sip-roe-FLOKS-a-sin hye-droe-KOR-ti-sone oh-TIK)
*Brand: **Cipro-HC***

Ciprofloxacin-hydrocortisone otic (an ear drug) is a combination drug made up of a fluoroquinolone antibiotic (ciprofloxacin) and steroid (hydrocortisone). It is used to fight bacterial infection and reduce inflammation caused by COM. Together, ciprofloxacin and hydrocortisone are used to treat ear infections. In general, after applying ciprofloxacin-hydrocortisone otic, the ears should remain tilted for approximately 30 seconds to 60 seconds to allow the drug to penetrate the ear.

In a clinical study conducted in Spain involving patients with COM, topical ciprofloxacin solution alone was beneficial and well tolerated compared with the group that received a combination treatment consisting of polymyxin B, neomycin, and hydrocortisone. In another study, ciprofloxacin otic solution, ciprofloxacin otic solution with hydrocortisone, and polymyxin B-neomycin hydrocortisone were compared. Researchers concluded that results showed that all drugs were found to be equally effective for ear infection. Time to end of pain was significantly shorter in patients treated with the ciprofloxacin-hydrocortisone combination or with polymyxin B-neomycin hydrocortisone (3.8 days) than with ciprofloxacin alone (4.8 days).

For more information see page 1094.

Inner Ear Infection

See Labyrinthitis

Labyrinthitis

Labyrinthitis, or inner ear infection, is an infection of the inner ear that affects hearing and causes motion disturbance. Medical experts think that labyrinthitis is caused by viral infections. In this ear disorder, hearing may be reduced or distorted, and patients may experience vertigo (a sense of spinning and/or dizziness). Nausea and vomiting may also accompany it and be quite difficult to control. Another complication of labyrinthitis is middle ear infection (otitis media). Recovery from infection may take three weeks since the body has to fight off the infection, and the brain needs to recover from the imbalances. Persistent vertigo and nausea may endure for more than three weeks in some people.

Commonly Prescribed (On-Label) Drugs: *None*

OFF-LABEL PRESCRIPTION DRUGS
BREAKTHROUGH OPTIONS

Generic: **Diazepam** *(dye-AZ-e-pam)*
Brands: **Diastat, Diazepam Intensol, Valium**

Diazepam, which is a benzodiazepine derivative, induces calming effects on the central nervous system (CNS). It is usually given for anxiety-related disorders and alcohol withdrawal. Common side effects associated with the use of diazepam include drowsiness and fatigue; chemical dependence on this drug and symptoms of withdrawal are also possible. Diazepam is used to reduce dizziness in labyrinthitis. Since diazepam depresses CNS functions, it is helpful in the primary reduction of dizziness and nausea in acute labyrinthitis.

Researchers do not know whether the positive effects of diazepam in labyrinthitis occur in the ear or through the CNS. Compared with other CNS-type drugs, diazepam has provided superior results with fewer side effects. In people with liver impairment, and in those taking other benzodiazepines, this drug should be taken cautiously.

For more information see page 1139.

Generic: **Lorazepam** *(Lore-AZ-ee-pam)*
Brands: **Ativan, Lorazepam Intensol**

Lorazepam, an anti-anxiety drug, belongs to a class of drugs known as benzodiazepines. This drug produces calming effects of the central nervous system (CNS) functions, and is used to treat anxiety-related disorders and alcohol withdrawal. Common side effects associated with lorazepam include drowsiness and fatigue; chemical dependence on this drug and symptoms of withdrawal are also possible.

Since lorazepam acts on CNS functions, it has been useful for the symptomatic treatment of vertigo in acute labyrinthitis. The medical literature notes that anxiety may occur with acute labyrinthitis, which is precipitated by vertigo spells. In people with vertigo and anxiety, benzodiazepine drugs, such as lorazepam, may offer multiple benefits. Finally, lorazepam is a preferred drug by physicians for elderly persons because of its short-acting duration.

For more information see page 1287.

Ménière's Disease

Ménière's disease a disorder of the inner ear causing vertigo, which is a sense of spinning/dizziness and ringing in the ears, fluctuating hearing loss, and pressure or pain in the ear. Usually it affects only one ear and is a common cause of hearing loss. Causes of the disease remain unknown. The symptoms of Ménière's disease are associated with a change in fluid volume in a portion of the inner ear. Some experts think a rupture of the inner ear area allows certain lymphatic substances to mix, causing the symptoms of Ménière's disease. Researchers believe that a low-salt diet and a water pill may reduce the frequency of Ménière's disease attacks.

Commonly Prescribed (On-Label) Drugs: *None*

OFF-LABEL PRESCRIPTION DRUGS
BREAKTHROUGH OPTIONS

Generic: **Acetazolamide** *(a-set-a-ZOLE-a-mide)*
Brands: **Diamox, Diamox Sequels**

Acetazolamide is an anticonvulsant drug. This drug may be used in the treatment of glaucoma, seizure disorders, and motion sickness. Acetazolamide has been studied in cats, and had been noted to decrease lymph pressures of the inner ear. In one analysis in *The American Journal of Otology*, people with Ménière's disease were given acetazolamide or chlorthalidone and the short-term and long-term effects on the rate of hearing loss were evaluated. Treatment with acetazolamide or chlorthalidone was useful in the testing of hearing function and in managing of vertigo attacks. However, these treatments were not useful in the long-term prevention of hearing loss that occurs with Ménière's disease. In an earlier study, the immediate effects of acetazolamide were evaluated in 30 patients with Ménière's disease, where it caused fluid shifts in the inner ear.

In another study from the University of Budapest, 60 patients suffering from Ménière's disease for more than eight years were treated with acetazolamide in varying doses. This study evaluated the drug's effects on hearing function and symptoms of tinnitus. Researchers observed successful response to therapy in newly diagnosed patients and those younger than age 50.

For more information see page 985.

Generic: **Dexamethasone** *(deks-a-METH-a-sone)*
Brands: **Decadron, Dexameth, Dexone, Hexadrol**

Dexamethasone belongs to a class of drugs known as glucocorticosteroids. These drugs resemble natural steroids found in the body. In general, steroids host a number of functions in the body including the maintenance of minerals and fluids, fat storage, glucose metabolism, cell growth, and inflammation. Glucocorticosteroids are used in a number of conditions such as cancer, gastrointestinal (GI) disorders, arthritis, and autoimmune disorders. In Ménière's disease, use of dexamethasone has been successful, perhaps because of its anti-inflammatory properties.

One study at the Hacettepe University Medical Faculty in Turkey involving 24 patients evaluated the use of dexamethasone administered through a tube into the ear for intractable vertigo. After treatment, vertigo was controlled in 72% of cases. One person experienced an ear infection and required the removal of the tube. Two percent of the patients experienced complete resolution of tinnitus, 10% experienced decreased tinnitus, and 12% experienced no change with dexamethasone.

Another study involving 34 patients with intractable Ménière's disease evaluated the use of intratympanic (inside the ear) injections of dexamethasone for the long-term control of vertigo. Almost one-half of patients (47%) experienced control of vertigo with one or more courses of treatment. However, only 24% of patients experienced long-term control of vertigo. Based on these findings, researchers determined that multiple courses of injections of corticosteroids in the eardrum, along with other treatments, are necessary in patients with Ménière's disease and intractable vertigo. Additionally, investigators in Spain found that combination therapy with dexamethasone administered in the eardrum via IV in a small study revealed improved vertigo in all patients, and hearing improvement in some.

For more information see page 1138.

Generic: **Diazepam** *(dye-AZ-e-pam)*
Brands: **Diastat, Diazepam Intensol, Valium**

Diazepam, which is a benzodiazepine-type drug, induces a calming effect of the central nervous system (CNS) functions. It is usually prescribed for anxiety-related disorders and alcohol withdrawal. Common side effects of diazepam include drowsiness and fatigue; however, similar to most drugs containing benzodiazepine, dependence and withdrawal effects are possible.

Recent studies have shown that diazepam is helpful in controlling vertigo in Ménière's disease following a trial of failed diet and diuretic ("water pills") therapy. Researchers believe that diazepam has a selective sedative effect within inner ear cells. Treatment with diazepam should be short term and discontinued when the symptoms improve or subside. Medical literature states that diazepam has been found to be particularly effective for the relief of nausea, which can accompany vertigo in Ménière's disease. People who suffer from vertigo attacks should have a prescription of diazepam at hand if an attack should occur. Some experts consider benzodiazepines as a short-term treatment because it only masks disease symptoms and does not treat the actual disease. If your vertigo attacks are not resolved by standard measures and are debilitating, surgical interventions may be the next step of treatment.

For more information see page 1139.

Generic: **Droperidol** *(droe-PER-i-dole)*
Brand: **Inapsine**

Droperidol belongs to a class of drugs called butyrophenones, and may be prescribed as an antiemetic, antipsychotic, and along with anesthesia. It blocks dopamine, which triggers receptors in the brain stem, and thereby relieves nausea and vomiting. The warnings for treatment with droperidol include abnormal heartbeats and increased sedation.

Droperidol has been researched in the treatment of acute symptoms of Ménière's disease and vestibular neuronitis. In a Canadian study, 20 patients were treated with an IV mixture of droperidol and fentanyl (a pain drug) during acute episodes of vestibular disease. Symptoms including nausea, vertigo, uncontrolled eye movements, and vomiting had improved with treatment. The mixture had no effect on hearing function and no significant effects on tinnitus. Some patients reported symptom improvement within 10 minutes after injection, others demonstrated responses after one hour. The duration of symptom relief ranged from under three hours to more than 24 hours. The investigators also studied 12 patients in a trial to compare the efficacy of droperidol with placebo. All six patients who received droperidol experienced symptom control within 60 minutes after injection. None of the placebo-injected patients had symptom control.

Additional medical literature suggests that treatment with IV droperidol is useful in managing acute episodes of Ménière's disease. A study from the University of Washington evaluated the treatment of intractable vertigo in Ménière's disease with droperidol and fentanyl in patients who failed conventional medical therapy. Although hearing function was not affected, 58% of patients treated with this combination had long-term relief of vertigo after a follow-up of two to eight years. Researchers concluded combined droperidol and fentanyl is safe, second-line treatment for those with Ménière's disease who have failed conventional first-line medical therapy.

For more information see page 1161.

Generic: *Gentamicin* (jen-ta-MYE-sin)
Brands: *Garamycin, Genoptic, Gentacidin, Gentak*

Gentamicin is an antibiotic that belongs to the class of drugs called aminoglycosides. It is used to treat many types of infections including lung, skin, bone, joint, stomach, blood, and urinary tract infections. In treatment of infection, and in persons with normal ear function, dosing with gentamicin may cause toxic effects to the ear (ototoxicity) and lead to permanent hearing loss.

In patients with Ménière's and vertigo attacks that have not been responsive to treatment with drugs, other interventions include the instillation of gentamicin into the inner ear, which allows for high drug concentrations to be administered safely. The chemical administration of gentamicin causes a partial loss of balance function in the treated ear, controlling vertigo in about 75% of cases. Patients undergoing treatment may experience a period of disequilibrium (imbalance), yet usually tolerate the drug. Deafness is possible in 10% of patients and significant hearing loss in another 25%; yet, vertigo relief is achieved in 85% of patients. The drug's positive effects have been noted to last about two to five years.

Researchers feel that intravenous gentamicin in small doses has shown positive effects in the treatment of bilateral Ménière's disease. In bilateral Ménière's disease, treatment and preservation of hearing function are challenging, yet IV gentamicin does not cause severe equilibrium problems afterward, so therapy can be safely repeated, if needed. Since gentamicin has the potential to permanently damage inner ear components and functions and the tendency to relieve symptoms in Ménière's disease, the use of this antibiotic remains controversial. In general, research has found that large amounts of gentamicin over a short amount of time produce the highest rates of hearing loss.

For more information see page 1212.

*Generic: **Glycopyrrolate** (glye-koe-PYE-roe-late)*
*Brands: **Robinul, Robinul Forte***

Glycopyrrolate is an anticholinergic drug used in combination with other drugs to treat stomach ulcers. It decreases stomach acid production. Side effects include dry mouth; this drug should be avoided by patients with heart disease, hepatitis, and glaucoma. It has also been used as add-on treatment in Ménière's disease.

In a clinical trial conducted at Columbia University in New York City, 37 patients with Ménière's disease who had been receiving treatment with a diuretic ("water pill") and adhering to a 1500-mg sodium–restricted diet for six weeks were evaluated. Researchers sought to evaluate vestibular suppression with glycopyrrolate treatment. Patients treated with glycopyrrolate at the onset of a vertigo attack experienced a statistically significant reduction in dizziness, depression, and somatic perception. In the placebo group, no score improvements were noted. This study confirmed the use of glycopyrrolate as an add-on drug to diuretics and a low-sodium diet in the treatment Ménière's disease. Also, glycopyrro-late was effective in reducing breakthrough vertigo attacks.

For more information see page 1214.

Generic: **Meclizine** *(meh-cle-zeen)*
Brand: **Antivert**

Meclizine, an antihistamine, is also classified as a vestibulosup-pressant (suppresses vertigo). This drug is used for the manage-ment of nausea, vomiting, vertigo attacks, and dizziness associated with motion sickness. Meclizine works by decreasing the excitability of the middle ear and blocking conduction in the middle ear thereby decreasing the symptoms of an acute vertigo attack by dulling the brain's signal and response. Medical litera-ture notes that meclizine provides only temporary relief from ver-tigo. Side effects associated with this drug include drowsiness, dry mouth, and blurry vision. This drug is not recommended for chil-dren younger than 12 years. In general, drug therapy such as meclizine usually provides only symptomatic relief of Ménière's disease.

For more information see page 1294.

Generic: **Methazolamide** *(meth-a-ZOE-la-mide)*
Brand: **Neptazane**

Methazolamide is a carbonic anhydrase inhibitor, and its func-tion is similar to a diuretic or "water pill." It is usually pre-scribed for the treatment of glaucoma by reducing the amount of fluid produced in the eyes, thereby reducing pressure. Since some persons have a severe allergy to sulfa drugs, this drug should be used with caution since it is a sulfa-derivative. Methazolamide side effects include nausea, loss of appetite, constipation, frequent urination, drowsiness, weakness, and headache. In Ménière's disease, this methazolamide decreases fluid pressure in the ear.

Methazolamide may prevent Ménière's disease attacks; however, the drug does not provide additional benefit after the onset of at-tack. Treatment with methazolamide is usually considered a con-servative management along with a low-salt diet.

For more information see page 1309.

*Generic: **Propantheline** (proe-PAN-the-leen)*
*Brand: **Pro-Banthine***

Propantheline bromide belongs to a class of drugs known as anticholinergics; it is also classified as an antispasmodic, used to treat cramps or spasms of the stomach, intestines, and bladder and in conditions such as peptic ulcers in adults and urinary incontinence in children. Propantheline, in combination with other treatments, has shown sufficient results in reducing the symptoms of vertigo and nausea associated with Ménière's disease.

In general, propantheline is added to other drugs to treat this ear disorder. Propantheline may be used in conjunction with a low-salt diet and a diuretic ("water pill"). About 80% of patients have experienced a longer remission or less severe symptoms with the use of combination therapy in Ménière's disease. Side effects of propantheline include dry mouth, blurry vision, and photosensitivity (sensitivity to light). Clinical studies evaluating the use of propantheline for the treatment of Ménière's disease are limited in the medical literatures. In one patient case study, symptoms of nausea and vertigo were relieved with the use of propantheline.

For more information see page 1437.

*Generic: **Streptomycin** (strep-toe-MY-sin)*
*Brand: **Streptomycin Sulfate***

Streptomycin belongs to a group of antibiotics called aminoglycosides. It is a very strong drug used to treat very serious infections including tuberculosis, certain types of pneumonia, blood infections, and meningitis (inflammation of the membranes covering the brain and spinal cord). In general, this drug is reserved for use in people who do not respond to standard Ménière's disease treatments.

This drug has the potential to cause harmful effects on ear functioning (ototoxicity). Dysfunctions of the ear can occur from the use of streptomycin; the degree of impairment is usually proportional to the dose and duration of drug, to patient age, to the functioning of the kidneys, and to the amount of existing hearing dysfunction. Ear dysfunction associated with the use of strepto-mycin may worsen in those also receiving diuretics ("water pills"). Streptomycin selectively destroys balance, and in higher doses, hearing may be affected.

Streptomycin is given as an injection into the muscle for five days until symptoms decrease or hearing and balance dysfunction de-creases. Hearing and balance measurements must be monitored. In one-third of cases, unexplained improvement in hearing or balance occurs. In one British study, 17 patients were treated with streptomycin perfusions into the ear for incapacitating vertigo. Eighty-eight percent of patients achieved symptom control of vertigo, and hearing was preserved in 55% of patients. In another British study, 47 patients were given streptomycin perfusions into the inner ear, but patients who had poor hearing prior to the pro-cedure had poor hearing preservation after treatment with strep-tomycin.

For more information see page 1481.

Generic: **Triamterene-hydrochlorothiazide**
(trye-AM-ter-een hye-droe-klor-oh-THYE-a-zide)
Brands: **Dyazide, Maxide**

Triamterene-hydrochlorothiazide is a potassium-sparing (con-serves potassium) diuretic ("water pill"). This drug is used to treat high blood pressure, congestive heart failure, and pulmonary edema (excess fluid in the lungs). Elevated potassium levels are a serious side effect of this drug; therefore people with diabetes or impaired kidney function should be carefully monitored when using this drug.

Triamterene-hydrochlorothiazide is used in Ménière's disease to decrease fluid pressure in the inner ear and to help prevent at-tacks. This drug does not help once the attack has begun. Diuretic drugs require that you monitor sodium and potassium levels in the body. In one study, 33 patients were treated with triamterene and hydrochlorothiazide or placebo for Ménière's disease. After treatment, 17 patients preferred treatment with triamterene-hydrochlorothiazide, three patients chose placebo, and the re-maining 13 had no preference for any treatment. Typically, in treating Ménière's disease, diuretics are used in combination with a low-salt diet to decrease fluid, thereby decreasing pressures of the inner ear and decreasing the number of attacks.

For more information see page 1525.

Otitis Externa

Otitis externa, also known as swimmer's ear, is a common disorder that is usually represented by an acute bacterial infection of the skin inside the ear canal. This ear disorder also can be caused by a fungal infection contracted through swimming or bathing in contaminated water. Otitis externa is more common in hot and humid weather, in instances of local injury, for example with cotton swabs or hearing aids, and in the absence of earwax. Edema, redness, fluid, and pus often appear in the ear canal. Symptoms of otitis externa include ear pain and pressure, temporary hearing loss, fever, and tinnitus (ringing or roaring in the ears).

Commonly Prescribed (On-Label) Drugs: *Boric Acid, Ciprofloxacin, Ciprofloxacin/Dexamethasone, Desonide, Neomycin/Polymyxin/Hydrocortisone, Ofloxacin*

OFF-LABEL PRESCRIPTION DRUGS
BREAKTHROUGH OPTIONS

Generic: **Betamethasone** *(bay-ta-METH-a-sone)*
Brand: ***Celestone***

Betamethasone belongs to a class of drugs known as steroids, which reduce edema (swelling) and decrease the body's immune responses. Betamethasone is used to treat many different conditions including arthritis, lupus, psoriasis, asthma, and ulcerative colitis. In otitis externa, small doses of topical antibiotic solutions can help to reduce pain and edema commonly seen with this ear infection.

Betamethasone may be mixed with gentamicin (an antibiotic drug) to create an eardrop compound to treat otitis externa. In more difficult to treat otitis externa infections, such as those that are resistant to common antibiotic therapies, betamethasone cream can be combined with other drugs and applied topically. Use of betamethasone for otitis media is documented in the medical literature. In a study conducted in Ireland, the use of combined treatment of otitis externa was examined. In this study, 239 patients with antibiotic-resistant otitis externa were treated with betamethasone cream combined with fusidic acid. All patients responded well to this combined treatment.

For more information see page 1044.

Generic: **Clotrimazole** (kloe-TRIM-a-zole)
Brand: **Clotrimazole**

Clotrimazole is an antifungal drug used to treat yeast infections of the vagina, mouth, and skin. Clotrimazole is available in creams, lotions, and solutions. Some side effects of clotrimazole include itching, burning, redness, and irritation. Although only a small number of otitis externa infections are caused by fungi, clotrimazole ear drops have been shown to be useful in the treatment of this ear disorder. Otitis externa is treated by the inhibited growth and death of fungal cells.

Researchers from Johns Hopkins University in Baltimore, Maryland, reported the use of topical clotrimazole in a patient case study. In this analysis, an eight-year-old boy infected with fungal otitis media and otitis externa infection was given topical clotrimazole and the infected tissue surgically removed, a combination deemed successful. In another patient case study, a 28-year-old man with fungal otitis externa resulting from a previous fungal infection of the foot, was given topical clotrimazole, which relieved ear inflammation and treated the infection within two weeks. Lastly, in a study involving 79 patients, a number of fungal types were examined. Patients in this study were treated with topical clotrimazole, and all patients had a beneficial response.

For more information see page 1110.

Generic: **Gentamicin** (jen-ta-MYE-sin)
Brands: **Garamycin, Genoptic, Gentacidin, Gentak**

Gentamicin, an antibiotic, belongs to the class of drugs called aminoglycosides. It is used to treat many types of infections, including lung, skin, bone, joint, stomach, blood, and urinary tract. In the treatment of infections, and in patients with normal ear function, the duration of dosing with gentamicin should be closely monitored since the drug can cause toxic effects to the ear (ototoxicity) and lead to permanent hearing loss. Side effects associated with the use of this drug include dizziness, increased thirst, loss of balance, muscle weakness, nausea, skin irritation, pain or difficulty passing urine, and ringing in the ears.

In a study conducted in Israel, the duration of effectiveness of gentamicin eardrops in external otitis was examined in 17 patients with otitis externa. Researchers found that the concentration of gentamicin started to decrease only after 12 hours; a more significant decrease was detected after 14 hours of treatment. Based on these findings, routine otitis externa treatment should include eardrops twice daily.

In another study by researchers in Spain, topical ciprofloxacin and topical gentamicin were evaluated in otitis externa and other ear disorders. In this study, topical ciprofloxacin was compared with topical gentamicin. Both drugs were well tolerated and there was no significant change in ear diagnostic test measurements with either medication in either group. Investigators concluded that ciprofloxacin was as effective as gentamicin in such ear infections, including otitis externa.

For more information see page 1212.

Otitis Media, Prevention of Recurrent

To prevent recurrent otitis media, medical treatment should follow soon after awareness of symptoms and diagnosis. Prompt treatment of acute ear infections may reduce the risk of developing recurrent or chronic otitis media. Follow-up examinations after treatment can ensure resolution. Some goals to successful prevention of otitis media include decreasing exposure to common ear pathogens, boosting immunity, and improving the ear function. To decrease exposure in children, smaller day care and class sizes, especially in the winter months, can reduce the number of outbreaks.

Commonly Prescribed (On-Label) Drugs: *None*

OFF-LABEL PRESCRIPTION DRUG
BREAKTHROUGH OPTION

Generic: **Sulfasoxazole** *(sul-fa-SOX-a-zole)*
Brand: **Gantrisin**

Sulfasoxazole belongs to a class of drugs known as sulfonamide antibiotics. This antibiotic drug contains a sulfa derivative and is used to treat different types of acute otitis media, sexually transmitted diseases, and some urinary tract infections. Side effects associated with sulfasoxazole include itching, skin rash, sensitivity to light, muscle aches, fatigue, and yellowing of the eyes or skin. To minimize side effects, you should drink eight ounces of water each day of treatment.

One medical report suggested that sulfasoxazole should be used in the prevention of recurrent otitis media in children with impaired immune systems and complications from acute otitis media infections. In the same report, researchers considered sulfasoxazole as a suggested therapy to prevent recurrence in patients who maintained adherence during primary treatment of otitis media.

In a trial by researchers in Israel, the efficacy of sulfasoxazole was evaluated. Patients in this study included 32 children who were susceptible to otitis media. During therapy, 22% of patients had nine episodes of acute otitis media, while 63% of patients in the placebo group had 36 episodes of acute otitis media. Even though these percentages from the sulfasoxazole group were statistically significant, the efficacy of this drug was noted only in children younger than two years of age. Despite the success, 31% of patients treated with sulfasoxazole experienced fluid collection in the inner ear. Researchers concluded that sulfasoxazole treatment prevented recurrent symptomatic acute otitis media, but did not reduce persistent otitis media with fluid collection in the inner ear.

For more information see page 1484.

Sudden Hearing Loss

Sudden hearing loss (SHL) is greater than 30 decibel hearing reduction, over at least three consecutive frequencies, and occurring during 72 hours or less. In general, SHL most often affects persons in the 30- to 60-year-old age range. Although this hearing loss is termed "sudden," it usually occurs during a few hours. Hearing loss is generally limited to one ear, and is accompanied with vertigo (problems with balance) and/or tinnitus (ringing in the ears). SHL may be severe, and involve different parts of the hearing frequency range. Causes of SHL include viral diseases and unknown causes. Steroids have been the drugs of choice for moderate to profound hearing loss.

Commonly Prescribed (On-Label) Drugs: *None*

OFF-LABEL PRESCRIPTION DRUGS
BREAKTHROUGH OPTIONS

---

*Generic: **Dexamethasone** (deks-a-METH-a-sone)*
*Brands: **Decadron, Dexameth, Dexone, Hexadrol***

Dexamethasone belongs to a drug class known as corticosteroids and is similar to a natural hormone produced by the adrenal glands in the body. It is used to replace this hormone when the body does not make enough of it. Dexamethasone has been found to relieve inflammation. It is used to treat certain forms of arthritis; skin, blood, kidney, eye, thyroid, and intestinal disorders; severe allergies; and asthma. Common side effects associated with the use of dexamethasone include upset stomach, vomiting, headache, dizziness, insomnia, depression, and anxiety, among others. Dexamethasone can make you more susceptible to certain illnesses and infections.

Topical application of this drug in the ear resulted in increased blood flow to the ear in animal studies. Other studies have noted that this drug alters production of proteins responsible for immune cell communication and volume regulation of the ear. In a study in Taiwan, the efficacy of intratympanic (ear injections) dexamethasone was examined in patients with SHL. In this study, patients were assigned to the dexamethasone group or a control group. Injections were given once weekly for three consecutive weeks. Results from this study showed that with dexamethasone, 26% of patients had a hearing improvement, whereas the remaining 74% of patients in this group had a hearing improvement of less than 30 decibels. Factors such as age, treatment delay time, and sex did not significantly affect patient response to treatment. Researchers concluded that dexamethasone injection improves hearing in patients with severe SHL after treatment failure with standard therapies.

A study conducted in Germany concluded that intratympanic injection of dexamethasone results in significant improvement of hearing in patients with SHL. Moreover, they noted that this drug improves hearing at specific frequencies, and does not cause body system or local side effects.

For more information see page 1138.

Generic: *Low Molecular Weight Heparin* (HEP-a-rin)
Brand: *Hep-Lock*

Heparin (low molecular weight) belongs to a class of drugs known as anticoagulants, or "blood thinners." It is used to prevent blood clots from forming and stops clots from increasing in size and is used to prevent or treat blood clots in the arteries, veins, lungs, and heart. Side effects of heparin include burning or itching on the bottoms of feet, irritation at the site of injection, bleeding gums, heavy bleeding or oozing from cuts or wounds, bruising, nosebleeds, heavy or unexpected periods, back or rib pain, changes in skin color, and chest pain, among others. In sudden hearing loss (SHL), the way low molecular weight heparins works is not completely clear, but researchers believe that it might improve blood circulation to the ear or lower the effects of blood cholesterol thereby increasing blood flow.

Researchers in China evaluated low molecular weight heparin for the treatment of SHL. Of 100 patients with SHL, 50 received standard treatment plus low molecular weight heparins (group 1) and 50 patients received standard treatment (group 2). Results showed significant improvement for early or late audiometric outcomes in group 1 (low molecular weight heparins) compared with group 2 (standard treatment). Eight-six percent of patients had recovery or good improvement in SHL in group 1, which was higher than group 2. Researchers in this study concluded that the use of low-molecular-weight heparins improved the cure rates in SHL. Another study in Germany evaluated the use of low molecular weight heparin in SHL and found that it resulted in rapid improvement in hearing thresholds within 24 hours of treatment in six of seven patients in this study.

There is no drug profile for this drug as data are pending.

Generic: **Methylprednisolone** *(meth-il-pred-NIS-oh-lone)*
Brands: **Depo-Medrol, Medrol, Solu-Medrol**

Methylprednisolone belongs to a class of drugs known as corticosteroids. It is similar to a natural hormone produced in the body; doctors prescribe this drug to replace this hormone when the body does not produce enough. This corticosteroid relieves inflammation and is used in a number of conditions such as asthma, arthritis, and in severe allergies. Side effects of methylprednisolone are uncommon, but may occur and include: headache, dizziness, difficulty sleeping, restlessness, anxiety, unusual moods, increasing sweating, increased hair growth, reddened face, acne, and thinned skin, among others.

Glucocorticosteroids are thought to influence the course of SHL by decreasing inflammation from viral infection or by changing immune cell responses in the ear. In a study conducted by researchers affiliated with the University of Maryland in Baltimore, six patients with SHL were treated with an infusion of methylprednisolone in the ear for eight to 10 days. Results from this study showed that all six patients had hearing improvements, ranging from 16.25 decibels to 25 decibels. Additionally, all patients had a dramatic improvement in speech discrimination. Researchers concluded that methylprednisolone provides significant recovery of hearing in those who fail to respond to standard SHL drugs.

A study at the Ear Research Foundation in Sarasota, Florida, supported the use of methylprednisolone for sudden hearing loss. They noted that people with severe, profound SHL who fail to respond to standard drugs do respond to methylprednisolone.

For more information see page 1316.

Generic: **Prednisone** *(pred-NIS-zone)*
Brands: **Deltasone, Liquid Pred, Meticorten, Orasone, Sterapred**

Prednisone is an immunosuppressant, part of a class of drugs known as corticosteroids. It resembles a natural hormone that is produced by the adrenal glands in the body and is given to replace that hormone when the body does not produce enough. Prednisone is frequently used to treat inflammation and prevent rejection of transplanted organs; it is also used to treat certain types of cancer. Side effects associated with prednisone include upset stomach, vomiting, headache, dizziness, insomnia, and depression, among others. Additionally, the use of prednisone increases your risk for infection.

Corticosteroids, such as prednisone, are the most commonly used drugs, and are among the few treatments used in SHL. A number of studies support their use for this condition by influencing the course of SHL by decreasing inflammation from viral infection or by changing immune cell responses in the ear. In a review by researchers at the House Ear Institute in Los Angeles, California, prednisone provided numerous treatment benefits. Patients with SHL were treated with various prednisone regimens. Researchers noted that SHL recovery was associated with prednisone given within two weeks of symptom onset, better hearing at the start of treatment, and treatment with higher doses of prednisone in patients with only one additional symptom (dizziness or tinnitus). After four months of treatment, patients continued to have some hearing recovery. These researchers concluded that immediate treatment of SHL along with additional symptoms (dizziness or tinnitus) with a 14-day course of prednisone is recommended.

For more information see page 1429.

Tinnitus

See Brain and Nervous System Disorders Chapter

NOSE DISORDERS

In general, disorders of the nose are not fatal; however, they can be debilitating. The nose is the primary point of entry for air for the lungs. Inhaled air is cleansed and moisturized by cilia (hairlike projections) and mucus that line the nasal passages. Mucus is produced in the nose, lungs, and sinuses. Nose disorders include allergic rhinitis, nasal polyps, and sinusitis; persons affected with these ailments may have difficulty breathing or speaking. A number of drug treatments are available for each nasal disorder. For some, drug therapy may be ineffective and surgery may be necessary.

Allergic Rhinitis

See Lung and Airway Disorders Chapter

Nasal Polyps

Nasal polyps are soft, noncancerous growths in the lining of the nose and sinuses. Small nasal polyps cause very few problems; however, larger ones can affect breathing, diminish sense of smell, and lead to headaches and snoring. Causes of nasal polyps include inflammation from viral, bacterial, or fungal infections, and allergies. Chronic inflammation causes blood vessels in the lining of the nose and sinuses to become permeable. Over time, water accumulates and gravity pulls down these drenched tissues to form polyps. Symptoms of nasal polyps include runny nose, persistent stuffiness, chronic sinus infections, loss of smell, dull headaches, and snoring.

Commonly Prescribed (On-Label) Drugs: Budesonide, Fluticasone, Mometasone

---

OFF-LABEL PRESCRIPTION DRUGS
BREAKTHROUGH OPTIONS

Generic: **Betamethasone** *(bay-ta-METH-a-sone)*
Brands: **Bet-Val, Diprosone, Luxiq, Maxivate, Teladar**

Betamethasone belongs to a class of drugs known as corticosteroids. It is typically used to reduce swelling, redness, itching, and allergic reactions. Betamethasone was originally approved to treat allergies, skin problems, asthma, arthritis, Crohn's disease, ulcerative colitis, and a variety of other conditions. Off-label, corticosteroids, such as betamethasone, are considered the only drugs effective in shrinking nasal polyps. These drugs work by providing a nonspecific anti-inflammatory response that reduces the size of the polyps and improves symptoms related to nasal obstruction. Caveats to use of corticosteroid-type drugs such as betamethasone are their short-lasting effects and polyps grow back within weeks to months. Side effects associated with betamethasone include diarrhea, constipation, headache, increased appetite, increased sweating, nervousness, unusual hair growth on face and body, and upset stomach, among others. Additionally, long-term betamethasone use may increase the risk of infection.

In a study conducted in Japan on betamethasone for treatment of nasal polyps all cases showed blocked cell growth when betamethasone was added to cell cultures taken from nasal polyps. Researchers concluded that topical use of steroids in patients with nasal polyps stops the multiplication of connective tissue cells in polyps and provides favorable outcome in affected patients.

In general, topical use of betamethasone can lead to systemic absorption by the nasal mucosa and by the gastrointestinal system. This effect was validated in a study conducted by researchers in England where the use of topical betamethasone suppressed the hypothalamo-pituitary-adrenal axis in patients with nasal polyps, whereas fluticasone (a steroid drug) did not.

For more information see pages 1042 and 1044.

Generic: *Montelukast* (mon-te-LOO-kast)
Brand: *Singulair*

Montelukast belongs to a class of drugs known as leukotriene receptor antagonists, and is used in mild to moderate asthma to decrease the symptoms of asthma and the number of acute asthma attacks. Montelukast is also typically used to treat the symptoms of seasonal allergies. It has been found that leukotrienes, powerful chemical substances produced by the body that promote the inflammatory response caused by allergens, are associated with the development of nasal polyps. Early studies of leukotriene-type drugs, such as montelukast, have shown improved nasal airflow and reduction in nasal polyps.

Researchers in England evaluated the use of montelukast in patients with nasal polyps and asthma who were both aspirin-sensitive and aspirin-tolerant. In this study, patients received a three-month regimen consisting of montelukast in addition to intranasal and inhaled corticosteroid. Results from this study showed a clinical improvement in nasal polyps in 64% of aspirin-tolerant patients and 50% of aspirin-sensitive patients. Asthma improved in both groups of patients. Montelukast improvements were not related to age, sex, disease duration, or aspirin sensitivity. Researchers concluded that in some people leukotriene receptor antagonists, such as montelukast, are effective.

For more information see page 1340.

*Generic: **Prednisolone** (pred-NISS-oh-lone)*
*Brands: **Predalone, Prelone***

Prednisolone belongs to a class of drugs known as synthetic adrenal corticosteroids. In general, corticosteroids have strong anti-inflammatory properties and are used in inflammatory diseases such as arthritis, asthma, and bronchitis, among others. Side effects associated with the use of this drug include diarrhea, constipation, headache, increased or decreased appetite, increased sweating, nervousness, restlessness, and upset stomach, among others. Prednisolone can impair the immune system's ability to fight infections.

Researchers in France evaluated the use of corticosteroids for the treatment of nasal polyps in a review of medical records. One hundred patients were treated with a combination of short-term oral prednisolone and daily intranasal spray of beclomethasone (a steroid drug). During the three-year follow-up of these patients, both drugs proved to be successful in 85% of the patients. In this medical chart review, only 15% of patients needed surgery because of treatment failure. The daily dosage of prednisolone and beclomethasone was progressively decreased while the nasal comfort continued. Researchers concluded that use of drugs, such as prednisolone, for the management of nasal polyps is recommended over surgery. These findings were validated in another study conducted in Sweden. In this study, patients' sense of smell improved with the use of local and oral steroids (prednisolone and budesonide). Surgery provided no additional effect, and symptom scores improved significantly with the use of steroids alone.

For more information see page 1428.

Generic: **Prednisone** (pred-NIS-zone)
Brands: **Deltasone, Liquid Pred, Meticorten, Orasone, Sterapred**

Prednisone is an immunosuppressant and belongs to a class of drugs known as corticosteroids. It resembles a natural hormone that is produced by the adrenal glands in the body; this drug is given to replace this hormone when the body does not produce sufficient amounts. This corticosteroid is frequently used to treat inflammation and prevent rejection of transplanted organs and treat certain types of cancer.

Oral corticosteroids, such as prednisone, are the only effective drugs in shrinking nasal polyps; these drugs provide a nonspecific anti-inflammatory response that reduces the size of the polyps and improves symptoms related to nasal obstruction. It is also noted to be cost-effective in the treatment of nasal polyps, since a generic formulation is available. Side effects associated with prednisone include upset stomach, vomiting, headache, dizziness, insomnia, and depression, among others. Additionally, the use of prednisone increases the risk for infection.

In a study conducted in Spain, approximately 53 patients with nasal polyps were given oral prednisone for two weeks and 56 patients were selected for surgery. After six and 12 months, significant quality-of-life improvements were seen with both medical and surgical treatment. Nasal symptoms and polyp size improved after both medical and surgical treatment at six and 12 months. Researchers concluded that both medical and surgical treatment resulted in similar quality-of-life improvements.

For more information see page 1429.

Sinus Infection

See Sinusitis

Sinusitis

Sinusitis is inflammation of the sinuses (moist air spaces within the bones of the face surrounding the nose) generally caused by viral or bacterial infections. Signs and symptoms of sinusitis include a stuffy or runny nose with daytime cough that persists for 10 days to 14 days; mucus discharge from the nose; persistent dull pain or swelling around the eyes; pain or tenderness in or surrounding the cheekbones; a feeling of pressure in the head; a headache upon awakening; bad breath; pain in the upper teeth; and a fever greater than 102 degrees Fahrenheit (39 degrees Celsius).

Commonly Prescribed (On-Label) Drugs:
Amoxicillin/Clavulanic Acid, Azithromycin, Cefdinir, Cefpodoxime, Cefprozil, Cefuroxime, Ciprofloxacin, Gatifloxacin, Levofloxacin, Loracarbef, Moxifloxacin, Telithromycin

---

OFF-LABEL PRESCRIPTION DRUG
BREAKTHROUGH OPTION

Generic: **Trimethoprim-sulfamethoxazole**
(try-METH-oh-prim – sul-fah-meth-OX-ahzole)
Brands: **Bactrim, Septra**

Trimethoprim-sulfamethoxazole is an antibiotic that contains a combination of two drugs: trimethoprim and sulfamethoxazole. It is used in several different types of infections including pneumonia, bronchitis, ear infections, and urinary tract infections. For the treatment of sinusitis, antibiotics such as trimethoprim-sulfamethoxazole are the mainstay medical treatment. In general, antibiotics are selected by the type of sinusitis such as acute, chronic, or recurrent.

Trimethoprim/sulfamethoxazole for sinusitis was evaluated in a trial conducted by researchers affiliated with a number of U.S.-based medical schools. In this study, patients received double-strength trimethoprim/sulfamethoxazole (one tablet twice daily for 10 days or one tablet twice daily for three days followed by seven days of placebo). Results showed that, at two-week follow-up, clinical symptoms and diagnostic scores of sinusitis improved equally after three or ten days of trimethoprim/sulfamethoxazole. Seventy-seven percent of patients in the three-day group and 76% of patients in the 10-day group rated their sinus symptoms as "cured" or "much improved." Researchers concluded that three days of antibiotic drug treatment was as effective as ten days of treatment.

For more information see page 1530.

THROAT DISORDERS

Disorders of the throat are not usually fatal; but, they can make it difficult to eat, breathe, and talk. The throat has three components: the pharynx, epiglottis, and larynx (voice box). Food travels through the pharynx to the esophagus and stomach. Air passes through the pharynx on the way to the trachea and lungs. The epiglottis covers the voice box and prevents food from entering lungs. Throat disorders include, but are not limited to, pharyngitis, tonsillitis, and the need for tonsillectomy.

Inflammation of the Larynx

See Laryngitis

Laryngitis

See Lung and Airway Disorders Chapter

Pharyngitis

Pharyngitis, also known as sore throat, is one of the most common medical complaints. Pharyngitis is caused by viral infections about 90% of the time and so there are no drugs to treat it since antibiotics only work against bacterial infections. But pharyngitis can also be caused by bacteria—the bacteria known as *streptococcus* are responsible for strep throat in one in 10 Americans each year. Symptoms of pharyngitis include difficulty swallowing, soreness, and a feeling of having a lump in the throat. These symptoms may be accompanied by headache, muscle and joint pain, and fever.

Commonly Prescribed (On-Label) Drugs: *Azithromycin, Benzocaine, Cefadroxil, Cefdinir, Ceftibuten, Cefuroxime, Cephalexin, Clarithromycin, Dirithromycin, Loracarbef, Penicillin G*

OFF-LABEL PRESCRIPTION DRUGS
BREAKTHROUGH OPTIONS

Generic: **Clindamycin** *(klin-da-MYE-sin)*
Brands: **Cleocin, Clindamycin**

Clindamycin belongs to a class of drugs known as antibiotics, and is usually reserved for use in more serious infections because it is associated with colitis (inflammation of the large intestine). Clindamycin works by blocking bacterial protein production and stopping bacterial growth; it is often used to treat recurrent pharyngitis. Possible side effects of clindamycin include colitis, diarrhea, stomach cramps, fever, and increased thirst.

Researchers in Venezuela evaluated two doses of clindamycin in 164 patients with throat disorders. Patients received either clindamycin hydrochloride capsules four times per day or clindamycin hydrochloride capsules two times per day and placebo capsules twice daily for 10 days. After 12 days, 92.8% of patients who received clindamycin four times per day were cured; 7.2% of patients improved. In patients who received clindamycin twice daily, 93.1% were cured, and 6.9% improved. There were no significant differences between the groups, and both regimens were well tolerated with only one patient discontinuing therapy because of skin rash.

For more information see page 1099.

Generic: **Dexamethasone** *(deks-a-METH-a-sone)*
Brands: **Decadron, Dexameth, Dexone, Hexadrol**

Dexamethasone belongs to a drug class known as corticosteroids. It is similar to a natural hormone produced by the adrenal glands in the body and is used to replace this hormone when the body does not make enough. Dexamethasone has been found to relieve inflammation; it is used to treat certain forms of arthritis; skin, blood, kidney, eye, thyroid, and intestinal disorders; severe allergies; and asthma.

In pharyngitis, dexamethasone may be used as an add-on to antibiotic drug therapy to improve pain relief. Common side effects associated with dexamethasone include upset stomach, vomiting, headache, dizziness, insomnia, depression, and anxiety, among others. It can also make persons more susceptible to certain illnesses and infections.

In a study in children with pharyngitis, a single oral dose of dexamethasone did not decrease the time to onset of clinically significant pain relief or the time to complete pain relief. In those children with positive strep test results, improvement in the time to onset of pain relief was statistically significant. In another study, researchers at the Orlando Regional Medical Center evaluated dexamethasone added to oral penicillin or erythromycin in patients with pharyngitis. Researchers found that dexamethasone was effective as an add-on treatment in this study. Improvements in pain scores were greater in the dexamethasone-treated group; also time to onset of pain relief was faster in those patients that received dexamethasone.

For more information see page 1138.

Generic: *Rifampin* *(rif-AM-pin)*
Brand: *Rifadin*

Rifampin is an antibiotic that is approved to prevent and treat tuberculosis (a lung disease) or other infections. In patients who are severely ill or have decreased immunity, IV rifampin may be added at the start of treatment. Off-label, rifampin is often used in conjunction with penicillin (an antibiotic drug) for recurrent pharyngitis. This drug works by blocking bacterial genetic material used in growth. Side effects associated with rifampin include diarrhea; stomach cramps; sores on the mouth or tongue; and discolored urine, stool, saliva, sputum, sweat, and tears.

Researchers at the Children's Memorial Hospital in Chicago, Illinois examined the efficacy of rifampin in children with pharyngitis. In this study, 38 patients were divided into three groups: group one received no treatment, group two received penicillin; and group three received penicillin plus oral rifampin. This study showed that penicillin plus rifampin were effective in 89% of treatment courses and superior to no therapy and penicillin alone.

For more information see page 1450.

Tonsillectomy

Tonsillectomy is surgical removal of the tonsils from the throat. This procedure is recommended in persons with frequent tonsillitis, particularly if the infections interfere with daily activities, hearing, or breathing and cannot be effectively treated with antibiotics. The guidelines for tonsillectomy include seven or more episodes of tonsillitis in one year; five or more episodes per year during a two-year period; enlarged tonsils that interfere with breathing; an abscess in the tonsils; and grossly uneven tonsils. Antibiotics are one of the drug classes that are used to treat tonsillitis, and these types of drugs may be helpful after tonsillectomy to prevent complications and infection.

Commonly Prescribed (On-Label) Drugs: None

OFF-LABEL PRESCRIPTION DRUGS
BREAKTHROUGH OPTIONS

Generic: **Amoxicillin** *(a-moks-i-SIL-in)*
and **Clavulanate** and *(klav-yoo-LAN-ate)*
Brands: **Augmentin, Augmentin ES-600, Augmentin XR**

Amoxicillin and clavulanate belong to a class of drug known as penicillin antibiotics, that are approved to treat a variety of bacterial infections including those that invade the ears, kidney, respiratory tract, sinuses, and skin. Amoxicillin and clavulanate stops the growth of bacteria that cause infection. Clavulanic acid is added to improve the efficacy of amoxicillin. Amoxicillin and clavulanate has specific activity against penicillin-resistant organisms. Side effects associated with amoxicillin and clavulanate include diarrhea, appetite loss, nausea, vomiting, stomach gas, and heartburn.

A trial in Ireland examined the effects of amoxicillin and clavulanate after tonsillectomy in children. Researchers noted that the decision to prescribe antibiotics post-tonsillectomy still remains controversial, although there is evidence of bacterial infiltration and there may be a need for drugs after this procedure. Two groups of children were treated: group A received amoxicillin and clavulanic acid for one-week post tonsillectomy; group B did not receive treatment. There were fewer complications in those children receiving postoperative antibiotics compared with those who did not based on pain drug used, time to normal eating, and pain scales. They concluded that treating children with amoxicillin and clavulanic acid that have undergone tonsillectomy significantly reduces postoperative complications.

For more information see pages 1012 and 1013.

Generic: **Dexamethasone** *(deks-a-METH-a-sone)*
Brands: **Decadron, Dexameth, Dexone, Hexadrol**

Dexamethasone belongs to a drug class known as corticosteroids. It is similar to a natural hormone produced by the adrenal glands in the body and is used to replace this hormone when the body does not make enough. Dexamethasone has been found to relieve inflammation. It is used to treat certain forms of arthritis; skin, blood, kidney, eye, thyroid, and intestinal disorders; severe allergies; and asthma. Common side effects associated with the use of dexamethasone include upset stomach, vomiting, headache, dizziness, insomnia, depression, and anxiety, among others. The use of dexamethasone can make you more susceptible to certain illnesses and infections.

Dexamethasone may be used before tonsillectomy to reduce the risk of surgical complications. Researchers at the State University of New York at Stony Brook evaluated the use of IV dexamethasone in 80 children undergoing tonsillectomy. In this study, 41 children received IV dexamethasone and 39 children received placebo before surgery. Results showed that patients who received IV dexamethasone had less vomiting, fewer temperature increases, and less lockjaw compared with placebo. Additionally, these patients were able to eat and drink at 24 hours more easily than others. Researchers concluded that IV dexamethasone before tonsillectomy is a safe treatment that decreases complications.

For more information see page 1138.

Tonsillar Abscess

See Tonsillitis/Peritonsillar Abscess

Tonsillitis/Peritonsillar Abscess

Tonsillitis is inflammation of the tonsils (lymph nodes at the back of the mouth and top of the throat). Tonsils filter out bacteria and other organisms to prevention infection in the body; when they become overwhelmed by infection, they swell and become inflamed. Symptoms of tonsillitis include sore throat, difficulty swallowing, headache, fever, and chills, among others. A complication of tonsillitis is peritonsillar abscess, or a collection of infected material surrounding the tonsils. In this condition, one or both of the tonsils become infected; the infection can spread to other areas of the body (neck, chest, and lungs). Antibiotics are one of the drug classes that are used to treat tonsillitis. In order for these types of drugs to work, they must be able to kill all types of suspected bacteria.

Commonly Prescribed (On-Label) Drugs: *Azithromycin, Cefdinir, Cefditoren, Cefuroxime, Clarithromycin, Loracarbef*

OFF-LABEL PRESCRIPTION DRUGS
BREAKTHROUGH OPTIONS

Generic: **Amoxicillin** *(a-moks-i-SIL-in)* and **Clavulanate** *(klav-yoo-LAN-ate)*
Brands: **Augmentin, Augmentin ES-600, Augmentin XR**

Amoxicillin and clavulanate belong to a class of drugs known as penicillin antibiotics, and are approved to treat a variety of bacterial infections including those that invade the ears, kidney, respiratory tract, sinuses, and skin. Amoxicillin and clavulanate stop the growth of bacteria that cause infection. Clavulanic acid is added to improve the efficacy of amoxicillin.

In combination amoxicillin and clavulanate have specific activity against penicillin-resistant organisms. Side effects include diarrhea, appetite loss, nausea, vomiting, stomach gas, and heartburn.

A number of studies have evaluated amoxicillin and clavulanate for tonsillitis. In a study in Poland, the efficacy and safety of amoxicillin and clavulanate were compared with another antibiotic drug, cefaclor. In this study, 100 children were treated with either amoxicillin and clavulanate or cefaclor. This study showed that both antibiotic drugs provided nearly 98% efficacy; however, amoxicillin and clavulanate was associated with more tonsillitis relapses and recurrences compared with cefaclor.

A study conducted in Greece found that five days of amoxicillin and clavulanate and clarithromycin (an antibiotic drug) were effective compared with penicillin 10-day treatment. However, amoxicillin and clavulanate and penicillin were more effective against bacteria compared with clarithromycin, so researchers concluded that clarithromycin regimens should not be used to treat streptococcal tonsillitis.

For more information see pages 1012 and 1013.

Generic: *Clindamycin* (klin-da-MYE-sin)
Brands: *Cleocin, Clindamycin*

Clindamycin is an antibiotic usually reserved for use in more serious infections (bone, blood, joint, lung, urinary tract, and pelvic infections) because it is associated with colitis (inflammation of the large intestine). It works by blocking bacterial protein production and stopping bacterial growth and works against a number of bacterial species; it is also considered to have good absorption into the blood stream in both the oral and IV formulation. Possible side effects of clindamycin include colitis, itching in the rectal or genital area, nausea, and vomiting.

In a clinical study in Venezuela, two regimens of clindamycin were evaluated in patients with tonsillitis. Researchers gave clindamycin in one of two ways: 150 mg four times a day (group one) or 300 mg two times a day (group two) and placebo capsules twice daily for 10 days. Results showed that 92.8% of patients in group one were cured, and 7.2% were improved. In group two, 93.1% of patients were cured, and 6.9% of patients were improved. Additionally, there was no significant difference between the treatment groups, and both clindamycin drug regimens were well tolerated. Only one patient discontinued treatment because of skin rash. According to researchers, clindamycin 300 mg twice daily was as effective as the 150-mg dose given four times daily for this throat condition.

For more information see page 1099.

Generic: **Dexamethasone** *(deks-a-METH-a-sone)*
Brands: **Decadron, Dexameth, Dexone, Hexadrol**

Dexamethasone belongs to a drug class known as corticosteroids. It resembles a natural hormone produced by the adrenal glands in the body, and is used to replace this hormone when the body does not make enough of it. Dexamethasone relieves inflammation; it is used to treat certain forms of arthritis; skin, blood, kidney, eye, thyroid, and intestinal disorders; severe allergies; and asthma.

Dexamethasone is used for tonsillitis to relieve this throat condition by reducing inflammation, which may impair breathing and swallowing. Common side effects associated with the use of dexamethasone include upset stomach, vomiting, headache, dizziness, insomnia, depression, and anxiety, among others. The use of dexamethasone can make you more susceptible to certain illnesses and infections.

In a study in Turkey, the effects of dexamethasone, bupivacaine (a drug for pain), and topical lidocaine (a drug for pain) were compared with placebo in children who had their tonsils removed. The first group of children received bupivacaine, the second group received dexamethasone on each tonsil, the third received lidocaine sprayed on the throat four times daily, and the fourth received placebo. Based on patient ratings of pain, all three drugs were effective in reducing pain after the tonsil surgery, but lidocaine was more preferred after surgery compared with bupivacaine.

For more information see page 1138.

Generic: **Immune Globulin** *(EH-mune GLOB-ewe-lyn)*
Brands: **Gamimune N, Gamunex, Octagam, Polygam S/D, Venoglobulin S**

Immune globulin belongs to a class of drugs known as immunoglobulins or immunizing agents and is used to improve immune function in the presence of viral auto-antibodies. It prevents or reduces the severity of certain infections in patients at an increased risk of infection and is used as a replacement drug in people whose bodies do not produce enough immune globulin.

Researchers in Japan examined the production of immunoglobulins against *H. parainfluenzae* in tonsil cells of patients with tonsillitis. In this study, researchers found that *H. parainfluenzae* antigens stimulate tonsil immune cells in patients with IgA nephropathy. Additionally, these patients have activation of immune cells against *H. parainfluenzae* antigens. Researchers concluded that immune globulin could be helpful in fighting severe infections in patients with tonsillitis.

For more information see pages 1234 and 1235.

Generic: **Rifampin** (rif-AM-pin)
Brand: **Rifadin**

Rifampin is an antibiotic and approved to treat certain bacterial infections. This drug is also used with other medicines to treat tuberculosis (a lung infection). Rifampin is also taken by itself by people who may carry meningitis bacteria and may spread these bacteria to others.

In tonsillitis/peritonsillar abscess, rifampin is among a number of off-label drugs a doctor may use. It works by blocking the genetic material used in bacterial growth and spread. This drug is mainly used in children with tonsillitis. Side effects associated with rifampin include diarrhea, stomach cramps, sores on the mouth or tongue, and discolored urine, stool, saliva, sputum, sweat, and tears.

Use of rifampin for tonsillitis was documented in a case study reported by researchers at UCLA School of Medicine in Los Angeles, California. In this instance, a 27-year-old man with a six-week history of sore throat had been unsuccessfully treated with the antibiotic drugs penicillin and ampicillin. He was then given rifampin once daily. After two weeks of treatment with rifampin, his sore throat resolved and the inflamed tonsil appeared normal on examination.

For more information see page 1450.

Generic: **Vancomycin** (vank-coe-MY-sin)
Brands: **Vancocin, Vancoled**

Vancomycin belongs to a class of drugs known as glycopeptide antibiotics. This drug is most commonly used to treat colitis (inflammation of the intestine caused by certain bacteria) by killing bacteria in the intestines. Vancomycin is among a number of drugs that doctors may use to treat tonsillitis/peritonsillar abscess; it is indicated for patients who cannot receive or have failed to respond to other antibiotic drugs. The use of vancomycin may cause upset stomach.

Researchers in Japan conducted a nationwide evaluation of ear, nose, and throat disorders treated at a variety of treatment centers in their country. Among the studied disorders, 724 patients with acute tonsillitis and 141 patients with peritonsillar abscess were included. In this study, vancomycin was shown to have the highest antimicrobial activity against methicillin-resistant *Staphylococcus aureus* bacteria; resistance to this drug was not detected.

For more information see page 1537.

EYE
DISORDERS

EYE DISORDERS

Some consider sight the most important of our five senses, because vision tells us more about the world around us than other senses. Eyes are complex, intricate, and delicate. Eye disorders include: errors of refraction, such as nearsightedness; problems with the parts of the eye you can see, such as the lens and the iris; the two forms of glaucoma; disorders that affect the structures in the inner layer of the eye, including the retina; as well as problems with the muscles and other tissues that surround the eye.

Blepharitis

Blepharitis is a common inflammatory condition that affects the eyelids. Some people have no symptoms, but most experience eyelid burning, itching, and irritation. In severe cases, blepharitis may cause styes and irritation and inflammation of the cornea and conjunctiva, called keratitis and conjunctivitis, respectively. People who have blepharitis often have systemic diseases, such as rosacea and seborrheic dermatitis, as well as eye diseases, such as dry eye syndromes, chalazion, or trichiasis.

Commonly Prescribed (On-Label) Drugs: *Gentamicin, Natamycin, Neomycin, Sulfacetamide*

OFF-LABEL PRESCRIPTION DRUGS
BREAKTHROUGH OPTIONS

*Generic: **Acetylcysteine** (a-se-teel-SIS-teen)*
*Brands: **Acetadote, Mucomyst***

Acetylcysteine is typically given to patients with thick mucus secretions in the lungs, such as those with chronic emphysema, chronic bronchitis, pneumonia, and cystic fibrosis, in which case it is inhaled through a nebulizer. It is believed that acetylcysteine breaks up mucus in the lungs by blocking the oxidation of lipids (fats). Researchers at Okmeydani Training Hospital in Turkey developed a study to see if acetylcysteine would work in a similar way to break up mucus in the eye. As reported in *Cornea*, results indicated acetylcysteine would be of value to people with blepharitis. The study included 79 eyes of 40 people with chronic posterior blepharitis. During the study, a topical steroid, a topical antibiotic, and artificial tears were given in 36 eyes of 18 patients; then three daily doses of oral acetylcysteine were given to the other 22 patients (43 eyes). All groups were examined weekly for one to four months. All patients with acetylcysteine showed significant improvement.

For more information see page 986.

*Generic: **Itraconazole** (i-tra-KOE-na-zole)*
*Brand: **Sporanox***

In some instances, the cause of blepharitis is not clear. Itraconazole is an antifungal drug that is FDA-approved for a wide range of fungal diseases. In *Japanese Journal of Medical Mycology,* physicians reported a patient who had a clear case of fungal disease of his finger and toenails and scales on the margins of his upper and lower eyelids and his ear, which they diagnosed as seborrheic blepharitis with swelling along the margin of the eyelid. When his lids and ear were examined closely with a special tool, they were revealed to have the spores of a related fungus, a yeast named *Malassezia*. The physician prescribed oral itraconazole as a treatment for both infections. Soon after administering itraconazole the scales and itching of the eyelids ceased. Two months after treatment was discontinued, there was no recurrence of blepharitis and oral itraconazole was deemed curative. The physicians concluded that *Malassezia* is one of the major causes of seborrheic blepharitis, a conclusion with which other researchers have agreed.

For more information see page 1256.

Generic: **Tacrolimus** *(ta-KROE-li-mus)*
Brands: **Prograf, Protopic**

Tacrolimus is an immunosuppressive drug that, in its oral form, is commonly used to prevent organ rejection in transplant patients. In its topical form, it is used to treat atopic dermatitis. It interferes with the ability of certain white blood cells, called T-helper lymphocytes, to become activated—an important step in immune system function. This makes it particularly useful for helping suppress inflammation.

Severe blepharitis is often treated with topical corticosteroids to suppress the inflammation, but they provide limited benefit that decreases over time. A study at Heinrich Heine University in Düsseldorf, Germany, included 14 patients with severe blepharitis. Tacrolimus ointment was applied to their eyelids twice daily, and the eyelids were examined regularly over the course of five months to assess redness, swelling, scaling, oozing, crusting, and any abrasion due to scratching. Skin, eyelid and itching scores all dropped markedly, although the authors concluded that long-term efficacy and safety still had to be evaluated in follow-up studies.

For more information see page 1489.

Chilaza

See Chalazia

Chalazia

A chalazion is a small mass in the eyelid, caused by a blockage of a tiny oil gland in the eyelid. These chalazia develop within the eyelid's Meibomian glands, the sebaceous glands that produce the tear film that lubricates the eyes. The eyelid has about 100 of these glands, located near the eyelashes. A chalazion begins as diffuse swelling and tenderness and later forms a cyst-like localized swelling.

Commonly Prescribed (On-Label) Drugs: None

OFF-LABEL PRESCRIPTION DRUGS
BREAKTHROUGH OPTIONS

---

*Generic: **Triamcinolone Acetonide***
(trye-am-SIN-oh-lone ah-SIT-oh-nide)
*Brand: **Kenalog 10, Tac 40, Tri-Kort, Trilog***

Triamcinolone is a corticosteroid drug, one of the most powerful anti-inflammatories available, used to treat a wide range of inflammatory problems, allergic, and autoimmune disorders. However, because irritation and inflammation typically accompany chalazia and may lead to its prolongation, local injections of triamcinolone directly into the chalazia can be useful to their resolution.

Ophthalmology reported on a study of 147 patients with new or recurrent chalazia treated at the Jules Stein Eye Institute who received an injection of triamcinolone directly into the chalazia. Success was defined as at least an 80% decrease in size with no recurrence. If it recurred, or the chalazion did not shrink at least 50%, further injections were given. Eighty percent of people were healed with only one or two injections. The investigators concluded that triamcinolone may be considered as a first treatment in cases where diagnosis is straightforward.

Another study in the *Journal of French Ophthalmology* was conducted at the University of Kinshasa, in the Democratic Republic of the Congo. Twenty-five black African patients received injections of triamcinolone directly into their chalazia. Improvement was achieved in 72% of the patients.

For more information see page 1524.

Cystoid Macular Edema

Cystoid macular edema (CME) is swelling of the macula—the central retina at the back of the eye—that typically occurs as a result of diseases such as uveitis or diabetes, injury or, more commonly, eye surgery, especially cataract surgery. Fluid collects within the layers of the macula, causing blurred, distorted central vision. CME rarely causes permanent loss of vision, but recovery is often slow and gradual over the course of months.

Commonly Prescribed (On-Label) Drugs: None

OFF-LABEL PRESCRIPTION DRUGS
BREAKTHROUGH OPTIONS

Generics: **Diclofenac Sodium** *(dy-KLOE-fen-ak)* and **Ketorolac (Ophthalmic)** *(KEE-toe-role-ak)*
Brands: **Voltaren ophthalmic (diclofenac sodium), Acular, Acular LS (ketorolac)**

Diclofenac and ketorolac are nonsteroidal anti-inflammatory drugs (NSAIDs). In their oral forms they are prescribed for such inflammatory conditions as arthritis. Diclofenac ophthalmic and ketorolac ophthalmic are topical drugs normally prescribed for ocular irritation, postoperative ocular pain, and photophobia (sensitivity to light). However, because inflammation typically accompanies CME, diclofenac and ketorolac can play a key role in helping reduce the inflammation and, hence, the swelling.

In a study in the *Journal of Cataract Refractory Surgery*, 34 patients had their cataracts extracted, had intraocular lenses implanted, and subsequently developed CME. Half were treated with diclofenac ophthalmic and half with ketorolac ophthalmic. Within six months, diclofenac resolved the CME in 89% of patients and ketorolac in 88%. The researchers considered them equally effective and said either solution may be considered for CME after cataract surgery, especially in those who may not tolerate corticosteroid treatment.

For more information see pages 1142, 1143, and 1262.

Generic: **Triamcinolone Acetonide** *(trye-am-SIN-oh-lone ah-SIT-oh-nide)*
Brand: **Kenalog 10, Tac 40, Tri-Kort, Trilog**

Triamcinolone is one of the most powerful anti-inflammatories available. In high doses it also acts as an immune suppressant. It is used to treat a wide range of inflammatory problems, allergic, and autoimmune disorders. However, because inflammation typically accompanies CME, local injections of triamcinolone acetonide directly into the vitreous can be useful when systemic steroids (medications given by pill that affect the whole body) need to be avoided. By helping reduce the inflammation, triamcinolone can help reduce the swelling.

A report from the Keio University School of Medicine in Tokyo discussed eight eyes of seven patients who had CME due to various causes. After intravitreal injections of triamcinolone, all cases of CME resolved within a month.

The American Journal of Ophthalmology reported on another study of 18 patients with CME due to central retinal vein occlusion. They received intraocular injections of triamcinolone and were followed for one year. The investigators concluded that triamcinolone injections were very effective in reversing CME and improving visual acuity in the first six months, but the improvement was not sustained at one year.

For more information see page 1524.

Endophthalmitis

Endophthalmitis is an inflammation of the intraocular cavities. It may be noninfectious, as a result of a retained contact lens, surgery, trauma, or a toxic agent. But it is usually due to an infection, such as virus, bacteria, or fungus.

Commonly Prescribed (On-Label) Drugs: *None*

OFF-LABEL PRESCRIPTION DRUGS
BREAKTHROUGH OPTIONS

Generic: **Fluconazole** *(floo-KOE-na-zole)*
Brand: **Diflucan**

Fluconazole is an oral antifungal medication that is used to treat a wide range of fungal diseases. Although a drug called amphotericin B is currently the FDA-approved drug to treat endophthalmitis caused by fungal infection, there are concerns about its potential to cause renal damage and the need to administer it by intravenous infusion, as reported in the *Archives of the Spanish Society of Ophthalmology*. Those risks are raised when it is given in conjunction with certain other drugs that the patient may be taking. In those instances, the physician may look to off-label anti-fungal drugs, such as fluconazole.

The Spanish Society reported on the case of a patient with endophthalmitis due to the fungus *Candida parapsilosis*. The person was treated with amphotericin without success. Subsequently, the person was treated simultaneously with two off-label drugs—topical fluconazole and oral itraconazole—and they appeared to be effective in controlling the infection.

Additionally, oral fluconazole may be administered as reported by Indian researchers at the Joseph Eye hospital. They reported at a recent conference that in some cases oral fluconazole may be more effective than oral itraconazole because of its high water-soluble properties, which allows it to be absorbed into the body faster.

An earlier study reported in the *Journal of Ocular Pharmacological Therapy* had shown no retinal toxicity with fluconazole infusion and that it was effective in the treatment of experimental endophthalmitis due to the fungus *candida*.

For more information see page 1188.

Generic: **Itraconazole** (i-tra-KOE-na-zole)
Brand: **Sporanox**

Itraconazole is an orally administered anti-fungal medication that is effective against fungal causes of endophthalmitis. Currently, amphotericin B is FDA-approved to treat endophthalmitis caused by fungal infection. However a report published in the *Archives of the Spanish Society of Ophthalmology* raised concerns about its potential to cause renal damage and the need to administer it by intravenous infusion. These effects are greater when used in conjunction with certain other drugs that the patient may be taking. In such cases, the physician may treat endophthalmitis with itraconazole.

In a case report published by the Spanish Society, doctors treated a patient with endophthalmitis due to the fungus *Candida parapsilosis*. The patient was treated with amphotericin with no success.

The patient was then treated simultaneously with topical flucona-zole and oral itraconazole, which proved to be effective in control-ling the infection.

An article in *Reviews of Infectious Diseases* discussed the case of a patient suffering with AIDS. It is known to be very difficult to treat fungal infections in such people. The investigators reported a case of presumed endophthalmitis in their patient. Treatment with oral itraconazole resulted in complete resolution of his illness, with restoration of normal vision.

For more information see page 1256.

Inflammation of the Eyelids

See Blepharitis

Keratoconjunctivitis Sicca

Keratoconjunctivitis sicca is dry eye—inadequate protection of the cornea because of either inadequate tear production or abnor-mal constitution of the tears, which results in excessively fast evaporation or premature destruction of the tear film. The tear film is normally composed of three layers: a lipid (fat) layer; an aqueous (water) layer (produced by the lacrimal glands); and a mucin layer. Any abnormality in these layers can produce dry eye symptoms.

Commonly Prescribed (On-Label) Drugs: *Cyclosporine, Rose Bengal*

OFF-LABEL PRESCRIPTION DRUGS
BREAKTHROUGH OPTIONS

Generic: ***Acetylcysteine*** *(a-se-teel-SIS-teen)*
Brands: ***Acetadote, Mucomyst***

Acetylcysteine is typically given to those with thick mucus secre-tions, such as those with chronic emphysema, in which case it is inhaled through a nebulizer. Researchers suspected that the way in which acetylcysteine breaks up mucus by blocking the oxidation of lipids (fats) in chronic emphysema would be of value to people with dry eye.

Researchers at Bristol Eye Hospital in the United Kingdom conducted a trial in 30 patients, published in the *British Journal of Ophthalmology*, comparing the benefits of therapy with drops every two hours of either acetylcysteine or artificial tears. After two months, patients were switched and given the other preparation. The researchers found that treatment with acetylcysteine produced significantly better results than treatment with artificial tears.

Another report from the Bolivian National Institute of Ophthalmology notes that acetylcysteine drops can be used successfully in patients with corneal filaments secondary to extreme keratitis sicca, but that they should not be used at the same time as contact lenses. Further, this drug should not be used at the same time as topical antibiotics.

For more information see page 986.

Generic: *Tacrolimus* (ta-KROE-li-mus)
Brands: *Prograf, Protopic*

Tacrolimus is commonly used to prevent organ rejection in transplant patients. The immunosuppressive power of tacrolimus has been shown to be more pronounced than cyclosporine, although it is not as widely used because it can be more toxic to the kidney.

Two patients, described in *Cornea* by physicians at the Keio University School of Medicine in Tokyo, had severe dry eye with chronic graft vs. host disease after stem cell transplantation. One had received such transplantation for chronic myelogenous leukemia. He developed rejection problems after transplantation and dry eye. Despite treatment with cyclosporin A, a potent immunosuppressive A and prednisolone (another corticosteroid), he did not improve sufficiently. Subsequently, both were discontinued and tacrolimus was instituted; the dry eye and graft vs. host disease showed marked improvement.

In the second case, a woman had stem cell transplantation for myelodysplastic syndrome. She had mild dry eye beforehand, which worsened significantly when her tacrolimus was being tapered. When the dose was increased, her dry eye symptoms markedly improved.

The investigators concluded that systemic tacrolimus with corticosteroids is an effective treatment for severe dry eyes in patients with graft vs. host disease, but long-term administration may be required to achieve lasting remission. They suggested exploring topical tacrolimus as maintenance therapy.

For more information see page 1489.

Meibomian Cyst

See Chalazia

Neuromyelitis Optica

See Optic Neuritis

Oculogyric Crisis

An oculogyric crisis is a spasmodic movement of the eyeballs into a fixed position, usually upward, that persists for several minutes or hours. It is an acute dystonia—sudden, uncoordinated muscle movements—the eye muscle is holding too much tension. It most commonly occurs as a side effect of treatment with certain drugs, especially those of the class called neuroleptics, used to treat psychosis, tic disorders, hallucinations, and various disorders of excess involuntary movement. It may also occur with other drugs to treat psychiatric and neurological conditions, as well as head trauma and brain infections.

Commonly Prescribed (On-Label) Drugs: None

OFF-LABEL PRESCRIPTION DRUGS
BREAKTHROUGH OPTIONS

---

*Generic: **Benztropine** (BENZ-troe-peen)*
*Brand: **Cogentin***

Benztropine is used in the treatment of Parkinson's disease, both in oral form and as an injection for acute dystonia, sudden, uncoordinated muscle movements. This medication blocks nerve impulses that help control the muscles and also reduce levels of acetylcholine, an important chemical messenger in the brain that controls muscle movement and other functions. These benefits help ease the muscle spasms of oculogyric crisis.

Annals of Pharmacotherapy reported on a case from the California Clinical Trials Medical Group of delayed-onset dystonic reactions and oculogyric crisis in a woman who received an intramuscular injection of a psychiatric drug. She did not develop symptoms until 26 hours later, at which point she became unable to lower her gaze and reported her neck was stiff. She was given an intramuscular injection of benztropine, and her symptoms almost completely disappeared within 15 minutes.

In oculogyric crisis, benztropine can be given as an intravenous infusion or an intramuscular injection, according to the Canadian Movement Disorder Group. It is also available in oral form.

For more information see page 1041.

Generic: **Diazepam** *(dye-AZ-e-pam)*
Brands: **Diastat, Diazepam, Intensol, Valium**

Diazepam belongs to a class of drugs called benzodiazepines. They are used to treat anxiety and are also used as sedatives and muscle relaxants. This last characteristic is beneficial in treating oculogyric crisis. Their action of increasing a major inhibitory chemical messenger in the brain also helps this condition.

If you tend to have low blood pressure, diazepam can aggravate it, and diazepam should not be given if you have glaucoma. In oculogyric crisis, diazepam can be given as an intravenous infusion or an intramuscular injection, according to the Canadian Movement Disorder Group. It is also available in oral form for maintenance treatment.

For more information see page 1139.

Generic: **Lorazepam** *(lore-AZ-ee-pam)*
Brands: **Ativan, Lorazepam Intensol**

Lorazepam, a benzodiazepine, is used to treat anxiety and anxiety with depression, as well as insomnia. It is also a muscle relaxant, which benefits the treatment of oculogyric crisis.

In *Epilepsia,* neurologists at the Mayo Clinic in Rochester, Minnesota, reported a case of oculogyric crisis and unusual movements in a patient being treated with the drug gabapentin, used to treat epilepsy. Although discontinuation of the drug led to rapid resolution of the movements, a single dose of lorazepam was needed to end the oculogyric crisis.

In oculogyric crisis, lorazepam can be given as an intravenous infusion or an intramuscular injection, according to the Canadian Movement Disorder Group. As a maintenance dose it is available in oral form.

For more information see page 1287.

Optic Neuritis

Optic neuritis is an inflammation of the optic nerve that causes pain and vision loss by damaging to the sheath around the nerve. It often occurs as the first symptom of multiple sclerosis although it may occur on its own. You must receive prompt treatment to help prevent permanent vision damage.

Commonly Prescribed (On-Label) Drugs: *Betamethasone, Cortisone, Dexamethasone, Prednisolone, Prednisone, Triamcinolone*

OFF-LABEL PRESCRIPTION DRUG
BREAKTHROUGH OPTION

Generic: **Methylprednisolone**
(meth-il-pred-NIS-oh-lone)
Brands: **Depo-Medrol, Medrol, Solu-Medrol**

Methylprednisolone is a corticosteroid drug, one of the most potent anti-inflammatory drugs available and, when given in high doses, is also a potent immunosuppressive.

A study explored treatments for optic neuritis, as well as the association between optic neuritis and multiple sclerosis. A total of 435 patients received one of three treatments: oral prednisone, intravenous methylprednisolone followed by oral prednisone, or oral placebo.

Intravenous methylprednisolone was chosen because recent experience at the time had demonstrated promising results, despite the fact that prednisone was then the treatment most commonly used. The study showed that the second regimen, intravenous methylprednisolone for three days followed by an oral prednisone taper, decreased the short-term risk of developing multiple sclerosis in patients with certain lesions in the central nervous system. Intravenous methylprednisolone does little to affect the ultimate visual acuity of optic neuritis patients, but it does speed the rate of recovery.

While intravenous methylprednisolone is usually administered in a hospital, it is sometimes given in outpatient settings.

For more information see page 1316.

Outer Retinal Necrosis

Outer retinal necrosis is a very serious form of retinopathy—damage to the retina at the back of the eye. It has been theorized that this disorder may be caused by viruses, such as chickenpox or herpes. Progressive outer retinal necrosis is most commonly seen in people with AIDS.

Commonly Prescribed (On-Label) Drugs: None

OFF-LABEL PRESCRIPTION DRUGS
BREAKTHROUGH OPTIONS

Generic: **Acyclovir** *(ay-SYE-kloe-veer)* and
Foscarnet *(fos-KAR-net)*
Brands: **Zovirax (acyclovir), Foscavir (foscarnet)**

Acyclovir is an anti-viral drug typically used to treat chickenpox and different types of herpes. *Journal of French Ophthalmology* reported on a study done at the Pitié Salpêtrière Hospital in Paris in which intraocular specimens from 33 patients admitted with acute retinal necrosis or progressive outer retinal necrosis were discussed to determine the viral cause. Sophisticated techniques found viruses and detected herpes virus in 80.5% of the patients. In the acute retinal necrosis group, they found herpes in 34.4%, varicella-zoster virus (chickenpox) in 28.1%, cytomegalovirus in 12.5%, and Epstein-Barr virus in 3.1%. In the progressive outer retinal necrosis group, all had the chickenpox virus. All patients had been treated with antiviral drugs, including two with intravenous acyclovir, and 10 with an intravenous combination of acyclovir and foscarnet. Vision was improved by intensive antiviral therapy.

European Journal of Ophthalmology reported on a person with progressive outer retinal necrosis also treated with a combination of antiviral drugs, in his case intravenous acyclovir, three injections of foscarnet directly into the vitreous of the eye, and a ganciclovir implant in the right eye. The improvements were dramatic within two weeks and continued at three months' follow-up.

For more information see pages 989 and 1203.

Generic: Immune Globulin IgG *(EH-mune GLOB-ewe-lyn)* Brands: Gamimune N, Gamunex, Octagam, Polygam S/D, Venoglobulin S

Immune globulin is the part of blood that contains the most antibodies. They attach to foreign substances, such as bacteria, and help destroy them. As a medication, immune globulin is obtained from plasma pooled from about a thousand donors. Its normal use is to provide short-term protection to people exposed to infections for which they have not received immunization, such as pregnant women exposed to German measles who have not received the rubella vaccine.

American Journal of Ophthalmology reported on a man with lymphocytic lymphoma who was diagnosed with progressive outer retinal necrosis in one eye. For his lymphoma, over the course of four years, he was treated with a variety of chemotherapy drugs including chlorambucil, cyclophosphamide, and high-dose corticosteroids. At the end of this period, he developed progressive outer retinal necrosis. He received intensive therapy with intravenous foscarnet, ganciclovir, and immune globulin, and oral decadron. The chlorambucil dose for his lymphoma was continued. Despite this immunosuppression, no further vision loss occurred. Within two weeks, his retinitis began to resolve. He remained stable when his eye doctor last saw him ten months later. The investigator of the study suggests that, given the rapid improvement seen in this patient, it may be reasonable to consider using immunoglobulin in immunocompromised patients as an accompaniment to antiviral therapy.

For more information see pages 1234 and 1235.

Papillitis

See Optic Neuritis

Pterygium, Prevention of Recurrence

A pterygium is a mass that forms on the conjunctiva and extends onto the cornea. They vary from small, quiet lumps to large, rapidly growing ones that can severely distort the cornea and distort the optical center. They may become inflamed, causing redness and irritation, cosmetic problems, or damaged vision, all of which may be cause for surgical removal.

Commonly Prescribed (On-Label) Drugs: None

OFF-LABEL PRESCRIPTION DRUG
BREAKTHROUGH OPTIONS

Generic: Cyclosporine (ocular) (si-klo-SPOR-een)
Brand: Restasis

Cyclosporine is an immunosuppressive drug commonly used to prevent organ rejection in transplant patients and to treat autoimmune diseases such as lupus. Among its effects, cyclosporine interferes with the ability of certain white blood cells, called T-helper lymphocytes, to become activated—an important step in immune system function. This makes it particularly useful for ocular inflammatory disease.

A study performed at the Sun Yat-sen University of Medical Sciences in Guangzhou, China, evaluated the efficiency of cyclosporine A and thiotepa to decrease the postoperative recurrence of pterygium. Thiotepa is a cytotoxic drug that slows or stops the growth of cancer cells. After 50 patients had their pterygia removed, half were treated with cyclosporine eye drops and the other group used thiotepa eye drops. After an average of 10 months' follow-up, the recurrence rate was only 5% in the cyclosporine group and 10% in the thiotepa group. The researchers concluded that both drugs can inhibit the hyperplasia (tissue overgrowth) seen in pterygium and decrease recurrence.

For more information see pages 1125 and 1127.

Generic: **Doxorubicin** (*dox-oh-ROOB-eh-sin*)
Brand: **Adriamycin**

Doxorubicin is a type of antibiotic used only to treat cancer, not to treat infections. It slows or stops the growth of cancer cells. That inhibition of cell growth is what makes it of value in helping to prevent the return of pterygia after surgery.

Ophthalmic Research reported on a study comparing doxorubicin and mitomycin C in preventing pterygia recurrences. Mitomycin is similar to doxorubicin in that it is also an antibiotic used only in cancer medicine to slow or stop the growth of cancer cells. However, doxorubicin is a newer drug and is considered more potent in reducing cellular viability. Fifty-six patients at several hospitals in India were divided into two groups. During the operation to remove their pterygia, half received doxorubicin, and half received mitomycin, both placed directly into the eye. Instilling the drugs directly in the eye, rather than giving them orally or intravenously, aimed to reduce side effects. All were seen regularly for a year after the operation. Although the patients experienced a variety of side effects, pterygia recurred in only three people in the doxorubicin group and four people in the mitomycin C group, making the drug benefits comparable in the researchers' opinion.

For more information see page 1156.

Generic: **Mitomycin** (*mye-toe-MYE-sin*)
Brand: **Mutamycin**

Mitomycin is a type of antibiotic used only to treat cancer, not to treat infections. It slows or stops the growth of cancer cells, which makes it helpful in preventing the return of pterygia after surgery.

Cornea reported on 46 patients seen at Sapir Medical Center in Israel who had pterygium surgery combined with mitomycin to their eye during surgery. Patients were followed for an average of 29.2 months, and pterygium recurred to a small extent in only one person.

A slightly different approach was taken in another Israeli study reported in *Cornea*. Instead of intraoperative installation, a pre-operative injection of mitomycin was given four weeks before combined pterygium and cataract surgery and compared to no preoperative surgery. Mitomycin-treated patients had no recurrences compared to recurrences in 50% of the untreated patients. The investigators recommended this approach over instillation at the time of surgery to prevent side effects and excess costs.

In a third *Cornea* article, physicians at the Centro Klinik studied 101 patients who underwent pterygium surgery using a laser to smooth the bare sclera (the outer tissue that covers the eye). Mitomycin was applied to the eyes at the time of surgery and twice daily for four days. Patients were followed for an average of 53 months. Among those who had been treated for their first round of pterygia, only 2.9% experienced recurrences; in the group with prior surgeries, the recurrence rate was 6.4%.

For more information see page 000.

Generic: **Thiotepa** *(thye-oh-TEP-a)*
Brand: **Thioplex**

Thiotepa is in a class of drugs called cytotoxic drugs typically used to treat cancer because they slow or stop the growth of rapidly dividing cells, such as cancer cells.

American Journal of Ophthalmology reported on a study in Puerto Rico with patients who had pterygia in both eyes. After surgery, during the six-week follow-up period, patients applied thiotepa drops every three hours to only one eye. Researchers found that 48 patients had a recurrence rate of 31.3% in those eyes not treated with thiotepa and only 8.3% in the treated eyes. They concluded that thiotepa was safe and effective in attempting to reduce recurrence rates after operations for pterygium.

French Journal of Ophthalmology reported on a study at the Font-Pre Hospital in Toulon, France of its 18 years of experience using thiotepa eye drops for the prevention of pterygium recurrence. It reviewed 64 cases, of which eight were cases of a second round of surgery. Following surgery, patients took thiotepa eye drops four times a day for six to eight weeks. There were only two cases of recurrence.

A study at Sun Yat-sen University of Medical Sciences in Guangzhou, China, evaluated the efficiency of thiotepa and cyclosporine A to decrease the postoperative recurrence of pterygium. After 50 patients had their pterygia removed, half were treated with cyclosporine eye drops and the other group used thiotepa eye drops. The researchers concluded that both drugs can inhibit the hyperplasia (tissue overgrowth) seen in pterygium and decrease recurrence.

For more information see page 1508.

Pterygium Unguis

See Pterygium

Retrobulbar Neuritis

See Optic Neuritis

Tarsal Cyst

See Chalazia

Uveitis

The outer layer of the eyeball is the tough sclera, the inner coat is the thin retina, and the middle layer is the uvea. The uvea is composed of the choroid (a layer rich in blood vessels that supply the eye with oxygen and nutrients), and the ciliary body (an area toward the front of the eye where the choroid thickens), and the iris (which gives the eye color and in the center of which is an opening, the pupil, which looks like a black disc). Inflammation of any part of the uvea is called uveitis. It may be caused by infection, autoimmune disease, trauma, or unknown causes.

Commonly Prescribed (On-Label) Drugs: Betamethasone, Cortisone, Dexamethasone, Homatropine, Prednisolone, Prednisone, Rimexolone, Scopolamine, Triamcinolone

---

OFF-LABEL PRESCRIPTION DRUGS
BREAKTHROUGH OPTIONS

---

*Generic: **Azathioprine*** *(ay-za-THYE-oh-preen)*
Brand: **Imuran**

Azathioprine is a drug that suppresses inflammation by tamping down the immune system. It is approved for use in the treatment of rheumatoid arthritis and for preventing rejection of transplanted organs. Its anti-inflammatory effects are a direct benefit in treating uveitis of all types, and its immunosuppressive action is specifically valuable when the uveitis has autoimmune causes. An article from the Brown University Medical School notes that azathioprine is specifically recommended for chronic uveitis, particularly in conjunction with oral corticosteroids. *Optometric Management* notes that antimetabolite drugs such as azathioprine are needed when severe inflammation associated with a specific systemic disease occurs and corticosteroids alone are not effective.

According to an article in *Pediatric Drugs*, the efficacy of azathioprine for treating uveitis in adults has been well demonstrated, although it has been used safely and effectively in treating other diseases in children. The investigators of the article recommended it for treating uveitis in children.

For more information see page 1033.

---

*Generic: **Chlorambucil*** *(khlor-AM-byoo-sil)*
Brand: **Leukeran**

Chlorambucil is one of a group of drugs that act on the immune system and used to treat certain types of leukemia, lymphoma, and Hodgkin's disease, and amyloidosis complicating juvenile chronic arthritis. It is a cytotoxic drug (similar to cyclophosphamide) that leads to a decrease in cell replication.

Studies have suggested that chlorambucil may be effective for various sight-threatening uveitic syndromes, such as those caused by Behcet's disease and sympathetic ophthalmia, according to a report from the Brown University Medical School. Treatment is usually continued for six to 12 months after the inflammation is suppressed. It can be used in both adults and children, according to *Pediatric Drugs*.

A study in the *American Academy of Ophthalmology* reviewed the records of 28 patients with chronic noninfectious uveitis due to various systemic diseases, who were treated with chlorambucil at the Massachusetts Eye & Ear Infirmary. All had not responded to corticosteroids and other drugs that modulated the immune system, and were subsequently treated with chlorambucil for an average of 12 months, although seven discontinued because of side effects. Visual acuity was improved in 43%, stable in 39%, and worsened in 18%. Fourteen patients were free of inflammation at the end of follow-up (up to 166 months) without any medication. The investigators of the report concluded that chlorambucil can be a safe and effective alternative for preserving vision in people with otherwise treatment-resistant uveitis.

For more information see page 1079.

*Generic: **Cyclopentolate** (sye-cloe-PEN-toe-late)*
*Brands: **AK-Pentolate (DSC), Cyclogyl, Cylate***

Cyclopentolate ophthalmic is usually used to dilate (enlarge) the pupil before eye examinations when your eye doctor wants to see the back of your eye, such as for a retinal exam. Cyclopentolate blocks the receptors in the muscles of the eye that are involved in controlling the size of the pupil and the shape of the lens. As a result, cyclopentolate produces mydriasis, the dilation of the pupil. Further, it relaxes the muscles that inflame and over-contract in uveitis.

As reported in the *British Journal of Ophthalmology*, physicians at St. Thomas's Hospital in the United Kingdom have observed resolution of acute anterior uveitis, which affects the front of the eye (normally the iris or the ciliary body), upon treatment with dexamethasone and cyclopentolate drops. Physicians at Brown University Medical School report that cyclopentolate can be used to alleviate the symptoms and complications of inflammation in uveitis, in particular by decreasing photophobia (reactions to light) caused by spasm of the iris and ciliary body. The effects of the drug begin in 30 to 60 minutes and last up to 24 hours. It should not be used in those who have narrow-angle glaucoma, and its safety for use during pregnancy has not been established.

For more information see page 1122.

Generic: **Cyclophosphamide** *(sye-kloe-FOS-fa-mide)*
Brands: **Cytoxan, Neosar**

Cyclophosphamide interferes with the growth of both normal and rapidly dividing (likely to be cancerous) cells, and is most likely to be used in the treatment of malignancies. But because it suppresses the immune system, it is also used in the treatment of autoimmune diseases such as lupus. Cyclophosphamide is useful as a sole therapy for various uveitis conditions, according to a report from the Brown University Medical School. Such a powerful immunosuppressive is only used, however, when steroids have not been effective or if the uveitis results in severe inflammation associated with a specific systemic disease, according to *Optometric Management*.

For more information see page 1123.

Generic: **Cyclosporine** *(si-klo-SPOR-een)*
Brands: **Gengraf, Neoral, Sandimmune**

Cyclosporine is an immunosuppressive drug commonly used to prevent organ rejection in transplant patients as well as in the treatment of autoimmune diseases such as lupus. According to a report from the Brown University Medical School, cyclosporine is useful as a therapy for various uveitis conditions. Since cyclosporine is such a powerful immunosuppressive, it is only used when steroids have not been effective or if the uveitis results in severe inflammation associated with a specific systemic disease, according to *Optometric Management*.

Among its effects, cyclosporine interferes with the ability of certain white blood cells, called T-helper lymphocytes, to become activated—an important step in immune system function. This effect makes it a particularly useful drug for vision-threatening atopic ocular inflammatory disease. According to *British Journal of Ophthalmology*, when cyclosporine was used in children with noninfectious uveitis that had not responded to other therapies, 92% maintained or improved their visual acuity. Further, the children's growth was not impaired because systemic corticosteroids were tapered without uveitis recurring.

For more information see pages 1125 and 1127.

Generic: **Diclofenac Ophthalmic** *(dye-KLOE-fen-ack)*
Brand: **Voltaren Ophthalmic**

Diclofenac is a nonsteroidal anti-inflammatory drug (NSAID). In its oral form, it is prescribed for inflammatory conditions such as arthritis and has been proven useful for inflammation of the uvea seen in uveitis.

In addition to diclofenac as an oral medication, studies have shown that diclofenac as eye drops is also a successful local anti-inflammatory treatment. Diclofenac ophthalmic is a topical drug normally prescribed for ocular irritation, postoperative ocular pain, and photophobia (sensitivity to light). *The International Ophthalmology Clinics* reports that diclofenac is among the most commonly used topical optical preparations and provides anti-inflammatory therapeutic effect in the treatment of Fuchs heterochromic uveitis. Ocular diclofenac is well tolerated, however, it may cause a mild burning sensation.

Interestingly, studies have shown that the penetration of diclofenac into eye tissue is actually enhanced by the presence of inflammation, according to *Investigational Ophthalmology and Vision Science*.

For more information see page 1142.

Generic: **Ketorolac** *(KEE-toe-role-ak)*
Brands: **Acular, Acular LS**

Ketorolac is a nonsteroidal anti-inflammatory drug (NSAID), a type of drug that can reduce pain, fever, and inflammation. NSAIDs do not cause sedation, respiratory depression, or addiction. Ketorolac in its oral form is prescribed for inflammatory conditions such as arthritis and may also be useful for inflammation of the uvea seen in uveitis. Ketorolac ophthalmic, a topical drug, is normally prescribed for ocular irritation, postoperative ocular pain, and photophobia (sensitivity to light). It works by inhibiting the release of lipids that cause inflammation.

The *International Ophthalmology Clinics* reports that ketorolac is among the most commonly used topical optical preparations.

A study showed that ketorolac was successful in treating uveitis induced by tumors. Ketorolac is generally used in older people, but successful clinical trials have led doctors and researchers to treat newborns, children, and middle-aged patients with it. Patients experienced significantly greater pain relief and uveitis was alleviated.

For more information see page 1262.

Generic: **Methotrexate** (meth-oh-TREKS-ate)
Brands: **Rheumatrex, Trexall**

Methotrexate suppresses the immune system by affecting the metabolism of cells. It was first used in the treatment of leukemia because it suppresses rapidly dividing cancerous cells. It was later used in diseases such as rheumatoid arthritis, psoriasis, and lupus. It was first used to treat inflammation of the eye in 1965. According to a report by the Brown University Medical School, it is now commonly used to treat a variety of inflammatory diseases of the eye, including panuveitis and intermediate uveitis.

In a study in the *American Academy of Ophthalmology*, 160 patients with chronic noninfectious uveitis were treated with methotrexate at the Massachusetts Eye & Ear Infirmary. Inflammation was controlled in 76.2% of the patients, with visual acuity maintained or improved in 90%, and steroids discontinued in most. Potentially serious adverse reactions occurred in only 8.1%. The researchers concluded that methotrexate is effective for chronic noninfectious uveitis that fails to respond to conventional steroid treatment. Methotrexate is taken together with the vitamin folate, which helps minimize side effects.

For more information see page 1312.

Generic: **Methylprednisolone** (meth-il-pred-NIS-oh-lone)
Brands: **Depo-Medrol, Medrol, Solu-Medrol**

Methylprednisolone is a corticosteroid drug typically prescribed to treat inflammatory and allergic diseases, as well as certain malignancies, such as some types of leukemia and Hodgkin's lymphoma. Uveitis is usually treated with topical corticosteroids, although injections into the eye are also sometimes used.

Systemic corticosteroids, in contrast to topical or intraocular, are more likely to be prescribed for people who have anterior uveitis that is associated with a systemic inflammatory disorder, according to *Optometric Management*, which also noted that methylprednisolone comes in a formulation, that starts out with a high dose and then provides the patient with a progressively lower dose of the drug for a six-day course of therapy. This may be added to a steady dose to quickly increase the therapeutic result. Methylprednisolone may also be given intravenously in a form known as bolus steroids, perhaps on a monthly basis.

For more information see page 1316.

Generic: *Mycophenolate Mofetil*
(mye-koe-FEN-oh-late MAH-feh-till)
Brands: *CellCept, Myfortic*

Mycophenolate mofetil modulates the immune system through multiple mechanisms, which include preventing the proliferation of certain white blood cells, suppressing the synthesis of antibodies, and decreasing the recruitment of other white blood cells to the sites of inflammation, thus suppressing inflammation overall. It was developed to prevent the rejection of transplanted organs and is now also used in the treatment of certain autoimmune and inflammatory diseases such as lupus.

According to a report from the Brown University Medical School, mycophenolate mofetil is used in combination with other drugs (particularly oral corticosteroids) to treat uveitis. It may be especially useful in those who cannot tolerate azathioprine or methotrexate.

Pediatric Drugs reported on its use in children in uveitis but urged caution on dosing; although the low doses needed to treat uveitis are not comparable to the very high doses used in transplantation medicine, the article noted toxicity in children receiving such doses after kidney transplants.

For more information see page 1344.

Generic: **Tacrolimus** *(ta-KROE-li-mus)*
Brands: **Prograf, Protopic**

Tacrolimus is used to prevent organ rejection in transplant patients. It has similar immunosuppressive activity to cyclosporine, interfering with the ability of certain white blood cells, called T-helper lymphocytes, to become activated—an important step in immune system function. This effect makes it particularly useful for vision-threatening ocular inflammatory disease.

According to a report from the Brown University Medical School, a small case series suggested that tacrolimus might be useful for treating noninfectious uveitis. However, such powerful immunosuppressives are only used when steroids have not been effective or if the uveitis results in severe inflammation associated with a specific systemic disease, according to *Optometric Management.*

American Journal of Ophthalmology reported on a study in which tacrolimus was given to 53 adults with uveitis that had not responded to other therapies. After 12 weeks, 76.5% had reduced inflammation with vision remaining stable or improving.

For more information see page 1489.

Generic: **Triamcinolone Acetonide Injection**
(trye-am-SIN-oh-lone ah-SIT-oh-nide)
Brands: **Kenalog 10, Tac 40, Tri-Kort, Trilog**

Triamcinolone is a corticosteroid drug that is an anti-inflammatory. In high doses it also acts as an immune suppressant. Its anti-inflammatory effects help treat uveitis of all types and its immunosuppressive action is specifically valuable for uveitis with autoimmune causes. In cases of anterior uveitis that are severe, chronic, recurrent, or resistant to topical corticosteroid therapy, and in situations when systemic steroids (medications given by pill that affect the whole body) need to be avoided, the physician may inject periocular corticosteroids that affect only the eye area. In such cases, triamcinolone may be especially helpful, according to *Optometric Management.*

A report from the Brown University Medical School in *eMedicine* notes that such injections should not be used in people with infectious uveitis or scleritis. A report from the General Hospital of Athens in the *American Journal of Ophthalmology* indicated success in closing a macular hole after such a triamcinolone injection in a patient with anterior uveitis.

For more information see page 1524.

HEMATOLOGICAL DISORDERS

ANEMIA

Human blood is composed of three types of cells (red blood cells, white blood cells, and platelets) that circulate throughout the body. Red blood cells contain hemoglobin (Hb) that carries oxygen from the lungs to all of the body's muscles and organs. Oxygen provides the energy the body needs for all of its normal activities. Anemia occurs when the number of red blood cells falls below normal and the body gets less oxygen and therefore has less energy than it needs to function properly.

Aplastic Anemia

Aplastic anemia occurs when the bone marrow stops making enough blood cells. When this happens, the bone marrow is almost empty of blood forming cells and is described as *hypoplastic* or *aplastic* (meaning low- or no growth). Anemia results from reduced red cell production. It is estimated that there are approximately 1,000 new cases of aplastic anemia each year in the United States.

Commonly Prescribed (On-Label) Drugs: *Lymphocyte Immune Globulin, Oxymetholone*

OFF-LABEL PRESCRIPTION DRUGS
BREAKTHROUGH OPTIONS

*Generic: **Antithymocyte Globulin***
(an-te-THY-moe-site GLOB-yu-lin)
*Brand: **Thymoglobulin (Immune Globulin)***

Antithymocyte globulin is an immunosuppressive drug most commonly used to treat rejection after organ transplant. A study conducted at the Children's Hospital in Denver, Colorado, examined the outcomes of a therapy regimen for severe aplastic anemia (SAA) using antithymocyte globulin and cyclosporine A in combination. Researchers concluded that the overall response to immunosuppressive therapy was 100%, without any relapses. According to researchers, this report documents excellent outcome using combination antithymocyte globulin and cyclosporine A for pediatric SAA.

Additionally, researchers in Germany reported on an 11-year study involving patients treated with immunosuppressions for aplastic anemia. The treatments included antithymocyte globulin, methylprednisolone, and cyclosporin A. The researchers found that the treatment was effective in 70% of all patients treated and 65% effective for patients with severe aplastic anemia. Researchers observed that patients responded more rapidly after treatment with cyclosporine. Most patients treated with cyclosporine needed only one course of immunosuppression, whereas many patients treated without cyclosporine required repeated immunosuppressive treatment. According to researchers, the overall survival was not different between the two treatment groups. Researchers stated that these data demonstrate that antithymocyte globulin, methylprednisolone, and cyclosporin A are an effective regimen for the treatment of aplastic anemia.

For more information see page 1021.

*Generic: **Cyclosporine** (si-klo-SPOR-een)*
*Brands: **Gengraf, Sandimmune, Neoral***

Cyclosporine is used most commonly to prevent or treat organ rejection if you have had a transplant. This medication works by suppressing the immune system. In a study conducted in Mexico, 61 individuals with severe aplastic anemia (SAA) were identified. Of these, 33 were followed for at least three months. Researchers observed that 26 patients could be treated with immunosuppression, 20 with combination antithymocyte globulin and cyclosporin A, and six with cyclosporin A alone. In the patients treated with immunosuppression a complete remission was achieved in 12 and a partial remission in six. The overall survival was 54%. Researchers observed it was superior for the patients who received both antithymocyte globulin and cyclosporin A (58 vs. 50%). Researchers believed that immunosuppression was a good therapeutic choice for some patients with SAA.

For more information see pages 1125 and 1127.

Generic: *Epoetin Alpha* (e-POE-e-tin AL-fa)
Brands: *Epogen, Procrit*

Epoetin Alpha stimulates the body to make red blood cells. It is used in the treatment of various anemia conditions. In a study published in the *International Journal of Hematology*, approximately 60% of aplastic anemia (AA) and refractory anemia (RA) (a type of anemia resistant to therapy) patients treated with recombinant human granulocyte colony-stimulating factor (rhG-CSF) and epoetin alpha showed a response. Researchers analyzed the long-term follow-up of 10 patients who suffered from multiple symptoms stemming from various sources or disorders (known as multilineage responders). One AA and one RA patient among the multilineage responders developed acute leukemia. Of seven living multilineage responders, three AA and two RA patients did not need a transfusion. Four of them maintained a suitable blood count for quality-of-life benefit. Researchers suggest that this result is an important advantage of this treatment.

For more information see page 1169.

Generic: *Sargramostin* (sar-GRAM-oh-stim)
Brand: *Leukine*

Sargramostin is a medication that stimulates the body to make white blood cells. It is used after bone marrow transplants and has also been used to improve blood conditions due to certain types of anemia or drug therapy. A recent study demonstrated that all patients treated with sargramostin had improved white blood cell counts.

For more information see page 1464.

Autoimmune Hemolytic Anemia

Autoimmune hemolytic anemia (AIHA) is a group of disorders characterized by a malfunction of the immune system that produces autoantibodies (proteins that attack other proteins or substances found in organs of the body), which attack red blood cells as if they were substances foreign to the body. Autoimmune hemolytic anemia is an uncommon group of disorders that can occur at any age. These disorders affect women more often than men. About half of the time, the cause of AIHA cannot be determined, which is referred to as idiopathic autoimmune hemolytic anemia. AIHA can also be caused by or occur with another disease, such as lupus.

Commonly Prescribed (On-Label) Drugs: *Betamethasone, Cortisone, Dexamethasone, Fludarabine, Methylprednisolone, Prednisolone, Prednisone*

OFF-LABEL PRESCRIPTION DRUGS
BREAKTHROUGH OPTIONS

Generic: **Cyclophosphamide** *(sye-kloe-FOS-fa-mide)*
Brands: **Cytoxan, Neosar**

Cyclophosphamide inhibits abnormal cell growth. High-dose cyclophosphamide has been used successfully to treat aplastic anemia and other autoimmune disorders. To determine the safety and efficacy of high-dose cyclophosphamide with granulocyte colony-stimulating factor (GCSF) among patients with severe therapy-resistant autoimmune hemolytic anemia, researchers at Sidney Kimmel Comprehensive Cancer Center at Johns Hopkins University treated nine patients who had failed other treatments with cyclophosphamide. Six patients achieved complete remission and none relapsed after a follow-up of 15 months. Three patients are in partial remission. Researchers concluded that high-dose cyclophosphamide was well tolerated and induced remissions in patients with severe, therapy-resistant AIHA.

For more information see page 1123.

Generic: **Cyclosporine** *(si-klo-SPOR-een)*
Brands: **Gengraf, Sandimmune, Neoral**

Cyclosporine is a medication used to suppress the immune system. Cyclosporine A has long been successfully used in organ transplants and bone marrow transplants. The strong immunosuppressive effect of cyclosporine A makes this drug useful in treating various autoimmune diseases. According to researchers, treatment with cyclosporine A for certain blood diseases, such as AIHA, has recently been expanding. Researchers consider cyclosporine A in the treatment of AIHA due to the drug's influence on small proteins that regulate immunity, inflammation, and blood cell production.

In a case report a patient who suffered from steroid-resistant AIHA received a low dose of cyclosporine A combined with prednisone. Researchers observed that within nine months of starting this combination drug therapy, the patient made a complete recovery from AIHA.

For more information see pages 1125 and 1127.

Generic: **Danazol** *(DA-na-zole)*
Brand: **Danocrine**

Danazol is a synthetic form of testosterone with weak steroid properties; however, it does not change or affect the levels of the hormones estrogen and progesterone. Investigators in France documented a case of ten adult patients with AIHA and seven patients with therapy-resistant AIHA. Both groups were treated with both danazol and prednisone. Eighty percent of the first group and 60% of the second group, displayed long-lasting responses with minimal side effects. Researchers believe that danazol therapy in the treatment of AIHA may decrease the duration of prednisone therapy and reduce the necessity of an operation to remove the spleen, which is often required in many patients.

Another report included a patient with systemic lupus erythematosus (SLE) complicated by severe AIHA. The patient responded to danazol. Thus, researchers concluded that danazol may represent an important therapeutic option in the treatment of autoimmune hemolytic anemia in some patients.

For more information see page 1129.

*Generic: **Rituximab** (ri-TUK-si-mab)*
*Brand: **Rituxan***

Rituximab is a type of medication called a monoclonal antibody (MoAb). It is used to treat certain types of cancer such as non-Hodgkin's lymphoma. In recent years, clinical studies have been undertaken with selected MoAbs in the treatment of several hematological diseases. However, according to researchers, some clinical observations indicate that MoAbs may be an important alternative for the conventional therapy of some autoimmune disorders such as autoimmune hemolytic anemia.

Rituximab may be an effective and safe drug for the treatment of AIHA. According to investigators, preliminary results indicate that further studies with rituximab are warranted. A longer follow-up and studies on larger number of patients are needed to determine the real value of these new approaches in AIHA.

For more information see page 1457.

Therapy-resistant Anemia

Therapy-resistant anemia is a subgroup in the myelodysplastic syndromes (MDS), also called pre-leukemia or "smoldering" leukemia. These are disorders in which the bone marrow—the spongy tissue inside the large bones—does not function normally. Bone marrow cells called "blast" develop or mature into several different types of blood cells including red blood cells that carry oxygen and other materials to all tissues of the body. The marrow cells that produce red cells appear abnormal. The white cell and producing cells may also appear abnormal. The proportion of blast cells is near normal levels. Therapy-resistant anemia accounts for about 20 to 30 percent of MDS cases. This form of the disease rarely transforms to acute leukemia.

Commonly Prescribed (On-Label) Drugs: *None*

OFF-LABEL PRESCRIPTION DRUGS
BREAKTHROUGH OPTIONS

Generic: **Epoetin Alpha** *(e-POE-e-tin AL-fa)*
Brands: **Epogen, Procrit**

Epoetin alpha affects production of red blood cells. Epoetin alpha has been used in a limited number of patients with myelodysplastic syndromes, which are classified as a group of closely related bone marrow disorders. In a study conducted by researchers at the University of Washington, a trial was designed to assess the efficacy and safety of therapy with granulocyte-macrophage colony-stimulating factor (GM-CSF) and epoetin alpha in 66 anemic patients with low white blood cell counts. The percentages of patients in the epoetin alpha and the placebo groups requiring transfusions of red blood cells were 60% and 92%, respectively. Researchers noted that treatment was well tolerated in most patients, though 10 withdrew from the study for reasons related to toxicity.

For more information see page 1169.

Generic: **Sargramostim** *(sar-GRAM-oh-stim)*
Brand: **Leukine**

Sargramostim is a drug that affects the production of a variety of blood cells. Sargramostim has been used to increase white blood cell counts in some adults with myelodysplastic syndrome (MDS) classified as refractory anemia (RA) (anemia resistant to therapy).

Use of sargramostim in patients with MDS generally results in an increase in the number of white blood cells in most patients and an increase in the number of eosinophils (types of white blood cells that turn red when stained for testing) and lymphocytes (types of white blood cells involved in the body's immune system) in many patients. In a few patients with MDS receiving sargramostim, platelet and immature red blood cell counts were unaffected and the need for red blood cell transfusions generally was unchanged during therapy with the drug. Researchers believe that prolonged maintenance therapy with sargramostim appears necessary in patients with MDS.

For more information see page 1464.

Thalassemia

Thalassemia includes a number of different forms of anemia (red blood cell deficiency). The two main types are called alpha and beta thalassemias, depending on which part of an oxygen-carrying protein (called hemoglobin) is lacking in the red blood cells. Thalassemia consists of a group of inherited blood diseases. About 100,000 babies worldwide are born with severe forms of the disease each year. Thalassemia occurs most frequently in people of Italian, Greek, Middle Eastern, Southern Asian, and African ancestry.

Commonly Prescribed (On-Label) Drugs: None

OFF-LABEL PRESCRIPTION DRUG
BREAKTHROUGH OPTION

---

*Generic: **Hydroxyurea** (hye-droks-ee-yoor-EE-a)*
*Brands: **Droxia, Hydrea, Mylocel***

Hydroxyurea inhibits abnormal cell growth. Hydroxyurea is a well-known chemotherapeutic drug that has been used largely for the treatment of various disorders where cancerous bone marrow cells multiply and spread to the blood. Researchers state that in beta-thalassemia, the role for hydroxyurea is much less clear. A study published in the *Journal of Pediatric Hematology/Oncology* was undertaken to describe the clinical responses of 163 thalassemia patients to hydroxyurea treatment during six years in southern Iran. Of the 163 patients in the study, 149 tolerated hydroxyurea well and showed a dramatic response to the drug. Eighty-three of 106 transfusion-dependent patients became completely transfusion free and 23 had one or two transfusions throughout the study.

After treatment, 97% of patients described an increase in exercise tolerance. Researchers concluded that hydroxyurea may be administered to thalassemia patients to minimize or even prevent the need for regular transfusions. Hydroxyurea therapy appears to be safe and effective when administered in thalassemic patients.

For more information see page 1226.

BLEEDING DISORDERS

Hemophilia

Hemophilia is a bleeding disorder caused by a deficiency in one of the blood clotting factors. Hemophilia A (often called classic hemophilia) accounts for about 80% of all hemophilia cases. It is a deficiency in clotting factor VIII. Hemophilia A is a hereditary disorder in which the clotting ability of the blood is impaired and excessive bleeding results. Small wounds and punctures are usually not a problem, but uncontrolled internal bleeding can result in pain and swelling and permanent damage, especially to joints and muscles. Severity of symptoms can vary and severe forms become apparent early on.

Commonly Prescribed (On-Label) Drugs: *Anti-Inhibitor Coagulant Complex, Antihemophilic Factor, Desmopressin, Factor IX, Factor VII, Tranexamic Acid*

OFF-LABEL PRESCRIPTION DRUG
BREAKTHROUGH OPTION

Generic: **Aminocaproic Acid** *(a-mee-noe-ka-PROE-ik AS-id)*
Brand: **Amicar**

Aminocaproic acid is medication used to treat excessive bleeding caused by problems with the blood clotting system. A study by researchers at the University of Washington analyzed the management of bleeding crises in 10 patients with hemophilia. Aminocaproic acid was used by local, oral, or intravenous routes either in combination or separately. In all the patients, the use of aminocaproic acid to manage bleeding resulted in stoppage and/or reduced frequency of bleeding. According to researchers, in six of 10 patients, the results were excellent. No patient needed to stop the medicine because of the side effects of aminocaproic acid.

Symptoms such as mild nausea and vertigo were seen as the side effects of this medicine when a high intravenous dosage was administered. According to researchers, aminocaproic acid thus appears to be an effective therapy for hemophilic patients. Researchers believe more extensive use of this inexpensive and safe product is warranted. It is also especially useful if you are a hemophilic patient undergoing dental procedures.

For more information see page 1006.

Impaired Hemostasis

Hemostasis, the stopping of bleeding from an injured blood vessel, requires the process of several steps involving the constriction of blood vessels, platelets, and clotting actions. Hemostatic abnormalities can lead to excessive bleeding or thrombosis (clotting) when abnormalities occur in response to injury. This may reduce blood flow from trauma by local vasoconstriction (an immediate reaction to injury) and platelet factors cause platelets to adhere to the site of vessel wall injury and form aggregates or "plugs".

Commonly Prescribed (On-Label) Drugs: None

OFF-LABEL PRESCRIPTION DRUGS
BREAKTHROUGH OPTIONS

Generic: Aprotinin (a-proe-TYE-nin)
Brand: Trasylol

Aprotinin is a naturally occurring protease inhibitor, meaning that it stops the protease enzyme that enables viruses to make copies of themselves. In a study conducted by researchers in Germany, 254 of 5,649 patients scheduled for surgery were identified preoperatively as having either acquired or inherited impaired primary hemostasis. All patients were initially pretreated with desmopressin. The non-responders were additionally treated with tranexamic acid or aprotinin. Those still unresponsive to therapy received estrogens and as a last attempt, a platelet transfusion. The administration of desmopressin led to a correction of platelet dysfunction in 229 of the 254 patients treated (90.2%). Tranexamic acid was effective in 12 of 16, and aprotinin was effective in three of five. Researchers concluded that preoperative correction of impaired hemostasis is possible in nearly all patients affected and results in a reduction of blood transfusions.

For more information see page 1024.

Generic: **Desmopressin** *(dez-mow-PREZ-in)*
Brands: **DDAVP, Minrin, Stimate**

Desmopressin is used for the prevention and treatment of bleeding if you have von Willebrand disease or mild hemophilia A. It is also used if you have a problem with hemostasis due to uremia, liver cirrhosis, or aspirin-associated bleeding. Researchers state that the administration of desmopressin results in an increase in the concentration of the factor responsible for blood clotting.

For more information see page 1134.

MISCELLANEOUS BLOOD DISEASES

Hemosiderosis

Hemosiderosis is a rare, often fatal, condition in which iron builds up in the lungs. The iron is in the form of hemosiderin, a pigment in blood. Hemosiderosis results from bleeding into the lungs, also known as pulmonary hemorrhage. Pulmonary hemosiderosis is often broken down into four categories: (1) idiopathic (unknown cause), (2) occurs along with pancreatic or heart disease, (3) occurs along with a milk sensitivity, and (4) occurs along with a kidney disease called glomerulonephritis.

Commonly Prescribed (On-Label) Drugs: None

OFF-LABEL PRESCRIPTION DRUG
BREAKTHROUGH OPTION

Generic: **Prednisone** *(pred-NIS-zone)*
Brands: **Deltasone, Liquid Pred, Meticorten, Orasone, Sterapred**

Prednisone is used for its anti-inflammatory or immunosuppressant effects. A study conducted by researchers from the Children's Hospital, Los Angeles, and the University of Southern California

School of Medicine was performed to determine a therapy regime for idiopathic pulmonary hemosiderosis (IPH) patients. Seventeen patients in whom IPH was diagnosed between 1972 and 1998 were included.

Initial treatment consisted of prednisone only in 14 patients and prednisone and hydroxychloroquine in two patients. Thirteen patients required long-term corticosteroids. Eight patients required other immunosuppressants (hydroxychloroquine or azathioprine) in addition to prednisone to control their disorder. One patient who was not treated with prednisone did not have symptoms for 1.8 years. Five-year survival for IPH patients in the study was 86%. Researchers concluded that the IPH patients who received long-term treatment had a better outcome than those who were not treated with immunosuppressive therapy. They believe that immunosuppression therapy may improve the survival of patients with IPH.

For more information see page 1429.

Sickle Cell Anemia

See Sickle Cell Disease

Sickle Cell Disease

Sickle cell disease affects the red blood cells. Normal red blood cells are smooth and round like doughnuts. They move easily through blood vessels to carry oxygen to all parts of the body. In sickle cell anemia, the red blood cells become hard, sticky, and shaped like sickles or crescents. When these hard and pointed red cells go through the small blood vessels, they tend to get stuck and block the flow of blood. This can cause pain, damage, and a low blood count or anemia.

Commonly Prescribed (On-Label) Drugs: *Hydroxyurea*

OFF-LABEL PRESCRIPTION DRUG
BREAKTHROUGH OPTION

Generic: **Ticlopidine** *(tye-KLOE-pi-deen)*
Brand: **Ticlid**

Ticlopidine works by making blood less likely to clot. The drug improves abnormalities of blood cell function. The effectiveness of ticlopidine has been investigated in patients at high risk for developing blood clots in their arteries and veins. Data from several large studies have shown that ticlopidine has a substantial benefit in patients who have experienced a stroke or heart disease. Ticlopidine reduces the incidence of further stroke, heart attack, or vascular death and is better than placebo and aspirin in this regard. Ticlopidine is equally effective in both men and women and also improves symptoms of pain in the calf or thighs after walking a certain distance in patients with artery disease and appears to reduce angina (chest pain).

Researchers state that patients with sickle cell disease have shown some improvement when treated with ticlopidine. Most adverse effects of ticlopidine do not require withdrawal of treatment. Gastrointestinal symptoms (particularly diarrhea) are most common, occurring almost twice as frequently with ticlopidine as with aspirin.

For more information see page 1512.

Uremic Pruritus

Pruritus affects 50-90% of patients undergoing dialysis. Symptoms such as mild itching usually begin about six months after the start of dialysis and range from localized and mild to generalized and severe. Uremic pruritus is poorly understood; possibilities include thyroid disorder, allergy, and iron-deficiency anemia, or some combination of these.

Commonly Prescribed (On-Label) Drugs: *None*

OFF-LABEL PRESCRIPTION DRUGS
BREAKTHROUGH OPTIONS

*Generic: **Epoetin Alpha** (e-POE-tin-AL-fa)*
*Brands: **Epogen, Procrit***

Uremic pruritus is one of the most bothersome symptoms in patients with chronic renal failure. According to investigators, the improvement of pruritus in several patients receiving epoetin alpha therapy raised the possibility that epoetin alpha affects uremic pruritus directly. A study performed in Italy involved a group of patients receiving hemodialysis (kidney dialysis) who had severe pruritus. They wanted to determine the effects of epoetin alpha on the patients' pruritus. Twenty patients with uremia, of whom 10 had severe pruritus and 10 did not, received epoetin alpha and placebo each for five weeks. Eight of the 10 patients with pruritus had improved symptoms during epoetin alpha therapy. However, the pruritus returned within one week after the discontinuation of therapy. These eight patients were successfully treated again with low doses of epoetin alpha and the effect persisted for six months. Researchers observed that epoetin alpha therapy can result in improvement of pruritus.

For more information see page 1169.

*Generic: **Ondansetron** (on-DAN-se-tron)*
*Brands: **Zofran, Zofran** ODT*

Ondansetron is a medication commonly used to prevent nausea and vomiting caused by cancer chemotherapy or in the post-surgery recovery period. It works by blocking the hormone (serotonin) that causes vomiting. Serotonin is known to enhance pain perception and pruritic symptoms through nerve endings. In a study conducted at St James's University Hospital in the United Kingdom, 16 hemodialysis (kidney dialysis) patients with persistent pruritus received treatment with either ondansetron or placebo three times daily for two weeks each. Patients scored their intensity of pruritus daily on a 0-to-10 visual analogue scale (0 = no pruritus, 10 = maximal pruritus). They also recorded the daily use of antihistamines as escape medication.

The daily pruritus score did not change significantly during active or placebo treatment. The percentage of escape medication use decreased from 21% to 9% with ondansetron and from 53% to 5% with placebo. Based on these results, investigators concluded that ondansetron does not improve pruritus in hemodialysis patients.

For more information see page 1387.

MYELOPROLIFERATIVE DISEASES

Myelodysplastic/myeloproliferative diseases (MDS/MPD) are diseases of the bone marrow. They share characteristics of myeloproliferative disorders and myelodysplastic syndromes.

Myeloproliferative disorders are diseases in which too many of certain types of blood cells are made in the bone marrow. The bone marrow, the tissue inside the large bones in the body, makes red blood cells (which carry oxygen to all the tissues in the body), white blood cells (which fight infection), and platelets (which make the blood clot). Myelodysplastic syndromes, also called preleukemia or "smoldering" leukemia, are diseases in which the bone marrow does not function normally and not enough normal blood cells are made.

Erythremia

See Polycythemia Vera

Myelofibrosis

Myelofibrosis is a disease of the bone marrow where collagen creates scar tissue inside the marrow cavity. It is caused by a disturbance of the immune system. You may also know this disorder as primary or idiopathic myelofibrosis or agnogenic myeloid metaplasia. These names describe a situation where myelofibrosis is the primary disorder. It is also possible to have myelofibrosis as a consequence of another disease such as polycythemia vera (PV) or essential thrombocythemia (ET).

Commonly Prescribed (On-Label) Drugs: *None*

OFF-LABEL PRESCRIPTION DRUGS
BREAKTHROUGH OPTIONS

*Generic: **Interferon Alfa-2b** (in-ter-FEER-on AL-fa-too-bee)*
*Brand: **Intron A***

According to researchers, interferon alpha has had positive results in other chronic myeloproliferative diseases and is now being tested for idiopathic myelofibrosis. In a study conducted by researchers in, Spain, four patients with idiopathic myelofibrosis were selected for interferon treatment. The researchers administered interferon alpha-2b at an initial dose and then increased the dosage at 4 to 6 weeks in cases where insufficient response existed.

In patients who exhibited a favorable response, a maintenance schedule was initiated with low doses of interferon. Because of bad tolerance in two patients, treatment was discontinued at six and eight weeks of initiation of treatment with no response having been observed until that time. The other patients had favorable responses with disappearance of the symptoms after administration of interferon. Due to the positive results of this trial, researchers concluded that interferon alpha-2b may be an effective therapy for patients with idiopathic myelofibrosis.

For more information see page 1243.

*Generic: **Thalidomide** (tha-LI-doe-mide)*
*Brand: **Thalomid***

In a study conducted at the Heinrich-Heine University in Germany, investigators administered thalidomide to 16 patients with idiopathic myelofibrosis (IMF) who had anemia, thrombocytopenia (a reduced platelet count), or splenomegaly (enlargement of the spleen). Adverse effects were severe constipation, fatigue, and edema. Researchers concluded that thalidomide appears useful in the treatment of IMF.

For more information see page 1505.

Polycythemia Rubra Vera

See Polycythemia Vera

Polycythemia Vera

Polycythemia vera (PV) is a myeloproliferative disorder (MPD). In this type, there is uncontrolled production of mature red blood cells leading to an increase in red blood cells. If not controlled, this can lead to complications involving clotting or bleeding episodes. PV is fairly rare, occurring in approximately 1 in 100,000 and is considered an orphan disease (a disease that pharmaceutical companies do not dedicate much research time to).

Commonly Prescribed (On-Label) Drugs: Mechlorethamine

OFF-LABEL PRESCRIPTION DRUGS
BREAKTHROUGH OPTIONS

Generic: **Anagrelide** *(an-AG-gre-lide)*
Brand: **Agrylin**

Anagrelide is typically used to treat a blood disorder (high platelet count) that can cause blood clots to form. The drug reduces the number of platelets in the bloodstream. A study was conducted to analyze 3,660 anagrelide-treated patients. The study conducted at Mount Sinai Medical Center included myeloproliferative disease (MPD) patients with thrombocytosis (a condition where the body produces a surplus of platelets).

The safety of 3,660 patients, including 2,251 with essential thrombocythemia (ET), 462 with polycythemia vera (PV), and 947 with chronic myeloid leukemia (CML) and other MPDs, was analyzed to establish the incidence of leukemia in patients with ET and PV. Acute leukemia/myelodysplasia developed in 2.1% of ET patients. Of the PV patients, 2.8% developed acute leukemia/myelodysplastic syndrome. There were no ET or PV patients in the study who transformed to leukemia exposed solely to anagrelide.

For more information see page 1017.

Generic: **Hydroxyurea** *(hye-droks-ee-yoor-EE-a)*
Brands: **Droxia, Hydrea, Mylocel**

Hydroxyurea is often used to treat certain types of cancer as well as blood disorders. Currently, there are three drugs used for the treatment of polycythemia vera: hydroxyurea, interferon-alfa, and anagrelide. These medications work differently, and there is a potential role for combination therapy as well. They also differ widely in side effects profiles and severity. Because of the different risks for long-term complications associated with these drugs, your age is an important variable in selecting treatments. Hydroxyurea is used sparingly in younger patients because of the long-term increased risk of genetic mutations and possible association with increased risk of leukemia. Researchers have found that patients taking hydroxyurea had lower incidences of early blood clots in the arteries and acute leukemia.

For more information see page 1226.

Generic: ***Interferon Alfa-2b*** *(in-ter-FEER-on AL-fa-too-bee)*
Brand: ***Intron A***

Interferon alfa-2b is a medication used for the treatment of leukemia, certain types of cancer, and viral infections. The therapeutic efficacy of interferon alfa-2b has been evaluated in seven patients with polycythemia vera (PV). There were six complete responses and one partial response. Itching significantly improved in 80% of the cases. Researchers concluded that interferon alfa-2b seems to be an effective treatment for the myeloproliferation of PV and pruritus complaints.

During a six-year study, researchers examined 11 patients with PV. Although the duration of disease differed, all patients had active disease as indicated by the need for therapeutic bloodletting. For the 11 patients, the number of required bloodletting per year was 4.5. According to researchers, results indicate that red blood cell values can be controlled with interferon alfa-2b within six to 12 months, eliminating the need for blood letting. The side effects of interferon alfa-2b were tolerable and could be alleviated during the first year of therapy. Thus, investigators concluded that interferon alfa-2b may be an important new treatment. Because PV is a disease of long duration, additional follow-up is required.

For more information see page 1243.

Thrombocythemia

Platelets (thrombocytes) are normally produced in the bone marrow by cells called megakaryocytes. In thrombocythemia, megakaryocytes increase in number and produce too many platelets. Thrombocythemia usually occurs in people older than 50 and more frequently in women. The cause of thrombocythemia is unknown.

Commonly Prescribed (On-Label) Drugs: *Anagrelide*

OFF-LABEL PRESCRIPTION DRUGS
BREAKTHROUGH OPTIONS

Generic: **Hydroxyurea** *(hye-droks-ee-yoor-EE-a)*
Brands: **Droxia, Hydrea, Mylocel**

Hydroxyurea is used to treat certain types of cancer or blood disorders. One study published in *New England Journal of Medicine* compared the use of hydroxyurea with anagrelide for the treatment of essential thrombocythemia (ET). A total of 809 patients with ET who were at high risk for vascular events received low-dose aspirin plus either anagrelide or hydroxyurea. After a follow-up of 39 months, patients in the anagrelide group were significantly more likely than those in the hydroxyurea group to have a serious complication due to ET. As compared with hydroxyurea plus aspirin, anagrelide plus aspirin was associated with increased rates of other blood and heart complications. The investigators concluded that hydroxyurea plus low-dose aspirin is superior to anagrelide plus low-dose aspirin for patients with essential thrombocythemia at high risk for vascular events.

For more information see page 1226.

Generic: **Interferon Alfa-2b**
(in-ter-FEER-on AL-fa-too-bee)
Brand: **Intron A**

Essential thrombocythemia (ET) can be treated with a variety of medications, including interferon alfa-2b. Interferon was found to control symptoms, reduce platelet counts, and reduce bone marrow mass. In a study involving 11 patients, none had symptoms of blood clotting while undergoing treatment. The study concluded that interferon alfa-2b is very effective for long-term use in treating essential thrombocythemia and has not been associated with an increased risk of causing leukemia.

For more information see page 1243.

Generic: **Peginterferon Alfa-2b**
(peg-in-ter-FEER-on AL-fa-too-bee)
Brand: **PEG-intron**

A study from MD Anderson Cancer Center reported on the effectiveness of peginterferon alfa-2b for thrombocythemia. Interferon-alpha is known to control symptoms, reduce platelet counts and reduce the bone marrow of large blood cell mass in patients with essential thrombocythemia (ET). The 11 patients who were treated with peginterferon alfa-2b experienced rapidly controlled platelet counts and symptoms were resolved. After two months of therapy, 10 patients (91%) were in complete remission and 11 (100%) after four months. The investigators concluded that peginterferon alfa-2b has significant efficacy in patients with ET.

For more information see page 1399.

Thrombocytosis

See Thrombocythemia

Vaquez disease

See Polycythemia Vera

PURPURA

Immune Thrombocytopenic Purpura

See Therapy-resistant Idiopathic Thrombocytopenic Purpura

Therapy-resistant Idiopathic Thrombocytopenic Purpura

Idiopathic thrombocytopenic purpura (ITP) is a bleeding disorder in which the blood does not clot properly. The bleeding is due to a low number of platelets, which helps the blood clot and prevents bleeding. ITP is also accompanied by bruises that appear on the skin due to bleeding that has occurred in small blood vessels under the skin. Therapy-resistant idiopathic thrombocytopenic purpura does not respond to conventional treatment.

Commonly Prescribed (On-Label) Drugs: *Cortisone, Immune Globulin, Methylprednisolone, Prednisolone, Prednisone, Triamcinolone*

OFF-LABEL PRESCRIPTION DRUGS
BREAKTHROUGH OPTIONS

Generic: ***Azathioprine*** *(ay-za-THYE-oh-preen)*
Brand: ***Imuran***

Azathioprine is typically used to prevent rejection of transplanted organs and for cases of severe arthritis that do not respond to other therapies. If you have therapy-resistant ITP, azathioprine is used in cases with dangerously low platelet counts. Your response to azathioprine may occur slowly over a 3- to 6-month period. Physicians advise that while undergoing treatment with azathioprine your blood counts should be monitored.

For more information see page 1033.

Generic: ***Cyclophosphamide*** *(sye-kloe-FOS-fa-mide)*
Brands: ***Cytoxan, Neosar***

Cyclophosphamide is used to treat different types of cancer. In a report from the National Institutes of Health (NIH), 14 patients with chronic ITP were treated with cyclophosphamide and autologous granulocyte colony-stimulating factor (G-CSF). Treatment-related complications included vaginal bleeding, gastrointestinal bleeding, nosebleed, antibiotic-responsive fever and low circulation. Six patients obtained complete responses. Two additional patients obtained partial responses. Researchers believe this therapeutic approach is feasible for patients with severe chronic idio-pathic thrombocytopenia purpura.

For more information see page 1123.

Generic: **Cyclosporine** *(si-klo-SPOR-een)*
Brands: **Gengraf, Neoral, Sandimmune**

Cyclosporine is typically used to prevent or treat organ re-jection in transplant patients. Treatment of severe, chronic idiopathic thrombocytopenic purpura resistant to most usual therapies is a difficult challenge. A report documented the long-term treatment with cyclosporine in 12 adult patients with resistant ITP. Cyclosporine used in relatively low doses led to a clinical improvement in 10 patients. Five had a complete response, four a complete response to maintenance therapy, and one a partial response. Two patients had no response. Most patients with a response had a long-term remission after dis-continuation of cyclosporine. Side effects were moderate, even in patients dependent on continued cyclosporine treatment. Researchers believe cyclosporine seems to be a reasonable treat-ment in severe, potentially life-threatening, therapy- resistant ITP.

For more information see pages 1125 and 1127.

Generic: **Danazol** *(DA-na-zole)*
Brand: **Danocrine**

Danazol is a synthetic hormone. If you have chronic ITP and stan-dard-dose corticosteroids and spleen removal have failed or who have contraindications to these therapies you may require further treatment for life-threatening thrombocytopenia or bleeding. Re-searchers in France conducted a study on whether danazol is use-ful in the treatment of chronic, therapy-resistant ITP. The study included 57 patients who had chronic ITP and who were unre-sponsive to spleen removal or corticosteroids. Thirty-eight pa-tients experienced a partial or complete response to therapy, among whom 27 remained in remission. Treatment tolerance was acceptable, although severe adverse effects were reported in nine patients. Researchers concluded that the findings suggest that danazol therapy may be beneficial in the management of therapy-resistant chronic ITP.

For more information see page 1129.

Generic: **Dexamethasone** *(deks-a-METH-a-sone)*
Brands: **Decadron, Desmeth, Dexone, Hexadrol**

Dexamethasone is used principally as an anti-inflammatory drug. High-dose dexamethasone has been used in treatment of patients with ITP who are resistant to other treatments such as prednisone and spleen removal. Different studies show variable success rates. One study performed in Mexico evaluated the effectiveness of high dose dexamethasone in 19 Mexican mestizo adult patients diagnosed with ITP. Patients received dexamethasone intravenously during four consecutive days every four weeks until six cycles were completed. Of 19 patients, nine achieved a favorable response. Nevertheless, after six months only four patients maintained a favorable response. Researchers concluded that high-dose dexamethasone therapy appears to be useful for patients with ITP and high-dose dexamethasone appears to be a good alternative therapy for relapse patients. However, duration of favorable response to treatment was brief; therefore, other treatment plans might be required to achieve a longer remission.

For more information see page 1138.

Generic: **Mycophenolate Mofetil**
(my-koe-FEN-oh-late MOE-feh-till)
Brands: **CellCept, Myfortic**

Mycophenolate mofetil suppresses the body's immune system. It is used in combination with other medications to prevent rejection of transplanted kidneys or other organs. A study was conducted in China to determine whether mycophenolate mofetil has beneficial effects on therapy-resistant ITP. Twenty therapy-resistant ITP patients who did not respond to corticosteroid and/or spleen removal and chemical therapy were given mycophenolate mofetil orally for a two- to four-month period. Sixteen of the 20 patients had responses to mycophenolate mofetil treatment; nine achieved a complete response, four achieved a partial response, and three achieved a minor response. Researchers observed that the therapeutic effects were found to be better in male patients than female patients. They concluded that therapy for a period of eight to 16 weeks of mycophenolate mofetil was valuable for the treatment of therapy-resistant ITP.

For more information see page 1344.

Generic: **Rituximab** *(ri-TUK-si-mab)*
Brand: **Rituxan**

Rituximab is most commonly used for cancer treatment. Management of patients with therapy-resistant ITP is difficult. Recent studies have shown that rituximab is useful in the treatment of these patients, with overall response rates of about 50%. A study conducted in Denmark of rituximab evaluated the treatment of 35 adult patients with therapy-resistant ITP. Based on the results of the study, investigators concluded that rituximab may be a useful alternative therapy in patients with severe ITP resistant to conventional treatment.

For more information see page 1457.

Generic: **Vincristine** *(ven-CHRIS-teen)*
Brand: **Vincasar PFS**

Vincristine sulfate is a drug used to inhibit the growth of malignant cells. Intravenous (IV) injections or slow IV infusions of vincristine have reportedly been effective in some cases for the treatment of therapy-resistant idiopathic thrombocytopenic purpura.

A study conducted at the Institute of Hematology and Blood Transfusion in Poland evaluated the use of vincristine or vinblastine in 22 patients with chronic ITP, resistant to corticosteroids. Eight of these patients were additionally administered prednisone in an oral dose. Two-hour intravenous infusions of drugs were made once a week, at least three times. In every patient, the platelet count was evaluated before and after the three infusions. A rise of the platelet count was assumed to signify improvement. Significant improvement was obtained in nine. Researchers concluded that vinca alkaloids like vincristine could be used in situations requiring short-term increase of the platelet count in patients with ITP who are resistant to corticosteroids.

For more information see page 1546.

Therapy-resistant Thrombotic Thrombocytopenic Purpura

Patients with Thrombotic Thrombocytopenic Purpura (TTP) have low numbers of platelets (thrombocytopenia), abnormal red cells, and a tendency to develop tiny clots in small blood vessels. TTP is caused by an immune reaction when your body makes an antibody that inactivates an important protein (ADAMTS13) whose function is to prevent platelets from sticking together and plugging blood vessels. You may have easy bruising, rashes with many little dots or large purple patches (purpura), fever, belly pain, small clots in the brain or kidneys, or bleeding due to few platelets.

Commonly Prescribed (On-Label) Drugs: *None*

OFF-LABEL PRESCRIPTION DRUGS
BREAKTHROUGH OPTIONS

Generic: **Azathioprine** *(ay-za-THYE-oh-preen)*
Brand: **Imuran**

Azathioprine is a medication used to suppress the immune system. Multiple relapses of thrombotic thrombocytopenic purpura (TTP) occur in a minority of patients but pose a significant therapeutic challenge. Suppression of the immune system may be a possible alternative if you have experienced relapses. A study evaluated immunosuppressive therapy with either cyclophosphamide or azathioprine in three patients with relapsing TTP. All three patients maintained remissions of eight to 10 months without recurrence. Researchers believe that immunosuppressive therapy may have a role in inducing long-term remissions in recurrent TTP.

For more information see page 1033.

Generic: **Cyclophosphamide** *(sigh-kloe-FOS-fuh-mide)*
Brands: **Cytoxan, Neosar**

Cyclophosphamide is a drug that inhibits growth of malignant cells. A case from Washington University School of Medicine in Missouri examined the efficacy of intensive immunosuppressive treatments in therapy-resistant TTP. A 42-year-old woman with relapsing TTP participated. For 19 months, she had relapsing bleeding of small blood vessels despite transfusion, spleen removal, and therapy with vincristine, prednisone, and cyclosporine. After treatment with rituximab and cyclophosphamide, the disease went into remission for 13 months. Therefore, investigators concluded that intensive therapy with cyclophosphamide may lead to remission in patients with therapy-resistant TTP.

For more information see page 1123.

*Generic: **Rituximab** (ri-TUK-si-mab)*
*Brand: **Rituxan***

Rituximab is an antibody used most commonly for the treatment of cancer. Researchers in France conducted a clinical trial to determine the efficacy of rituximab as a curative and preventive treatment in patients with TTP. Six patients were included during a therapy-resistant TTP episode. Five patients with severe relapsing TTP were preventively treated during remission. All patients received four weekly infusions of rituximab. Researchers observed that treatment with rituximab led to clinical remission in all cases of therapy-resistant TTP. Tolerance of rituximab was good. Researchers concluded that rituximab may be a promising first-line immunosuppressive treatment in patients with acute therapy-resistant and severe relapsing TTP.

For more information see page 1457.

*Generic: **Vincristine** (ven-CHRIS-teen)*
*Brand: **Vincasar PFS***

Vincristine is used most commonly for the treatment of cancer. It has been generally reserved for therapy-resistant TTP. Researchers from Cedars-Sinai Medical Center reported improved survival when vincristine and transfusion were administered to patients at the early stages of diagnosis. The researchers reviewed medical records of all patients with a diagnosis of TTP treated between 1995 and 2002. Transfusion was performed daily. Additionally, patients received vincristine after the first transfusion. All patients achieved remission. Patients tolerated vincristine without significant complications. Researchers believe that the 100% survival rate, as well as evidence gained from literature review, suggests that combination therapy with vincristine and transfusion at first appearance of TTP might be more effective than transfusion alone and therefore warrants consideration as first-line therapy for TTP patients.

For more information see page 1546.

Thrombocytopenic Purpura

See Therapy-resistant Idiopathic Thrombocytopenic Purpura

Thrombopenic purpura

See Therapy-resistant Thrombocytopenic Purpura

Thrombotic Thrombocytopenic Purpura

Patients with thrombotic thrombocytopenic purpura (TTP) have low numbers of platelets (thrombocytopenia), abnormal red cells and a tendency to develop tiny clots (thrombi) in small blood vessels. TTP is caused by an immune reaction when your body makes an antibody that inactivates an important protein (ADAMTS13) whose function is to prevent platelets from sticking together and plugging blood vessels. TTP may be accompanied by easy bruising, rashes with many little dots or large purple patches (purpura), fever, belly pain, thrombi in the brain or kidneys, or bleeding due to few platelets.

Commonly Prescribed (On-Label) Drugs: None

OFF-LABEL PRESCRIPTION DRUGS
BREAKTHROUGH OPTIONS

Generic: **Prednisone** (pred-NIS-zone)
Brands: **Deltasone, Liquid Pred, Meticorten, Orasone, Sterapred**

Prednisone is usually used for its anti-inflammatory or immuno-suppressant effects. It is used to treat conditions such as arthritis, blood disorders, breathing problems, certain cancers, eye problems, immune system diseases, and skin diseases.

A study conducted by the Department of Medicine at Johns Hopkins University School of Medicine and Hospital examined 108 patients with thrombotic thrombocytopenic purpura-hemolytic uremic syndrome (TTP-HU), a disease with symptoms of thrombocytopenia, fever, central nervous system abnormalities, and kidney dysfunction. Patients with minimal symptoms and no central nervous system complications received prednisone. Patients with severe cases of TTP-HU and who did not respond to initial treatment of prednisone received prednisone in addition to transfusion. Of the 108 patients receiving treatment, 91% survived. For patients with minimal symptoms, investigators concluded that prednisone alone was effective in 30 patients with mild TTP-HU. In 78 patients with severe TTP-HU who received prednisone and transfustion, treatment resulted in 67 relapses and 8 deaths. Researchers determined that prednisone is an effective treatment in patients with mild cases of TTP-HU.

For more information see page 1429.

Generic: **Vincristine** *(ven-CHRIS-teen)*
Brand: **Vincasar PFS**

Vincristine is a medication often used alone or with other drugs to treat cancer.

In a report published in *Transfusion*, improved survival was noted when both vincristine and transfusion were administered in patients treated from 1979 to 1994. Medical records of all patients with a diagnosis of TTP treated between 1995 and 2002 at Cedars-Sinai Medical Center were reviewed. Patients tolerated vincristine without significant complications. Researchers concluded that the 100% survival rate, as well as evidence garnered from the literature review, suggests that combination therapy with vincristine and transfusion at the time of TTP's appearance might be more effective than transfusion alone and therefore warrants consideration as first-line therapy for TTP patients.

For more information see page 1546.

WHITE BLOOD CELL DISORDERS

White blood cell disorders are those diseases affecting the cells in blood that fight infection. White blood cells are produced by bone marrow. Disorders involving white blood cells include leukemia, a cancer of the blood, and neutropenia, a disorder that causes lower than normal levels of neutrophils, a type of white blood cell.

Agranulocytic Angina

See Agranulocytosis

Agranulocytosis

Agranulocytosis is a condition characterized by an insufficient number of white blood cells called neutrophils or granulocytes. This can be caused by a failure of the bone marrow to make sufficient neutrophils, or when white blood cells are destroyed faster than they can be produced. You may be more susceptible to infections due to this disorder.

Commonly Prescribed (On-Label) Drugs: *None*

OFF-LABEL PRESCRIPTION DRUGS
BREAKTHROUGH OPTIONS

*Generic: **Filgrastim** (fil-GRA-stim)*
*Brand: **Neupogen***

Filgrastim is a medication that stimulates the blood system (bone marrow) to make white blood cells. White blood cells help patients fight infections, and it is given if your ability to make white bloods cells has been reduced. A study evaluated the effectiveness of filgrastim and pegfilgrastim in reducing the risk and incidence of white blood cell complications with chemotherapy. Reviews of the data were performed by investigators at the UPMC Cancer Pavilion in Pittsburgh, Pennsylvania, for both pegfilgrastim and filgrastim. Researchers concluded that pegfilgrastim and filgrastim are safe and effective in reducing both the incidence and duration of white blood cell destruction in patients who have been treated with chemotherapy. Approximately 11 daily injections of filgrastim per chemotherapy cycle are required to achieve results. Pegfilgrastim provides the same benefits of daily filgrastim but with a single dose per chemotherapy cycle.

For more information see page 1185.

Generic: **Sargramostim**
(sar-GRAM-oh-stim)
Brand: **Leukine**

Sargramostim is a medication that stimulates the body to make white blood cells. It is used after bone marrow transplants and has also been used to improve blood conditions due to certain types of anemia or drug therapy. Part one of a two-part study by UCLA School of Medicine focused on the use of sargramostim and filgrastim to shorten the duration of chemotherapy-induced neutropenia (an abnormally low number of white blood cells that fight infection in the blood) and thus prevent infection in cancer patients. In trials, researchers concluded that filgrastim may be more effective in decreasing the duration of neutropenia during all cycles of chemotherapy and reduced the risk of infection by 50% or more.

For more information see page 1464.

Angina Lymphomatosa

See Agranulocytosis

Neutropenia

Neutropenia is an abnormally low number of neutrophils (white blood cells that fight infection) in the blood. Neutrophils serve as the major defense of the body against acute bacterial and certain fungal infections. Neutrophils usually constitute about 45 to 75% of all white blood cells in the bloodstream. When the neutrophil count falls below 1,000 cells per microliter of blood, the risk of infection increases somewhat; when it falls below 500 cells per microliter, the risk of infection increases greatly. Without the key defense provided by neutrophils, you may have problems controlling infections and are at risk of dying from an infection.

Commonly Prescribed (On-Label) Drugs: *Cefepime, Ciprofloxacin, Filgrastim, Itraconazole, Mezlocillin, Pegfilgrastim, Sargramostim*

OFF-LABEL PRESCRIPTION DRUG
BREAKTHROUGH OPTION

Generic: **Lithium** *(LITH-ee-um)*
Brands: **Eskalith, Eskalith CR, Lithobid**

Lithium is most commonly used to treat manic-depressive disorder (bipolar disorder). It works to stabilize the mood and reduces extremes in behavior. Lithium leads to a release of blood cell growth factors and therefore to proliferation of white blood cells.

Lithium has also been used to treat neutropenia. In a limited number of patients with neutropenia, the addition of lithium to the treatment has decreased the number of days neutropenia is present. The number of hospitalizations related to infection or fever and the number of infection-related deaths also have been reduced when lithium was added to a chemotherapy regimen.

If you are receiving chemotherapy you may be debilitated and generally are more susceptible to the adverse effects of lithium. Therefore, the benefit-to-risk ratio of lithium therapy for you remains to be established. Some clinicians recommend short-term lithium therapy when you have had severe neutropenic episodes during previous courses of chemotherapy or when a patient is undergoing treatment with combination chemotherapy known to be severely inhibiting to blood cell formation.

For more information see page 1286.

Neutropenic Angina

See Agranulocytosis

Neutrophilic Leukopenia

See Neutropenia

Neutrophilopenia

See Neutropenia

HORMONAL DISORDERS

ADRENAL DISORDERS

We have two adrenal glands, each about the size of a grape. Each sits on top of one of our kidneys, one on each side of the body. Each adrenal gland has two parts—the central core, called the medulla, and the outer layer, called the cortex. The medulla produces two hormones: epinephrine (adrenaline) and norepinephrine (noradrenaline), which play an important part in controlling heart rate and blood pressure. The cortex produces three groups of steroid hormones that control a wide range of other body processes. The most important include aldosterone, hydrocortisone, and the sex hormones—androgens, estrogen, and progesterone—which influence sexual development.

Aldosteronism

See Hyperaldosteronism

Cushing's Syndrome

In Cushing's syndrome, there is an excess of steroid hormones in your blood. In the majority of cases, it is caused by large doses of such hormones, like prednisone, that are being taken for another illness, such as an autoimmune disease or asthma. Rarely, Cushing's syndrome is caused because the cortex of one or both of the adrenal glands is producing too much hydrocortisone; such overproduction could be due to a tumor in the gland or a tumor elsewhere in your body that is over-stimulating the gland. If the tumor is in the pituitary gland, the condition is called Cushing's disease rather than Cushing's syndrome.

Commonly Prescribed (On-Label) Drugs: *Amino-glutethimide, Dexamethasone, Trilostane*

OFF-LABEL PRESCRIPTION DRUGS
BREAKTHROUGH OPTIONS

Generic: **Ketoconazole** *(kee-toe-KOE-na-zole)*
Brand: **Nizoral**

Ketoconazole belongs to a class of drugs called imidazole derivatives, normally used to treat fungal infections. It also inhibits key steps in the syntheses of mineralocorticoids and glucocorticoids, the first step in cortisol synthesis, according to a report from Harvard Medical School. As an adrenal steroid inhibitor, it is recommended in the treatment of Cushing's syndrome.

Endocrinology Journal reported from Chang Gung University in Taiwan on three patients who had residual or recurring Cushing's disease after surgical treatment. Ketoconazole was administered orally and adjusted according to individual response based on lab testing. Based on follow-up periods up to 83 months, the researchers concluded that ketoconazole was a valuable therapy when surgery is contraindicated or unsuccessful.

A report from the University of Montreal in Canada on Cushing's syndrome noted that ketoconazole is one of various drugs that inhibits steroid synthesis and can be effective for rapidly controlling hypercortisolism either in preparation for surgery, after unsuccessful removal of the causative tumor, or while awaiting the full effect of radiotherapy or more definitive therapy.

Clinical and Experimental Pharmacology and Physiology reported on eight patients with Cushing's disease who were given ketoconazole for two weeks. Large reductions in urine excretion of free cortisol and cortisol metabolites were seen, and the researchers concluded it was clinically useful.

For more information see page 1259.

Generic: **Mifepristone** *(mi-FE-pris-tone)*
Brand: **Mifeprex**

Mifepristone, also known as RU486, was developed to aid in early abortion, for which it is used in combination with another drug that stimulates uterine contractions a few days later.

Because mifepristone is a potent antiglucocorticoid agent, it can be used to treat types of Cushing's syndrome that are ACTH- (adrenocorticotropic hormone) independent, according to an article in Steroids from the Shaare Zedek Medical Center in Jerusalem, Israel.

Journal of Clinical Endocrinology and Metabolism reported on a severely ill patient with Cushing's syndrome caused by an ACTH-secreting pituitary macroadenoma. He had been treated unsuccessfully by a combination of conventional surgical, medical, and radiotherapeutic approaches. Subsequently, he responded dramatically to high-dose long-term mifepristone therapy, with significant reversal of his heart failure and resolution of his psychotic depression. Nonetheless, the case demonstrated the potential need for concomitant mineralocorticoid receptor blockade in mifepristone-treated Cushing's disease because cortisol levels may rise markedly.

For more information see page 1328.

Generic: **Mitotane** *(MYE-toe-tane)*
Brand: **Lysodren**

Researchers at the University of Montreal in Canada have noted that mitotane inhibits steroid synthesis and is useful for rapidly controlling hypercortisolism either in preparation for surgery, after unsuccessful removal of the causative tumor, or while waiting for radiotherapy or another treatment to take full effect.

The University School of Medicine in Kawasaki, Japan reported in *The Lancet* on the efficacy of mitotane in a woman with massive alternariosis, a fungal infection, as well as Cushing's syndrome. Not only did the mitotane effectively treat the Cushing's, but also the fungal infection disappeared. The researchers believe that immunosuppression due to the high blood cortisol from the Cushing's syndrome is what caused the fungal infection, because a direct action of the mitotane on the fungus itself seems unlikely. Once the immunosuppression stopped, the patient's immune system took over and eliminated the fungus.

For more information see page 1337.

Hyperaldosteronism

Hyperaldosteronism is a rare disease caused by an excess production of aldosterone by the adrenal gland. This hormone is responsible for sodium and potassium balance, which then directly controls water balance to maintain appropriate blood pressure and blood volume. Primary hyperaldosteronism is caused by an abnormality within the gland. Secondary hyperaldosteronism is caused by something outside the gland that mimics the primary condition.

Hyperaldosteronism causes high blood pressure and a low serum potassium level.

Commonly Prescribed (On-Label) Drug: Spironolactone

OFF-LABEL PRESCRIPTION DRUGS
BREAKTHROUGH OPTIONS

Generic: **Amiloride** (a-MIL-oh-ride)
Brand: **Midamor**

Amiloride belongs to a class of drugs called potassium-sparing diuretics, which have been recommended for the treatment of hypokalemic disorders—that is, conditions in which the body fails to retain enough potassium to maintain health. Diuretics are often the first line of drugs prescribed for hypertension because they reduce fluid volume in the body, thus reducing the pressure on blood vessels. But a significant number of diuretics tend to drain the body of potassium. And hyperaldosteronism causes both problems—high blood pressure and low potassium levels. Hence, a drug that will act as a diuretic but not drain potassium is ideal.

In the *Journal of Clinical Pharmacology*, experts from Boston University School of Medicine explained that amiloride acts on distal tubular cells in the kidney to reduce the urinary excretion of potassium, while augmenting the excretion of sodium and chloride. They called the drug a significant advancement in hypokalemic therapy since it is more potent than two other potassium-sparing diuretics, spironolactone and triamterene, and has fewer side effects.

In 10 patients with primary hyperaldosteronism treated with amiloride over 24 weeks, blood pressure fell significantly and plasma potassium and aldosterone increased, as did plasma renin activity. The study concluded that amiloride therapy is efficacious in correcting the hypokalemia of primary hyperaldosteronism.

For more information see page 1004.

Generic: **Captopril** (KAP-toe-pril)
Brand: **Capoten**

Captopril belongs to a class of drugs called angiotensin converting enzyme (ACE) inhibitors. It inhibits an enzyme needed to produce a substance that causes blood vessels to tighten. With captopril, blood vessels relax, lowering blood pressure. Captopril is typically prescribed to treat hypertension or treat heart failure.

Physicians at Laval University in Quebec, Canada believed that captopril could be equally effective in the diagnosis of salt loading, which is defined as a sodium administration of a minimum of 77 mmol in addition to daily intake. In 49 patients with a presumed diagnosis of primary aldosteronism, with baseline values taken on all, captopril was given with blood samples taken at baseline and again two hours later. Then they were placed on a salt-loading diet for three days. Of the 59, 44 had nonsuppressible aldosterone concentrations with all the clinical characteristics of primary aldosteronism: 22 had surgically confirmed unilateral adenoma, and 22 had presumed bilateral hyperplasia. There was a significant correlation between plasma aldosterone values of salt-loaded patients and the values two hours after captopril administration. The physicians concluded that their results showed that the captopril suppression test is as effective as sodium loading in confirming the diagnosis of primary aldosteronism, but results are available in two hours rather than in three days.

Experts at the University of Oklahoma wrote in *Hypertension* that the addition of the post-captopril test enhances the accuracy for diagnosing patients with primary aldosteronism.

For more information see page 1066.

*Generic: **Triamterene** (trye-AM-ter-een)*
*Brand: **Dyrenium***

Triamterene is in a group of drugs called potassium-sparing diuretics, which play an important role in the treatment of hyperaldosteronism because the disease involves hypertension, and diuretics reduce fluid volume in the body, thus reducing the pressure on blood vessels. But a significant number of diuretics tend to drain the body of potassium, so one that does not drain potassium can be helpful.

According to the MedStar Research Institute and the Washington Hospital Center on *eMedicine*, potassium-sparing agents are second-line drugs for treatment of primary hyperaldosteronism when surgery is contraindicated or refused. They often must be used together with other drugs for ideal blood pressure control because they are not potent antihypertensives.

Researchers from Indiana University explored using a combination of triamterene with a thiazide diuretic. Although thiazides do deplete potassium, it could be used in a lower dose because it was being used in combination with triamterene. It was hoped that the two together would achieve adequate blood pressure control without draining the body of potassium. A group of eight patients with hyperaldosteronism were tested and the combination successfully reduced fluid volume in the body. Physicians increased potassium concentration to the normal range in all but one patient and concluded that this combination may offer an alternative for patients who cannot tolerate spironolactone.

For more information see page 1525.

Pheochromoblastoma

See Pheochromocytoma

Pheochromocytoma

Pheochromocytoma is a tumor of the adrenal gland that arises in the medulla, the center of the adrenal gland. 80% are found in only one adrenal gland. Ten percent occur on both kidneys, and 10% occur outside the adrenal glands. Pheochromocytomas can cause headaches, sweating, rapid changes in blood pressure—up and down—rapid heartbeat, and other symptoms. Those that arise in the medulla can cause a serious rise in blood pressure.

Commonly Prescribed (On-Label) Drugs: *Iobenguane I-131, Metyrosine, Phenoxybenzamine, Phentolamine, Propranolol*

OFF-LABEL PRESCRIPTION DRUGS
BREAKTHROUGH OPTIONS

Generic: Alpha blockers such as **Doxazosin** *(doks-AY-zoe-sin)* and **Prazosin** *(PRA-zoe-sin)*
Brands: **Cardura (doxazosin), Minipress (prazosin)**

Doxazosin and prazosin are part of a class of drugs called alpha-blockers used to treat hypertension. In pheochromocytoma patients, it is particularly important to get the blood pressure down prior to surgical removal of the tumor, and alpha-blockers are potent hypertensives. According to *eMedicine*, the first line of pre-operative therapy usually is an alpha-blocking agent, with a beta blocker as an add-on therapy. At higher doses, alpha blockers may cause sodium and fluid to accumulate. Therefore, using the two together can maintain the hypotensive effects of the alpha-blockers.

An article in the *American Heart Journal* from the Tohoku University School of Medicine in Sendai, Japan, compared doxazosin alone or in conjunction with a beta-blocker in 24 patients in pre-operative patients with pheochromocytoma. Excellent or good antihypertensive efficacy was assessed in 19 of 24 patients. Doxazosin was effective in 66.7% and combined therapy was effective in 91.7%. Overall, doxazosin was considered very useful or useful in 83.3%.

An article in the *Annals of Internal Medicine* from the New York Hospital–Cornell University Medical Center presented four cases in which prazosin was used to control signs and symptoms of pheochromocytomas, although intravenous phentolamine was required during surgery to manage pressure surges. *eMedicine* notes that prazosin decreases blood pressure with minimum risk of reflex tachycardia, an increase in a normal heart rhythm.

For more information see pages 1152 and 1426.

Generic: Beta-blockers such as ***Atenolol*** *(a-TEN-oh-lole)*, ***Esmolol*** *(ES-moe-lole)*, ***Labetalol*** *(la-BET-a-lole)*, and ***Metoprolol*** *(me-toe-PROE-lole)*
Brands: ***Tenormin (atenolol), Brevibloc (esmolol); Normodyne, Trandate (labetalol), Lopressor, Toprol-XL (metoprolol)***

Atenolol, esmolol, labetalol, and metoprolol are beta-blockers that are used to treat hypertension, angina, heart attacks, and heart failure. Because pheochromocytomas often cause high blood pressure, patients often need medications to control it. Usually, the first line of therapy is an alpha blocking agent used along with a beta-blocker.

An article in *Anesthesia and Analgesia* from the Johns Hopkins Medical Institutions in Baltimore, Maryland, reported on the first use of esmolol in the management of pheochromocytoma during an operation. They conclude that esmolol has significant potential for the treatment of cardiovascular abnormalities associated with excess beta-stimulation of the patient undergoing removal of pheochromocytoma.

An article in *Anesthesiology* from the Stanford University School of Medicine in California reported on a woman who was diagnosed with pheochromocytoma while in an intensive care unit for multisystem organ failure after knee arthroscopy. Therapy was begun with metoprolol and phenoxybenzamine. She slowly recovered, and her surgery was postponed because of her kidney problems.

According to *eMedicine*, labetalol actually blocks both alpha- and beta-adrenergic receptor sites, whereas esmolol is excellent for people at risk for experiencing complications from beta-blockers, especially those with reactive airway disease, mild-to-moderate left ventricular dysfunction, and/or peripheral vascular disease.

For more information see pages 1027, 1174, 1265, and 1329.

*Generic: **Clonidine** (KLON-i-deen)*
*Brands: **Catapres, Catapres-TTS, Duraclon***

Clonidine is an antihypertensive drug. It normally lowers blood levels of the hormone adrenaline. However, if a tumor is present, adrenaline levels do not decrease with clonidine.

Various tests are used to diagnose and locate pheochromocytomas, including urine tests, x-ray tests (such as CT and MRI scans), and blood tests. Clonidine is used in one of the blood tests. As described in a National Institute of Health (NIH) patient information publication, a patient takes a tablet of clonidine and, over the next three hours, blood samples are drawn and checked in the lab. Blood pressure and heart rate are also checked during this period. If adrenaline levels do not decrease, that is one confirmatory sign that a patient has a pheochromocytoma. This is called the clonidine suppression test.

In the *Archives of Internal Medicine*, doctors at the Fitzsimons Army Medical Center in Aurora, Colorado confirmed that the clonidine suppression test is 92% accurate in diagnosing pheochromocytoma. Its accuracy diminishes in patients with low baseline plasma catecholamine levels, who may be better tested with a stimulatory test, such as glucagon. The use of diuretics, beta-blockers, and antidepressants may cause false-positive results or severe hypotension during this test. The physicians concluded that although it is rarely necessary for the diagnosis of pheochromocytoma, the clonidine suppression test is an accurate and safe test in a select group of patients.

For more information see page 1108.

DIABETES, TYPE 1 AND TYPE 2

Diabetes consists of serious diseases characterized by high blood sugar levels that result from defects in the body's ability to produce and/or use insulin. Type 1 is an autoimmune disorder in which the body destroys the beta cells in the pancreas, leading to a total inability to produce insulin. Type 2 diabetes involves insulin resistance—the body's inability to properly use its own insulin supply. Some people have a form of diabetes that is in between the two types.

Arteriosclerosis

See Prevention of Peripheral Vascular Disease and Atherosclerosis in Type 2 Diabetes

Chronic Peripheral Arterial Occlusive Disease

See Prevention of Peripheral Vascular Disease and Atherosclerosis in Type 2 Diabetes

Diabetic Glomerulosclerosis

See Diabetic Nephropathy

Diabetic Kidney Disease

See Diabetic Nephropathy

Diabetic Nephropathy

Diabetic nephropathy is a complication of diabetes involving damage to the kidneys, impairing their ability to filter blood and form urine properly. At its earliest stages, called microalbuminuria, small amounts of protein appear in the urine—and this may persist for many years before proteinuria, signaling high protein levels in the urine, occurs. Over time, diabetic nephropathy may eventually lead to chronic kidney failure and end-stage kidney disease.

Commonly Prescribed (On-Label) Drugs: *Irbesartan, Losartan*

OFF-LABEL PRESCRIPTION DRUGS
BREAKTHROUGH OPTIONS

Generic: ACE inhibitors such as ***Enalapril*** *(e-NAL-a-pril),*
Lisinopril *(lyse-IN-oh-pril),* and ***Ramipril*** *(ra-MI-pril)*
Brands: ***Vasotec, Vasotec I. V. (enalapril), Prinivil, Zestril***
(lisinopril), Altace (ramipril)

Enalapril, lisinopril, and ramipril are three of many drugs that
are angiotensin converting enzyme (ACE) inhibitors. They
block an enzyme needed to produce a substance that causes
blood vessels to tighten. As a result, blood vessels relax, lowering
blood pressure. Therefore, they are normally prescribed widely
to treat hypertension.

As reported in *Diabetes Care,* a number of large trials in people
with type 1 diabetes have demonstrated that lowering systolic
blood pressure to under 140 mmHg with ACE inhibitors provides a selective benefit not found when using other antihypertensive drugs. For example, the Collaborative Study Group
reported in the *New England Journal of Medicine* that ACE inhibitors can slow the decline in glomerular filtration rate (a
measure of kidney damage).

Experts from the University of the Sciences in Philadelphia reported in *Clinical Therapy* that ACE inhibitors are the drug of
choice for patients with type 1 diabetes and evidence of incipi-
ent or overt nephropathy. The American Diabetes Association
considers treatment with ACE inhibitors a standard of care for
type 1 or 2 patients with diabetic nephropathy, and the National
Kidney Foundation has achieved the same consensus. If ACE inhibitors are not tolerated, an alternative may be angiotensin II
receptor blockers.

For more information see pages 1166, 1284, and 1355.

Generic: Angiotensin II receptor blockers such as **Candesartan** *(kan-de-SAR-tan)*, **Telmisartan** *(tell-miss-SAR-tan)*, and **Valsartan** *(val-SAR-tan)*
Brands: **Atacand (candesartan), Micardis (telmisartan), Diovan (valsartan)**

Candesartan, telmisartan, and valsartan belong to a class of drugs called angiotensin II receptor blockers (ARBs) or angiotensin II receptor antagonists. They are a newer class of antihypertensive agents than the ACE inhibitors, although they aim at that same troublesome substance—angiotensin—that plays a role in hypertension.

According to a series of reports in the *New England Journal of Medicine,* ARBs have been shown to reduce the rate of progression from micro- to macroalbuminuria, as well as end-stage renal disease in patients with type 2 diabetes.

According to the American Diabetes Association, published in its journal *Diabetes Care,* ARBs have clearly been shown to delay the progression to macroalbuminuria in patients with type 2 diabetes. Further, in patients with type 2 diabetes, hypertension, macroalbuminuria and renal insufficiency, ARBs have been shown to delay the progression of nephropathy.

Medscape confirms that angiotensin II receptor antagonists such as valsartan have been shown to slow the rate of progression of kidney disease in people with hypertension and diabetes.

For more information see pages 1065, 1497, and 1536.

Diabetic Neuropathy

Diabetic neuropathy is a complication of diabetes due to nerve damage throughout the body. Neuropathy can cause sensations ranging from numbness to "pins and needles" to severe pain to weakness in the hands, arms, feet, and legs. Problems can also occur in every organ of the body including the digestive tract, heart, urinary tract, and sex organs. Although a wide range of drugs may help somewhat, a single drug has not been found for everyone.

Commonly Prescribed (On-Label) Drugs: *Capsaicin, Duloxetine, Pregabalin*

OFF-LABEL PRESCRIPTION DRUGS
BREAKTHROUGH OPTIONS

*Generic: **Bupropion** (byoo-PROE-pee-on)*
*Brands: **Wellbutrin, Wellbutrin SR, Wellbutrin XL, Zyban***

Bupropion is an antidepressant in a class by itself, somewhat different from other antidepressants (tricyclic antidepressants and selective serotonin reuptake inhibitors). However, like other antidepressants, bupropion's effect in neuropathy has nothing to do with depression. Rather, it has to do with bupropion's ability to interfere with chemical messengers, called neurotransmitters, in the brain. Bupropion affects dopamine and norepinephrine, which in turn affects the way the brain perceives pain.

Bupropion demonstrated greater effectiveness than placebo in a study in 46 patients with neuropathy due to various causes, according to *Neurology*. Nearly 75% of patients rated their pain as improved or much improved with bupropion compared to no significant change with placebo. A major benefit of bupropion compared to selective serotonin reuptake inhibitors (SSRIs) is that it is less likely to cause negative sexual side effects.

For more information see page 1058.

*Generic: **Carbamazepine** (kar-ba-MAZ-e-peen)*
*Brands: **Carbatrol, Epitol, Tegretol, Tegretol XR***

Carbamazepine has multiple applications. It is an anticonvulsant used for treating epilepsy, and is also chemically related to the tricyclic antidepressants. Both classes of drugs are also used to treat diabetic neuropathy because they affect chemical messengers in the brain that affect the perception of pain.

The first study demonstrating the effectiveness of carbamazepine in diabetic neuropathy was in 1969, in which 28 of 30 patients experienced relief within two weeks, as published in *Diabetologia*. However, another study shortly thereafter, published in *Drugs*, was equivocal, but some experts thought the problem was due to the crossover study design. More recently, a study compared carbamazepine to a combination of nortriptyline and fluphenazine. While both yielded benefits in diabetic neuropathy, with no significant differences in those benefits, fewer adverse effects were reported with carbamazepine, according to *Archives of Medical Research*.

For more information see page 1068.

Generic: **Clonidine** (KLON-i-deen)
Brands: **Catapres, Catapres-TTS, Duraclon**

Clonidine is an antihypertensive drug. Often, diabetic neuropathy refers to peripheral neuropathy—that is the pain or numbness that affects the hands and feet. But diabetic neuropathy can also mean autonomic neuropathy, which can cause, among other problems, heart disease.

An article in the *Cleveland Clinic Journal of Medicine* pointed out that orthostatic hypotension is a significant sign of autonomic neuropathy. In this problem, a patient gets dizzy or faints when he or she stands up suddenly from a reclining or sitting position. Experts recommend clonidine as a potential treatment for this type of autonomic neuropathy, but warn that it can worsen the problem in some patients. Therefore the initial dose should be small and increased gradually. According to the *Journal of Endocrinology & Metabolism*, clonidine is one of the many third-line treatments for diabetic neuropathy.

For more information see page 1108.

Generic: **Gabapentin** (GA-ba-pen-tin)
Brand: **Neurontin**

Gabapentin is an anticonvulsant originally developed to treat epilepsy. It has also since been FDA-approved for treating a neuropathic form of pain called post-herpetic neuralgia which occurs in adults who have had chicken pox as children and develop shingles; the virus remains latent in their systems for many years and then reactivates to cause this pain. Gabapentin works on chemical pain messengers in the brain that affect the way we perceive pain.

Considerable evidence supports its use for painful diabetic peripheral neuropathy, according to *Formulary*. Gabapentin was superior in a variety of measures of pain and quality of life (including improved sleep quality) in diabetic neuropathy in a study in the *Journal of the American Medical Association;* 26% of the gabapentin group reported no pain and 60% had at least moderate improvement, compared to 15% and 33% in the placebo group.

Even with relatively low doses, gabapentin was superior to placebo for diabetic neuropathy in a study in the *Journal of Neurology, Neurosurgery and Psychiatry.*

In another trial in the Archives of Internal Medicine, gabapentin had equivalent pain relief to the previously established therapy for diabetic neuropathy—amitriptyline. In this study, the gabapentin dose was also relatively low.

For more information see page 1206.

Generic: **Lamotrigine** *(la-MOE-tri-jeen)*
Brand: **Lamictal**

Lamotrigine is an anticonvulsant drug widely prescribed for the treatment of epilepsy and bipolar disorder, a psychiatric problem with mood swings from mania to depression. Lamotrigine's benefits in diabetic neuropathy have nothing to do with depression or epilepsy, but rather its ability to affect chemical messengers in the brain called neurotransmitters, which affect the way the brain perceives pain.

At a presentation at the World Congress of Pain, researchers from Nevada Neurological Consultants discussed a series of 80 patients with various types of neuropathy, including five with diabetic neuropathy. All had failed to respond to at least two or more other medications including those most commonly prescribed, such as tricyclic antidepressants and the anticonvulsant gabapentin. Thirty eight percent of their patients responded to lamotrigine, and it was most effective in those with diabetic neuropathy.

In another study of 59 people with diabetic neuropathy, nearly one-third of the 27 who received lamotrigine considered it highly efficacious, according to *Neurology.* However, *Formulary* warns of the serious risk of rash.

For more information see page 1268.

Generic: **Lidocaine** *(LYE-doe-kane)*
Brand: **Lidoderm**

Lidocaine is a topical anesthetic. Your dentist may use it as an injected drug but it is also used topically as a pain killer. When applied to the skin, it produces pain relief by blocking the signals at the nerve endings. Topically applied lidocaine is usually used to relieve the pain of post-herpetic neuralgia, or, shingles, which occurs in people who have had chicken pox years ago. The virus remains dormant in the body for years, and then reactivates to cause pain along nerves. Thus, it is a "nerve"-related pain and might be considered similar to diabetic neuropathy.

Topical lidocaine can be used in a pain "patch" applied to the skin that gradually releases lidocaine into the local area and is not associated with systemic accumulation of the drug. In one study, the lidocaine patch was applied to the area of maximal pain, and patients were told to use no more than four patches changed every 24 hours, for two weeks. The diabetic neuropathy patients reported significant improvement in four measures of the quality of pain on the Neuropathic Pain Scale, according to *Current Medical Research and Opinions.*

For more information see page 1283.

Generic: **Memantine** *(me-MAN-teen)*
Brand: **Namenda**

Memantine is used to treat Alzheimer's disease. Overstimulation of a receptor in the brain called NMDA by a substance called glutamate has been implicated in neurodegenerative disorders, and memantine is an NMDA receptor-antagonist.

In a study reported in *Anesthesiology,* memantine was compared to dextromethorphan and an active placebo (lorazepam) in a trial of patients with diabetic neuropathy and post-herpetic neuralgia. Of the 19 diabetic neuropathy patients who completed the trial, memantine only reduced pain intensity on average by 17%, compared to a reduction of 33% by dextromethorphan and 16% by the placebo.

In *European Journal of Neurology,* studies of memantine are associated with hallucinations, particularly visual hallucinations. The incidence is low and mild and does not seem to be a problem in Alzheimer's disease.

For more information see page 1304.

Generic: **Mexiletine** *(MEKS-i-le-teen)*
Brand: **Mexitil**

Mexiletine is used in the treatment of a life-threatening abnormal heart rhythm called ventricular arrhythmia. In diabetic neuropathy, mexiletine is thought to have analgesic effects by stabilizing how cells handle sodium. Mexiletine is the oral form of lidocaine.

Mexiletine has been evaluated in three clinical trials involving a total of about 250 people. Although most studies reported substantial reductions in pain scores, statistically significant differences compared to placebo were documented only in one small trial with fewer than 20 patients, as reported in *The Lancet.* In a larger study, mexiletine was superior to placebo only for those with specific types of pain, including burning and stabbing, as reported in *Diabetes Care.*

American Journal of Health-System Pharmacists concluded, based on four studies, that mexiletine failed to show a statistically significant improvement in pain compared with placebo, and it can be recommended only as an alternative treatment for those with extreme symptoms who have not responded to multiple other drugs and who have no cardiac risks.

The website, *Medscape,* also refers to studies with mexiletine as "equivocal" for diabetic neuropathy and says its role remains to be established. Their experts recommend that its use in diabetic neuropathy "should be limited to patients who do not respond to, or who cannot tolerate, more established therapies."

For more information see page 1324.

Generic: **Oxcarbazepine** *(ox-car-BAZ-e-peen)*
Brand: **Trileptal**

Oxcarbazepine is an anticonvulsant used for treating the seizures of epilepsy. It is chemically related and has a mechanism of action similar to carbamazepine, but may have fewer adverse effects and drug interactions, according to *The New England Journal of Medicine and Pain*. Oxcarbazepine is used to treat diabetic neuropathy because it affects chemical messengers in the brain, called neurotransmitters, that affect the perception of pain.

Clinical Journal of Pain reported on a study of oxcarbazepine in 30 patients with painful diabetic neuropathy. After one week of screening, the dose was increased for four weeks and then maintained for another four weeks. The mean pain scores dropped 48.3%. The researchers concluded that oxcarbazepine was efficacious and safe as a sole therapy for diabetic neuropathy, although they acknowledged that this was an open study and results would need to be confirmed in a more precise trial.

For more information see page 1390.

Generic: Selective serotonin reuptake inhibitors such as **Citalopram** *(sye-TAL-oh-pram)* and **Paroxetine** *(pa-ROKS-e-teen)*
Brands: **Celexa (citalopram), Paxil, Paxil CR (paroxetine)**

Citalopram and paroxetine belong to a larger class of drugs known as selective serotonin reuptake inhibitors (SSRIs). Most commonly prescribed for depression, these drugs' beneficial impact on neuropathy has nothing to do with depression, but instead with the transmission of physical pain messages to the brain. SSRIs interfere with chemical messengers in the brain called neurotransmitters. SSRIs inhibit the reuptake of serotonin and so the brain does not perceive pain messages because that chemical messenger does not convey the message.

In general, SSRIs have fewer side effects than tricyclic antidepressants but are somewhat less effective, and therefore should not be considered as the sole therapy, according to *New England Journal of Medicine*. Indeed, some of the reports on these drugs showed them to be no better than placebo, but there is strong variation from one individual to another. An article in *American Family Physician* calls evidence for their use fair and indicates that SSRIs may be "only possibly effective."

For more information see pages 1096 and 1395.

*Generic: **Topiramate** (TOE-pie-rah-mate)*
*Brand: **Topamax***

Topiramate is an anticonvulsant drug normally used in the treatment of epilepsy. Although a variety of anti-epileptics are used off-label for neuropathy because they may affect the way pain messages travel to the brain, their benefits may fade over time. However, topiramate may also affect underlying causative mechanisms of diabetic neuropathy.

In an eight-week study of topiramate reported at the 2005 American Diabetes Association's annual meeting, lab tests showed not only a decrease in total neuropathy scores but a healing of the underlying nerves. Further, decreases were seen in total cholesterol, diastolic blood pressure, and hemoglobin A1C (a measure of long-term blood control), and the drug also promotes weight loss. These are all components of the metabolic syndrome that often precede type 2 diabetes, and their reversal could prolong the onset of the disease and, thus, lead to a reversal in diabetic neuropathy. The lead researcher concluded that topiramate may be the first drug to change the biology of diabetic neuropathy. In another study he observed that the reduction in pain was comparable to that seen with gabapentin, another anti-epileptic drug.

For more information see page 1516.

*Generic: **Tramadol** (TRAM-a-dole)*
*Brand: **Ultram***

Tramadol is an analgesic that is related to the opioids. While its mode of action resembles that of narcotics and it is as effective as many narcotics in relieving pain, it is not a narcotic and does not depress breathing, a side effect of most narcotics. Tramadol is also not a nonsteroidal anti-inflammatory drug (NSAID) and does not have the increased risk of stomach ulceration and internal bleeding that can occur with the use of NSAIDs. It does affect serotonin neurotransmitters—chemical messengers—in the brain that may help change the perception of pain in diabetic neuropathy.

Two key studies have demonstrated the efficacy and safety of tramadol in diabetic neuropathy. A clinical study in 131 diabetes patients showed a significant reduction in pain intensity compared to placebo, according to *Neurology*. A second study compared tramadol to placebo for the treatment of pain, paresthesia, and touch-evoked pain associated with polyneuropathies. The drug again proved to be more effective than placebo, although the improvement was modest, according to *Pain*.

An article in the *American Journal of Health System Pharmacists* concluded that tramadol is safe and effective for diabetic neuropathy, although the dose required for benefits is relatively high.

For more information see page 1518.

Generic: Tricyclic antidepressants such as ***Amitriptyline*** *(a-mee-TRIP-ti-leen)*, ***Clomipramine*** *(kloe-MI-pra-meen)*, ***Desipramine*** *(des-IP-ra-meen)*, ***Imipramine*** *(im-IP-ra-meen)*, and ***Nortriptyline*** *(nor-TRIP-ti-leen)* ***Brands: Elavil (amitriptyline), Anafranil (clomipramine), Norpramin (desipramine), Tofranil, Tofranil-PM (imipramine); Aventyl, Pamelor (nortriptyline)***

Amitriptyline, clomipramine, desipramine, imipramine, and nortriptyline are five drugs that belong to a large class of agents called tricyclic antidepressants or TCAs. Their effect in neuropathy has nothing to do with depression but rather their ability to interfere with certain chemical messengers in the brain and the way the brain perceives pain.

Studies in *Pain* and *Annals of Pharmacotherapy* suggest that amitriptyline, clomipramine, desipramine, and imipramine have the best efficacy in diabetic neuropathy among all the TCAs. One study reported in *New England Journal of Medicine* of desipramine and amitriptyline showed no difference in effectiveness but suggested that desipramine was better tolerated. Evaluation of nortriptyline is difficult because it was given in combination with other medications in existing trials. *Journal of Clinical Endocrinology and Metabolism* calls the TCAs the mainstays of treatment for painful diabetic neuropathy. A report from *eMedicine* states that until new therapies are proven to relieve symptoms in appropriately designed trials, tricyclic drugs will remain first-line drugs for the relief of painful neuropathic symptoms.

For more information see pages 1009, 1105, 1132, 1230, and 1378.

Generic: **Venlafaxine** *(ven-la-FAX-een)*
Brands: **Effexor, Effexor XR**

Venlafaxine is a new antidepressant with a novel chemical structure that does not resemble those of any antidepressants currently used. It is not a tricyclic antidepressant, but does have the same type of effect on two chemical messengers in the brain—serotonin and norepinephrine—associated with the tricyclic antidepressant drugs. Therefore, it does the same type of thing—that is, it blocks pain messages from getting through to the brain, thereby helping diabetic neuropathy.

In a series of eight patients with diabetic neuropathy reported in *Diabetes Care,* venlafaxine provided dramatic relief within two to eight days after the start of therapy. In another series of 11 people with diabetic neuropathy reported in the same journal, 75% to 100% pain relief was experienced within three to 14 days. All of these patients, in both reports, had not responded to conventional treatment regimens with other antidepressants, narcotics, or analgesics.

For more information see page 1542.

Diabetic Retinopathy

Diabetic retinopathy is a complication of the high blood glucose levels of diabetes in which tiny blood vessels inside the retina, the light-sensitive tissue at the back of the eye, are damaged. Initially, it causes no symptoms, although it can be diagnosed by an eye doctor. However, if poor glucose control allows diabetic retinopathy to progress, it will eventually lead to loss of vision. It is the leading cause of blindness in adults in the United States.

Commonly Prescribed (On-Label) Drug: *Indocyanine green*

OFF-LABEL PRESCRIPTION DRUG
BREAKTHROUGH OPTION

Generic: **Lisinopril** *(lyse-IN-oh-pril)*
Brands: **Prinivil, Zestril**

Lisinopril is widely prescribed to treat hypertension, left ventricular failure, and chronic heart failure, especially after a heart attack. It belongs to a class of drugs called angiotensin converting enzyme (ACE) inhibitors. It blocks an enzyme needed to produce a substance that causes blood vessels to tighten. As a result, blood vessels relax. This lowers blood pressure and increases the supply of blood and oxygen to the heart.

Clinical studies discovered that diabetes patients taking ACE inhibitors, including lisinopril, for hypertension or other prescribed therapy also saw inhibition of diabetic retinopathy. For example, in the EURODIAB Controlled Trial of Lisinopril in Insulin-Dependent Diabetes, lisinopril reduced progression of retinopathy in nonhypertensive patients by 50% over two years, according to *Heart*. Studies were done to discern what might be the causative mechanisms.

The enzyme angiotensin II is involved in diabetic complications of the large blood vessels. Scientists at the University of Melbourne in Australia undertook studies in animal models and determined that the same enzyme system is also involved in the tiny blood vessels of the eye. They then treated the animals with lisinopril in their drinking water and were able to inhibit the progression of their retinopathy, as reported in the *American Journal of Pathology*. In another study conducted by Case Western Reserve University in Ohio, lisinopril inhibited the accumulation of glucose in the retinal cells of diabetic animals, another potential mechanism for its benefits.

For more information see page 1284.

Diabetic Sclerosis

See Diabetic Nephropathy

Fundus Diabeticus

See Diabetic Retinopathy

Peripheral Atherosclerosis

See Prevention of Peripheral Vascular Disease and Atherosclerosis in Type 2 Diabetes

Peripheral Vascular Disease (PVD)

See Prevention of Peripheral Vascular Disease and Atherosclerosis in Type 2 Diabetes

Prevention of Type 2 Diabetes

Because type 2 diabetes is associated with being overweight, having a poor diet, and not getting adequate exercise, along with a gradual escalation in blood sugar levels over a period of years, several large studies have explored the feasibility of preventing it with lifestyle modification or glucose-lowering drugs approved for treating diabetes. According to the American Diabetes Association, intensive lifestyle modification was more effective than any of the drugs discussed below, yielding a 58% reduction in diabetes incidence in one study.

Commonly Prescribed (On-Label) Drugs: None

OFF-LABEL PRESCRIPTION DRUGS
BREAKTHROUGH OPTIONS

*Generic: **Acarbose** (AY-car-bose)*
*Brand: **Precose***

Acarbose is used to treat type 2 diabetes. It reduces the body's secretion of extra insulin after a meal and also improves insulin resistance

The STOP-NIDDM (stop non-insulin dependent diabetes mellitus) was a clinical trial seeking to identify and treat people at high risk of developing diabetes. As reported in *The Lancet*, in the

STOP-NIDDM trial, 714 people with impaired glucose tolerance received either acarbose or a placebo three times daily. After an average follow-up of 3.3 years, 42% in the placebo group but only 31% of those in the acarbose group progressed to diabetes, yielding a 32% relative risk reduction of progression to diabetes in those taking the acarbose. To delay development of type 2 diabetes, the researchers recommended that acarbose be used either as an alternative or in addition to changes in lifestyle.

For more information see page 982.

Generic: **Metformin** *(met-FOR-min)*
Brands: **Glucophage, Glucophage XR, Riomet**

Metformin belongs to a class of drug called biguanides and has long been used successfully to treat type 2 diabetes. It decreases the liver's output of glucose and, to a lesser extent, increases utilization of glucose. Thus, it lowers insulin resistance. Off-label metformin was evaluated as a way to help prevent diabetes in people who already have impaired glucose tolerance in the largest and most important study of its kind, the Diabetes Prevention Program (DPP), co-sponsored by the National Institutes of Health; numerous articles about the program's success have appeared in *New England Journal of Medicine* and other journals.

The DPP enrolled more than 3,000 obese adults, about half of whom were from minority groups (African-American or Hispanic) and randomly assigned them to one of three intervention groups, which included the intensive nutrition and exercise counseling ("lifestyle") group or either of two medication treatment groups: the metformin group or the placebo group. The medication interventions were combined with standard diet and exercise recommendations. After an average follow-up of 2.8 years, the lifestyle group did best with a 58% relative reduction in progression to diabetes compared to the placebo group. However, the metformin group also did well with a 31% relative reduction in progression to diabetes.

For more information see page 1308.

*Generic: **Orlistat** (OR-li-stat)*
*Brand: **Xenical***

Orlistat is an anti-obesity drug normally prescribed to people to help them lose weight. It has well documented effectiveness in both weight reduction and maintenance of that weight loss. Further, weight loss with the use of orlistat has been associated with a decrease in obesity-related cardiovascular risk factors. Because type 2 diabetes most commonly occurs in people who are over 40 and overweight, and because the risk of type 2 declines when people lose weight, a drug that helps people lose weight can help prevent type 2 diabetes.

According to *Diabetes and Metabolism,* treatment with orlistat reduces the incidence of type 2 diabetes in people who already have impaired glucose tolerance. And in those who already have type 2 diabetes, it has enabled them to lower their required dose of metformin, sulfonylureas, and/or insulin. Of concern, because diabetes patients are at greater risk of cardiovascular disease, it was also noted that it helped reduce their total and LDL cholesterols and other lipid markers and decreased inflammation associated with heart attack risk.

In the Prevention of Diabetes in Obese Subjects study, orlistat reduced the incidence of diabetes from 9% to 6% compared to placebo, according to Diabetes Care. However, analysis of three other trials reported a nonsignificant reduction in the incidence of type 2 from 2% to 0.6% with orlistat, as reported in the *Archives of Internal Medicine.*

Nonetheless, a report in the *Journal of the American Board of Family Practitioners* noted the benefits of orlistat in helping prevent diabetes in obese patients.

For more information see page 1388.

Generic: Thiazolidinediones such as ***Pioglitazone***
(pye-oh-GLI-ta-zone), and ***Rosiglitazone***
(roh-si-GLI-ta-zone)
*Brands: **Actos** (pioglitazone), **Avandia** (rosiglitazone)*

Thiazolidinediones are a class of drugs used successfully to help lower blood sugar levels in the treatment of diabetes. The first of these drugs to be introduced was troglitazone. In the Troglitazone in Prevention of Diabetes (TRIPOD) study, reported in *Diabetes*, women who had previously had gestational diabetes (a type of diabetes that occurs only during pregnancy and then disappears but increases your risk of subsequent type 2) received either placebo or troglitazone. After an average follow-up of 30 months, troglitazone treatment was associated with a 56% relative reduction in progression to diabetes.

Although troglitazone is no longer on the market, two second-generation thiazolidinediones are available—rosiglitazone and pioglitazone—and the TRIPOD study was part of the model for considering their use in preventing type 2 diabetes. The theory is that the thiazolidinediones, also called glitazones, improve insulin secretion and help preserve beta cells in the pancreas.

A study in *Diabetes, Obesity and Metabolism* examined 172 adults with impaired glucose tolerance and insulin resistance who had been taking troglitazone. When it was taken off the market, 71 no longer took any glucose-lowering drug and became the control group; the other 101 were switched to either rosiglitazone or pioglitazone. After two years, none of the patients receiving either rosiglitazone or pioglitazone had developed diabetes, while 11 of the controls had done so; after another year, 3 of the patients taking either rosiglitazone or pioglitazone had developed diabetes and a total of 19 in the control group had done so. The incidence of diabetes was 88.9% lower in the rosiglitazone or pioglitazone group compared to controls.

For more information see pages 1419 and 1462.

Prevention of Cardiovascular Disease in Type 2 Diabetes

Heart disease and stroke are the most life-threatening consequences of diabetes and occur to people with diabetes more than twice as often as to others. High blood glucose levels damage artery walls and contribute to premature atherosclerosis (hardening of the arteries). People with diabetes also seem to have high levels of inflammation in their bodies, high cholesterol levels, and central obesity (apple shapes), all of which increase the risk of cardiovascular disease.

Commonly Prescribed (On-Label) Drugs: *Atorvastatin, Pravastatin, Simvastatin*

OFF-LABEL PRESCRIPTION DRUGS
BREAKTHROUGH OPTIONS

Generic: Thiazolidinediones, such as ***Pioglitazone***
(pye-oh-GLI-ta-zone) and ***Rosiglitazone*** *(roh-si-GLI-ta-zone)*
Brands: ***Actos (pioglitazone), Avandia (rosiglitazone)***

Thiazolidinediones are a class of drugs approved to help lower blood sugar levels in the treatment of diabetes. The first of these drugs to be introduced was troglitazone, but it has been removed from the market because of hazards to the liver. The second generation drugs, pioglitazone and rosiglitazone, have been proven to be safe. Off-label, the drugs have been found to help prevent heart disease in people with type 2 diabetes.

The Diabetes Control and Complications Trial, sponsored by the National Institute of Health (NIH), showed that a greater than 50% lower risk of heart disease is one of the proven long-term benefits of tight glucose control in people with type 1 diabetes. This effect was achieved with insulin injections.

An article in *Diabetic Medicine* from the University of Turku, Finland, reported on the effects of rosiglitazone on heart glucose uptake in patients with type 2 diabetes, using placebo and metformin as control treatments. Researchers concluded that in addition to improving whole body insulin sensitivity, rosiglitazone enhances insulin-stimulated myocardial glucose uptake.

For more information see pages 1419 and 1462.

Prevention of Peripheral Vascular Disease and Atherosclerosis in Type 2 Diabetes

Atherosclerosis (hardening of the arteries) and peripheral vascular disease (damaged blood vessels other than those immediately surrounding the heart) occur twice as often and at an earlier age in people with diabetes as in those without. This higher risk is due to multiple risk factors including: high blood glucose levels that damage artery walls; high levels of inflammation in the body, high cholesterol levels; and central obesity (apple shapes).

Commonly Prescribed (On-Label) Drugs: *None*

OFF-LABEL PRESCRIPTION DRUG
BREAKTHROUGH OPTION

Generic: **Cilostazol** *(sil-OH-sta-zol)*
Brand: **Pletal**

Cilostazol is a drug that has been FDA-approved for the treatment of intermittent claudication, a form of peripheral arterial disease (PAD). It enables people with PAD to walk longer distances before developing the pain in the legs characteristic of this condition. Cilostazol dilates blood vessels and inhibits blood clotting, but other drugs with those benefits do not help PAD, so some other action must be involved, according to a report submitted to the FDA for approval of the drug. These actions have a direct effect on prevention of atherosclerosis and peripheral vascular disease since the drug is used to treat one form of such disease.

Clinical and Experimental Medicine noted that cilostazol affected lipid levels and composition. In 17 patients with type 2 diabetes, after six months of treatment with cilostazol, fat concentrations were significantly decreased and plasma docosahexaenoic acid levels significantly increased. Triglycerides are a significant contributor to cardiovascular disease, whereas docosahexaenoic acid is beneficial. The researchers concluded that cilostazol can induce positive changes in the serum lipid profile and fatty acid composition.

For more information see page 1089.

Prevention of Proteinuria in Type 2 Diabetes

About 50% of people who have diabetes develop diabetic nephropathy, one of its major complications, which involves damage to the kidneys that impairs their ability to filter blood and form urine properly. At its earliest stages, called microalbuminuria, small amounts of protein appear in the urine. If this persists unchecked for many years, eventually proteinuria develops, which signals high protein levels in the urine. Proteinuria leads to chronic kidney failure and end-stage kidney disease.

Commonly Prescribed (On-Label) Drugs: *None*

OFF-LABEL PRESCRIPTION DRUG
BREAKTHROUGH OPTION

Generic: **Eplerenone** *(e-PLER-en-one)*
Brand: **Inspra**

Eplerenone is normally used to treat hypertension or congestive heart failure in people who have had a heart attack. It blocks a hormone in the body called aldosterone. High levels of aldosterone and other hormones can lead to heart failure. By blocking aldosterone, eplerenone helps prevent or slows worsening of the heart failure.

A study at the University of Miami found that eplerenone can also help prevent proteinuria (an abnormal amount of protein in the urine) by helping prevent damage to the cells that line the inner surface of blood vessels, thus keeping the kidneys working properly. The researchers divided 270 people with albuminuria into four groups; half received one of two doses of eplerenone, and all received other drugs as needed to control blood pressure. By the 12th week, lab tests showed more than 50% less protein in the urine of those who had been on eplerenone, compared to only a 13% decrease in those who had not.

For more information see page 1168.

DIABETES INSIPIDUS

There are several types of diabetes insipidus (DI), an uncommon condition that occurs when the kidneys are unable to conserve water during their job of filtering blood. Therefore, excessive urination (polyuria) occurs; the amount of water conserved is controlled by antidiuretic hormone (ADH), also called vasopressin. People experience extreme thirst (polydipsia). Diagnosis may be straightforward or may require special blood and urine tests.

Central Diabetes Insipidus

Diabetes insipidus caused by a lack of ADH—antidiuretic hormone produced in the hypothalamus in the brain and then released by the pituitary—is called central diabetes insipidus and is determined by testing. One test involves an infusion of a synthetic analog of AVP called desmopressin acetate (DDAVP). Patients who show more highly concentrated urine in response to DDAVP may have central or neurogenic diabetes insipidus or pituitary diabetes insipidus. Those who don't respond to DDAVP may have nephrogenic diabetes insipidus.

Commonly Prescribed (On-Label) Drugs: None

OFF-LABEL PRESCRIPTION DRUGS
BREAKTHROUGH OPTIONS

Generic: **Carbamazepine** (kar-ba-MAZ-e-peen)
Brands: **Carbatrol, Epitol, Tegretol, Tegretol XR**

Carbamazepine belongs to a class of drugs called anticonvulsants, developed for treating epilepsy. However, carbamazepine is also chemically related to the tricyclic antidepressants. Both classes of drugs are also used to treat diabetic neuropathy because they affect chemical messengers in the brain that affect the perception of pain. Hence, one of carbamazepine's off-label uses is to treat painful diabetic neuropathy.

According to an article in *Diseases of Water Metabolism,* central diabetes may be treated with hormone replacement drugs, and carbamazepine can potentiate the release of antidiuretic hormone in such patients.

However, in clinical practice, it is sometimes found that one drug works just as well as two, as reflected by a study in the *Journal of the Association of Physicians of India.* Doctors from CMC Hospital in Tamil Nadu reported on 20 patients seen over an eight-year period, of whom 18 had central diabetes insipidus, and 61% responded to carbamazepine.

For more information see page 1068.

*Generic: **Indapamide** (in-DAP-ah-mide)*
*Brand: **Lozol***

Indapamide is called a "thiazide-like" diuretic. It is one of the many drugs that have been in use for more than 20 years that continue to find new applications. Although originally developed as a drug for hypertension, its chemical actions make it useful in other areas: it inhibits reabsorption of sodium and chloride in the kidney, thus increasing excretion of sodium and water. It is also believed to reduce the sodium in the smooth muscle lining of blood vessels, promoting its loss in the urine; the salt dissipation causes the muscle to relax, one of the mechanisms in blood pressure reduction.

An article in the *Archives of Internal Medicine* from researchers at Balcali Hospital in Adana, Turkey, reviewed the treatment of 20 patients with central diabetes insipidus with indapamide, which proved to be as effective as chlorpropamide. The researchers concluded that because of its low cost and lack of significant side effects, indapamide may be a suitable, easy-to-use alternative to the current standard of desmopressin for some patients.

Researchers at Hunan Medical University in Changsha, China, reported on eight patients with central diabetes treated with indapamide, dihydrochlorothiazide, or carbamazepine for eight days with therapy changed twice after four days without treatment. Based on changes in urine output and serum potassium and chloride concentrations, they concluded that indapamide has antidiuretic action on central diabetes insipidus. Their theory is that this may result from changes of hydroelectrolytes and the renin-angiotensin-aldosterone system

For more information see page 1237.

Nephrogenic Diabetes Insipidus

When diabetes insipidus is caused by failure of the kidneys to respond to ADH, the condition is called nephrogenic diabetes insipidus. ADH is produced in a region of the brain called the hypothalamus, then stored and released from the pituitary gland, at the base of the brain. Many tests are performed to diagnose nephrogenic diabetes insipidus. Experts from the Kutato Laboratorium wrote in *Orv Hetil* that the differential diagnostics of central diabetes, nephrogenic, and dipsogenic diabetes insipidus sometimes seems enigmatic.

Commonly Prescribed (On-Label) Drugs: *None*

OFF-LABEL PRESCRIPTION DRUGS
BREAKTHROUGH OPTIONS

Generic: **Amiloride** *(a-MIL-oh-ride)*
Brand: **Midamor**

Amiloride, a potassium-sparing diuretic, inhibits the sodium/potassium pump by reducing sodium entry into cells. Its main use is in congestive heart failure to counteract the potassium-draining effects of other diuretics, although it is used off label in primary hyperaldosteronism, according to *The Drug Monitor*.

The Nephrogenic Diabetes Insipidus Foundation's Facts & Statistics notes that combining a thiazide (such as hydrochlorothiazide) with a potassium-sparing diuretic (such as amiloride) may be more effective than using a thiazide alone. The combination of thiazides and amiloride may be preferable because they have fewer potent side effects than the indomethacin-thiazide combination.

For more information see page 1004.

Generic: **Ethacrynic acid** *(eth-a-KRIN-ik AS-id)*
Brand: **Edecrin**

Ethacrynic acid is called a loop diuretic because it inhibits the sodium, potassium and chloride cotransport system. It treats hypertension, congestive heart failure in the presence of renal insufficiency and peripheral and pulmonary edema due to congestive heart failure.

Medline Plus, a publication of the National Institutes of Health (NIH), reports that ethacrynic acid is usually used to treat a type of diabetes insipidus that does not respond to other medicines. An article in *Pediatrics* emphasized the value of ethacrynic acid over thiazide diuretics because patients do not have to be maintained on low sodium diets. Like amiloride, however, ethacrynic acid can be toxic to the auditory nerve when given intravenously for crises such as acute hypertensive crisis, warns the South Shore Chapter of Help for Hard of Hearing People in New York.

For more information see page 1175.

*Generic: **Indapamide** (in-DAP-a-mide)*
*Brand: **Lozol***

Indapamide is a thiazide-like diuretic (water pill) that has been in use since the early 1980s, primarily for the treatment of high blood pressure. Although it is an antihypertensive, it blocks reabsorption of sodium and chloride in the distal tubule of the kidney, increasing excretion of sodium and water by the kidney. Its indications are for hypertension, alone or in combination with another hypertensive, but its off-label use is for diabetes insipidus, especially nephrogenic diabetes insipidus. Indapamide is a key drug mentioned for stopping the cascade of diabetes insipidus in an article in *Nursing*.

Indapamide works by preventing the kidney from retaining salt and water in the body that is really destined to be eliminated in the urine. This results in increased urine output (diuresis). Indapamide also is thought to reduce the salt in the smooth muscular walls of the blood vessels ultimately destined to be eliminated in urine. The loss of salt from the muscle causes the muscular walls of the blood vessels to relax, and the relaxation of the vessels results in reduced blood pressure.

For more information see page 1237.

*Generic: **Indomethacin** (in-doe-METH-a-sin)*
*Brands: **Indocin, Indocin I. V., Indocin SR***

Indomethacin belongs to a class of drugs called nonsteroidal anti-inflammatory drugs (NSAIDs), which are most commonly used to treat the inflammation of arthritis. The Nephrogenic Diabetes Insipidus Foundation's Facts & Statistics notes that sometimes thiazides are used in combination with a nonsteroidal anti-inflammatory drug like indomethacin, which also acts as a prostaglandin inhibitor. By inhibiting elevated levels of prostaglandin E2 that have been reported in these patients, excess urination is reduced.

Clinical Investigator noted that indomethacin had an antidiuretic effect and normalized prostaglandin levels in a person who had nephrogenic diabetes insipidus that they believed had been induced by treatment with amphotericin B, an antifungal medication. Hormone Research reported on a patient with nephrogenic diabetes insipidus believed to have been induced by lithium treatment; therapy with a indomethacin was successful. Researchers pointed to its benefits as a prostaglandin inhibitor as the underlying mechanism.

Acta Paediatrica reported on a study comparing hydrochlorothiazide versus hydrochlorothiazide and indomethacin combined on kidney function in four boys, two with nephrogenic diabetes insipidus and two with partial nephrogenic diabetes insipidus. While hydrochlorothiazide had the desired effect of reducing urine flow and lithium clearance, these benefits were further potentiated by the addition of indomethacin.

For more information see page 1238.

Generic: Thiazide diuretics such as **Bendroflumethiazide** (ben-dro-FLU-meth-a-zide), **Chlorthalidone** (klor-THAL-i-done), **Chlorothiazide** (klor-oh-THYE-a-zide), **Hydrochlorothiazide** (hye-droe-klor-oh-THYE-a-zide), **Hydroflumethiazide** (hi-dro-FLU-meth-a-zide), and **Metolazone** (me-TOLE-a-zone)
Brands: **Naturetin (bendroflumethiazide), Thalitone (chlorthalidone), Diuril (chlorothiazide), Esidrix, HydroDIURIL, Microzide, Ezide (hydrochlorothiazide), Diucardin (hydroflumethiazide), Mykrox, Zaroxolyn (metolazone)**

Thiazide diuretics are the mainstays of antihypertensive care in the United States. They have been used for at least 40 years. Although new thiazide diuretics have been developed in recent years, doctors still rely on many of the original ones. Their primary use is in hypertension and congestive heart failure, although they are used off-label in nephrogenic diabetes insipidus to prevent further urine dilution from taking place, according to *The Drug Monitor.*

Thiazide diuretics can reduce a person's excess urination (polyuria), but they may also drain the body's stores of potassium, causing dangerous symptoms. So your potassium levels must be monitored, and perhaps potassium boosted with supplements or amiloride—but not both, according to the Nephrogenic Diabetes Insipidus Foundations Facts & Statistics.

The ALLHAT study, the largest of its kind in the world, sought to compare therapies in 40,000 hypertensive people to discern what is the ideal hypertensive. Ultimately, as reported in *The New Zealand Medical Journal,* this effort concluded that physicians should start with a diuretic and, if necessary, build from there based on the patient's accompanying conditions and symptoms. But thiazide diuretics remain the mainstay.

Chlorothalidone, according to the ALLHAT study, was a standout thiazide. Interestingly, doxazosin was found to be inferior to the diuretic chlorothalidone, and the trial was terminated early after an average of 3.2 years. Subsequent analysis showed that the doxazosin patients had higher rates of stroke and heart failure.

For more information see pages 1040, 1083, 1085, 1221, 1224, and 1319.

Partial Diabetes Insipidus (Dipsogenic)

Experts from Northwestern University note in an article in *Diabetes Insipidus* that a patient may have a partial form of any one of the types of diabetes insipidus. This has led to the creation of another category of partial central diabetes insipidus. The demarcation—and name—of the third category seems to change depending on which study one is reading.

Commonly Prescribed (On-Label) Drug: Phenobarbital

OFF-LABEL PRESCRIPTION DRUGS
BREAKTHROUGH OPTIONS

Generic: **Carbamazepine** *(kar-ba-MAZ-e-pēen)*
Brands: **Carbatrol, Epitol, Tegetrol, Tegretol XR**

Carbamazepine belongs to a class of drugs called anticonvulsants, which were developed for treating epilepsy. However, carbamazepine is interesting in that it is also chemically related to the tricyclic antidepressants. Both these classes of drugs are also used to treat diabetic neuropathy because they affect chemical messengers in the brain that affect the perception of pain. Hence, one of carbamazepine's off-label uses is to treat painful diabetic neuropathy.

Carbamazepine may stimulate antidiuretic hormone secretion in people with partial pituitary insipidus and may be tried as a treatment, according to a report from the University of Minnesota in *American Family Physician*.

According to a report in *The Lancet* from the University of Colorado School of Medicine, in partial diabetes insipidus, carbamazepine is beneficial because it helps in the release of antidiuretic hormone. However, they recommend that it be prescribed in combination with hormonal therapy, decreased amount of solution, or a diuretic.

In a study in *Pediatric Pharmacology and Therapeutics* from the Children's Hospital of Pittsburgh, the effectiveness of therapy with carbamazepine and clofibrate (another oral), intramuscular pitressin, and intranasal DDAVP was compared in 15 children with partial or complete central diabetes insipidus. Oral drugs decreased the daily urine volume in patients with partial diabetes insipidus with good symptomatic control except for some night urination.

For more information see page 1068.

Generic: **Chlorpropamide** *(klor-PROE-pa-mide)*
Brand: **Diabinese**

Chlorpropamide, together with three other drugs, belongs to a group called the first-generation sulfonylureas. That is, they were the first four oral blood sugar-lowering drugs in a class of medications for diabetes called sulfonylureas, and they all worked by the same mechanism to treat type 2 diabetes. They stimulate the pancreas to release more insulin. But one problem in using the drug, whether in someone with diabetes or, especially, in someone without diabetes, is that it may prompt hazardous low blood sugar levels.

People with partial pituitary insipidus may respond to chlorpropamide, which also stimulates antidiuretic hormone secretion and its effect on the kidneys, according to a report from the University of Minnesota in the *American Family Physician.*

LifeScan Diabetes Care also notes that when some antidiuretic hormone secretion is still present, mild (partial) diabetes insipidus can be treated with chlorpropamide.

An *eMedicine* article from Temple University notes that nonhormonal drugs usually are more effective in treating nephrogenic diabetes insipidus and chlorpropamide promotes the kidney to respond to antidiuretic hormone.

American Journal of Physiology and Renal Physiology reports on studies that examine the mechanism by which chlorpropamide promotes antidiuresis. Its impact on different receptors led to a theory that it helps partial central diabetes insipidus but not nephrogenic diabetes insipidus.

For more information see page 1088.

HAIR LOSS IN WOMEN

Hair loss (alopecia) in women is common. There are several different types of hair loss including androgenetic alopecia, alopecia areata, and telogen effluvium. Androgenetic alopecia is the most common type of hair loss in women. Another type is alopecia areata that causes small patches of baldness, although it can cause total hair loss, and is usually an immune disorder. Telogen effluvium, a sudden thinning of hair that is not total and usually not permanent, is usually caused by stress (even high fever), and hair growth will normalize in a month or two. Traumatic alopecia is due to hair care practices, such as pulling it back or braiding too tightly.

Androgenetic Alopecia

Androgenetic alopecia is similar to the type of hair loss that occurs in men, with hair lost above the forehead and on the top and back of the head. In women, instead of baldness developing as it does in men, the hair slowly thins in these areas, starting at the crown.

Commonly Prescribed (On-Label) Drugs: Finasteride

OFF-LABEL PRESCRIPTION DRUG
BREAKTHROUGH OPTION

*Generic: **Spironolactone** (speer-on-oh-LAK-tone)*
*Brand: **Aldactone***

Spironolactone belongs to a class of drugs called potassium-sparing diuretics. Diuretics are used to remove surplus fluid from the body's bloodstream or tissues and are prescribed to treat hypertension. Spironolactone inhibits the hormone aldosterone, thus preventing salt retention and is used to treat advanced heart failure when symptoms persist after other drug therapies are maximized.

Spironolactone also seems to have antiandrogen potential and has been used to treat hormonal hair loss in women. A report from the University of Bologna, Italy in the *Journal of the European Academic Dermatology* and *Venereology* indicated that mild to moderate androgenetic alopecia in women responds to therapy with spironolactone with good results in many cases.

British Journal of Dermatology had a study from the University of Melbourne in Australia on the efficacy of oral antiandrogen therapy in women with female pattern hair loss. In an open study of 80 women aged 12 to 79 years, 40 received spironolactone and 40 received cyproterone. There were no significant differences in the results between the two drugs: 44% had hair regrowth; 44% had no change in hair density; and 12% had continuing hair loss. There was no pattern based on age, menopause status, hormone levels, clinical stage or other parameters, other than high midscalp clinical grade, which predicted a greater response.

For more information see page 1478.

Baldness

See Hair Loss in Women

MULTIPLE ENDOCRINE NEOPLASIA

Multiple endocrine neoplasia are defined by type. Type 1 affects the parathyroid glands, the pancreatic islets and the anterior pituitary. Associated tumors include lipomas, angiofibromas, or those located in the adrenal gland cortex. Type 2 A is defined by medullary thyroid carcinoma, pheochromocytoma (about 50%), and hyperparathyroidism caused by parathyroid gland hyperplasia (about 20%). Type 2B is defined by medullary thyroid tumor and pheochromocytoma. Associated abnormalities include mucosal neuromas, medullated corneal nerve fibers, and marfanoid habitus.

Insulinomas

Insulinomas are rare, insulin-secreting tumors that cause low blood sugar levels that derive from the beta cells of the pancreas. About 99% of insulinomas arise in the pancreas, with 1% arising outside it, but always nearby, such as the duodenum. Nearly 95% are benign. Although called insulinomas, they are often capable of secreting other hormones in addition to insulin. These tumors also occur as part of the type 1 Multiple Endocrine Neoplasia syndrome.

Commonly Prescribed (On-Label) Drugs: None

OFF-LABEL PRESCRIPTION DRUG
BREAKTHROUGH OPTION

Generic: **Diazoxide** *(dye-az-OKS-ide)*
Brand: **Hyperstat IV**

Diazoxide is a drug used in hypertensive emergencies to lower blood pressure. A report from the Yale University School of Medicine explains that diazoxide works differently when given intravenously compared to when it is given orally. When people take diazoxide orally for hypertension, it has no effect on blood glucose levels. However, when it is given intravenously for rapid administration, diazoxide increases blood sugar within one hour by blocking insulin release from the insulinoma.

The University Hospital in Zagreb, Croatia, reported on a young woman with multiple endocrine neoplasia who required surgery and noted that both diazoxide and octreotide inhibit insulin secretion, and that both drugs also have other effects. They urge consultation with a physician experienced in their use, confirming the *eMedicine* article which urged that diazoxide be initiated under close clinical supervision and that prolonged treatment required regular monitoring of urine and blood sugar levels.

For more information see page 1141.

PITUITARY DISORDERS

The pituitary gland is a peanut-sized organ located in the brain. The pituitary is sometimes called the master gland because it regulates many aspects of growth, development, and everyday functioning. Its anterior lobe produces six hormones: growth hormone, prolactin (which stimulates breasts to produce milk), and four that stimulate other glands. The posterior lobe produces antidiuretic hormone, which acts on the kidneys, and oxytocin, which plays a role in childbirth.

Acromegaly

Acromegaly is a rare condition in adults in which the pituitary gland produces too much growth hormone, yielding excessive growth. However, an adult cannot grow taller, because vertical growth stops at the end of adolescence when the bone ends seal. Therefore, the excess growth hormone causes bones to thicken and all other structures and organs grow larger. Overproduction of the growth hormone is usually caused by a pituitary tumor.

Commonly Prescribed (On-Label) Drugs: Bromocriptine, Octreotide, Pegvisomant

---

OFF-LABEL PRESCRIPTION DRUGS
BREAKTHROUGH OPTIONS

Generic: **Cabergoline** (ca-BER-goe-leen)
Brand: **Dostinex**

Cabergoline is a drug approved to treat hyperprolactinemia—that is, an excess production of the hormone prolactin. It stops the brain from making and releasing the prolactin hormone from the pituitary. Off-label, the drug has been successful in helping shrink pituitary tumors and in reducing growth factor blood levels.

Journal of Clinical Endocrinology and Metabolism reported on the experiences of physicians in Antwerp, Brussels, Aalst, Hasselt, and Liege, Belgium in treating acromegaly in 64 patients in an study. Ideal insulin-like growth factor blood factor levels (an indicator of tumor acromegaly activity) was achieved in a significant number of cases, as was tumor shrinkage. Except for slight gastrointestinal discomfort and orthostatic hypotension at the beginning of therapy in a few patients, the drug was well tolerated; only two stopped taking it because of side effects. Researchers concluded that cabergoline is an effective, well-tolerated therapy. They urged that it be considered in the management of acromegaly, particularly if the pituitary adenoma cosecretes certain hormones.

Medscape cited studies from the UCLA School of Medicine that indicated the superior efficacy and tolerability of cabergoline compared with older agents (bromocriptine and quinagolide) in treating hyperprolactinemia. One study showed efficacy of cabergoline in normalizing insulin growth factor-1 levels in 35% of patients and suppression of growth hormone in 44% of patients, with some tumor shrinkage, especially in those whose tumors secreted both prolactin and growth hormone.

For more information see page 1062.

Generic: **Pergolide** *(PER-go-lide)*
Brand: **Permax**

Pergolide has a wide range of effects on the human body, including on blood circulation and neurotransmission in the brain. It belongs to a class of medications called dopamine agonists that act in place of dopamine, a natural substance in the brain needed to control movement. Pergolide is used as an add-on drug with levodopa or carbidopa in the treatment of Parkinson's disease.

Clinical Endocrinology reported that pergolide given once daily was an effective long-term treatment of acromegaly. Six patients showed a statistically significant reduction in growth hormone, with four getting below 75% of pretreatment levels. Increases in dosage yielded increased benefits for all eight patients. The authors conclude that pergolide given once daily has a beneficial effect in acromegaly, with a significant reduction in growth hormone.

A report in *Medscape* from the UCLA School of Medicine indicated that a number of dopamine antagonists, despite being used off-label, such as pergolide, are useful as ancillary medical therapy for acromegaly patients.

For more information see page 1406.

Hyperprolactinemia

Hyperprolactinemia is a disorder in which the level of the hormone prolactin is elevated in the blood. The primary role of prolactin is to enhance the development of the breasts during pregnancy to induce lactation when the baby is born. However, prolactin also binds to specific receptors in the gonads, lymphoid cells, and liver. Hyperprolactinemia often leads to reproductive dysfunction and galactorrhea.

Commonly Prescribed (On-Label) Drugs: Bromocriptine, Cabergoline

OFF-LABEL PRESCRIPTION DRUG
BREAKTHROUGH OPTION

Generic: **Pergolide** *(PER-go-lide)*
Brand: **Permax**

New England Journal of Medicine provided a study from the New York Veterans Administration Medical Center on pergolide for the treatment of pituitary tumors secreting prolactin or growth hormone. Among 41 patients with hyperprolactinemia who took pergolide for three months or more, prolactin levels fell to normal and remained slightly elevated in two. The researchers concluded that pergolide may be superior to surgery and x-ray treatment in some patients.

British Medical Journal reported on 25 patients with hyperprolactinemia treated with pergolide, 23 of whom received therapy for six to 20 months. In most, prolactin concentrations were maintained in the normal range by a once-daily dose and reproductive disorders were reversed and tumor sizes reduced. The researchers consider it a useful addition to currently available drugs.

Experts from the Massachusetts General Hospital in Boston, writing in the *International Journal of Fertility and Women's Medicine,* reported that the treatment of choice for nearly all patients with hyperprolactinemic disorders is medical and, in most cases, dopamine agonists such as pergolide are extremely effective because they lower prolactin levels, decrease tumor size, and restore reproductive function.

For more information see page 1406.

THYROID DISORDERS

The thyroid gland straddles your windpipe in the lower part of your neck. It is butterfly-shaped, with two lobes connected by a thin strand of tissue. The thyroid makes the hormone thyroxine. On the four corners of the thyroid gland are the four small parathyroid glands, each about the size of a sesame, which produce parathyroid hormone. Problems with these glands often involve over- or under-production of the hormones.

Hyperparathyroid Crisis

Most people who show up at their doctor's office with symptoms of hyperparathyroidism are chronically ill with symptoms arising from the kidneys or the skeleton. Rarely, however, they arrive acutely ill with urgent symptoms that sometimes prove fatal. The terms acute hyperparathyroidism and hyperparathyroid crisis describe a simple episode of life-threatening high levels of calcium in the blood, causing symptoms such as nausea and vomiting, weakness, and mental changes.

Commonly Prescribed (On-Label) Drugs: None

OFF-LABEL PRESCRIPTION DRUGS
BREAKTHROUGH OPTIONS

Generic: Cimetidine (sye-MET-i-deen)
Brand: Tagamet

Cimetidine is one of a group of drugs called histamine H2-receptor antagonist. Histamine blockers were originally developed to treat stomach ulcers, but they are also used to treat GERD (gastroesophageal reflux disease), a type of endocrine adenoma, and other conditions. Because histamine increases stomach acid, blocking secretion helps heal and prevent ulcers. Histamine also stimulates parathyroid hormone (PTH) production and cyclic adenoside monophosphate, a reaction inhibited by cimetidine.

Massachusetts General Hospital researchers have identified H2-receptors in the parathyroid glands, which supports the theory that there is an H-2 related response in hyperparathyroidism.

American Surgery reports on three patients with severe hyperparathyroid syndrome. Effective control of acute hyperparathyroid crisis was achieved with the use of cimetidine in all three cases and was followed by surgical removal of a solitary parathyroid adenoma. The authors wrote that, "The intimate relationship of the bioavailability of cimetidine and its effect in primary hyperparathyroidism is clearly demonstrated." They compare it to Zollinger Ellison syndrome, another endocrinopathy requiring a dose of cimetidine in excess of that normally considered therapeutic for peptic ulcer disease. They conclude that cimetidine is an important aid in the treatment of hyperparathyroid crisis.

For more information see page 1091.

*Generic: **Pamidronate** (pa-mi-DROE-nate)*
*Brand: **Aredia***

Pamidronate belongs to a class of agents called bisphosphonates, which inhibit resorption (breakdown) of bone. Oral bisphosphonates are sometimes used in the treatment of osteoporosis, a disease of low bone density that primarily occurs in women after menopause. But pamidronate is given intravenously and is a more intense inhibitor. It is used to treat Paget's disease, to slow bone metastases in cancer, and to lower the hypercalcemia that occurs in people with some types of cancer.

Off-label, it is used in primary and secondary hyperparathyroidism when severe hypercalcemia occurs, and some physicians also have come to rely on it in hyperparathyroid crisis. *Surgery* reported on six patients who benefited when treated with pamidronate preoperatively to lower their serum calcium levels before parathyroid levels. The researchers concluded treatment with pamidronate is effective and suggests that the hypercalcemia of primary hyperparathyroidism is mainly due to osteoclasts (cells that break down bone).

For more information see page 1391.

Hyperthyroidism

Hyperthyroidism is overactivity of the thyroid gland, resulting in the production of too much of the hormone thyroxine. The gland is normally controlled by thyroid-stimulating hormone (TSH), which is made in the pituitary gland. In hyperthyroidism, something has gone wrong with the control mechanism. Despite normal or low levels of TSH, the thyroid gland itself produces large quantities of thyroxine. Why this happens is not well understood, but it speeds up all chemical reactions in the body affecting physical and mental processes.

Commonly Prescribed (On-Label) Drugs: Methimazole, Potassium Iodide, Propylthiouracil

OFF-LABEL PRESCRIPTION DRUG
BREAKTHROUGH OPTION

*Generic: **Propranolol** (proe-PRAN-oh-lole)*
*Brands: **Inderal, Inderal LA, InnoPran XL, Propranolol Intensol***

Propranolol belongs to a class of drugs called beta-blockers. It was originally developed as a drug for hypertension, although it is now also given to help prevent angina, migraine, heart attack, and a type of heart arrythmia. According to the Mayo Clinic, propranolol does not reduce the high levels of thyroxine but can reduce the rapid heart rate and palpitations induced by the high thyroxine. *American Journal of Medicine* reports that it reduces the oxygen requirements of the heart and improves the heart's efficiency in people with hyperthyroidism. So it may be prescribed until other medications normalize your thyroxine levels. Thus, propranolol is a drug prescribed for the acute symptoms of hyperthyroidism, until a doctor figures out what the underlying cause is and determines whether further medication is necessary, according to the *American Family Physician*.

According to EndocrineWeb.com, propranolol blocks the effect of the thyroid hormone but does not have an effect on the thyroid itself. It can reduce the symptoms of hyperthyroidism within hours. *EndocrineWeb* points out that propranolol may be the only treatment needed for people with such temporary forms of hyperthyroidism as thyroiditis due to inflammation of the gland or the result of taking excess thyroid medication; once the inflammation resolves, the patient can be tapered off the propranolol.

For more information see page 1438.

Primary Hyperparathyroidism

Hyperparathyroidism occurs when excessive amounts of parathyroid hormone (PTH) are produced. PTH helps control bone growth by regulating calcium and phosphorus balance in the body. In primary hyperparathyroidism, the glands secrete too much PTH because one or more of them have become enlarged. This may affect the skeletal, gastrointestinal, renal (kidney), muscular, and central nervous system. It is most likely to occur in those over 60 but younger adults can develop the disorder.

Commonly Prescribed (On-Label) Drugs: None

OFF-LABEL PRESCRIPTION DRUGS
BREAKTHROUGH OPTIONS

Generic: **Cimetidine** *(sye-MET-i-deen)*
Brand: **Tagamet**

Cimetidine belongs to a class of drugs called histamine H2-receptor antagonists. They were originally developed to treat duodenal and gastric ulcers. Histamine increases stomach acid secretion; hence, blocking it yields benefits for patients with ulcer disease. But various types of histamine also play a role in dilation of blood vessels, smooth muscle constriction such as in the bronchi, and mucus production, tissue swelling, and itching (during allergic reactions). Histamine also stimulates parathyroid hormone (PTH) production and cyclic adenoside monophosphate, a reaction which is inhibited by cimetidine.

Researchers at the Massachusetts General Hospital have identified H2-receptors in the parathyroid glands and believe that H-2-receptors have a role in the development of hyperparathyroidism. Researchers recommend very high doses of oral cimetidine in primary hyperparathyroidism due to adenomatous disease, according to their report in *The Lancet*. However they emphasize that it is important to distinguish this type of hyperparathyroidism from elevated PTH due to other causes; in their series of 97 cases, they were unable to detect any effect by cimetidine in any condition other than primary hyperparathyroidism due to adenomatous disease.

For more information see page 1091.

Generic: **Pamidronate** *(pa-mi-DROE-nate)*
Brand: **Aredia**

Pamidronate belongs to a class of drugs called bisphosphonates. It is used to treat Paget's disease of bone and the spread of cancer from other organs to bone. Pamidronate is given intravenously. Bisphosphonates reduce the breakdown of bone, which is why oral versions are also used to treat osteoporosis, a disease of low bone density. However, pamidronate is also used to help reduce the high levels of calcium in blood (hypercalcemia) that may occur in people with some types of cancer. This led to consideration of its use in the severe hypercalcemia of primary hyperparathyroidism.

Bone reported on a study in Sweden on surgery planned for 20 patients with hypercalcemia due to primary hyperparathyroidism. One to two months beforehand, they were given an infusion of pamidronate. A significant reduction in calcium occurred during the following month, and the researchers considered it effective for preparing patients for surgery.

Surgery reported a similar study in six patients treated preoperatively. The researchers concluded that the effectiveness of treatment with pamidronate suggests that the hypercalcemia of primary hyperparathyroidism is mainly due to osteoclasts (cells that break down bone). They also use it after unsuccessful parathyroid surgery as a long-term treatment before reoperation and in aged and fragile patients treatments as an alternative to surgery.

For more information see page 1391.

Secondary Hyperparathyroidism

The production of excessive amounts of parathyroid hormone (PTH) by the parathyroid gland produces hyperparathyroidism. The parathyroid glands help control bone growth because PTH regulates calcium and phosphorus balance in the body. When this occurs in response to low blood calcium caused by another disorder, it is called secondary hyperparathyroidism. The most common causes are: disorders of vitamin D (such as osteomalacia and vitamin D deficiency or malabsorption); children or the elderly with little sun exposure; those with disorders of phosphate metabolism (due to malnutrition, malabsorption, kidney disease, cancer); calcium deficiency.

Commonly Prescribed (On-Label) Drugs: Cinacalcet, Paricalcitol

OFF-LABEL PRESCRIPTION DRUG
BREAKTHROUGH OPTION

Generic: **Pamidronate** *(pa-mi-DROE-nate)*
Brand: **Aredia**

Pamidronate is one of a group of drugs called bisphosphonates, which reduce the breakdown (resorption) of bone. It is used to treat Paget's disease and to slow bone metastases in cancer. Although pamidronate is given intravenously, oral bisphosphonates are prescribed to treat osteoporosis, a disease of low bone density. Pamidronate is also approved for use in lowering the hypercalcemia that occurs in people with some types of cancer. This application led to its consideration in secondary hyperparathyroidism when severe hypercalcemia occurs.

Kidney International discussed the usefulness of pamidronate in patients with severe secondary hyperparathyroidism who were undergoing hemodialysis. The University of Barcelona conducted a study with 13 patients who were given pamidronate intravenously every two months for one year. Pamidronate was effective in controlling the hypercalcemia and allowed for a more aggressive use of needed intravenous calcitrol.

For more information see page 1391.

Thyroid Crisis

Thyroid crisis, also known as thyroid storm or thyrotoxic crisis, is a medical emergency. It usually occurs in patients with poorly controlled or unrecognized hyperthyroidism. It may be precipitated by some other illness, such as an infection, surgery, uncontrolled diabetes, trauma (such as an automobile accident), or eclampsia or labor in a pregnant woman. Thyroid storm is rare, characterized by hypertension, hyperthermia, and abnormalities in multiple organs of the body.

Commonly Prescribed (On-Label) Drugs: *None*

OFF-LABEL PRESCRIPTION DRUGS
BREAKTHROUGH OPTIONS

Generic: **Methimazole** *(meth-IM-a-zole)*
Brand: **Tapazole**

Methimazole belongs to a class of drugs called thioamide antithyroid agents. It is normally used to treat hyperthyroidism associated with Grave's disease until spontaneous remission occurs, which generally takes a year or two. Thioamide antithyroid agents do not modify the underlying cause of hyperthyroidism and are not used for long-term treatment of the disease. Since spontaneous remission does not occur in all patients, alternative treatments may be required. However, according to *Medscape,* methimazole is also used to manage a thyroid crisis by inhibiting thyroid hormone synthesis.

American Journal of Medicine reported from the Polyclinic University of Messina, Italy, on the successful use of low doses of methimazole together with L-carnitine in the treatment of three successive thyroid storms that were associated with potentially life-threatening precipitating factors—post-influenza myocarditis and thrombophlebitis.

ThyroidManager.Org recommends immediate therapy for thyroid storm with an antithyroid drug such as methimazole, and notes that it can be given orally, by injection, or as a rectal suppository.

For more information see page 1311.

Generic: **Propranolol** *(proe-PRAN-oh-lole)*
Brands: **Inderal, Inderal LA, InnoPran XL, Propranolol Intensol**

Propranolol belongs to a class of drugs called beta-blockers. Originally developed for hypertension, it is also prescribed to help prevent angina, heart attack, a type of heart arrythmia, and migraine.

Propranolol does not reduce high levels of thyroxine, according to the Mayo Clinic, but it can reduce the rapid heart rate and palpitations induced by the high thyroxine. Hence, propranolol is valuable for treating the acute symptoms of hyperthyroidism and especially useful in thyroid storm. When methimazole is given in the management of thyroid crisis, a beta-blocking agent such as propranolol is usually given simultaneously to manage the signs and symptoms of hyperthyroidism, especially the cardiovascular effects, such as tachycardia, according to *Medscape*.

An article in ThyroidManager.org on thyroid storm recommends immediate therapy with an antithyroid drug and emphasizes that, unless congestive heart failure is present, propranolol or another beta blocker should be given immediately, either orally or by injection.

For more information see page 1438.

IMMUNE SYSTEM DISORDERS

ANAPHYLAXIS

Anaphylaxis is a severe allergic reaction that affects the entire body and can be fatal. Your immune system becomes sensitized upon first exposure to a substance such as insect toxin, certain drugs or foods. On subsequent exposure, a sudden, severe body-wide allergic reaction occurs as various tissues in the body release histamine and other substances. This release results in breathing difficulties, lowered blood pressure and blood volume, pulmonary swelling, and possibly gastrointestinal symptoms. Anaphylaxis is generally treated with a combination of epinephrine (adrenalin), an antihistamine (such as diphenhydramine) and corticosteroids (cortisone, prednisone).

Chemotherapy-induced Anaphylaxis (Prevention)

Chemotherapy-induced anaphylaxis is most commonly associated with medicine and chemotherapy. Reactions to chemotherapy may occur within seconds or minutes, particularly if you have been exposed to the anti-cancer treatment. Hypersensitivity reactions have been reported with most chemotherapy drugs, although generally infrequently. Reactions more often occur with L-asparaginase, paclitaxel, docetaxel, teniposide, procarbazine, and cytarabine. Common chemotherapy-induced anaphylactic symptoms include hives, swelling, itching, flushing, and skin rash.

Commonly Prescribed (On-Label) Drugs: *None*

OFF-LABEL PRESCRIPTION DRUGS
BREAKTHROUGH OPTIONS

Generic: **Cetirizine** *(se-TI-ra-zeen)*
Brand: **Zyrtec**

Cetirizine belongs to a second generation of allergy medications called "nonsedating antihistamines." It blocks the effects of histamines that produce allergy symptoms such as sneezing, hives, itchy nose, or itchy eyes. Based on its favorable efficacy and safety profile, cetirizine has been studied in a wide variety of allergic disorders, including chemotherapy-induced anaphylaxis.

In one case, a person experienced a hypersensitivity reaction that included hives, facial swelling, cough, and chest tightness due to high-doses of chemotherapy. Once the chemotherapy infusion was discontinued, the patient's symptoms stopped. The patient, in this instance, received a pre-chemotherapy regimen consisting of a corticosteroid and cetirizine. Once methotrexate was re-started, the patient did not experience chemotherapy-induced anaphylaxis. Preventive treatments including cetirizine allow people to continue with required chemotherapy regimes. Physicians will often prescribe or recommend drugs such as cetirizine to minimize the effects of chemotherapy allergic reactions.

For more information see page 1078.

Generic: **Cimetidine** *(sye-MET-i-deen)*
Brand: **Tagamet**

Cimetidine blocks the action of histamine, a natural chemical in the body, on the stomach cells, thereby decreasing stomach acid production in heartburn, ulcer, or acid reflux disease. In other instances, cimetidine may be prescribed to treat allergic reactions such as hives and itching.

In prevention of chemotherapy-induced anaphylaxis, cimetidine is often given to prevent hypersensitivity reactions. Several clinical studies and case study reports demonstrate efficacy with preventive cimetidine therapy. Researchers observed that single-dose IV regimens of cimetidine, along with dexamethasone (a corticosteroid) and diphenhydramine (an antihistamine) can be given before paclitaxel chemotherapy, and are a safe, convenient alternative in the prevention of hypersensitivity reactions to chemotherapy. In another study, researchers at the Medical University in Gdansk, Poland used a premedication regimen of IV dexamethasone, diphenhydramine, and cimetidine before paclitaxel chemotherapy and noticed that no hypersensitivity reactions occurred during the first or following administrations. People who develop mild-to-moderate hypersensitivity to chemotherapy may be successfully pretreated with cimetidine 30 minutes before chemotherapy is received.

For more information see page 1091.

Generic: *Famotidine* (fa-MOE-ti-deen)
Brand: *Pepcid*

Famotidine inhibits the action of histamine on stomach cells and reduces the production of stomach acid in ulcers, acid reflux, and heartburn. Researchers from the Cleveland Clinic Cancer Center in Ohio evaluated pretreatment with IV diphenhydramine, famotidine, and dexamethasone before paclitaxel chemotherapy in more than 200 patients. They found that only 9% of patients developed hypersensitivity reactions. Researchers concluded that this pretreatment regimen, which was administered 30 minutes prior to paclitaxel therapy, was as effective as and more convenient than standard regimens.

In a study comparing cimetidine and famotidine and the effects of paclitaxel, researchers found that cimetidine and famotidine did not differ in the way they affect the use of paclitaxel when used to prevent chemotherapy-induced anaphylaxis.

For more information see page 1181.

Generic: *Hydroxyzine* (hye-DROKS-i-zeen)
Brands: *Atarax, Vistaril*

Hydroxyzine is an antihistamine commonly used to treat symptoms of allergic reactions and viral infections. Once hydroxyzine is ingested, it becomes cetirizine, another antihistamine that is less sedating. Hydroxyzine is also used to treat insomnia and promote sedation before diagnostic or therapeutic procedures.

In a case study of a person with a history of methotrexate anaphylaxis, doctors recommended a preventive treatment of hydroxyzine prior to methotrexate chemotherapy. Consequently, the person received methotrexate chemotherapy without repeated anaphylactic reaction.

Common side effects of hydroxyzine include sedation, tiredness, sleepiness, dizziness, disturbed coordination, drying and thickening of mouth or respiratory fluids, and stomach distress. Caution must be exercised when hydroxyzine is administered if you have narrow-angle glaucoma, enlarged prostate gland, cardiovascular disease, high blood pressure, or asthma. Hydroxyzine adds to the sedating effects of alcohol and other drugs such as anti-anxiety medications, narcotic pain medications, tricyclic antidepressants, and certain blood pressure medications.

There is no drug profile for this drug as data are pending.

Generic: **Ranitidine** *(rah-NIT-a-deen)*
Brands: **Zantac, Zantac EFFERdose**

Ranitidine blocks the action of histamine on stomach cells, thereby decreasing stomach acid production in ulcers, heartburn, and acid reflux. Antihistamines, such as ranitidine, are often used to prevent chemotherapy-induced anaphylaxis. In fact, in some instances, premedication with ranitidine, dexamethasone, and clemastine is mandatory to certain chemotherapy treatments.

A study by the Fox Chase Cancer Center in Philadelphia examined the incidence of chemotherapy-induced anaphylactic reactions. Researchers reviewed a database of patients who received paclitaxel 30 minutes after ranitidine, dexamethasone, and diphenhydramine IV infusion. Of the 283 cases reviewed, all patients received pretreatment with the previously mentioned drugs before paclitaxel chemotherapy. Only 13 patients during the first or second cycle of chemotherapy experienced anaphylaxis, which was quickly resolved and the patient did not require hospitalization. Researchers concluded that pretreatment consisting of ranitidine, dexamethasone, and diphenhydramine provided a safe option for the prevention of chemotherapy-induced anaphylaxis.

Ranitidine has also been used as a "premedication" to chemotherapy in various forms of cancer such as breast, ovarian, cervical, gastric, and lung cancer. Ranitidine has been used in both adults and children with chemotherapy-induced anaphylaxis, although the drug's safety for children has not been established.

For more information see page 1443.

Drug-induced Anaphylaxis

Drugs such as antibiotics, anesthetics, anti-seizure medications, and x-ray dye may cause an anaphylactoid reaction, which is another type of immediate reaction that mimics anaphylaxis, although it is toxic. Risk factors for drug allergies include frequent exposure to the offending drug, large drug doses, drugs given by injection, and family history of allergic reactions. Drug-induced anaphylactic symptoms often occur within seconds or minutes and include difficulty breathing, rapid or weak pulse, fainting, heart palpitations, and gastrointestinal symptoms.

Commonly Prescribed (On-Label) Drugs: None

OFF-LABEL PRESCRIPTION DRUGS
BREAKTHROUGH OPTIONS

---

*Generic: **Methylprednisolone** (meth-il-pred-NIS-oh-lone)*
*Brands: **Depo-Medrol, Medrol, Solu-Medrol***

Methylprednisolone is used in a variety of inflammatory disorders, such as arthritis, asthma, and severe allergies, to block symptoms of inflammation. Although corticosteroids do not have an immediate effect on anaphylaxis, physicians recommend that they be given as a secondary measure early on in the reaction.

In a study, a patient who was exposed to furosemide (a diuretic) experienced symptoms of drug-induced anaphylaxis. Researchers observed that complete recovery was achieved through the administration of adrenaline, methylprednisolone, and diphenhydramine. In another instance, a French team of researchers studied an elderly patient who experienced anaphylaxis symptoms after high doses of aprotinin. Immediate treatment involved IV adrenaline and methylprednisolone, and after 10 minutes, cardiovascular stability was restored.

Interactions can occur when methylprednisolone is used with certain antibiotics, antifungals, and birth control pills. In these instances, a lower dose of methylprednisolone may be required to avoid adverse reactions.

For more information see page 000.

Generic: **Prednisone** (pred-NIS-zone)
Brands: **Deltasone, Liquid Pred, Meticorten, Orasone, Sterapred**

Prednisone is used to suppress the immune system and inflammation in conditions such as arthritis, asthma, and other allergic or inflammatory conditions. Prednisone provides strong anti-inflammatory effects and mimics a naturally occurring corticosteroid produced by the adrenal glands in the body known as cortisol.

For some people, doctors may recommend pretreatment with prednisone to prevent an allergic reaction to a certain drug. Once prednisone is administered, the offending medication may then be given. In the prevention of anaphylaxis, pretreatment with prednisone administered 13, seven, or one hour before procedure, along with diphenhydramine and ephedrine, is a well-recognized regimen to prevent reaction.

For more information see page 1429.

HIV

Human immunodeficiency virus (HIV) is the virus that causes acquired immunodeficiency syndrome (AIDS), a chronic, life-threatening condition. HIV affects the body by damaging or destroying immune system cells that prevent viral, bacterial, and fungal infections. People with HIV are more prone to certain cancers and infections than healthy individuals. HIV transmission most commonly occurs through sexual contact with an infected person. Other modes of HIV infection include exposure to infected blood, sharing needles or syringes contaminated with the virus, or transmission from an untreated infected mother to infant during pregnancy, delivery, or through breast milk.

Commonly Prescribed (On-Label) Drugs: *Abacavir/ Lamivudine, Abacavir/Lamivudine/Zidovudine, Amprenavir,*

Atazanavir, Didanosine, Efavirenz, Fosamprenavir, Lamivudine, Lopinavir/Ritonavir, Pneumococcal Vaccine, Tenofovir, Zalcitabine, Zidovudine

OFF-LABEL PRESCRIPTION DRUGS
BREAKTHROUGH OPTIONS

Generic: **Filgrastim** *(fil-GRA-stim)*
Brand: **Neupogen**

Filgrastim affects the production of neutrophils, or white blood cells, in the bone marrow and potentially other areas of the body. This drug is typically used to decrease the risk of infection, reduce the time to white blood cell recovery and duration of fever in a variety of disease or drug-induced immune deficiencies.

Filgrastim has been used in patients with HIV to correct or minimize HIV-associated and/or drug-induced neutropenia, or low levels of white blood cells. In these patients, filgrastim has been demonstrated to increase white blood cells. Use of filgrastim in patients with HIV may reduce the risk of bacterial infections. In adults who have progressed to AIDS or AIDS-related complex, filgrastim has been effective alone or in combination with another hematopoietic drug, epoetin alfa, in reducing bone marrow toxicity associated with the anti-infective therapy zidovudine. Filgrastim does not appear to adversely affect HIV replication or interfere with the antiretroviral effects of zidovudine, although researchers note that there is a lack of data on the use of filgrastim in HIV.

For more information see page 1185.

Generic: **Foscarnet** *(fos-KAR-net)*
Brand: **Foscavir**

Like other antivirals, foscarnet interferes with the virus life cycle by blocking the action of an enzyme known as DNA polymerase. This interference likely slows down or stops viral replication in the body. Test tube studies have shown that foscarnet is effective against all known herpes viruses. In a study of 18 cases of acyclovir-resistant zoster in people with HIV, of the 13 patients who received intravenous (IV) foscarnet for more than two weeks, complete healing was noted in 10 patients. Once foscarnet treatment was stopped, half of the patients who previously responded to therapy experienced zoster relapse.

Researchers use foscarnet in cases where zoster is strongly suspected or proven to be caused by acyclovir-resistant complications. Therapy should continue for a minimum of 10 days or until lesions are fully healed. It is thought that since people who have received multiple acyclovir treatments appear to be at the highest risk of having acyclovir-resistant strains, and acyclovir-resistant zoster responds well to therapy with foscarnet, this antiviral may be an effective treatment for HIV patients with varicella-zoster.

For more information see page 1204.

Generic: Sargramostim (sar-GRAM-oh-stim)
Brand: Leukine

Sargramostim helps bone marrow produce new white blood cells. Sargramostim is a man-made version of chemicals that are naturally produced by the body to help fight infection. It is often used to treat suppression of bone marrow function due to HIV infection or certain drugs.

Evidence from clinical studies demonstrates that sargramostim may be beneficial alone or in combination with other drugs in patients with HIV. In a study conducted by the Leukine/HIV Study Group comparing injections of sargramostim with placebo three times weekly for 24 weeks in patients with advanced HIV disease, sargramostim significantly increased immune cells and decreased virus breakthrough and overall infection rates more than placebo. In patients with oral fungal infections that are resistant to the antifungal therapy fluconazole, sargramostim appears to activate inflammatory cells, enhance ingestion and destruction of microorganisms, and kill the species of fungal bug known as *Candida*. According to researchers, in those who received fluconazole and sargramostim for two weeks, sargramostim showed a positive effect on oral mucosal organisms, further supporting the role of this therapy as an alternative treatment in patients with advanced HIV and oral fungal infections that are resistant to fluconazole.

For more information see page 1464.

MISCELLANEOUS AUTOIMMUNE DISORDERS

There are more than 80 autoimmune disorders/reactions, including autoimmune hepatitis, urticaria, food allergy, and seasonal allergic rhinitis. In autoimmune disease, the immune system attacks itself, unintentionally resulting in illness. The effects of autoimmune diseases can be present in connective tissues of the body, nerves, muscles, endocrine system, and the digestive system. Certain autoimmune disorders have similar symptoms, so diagnosing a particular disease may be a challenge. Autoimmune disorders often affect women more than men, and the diseases tend to be genetic.

Autoimmune Hepatitis

Autoimmune hepatitis is a serious disease in which the immune system attacks cells in the liver, which causes the liver to become inflamed. If autoimmune hepatitis is not treated, the disease worsens and leads to scarring or hardening of the liver, known as cirrhosis. Liver failure and death are the end results of autoimmune hepatitis. Autoimmune hepatitis is classified as type I or type II, with type I being the most common form in North America.

Commonly Prescribed (On-Label) Drugs: None

OFF-LABEL PRESCRIPTION DRUGS
BREAKTHROUGH OPTIONS

*Generic: **Azathioprine*** (ay-za-THYE-oh-preen)
*Brand: **Imuran***

Azathioprine is an immunosuppressive drug that blocks the synthesis of DNA, RNA, and proteins, and may also decrease the growth of immune cells. Researchers suggest that starting azathioprine with prednisone at the beginning of treatment may be effective. Starting azathioprine early in autoimmune hepatitis enables the steroid dose to be lowered more quickly, thereby avoiding side effects. In an article on autoimmune hepatitis, the researchers regarded corticosteroids alone or in combination with azathioprine, the treatment of choice in autoimmune hepatitis.

Several clinical studies support the use of azathioprine in autoimmune hepatitis. When combined with prednisone, one scientific paper reported a remission of disease in 65 to 87% of patients within three years. Additionally, other researchers reported that azathioprine should be combined with prednisone whenever possible because of the favorable side effect profile and the infrequent occurrence of disease relapse. Based on the numerous reports and recommendations by the medical community, the use of azathioprine for autoimmune hepatitis is an acceptable treatment option for most people.

For more information see page 1033.

Generic: *Cyclosporine* (si-klo-SPOR- een)
Brands: *Gengraf, Neoral, Sandimmune*

Cyclosporine belongs to the class of drugs known as immunosuppressive agents and suppresses immune reactions in different body organs, such as the liver. Since cyclosporine is a strong drug, it has the potential to cause serious side effects such as high blood pressure and kidney and liver problems. It may also reduce the body's ability to fight off infections.

Cyclosporine may be given instead of corticosteroids and azathioprine in an effort to reduce treatment-related side effects or to achieve response. In a review of medical records of 12 patients treated in a healthcare facility between 1987 and 2001, researchers in Italy noted that eight of the patients had autoimmune hepatitis. The remaining patients had other autoimmune disorders of the liver. Medical record data showed that cyclosporine was prescribed for patients who failed to respond to other treatments, patients who refused steroid treatment, or patients who were contraindicated to receive steroids. Cyclosporine was administered in five untreated patients and seven patients during relapse. All patients in this review achieved complete remission within 4.5 weeks, without treatment withdrawal due to side effects. Researchers noted that tolerability to cyclosporine was "excellent."

For more information see pages 1125 and 1127.

Generic: **Mercaptopurine** *(mer-kap-toe-PYOOR-een)*
Brand: **Purinethol**

Mercaptopurine was originally developed to treat leukemia and is often used to treat autoimmune diseases since the drug interacts with the immune system. It can be used for a long time; however, a physician will need to evaluate your blood periodically.

In an effort to avoid treatment-related side effects with other drugs for autoimmune hepatitis, a physician may administer mercaptopurine as an alternative treatment. In three instances, researchers in Boston noted that patients with autoimmune hepatitis could not tolerate or failed treatment with azathioprine, an immunosuppressive drug. Patients were then given mercaptopurine and responded well to treatment. Mercaptopurine is a possible treatment alternative for people with autoimmune hepatitis that is resistant to conventional therapy such as steroids and azathioprine.

For more information see page 1305.

Generic: **Mycophenolate mofetil**
(my-koe-FEN-oh-late MOE-feh-till
Brands: **CellCept, Myfortic**

Mycophenolate mofetil, which belongs to a class of drugs known as immunosuppressants, acts to decrease the actions of the body's immune system. Mycophenolate mofetil is primarily used to prevent the body from rejecting a transplanted organ. Other drugs such as prednisone, a steroid, and azathioprine, an immunosuppressant, are mainly used to treat autoimmune hepatitis. When people are resistant to one or all of these drugs, mycophenolate mofetil may be used. It is noted that the use of mycophenolate mofetil increases the risk of immune system cancer.

In a case series of five Canadian patients with autoimmune hepatitis who were unresponsive to or unable to take other drugs, mycophenolate mofetil normalized liver enzyme levels or retained normalized levels in all patients. Remission of autoimmune hepatitis was shown in one patient after seven months of therapy. One patient experienced a case of kidney infection. Based on these data, researchers concluded that mycophenolate mofetil can induce and maintain remission in patients with autoimmune hepatitis that is resistant to other drugs.

For more information see page 1344.

*Generic: **Prednisone** (pred-NIS-zone)*
*Brands: **Deltasone, Liquid Pred, Meticorten, Orasone, Sterapred***

Prednisone is a corticosteroid typically used to reduced swelling, redness, itching, and allergic reactions, and may be used to treat other immune disorders. In autoimmune hepatitis, prednisone suppresses an overactive immune system and may decrease inflammation.

Prednisone is the preferred treatment for autoimmune hepatitis because it is effective in achieving disease remission and may be used alone or in combination with other drugs. Doctors may start treatment with a high dose and lower the dose of prednisone as the disease is controlled. In clinical studies, low doses of prednisone, in combination with azathioprine, an immunosuppressive drug, were sufficient to maintain response to treatment for autoimmune hepatitis. Researchers observed that the combination of prednisone and azathioprine reverses the disease course. In general, a large majority of patients with autoimmune hepatitis demonstrate a satisfactory response to prednisone therapy. Although prednisone is the cornerstone therapy for autoimmune hepatitis, however, not all patients respond to this treatment. According to researchers, about 15 to 20% of patients with severe autoimmune hepatitis continue to have liver deterioration despite treatment with steroids such as prednisone.

For more information see page 1429.

Food Allergy

About one percent of adults and five percent of children have food allergies—adverse reactions to certain foods triggered by the immune system. In food allergy, the immune system mistakes the ingested food as harmful and activates certain cells to produce antibodies to fight the food or food component. These antibodies release chemicals such as histamine into the blood, and cause allergic symptoms such as dry throat, itchy eyes, dripping nose, hives, and difficulty breathing.

Commonly Prescribed (On-Label) Drugs: *None*

OFF-LABEL PRESCRIPTION DRUGS
BREAKTHROUGH OPTIONS

Generic: **Cromolyn** *(KROE-moe-lin)*
Brands: **Crolom, Gastrocrom, Intal, Opticrom**

Cromolyn is an antihistamine often used to prevent the start of an allergic reaction, since it prevents the release of chemicals that cause allergic symptoms.

In a Polish study, 25 and 29 children ranging in age from six months to three years, were given oral cromolyn sodium or ketotifen, respectively, during a period of four to 20 weeks. Skin, digestive, respiratory, and behavior symptoms were monitored in both groups of children. Cromolyn and ketotifen use resulted in a significant decrease in total food allergy symptoms. Researchers observed that cromolyn was well tolerated, and there were no serious side effects. In this study, skin rash, night symptoms, diarrhea, and itching were noted in only 8% of children. Researchers concluded that cromolyn was safe and effective for food allergy in children. In another study, Italian researchers attempted to desensitize patients to their respective food allergy. During treatment, 51.1% of patients experienced mild side effects that were easily controlled by cromolyn. Cromolyn has been demonstrated to be safe and effective in both adults and child patients.

For more information see page 1120.

Food Hypersensitivity

See Food Allergy

Hay fever

See Seasonal Allergic Rhinitis

Seasonal Allergic Rhinitis

See Lung and Airway Disorders

Urticaria

See Skin Disorders

INFECTIOUS DISEASES

BACTERIAL DISEASES

Bacteria are microscopic, single-celled organisms. Although there are thousands of different types of bacteria throughout the world, only a few kinds actually cause disease. Some bacteria are present in the environment; others live on the skin, in the airways, mouth, or digestive tract of people and animals. Certain bacteria give off toxins (poisons) that invade and multiply in your tissues, causing infection. A bacterial disease occurs when the affected cells or molecules in a person's body stop working properly due to an infection.

Asiatic Cholera

See Cholera

Bacterial Endocarditis, Prevention of

Bacterial endocarditis is a bacterial disease in which microbes infect the endothelial surface (layer of flat cells) of the heart. Since the signs and symptoms of bacterial endocarditis vary, doctors must have a high degree of suspicion to make an early, accurate diagnosis. Risk factors for bacterial endocarditis are classified as those associated with high-risk conditions such as congenital heart disease, intravenous (IV) drug use, and valve disease, and high-risk procedures such as dental surgery, respiratory tract surgeries, and gastrointestinal surgeries.

Commonly Prescribed (On-Label) Drugs: *Erythromycin*

OFF-LABEL PRESCRIPTION DRUGS
BREAKTHROUGH OPTIONS

Generic: **Azithromycin** *(az-ith-roe-MYE-sin)*
Brands: **Zithromax Tri-Pak, Zithromax Z-Pak**

In bacterial endocarditis, complete eradication of the organism causing the disease is necessary. Prolonged therapy with an antibacterial drug is the only way to kill all bacteria that are present in the endocarditis (inner lining of the heart). In instances where bacterial endocarditis may occur such as during surgery, doctors will give you a macrolide antibiotic, such as azithromycin, prior to the procedure to prevent the disease. In general, treatment of bacterial endocarditis is tailored to the type of antibiotic used.

Azithromycin has been recommended by doctors to prevent streptococcal such as congenital heart disease, heart valve surgery, and dental surgery. In a study conducted in Greece, two microorganisms, *Streptococcus oralis* and *Staphylococcus aureas,* were taken from blood cultures of patients with bacterial endocarditis. These microorganism samples were, in turn, given to rabbits to induce endocarditis. Rabbits were then given a single IV dose of azithromycin, vancomycin (an antibiotic), or ampicillin (an antibiotic). Results from this study demonstrated that azithromycin was effective in preventing streptococcal endocarditis.

For more information see page 1034.

Generic: **Clarithromycin** *(kla-RITH-roe-mye-sin)*
Brands: **Biaxin, Biaxin XL**

Clarithromycin, an antibiotic used in a wide variety of bacterial infections, blocks bacterial growth in bacterial endocarditis and is given preventively before medical procedures. In those adults and children with risk factors for the disease such as congenital heart disease, heart valve surgery, dental surgery along with an allergy to penicillin (an antibiotic) clarithromycin has been recommended by doctors to prevent streptococcal bacterial endocarditis. In a U.S. study conducted at the Mayo Clinic in Minnesota, the efficacy of clarithromycin and azithromycin was compared with other antibiotics including amoxicillin, clindamycin, and erythromycin in the prevention of endocarditis. In this study, rabbits induced with endocarditis were given one of the following regimens: no antibiotics or two doses of the following antibiotics: amoxicillin, azithromycin, clarithromycin. In this study, clarithromycin and azithromycin were as effective as amoxicillin, clindamycin, or erythromycin for the prevention of endocarditis.

For more information see page 1098.

Cerebrospinal Meningitis

See Meningitis

Cholera

Cholera is an acute diarrheal illness caused by infection in the intestine with the bacterium known as *Vibrio cholerae*. Oftentimes, cholera is mild or without symptoms, but it can be severe. It is estimated that one in 20 infected people experience severe disease characterized by watery diarrhea, vomiting, and leg cramps. Rapid loss of body fluids can lead to dehydration, shock, and possibly death. You can contract cholera by eating food or drinking water that is contaminated with cholera bacteria.

Commonly Prescribed (On-Label) Drugs: *Cholera Vaccine, Doxycycline, Furazolidone, Tetracycline*

OFF-LABEL PRESCRIPTION DRUGS
BREAKTHROUGH OPTIONS

Generic: **Ampicillin** *(am-pi-SIL-in)*
Brand: **Principen**

Antibiotics, such as ampicillin, can reduce the volume of diarrhea in patients with severe cholera. Antibiotics can also shorten the excretion time of the microorganism involved with cholera known as *Vibrio cholerae*. In general, antibiotic therapy for cholera is considered in addition to fluid therapy. However, since antibiotics such as ampicillin reduce diarrhea volume and duration by about 50 percent, they can shorten hospitalization time.

In a clinical trial conducted at the International Centre for Diarrhoeal Disease in Bangladesh, researchers compared the efficacy of ampicillin and two other antibiotics (erythromycin and tetracycline) in children with cholera. Ampicillin was also used since many patients with diarrhea symptoms also have respiratory tract infection. In this study, 184 children with diarrhea (less than 48 hours' duration), symptoms of dehydration, and evidence of the organism *Vibrio cholerae* received placebo or the antibiotics ampicillin, tetracycline, or erythromycin by mouth every six hours for three days. After three days, diarrhea volume was reduced in all treatment groups. Compared with tetracycline, the clinical recovery rates by 96 hours were: 75% with placebo, 91.3% with ampicillin, and 95.7% with erythromycin. In comparison with tetracycline, the total mean times to recovery were increased as follows: 66% with placebo, 25% with ampicillin, and 9% with erythromycin. According to researchers, results from this study showed comparable efficacy with tetracycline, ampicillin, and erythromycin.

For more information see page 1015.

Generic: **Ciprofloxacin** *(sip-roe-FLOKS-a-sin)*
Brands: *Ciloxan, Cipro, Cipro XR*

Ciprofloxacin, a type of antibiotic known as a fluoroquinolone, blocks bacterial production and growth. It is used off label for the treatment of cholera. It is approved in a wide variety of bacterial diseases that affect the skin, lungs, airways, bones, and joints. An article reviewing current cholera treatments, noted the utility of ciprofloxacin as an add-on treatment to rehydration therapy, particularly in patients with severe diarrhea. Moreover, the use of ciprofloxacin may result in shortened hospital stays, reduced excretion of the organism *Vibrio cholerae* in the stool, and minimize the need for fluids; although resistance to antibiotics has been seen. In a study of 74 adults with cholera, a single dose ciprofloxacin for three days showed similar efficacy when compared with another antibiotic, doxycycline. More clinical advantages were seen by researchers with ciprofloxacin because of the single-dose formulation and shortening the duration of diarrhea.

For more information see page 1091.

Generic: **Erythromycin** *(er-ith-roe-MYE-sin)*
Brands: **Akne-Mycin, E.E.S., Eryc, Ery-Tab, Erythrocin**

Erythromycin is used in a wide variety of infections since it prevents bacterial production and growth. Researchers at the U.S. Naval Medical Research Unit in Cairo, Egypt compared the efficacy of twice-daily erythromycin, trimethoprim-sulfamethoxazole (an antibiotic), and placebo in 47 people with tetracycline-resistant cholera. After treatment, patients who received erythromycin or trimethoprim-sulfamethoxazole had a decrease of the microorganism *Vibrio cholerae* in their stool, whereas organisms persisted in those who received placebo. Also, people who received erythromycin had a significant decrease in the number of diarrhea-like stools per day and duration of diarrhea versus placebo. A strain of *Vibrio cholerae* that was resistant to trimethoprim-sulfamethoxazole but sensitive to erythromycin was seen. Researchers concluded that in addition to oral rehydration treatment, erythromycin may be an effective treatment alternative for cholera, particularly in instances of trimethoprim-sulfamethoxazole resistance.

For more information see page 1170.

Generic: **Trimethoprim-sulfamethoxazole**
(try-METH-oh-prim–sul-fuh-meth-OX-ahzole)
Brands: **Bactrim, Septra**

Trimethoprim-sulfamethoxazole consists of a combination of trimethoprim and sulfamethoxazole, and inhibits bacterial growth in cholera. Researchers conducted a study to evaluate the efficacy of trimethoprim-sulfamethoxazole and erythromycin in children with cholera. Fifteen children received erythromycin; 18 children received trimethoprim and sulfamethoxazole; and 15 children received no treatment. All children in this study also received fluids for dehydration. In this study by the International Centre for Diarrhoeal Research in Bangladesh, 67% of the children in the erythromycin group and 82% in the trimethoprim-sulfamethoxazole group recovered within 72 hours compared with 33% in the no-treatment group. Cures were 80% in the erythromycin group and 83% in the trimethoprim-sulfamethoxazole group compared with 27% in the no-treatment group. Researchers in this study noted that erythromycin or trimethoprim-sulfamethoxazole was effective in the treatment of cholera.

For more information see page 1530.

Food Poisoning

Food poisoning is an acute illness caused by ingestion of food contaminated with bacteria, bacterial toxins (poisons), or harmful chemical substances. Nearly 76 million people suffer from food poisoning in the United States each year. Symptoms of food poisoning vary in severity and can include stomach pain, vomiting, diarrhea, headache, and may result in life-threatening neurologic, liver, and kidney syndromes. Bacteria are responsible for the following five foodborne diseases: botulism, campylobacteriosis, E. coli, salmonellosis, and shigellosis.

Commonly Prescribed (On-Label) Drugs: None

OFF-LABEL PRESCRIPTION DRUGS
BREAKTHROUGH OPTIONS

---

*Generic: **Ampicillin** (am-pi-SIL-in)*
*Brand: **Principen***

Ampicillin is in the family of antibiotics known as penicillins. The drug blocks the formation of the bacterial cell wall and is approved in a number of bacterial infections, other than food poisoning, caused by streptococci, pneumococci, Listeria, Salmonella, Shigella, and E. coli, among others. In a review article published by a researcher in the Netherlands, ampicillin, among other traditional antibiotics, was mentioned as the mainstay therapy for the management of bacterial Salmonella infections from food. Also mentioned was that the increasing resistance to these traditional antibiotic drugs necessitates the use of different types of antibiotics for this type of bacterial disease.

Case reports also document the use of ampicillin for Salmonella infections. In one instance, a pregnant woman came down with gastroenteritis one week before delivery. The newborn infant was subsequently treated with ampicillin, gentamicin (an antibiotic), and amoxicillin (an antibiotic); however, five months later, Sal-

monella was still present. In this case, researchers discussed the potential route of infection and the guidelines for treatment and management of this type of bacterial infection in pregnancy and post-partum.

For more information see page 1015.

Generic: **Methotrexate** *(meth-oh-TREKS-ate)*
Brands: **Rheumatrex, Trexall**

Methotrexate belongs to a class of drugs known as antimetabolite drugs. As a drug class, antimetabolites block the metabolism of cells; so, they are helpful in treating diseases associated with rapid, abnormal cell growth like cancer. Methotrexate is also used to treat a skin condition known as psoriasis and in rheumatoid arthritis. In some people affected with food poisoning, antibiotic drugs are not effective. Moreover, a condition known as reactive arthritis can arise from infections with certain strains of *Salmonella* and *Shigella*. Reactive arthritis, also known as Reiter's syndrome, is a type of inflammatory arthritis. Researchers noted a 1984 outbreak of *Salmonella typhimurium* food poisoning affecting Canadian police officers that resulted in acute arthritis. Researchers mentioned that those who have food poisoning and develop arthritis often have more prolonged episodes of diarrhea. Recommended treatment was identified as methotrexate.

For more information see page 1312.

Lockjaw

See Tetanus

Lyme Borreliosis

See Lyme Disease

Lyme Disease

Lyme disease is a disease caused by the bacteria known as *Borrelia burgdorferi*. Within one to two weeks of being infected, you may have a "bull's-eye" rash accompanied with fever, headache, and muscle or joint pain. However, some people do not have any early symptoms. Other people may experience fever and other flu-like symptoms without a rash. After several days or weeks, the bacteria may spread throughout the body. If the disease is not treated, swelling and pain in major joints or mental changes can occur months after initial infection.

Commonly Prescribed (On-Label) Drugs: Cefuroxime, Lyme Disease Vaccine

---

OFF-LABEL PRESCRIPTION DRUGS
BREAKTHROUGH OPTIONS

---

*Generic: **Amoxicillin*** *(a-moks-i-SIL-in)*
*Brands: **Amoxil, Trimox***

Amoxicillin is an antibiotic that belongs to a class of drugs known as penicillins. Amoxicillin stops the growth and multiplication of bacteria by preventing the formation of bacterial cell walls. Efficacy of amoxicillin has been demonstrated among bacteria such as *E. coli* and *streptococci.* This antibiotic is often used in middle ear, tonsil, throat, urinary, skin, and respiratory bacterial infections. Oral amoxicillin is considered, along with some other antibiotics (doxycycline, cefuroxime), as first-line treatment for the early stages of Lyme disease. In a study conducted by Japanese researchers, seven *Ixodes persulcatus* (a microorganism) strains were susceptible to antibiotics, including amoxicillin. Additionally, amoxicillin in this analysis provided good protection against borreliosis in mice; and higher doses of the drug eliminated Lyme disease from all mice receiving the drug. In children with early Lyme disease, researchers compared amoxicillin with cefuroxime axetil (a broad-spectrum antibiotic) and found that both treatments were safe and effective.

For more information see page 1012.

*Generic: **Clarithromycin*** *(kla-RITH-roe-mye-sin)*
*Brands: **Biaxin, Biaxin XL***

Clarithromycin is an antibiotic approved for a wide variety of infections including middle ear, throat, skin, and respiratory infections. In general, clarithromycin is well tolerated; reported side effects include nausea, diarrhea, and stomach pain, among others.

In early Lyme disease, antibiotics such as clarithromycin have been effective; however, certain antibiotics may be less effective than penicillin-type or tetracycline-type drugs. Experts associated with the Infectious Disease Society of America (IDSA) and the American Academy of Pediatrics (AAP) recommend that macrolide-type antibiotics not be used as a first-line treatment for early Lyme disease.

In a study conducted at the Lyme Disease Center at the State University of New York at Stony Brook, researchers enrolled 41 patients with symptoms of early Lyme disease and administered clarithromycin. Immediately following therapy, signs and symptoms of Lyme disease resolved in 91% of the 33 evaluable patients. After six months, all 28 evaluable patients responded well to treatment. Researchers concluded that clarithromycin for Lyme disease is effective.

For more information see page 1098.

Generic: **Doxycycline** (doks-I-SYE-kleen)
Brands: **Adoxa, Doryx, Doxy-100, Monodox, Periostat, Vibramycin, Vibra-Tabs**

Doxycycline belongs to a class of drugs known as tetracycline antibiotics. It works by preventing the growth and spread of bacteria, and physicians recommend the oral formulation as a first-line treatment for stages of Lyme disease without nervous system or cardiac involvement.

In a clinical survey, doxycycline was among the most frequently used antibiotics in people with Lyme disease. In this analysis, 50.4% of patients received this antibiotic. In another study, researchers evaled oral doxycycline or placebo in 482 patients who had removed an attached tick from their bodies within 72 hours. In patients treated with doxycycline, the characteristic skin rash at the bite site developed significantly less compared with the placebo group. Treatment with doxycycline was associated with more frequent adverse effects compared with placebo. The adverse effects included nausea and vomiting. Researchers concluded that a single dose of doxycycline given within 72 hours of an *Ixodes scapularis* tick bite may prevent the development of Lyme disease.

For more information see page 1158.

Generic: **Erythromycin** *(er-ith-roe-MYE-sin)*
Brands: **Akne-Mycin, E.E.S., Eryc, Ery-Tab, Erythrocin**

Erythromycin is used to prevent bacteria from producing proteins and to prevent growth and multiplication of bacteria. Erythromycin is typically used in bacterial infections including throat and respiratory infections.

Antibiotics such as erythromycin have been used off label in the treatment of early Lyme disease. There is some evidence that macrolide antibiotics such as erythromycin may be less effective than penicillin-type or tetracycline-type drugs. Experts recommend that macrolide-type antibiotics not be used as a first-line treatment for early Lyme disease. According to physicians, macrolide antibiotics, such as erythromycin, should be reserved for people who are intolerant to other antibiotics such as amoxicillin, doxycycline, and cefuroxime axetil.

In a study conducted in Japan, the antibiotic susceptibilities of seven strains of *Ixodes persulcatus* were tested. All strains in this study were susceptible to erythromycin along with other antibiotics (amoxicillin and minocycline-erythromycin was prescribed in 4.2% of patients). In a review of the treatment of early Lyme disease, Canadian researchers identified erythromycin among the many antibiotic treatments used for this bacterial disease. For second-line treatment of early Lyme disease, macrolide antibiotics, such as erythromycin, are considered.

For more information see page 1170.

Generic: **Minocycline** *(min-OH-sik-leen)*
Brands: **Dynacin, Minocin**

Minocycline belongs to a class of drugs known as tetracycline antibiotics. It is used in a wide variety of bacterial diseases, and has been found to be useful in Lyme disease. In a study, seven strains were susceptible to minocycline and other antibiotics (amoxicillin and erythromycin). Moreover, in this analysis, minocycline provided good protection against borreliosis (an infection caused by a tick bite) when given to mice infected with Lyme disease. Higher doses of minocycline resulted in elimination of Lyme disease in all mice receiving the drug. Researchers concluded that minocycline could be helpful in the treatment of

Lyme disease. In a review conducted by researchers, it was noted that oral tetracycline antibiotics are effective first-line treatments for patients with early stage Lyme disease and was found to be effective in the treatment of Lyme disease. In this study, 14 people with Lyme disease skin rashes received minocycline. Researchers then evaluated the presence of *Borrelia burgdorferi*. After treatment with minocycline, there was no presence of the microorganism.

For more information see page 1331.

Generic: **Penicillin** *(pen-eh-SILL-in)*
Brands: **Bicillin, Penicillin VK, Pfizerpen, Veetids**

Discovered in 1928, penicillin V is still used today in a variety of bacterial diseases since this blocks the growth of bacteria. In general, penicillin is a well-tolerated drug. Researchers note that seven percent of patients receive penicillin for Lyme disease. Additionally, in another study, penicillin V along with other antibiotics was noted to be effective for tick-borne relapsing fever in children with Lyme disease.

Alternatively, in a study of 65 patients with skin symptoms of early Lyme disease, researchers compared penicillin V with oral azithromycin for 10 days. They found that 62% of patients given azithromycin and 51% of patients given penicillin V were completely free of all Lyme disease signs and symptoms. Azithromycin use was associated with a significantly faster resolution of skin rash compared with penicillin. Although, researchers state that penicillin-type antibiotics are considered among the first-line treatments in patients with Lyme disease.

For more information see page 1403.

Meningitis (Prevention of Meningococcal Meningitis)

An infection of the meninges (the membranes that surround the brain and spinal cord) is called meningitis. It is generally caused by bacterial or viral infection; bacterial meningitis is a rare but potentially fatal disease, and can be caused by several different forms of bacteria that may initially cause an upper respiratory tract infection and then travel through the blood to the brain. Bacterial meningitis can also happen when certain bacteria invade the meninges directly. The disease can block blood vessels in the brain, causing stroke and permanent brain damage. Symptoms of meningitis include sudden fever, severe headache, and stiff neck.

Commonly Prescribed (On-Label) Drugs: Minocycline, Penicillin G

OFF-LABEL PRESCRIPTION DRUGS
BREAKTHROUGH OPTIONS

Generic: **Ceftriaxone** *(sef-trye-AKS-one)*
Brand: **Rocephin**

Ceftriaxone works by fighting bacteria in the body, and is used in a wide variety of bacterial infections including stomach infections, skin infections, ear infections, and urinary tract infections, among others. Ceftriaxone is used in the treatment of invasive infections like meningitis, which are caused by the microorganism known as *Neisseria meningitidis.* The first-line drug for the treatment of meningitis is IV penicillin G (an antibiotic); however, ceftriaxone is considered an acceptable alternative.

Patients with invasive meningitis who have been treated with penicillin G or another anti-infective drug may still be carriers of *Neisseria meningitides* in the nasopharynx (the space within the skull that is above the roof of the mouth and behind the nose). Therefore, researchers recommend that these people receive an anti-infective drug to eradicate these bacteria before discharge from a hospital. Ceftriaxone or other drugs are helpful in this instance. The recommended regimen to prevent meningitis includes a single IM dose of ceftriaxone. Based on its efficacy, ease of use, and low cost as identified in a recent study; ceftriaxone appears to be an alternate drug for the treatment of meningitis.

For more information see page 1076.

Generic: **Ciprofloxacin** *(sip-roe-FLOKS-a-sin)*
Brands: **Ciloxan, Cipro, Cipro XR**

Ciprofloxacin is an antibiotic. It works by blocking the reproduction and multiplication of bacteria and is used to treat a wide variety of bacterial infections of the skin, lungs, airways, bones, and joints. In adults, ciprofloxacin is used to eliminate *Neisseria meningitides* from the nasopharynx (the space within the skull that is above the roof of the mouth and behind the nose). This antibiotic has been shown to be effective when given as a single oral adult dose, or in multiple oral doses. Even though rifampin (an antimycobacterial drug) has been considered the first-line treatment for eradicating *Neisseria meningitides* from the nasopharynx, ciprofloxacin is considered to be an effective treatment alternative. Besides its use in the treatment of meningitis, oral ciprofloxacin is also used to prevent this bacterial disease in uninfected individuals who have been in contact with a person with meningitis. If an individual has received ciprofloxacin to prevent meningitis and is re-exposed to the bacteria more than two weeks after initial treatment, another course of the drug should be given. Ciprofloxacin can also be given before hospital discharge to prevent infection.

For more information see page 1093.

Mycobacterium Avium Complex in AIDS

Mycobacterium Avium Complex, or MAC, is a serious illness caused by common bacteria found in water, soil, dust, and food. MAC infection can be limited to one part of the body or spread throughout the entire body. Oftentimes, MAC infection occurs in the lungs, intestines, bone marrow, liver, and spleen. A person with a healthy immune system can control MAC, but people with weakened immune systems can develop MAC disease. In persons with acquired immune deficiency syndrome (AIDS) up to 50 percent may develop MAC, particularly if their white blood cell count (T-cells) is below 50. Symptoms of MAC may include night sweats, fever, unintentional weight loss, diarrhea, and low level red and white blood cell counts. A doctor can diagnose MAC through blood or bone marrow testing.

Commonly Prescribed (On-Label) Drugs: Azithromycin, Clarithromycin, Rifabutin

OFF-LABEL PRESCRIPTION DRUG
BREAKTHROUGH OPTION

*Generic: **Ethambutol** (e-THAM-byoo-tole)*
*Brand: **Myambutol***

Ethambutol is classified as an antibiotic drug and is typically used to treat tuberculosis (respiratory infection). It may also be used to treat MAC. Although the first-line treatments of MAC involve other antibiotics like clarithromycin and azithromycin, ethambutol is recommended as the second-line drug for this bacterial disease.

In the treatment of MAC, ethambutol is used in combination with other antituberculosis drugs. Experts recommend that therapy for disseminated (spread throughout the body) MAC in patients with AIDS include clarithromycin or azithromycin combined with ethambutol or rifabutin. In a study, researchers noted the added benefits of combination drugs in patients with AIDS and disseminated MAC. In this study by the University of Colorado Health Sciences Center in Denver, Colorado, 160 patients were given ethambutamol and clarithromycin; clarithromycin and rifabutin; or ethambutamol, clarithromycin, and rifabutin for 48 weeks. Patients that received all three drugs had improved survival compared with the ethambutamol and clarithromycin and the clarithromycin and rifabutin groups.

For more information see page 1176.

Nocardiasis

See Nocardiosis

Nocardiosis

Nocardiosis, or nocardia infection, is a rare disorder caused by the *Nocardia* bacteria. It often affects individuals with weakened immune systems. The infection generally starts in the lungs and has a tendency to spread to other organ systems; nocardiosis can also involve the kidneys, the joints, the ear, the eyes, and the bones. *Norcardia* bacteria are found in soil all over the world, therefore the infection can be contracted by breathing in contaminated dust or through direct contact with contaminated soil such as through an open wound.

Commonly Prescribed (On-Label) Drugs: *Sulfadiazine, Sulfamethoxazole*

OFF-LABEL PRESCRIPTION DRUGS
BREAKTHROUGH OPTIONS

Generic: **Amikacin** *(am-i-KAY-sin)*
Brand: **Amikin**

Amikacin belongs to a class of drugs known as aminoglycoside antibiotics, which are used to treat serious bacterial infections and is used off label for nocardiosis. In nocardiosis, amikacin helps to block protein synthesis and inhibits the growth of bacteria. Currently, along with imipenem (an antibiotic), amikacin is the most active IV drug against nocardiosis, with 90% to 95% efficacy against all strains. Adverse effects associated with this drug, such as hearing loss, clumsiness, dizziness, urination increase or decrease, and nausea and vomiting, may limit long-term use. It is recommended that amikacin be reserved for use in more severe infections when other drugs have not worked.

In a review by researchers in Valencia, Spain of 10 patients with pulmonary nocardiosis who were diagnosed and treated in the hospital, antimicrobial susceptibility testing showed 100% sensitivity for amikacin, 83% sensitivity for imipenem, and 71% sensitivity for cefotaxime (an antibiotic). Pulmonary nocardiosis remained in five of the 10 patients. Researchers noted that antibiotic combinations with proven effectiveness, such as amikacin and imipenem, are recommended for initial therapy. In general, amikacin is considered an alternative treatment to cotrimoxazole (an antibiotic) or sulfonamide antibiotics, which are the drugs of choice for nocardiosis.

For more information see page 1003.

*Generic: **Amoxicillin-Clavulanate***
(a-moks-i-SIL-in klav-yoo-LAN-ate)
*Brands: **Augmentin, Augmentin ES-600, Augmentin XR***

Amoxicillin and clavulanate belong to the class of drugs known as penicillin-type antibiotics, and are approved in a wide variety of bacterial infections. This drug combination treats bacteria that are resistant to certain types of drugs known as beta-lactam antibiotics. Amoxicillin works by making the cell wall of bacteria leaky; it also kills bacteria. Clavulanate protects amoxicillin from being destroyed by certain bacteria. Therefore, this drug combination kills more kinds of bacteria and is generally used in more difficult bacterial infections. Amoxicillin and clavulanate potassium are considered to be an alternative oral treatment in mild to moderately severe nocardiosis. Additionally, this drug combination may be used after IV therapy is given. The efficacy of amoxicillin and clavulanate potassium in nocardiosis has been documented in various case studies of affected people.

For more information see page 1013.

*Generic: **Cefotaxime** (sef-oh-TAKS-eem)*
*Brand: **Claforan***

Cefotaxime is a type of antibiotic. In nocardiosis, cefotaxime stops bacterial cell wall production, which in turn stops growth of bacteria. High levels of resistance to *Nocardia farcinica* (a microorganism) have been seen with the use of third-generation antibiotics such as cefotaxime. Additionally, researchers found that 95% of *Nocardia asteroides* had one of five antibiotic resistance patterns. Researchers found this pattern of resistance to cefotaxime and another drug in 19% of 200 *Nocardia asteroides* strains. This was the first recognition that *Nocardia farcinica* has a specific drug resistance pattern and confirms the concept that drug resistance patterns of *Nocardia asteroides* may be associated with specific bacteria groups. Alternatively, in a study conducted at the University of Texas Health Center reviewing the susceptibility of *Nocardia asteroides* to a variety of antibiotics, researchers noted that the most active IV drugs for this microorganism included cefotaxime.

For more information see page 1037.

Generic: **Ceftriaxone** *(sef-trye-AKS-one)*
Brand: **Rocephin**

Ceftriaxone is a type of antibiotic that is highly effective against resistant organisms in nocardiosis. In patients with nocardiosis, alternative IV therapies included third-generation cephalosporins, such as ceftriaxone. Side effects are not common; however, they may include diarrhea, stomach pain, upset stomach, and vomiting.

The use of ceftriaxone has been primarily documented in case studies of patients with nocardiosis. In one case study conducted in Switzerland, an 85-year-old woman with disseminated *Nocardia asteroides* infection and brain abscess (a mass of immune cells, pus, and other material that can occur in brain infections) was treated with amikacin (an antibiotic) for two weeks and ceftriaxone for six weeks. Treatment with both of these drugs resulted in complete recovery, and there was no recurrence of infection after 12 months. Researchers noted that the use of ceftriaxone with amikacin might vastly decrease the duration of treatment in patients with disseminated nocardiosis. In a different case study, researchers evaluated a 56-year-old man with a brain abscess involving *Nocardia asteroides* and neurologic symptoms such as confusion and sluggishness of the body. A combination of IV antibiotics, including ceftriaxone, was given along with surgery. Two weeks after surgery, the man's neurological status improved.

For more information see page 1076.

Generic: **Imipenem-cilastatin** *(i-mi-PEN-em sye-la-STAT-in)*
Brand: **Primaxin**

Imipenem-cilastatin is classified as a broad-spectrum antibiotic. In nocardiosis, imipenem-cilastatin works by blocking the synthesis of the bacteria cell wall.

Imipenem-cilastatin is among the alternative IV therapies for nocardiosis. Futhermore, imipenem-cilastatin and amikacin (an antibiotic) may be the preferred drug regimen in this nocardiosis. In a review of 10 patients with pulmonary nocardiosis who were diagnosed and treated in a hospital, antimicrobial susceptibility testing showed 100% sensitivity for amikacin (an antibiotic), 83% sensitivity for imipenem, and 71% sensitivity for cefotaxime (an antibiotic). Pulmonary nocardiosis remained localized in five of the 10 patients in this study conducted in Spain. Researchers noted that antibiotic combinations with proven effectiveness, such as amikacin and imipenem, are recommended for initial therapy.

For more information see page 1229.

Generic: **Meropenem** (MIRO-pen-em)
Brand: **Merrem IV**

Meropenem belongs to a class of drugs known as broad-spectrum antibiotics. In nocardiosis, meropenem blocks bacterial cell wall synthesis. Alternative IV antibiotics used in nocardiosis include the carbapenems, such as meropenem. Meropenem may offer an advantage compared with imipenem (an antibiotic); however, this drug has not been well studied for this bacterial disease. Overall, meropenem use and efficacy is limited to a number of international patient case reports. In a kidney transplant patient with disseminated nocardiosis, researchers reported improvement with combination antibiotic therapy consisting of IV meropenem, cefotaxime, and minocycline.

In another case, a 50-year-old woman with convulsions after kidney transplant was identified to have *Nocardia* infection. Subsequent treatment consisted of meropenem, rifampicin (an antibiotic), ciprofloxacin (an antibiotic), tacrolimus (immunosuppressive drug), and a steroid. At five months from the termination of antibiotic therapy, the woman regained normal strength and function on the left side of her body. In another case, a 22-year-old man with *Nocardia* bacterial infection and fungal infection was treated with liposomal amphotericin B (antifungal), amikacin (antibiotic), meropenem, and cotrimoxazole (antibiotic). After treatment with this drug combination, he fully recovered.

For more information see page 1307.

Generic: **Minocycline** (min-OH-sik-leen)
Brands: **Dynacin, Minocin**

Minocycline belongs to a class of drugs known as tetracycline antibiotics. Oral therapies for nocardiosis include minocycline, which can be used initially in mild to moderately severe disease or after IV antibiotic therapy is completed. According to investigators, minocycline has excellent activity against most species of *Nocardia*, particularly *Nocarida farcinica* (4% resistance). *Nocardia transvalensis* is the only microorganism that is significantly resistant to this antibiotic (46% resistant).

The use of minocycline in the medical literature is primarily documented in patient case study reports. In one instance, researchers in the United Kingdom described a patient case involving a disseminated *Nocardia farcinica* infection possibly acquired from a road traffic accident. Minocycline was given for 12 months, and the patient improved. In another case, researchers noted that in two patients with lung infection due to *Nocardia*, minocycline was not sufficient to prevent the spread of the bacterial infection to the central nervous system.

For more information see page 1331.

Generic: **Trimethoprim-sulfamethoxazole**
(try-METH-oh-prim–sul-fah-meth-OX-ahzole)
Brands: **Bactrim, Septra**

Trimethoprim-sulfamethoxazole belongs to a class of drugs known as sulfonamide antibiotics. Trimethoprim-sulfamethoxazole contains a combination of two antibiotic drugs: trimethoprim and sulfamethoxazole, and is approved for a wide variety of bacterial infections. As an off-label treatment, this drug combination is considered first-line therapy for both skin and body-system nocardiosis; it works by blocking bacterial growth.

A variety of patient case study reports document the efficacy of trimethoprim-sulfamethoxazole in nocardiosis. In a study by researchers from the Czech Republic, trimethoprim-sulfamethoxazole in combination with antibiotics drugs such as cefotaximine, amikacin, chloramphenicol, and doxycycline successfully treated disseminated nocardiosis in the skin, right kidney, liver, peritoneal cavity, lungs, and thigh in a 55-year-old woman with mild trauma to the arm. The researchers noted that the combination of trimethoprim-sulfamethoxazole and doxycycline was beneficial. In another study, five cases of *Nocardia* infection were noted among 301 patients who received bone marrow transplant. Treatment consisted of trimethoprim-sulfamethoxazole, ceftriaxone (an antibiotic), or carbapenem (an antibiotic). This regimen resulted in a one-year survival of 40%, and all patients who received more than two weeks of treatment were cured of their infections.

For more information see page 1530.

Tetanus

Tetanus is a disease that affects the nervous system and is caused by a bacteria known as *Clostridium tetani*. Tetanus is contracted through a cut or wound that becomes contaminated with tetanus bacteria; these bacteria, which are most often found in soil, dust, and manure, can get in through a tiny pinprick or scratch. Deep puncture wounds or cuts are especially susceptible to tetanus infection. Symptoms of tetanus infection include headache, muscular stiffness in the jaw, neck stiffness, difficulty swallowing, rigid stomach muscles, spasms, and fever. Approximately 11% of cases are fatal, with most deaths occurring in those 60 years or older.

Commonly Prescribed (On-Label) Drugs: Diphtheria, *Tetanus, Acellular Pertussis Vaccine, Diphtheria/Tetanus Toxoids, Tetanus Immune Globulin, Tetanus Toxoids*

OFF-LABEL PRESCRIPTION DRUGS
BREAKTHROUGH OPTIONS

Generic: **Diazepam** *(dye-AZ-e-pam)*
Brands: **Diastat, Diazepam Intensol, Valium**

Diazepam belongs to a class of drugs known as benzodiazepines, which are often used before surgery to relieve anxiety and provide sedation, and in alcohol withdrawal syndrome. In general, benzodiazepines such as diazepam are the main drugs used to control muscle spasms in tetanus.

Researchers feel that the use of diazepam is well documented in case study reports. In a report issued by researchers, high-dose diazepam was noted to work better than pancuronium bromide (a muscle-relaxant drug) and was proven to be a good muscle relaxant. In three instances of severe tetanus, researchers reported that two of the cases were managed with diazepam and pancuronium bromide, the third case was managed with high-dose diazepam. In a review article, researchers documented the diagnosis and treatment of tetanus in one healthcare facility between 2000 and 2002. During this time, 11 patients were diagnosed with tetanus and were given diazepam IV for muscle spasms. Of these 11 cases, 10 patients were eventually discharged from the hospital, and one patient died six days after hospital admission.

For more information see page 1139.

Generic: **Metronidazole** *(me-troe-NI-da-zole)*
Brands: **Flagyl, Flagyl ER, MetroCream, MetroGel, MetroLotion, MetroGel Vaginal**

Metronidazole, which belongs to a class of drugs known as antimicrobials, may be used off-label to treat the tetanus bacteria. Compared with the antibiotic penicillin, metronidazole has similar or better antimicrobial activity. In a study comparing oral metronidazole to penicillin, metronidazole showed better survival, shorter hospitalization, and less progression of disease.

Additionally, in four case studies by investigators in Saudi Arabia, people treated during 2001 and 2002 received both penicillin and metronidazole and had improved symptoms with these treatments. Despite the successful use of both drugs, researchers concluded that further scientific study should be conducted.

For more information see page 1322.

Toxic Shock Syndrome

Toxic shock syndrome is a rare, fatal bacterial infection most commonly associated with the use of superabsorbent tampons and occasionally with the use of contraceptive sponges. Symptoms occur suddenly and this disease can result in death. Other risk factors for toxic shock syndrome include the presence of skin wounds or surgical procedures. Toxins produced by the *Staphylococcus aureas* bacteria are primarily responsible for toxic shock syndrome. Even though this infection most often occurs in women, toxic shock syndrome can also affect children, men, as well as women who do not menstruate.

Commonly Prescribed (On-Label) Drugs: *None*

OFF-LABEL PRESCRIPTION DRUG
BREAKTHROUGH OPTION

*Generic: **Reteplase** (re-TE-plase)*
*Brand: **Retavase***

Reteplase is a drug used to improve blood flow to the heart, particularly after a heart attack. It may be used in instances of toxic shock syndrome that are accompanied with septic phlebitis (inflammation of a vein accompanied with fever and bacteria in the blood). Septic phlebitis can occur suddenly or is the result of infection by certain bacteria such as *Staphylococcus aureus*. The goal of this treatment in toxic shock syndrome with drugs such as reteplase is to dissolve an infected blood clot (thrombus) where resistant infection can reside and spread to other areas of the body; and potentially prevent the clot from traveling to other body systems.

According to a doctor at the Washington National Medical Center, reteplase appears to work faster than alteplase (a thrombolytic drug), and also may be more effective in patients with larger blood clots. Reteplase also has been reported to be more effective in people with larger clot burden and may be more effective than other drugs in the destruction of older blood clots.

For more information see page 1445.

Toxoplasmosis in AIDS

In persons with AIDS, infections like toxoplasmosis can cause significant sickness and result in death. Toxoplasmic encephalitis caused by the bacteria *Toxoplasma gondii* is the most common cause of central nervous system infection in persons with AIDS. Persons with white blood cell counts less than 50 cells/mcg are at greatest risk for this disease. Primary infection can occur after eating undercooked meat containing cysts or ingestion of unfertilized eggs found in cat feces that have been spread through the environment. The most common symptoms of this bacterial disease include headache, confusion, motor weakness, and fever.

Commonly Prescribed (On-Label) Drugs: *Pyrimethamine, Sulfadiazine, Sulfisoxazole*

OFF-LABEL PRESCRIPTION DRUGS
BREAKTHROUGH OPTIONS

Generic: **Clindamycin** *(klin-da-MYE-sin)*
Brands: **Cleocin, Clindamycin**

Clindamycin is an antibiotic. In toxoplasmosis in AIDS, clindamycin works by stopping the growth of bacteria such as *Toxoplasma gondii*. In patients with toxoplasmic infection in the presence of AIDS, clindamycin is often used as an add-on drug in combination with pyrimethamine (an antimalarial drug) and leucovorin (a folate drug).

According to researchers, clindamycin is an effective second-line treatment for toxoplasmic infection in AIDS patients who are unable to tolerate or fail to respond to first-line treatment. In patients who fail therapy with first-line antibiotics, common practice entails IV pentamidine (a drug used to prevent lung disease) and primaquine (an antimalarial drug) combined with clindamycin and leucovorin. According to the National Institute of Health (NIH), there is some evidence that high doses of injectable clindamycin used with pyrithemine may be as effective as pyrimethamine plus sulfadiazine (an antibiotic) in toxoplasmic encephalitis in patients with AIDS. Additionally, there is some indication that oral clindamycin may be effective for these people. Small studies and patient case reports have documented the efficacy of clindamycin combined with pyrimethamine and other drugs.

For more information see page 1101.

Trismus

See Tetanus

FUNGAL DISEASE

Fungal infections are more likely to occur if you have decreased immunity as the result of certain drugs such as steroids or immunosuppressants, in certain diseases like AIDS or diabetes, or as a result of physical trauma such as burns or other injuries. Fungal infection can occur when you come in contact with a certain fungus, such as *Candida*. Symptoms of fungal infections can include chronic infection, fever, chills, night sweats, anorexia, weight loss, tiredness and muscle weakness, and depression.

Chronic Mucocutaneous Candidiasis

Chronic mucocutaneous candidiasis (CMC) describes a group of syndromes that are characterized by persistent, recurrent, and sometimes severe superficial infections of the mucous membranes, nails, and skin caused by fungus known as *Candida*. CMC is generally confined to the skin surface and does not involve other body systems, and is associated with a weakened immune system (in children, in persons with diabetes, or in persons with thymic tumors). Fungal *Candida* infections of the mouth are characterized by white lesions; esophageal *Candida* infections are characterized by fever and burning pain or discomfort of the throat. Vaginal *Candida* infections are characterized by creamy white discharge, itching, and burning.

Commonly Prescribed (On-Label) Drugs: Ketoconazole

OFF-LABEL PRESCRIPTION DRUGS
BREAKTHROUGH OPTIONS

*Generic: **Cimetidine** (sye-MET-i-deen)*
*Brand: **Tagamet***

Cimetidine is an antihistamine. In chronic mucocutaneous candidiasis (CMC), antihistamines, such as cimetidine, are thought to increase cell immunity. The main treatment in CMC is systemic antifungals; however, these types of drugs do not affect the underlying immune deficiency, a characteristic of chronic fungal infections. Cimetidine boosts immunity and has been used in CMC with some success. A few reports by researchers in Italy document its use in individual patients. Cimetidine three times daily, along with zinc sulphate daily was given to a patient with CMC. After 16 months of treatment, a significant decrease in infectious events and an increase in immune cells were seen. Based on these results, researchers concluded that cimetidine and zinc sulphate are safe and cost-effective drugs for CMC.

For more information see page 1091.

*Generic: **Itraconazole** (i-tra-KOE-na-zole)*
*Brand: **Sporanox***

Itraconazole belongs to a class of drugs known as triazole antifungals. In general, chronic mucocutaneous candidiasis (CMC) is most commonly treated with systemic antifungals since they are effective; however, this type of drug does not affect the immune system. Itraconzole is thought to cause the fungal cell wall to leak thereby destroying the fungus. According to experts, itraconazole oral solution given for seven to 14 days is just as effective as oral fluconazole (an antifungal) but is less tolerated in patients with fungal infection of the mouth. Additionally, researchers believe that itraconazole capsules should be considered a second-line treatment for fungal mouth infections since this drug is less effective than fluconazole due to variations in its absorption in the body.

Researchers state that evidence of the efficacy, safety, and use of itraconazole for CMC is primarily limited to individual case studies. In one instance, researchers reported the use of itraconazole in two children with CMC of the mouth and fingernails. These children were given itraconazole for two months, and this antifungal produced a rapid cure in both children. This drug was well tolerated. In a review article, itraconazole was reported to cure more than 80% of patients with superficial fungal infections. According to these researchers, this antifungal may be used as a preventive treatment in patients with CMC.

For more information see page 1256.

SEXUALLY TRANSMITTED DISEASES

Sexually transmitted diseases (STDs) are bacterial or viral infections that are acquired through sexual contact with an infected person. Usually, STDs are passed through sexual intercourse;

however, they can also be passed through other forms of sex. Anyone who is sexually active is at risk for having an STD. The risk for STDs increases if a person has multiple sex partners or unprotected sex (without a condom). Symptoms of STDs vary according to the specific infection. STDs include chancroid, chlamydia, granuloma inguinale, herpes simplex, lymphoma venereum, and syphilis.

Chancroid

Chancroid is a sexually transmitted genital ulcer disease that is caused by the bacteria *Haemophilus ducreyi*. Chancroid is characterized by painful ulcers and swelling and/or inflammation of the lymph nodes in the groin, and is spread by sexual contact. Symptoms of chancroid generally appear within one week after exposure to the bacteria. They are often less noticeable in women and may be limited to painful urination or defecation, painful sexual intercourse, rectal bleeding, or vaginal discharge.

OFF-LABEL PRESCRIPTION DRUG
BREAKTHROUGH OPTION

*Generic: **Erythromycin** (er-ith-roe-MYE-sin)*
*Brands: **Akne-Mycin, E.E.S., Eryc, Ery-Tab, Erythrocin***

Erythromycin belongs to a class of drugs called macrolide antibiotics, and is used to prevent bacteria from producing proteins and to prevent growth and multiplication of bacteria. Antibiotic drugs, in general, are effective and well tolerated for chancroid; disease relapse after antibiotic use is around 5%. Repeating the original drug regimen is generally effective in disease relapse.

Erythromycin is typically used in a number of bacterial infections including throat and respiratory infections as well as other STDs such as syphilis and chlamydia. In patients with chancroid, oral erythromycin is used off-label to treat the ulcers caused by the bacteria *Haemophilus ducreyi*. In a clinical trial conducted in Nairobi, Kenya, researchers compared the antibiotic regimens of ciprofloxacin and erythromycin for chancroid. The cure rates in 111 patients treated for chancroid were 92% with ciprofloxacin and 91% for patients treated with erythromycin. In another study also conducted by researchers in Kenya, 219 patients with chancroid were treated with a low dose of erythromycin. In this study, low-dose erythromycin resulted in clinical cure in 88% of patients with HIV and 99% in patients without HIV. Researchers concluded that low-dose erthromycin is a cost-effective drug for chancroid; however, the healing process takes longer in patients with HIV.

For more information see page 1170.

Chlamydia

Chlamydia is a sexually transmitted diseases (STD) caused by the bacteria known as *Chlamydia trachomatis*. It is one of the most wide spread bacterial STDs in the United States and is acquired through oral, vaginal, or anal sexual contact with an infected person. The bacteria that cause chlamydia live in the semen and vaginal fluid, and infected persons may or may not have symptoms of infection. Symptoms generally occur within one to three weeks after infection and can include abnormal mucus or pus from the vagina or penis or pain during urination.

Commonly Prescribed (On-Label) Drugs: *Erythromycin, Ofloxacin, Sulfadiazine, Sulfamethoxazole, Sulfisoxazole*

OFF-LABEL PRESCRIPTION DRUGS
BREAKTHROUGH OPTIONS

*Generic: **Azithromycin** (az-ith-roe-MYE-sin)*
*Brands: **Zithromax Tri-Pak, Zithromax Z-Pak***

Azithromycin is a semi-synthetic (man-made) type of drug known as a macrolide antibiotic. Azithromycin is effective against a wide variety of bacterial organisms; in bacterial infections, azithromycin prevents bacteria from growing by interfering with its ability to produce proteins. It is commonly used to treat bacterial infections of the ear, throat, and sinuses; it is also used off label to treat chlamydia.

In a study conducted at University Hospital for Infectious Diseases in Croatia, 125 patients with chlamydia and chronic prostate infection were given either azithromycin or doxycycline (an antibiotic). Results from this study demonstrated that in people with chlamydia and chronic prostatitis, there was no significant difference between the eradication with either drug. In another study, researchers compared azithromycin with other antibiotics in pregnant women with chlamydia. Results from this study showed that use of azithromycin in these patients significantly improved cure rates and reduced drug side effects associated with other antibiotics. Another case noted that more obstetricians are using azithromycin in pregnant women with chlamydia because of its favorable side effect profile, improved treatment adherence, and efficacy.

For more information see page 1034.

Generic: **Doxycycline** *(doks-I-SYE-kleen)*
Brands: **Adoxa, Doryx, Doxy-100, Monodox, Periostat, Vibramycin, Vibra-Tabs**

Doxycycline belongs to a class of drugs known as tetracycline-type antibiotics, and is used to treat a wide variety of bacterial infections such as Lyme disease, acne, and STDs. In chlamydia, doxycycline is used off-label by preventing the growth and spread of bacteria.

When doxycycline is given for one week, it appears to be just as effective as a single-dose of azithromycin (an antibiotic) for chlamydia infections. In fact, clinical studies have continued to show that doxycycline and azithromycin have similar efficacy in curing chlamydia infections. A study of the activity of antibiotics on chlamydia, noted that the use of doxycycline for several years might be responsible for the high level of resistance to this drug in some regions of the world. When compared with other drugs (azithromycin or fluoroquinoline-type antibiotics) doxycycline showed the least activity on the *Chlamydia trachomatis* bacterium.

Researchers at the University Hospital for Infectious Diseases in Croatia conducted a study to examine 125 patients with chlamydia and chronic prostate infection. They were given either azithromycin or doxycycline. According to researchers, results demonstrated that there was no significant difference between the eradication or cure rates with either drug. However, a physician may prescribe doxycycline to you if you are resistant to other types of antibiotics.

For more information see page 1158.

Favre-Durand-Nicholas Disease

See Lymphogranuloma Venereum

Granuloma Inguinale

Granuloma inguinale is a bacterial sexually transmitted disease (STD) that is caused by the organism *Calymmatobacterium granulomatis*. Granuloma inguinale is often found in tropical and subtropical regions. Symptoms include a small, beefy-red bump on the genitals or perianal area that gradually eats away at the skin and forms an elevated, beefy-red, velvety nodule. Nodules are often painless and can bleed easily if traumatized. Other symptoms include spread of the disease to where the leg meets the torso and loss of skin color of the genitals. If untreated, granuloma inguinale can destroy the genital tissue.

Commonly Prescribed (On-Label) Drugs: *Streptomycin*

OFF-LABEL PRESCRIPTION DRUGS
BREAKTHROUGH OPTIONS

Generic: **Ciprofloxacin** *(sip-roe-FLOKS-a-sin)*
Brands: **Ciloxan, Cipro, Cipro XR**

Ciprofloxacin is an antibiotic that blocks the reproduction and multiplication of bacteria, and appears to stop tissue destruction seen in granuloma inguinale. According to investigators, in the treatment of granuloma inguinale, ciprofloxacin is considered a second-line treatment to the antibiotics trimethoprim-sulfamethoxazole or doxycycline, according to the Center for Disease Control (CDC). Antibiotics should be given for at least three weeks and continued until granuloma inguinale is completely gone. Researchers believe that evidence of the efficacy and safety of ciprofloxacin for the treatment of granuloma inguinale is limited to patient case studies. In one report, two researchers noted the successful treatment of granuloma inguinale with the treatment of ciprofloxacin. Despite effective treatment with antibiotic drugs, such as ciprofloxacin, granuloma inguinale can recur in six to 18 months.

For more information see page 1094.

Generic: **Erythromycin** *(er-ith-roe-MYE-sin)*
Brands: **Akne-Mycin, E.E.S., Eryc, Ery-Tab, Erythrocin**

Erythromycin is classified as a macrolide antibiotic, and is used to prevent bacteria from producing proteins used in bacterial growth and multiplication. In granuloma inguinale, erythromycin appears to stop the tissue destruction. Additionally, erythromycin is recommended in pregnant or breast-feeding women with granuloma inguinale. Antibiotics should be given for at least three weeks and continued until granuloma inguinale is completely gone.

In a review article, erythromycin was among the list of antibiotics that shows good activity and cellular penetration against bacteria associated with granuloma inguinale. In another review, researchers noted that treatment programs for granuloma inguinale involving erythromycin appear to be quite effective. Overall, despite effective treatment with antibiotics, such as erythromycin, granuloma inguinale can recur in six to 18 months.

For more information see page 1170.

Generic: **Trimethoprim-sulfamethoxazole**
(try-METH-oh-prim–sul-fah-meth-OX-ahzole)
Brands: **Bactrim, Septra**

Trimethoprim-sulfamethoxazole contains a combination of two drugs belonging to a class of drugs known as sulfonamide antibiotics. Together, trimethoprim and sulfamethoxazole inhibit bacterial growth in a variety of bacterial infections including ear, urinary, and respiratory infections, as well as some STDs.

A study conducted at the University of Zimbabwe evaluated the treatment of granuloma inguinale. Thirty seven patients with painless ulcers without involvement of the lymph nodes were treated and all patients responded well to a 14-day course of trimethoprim-sulfamethoxazole or a combination of other antibiotics. No new skin lesions formed after treatment was given. In another study, granuloma inguinale was safely and effectively treated with trimethoprim-sulfamethoxazole. Also, a 21-year-old man with penile sores for two months that were related to granuloma inguinale was successfully treated with trimethoprim-sulfamethoxazole. Despite effective treatment with antibiotic drugs, such as erythromycin, granuloma inguinale can recur in six to 18 months.

For more information see page 1530.

Lymphogranuloma Inguinale

See Lymphogranuloma Venereum

Lymphogranuloma Venereum

In lymphogranuloma venereum, a sexually transmitted disease (STD) caused by the bacteria *Chlamydia trachomatis*, inflammation and drainage of certain lymph nodes and destruction and scarring of surrounding tissue occurs. Symptoms of lymphogranuloma venereum include a small, painless ulcer on the genitals, swelling or redness of the skin in the groin, swollen groin lymph nodes, drainage from inguinal lymph nodes, drainage of blood or pus from the rectum, and pain during bowel movements. The main risk factor is having multiple sexual partners.

Commonly Prescribed (On-Label) Drugs: Doxycycline, Tetracycline

OFF-LABEL PRESCRIPTION DRUG
BREAKTHROUGH OPTION

Generic: ***Erythromycin*** (er-ith-roe-MYE-sin)
Brands: ***Akne-Mycin, E.E.S., Eryc, Ery-Tab, Erythrocin***

Erythromycin belongs to a class of drugs called macrolide antibiotics, and is used to prevent bacteria from producing proteins and to prevent growth and multiplication of bacteria. It is typically used in a number bacterial infections including throat, urinary, intestinal, and respiratory infections. In lymphogranuloma venereum, erythromycin is used off-label to cure the infection and prevent tissue damage. Although side effects are uncommon with erythromycin, upset stomach, diarrhea, vomiting, stomach cramps, mild skin rash, and stomach pain can occur.

Erythromycin is a well-recognized treatment for lymphogranuloma venereum. In a recent article, erythromycin was identified as a suitable treatment alternative for lymphogranuloma venereum. Use of erythromycin for lymphogranuloma venereum is further supported by the World Health Organization. Additionally, erthyromycin should be considered in women with lymphogranuloma venereum who are pregnant or breastfeeding, since tetracyclines are not indicated for use.

For more information see page 1170.

Nicolas-Favre Disease

See Lymphogranuloma Venereum

Soft Sore

See Chancroid

Soft Ulcer

See Chancroid

Tropical Bubo

See Lymphogranuloma Venereum

Venereal Sore

See Chancroid

Venereal Ulcer

See Chancroid

VIRAL DISEASES

A virus is a small, infectious organism that invades a cell to replicate (reproduce). Once the virus is in the body it will attach to a cell, enter it, and release its genetic material to produce new viruses. Viruses are spread through the air, through direct contact such as food, water or a handshake and through animal bites or parasites. Viral diseases include influenza, mononucleosis, varicella, and viral hemorrhagic fever.

Flu

See Influenza

Grip

See Influenza

Hemorrhagic Fever

See Viral Hemorrhagic Fever

Influenza

Influenza or "flu" is a viral infection of the lungs and airways that causes symptoms such as fever, runny nose, sore throat, cough, headache, muscle aches, and a feeling of illness. There are two types of influenza virus (type A and type B); however, within these types there are many different strains of the virus, which change each year. Influenza is spread by inhaling droplets that have been sneezed or coughed out by an infected person, or by having direct contact with an infected person's secretions.

Commonly Prescribed (On-Label) Drugs: *Amantadine, Oseltamivir, Rimantadine*

OFF-LABEL PRESCRIPTION DRUG
BREAKTHROUGH OPTION

Generic: **Ribavirin** *(rye-ba-VYE-rin)*
Brands: **Rebetol, Ribasphere, Virazole**

Ribavirin inhalation belongs to a class of drugs known as antivirals and is used to treat severe viral pneumonia in infants and children. This antiviral is generally given by breathing in the medicine as a fine mist through the mouth. In patients with influenza, ribavirin inhalation has been used for both influenza A and influenza B viruses. Additionally, the oral formulation of ribavirin has been used with some success for the treatment of infections caused by influenza A or B virus.

In studies involving adults with influenza A infection, ribavirin inhalation treatment was shown to decrease the degree and duration of fever, decrease the severity of body symptoms, and decrease the shedding of the virus in respiratory fluids. It also, increased the rate of symptomatic recovery. Alternatively, in another study, ribavirin inhalation did not significantly affect the degree and duration of the clinical manifestations of influenza A.

In clinical studies of patients with influenza B infection, ribavirin inhalation appeared to be effective in increasing the rate of symptom improvement as well as decreasing fever, the severity of systematic symptoms, and viral shedding in the respiratory fluids.

For more information see page 1446.

Influenza Prevention

Influenza or "flu" occurs in the lungs and airways and causes symptoms of fever, runny nose, sore throat, cough, headache, muscle aches, and a feeling of illness. There are several vaccines available as prevention against influenza; however, as they contain live virus, they should not be given to those with weak immune systems or to pregnant women. In such cases, other treatment options are available.

Commonly Prescribed (On-Label) Drugs: *Amantadine, Oseltamivir, Rimantadine*

OFF-LABEL PRESCRIPTION DRUG
BREAKTHROUGH OPTION

Generic: **Zanamivir** *(zan-AH-meh-vir)*
Brand: **Relenza**

Zanamivir, a type of antiviral known as a neuraminidase inhibitor, is approved by the U.S. FDA to treat influenza A and B viruses, the viruses responsible for the "flu." Zanamivir also prevents the spread of both of these viruses; however, it is used off label for influenza prevention. On average, zanamivir reduces the duration of symptoms by one day if treatment is started within 48 hours after symptoms begin.

Zanamivir is given by oral inhalation. The most common side effects include headaches, diarrhea, nausea, cough, vomiting, and dizziness, among others. People with respiratory diseases such as asthma may have difficulty breathing with the use of this drug. In a large study in healthy patients, preventive treatment with zanamivir for 28 days at the beginning of an influenza A outbreak resulted in 84% protective rate in preventing influenza with fever. In another study, nursing home patients received zanamivir during separate influenza A and B outbreaks. In those patients who used zanamivir, no influenza was detected by lab tests.

For more information see page 1550.

Mononucleosis/Epstein-Barr (Complicated)

Infectious mononucleosis is a syndrome caused by the Epstein Barr virus (a member of the herpes virus family), which is very common in children and adolescents. Symptoms of infectious mononucleosis include fever, sore throat, and swollen lymph glands. Transmission of the virus involves intimate contact with saliva of an infected person. Symptoms generally appear within four to six weeks after infection and include upper airway obstruction, splenic rupture, fatigue, and a number of other relatively rare manifestations.

Commonly Prescribed (On-Label) Drugs: *None*

OFF-LABEL PRESCRIPTION DRUGS
BREAKTHROUGH OPTIONS

Generic: **Acyclovir** *(ay-SYE-kloe-veer)*
Brand: **Zovirax**

Acyclovir belongs to a class of drugs known as antivirals. It is often used to treat herpes simplex viruses and block the replication of the Epstein Barr virus in affected people. According to experts, antivirals such as acyclovir are of no benefit in uncomplicated infectious mononucleosis. In clinical studies conducted by the Department of Infectious Diseases at Regional Hospital in Varese, Italy, acyclovir inhibited viral shedding. In an analysis of five trials involving 339 patients, acyclovir use resulted in less viral shedding at the end of therapy, however, this antiviral did not offer consistent or significant benefit. In general, antivirals for mononucleosis are not recommended for routine use.

For more information see page 989.

Generic: **Immune Globulin IV** *(EH-mune GLOB-ewe-lyn)*
Brands: **Gamimune N, Gamunex, Octagam, Polygam S/D, Venoglobulin S**

Immune globulin IV belongs to a class of drugs known as immunoglobulins or immunizing agents. Immune globulin IV is used to modulate immune function in the presence of viral autoantibodies. In the treatment of complicated infectious mononucleosis, this immune globulin has been used successfully to treat low blood platelet count (thrombocytopenia). In this viral disease, immune globulin IV regulates inflammatory cells, and suppresses specific immune cells.

In a small study, five patients with infectious mononucleosis-related severe thrombocytopenia were treated with intravenous immune globulin (IVIG) for two to five days. In this study at the University of Rochester Medical Center, four of the five patients rapidly developed significant increases in their platelet counts. Researchers concluded that immune globulin IV may also be effective in infectious mononucleosis-related severe thrombocytopenia.

For more information see page 1235.

Generic: **Prednisone** *(pred-NIS-zone)*
Brands: **Deltasone, Liquid Pred, Meticorten, Orasone, Sterapred**

Prednisone belongs to a class of drugs known as corticosteroids and is similar to a natural hormone produced in the body's adrenal glands. Corticosteroids are strong anti-inflammatory drugs that modify your body's immune response and are used in infectious mononucleosis to decrease tonsil size and lymph nodes in airway obstruction. Moreover, corticosteroids may be helpful in treating low blood platelets. Prednisone is thought to decrease inflammation.

In general, doctors will prescribe you prednisone to control the swelling of the throat and tonsils in infectious mononucleosis. Use of steroids, such as prednisone, have been reported to reduce the overall length and severity of illness. Additionally, corticosteroids, such as prednisone, may be helpful in other complications such as heart or brain inflammation.

For more information see page 1429.

Varicella

Varicella (also known as chickenpox) is caused by the varicella-zoster virus, a member of the human herpes virus. Varicella is a common and highly contagious virus and affects nearly all susceptible children before adolescence. The varicella virus enters through the respiratory system and colonizes the upper respiratory tract; it is characterized by a red, itchy rash that develops into blisters on the skin all over the body. Varicella's infectious period begins two days before skin lesions appear and ends when the lesions crust, usually five days later. A severe form of chicken pox involves a bacterial infection on the skin around the blisters, bones, lungs, joints, and blood.

Commonly Prescribed (On-Label) Drugs: *Acyclovir*

OFF-LABEL PRESCRIPTION DRUGS
BREAKTHROUGH OPTIONS

Generic: **Dexamethasone** *(deks-a-METH-a-sone)*
Brands: **Decadron, Dexameth, Dexone, Hexadrol**

Dexamethasone belongs to a class of drugs known as corticosteroids. It is similar to a natural hormone produced by the adrenal glands in the body and is used to replace this hormone when your body does not make enough. Dexamethasone has been found to relieve inflammation; it is used to treat certain forms of arthritis; skin, blood, kidney, eye, thyroid, and intestinal disorders; severe allergies; and asthma. Common side effects associated with the use of dexamethasone include upset stomach, vomiting, headache, dizziness, insomnia, depression, and anxiety, among others. The use of dexamethasone can make you more susceptible to certain illnesses and infections. It is recommended that you consult your doctor if you have been exposed to varicella or other infectious diseases prior to using this corticosteroid.

Researchers documented the use of dexamethasone or other corticosteroids in patients with inflammation of the cornea as a result of varicella. In one specific instance in this report, a patient with herpes infection of the eye was given dexamethasone three times daily. This drug was then terminated when the diagnosis was changed to varicella of the cornea. Corneal lesions then resolved; however, dexamethasone was reinstituted when lesions reappeared that did not test positive for varicella. Researchers concluded that most of the patients in this case report were given topical corticosteroids to control their eye symptoms, and these medications induced corneal inflammation in the presence of varicella.

For more information see page 1138.

Generic: **Tacrolimus** *(ta-KROE-li-mus)*
Brands: **Prograf, Protopic**

Tacrolimus belongs to a class of drugs known as immunosuppressants. Topical tacrolimus is often used to treat symptoms of a skin disease known as atopic dermatitis (also known as eczema); it can also be used in a wide variety of skin conditions. Tacrolimus works by stopping the immune system from making substances that cause atopic dermatitis. If you have been exposed to varicella while using tacrolimus, consult your physician immediately.

With the use of tacrolimus, isolated cases of adverse events that were considered serious included varicella that required hospitalization or visits to an emergency room. Particular attention has been paid to skin infections as a potential complication of topical treatment with an immunosuppressive agent, such as tacrolimus. Viral, fungal, and bacterial infections have all been reported. With the use of tacrolimus, herpes simplex infection is occasionally seen, and has been reported in 3 to 8% of people. Other viral infections seen with the use of tacrolimus include varicella. In a study, the incidence of varicella occurred in less than 5% of patients receiving topical tacrolimus. In the five cases of varicella in this study, the children were eight years or younger and had a normal course of the disease.

For more information see page 1498.

Viral Hemorrhagic Fever

Viral hemorrhagic fever consists of a diverse group of infections from various types of viruses (*Arenaviridae* and *Filoviridae* viral families). Viral hemorrhagic fever can cause mild illnesses, although many of these viruses are severe, often life-threatening in nature. Symptoms include fever, fatigue, dizziness, muscle weakness, and exhaustion; in severe illness, symptoms can include bleeding under the skin, in internal organs, or from the mouth, ears, and eyes. Viruses typically live in animals and can be spread by contact with urine, feces, or saliva from infected animals (rats) or from insect bites (ticks). In some instances, the virus can be contracted from the human secretions.

Commonly Prescribed (On-Label) Drugs: *None*

OFF-LABEL PRESCRIPTION DRUG
BREAKTHROUGH OPTION

*Generic: **Ribavirin** (rye-ba-VYE-rin)*
*Brands: **Rebetol, Ribasphere, Virazole***

Ribavirin belongs to a class of drugs known as antivirals and is used to treat a variety of viral hemorrhagic fevers such as Lassa fever and Hantavirus infections. Side effects associated with this drug include sour stomach, dizziness, feeling cold, irritability, and itching skin, among others. In Lassa fever, ribavirin has been effective when used orally or IV and is considered to be the drug of choice in treatment of this form of viral hemorrhagic fever.

In clinical studies conducted in Hamburg, Germany, use of ribavirin has been associated with decreased death in patients with naturally occurring Lassa fever. This antiviral was most effective when given early on in the infection (within six to seven days from onset of symptoms). In patients who are severely ill, experts support the use of this drug before diagnosis is confirmed. In a study, researchers found that ribavirin reduced the growth of the Crimean-Congo hemorrhagic fever virus in the liver, and significantly decreased the presence of the virus in the bloodstream of mice. Even though mice in this study had severe infection, the virus was not detected in the heart or brain in treated mice.

In another study, patients with Crimean-Congo hemorrhagic fever were treated with oral ribavirin. After treatment, the efficacy of oral ribavirin was noted to be 80% in patients with confirmed Crimean-Congo hemorrhagic fever and 34% in those suspected of having it. Researchers concluded that ribavirin is an effective treatment for the hemorrhagic fever of Crimean-Congo infection.

For more information see page 1446.
For more information see page 1446.

KIDNEY AND URINARY TRACT DISORDERS

BLADDER CONDITIONS

The bladder is the pouch where urine is kept before it exits the body. Urine is kept from draining out of the bladder by the urethral sphincter, which tightens or releases. Normally, you can consciously control the sphincter and, hence, the timing of when you urinate. But a variety of bladder conditions may cause loss of such control.

Bed-wetting

See Nocturnal Enuresis

Hunner Ulcer

See Interstitial Cystitis

Interstitial Cystitis

Also called painful bladder syndrome, interstitial cystitis causes symptoms ranging from mild discomfort and tenderness to intense pain in the bladder and surrounding pelvic area. In addition, you may experience changes in the degree of urgency and frequency of urination. Physicians believe that this condition is caused by the release of histamine from mast cells within the body. Mast cells are attached to the body's tissues and organs and are responsible for controlling many of the body's allergic reactions. When your body comes into contact with an allergen, your mast cells release histamine-containing granules, ultimately causing swelling. Symptoms vary over time. Because of the diversity of symptoms from one person to the next, physicians suspect that this is not one disease but rather several diseases that have yet to be sorted out.

Commonly Prescribed (On-Label) Drugs: Pentosan Polysulfate Sodium

---

OFF-LABEL PRESCRIPTION DRUGS
BREAKTHROUGH OPTIONS

Generic: **Amitriptyline** *(a-mee-TRIP-ti-leen)*
Brand: **Elavil**

In a study in *The Journal of Urology*, of 48 men and women suffering from interstitial cystitis, half were given amitriptyline and the other half a placebo. After four months, the patients taking amitriptyline saw their symptoms improve significantly, with the symptom score decreasing from 26.9 to 18.5 in that group. The placebo group saw a small improvement. Pain and urgency intensity lessened in a significant way. The investigators concluded that amitriptyline therapy is safe and effective for four months, although they noted that most of the patients taking it had expected anticholinergic side effects (actions of medications that reduce the spasms of smooth muscles), and many suffered dry mouth.

For more information see page 1009.

Generic: **Cimetidine** *(sye-MET-i-deen)*
Brand: **Tagamet**

Cimetidine reduces the release of acid in the stomach and is normally prescribed to treat or prevent ulcers. Because mast cells within the bladder wall has been identified as a contributing factor in the inflammatory process involved in interstitial cystitis, this condition may be related to the body's release of histamine. Based on this hypothesis, researchers suggested that the use of antihistaminic medications may possibly be beneficial.

In a clinical trial of 36 patients published in *British Journal of Urology International*, the cimetidine group had a significant improvement in overall symptoms, including less pubic pain and nocturia (night time urination). In a trial of 14 patients, published in the same journal, eight patients' symptoms improved. In another small open trial of nine patients, published in *Urology*, six had moderate to complete relief and were maintained on the drug for more than two years. No adverse reactions were observed in any of these studies.

While cimetidine would not be considered a first choice of treatment for interstitial cystitis, physicians may prescribe this drug if your problems seem resistant to other therapies.

For more information see page 1091.

Mixed Incontinence

People with mixed incontinence have symptoms of both urge incontinence (an overactive bladder) and stress incontinence (inability to control urination). In such situations, it can be difficult to distinguish exactly what is occurring, but in fact the two conditions are actually found together. Physicians maintain that the best treatment is to combine the treatments used for both disorders.

Commonly Prescribed (On-Label) Drugs: None

OFF-LABEL PRESCRIPTION DRUG
BREAKTHROUGH OPTION

Generic: **Imipramine** (im-IP-ra-meen)
Brands: **Tofranil, Tofranil-PM**

Imipramine is a tricyclic antidepressant, a class of drugs used for many health problems other than depression because they have numerous other therapeutic effects. Notably, they have several effects that help people suffering with mixed incontinence. Imipramine is the tricyclic antidepressant most often used for urge incontinence. It is prescribed for urge, stress, and mixed incontinence. Imipramine is often prescribed together with tolterodine or oxybutynin for this condition.

Experts at Virginia Mason Medical Center believe that imipramine inhibits unstable contractions and strengthens the urethral sphincter mechanism, that is, the muscles at the neck of the bladder. According to *Reviews in Urology*, imipramine can decrease bladder contractions. Researchers believe the main reason why imipramine and other tricyclic antidepressants are not more widely used to treat urge incontinence is because of their bothersome side effects such as dry mouth and sedation.

For more information see page 1230.

Nocturia

Nocturia refers to being awakened at night by the need to pass urine. While this is uncommon under the age of 60, it becomes more usual and frequent with aging due to reduced bladder capacity and function and, in men, prostate problems. It can occur in otherwise healthy elderly men and women or may be the first symptom of a variety of medical problems, such as diabetes or kidney disease. If no underlying disease is found and a reduction in fluid intake fails to solve the problem, you may need drug treatment to help.

Commonly Prescribed (On-Label) Drugs: *Desmopressin*

OFF-LABEL PRESCRIPTION DRUGS
BREAKTHROUGH OPTIONS

Generic: Diuretics such as **Bumetanide** *(byoo-MET-a-nide)* and **Furosemide** *(fyoor-OH-se-mide)*
Brands: **Bumex (bumetanide) and Lasix (furosemide)**

Bumetanide and furosemide are diuretics, commonly called "water pills." They block the reabsorption of sodium in the kidney, thus promoting the excretion of urine. Diuretics are widely prescribed to people with heart failure and hypertension as a way of reducing fluid volume in the body. In these cases, people generally take them first thing in the morning so that they can urinate on and off to get rid of the excess volume and then not worry about having to be near a toilet the rest of the day.

A report in *British Journal of Urology* on a clinical trial of bumetanide showed that the weekly number of nocturia episodes was 13.8 during the placebo period and was reduced by 3.8 during the bumetanide period. According to researchers, the nocturia episodes were reduced by four during the bumetanide period.

Since both furosemide and bumetanide tend to drain potassium from the body, your doctor may advise you to eat a diet rich in potassium from sources such as bananas and oranges or may prescribe potassium supplements.

For more information see pages 1057 and 1204.

*Generic: **Imipramine** (im-IP-ra-meen)*
*Brands: **Tofranil, Tofranil-PM***

Imipramine is one of a class of drugs called tricyclic antidepressants, but it has numerous therapeutic effects and is prescribed for many other health problems. Notably, it can help bladder problems. According to *Reviews in Urology*, imipramine is commonly prescribed for stress and urge incontinence because it can decrease bladder contractions but cause muscles at the bladder neck to contract, thus strengthening the exit. Based on these facts, physicians thought that imipramine would be useful in the elderly with nocturia even though the precise way that imipramine works is not fully understood. It may work at the neurotransmitter level (chemicals in the brain), by improving bladder capacity and/or by increasing an antidiuretic hormone. Physicians who prescribe imipramine for bladder disorders usually begin with a relatively low dose and increase it for the desired effect.

For more information see page 1230.

Nocturnal Enuresis

Enuresis means bed-wetting during sleep, and nocturnal enuresis refers to an inability to control the flow of urine at night. Since it is common for toddlers to wet the bed because they have not yet learned to control the flow of urine effectively, the usual definition of nocturnal enuresis is bed-wetting over the age of five years. The condition is also called urinary incontinence.

Commonly Prescribed (On-Label) Drugs: Belladonna, Scopolamine

OFF-LABEL PRESCRIPTION DRUGS
BREAKTHROUGH OPTIONS

*Generic: **Atomoxetine** (AT-oh-mox-e-teen)*
*Brand: **Straterra***

Atomoxetine belongs to a class of drugs called selective serotonin reuptake inhibitors (SSRIs), drugs that affect brain chemistry. Unlike others in its class, atomoxetine is primarily used to treat children who have attention deficit/hyperactivity disorder (ADHD). During clinical trials of the drug for that use, some of the parents reported that children who had bedwetting problems were having more dry nights. This led to another study to evaluate the drug for nocturnal enuresis. In a study, 35.7% of those treated with atomoxetine had an increase of at least two dry nights per week, compared with 14.6% of those who received a placebo. Researchers are unsure why atomoxetine works, but theorize that the drug likely stimulates the release of norepinephrine—a messenger of the sympathetic nervous system—that helps control the problem. Journal of Child and Adolescent Psychopharmacology reported on four children with attention deficit/hyperactivity disorder who were treated with atomoxetine. Like the children reported on in the American Psychiatric Association study, these four also had suffered with bedwetting and experienced resolution of their problems. It should be noted that in late 2004, the package labeling for this drug was revised to include a new warning regarding the potential for liver toxicity. Thus, according to physicians, other drug therapy may be more suitable.

For more information see page 1028.

Generic: Selective serotonin reuptake inhibitors such as
Fluoxetine *(floo-OKS-e-teen)* and **Fluvoxamine**
(floo-VOKS-a-meen)
Brands: **Prozac, Prozac Weekly, Sarafem (fluoxetine),**
Luvox (fluvoxamine)

Fluoxetine and fluvoxamine are of a class of drugs called selective serotonin reuptake inhibitors (SSRIs) that are now widely prescribed for major depressive disorder and certain other psychiatric problems. Because these drugs have other effects, they are also prescribed off-label for some non-psychiatric problems. Because psychiatrists have noted a cessation of bedwetting in youngsters being treated with SSRIs for other problems, studies were done testing these drugs for bed-wetting alone. Three case reports on fluoxetine show that benefits start within two to four weeks of beginning therapy. In all three of the published case reports, enuresis completely ended as long as patients remained on the drug.

Additionally, in a clinical trial of 18 children with bed-wetting reported in the *Journal of the American Academy of Child and Adolescent Psychiatry*, fluvoxamine was effective in 78%, completely halting the problem in 28% and reducing the frequency of the episodes in 50%. In two case reports in the same journal, the drug reduced the episodes in one patient and banished the problem in the other. A recent survey reported in *Pediatrics* showed that 10% of pediatricians and 20% of family practitioners had prescribed an SSRI for enuresis.

How fluoxetine works is unknown, but theories suggest it acts through a variety of brain messenger chemicals. Physicians suggest that because these drugs increase levels of serotonin throughout the body, they cause a relaxation of smooth muscle in the bladder, thus lowering any unwanted tendency to contract and lose urine.

For more information see pages 1192 and 1199.

Generic: Selective serotonin reuptake inhibitors such as **Paroxetine** *(pa-ROKS-e-teen)* and **Sertraline** *(SER-tra-leen)* Brands: **Paxil, Paxil CR (paroxetine) and Zoloft (sertraline)**

Paroxetine and sertraline are in a class of drugs called selective serotonin reuptake inhibitors (SSRIs) that are often prescribed for major depressive disorder and certain other psychiatric problems. In contrast to some SSRIs, published reports in the medical literature on the use of paroxetine and sertraline are limited. In one case of a teenage boy with bed-wetting reported in the *Journal of Developmental and Behavioral Pediatrics,* therapy with paroxetine was begun for psychiatric reasons, including depression and anxiety. Within two days, his bed-wetting ended. Over the next six months, it recurred only within 48 hours of missing his paroxetine doses.

Another case of a boy with bed-wetting reported in the *Journal of the American Academy of Child and Adolescent Psychiatry* who was treated with sertraline completely resolved his bed-wetting. Researchers observed that recurrence occurred only during a two-week period when the youngster was unable to take the drug due to a lack of supply, but the enuresis stopped as soon as he started taking it again.

For more information see pages 1395 and 1468.

Nycturia

See Nocturia

Polydipsia

Drinking lots of water is usually healthy, and doctors generally advise drinking eight glasses a day. However, if you have the urge to drink excessively it may reflect an underlying physical or emotional illness. Excessive thirst may be a symptom of high blood sugar (hyperglycemia) and can be an important clue in detecting diabetes.

Commonly Prescribed (On-Label) Drugs: *None*

OFF-LABEL PRESCRIPTION DRUGS
BREAKTHROUGH OPTIONS

Generic: Antihypertensives such as **Clonidine** *(KLON-i-deen)* and **Enalapril** *(e-NAL-a-pril)*
Brands: **Catapres, Catapres-TTS, Duraclon (clonidine) and Vasotec, Vasotec I.V. (enalapril)**

Clonidine and enalapril are angiotensin-converting enzyme (ACE) inhibitors. They block an enzyme in the body that is necessary to produce a substance that causes blood vessels to tighten. As a result, it relaxes blood vessels, lowers blood pressure, and increases the supply of blood and oxygen to the heart, so physicians widely use enalapril and clonidine to treat hypertension. According to the Columbia University College of Physicians and Surgeons, ACE inhibitors have been investigated in the treatment of polydipsia. A researcher reported that a study using enalapril helped dampen weight fluctuations in people with polydipsia.

In a study in *Neuropsychopharmacology*, enalapril and clonidine were tested on 14 people who suffered from psychogenic polydipsia. Researchers observed that improvement with either or both drugs in about 60% of the participants, although they recommended that further studies be done.

For more information see pages 1108 and 1166.

*Generic: **Clozapine** (KLOE-za-peen)*
*Brand: **Clozaril***

Clozapine is a drug normally prescribed for schizophrenia. These patients also often develop excessive thirst and experience hyponatremia, a condition known as "water intoxication," apathy, confusion, nausea, and fatigue and, eventually if untreated, coma and even death. *European Archives of Psychiatry and Clinical Neurosciences* reported on a physician's experience with patients with polydipsia in a U.S. psychiatric hospital over a five-year period. Two polydipsic patients worsened when switched from clozapine to other antipsychotic drugs, and the investigator urged that polydipsic patients be maintained on clozapine unless new prospective studies prove that other antipsychotics are as effective as clozapine for polydipsia.

Journal of Neuropsychiatry and Clinical Neuroscience found that switching eight schizophrenic men from another anti-schizophrenia drug to clozapine was an effective therapy for their hyponatremia. Based on these results, researchers concluded that this drug appears to be the first effective treatment for the severe water imbalance seen in this psychiatric disorder.

However, because clozapine has serious side effects such as seizures and cardiovascular and respiratory effects, it is unlikely that it would be prescribed for polydipsia due to other causes.

For more information see page 1111.

Stress Incontinence

Stress incontinence is a sudden involuntary loss of urine that occurs during physical activity, such as exercise, or simply due to coughing, sneezing, or laughing. It is the most common type of urinary incontinence in women. Stress incontinence occurs when the urethral sphincter is weakened and unable to prevent urine flow when pressure from the abdomen increases.

Commonly Prescribed (On-Label) Drugs: None

OFF-LABEL PRESCRIPTION DRUGS
BREAKTHROUGH OPTIONS

Generic: Tricyclic antidepressants such as **Desipramine** *(des-IP-ra-meen)*, **Imipramine** *(im-IP-ra-meen)*, and **Nortriptyline** *(nor-TRIP-ti-leen)*
Brands: Norpramin (desipramine), Tofranil, Tofranil-PM (imipramine) and Aventyl, Pamelor (nortriptyline)

Desipramine, imipramine, and nortriptyline are tricyclic antidepressants that are sometimes used for bladder problems because they can reduce unstable muscle contractions in the bladder. In a study in *British Journal of Obstetrics and Gynecology* on imipramine for women with stress incontinence, a majority of the 40 patients' symptoms were improved or cured, though treatment failed in 40%. Women were successfully treated with imipramine three times a day for three months.

According to physicians, the main reason why desipramine, imipramine, and nortriptyline are not more widely used to treat stress incontinence is because of their bothersome side effect profile such as dry mouth and sedation.

For more information see pages 1132, 1230, and 1378.

Urge Incontinence

Urge incontinence starts with a sudden strong need to urinate immediately followed by a bladder contraction, resulting in an involuntary loss of urine. It is also known as overactive bladder, irritable bladder, unstable bladder, or Detrusor instability. The Detrusor is the external longitudinal layer of muscle coating the bladder.

Commonly Prescribed (On-Label) Drugs: Estrogens, Tolterodine

OFF-LABEL PRESCRIPTION DRUGS
BREAKTHROUGH OPTIONS

Generic: Tricyclic antidepressants such as **Desipramine**
(des-IP-ra-meen), **Imipramine** *(im-IP-ra-meen)*, and
Nortriptyline *(nor-TRIP-ti-leen)*
Brands: **Norpramin (desipramine), Tofranil, Tofranil-PM
(imipramine) and Aventyl, Pamelor (nortriptyline)**

Desipramine, imipramine, and nortriptyline belong to a class of
drugs called tricyclic antidepressants that have many other therapeutic effects in the body. Most important for people with urge incontinence, according to *Reviews in Urology*, they can decrease
bladder contractions. Some experts believe it works because it
blocks the passage of impulses through the low back nerves that
inhibits unstable contractions and thereby helps reduce urge incontinence.

Imipramine is the tricyclic antidepressant most often mentioned
for urge incontinence in the research literature. However, one researcher believes that it is effective for urge incontinence only if
the problem occurs during sleep. Imipramine is often prescribed
together with tolterodine or oxybutynin. *European Urology* reported on the potency of nortriptyline, including a clinical trial of
low dosage therapy that benefited more than 70% of the patients
treated.

Physicians note that the main reason why desipramine, imipramine, and nortriptyline are not more widely used to treat urge
incontinence is because of their wide array of side effects.

For more information see pages 1132, 1230, and 1378.

NEPHROTIC CONDITIONS

Nephrotic conditions are damage to the tiny blood vessels of the
kidney that filter waste and excess water from the blood. They include nephrotic syndrome and membranous nephropathy.

Membranous Nephropathy

Membranous nephropathy involves inflammation of the tiny blood vessels (glomeruli) that filter waste and excess water in the kidneys. They disrupt kidney function due to thickening of the blood vessel walls in the glomerular basement membrane (the boundary between blood and urine). Usually, physicians do not know the cause, although in 30% of cases it may be secondary to some other disorder. It is an immunologically mediated disease. Membranous nephropathy is the most common cause of nephrotic syndrome in adults.

Commonly Prescribed (On-Label) Drugs: Prednisolone

OFF-LABEL PRESCRIPTION DRUGS
BREAKTHROUGH OPTIONS

Generic: Statins such as ***Atorvastatin*** *(a-TORE-va-sta-tin)* and ***Simvastatin*** *(SIM-va-stat-in)*
Brands: **Lipitor (atorvastatin), Zocor (simvastatin)**

People with membranous nephropathy tend to have high cholesterol levels, which must be reduced to help heal the disease. Atorvastatin and simvastatin are commonly called "statins." This class of drugs is widely prescribed to adults who have high cholesterol levels and are trying to reduce their risk of a heart attack. Atorvastatin is among the most commonly used of these statin drugs. According to the Department of Internal Medicine of the State University of New York at Stony Brook, statins inhibit cholesterol in the liver and increase cholesterol metabolism. Statins specifically treat the cholesterol problem associated with membranous nephropathy.

Although they are two of the most widely prescribed drugs in the United States, physicians advise that atorvastatin and simvastatin should not be used if you have liver disease, and liver function tests must be done regularly. Pregnant women should not use them.

For more information see pages 1030 and 1474.

Generic: **Chlorambucil** *(khlor-AM-byoo-sil)*
Brand: **Leukeran**

Chlorambucil is normally prescribed to treat cancers such as leukemia, certain lymphomas, and Hodgkin's disease. It suppresses the immune system, and such immune suppressive drugs can prolong periods of remission in children with underlying nephrotic syndrome who relapse frequently after initial treatment with a corticosteroid. Further, chlorambucil can help stop the proteinuria (abnormal amount of protein in the urine) associated with membranous nephropathy.

A group of researchers conducted a search of the Cochrane Central Register of Controlled Clinical Trials, and various other reference lists of articles and abstracts of proceedings from scientific meetings to find out about evaluations of non-corticosteroid drugs used in children with nephrotic syndrome. They found two trials in which a chlorambucil/corticosteroid regimen significantly reduced the risk of relapse at six to 12 months compared to a corticosteroid alone.

An Italian study showed that remission of nephrotic syndrome was favored with a six-month course of therapy that alternated every other month with the steroid methylprednisone or chlorambucil. This study suggested that this approach protected long-term kidney function.

Because of the serious risk of inducing a secondary malignancy due to the bone marrow suppressing properties of chlorambucil, you should discuss the use of this drug with your physician to assure that the benefits outweigh the risks.

For more information see page 1079.

Generic: **Cyclosporine** *(si-klo-SPOR-een)*
Brands: **Gengraf, Neoral, Sandimmune**

Cyclosporine is a drug normally used to treat cancer. However, since it suppresses the immune system it is also frequently prescribed off-label to treat some autoimmune diseases, such as lupus, a condition where the body is attacking itself. This drug helps treat membranous nephropathy by helping normalize the immune system and activating important white blood cells called T lymphocytes.

According to physicians at the Gambro Healthcare Reliant Dialysis Center in Houston, Texas, cyclosporine is highly effective for frequently relapsing, steroid-sensitive nephrotic syndrome; half the children treated with it enter a prolonged remission. A review carried out by the Cochrane Central Register of Controlled Trials found a trial in which eight weeks of treatment with cyclosporine was as effective as eight weeks of chlorambucil, another immunosuppressive, with the effects persisting over the course of two years. An Italian study showed cyclosporine to be effective in inducing partial or complete remission.

Because of the serious risks of inducing hypertension, infections, or a malignancy due to the immunosuppression of cyclosporine, you should discuss the use of this drug with your physician to assure that the benefits outweigh the risks.

For more information see pages 1125 and 1127.

Generic: Angiotensin-converting enzyme (ACE) inhibitors such as **Enalapril** *(e-NAL-a-pril)* and **Lisinopril** *(lyse-IN-oh-pril)*
Brands: **Vasotec, Vasotec I. V. (enalapril), Prinivil, Zestril (lisinopril)**

Enalapril and lisinopril are angiotensin-converting enzyme (ACE) inhibitors. They block an enzyme in the body that is necessary to produce a substance that causes blood vessels to tighten. As a result, they relax blood vessels, lower blood pressure, and increase the supply of blood and oxygen to the heart. Therefore, enalapril and lisinopril are widely used to treat hypertension, an important problem in membranous nephropathy. According to a report from the Department of Internal Medicine at the State University of New York at Stony Brook, by minimizing hypertension within the glomeruli (a part of the kidney that processes the filtration of the blood to form urine), ACE inhibition also decreases proteinuria (condition in which urine contains an abnormal amount of protein) in membranous nephropathy of unknown cause, thus specifically treating basic problems of the disorder.

ACE inhibitors are contraindicated in those who are hypersensitive to them or who develop angioedema (swelling of the ankles) in response. Enalapril must be used with caution if you have kidney impairment. Caution is advised in those with severe congestive heart failure or valvular stenosis for those taking enalapril. Safety for use in pregnancy has not been established.

Because of considerable interactions with other drugs, you should discuss the use of this drug with your physicians.

For more information see pages 1166 and 1284.

Generic: **Furosemide** *(fyoor-OH-se-mide)*
Brand: **Lasix**

Because people with membranous nephropathy have impaired kidney function, they suffer with fluid retention and have edema (swelling of an organ due to excess fluid). Therefore, according to the State University of New York at Stony Brook, one of the first drugs your physician is likely to prescribe is a diuretic—commonly known as a "water pill"—to promote the excretion of excess fluid and avoid excess fluid overload in the body. Furosemide is a potent diuretic because it blocks the reabsorption of sodium in the kidney. It also increases the therapeutic effect of other antihypertensive drugs, which may be prescribed for membranous nephropathy, so your doctor will want to monitor your blood pressure carefully.

According to physicians, caution is advised in prescribing this drug to people with kidney dysfunction, and, monitoring will be important. Further, since furosemide tends to drain potassium from the body, your doctor may advise a diet rich in potassium from sources such as bananas and oranges or may prescribe potassium supplements.

For more information see page 1204.

Generic: Non-steroidal anti-inflammatory drugs such as ***Ibuprofen*** *(eye-byoo-PROE-fen)*, **Ketoprofen** *(kee-toe-PROE-fen)*, and **Naproxen** *(na-PROKS-en)*
Brands: **Motrin, Ultraprin (ibuprofen), Oruvail (ketoprofen); Anaprox (DS), EC-Naprosyn, Naprelan, Naprosyn (naproxen)**

Ibuprofen, ketoprofen, and naproxen belong to a class called non-steroidal anti-inflammatory drugs (NSAIDs). They are

widely prescribed to inhibit pain and inflammation, especially
for arthritis. They work by decreasing the activity of cyclooxygenase, an enzyme responsible for synthesizing prostaglandin (a
hormone-like substance that affects contraction and relaxation
of smooth muscle) in the body. Interestingly, reduction of pain
and inflammation are beneficial in the management of kidney
pain, according to research reported from the University of
Michigan Medical Center. The Michigan Center for Minimally
Invasive Urology uses this oral NSAID for outpatient management but with a number of precautions.

For more information see pages 1228, 1261, and 1354.

*Generic: **Methylprednisolone** (meth-ill-pred-NIS-oh-lone)*
*Brands: **Depo-Medrol, Medrol, Solu-Medrol***

Methylprednisolone is a corticosteroid drug. It suppresses the
immune system and reduces inflammation. It is prescribed for a
wide range of diseases, including various types of arthritis,
blood disorders, skin diseases, allergic diseases, and much more.
According to a report from the Department of Internal Medicine at the State University of New York at Stony Brook methylprednisolone exerts an anti-inflammatory effect and thereby
induces remission of proteinuria (abnormal amounts of protein
in the urine). Italian research has also shown that it helps induce
remission of nephrotic syndrome, which is often the underlying
cause of membranous nephropathy.

In a typical regimen, methylprednisolone is given orally on alternate days with cyclophosphamide. Because both drugs place
patients at greater risk of infections, they should not be started
when patients have a viral, fungal or bacterial infection and patients should be monitored and let their doctors know right
away if they notice that they have developed such an infection.
Because of the potential serious toxicity of methylprednisolone,
you should discuss the use of this drug with your physician to assure that the benefits outweigh the risks. Once begun, it should
never be discontinued suddenly; it must be tapered off slowly
under your doctor's guidance.

For more information see page 1316.

Nephrosis

See Nephrotic Syndrome

Nephrotic syndrome

In nephrotic syndrome, people have very high levels of protein in the urine but very low levels of protein in the blood and high cholesterol. It results from damage to tiny blood vessels in the kidneys that filter waste and excess water from the blood and send them to the bladder as urine. The syndrome may be congenital in children, arise for no known cause, or develop secondary to some other disorder.

Commonly Prescribed (On-Label) Drugs: *Betamethasone, Bumetanide, Cortisone, Cyclophosphamide, Dexamethasone, Furosemide, Hydrocortisone, Methylprednisolone, Prednisolone, Prednisone, Spironolactone, Triamcinolone*

OFF-LABEL PRESCRIPTION DRUGS
BREAKTHROUGH OPTIONS

Generic: **Chlorambucil** (khlor-AM-byoo-sil)
Brand: **Leukeran**

Chlorambucil is a drug normally prescribed to treat such cancers as leukemia, certain lymphomas, and Hodgkin's disease. It suppresses the immune system, and such immune suppressive drugs can prolong periods of remission in those with nephrotic syndrome who relapse frequently after initial treatment with a corticosteroid. A group of researchers conducted a search of the Cochrane Central Register of Controlled Clinical Trials, and various other reference lists of articles and abstracts of proceedings from scientific meetings to find out about evaluations of non-corticosteroid drugs used in nephrotic syndrome. They found two trials in which chlorambucil significantly reduced the risk of relapse at six to 12 months compared to a corticosteroid alone.

In another trial, eight weeks of treatment with chlorambucil was as effective as eight weeks of cyclosporine, another immunosuppressive, with the treatment effect persisting over the course of two years. An Italian study showed that remission was favored with a six-month course of therapy that alternated every other month with the steroid methylprednisone or chlorambucil; the study suggested that this approach protected long-term kidney function.

Because of the serious risk of inducing a secondary malignancy due to the bone marrow suppressing properties of chlorambucil, you should discuss the use of this drug with your physician to assure that the benefits outweigh the risks.

For more information see page 1079.

*Generic: **Cyclosporine** (si-klo-SPOR-een)*
*Brands: **Gengraf, Neoral, Sandimmune***

Cyclosporine is normally used to treat cancer. However, since it suppresses the immune system it is also frequently prescribed to treat some autoimmune diseases, such as lupus, in which the body is attacking itself. According to physicians at the Gambro Healthcare Reliant Dialysis Center in Houston, Texas, cyclosporine is highly effective for frequently relapsing, steroid-sensitive nephrotic syndrome; half the children treated with it enter a prolonged remission. A review carried out by the Cochrane Central Register of Controlled Trials found a trial in which eight weeks of treatment with cyclosporine was as effective as eight weeks of chlorambucil, another immunosuppressive, with the treatment effect persisting over the course of two years. An Italian study showed cyclosporine to be effective in inducing partial or complete remission.

Because of the serious risks of inducing hypertension, infections, or a malignancy due to the immunosuppression of cyclosporine, you should discuss the use of this drug with your physician to assure that the benefits outweigh the risks.

For more information see pages 1125 and 1127.

*Generic: **Levamisole** (lee-VAM-i-sole)*
*Brand: **Ergamisol***

Levamisole is normally prescribed in the treatment of cancer. It is called an immunomodulator because it affects the immune system, although it does not tamp down the entire immune system in the way some other immune suppressants (such as corticosteroids) do. It even stimulates some aspects of the immune system, and has other therapeutic effects. Because it seems to regulate key steps of the immune system, researchers have found it useful for nephrotic syndrome.

The Cochrane Central Register of Controlled Trials found three trials in which levamisole was more effective than steroids alone, although the effect was not sustained. Researchers concluded that prolonged courses of levamisole reduce the risk of relapse in children with relapsing steroid-sensitive nephrotic syndrome compared with corticosteroids alone. A Serbian report suggested levamisole as one of useful alternatives for treatment of frequent relapses in children with steroid-dependent nephrotic syndrome.

Because of the potential serious toxicity of levamisole you should discuss the use of this drug with your physician to assure that the benefits outweigh the risks.

For more information see page 1275.

PREVENTION OF NEPHROTOXICITY

Nephrotoxicity refers in general to anything that can be toxic—that is, poisonous—to the kidney. However, in this section the topic is specifically situations in which medical treatment itself can create a threat to the kidney, either through diagnostic procedures or through therapy for disorders of other organs.

Nephrotoxicity Due to Coronary Procedures and CT Scan

Certain diagnostic procedures, such as CT scans and cardiac angiography, require that patients have substances called "radio-contrast agents" injected into their bloodstreams prior to the procedure. The contrast agents are essentially dyes that help to provide a clear picture during the diagnostic test. The contrast agents are injected into a vein. People who are at increased risk of radio-contrast agent-induced nephrotoxicity include those who have diabetes, kidney disease, or who are taking angiotensin-converting enzyme (ACE) inhibitors.

Commonly Prescribed (On-Label) Drugs: None

OFF-LABEL PRESCRIPTION DRUGS
BREAKTHROUGH OPTIONS

Generic: **Acetylcysteine** *(a-se-teel-SIS-teen)*
Brand: **Acetadote, Mucomyst**

Acetylcysteine is normally given as a nebulizing mist to people with abnormally sticky mucus secretions in such conditions as emphysema, chronic bronchitis, and tuberculosis. Or it may be given as a solution after acetaminophen overdose when it acts as a detoxifier to lessen liver injury. According to researchers, using acetylcysteine to prevent nephrotoxicity is based on its improving kidney function and preventing damage by enhancing oxidation.

In 10 trials involving more than a thousand patients, acetylcysteine has also been studied as a medication to protect the kidney when radio-contrast agents are used. The drug was given either orally or intravenously, together with intravenous infusions of saline started anywhere from two to 12 hours before the procedure and lasting up to 12 hours afterwards. Six of the 10 studies showed that acetylcysteine protected the kidney, while four found it to be no more effective than saline hydration alone. Researchers found that in the studies that showed acetylcysteine was effective, the drug was more effective than placebo in trials with the greatest number of high-risk patients, including those with more severe kidney damage and a higher incidence of diabetes, as well as in low-risk patients.

For more information see page 986.

Generic: **Sodium Bicarbonate**
(SOW-dee-um bye-KAR-bun-ate)
Brand: **Sodium Bicarbonate**

Sodium bicarbonate is widely used to de-acidify the stomach. It does this by altering the pH of the stomach contents. Researchers suggested that using sodium bicarbonate to prevent nephrotoxicity may work similarly, if added to the hydration solution given intravenously to patients before and after the procedure in order to increase the pH of the kidney.

In a trial of 119 patients, sodium bicarbonate infusion was given for one hour before and six hours after the contrast administration. The control group received sodium chloride. Participants were receiving diverse procedures such as cardiac catheterization, CT scans, and shunt placements. Tests of kidney function over the next two days showed that the group that received sodium bicarbonate experienced a significantly lower rate of radio-contrast induced nephropathy. Only one patient experienced an increase in blood pressure, indicating caution in use of this drug in people with hypertension.

For more information see page 1477.

Nephrotoxicity Due to Cyclosporine

Cyclosporine is used to treat a variety of autoimmune diseases, cancers, and to suppress rejection after some types of transplant surgery. However, it may damage the kidney by constricting and injuring the arteries and causing ischemia (inadequate blood flow) in the glomeruli (a part of the kidney that is responsible for the filtration of blood into urine). Medications can be given to help prevent such damage, notably those that reverse such constriction by relaxing the arteries in the kidneys.

Commonly Prescribed (On-Label) Drugs: *None*

OFF-LABEL PRESCRIPTION DRUGS
BREAKTHROUGH OPTIONS

Generic: Calcium channel antagonists such as **Diltiazem** *(dil-TYE-a-zem)*, **Felodipine** *(fe-LOE-di-peen)*, **Isradipine** *(iz-RA-di-peen)*, **Nifedipine** *(nye-FED-i-peen)*, and **Verapamil** *(vur-AP-ah-mill)*

Brands: **Cartia XT, Cardizem, Dilacor XR, Diltia XT, Taztia XT, Tiazac (diltiazem), Plendil (felodipine), DynaCirc, DynaCirc CR (isradipine), Adalat CC, Apo-Nifed (PA), Novo-Nifedin, Nu-Nifed, Procardia (nifedipine), Calan, Calan SR, Covera-HS, Isoptin SR, Verelan, Verelan PM (verapamil)**

Diltiazem, felodipine, isradipine, nifedipine, and verapamil are of a class of drugs called calcium channel antagonists and are usually prescribed to people with heart disease. By affecting the movement of calcium into the cells of the heart and blood vessels, they relax blood vessels and increase the supply of blood and oxygen to the heart while reducing its workload. Calcium channel blocking drugs, including diltiazem, felodipine, isradipine, nifedipine, and verapamil, are also prescribed to alleviate hypertension and angina, which they accomplish by alleviating ischemia (blockage of blood flow).

Similarly, diltiazem, felodipine, isradipine, nifedipine, and verapamil can relax the smooth muscle in the kidney's tiny blood vessels. These blood vessels' relaxation can help prevent kidney damage due to cyclosporine by allowing more blood and oxygen to reach all areas of the kidney. According to *Journal of Cardiovascular Pharmacology*, calcium channel blockers are the most frequently used drugs to help prevent such damage, due to their ability to dilate the tiny arterioles and reduce calcium within the cells.

In a Danish study of felodipine, reported in *Nephrology Dialysis and Transplant*, researchers concluded that these drugs showed improved kidney filtration rates following administration of felodipine despite cyclosporine use. However, of all the calcium channel blockers, the greatest experience has been with nifedipine.

For more information see pages 1146, 1182, 1255, 1360, and 1544.

STONES

Stones in the kidney and urinary tract are hard masses that form from crystals that separate from the urine. Those that develop in the kidney are called kidney stones. Those that are found in the ureters—the long tubes that carry urine from the kidneys to the bladder—are called ureteral stones. Stones usually contain chemicals, most commonly calcium, that are a normal part of our diet. Less commonly, they are caused by urinary tract infection or uric acid.

Calcinuric Diabetes

See Hypercalciuria

Cystinuria

Cystinuria is an inherited disorder. The kidneys filter the body's blood, keeping some substances (a process called reabsorption) and filtering out others for excretion. In cystinuria, certain important amino acids are not adequately reabsorbed, resulting in excess excretion. These amino acids may form crystals or stones in the kidneys, ureters, or bladder. Cystinuria is the least common cause of kidney stone formation, accounting for 3% or less of kidney stones.

Commonly Prescribed (On-Label) Drugs: Penicillamine, Tiopronin

OFF-LABEL PRESCRIPTION DRUG
BREAKTHROUGH OPTION

Generic: **Captopril** (KAP-toe-pril)
Brand: **Capoten**

Captopril belongs to a class of drugs called angiotensin-converting-enzyme (ACE) inhibitors. They block an enzyme in the body that is necessary to produce a substance that causes blood vessels to tighten. As a result, they relax blood vessels, lower blood pressure, and increase the supply of blood and oxygen to the heart. Therefore, these drugs are widely used to treat high blood pressure. Captopril is also used to treat kidney problems in some people with diabetes, and captopril may help slow down the further worsening of those kidney problems.

A study reported in *Journal of Endourology* found that captopril yielded significant improvement in urinary cystine capacity. Case reports in two non-U.S. professional journals of two children with cystinuria showed that after lithotripsy (a technique to break up stones using shock waves) to crush stones that were present or their surgical removal, captopril was given to prevent further stone formation. After a follow-up of up to 3-1/2 years, researchers found no stone recurrence in these youngsters.

For more information see page 1066.

Hypercalcinuria

See Hypercalciuria

Hypercalciuria

Hypercalciuria is the presence of an excessive amount of calcium in the urine. It is the most common cause of kidney stones caused by calcium that physicians have been able to identify. Medications used to reduce hypercalciuria include diuretics, bisphosphonates, vitamin D suppressors, and urinary macromolecules, alone or in combination in difficult cases. They should be used in conjunction with dietary therapy.

Commonly Prescribed (On-Label) Drugs: *Phosphates*

OFF-LABEL PRESCRIPTION DRUGS
BREAKTHROUGH OPTIONS

*Generic: **Amiloride*** *(a-MIL-oh-ride)*
*Brands: **Midamor***

Diuretics were originally intended to reduce fluid in the body and thereby reduce high blood pressure. According to the Kidney Stone Research Center at the Medical College of Ohio, they have become the primary medical treatment for hypercalciuria because of their ability to remove calcium from the urine and return it to the general circulation. They are useful in every type of hypercalciuria except resorptive hypercalciuria, where they can make the problem worse.

In contrast to the thiazide diuretics such as trichlormethiazide, amiloride is a potassium-sparing diuretic; that is, it does not drain the body of potassium. Therefore, patients usually do not have to take potassium citrate supplements or have diets with potassium-rich foods while taking these drugs. Although sometimes used alone, amiloride is generally used in combination with a thiazide. Amiloride reduces the magnesium loss caused by thiazide diuretics. According to physicians, it is the only potassium-sparing diuretic recommended for use in people who tend to form stones due to hypercalciuria. Triamterene, a chemical found in other potassium-sparing diuretics, is not advised because of its potential to trigger the formation of kidney stones.

Amiloride is not recommended in those who have hyperkalemia, kidney failure, diabetic kidney disease, or who have difficulty urinating. While it is generally considered safe in pregnancy, you and your doctor should decide if the benefits outweigh the risks.

For more information see page 1004.

Generic: Diuretics such as ***Indapamide*** *(in-DAP-ah-mide)* and ***Trichlormethiazide*** *(try-klor-met-THYE-a-zide)*
*Brands: **Lozol** (indapamide), **Diurese, Metahydrin, Naqua** (trichlormethiazide)*

Indapamide and trichlormethiazide are diuretics that reduce fluid in the body and are used to reduce hypertension. According to the Kidney Stone Research Center at the Medical College of Ohio, diuretics have become the primary medical treatment for hypercalciuria since they have a unique ability to remove calcium from the urine and return it to the general circulation. Diuretics can be useful in every type of hypercalciuria except resorptive hypercalciuria, where they can make the problem worse. They are especially useful in people with renal leak hypercalciuria, hypertension, or osteoporosis.

Trichlormethiazide is a long-acting thiazide diuretic that can be taken only once a day, and thiazides are one of the oldest types of diuretics in use. Indapamide, while not technically a thiazide, although its structure and function are very similar, can be taken only once daily; its effect on hypercalciuria is identical to the thiazides although side effects tend to be somewhat milder. However, because thiazide diuretics such as trichlormethiazide are sulfonamides, they can cause allergic reactions in people who have sulfa allergies.

For more information see pages 1237 and 1527.

Generic: **Ketoconazole** *(kee-toe-KOE-na-zole)*
Brand: **Nizoral**

Some types of hypercalciuria are vitamin D-dependent and, in those cases, drugs that suppress vitamin D can be useful in the diagnosis of the disease and in its treatment, according to experts at the Lorain Kidney Stone Research Center at the Medical College of Ohio. One such drug is ketoconazole, which is normally used as a broad-spectrum anti-fungal drug. However, since it interferes with the synthesis of vitamin D-3 by inhibiting a particular enzyme system, it has specific value in this type of hypercalciuria.

According to researchers, the long-term use of ketoconazole for hypercalciuria has to be balanced against its cost, adverse effects, and potential toxicity, especially on the liver, which requires careful monitoring. This must be carefully discussed with your physician, particularly since ketoconazole would not be a first-line choice.

Ketoconazole has documented hypersensitivity. It should not be used by those who have fungal meningitis, nor by those who are using the drugs terfenadine, astemizole, or cisapride. Caution should be used if you are taking certain other drugs because it may increase or decrease their effects or their toxicity, another subject to be discussed with your physician and which may require adjustment of other prescriptions.

For more information see page 1259.

Generic: **Pentosan Polysulphate**
(PEN-toe-san pol-i-SUL-fate)
Brand: **Elmiron**

Pentosan polysulphate is chemically and structurally similar to a form of carbohydrate called glycosaminoglycan, and it is normally used to treat a bladder problem called interstitial cystitis. In that disease, it is thought to help restore the glycosaminoglycans layers of the urinary bladder. Various studies have shown pentosan polysulphate to be potent inhibitors of crystal growth. Further, according to physicians at the Lorain Kidney Stone Research Center at the Medical College of Ohio, pentosan polysulphate occasionally may be helpful in inhibiting urinary crystal stone formation when other treatments are inadequate or unsuccessful. A study in *Renal Failure* in animals showed that in addition to reducing stone-forming constituents, it also decreased the extent of renal tubular damage.

Pentosan polysulphate is also a mild anticoagulant, which should be taken into consideration by those with bleeding problems or who take aspirin or anticoagulant drugs.

For more information see page 1404.

Generic: *Risedronate* (ris-ED-roe-nate)
Brand: *Actonel*

Risedronate is widely prescribed for the treatment of osteoporosis. It inhibits the activity of osteoclasts, cells that break down bone in the body. By inhibiting bone breakdown, the result is an increase in the amount of calcium that is deposited in bone. When more calcium is deposited in bone, less is left behind in the blood. When less is left behind in the blood, less goes into the kidneys to show up in the urine, thus directly treating hypercalciuria.

While diuretics are the first-line therapy for hypercalciuria, bisphosphonates such as risedronate, are a second-line therapy, according to physicians at the Lorain Kidney Stone Research Center of the Medical College of Ohio. The two classes of drugs may be used separately or together, and their effectiveness has been documented by research.

You should discuss carefully with your physician how to take this medication. Normally, it is taken first thing in the morning with water, and no food, beverages, or other medication is taken for 30 minutes, and you must remain in an upright position during that time. If this will be a problem, you must carefully work out some other regimen or plan an alternate medication. You should also discuss with your physician any history of ulcers or esophageal problems that might interfere with your ability to use this drug.

For more information see page 1454.

Hypercalcuria

See Hypercalciuria

Kidney Stones

Kidney stones are one of the most common disorders of the urinary tract. Most pass with no problem. But when larger ones get stuck in the ureter, they can cause enormous pain. The four main types are: stones that contain calcium that your kidneys have failed to flush out normally; struvite stones that may form after an infection; uric acid stones that may arise if you have too much acid in your urine; cystine stones, which are rare but tend to run in families.

Commonly Prescribed (On-Label) Drugs: None

OFF-LABEL PRESCRIPTION DRUGS
BREAKTHROUGH OPTIONS

Generic: Non-steroidal anti-inflammatory drugs such as **Ibuprofen** *(eye-byoo-PROE-fen)* and **Ketorolac** *(KEE-toe-role-ak)*
Brands: **Motrin, Ultraprin (ibuprofen), Toradol (ketorolac)**

Non-steroidal anti-inflammatory drugs (NSAIDs) such as ibuprofen and ketorolac are widely prescribed to inhibit pain and inflammation, especially for arthritis. The Michigan Center for Minimally Invasive Urology uses this oral NSAID for outpatient management but with a number of precautions. They also advise that ketorolac be intravenously administered since it is a much more powerful NSAID, as an inpatient treatment.

Ibuprofen, ketorolac, and other NSAIDs should not be taken by people with documented sensitivity to the drug, those with peptic ulcer disease, recent gastrointestinal (GI) bleeding or perforation, kidney insufficiency or at high risk of bleeding. It should also be used with caution by those who are pregnant (avoid in third trimester) or who have cardiovascular disease, including heart disease or who are at high risk of heart disease, including heart failure and hypertension and prior heart attack or stroke. Further caution is advised when taking ibuprofen and other

NSAIDs in conjunction with aspirin and a variety of other drugs, including hydralazine, captopril, beta-blockers, furosemide, thiazides, methotrexate, and phenytoin.

For more information see pages 1228 and 1263.

Generic: **Nifedipine** *(nye-FED-i-peen)*
Brands: **Adalat CC, Apo-Nifed (PA), Novo-Nifedin, Nu-Nifed, Procardia**

Nifedipine belongs to a class of drugs called calcium channel blockers that are commonly prescribed to people with heart disease. By affecting the movement of calcium into the cells of the heart and blood vessels, they relax blood vessels and increase the supply of blood and oxygen to the heart while reducing its workload. Calcium channel blocking drugs, including nifedipine, are also prescribed to relieve the chest pain called angina. These drugs are also used to treat high blood pressure. In the same way that nifedipine relaxes the lining of blood vessels, it can relax the smooth muscle in the ureters—the long tubes that carry urine from the kidneys to the bladder. When these tubes relax and loosen, it may be easier for a kidney stone to be released and pass out of the body.

Physicians at the Michigan Center for Minimally Invasive Urology advise that this therapy should be used for only five to 10 days. Further, because nifedipine itself can lower blood pressure, it should be used with great caution in conjunction with any other drug that can lower blood pressure, including beta-blockers and opioids (a type of pain killer).

For more information see page 1360.

Generic: **Prednisone** *(pred-NIS-zone)*
Brands: **Deltasone, Liquid Pred, Meticorten, Orasone, Sterapred**

Prednisone belongs to a class of drugs called corticosteroids that are widely prescribed for a variety of conditions to reduce inflammation. However, depending on the dose and how long they are given, they can have a wide range of effects on the body, especially suppression of the immune system, which can increase risk of infection. To minimize such risk and maximize effectiveness, the

Michigan Center for Minimally Invasive Urology uses a short course (five to 10 days) of relatively low-dose prednisone to reduce ureteral inflammation.

Nonetheless, physicians advise that prednisone should not be prescribed in the presence of documented hypersensitivity, peptic ulcers, or other gastrointestinal disease, liver disease, and certain infections. You should never discontinue prednisone suddenly and must consult your physician about tapering off your dose.

For more information see page 1429.

Renal Colic

Renal colic is intermittent, but often very severe, pain felt on the side of the abdomen that is most commonly caused by a tiny kidney stone passing down the ureter—the tube that connects the kidney to the bladder. Sometimes the stone gets stuck and remains in one place in the ureter. Another medical term for the condition is nephrolithiasis. It has been called one of the most severe types of pain. Treatment options are aimed at reducing the severity of pain.

Commonly Prescribed (On-Label) Drugs: *Dezocine*

OFF-LABEL PRESCRIPTION DRUGS
BREAKTHROUGH OPTIONS

Generics: **Ibuprofen** *(eye-byoo-PROE-fen)* and **Ketorolac** *(KEE-toe-role-ak)*
Brands: **Motrin, Ultraprin (ibuprofen), Toradol (ketorolac)**

Non-steroidal anti-inflammatory drugs (NSAIDs), such as ibuprofen are widely prescribed to inhibit pain and inflammation, especially for arthritis. The Michigan Center for Minimally Invasive Urology uses this oral NSAID for outpatient management but with a number of precautions. Also, according to research reported from the University of Michigan Medical Center patients are sometimes hospitalized for inpatient treatment and intravenously administered ketorolac, a much more powerful NSAID.

Ibuprofen, ketorolac, and other NSAIDs should not be taken by people with documented sensitivity to the drug, those with peptic ulcer disease, recent gastrointestinal (GI) bleeding or perforation, kidney insufficiency, or at high risk of bleeding. It should also be used with caution by those who are pregnant (avoid in third trimester) or who have cardiovascular disease, including heart disease or who are at high risk of heart disease, including heart failure and hypertension and prior heart attack or stroke. Further, caution is advised when taking ibuprofen and other NSAIDs in conjunction with aspirin and a variety of other drugs, including hydralazine, captopril, beta blockers, furosemide, thiazides, methotrexate, and phenytoin.

For more information see pages 1228 and 1262.

Ureteral Stones

Ureteral stones are those that form in the ureters—the long tubes that carry urine from the kidneys to the bladder. When a stone is in the ureters, as opposed to the kidneys, you may feel the need to urinate more often.

Commonly Prescribed (On-Label) Drugs: *None*

OFF-LABEL PRESCRIPTION DRUGS
BREAKTHROUGH OPTIONS

Generics: Non-steroidal anti-inflammatory drugs such as ***Ibuprofen*** *(eye-byoo-PROE-fen)* and ***Ketorolac*** *(KEE-toe-role-ak)*
Brands: ***Motrin, Ultraprin (ibuprofen), Toradol (ketorolac)***

Ibuprofen and ketorolac are in the class of drugs known as non-steroidal anti-inflammatory drugs (NSAIDS) that are used to reduce pain and inflammation. Ibuprofen and ketorolac's ability to reduce a particular enzyme is also helpful in treating kidney and ureter pain. In fact, research has shown that NSAIDs can be as effective as narcotics in relieving the pain of renal colic.

Additionally, in a study evaluating conservative therapy for ureteral stones, physicians at Metropolitan Hospital in Grand Rapids, Michigan, and Western Washington Medical Group in

Everett, Washington, concluded that ketorolac is the single most effective drug to treat renal colic. For hospitalized patients, physicians may prescribe an intravenous NSAID such as ketorolac.

For more information see pages 1228 and 1263.

Generic: **Nifedipine** *(nye-FED-i-peen)*
Brands: **Adalat CC, Apo-Nifed (PA), Novo-Nifedin, Nu-Nifed, Procardia**

Nifedipine belongs to a class of drugs called calcium channel blockers that are often prescribed to people with heart disease. By affecting the movement of calcium into the cells of the heart and blood vessels, they relax blood vessels and increase the supply of blood and oxygen to the heart while reducing its workload. In the same way that nifedipine relaxes the lining of blood vessels, it can relax the smooth muscle in the ureters—the long tubes that carry urine from the kidneys to the bladder. When these tubes relax and loosen, it may be easier for a kidney stone to be released and pass out of the body.

Physicians at the Michigan Center for Minimally Invasive Urology advise that this therapy should be used for only five to 10 days. Further, because nifedipine itself can lower blood pressure, it should be used with great caution in conjunction with any other drug that can lower blood pressure, including beta-blockers and opioids (a type of pain killer). Antihistamines such as cimetidine, given to reduce stomach acidity, may increase the side effects of nifedipine.

Investigators have used nifedipine in combination with a number of other drugs to encourage smaller stones to move relatively quickly through the ureters (within a week). Italian researchers reporting results in *Urology* found that nifedipine and deflazacort increased the rate of stone expulsion for a majority of patients (79%) with good pain control. In another Italian study published in *Urologia Internationalis,* researchers had good results with the combination of nifedipine and prednisolone, finding that 68% of patients with small stones and without overwhelming pain were able to use the drug therapy to pass their ureteral stones.

For more information see page 1360.

Generic: **Prednisone** *(pred-NIS-zone)*
Brands: **Deltasone, Liquid Pred, Meticorten, Orasone, Sterapred**

Prednisone belongs to a class of drugs called corticosteroids that are widely prescribed for a variety of conditions to reduce inflammation. However, depending on the dose and how long they are given, they can have a wide range of effects on the body, especially suppression of the immune system, which can increase risk of infection. To minimize such risk and maximize effectiveness, the Michigan Center for Minimally Invasive Urology uses a short course (five to 10 days) of relatively low-dose prednisone to reduce ureteral inflammation.

Nonetheless, prednisone is not advised in the presence of documented hypersensitivity, peptic ulcers or other gastrointestinal disease, liver disease, and certain infections. You should never discontinue prednisone suddenly but should taper off it under your physician's supervision.

For more information see page 1429.

Generic: **Tamsulosin** *(tam-SOO-loe-sin)*
Brand: **Flomax**

Tamsulosin is generally prescribed for men with benign enlarged prostate glands. It relaxes the muscle around the gland, freeing the flow of urine. In the treatment of stones, tamsulosin may relax the muscles of the ureters, enabling the stones to pass. In a study in *Journal of Urology,* patients received either supportive therapy (the control group) or treatment with nifedipine or tamsulosin. At the end of 4 weeks, 43% of the controls, 80% of those on nifedipine, and 85% of those on tamsulosin had passed the stones.

Another study published in *Journal of Urology* compared tamsulosin with floroglucine-trimetossibenzene (FTMB), a combination of antispasmodic drugs. In addition, all patients received a corticosteroid for anti-inflammatory benefits, an antibiotic, and a non-steroidal anti-inflammatory drug (NSAID) as needed for pain. After four weeks, all the tamsulosin patients had passed their stones, compared to 70% of the FTMB group.

In a trial published in *International Urology and Nephrology,* everyone received the local standard therapy, which included a painkiller, a tranquilizer, an NSAID, and an herbal; half also received tamsulosin. The stone expulsion rate was 80.4% in those on tamsulosin compared to 62.8% in those on standard therapy alone.

According to researchers, these studies suggest tamsulosin may have some benefit as an add-on therapy in treating ureteral stones; however, further study in needed. Physicians advise that it should be used with caution in those using other drugs that can lower blood pressure.

For more information see page 1494.

LIVER AND GALLBLADDER DISORDERS

GALLBLADDER DISORDERS

The gallbladder is a sac that is located under the liver. Its function is to store and concentrate bile—a fluid that helps in the digestion of fats—produced in the liver. Gallbladder disease arises when the flow of bile out of the gallbladder is slowed or obstructed. Gallbladder disease encompasses two types of conditions: cholecystitis and cholelithiasis. Cholecystitis is inflammation of the gallbladder; cholelithiasis a condition that results in gallstones. Symptoms of gallbladder disease include abdominal fullness, gas, abdominal pain, fever, nausea and vomiting, and heartburn, among others.

Acute Cholecystitis

Acute cholecystitis, also known as gallstones, involves a sudden inflammation of the gallbladder that causes severe abdominal pain. Approximately 90% of acute cholecystitis cases are caused by gallstones in the gallbladder; these gallstones obstruct the duct leading from the gallbladder to the common bile duct. Causes of acute cholecystitis include severe illness, alcohol abuse, and gallbladder tumors. Gallstones are more common in women than men; however, they become more common with age in both males and females. Symptoms include abdominal pain (especially after a fatty meal), nausea, vomiting, or fever.

Commonly Prescribed (On-Label) Drugs: *None*

OFF-LABEL PRESCRIPTION DRUGS
BREAKTHROUGH OPTION

*Generic: **Indomethacin** (in-doe-METH-a-sin)*
*Brands: **Indocin, Indocin I. V., Indocin SR***

Indomethacin, a prostaglandin (a hormone-type substance in the body) synthase inhibitor, belongs to a class of medications known as nonsteroidal anti-inflammatory drugs (NSAIDs). Indomethacin is used to relieve pain, tenderness, inflammation, stiffness caused by gout (a form of arthritis), arthritis, and other inflammatory conditions that affect the body. In acute cholecystitis, this drug can help to relieve symptoms of biliary colic, which is a syndrome of right upper quadrant abdominal pain accompanied with nausea that occurs after eating.

Researchers with Temple University School of Medicine in Philadelphia studied the effects of indomethacin in animals with acute cholecystitis. In this study, researchers sought to determine if the use of indomethacin reverses inflammation and gallbladder contractions. Researchers concluded that gallbladder inflammation and motor (contractile) dysfunction in acute cholecystitis can be improved with the early use of indomethacin.

Based on recent FDA recommendations, all NSAIDs have the risk to cause cardiovascular events (including heart attack and stroke) and serious or potentially life-threatening gastrointestinal (GI) bleeding. Also, if you have had heart surgery (cardiac bypass surgery) you should not take this class of drugs.

For more information see page 1238.

Biliary Colic

Biliary colic is a condition that is characterized by extreme cramping in the right upper part of the abdomen as a result of gallstones in the gallbladder or bile ducts. Approximately one third of people with gallstones develop biliary colic or other complications. Risk factors include overweight individuals, those with high cholesterol, pregnant women, women taking birth control pills or estrogen replacement therapy, and persons with diabetes, among others. Other symptoms include nausea after eating a fatty meal, indigestion, and gas.

Commonly Prescribed (On-Label) Drugs: None

OFF-LABEL PRESCRIPTION DRUG
BREAKTHROUGH OPTION

---

*Generic: **Diclofenac Sodium** (dye-KLOE-fen-ak)*
*Brands: **Voltaren, Voltaren-XR***

Diclofenac sodium belongs to a class of drugs known as NSAIDs and is used to relieve pain, inflammation, and tenderness associated with osteoarthritis, rheumatoid arthritis, and ankylosing spondylitis (a spine disease). In biliary colic, diclofenac sodium is believed to relieve inflammation and relax smooth muscle. Side effects of diclofenac sodium include stomach pain, diarrhea, heartburn, upset stomach, constipation, and gas, among others.

NSAIDs, such as diclofenac sodium, have been used to relieve biliary colic symptoms; however, the role of these types of drugs in this condition is not fully known. In one study, diclofenac sodium was shown to be more effective than papaverine (a vasodilator drug) and placebo in relieving biliary colic symptoms and possibly preventing gallstone production. Researchers with the University of Southern California Liver Unit in Downey, California and from Greece evaluated the effects of diclofenac sodium in 53 patients with gallstones and biliary colic. Results from this study showed that complete pain relief was achieved in 21 patients treated with diclofenac sodium and seven patients who received placebo. Four patients in the diclofenac-treated group developed gallstones compared with 11 patients in the placebo group. Researchers concluded that patients with gallstones who have biliary colic can achieve satisfactory pain relief from a single injection of diclofenac sodium. Moreover, diclofenac can significantly decrease the rate of progression to acute cholecystitis, which is a sudden inflammation of the gallbladder caused by gallstones. However, it should be noted that this drug is not available in injection formulation in the United States.

For more information see page 1143.

Gallstone Colic

See Biliary Colic

Hepatic Colic

See Biliary Colic

LIVER DISORDERS

A number of diseases can affect the liver. In some people, liver disease occurs without symptoms. Liver disease, in general, can manifest itself in several ways. Some symptoms that occur include a yellowish discoloration of the skin and the whites of eyes known as jaundice, a reduction or stopping of bile flow known as cholestasis, and liver enlargement. Other symptoms and conditions include abnormally high blood pressure in the veins of the liver (portal hypertension), a liver disorder where toxins accumulate in the blood and cause brain dysfunction (hepatic encephalopathy), and liver failure, among others.

Abdominal Dropsy

See Ascites in Liver Cirrhosis

Alcoholic Hepatitis

Inflammation of the liver from long-term, heavy alcohol use is known as alcoholic hepatitis. This condition results in widespread damage and destruction to the cells of the liver. Alcoholic hepatitis can affect heavy and moderate drinkers alike; a single episode of binge drinking can cause this liver disease. Signs and symptoms of alcoholic hepatitis generally arise during or after a drinking episode and include loss of appetite, nausea, vomiting, abdominal pain and tenderness, fever, jaundice, mental confusion, and abdominal swelling.

Commonly Prescribed (On-Label) Drugs: *None*

OFF-LABEL PRESCRIPTION DRUGS
BREAKTHROUGH OPTIONS

Generic: **Pentoxifylline** *(pen-TOKS-i-fi-leen)*
Brands: **Pentoxil, Trental**

Pentoxifylline improves blood flow through blood vessels and is used to reduce leg pain caused by poor circulation. Side effects associated with the use of pentoxifylline include dizziness, headache, nausea and vomiting, and stomach discomfort. In animal laboratory studies pentoxifylline has been shown to decrease the development of cirrhosis (a liver disease characterized by impaired liver function and liver scarring), and stop anorexia and muscle wasting that is seen in persons with alcoholic hepatitis.

Previous studies have shown that pentoxifylline decreases tumor necrosis factor (TNF) alpha levels, which are associated with increased death. In a clinical trial, researchers from the University of California Liver Unit evaluated the use of pentoxifylline in 49 patients with severe alcoholic hepatitis and its effect on TNF alpha levels. In this study, 49 patients received pentoxifylline whereas 52 patients received placebo for four weeks. In this analysis, the use of pentoxifylline was associated with improved survival. Based on these results, it has been rationalized that the benefit seen with pentoxifylline in patients with alcoholic hepatitis may be related to the significant decrease in the risk of developing liver and kidney failure. Researchers concluded that the use of pentoxifylline improves short-term survival in patients with severe alcoholic hepatitis.

For more information see page 1405.

Generic: **Prednisolone** *(pred-NISS-oh-lone)*
Brands: **Prelone, Predalone**

Prednisolone belongs to a class of drugs known as corticosteroids. As a drug class, corticosteroids have strong anti-inflammatory properties and are used in a number of inflammatory diseases such as arthritis, asthma, and bronchitis, among others. Prednisolone helps to reduce swelling, redness, itching in allergic reactions; in alcoholic hepatitis, prednisolone is used to reduce the inflammation associated with this disorder. Side effects associated with the use of this drug include diarrhea, constipation, headache, increased or decreased appetite, increased sweating, nervousness, restlessness, and upset stomach, among others. Prednisolone can also impair the immune system's ability to fight infections.

According to researchers in Austria, prednisolone should be used in eligible patients. In general, prednisolone is preferred to another steroid, prednisone, because prednisone must be broken down to prednisolone by the liver, which is often impaired in people with this condition.

In a clinical trial, researchers in France compared 28 days of prednisolone treatment with placebo in 61 patients with alcoholic hepatitis or spontaneous hepatic encephalopathy (a liver disorder where toxins accumulate in the blood and cause brain dysfunction). After 66 days, 16 of the 29 patients who received placebo had died compared with four of the 32 patients who received prednisolone. Moreover, there were no serious adverse events reported with the use of prednisolone. Researchers concluded that prednisolone improves the short-term survival in patients with severe alcoholic hepatitis.

For more information see page 1428.

Ascites in Liver Cirrhosis

Ascites is extra fluid in the space between the membranes that line the abdomen and the abdominal organs. Ascites is a common complication in liver cirrhosis and is associated with a grave prognosis; approximately 50% of patients die within two years of diagnosis. Causes of ascites include liver cirrhosis, alcoholic hepatitis, chronic hepatitis, and obstruction of the hepatic vein. Ascites, as a result of liver disease, generally accompany other disease characteristics such as high blood pressure. Symptoms of ascites can include a distended abdominal cavity, discomfort, and shortness of breath. Treatment goals for ascites include symptom relief, correction of the underlying abnormalities, and prevention of complications.

Commonly Prescribed (On-Label) Drugs: Spironolactone

OFF-LABEL PRESCRIPTION DRUGS
BREAKTHROUGH OPTIONS

Generic: **Amiloride** *(a-MIL-oh-ride)*
Brand: **Midamor**

Amiloride belongs to a class of drugs known as diuretics, which are used to increase the amount of urine passed so that the body gets rid of excess water and salt. Amiloride is a type of diuretic known as a potassium-sparing diuretic; it does not increase potassium loss. The mainstay treatment of ascites in liver cirrhosis is the use of diuretic drugs such as amiloride.

In a study conducted in London, patients with liver cirrhosis and ascites were treated with amiloride twice daily and furosemide (a diuretic drug). After treatment, 23 out of 24 patients with ascites and liver cirrhosis were controlled with a combination of amiloride and either furosemide or ethacrynic acid. The one treatment failure in this study occurred in those with terminal liver failure in which the use of diuretics is often unsuccessful. In this study, the amounts of fluid loss were unpredictable; therefore researchers recommended that low doses of furosemide or ethacrynic acid should be used with amiloride twice daily.

For more information see page 1004.

Generic: **Furosemide** *(fyoor-OH-se-mide)*
Brand: **Lasix**

Furosemide belongs to a class of drugs known as loop diuretics, and is used to increase the amount of urine so the body gets rid of excess water and salt. Furosemide helps to treat high blood pressure and also reduces water retention and swelling associated with heart, liver, and kidney diseases. Side effects associated with furosemide include dizziness, lightheadedness, increased sensitivity to the sun, upset stomach, stomach cramps, and appetite loss.

Diuretics, such as furosemide, have become the mainstay drug for the treatment of ascites associated with liver cirrhosis. Studies have shown that combining different types of diuretics such as furosemide with amiloride provide beneficial effects in patients with ascites. Adding furosemide to other diuretics to treat ascites in liver cirrhosis is well documented in the medical literature. French researchers proposed a regimen to treat ascites that included a decrease in salt intake and the use of spironolactone (a diuretic drug) combined with furosemide.

For more information see page 1204.

Chronic Hepatitis B

Chronic hepatitis B is a lifelong liver disease caused by the hepatitis B virus (HBV). Symptoms include tiredness, jaundice, stomach pain, vomiting, appetite loss, fever, and joint aches. In some persons, symptoms of HBV may not be present; however, this does not mean that the virus cannot be passed to others. Prevention of chronic HBV transmission to other persons includes vaccinations, practicing good hygiene and safe sex, and not sharing personal care items (razors, toothbrushes, and hypodermic needles). Long-term effects of chronic hepatitis include scarring of the liver tissue known as cirrhosis and liver cancer.

Commonly Prescribed (On-Label) Drugs: *Interferon alfa-2b, Lamivudine*

OFF-LABEL PRESCRIPTION DRUG
BREAKTHROUGH OPTION

Generic: ***Famciclovir*** *(fam-SYE-kloe-veer)*
Brand: ***Famvir***

Famciclovir belongs to a class of drugs known as antivirals and is used to treat herpes zoster (shingles) and genital herpes. In clinical trials, famciclovir has been shown to be effective against chronic HBV infection. However, treatment of chronic hepatitis B with a single antiviral for up to one year prevents the virus from copying itself in only 17% of patients. Therefore, a number of studies have examined the use of famciclovir combined with another antiviral, lamivudine, for the treatment of chronic hepatitis B. In a study conducted in China, 28 patients with chronic hepatitis B were treated with lamivudine and famciclovir for 24 weeks. In two other groups, 30 and 32 patients with chronic hepatitis B were treated with lamivudine and famciclovir alone, respectively. Results showed that the combination of famciclovir and lamivudine was superior and safer than either drug alone in patients with chronic hepatitis B.

In another study, researchers in Germany evaluated the use of famciclovir and lamivudine in patients after liver transplant and concluded that both antivirals are strong drugs to use for the treatment of HBV infection after liver transplant; however, the antiviral capacity of lamivudine is superior even after pretreatment with famciclovir although relapse is often seen with long-term use of the drug.

For more information see page 1180.

Chronic Hepatitis C

Chronic hepatitis C is a lifelong liver disease caused by the hepatitis C virus (HCV), and accounts for 60% to 70% of chronic hepatitis cases. Complications of HCV include cirrhosis, liver failure, and liver cancer. HCV is mainly spread by contact with blood or blood products; those at highest risk include injection drug users, people who have had blood transfusions before 1992, persons who have frequent exposure to blood products, infants born to HCV-infected mothers, healthcare workers, and persons who participate in high-risk sexual behavior. Symptoms can include fatigue, nausea, poor appetite, and muscle and joint pains.

Commonly Prescribed (On-Label) Drugs: *Interferon alfa-2b, Interferon alfa-N1*

OFF-LABEL PRESCRIPTION DRUG
BREAKTHROUGH OPTION

Generic: ***Amantadine*** *(a-MAN-to-deen)*
Brand: ***Symmetrel***

Amantadine belongs to a class of drugs known as antivirals and is used to prevent or treat influenza (flu) infections. This antiviral has shown activity against viruses that belong to the *Flaviviridae* family of viruses, to which HCV belongs. A recent review of studies in patients with chronic HCV infection showed that when amantadine was combined with interferon the response rate increased by 7% in patients.

In a clinical trial, researchers with the Pennsylvania State College of Medicine evaluated the use of amantadine or placebo for six months in patients with chronic hepatitis C. After six months of treatment, patients who received placebo were given amantadine for six months whereas patients treated with amantadine received an additional six months of treatment. Compared with placebo in this study, use of amantadine was associated with a significant decline in liver enzymes that doctors use to evaluate and follow up liver diseases. Nine percent of patients cleared the virus at the end of treatment and 6.8% of patients had a sustained response six months after amantadine was discontinued. Side effects were considered minimal in this study and quality of life improved with 12 months of amantadine therapy. Researchers concluded that oral amantadine may be a safe, alternative treatment for people with chronic hepatitis C who are unresponsive or intolerant to treatment with interferon.

For more information see page 1001.

Cirrhosis

See Liver Cirrhosis

Hanot Cirrhosis

See Primary Biliary Cirrhosis

Hepatic Encephalopathy

Brain and nervous system damage that occurs as a complication of liver diseases such as cirrhosis or hepatitis or conditions where blood circulation bypasses the liver is known as hepatic encephalopathy. This disorder is characterized by various neurologic symptoms including changes in consciousness, reflexes, and behavior that can range from mild to severe. Other symptoms and signs include confusion, forgetfulness, changes in mood, decreased alertness, muscle stiffness or rigidity, jaundice, and fluid collection in the abdomen, among others.

Commonly Prescribed (On-Label) Drugs: *Amino acid solutions, Kanamycin*

OFF-LABEL PRESCRIPTION DRUGS
BREAKTHROUGH OPTIONS

Generic: **Metronidazole** *(me-troe-NI-da-zole)*
Brands: **Flagyl, Flagyl ER, MetroCream, MetroGel,
MetroLotion, MetroGel Vaginal**

Metronidazole is an antibiotic used to kill or prevent the growth of bacteria or other microorganisms and is approved for the treatment of inflammatory lesions and rosacea, vaginosis and vaginitis. It is used off-label to treat hepatic encephalopathy by reducing the excessive amount of ammonia-producing bacteria in the body.

Metronidazole has been shown to be as effective as oral neomycin, another antibiotic. Metronidazole therapy should be used for no more than two weeks to avoid peripheral neuropathy (a nervous system condition). It also can cause side effects such as dark brown or reddish urine, diarrhea, dry mouth, metallic taste in the mouth, headache, appetite loss, nausea, and mild stomach pain or cramps.

In a study conducted at the Bristol Royal Infirmary, metronidazole and neomycin were evaluated for one week in 11 patients with acute or chronic hepatic encephalopathy. Improvement in mental state, and reduction in tremors and bad breath were seen with both antibiotic drugs. Results suggest that metronidazole may be as effective as neomycin for hepatic encephalopathy. The use of metronidazole is recognized by the American College of Gastroenterology for patients with hepatic encephalopathy, but they recommend close, careful monitoring of the kidneys, nervous system, and the ears.

For more information see page 1322.

Generic: **Vancomycin** *(vank-coe-MY-sin)*
Brands: **Vancocin, Vancoled**

Vancomycin is an antibiotic used in a wide variety of bacterial infections. It is useful in hepatic encephalopathy to decrease the amount of ammonia-producing bacteria in the body. Clinical studies have shown vancomycin to be effective in controlling hepatic encephalopathy in patients with cirrhosis.

Researchers from Japan evaluated the effects of vancomycin in patients with lactulose (a man-made sugar)-resistant chronic hepatic encephalopathy. During the first eight weeks of the trial, all 12 patients were given vancomycin by mouth twice daily. Six patients were later changed to lactose after the initial eight weeks on vancomycin while the remaining six patients continued to take vancomycin for another eight weeks. After this period, the medication was reversed and the study was continued for another eight weeks. Researchers found that hepatic encephalopathy improved in all 12 patients after vancomycin was given and this improvement was apparent after two to three days of treatment. Once patients were crossed over to lactulose, their mental status deteriorated and then improved when they were switched to vancomycin. Vancomycin also decreased the concentration of ammonia; once patients were changed to lactulose, ammonia levels increased. They observed that vancomycin also reduced bacteria in the stool. Vancomycin appears to be effective in the treatment of hepatic encephalopathy in patients who are not improved with lactulose.

For more information see page 1537.

Hydroperitoneum

See Ascites in Liver Cirrhosis

Liver Cirrhosis

Liver cirrhosis is a condition that results in irreversible scarring of the liver and liver dysfunction. Conditions that cause liver cirrhosis include alcohol abuse, chronic hepatitis B, chronic hepatitis C, autoimmune hepatitis, nonalcoholic fatty liver disease, inherited liver diseases (Wilson's disease), blocked or inflamed bile ducts, and prolonged exposure to toxic materials (certain drugs). Signs and symptoms of liver cirrhosis include appetite loss, weight loss, nausea, small red spider veins under the skin, weakness, fatigue, jaundice, and bleeding from veins in the esophagus or intestines, among others.

Commonly Prescribed (On-Label) Drugs: Indinavir

OFF-LABEL PRESCRIPTION DRUGS
BREAKTHROUGH OPTIONS

Generic: **Interferon Alfa-2a** *(in-ter-FEER-on AL-fa-2a)*
Brand: **Roferon-A**

Interferon alfa-2a belongs to a family of drugs known as interferons, which are naturally occurring proteins produced by cells of the immune system. Interferons direct the immune system's attack on viruses, bacteria, tumors, and other foreign substances that may invade the body; these drugs have both antiviral and immune-stimulating properties. Interferon alfa-2a is used to treat AIDS-related cancer, certain types of hepatitis, leukemia, and other cancers. Side effects associated with interferon alfa-2a include blurred vision, changes in taste, cough, diarrhea, dry or sore mouth, fever, chills, and headaches, among others.

Researchers in France evaluated the long-term effects of interferon alfa-2a in patients with chronic hepatitis C. In this analysis, 244 previously untreated patients with chronic hepatitis C without cirrhosis were given a standard interferon alfa-2a drug regimen three times a week for 24 weeks. Results from this study showed that sustained alanine aminotransferase (ALT) (a liver enzyme that plays a role in protein metabolism; elevated ALT levels signify liver damage from disease or drugs) response was seen in five patients. At 18 months, liver cirrhosis was seen in 10 patients. Researchers concluded that the standard regimen of interferon alfa-2a in patients with hepatitis C provides a minimal sustained response rate at 18 months and may not prevent liver cirrhosis.

For more information see page 1241.

Generic: **Interferon Alfa-2b** *(in-ter-FEER-on AL-fa-2b)*
Brand: **Intron A**

Interferon alfa-2b belongs to a family of drugs known as interferons, which are proteins produced by cells of the immune system. Interferons direct the immune system's attack on viruses, bacteria, tumors, and other foreign substances that may invade the body; these drugs have both immunostimulatory and antiviral properties. Side effects associated with interferon alfa-2b include blurred vision, changes in taste, cough, diarrhea, dry or sore mouth, fever, chills, hair loss, appetite loss, and headaches, among others. This drug may also decrease the body's ability to fight infection or may increase the risk of bruising or bleeding. Interferons are also associated with the exacerbation of neuropsychiatric disorders.

In a small case report published in *Clinical Gastroenterology and Hepatology*, researchers reported that interferon alfa-2b was effective in reversing liver cirrhosis due to chronic hepatitis B. Three patients with chronic hepatitis B and evidence of liver cirrhosis were treated with interferon alfa or lamivudine (an antiviral) and their mean ALT levels, bilirubin (a chemical in the body formed by hemoglobin breakdown), and liver fibrosis scores decreased.

For more information see page 1243.

Generic: **Lamivudine** *(la-MI-vyoo-deen)*
Brands: **Epivir, Epivir-HBV**

Lamivudine belongs to a class of drugs known as antivirals. Lamivudine is used to treat infections resulting from hepatitis B and HIV. In hepatitis B, lamivudine can slow liver damage; however, this drug will not cure or prevent hepatitis B infection. Moreover, lamivudine does not reduce the risk of infecting others with hepatitis B. Side effects associated with lamivudine include cough, diarrhea, nausea, vomiting, difficulty sleeping, and hair loss, among others.

In liver cirrhosis, lamivudine works by blocking viral DNA copying in the body. Clinical studies have found that lamivudine is safe and better tolerated than interferon alfa drugs in hepatitis B-related liver cirrhosis. In a study by researchers in Canada, up to 80% of 35 patients with liver cirrhosis due to hepatitis B experienced liver improvements with six-month use of this drug. Liver improvement was most evident after nine to 12 months of treatment.

In a study conducted by researchers in Japan, 54 patients with hepatitis B-related liver cirrhosis were treated with oral lamivudine each day for at least six months. Results showed that lamivudine suppressed hepatitis B DNA to undetectable levels in 77.8% of patients at 12 months and in 61.3% of patients at 24 months. Researchers concluded that, in some people, lamivudine can improve the course of liver cirrhosis.

For more information see page 1266.

Generic: **Ribavirin** *(rye-ba-VYE-rin)* and **Peginterferon Alfa-2b** *(peg-in-ter-FEER-on AL-fa-2b)*
Brands: **Rebetrol, Ribasphere, Virazole** *(ribavirin),* **PEG-intron** *(peginterferon Alfa-2b)*

Ribavirin is an antiviral used to treat hepatitis C in combination with another drug, peginterferon alfa-2b (a pegylated interferon drug). The beneficial effects of ribavirin combined with pegylated interferon were seen in an analysis of four major clinical trials involving 3,010 patients with chronic hepatitis C. Patients were treated with either interferon or pegylated interferon, with or without ribavirin. Combination therapy with ribavirin and either interferon or pegylated interferon yielded the most benefit, and reversal of liver cirrhosis was seen in 49% of 153 patients with liver cirrhosis. Researchers concluded that the combination of peginterferon alfa-2b and ribavirin has the potential to reduce death rates in those with hepatitis C and cirrhosis. A combination including a high-dose of ribavirin offered the most benefit to these patients.

Researchers at Massachusetts General Hospital in Boston studied the effects of ribavirin combined with peginterferon alfa-2b in patients with recurrent hepatitis C infection who underwent liver transplant. Results showed that ribavirin in combination with interferon or peginterferon alfa-2b offered a significant response in patients. Ribavirin and peginterferon alfa-2b were also shown to be effective in a majority of patients who did not respond to interferon and ribavirin treatment.

For more information see pages 1446 and 1399.

Liver Fibrosis

The accumulation of tough, fibrous scar tissue in the liver is known as liver fibrosis. Chronic infection with hepatitis C or hepatitis B can lead to liver fibrosis. In general, it occurs more rapidly in men than women, and in persons over age 50. Liver fibrosis appears to speed up once liver disease has progressed. Other conditions that can accelerate liver fibrosis include immune system dysfunction, HIV infection, use of immunosuppressive drugs, heavy alcohol intake, fatty liver diseases, and insulin resistance.

Commonly Prescribed (On-Label) Drugs: *None*

OFF-LABEL PRESCRIPTION DRUGS
BREAKTHROUGH OPTIONS

Generic: **Azathioprine** *(ay-za-THYE-oh-preen)*
Brand: **Imuran**

Azathioprine is used to reduce the body's natural immunity in patients who have undergone organ transplants. Azathioprine may also be used to treat rheumatoid arthritis, cirrhosis, and chronic active hepatitis. In liver diseases, azathioprine may be helpful in alleviating associated inflammation. Azathioprine has the potential to cause serious side effects such as low white blood cell count and a reduced number of blood platelets. Other side effects include increased risk of infection, delayed wound healing, liver problems, appetite loss, nausea, vomiting, and skin rash.

Researchers in Iran evaluated the effects of azathioprine on liver fibrosis rate in people with autoimmune hepatitis. In this study 19 patients were evaluated, of which seven patients were treated with cyclosporine (an immunosuppressive drug) for six months. These patients then had their treatment regimen switched to azathioprine. The other 12 patients were treated with prednisolone for three months, and then azathioprine was added and prednisolone was stopped. Fibrosis was compared before and after treatment. Results showed that, after treatment, enzymes released from liver cells, and fibrosis scores decreased. Researchers concluded that liver fibrosis regressed with the use of cyclosporine or a steroid drug in combination with azathioprine in autoimmune hepatitis.

For more information see page 1033.

Generic: **Cyclosporine** *(si-klo-SPOR-een)*
Brands: **Gengraf, Neoral, Sandimmune**

Cyclosporine belongs to a class of drugs known as immunosuppressive drugs, and is used to reduce the body's natural immunity in patients who have received a transplanted organ. It works by preventing white blood cells from rejecting the new organ. This drug is also used to treat rheumatoid arthritis and a skin condition known as psoriasis. Side effects associated with cyclosporine can be serious and include high blood pressure, kidney and liver problems, and a reduced ability to fight infection. Other less serious side effects include increased hair growth, trembling or shaking of the hands, acne, oily skin, headache, leg cramps, and nausea.

Researchers in Germany reported that the use of cyclosporine in patients with chronic hepatitis resulted in disease remission and a potential protective effect against liver fibrosis. In this same article, researchers presented results from a study of rats induced with liver cirrhosis and subsequent treatment with cyclosporine or placebo. After six weeks of treatment, excellent protective effects of cyclosporine against liver cirrhosis were found in the groups treated with cyclosporine.

For more information see page 1127.

Generic: *Interferon Alfa-2a* (in-ter-FEER-on AL-fa-2a)
Brand: *Roferon-A*

Interferon alfa-2a is a member of a family of drugs known as interferons, which are naturally occurring proteins produced by cells of the immune system. Interferons direct the immune system's attack on viruses, bacteria, tumors, and other foreign substances that may invade the body; these drugs have both antiviral and immune-stimulating properties. This drug is used to treat AIDS-related cancer, certain types of hepatitis, leukemia, and other cancers. This drug may also decrease the body's ability to fight infection or increase the risk of bruising or bleeding.

In an article by researchers in the United Kingdom, regression of scarring was reported after treatment with long-term interferon alfa treatment in patients with chronic hepatitis. In an article published in *Clinical Gastroenterology and Hepatology*, researchers reported the use of interferon alfa and lamivudine (an antiviral drug) in three patients with chronic hepatitis B and evidence of cirrhosis. Results revealed that the fibrosis score decreased with treatment. Researchers concluded that reversal of liver cirrhosis in chronic hepatitis B may occur after treatment with interferon alfa or lamivudine.

For more information see page 1241.

Generic: **Interferon Alfa-2b** *(in-ter-FEER-on AL-fa-2b)*
Brand: **Intron A**

Interferon alfa-2b is a type of interferon, which is a naturally occurring protein produced by cells of the immune system. Interferon alfa-2b is a man-made protein that has similar actions to interferon found naturally in the body. This drug is used to treat AIDS-related cancer, certain types of hepatitis, leukemia, and other cancers.

Researchers in the United Kingdom noted that the use of interferons or pegylated interferons (another type of interferon drug) with or without the addition of ribavirin (an antiviral drug) can provide major beneficial effects on liver fibrosis. This effect is particularly enhanced with the use of combination drug regimens. Additionally, researchers in Portugal evaluated the effects of interferon alfa-2b on fibrosis in patients with chronic hepatitis C. One hundred seventeen patients with chronic hepatitis C were treated with interferon alfa-2b three times a week for 12 months. Results from this study showed that out of 81 patients, a significant reduction in liver fibrosis was seen in 29.6% of patients. In this study, fibrosis worsened in 4.9% of patients. Researchers concluded that based on these findings, interferon alfa offers antifibrolytic activity separate from its antiviral properties.

In another study, researchers with the French Multicenter Study Group found that interferon alfa-2b in combination with ribavirin in patients with chronic hepatitis C significantly reduces the rate of liver fibrosis progression.

For more information see page 1243.

Generic: **Lamivudine** *(la-MI-vyoo-deen)*
Brands: **Epivir, Epivir-HBV**

Lamivudine belongs to a class of drugs known as antivirals, and is used to treat infection caused by the HIV or hepatitis B virus. In chronic hepatitis B, lamivudine blocks DNA replication of HBV and can slow liver damage. This drug is used off-label in the treatment of liver fibrosis much in the same way that it acts on chronic hepatitus B.

Researchers in Japan sought to determine factors that determine which patients are candidates for treatment with lamivudine for liver fibrosis and hepatitis B. Researchers found lamivudine to be an effective treatment.

An article in *Clinical Gastroenterology and Hepatology* noted the use of lamivudine and interferon alfa (an immunomodulator drug) in three patients with chronic hepatitis B and evidence of cirrhosis. The fibrosis score decreased drastically, and the mean grading score also decreased markedly. Researchers concluded that reversal of liver cirrhosis in chronic hepatitis B may occur after treatment with lamivudine or interferon alfa.

For more information see page 1266.

Generic: **Peginterferon Alfa-2b**
(peg-in-ter-FEER-on AL-fa-2b) and
Ribavirin *(rye-ba-VYE-rin)*
Brands: **PEG-intron (peginterferon Alfa-2b), Rebetol, Ribasphere, Virazole (ribavirin)**

Peginterferon alfa-2b (pegylated interferon) is a man-made protein. In the body, natural interferons (proteins) help the immune system fight off viral infections and certain types of cancers. Peginterferon alfa-2b works similarly to natural interferons and is used to treat hepatitis C infection. Ribavirin is an antiviral that treats lower respiratory tract infections.

Researchers from the United Kingdom reported that use of peginterferon alfa-2b with ribavirin (an antiviral drug) provides major beneficial effects in patients with liver fibrosis. In a study conducted by French researchers, the use of peginterferon alfa-2b with ribavirin in patients with HIV and HCV was found to be an effective treatment in people who failed standard interferon-based regimens; however, people with fibrosis or cirrhosis did not respond to treatment. In a study conducted by researchers in Spain, the use of once-weekly peginterferon alfa-2b combined with ribavirin resulted in a response rate of 38% compared with 7% for standard interferon treatment and ribavirin in those with HIV and HCV.

A German researcher noted that the use of peginterferon alfa-2b with ribavirin can eliminate HCV genetic material from the blood in approximately 60% of infected patients. And, there may be beneficial effects with this drug combination on disease progression and cancer risk in patients whose HCV genetic material is not eliminated. Overall, in liver disease, a reduction in the virus level in the blood to an undetectable level is correlated with improvement in liver fibrosis.

For more information see page 1399.

Generic: **Prednisolone** *(pred-NISS-oh-lone)*
Brands: **Prelone, Predalone**

Prednisolone is a corticosteroid that has strong anti-inflammatory properties and is used in inflammatory diseases such as arthritis, asthma, and bronchitis, among others. In liver fibrosis, prednisolone may help to alleviate liver inflammation and prevent progression of fibrosis. Prednisolone can also impair the immune system's ability to fight infections.

Researchers in Iran treated 19 patients with liver fibrosis and autoimmune hepatitis with either prednisolone or cyclosporine (an immunosuppressive drug) and azathioprine (an immunosuppressive drug). In this study, seven patients were treated with oral cyclosporine for six months. This treatment was then switched to tapering off low-dose prednisone together with azathioprine, and then changed to treatment with azathioprine alone. The other 12 patients in this study received prednisolone for three months and then azathioprine was added. Prednisolone was then gradually eliminated and only azathioprine was continued. Researchers found that in those patients who received cyclosporine or prednisolone and azathioprine had regression of liver fibrosis. In this study, improvement in liver fibrosis was associated with a reduction in inflammation; this suggests that liver inflammation is a trigger for liver fibrosis in acute hepatitis and immunosuppressive drugs may lead to regression of this condition.

For more information see page 1428.

Generic: **Ribavirin-interferon Alfa-2b**
(rye-ba-VYE-rin in-ter-FEER-on AL-fa-2b)
Brands: **Copegus, Rebetron**

Ribavirin-interferon alfa-2b is a combination drug containing the antivirals ribavirin (a nucleoside analogue) and interferon alfa-2b (a man-made protein and an immunomodulator). Interferon alfa-2b is similar to natural interferons that are produced by the immune system to fight viral infections. Side effects associated with ribavirin-interferon alfa-2b include flu-like symptoms, thinning hair, headache, heartburn, itching, nausea, skin rash, and vomiting. Blood monitoring by your physician is required during the first month of treatment, because use of this drug may also cause low red blood cell counts and increase the risk of infection.

Combination treatment with interferon and ribavirin has been found to be more effective than interferon alone. In an analysis of four major clinical studies involving 3,010 patients with chronic hepatitis C, combination therapy including interferon and ribavirin was shown to be effective in the treatment of liver fibrosis. Additionally, reversal of cirrhosis was observed in 49% of patients with chronic hepatitis C. Response to this combined drug has been shown to be better in people without cirrhosis compared with those with cirrhosis.

A number of scientific reports note the advantage of combination therapy for the treatment of liver diseases and the prevention of liver disease progression. A study by researchers in Kuwait and France concluded that patients with HCV type four showed a poor response to interferon treatment alone and therefore should be treated with interferon combined with ribavirin. In this study, 52% of patients treated with ribavirin-interferon alfa-2b had a sustained response compared with only 19% of patients receiving interferon alone.

For more information see page 1448.

Mallory Bodies

See Alcoholic Hepatitis

Portal Hypertension

An increase in the pressure in the portal vein, which carries blood from the digestive organs to the liver, is known as portal hypertension. This increased pressure in the portal vein is caused by a blockage of blood flow through the liver. Causes of portal hypertension include cirrhosis (scarring of the liver) and thrombosis (clotting in the portal vein). Symptoms and complications of portal hypertension include GI bleeding, black stools, vomiting blood, ascites (excess fluid in the abdomen), encephalopathy, reduced levels of blood platelets, and decreased white blood cell count.

Commonly Prescribed (On-Label) Drugs: None

OFF-LABEL PRESCRIPTION DRUGS
BREAKTHROUGH OPTIONS

Generic: **Carvedilol** *(KAR-ve-dil-ole)*
Brand: **Coreg**

Carvedilol belongs to a class of drugs known as beta-blockers, used to control high blood pressure and heart failure. Carvedilol may cause side effects including diarrhea, back pain, dry eyes, itchy skin, headache, insomnia, nausea, sore throat, and tiredness. It may also affect blood sugar levels.

Clinical studies have been conducted on the use of carvedilol for portal hypertension. A researcher at the University of Colorado School of Pharmacy in Denver reviewed studies involving the use of this drug for portal hypertension. In one study, 10 patients with mild to moderate liver disease were given a single dose of carvedilol. Researchers subsequently measured blood pressure at 60 minutes and 90 minutes. The average liver blood pressure was not significantly reduced at 60 minutes compared with before treatment but at 90 minutes, liver blood pressure was significantly reduced. Reductions were 20% or more in five patients at either 60 or 90 minutes.

For more information see page 1073.

Generic: **Nadolol** *(nay-DOE-lole)*
Brand: **Corgard**

Nadolol belongs to a class of drugs known as nonselective beta-blockers, and is used to reduce the workload of the heart and to help it beat more regularly. Nadolol is used to control high blood pressure, relieve chest pain, treat tremor, and relieve anxiety. Side effects associated with nadolol include darkened skin color, itchy skin, tiredness, and headache. It can also affect blood sugar levels.

A review article by a researcher at the University of Colorado School of Pharmacy in Denver noted that nonselective beta-blockers, such as nadolol, have been effective in reducing liver blood pressure; however, about two-thirds of patients do not attain a desired decrease in liver blood pressure to prevent further bleeding.

In a study conducted in Italy, 12 patients with cirrhosis and portal hypertension were treated with nadolol for one month. After treatment, cardiac output and an effective liver blood flow were found, although mean arterial pressure, liver function, and kidney blood flow were not affected. A significant correlation was found between decreases in blood pressure and cardiac output. Overall, in seven patients, nadolol reduced portal hypertension.

For more information see page 1347.

Generic: **Propranolol** *(proe-PRAN-oh-lole)*
Brands: **Inderal, Inderal LA, InnoPran XL, Propranolol Intensol**

Propranolol belongs to a class of drugs known as nonselective beta-blockers that reduces the workload of the heart and helps it to beat more regularly. Side effects associated with it include diarrhea, sore eyes, hair loss, nausea, sexual difficulties, weakness, and tiredness. It can also affect blood sugar levels.

Researchers in Spain evaluated the use of propranolol in 34 patients with portal hypertension and liver cirrhosis. Patients received oral propranolol twice daily. The dosage was increased every three days until the patient's resting heart rate was reduced by 25%. Once this was achieved, patients received combination therapy with oral molsidomine (a vein dilating drug). After treatment, researchers noted that propranolol significantly reduced liver vein pressure. The combination of propranolol and molsidomine offered a slight but significant decrease in liver vein pressure. Researchers concluded that the combination of drugs prevents some of the adverse effects of propranolol on liver and cardiopulmonary pressures; however, it does not offer a greater reduction in liver vein pressure compared with propranolol alone.

For more information see page 1438.

Portal-systemic Encephalopathy

See Hepatic Encephalopathy

Prevention of Bleeding in Cirrhosis

About one-third of people with liver cirrhosis experience bleeding and the mortality rate associated with the first bleeding episode can be as high as 50%. In liver cirrhosis, scar tissue blocks the flow of blood through the liver and results in liver dysfunction. This blockage results in large, swollen veins that can rupture and leak blood. Symptoms include vomiting blood, black stools, low blood pressure, rapid heart rate, and shock. Prevention of bleeding in high-risk patients is mandatory and involves nonselective beta-blocker drugs.

Commonly Prescribed (On-Label) Drugs: None

OFF-LABEL PRESCRIPTION DRUGS
BREAKTHROUGH OPTIONS

Generic: **Nadolol** *(nay-DOE-lole)*
Brand: **Corgard**

Nadolol belongs to a class of drugs known as nonselective beta-blockers. To prevent bleeding in liver cirrhosis, the standard treatment involves the use of nonselective beta-blockers such as nadolol. Nadolol reduces pressure in the portal vein in the liver by reducing portal and collateral blood flow. Although beta-blockers are the standard preventive measure, between 30% and 40% of people will not have sufficient protection against bleeding. Side effects associated with nadolol include shortness of breath; swelling of the legs, ankles, feet and hands; weight gain; and fainting. Suddenly stopping nadolol may result in chest pain or heart attack.

Researchers in China compared the use of nadolol and a medical procedure to prevent bleeding in patients with liver cirrhosis. One hundred patients were divided to receive either the medical procedure or treatment with nadolol once daily. At follow-up, 20% of patients in the medical treatment group and 32% of patients in the nadolol group had upper gastrointestinal bleeding. Esophageal bleeding occurred in 10% of patients in the procedure group and 18% of patients in the nadolol group. Minor complications were seen in 18% of patients in the procedure group and 8% of patients in the nadolol group. Researchers concluded that the medical procedure and nadolol treatment are similarly effective for the prevention of the first episode of bleeding in patients with liver cirrhosis.

For more information see page 1347.

Generic: **Propranolol** *(proe-PRAN-oh-lole)*
Brands: **Inderal, Inderal LA, InnoPran XL, Propranolol Intensol**

Propranolol belongs to a class of drugs known as nonselective beta-blockers, and is used to treat high blood pressure, prevent chest pain, and treat abnormal heart rhythms. The standard treatment to prevent bleeding in liver cirrhosis involves the use of nonselective beta-blockers such as propranolol. Side effects associated with propranolol include dizziness, lightheadedness, excessive tiredness, upset stomach, vomiting, diarrhea, constipation, and rash. Suddenly stopping propranolol may result in chest pain or heart attack.

In a study conducted in Germany, variceal band ligation (a medical procedure) was compared with propranolol treatment for the primary prevention of bleeding in 150 patients with liver cirrhosis. Patients received either treatment with propranolol twice daily and increased twice daily until resting heart rate was reduced by 20%; or variceal band ligation. Bleeding occurred in 25% of patients in the ligation group compared with 29% of patients in the propranolol group. Twelve percent of patients in the ligation group and 10% of patients in the propranolol group had fatal bleeding. Researchers concluded that variceal band ligation and propranolol are similarly effective for the primary prevention of bleeding in people with liver cirrhosis.

For more information see page 1438.

Primary Biliary Cirrhosis

Primary biliary cirrhosis is a liver disease that slowly destroys the liver bile ducts. When these ducts are damaged, bile, which aids in fat digestion, accumulates in the liver, damages surrounding tissue, and can cause cirrhosis. Primary biliary cirrhosis affects women more than men and occurs between the ages of 30 and 60 years. Symptoms of biliary cirrhosis include itchy skin, fatigue, jaundice, cholesterol deposits in the skin, fluid retention, dry eyes, and dry mouth.

Commonly Prescribed (On-Label) Drugs: *None*

OFF-LABEL PRESCRIPTION DRUGS
BREAKTHROUGH OPTIONS

Generic: **Azathioprine** *(ay-za-THYE-oh-preen)*
Brand: **Imuran**

Azathioprine belongs to a class of drugs known as immunosuppressives and is used to reduce the body's natural immunity in people who have undergone body organ transplants. Azathioprine may also be used to treat rheumatoid arthritis, cirrhosis, chronic active hepatitis, and biliary cirrhosis. It has the potential to cause serious side effects such as low white blood cell count and reduced number of blood platelets. Other side effects include increased risk of infection, delayed wound healing, liver problems, appetite loss, nausea, vomiting, and skin rash.

In a study, researchers from Britain reported on the use of azathioprine for the treatment of primary biliary cirrhosis. In this study, 124 patients with primary biliary cirrhosis were treated with azathioprine and 112 patients received placebo. Researchers found no significant effects on survival, clinical course of the disease, liver tissue, liver tests, or immunologic abnormalities with the use of azathioprine. There was some evidence that azathioprine positively affected the need for other drugs, jaundice, and cholesterol levels, among other variables; however, the results from this study were inconclusive.

For more information see page 1033.

Generic: **Budesonide (with UDCA)** *(byoo-DES-oh-nide)*
Brands: **Entocort EC, Pulmicort Respules, Pulmicort Turbohaler, Rhinocort Aqua**

Budesonide belongs to a class of drugs known as glucocortico-steroids, and is used to treat the inflammatory bowel disease known as Crohn's disease. Budesonide is thought to treat liver inflammation seen in primary biliary cirrhosis. Studies have shown that combination therapy with budesonide and ursodeoxycholic acid (UDCA) is superior to UDCA therapy alone. UDCA is a bile acid drug used to treat biliary cirrhosis, to dissolve gallstones, and is also used to treat other liver diseases.

In a clinical study, researchers in Finland examined the use of budesonide and UDCA versus UDCA alone in patients with primary biliary cirrhosis. Patients in this study received budesonide and UDCA or UDCA alone. Results from this study showed that disease stage improved 22% in the combination group but deteriorated 20% in the single-drug group. Liver fibrosis decreased 25% in the combination group, but increased 70% in the single-drug group. Inflammation decreased 34% in the combination group and 10% in the single-drug group. Bilirubin (a chemical in the body formed by hemoglobin breakdown) values increased in the single-drug group, but remained stable in the combination drug group. Researchers concluded that the combination of budesonide and UDCA improved liver tissue and function, and UDCA alone primarily affected laboratory values.

For more information see page 1055.

Generic: **Colestipol** *(koe-LES-ti-pole)*
Brand: **Colestid**

Colestipol belongs to a class of drugs known as bile acid resins. These drugs absorb bile acid in the intestines rather than letting it be reabsorbed and reused by the body. Colestipol absorbs and combines with bile acids, which increases the removal of cholesterol in the body through the stool. This drug lowers blood fats and cholesterol in patients at risk of heart attack or stroke. Since itching can be a bothersome symptom of primary biliary cirrhosis, one of the first drugs that may be prescribed by your doctor is colestipol to control this symptom. Side effects associated with colestipol include diarrhea, headache, dizziness, indigestion, upset stomach, gas, nausea, and vomiting.

In a review article, researchers in the United Kingdom noted the use of colestipol for people with itching related to primary biliary cirrhosis who could not tolerate treatment with another bile acid resin, cholestyramine. Another study reported that the bile acid drug, UDCA, improved primary biliary cirrhosis itching in up to 40% of people.

For more information see page 1116.

Generic: Cyclosporine (si-klo-SPOR-een)
Brands: Gengraf, Neoral, Sandimmune

Cyclosporine is used to reduce the body's natural immunity in people who have received a transplanted organ. Cyclosporine works by preventing white blood cells from rejecting the new organ. It is also used to treat rheumatoid arthritis and a skin condition known as psoriasis. In this liver disease, cyclosporine corrects immune cell dysfunction and affects immune system mechanisms, as well as provides short-term improvement in liver function tests. Side effects associated with cyclosporine can be serious, such as high blood pressure, kidney and liver problems, and a reduced ability to fight infection. Other less serious side effects include increased hair growth, trembling or shaking of the hands, acne, oily skin, headache, leg cramps, and nausea.

In a study conducted at the Mayo Clinic, the efficacy and safety of cyclosporine in primary biliary cirrhosis was evaluated. In this study, 29 patients with primary biliary cirrhosis were selected to receive cyclosporine or placebo. After one year of treatment, 17 of the 19 patients who were given cyclosporine had stability or improvement in primary biliary cirrhosis-related fatigue, and 18 had improvements in disease-related itching. Use of cyclosporine was also associated with improvements in liver function tests. Patients who received placebo were more tired and their disease-related itching worsened compared with the cyclosporine group. Long-term use of cyclosporine was associated with kidney toxicity and increased blood pressure.

For more information see pages 1125 and 1127.

Generic: **Methotrexate** *(meth-oh-TREKS-ate)*
Brands: **Rheumatrex, Trexall**

Methotrexate, a chemotherapy drug, belongs to a class of drugs known as immunosuppressives. It is used to treat certain types of cancer and inflammatory diseases such as rheumatoid arthritis. Immunosuppressive drugs, in general, block key factors that direct immune system reactions. In primary biliary cirrhosis, results from clinical trials suggest that methotrexate offers improvements in biochemical values and liver tissue after treatment. Side effects include hair loss, increased sensitivity to the sun, appetite loss, and nausea. Additionally, it may increase the risk of infection.

In a study conducted at Tufts University School of Medicine in Boston, five people with primary biliary cirrhosis were treated with low-dose oral methotrexate. All five completely responded to methotrexate treatment. Biochemical tests revealed that liver function returned to normal, disease-related symptoms stopped, and tissue analysis showed disease improvement. After five to 12 years of treatment with methotrexate, they had few signs of primary biliary cirrhosis, and three patients were considered close to normal. Researchers noted that use of methotrexate alone or in combination with other drugs may result in remission of primary biliary cirrhosis.

For more information see page 1312.

Generic: **Naloxone** *(nal-OKS-one)*
Brand: **Narcan**

Naloxone is used to reverse the effects such as difficulty breathing and coma that are produced by narcotic drugs. Narcotics may be used to reverse the effects of anesthesia once surgery is completed or to treat cases of narcotic drug overdose. Unrelieved itching in primary biliary cirrhosis may indicate the need for liver transplantation. In primary biliary cirrhosis, naloxone may be used as a last-line measure to relieve itching before your doctor considers liver transplantation. Side effects include diarrhea, fever, dizziness, lightheadedness, nausea, vomiting, nervousness, runny nose, and sweating, among others.

Researchers at the National Institute of Diabetes and Digestive and Kidney Diseases and the National Institutes of Health (NIH) in Bethesda tested the hypothesis that opioid agonist activity contributes to the itching seen in primary biliary cirrhosis. Patients with this liver disease were given one or two continuous IV infusions of naloxone or placebo solution. No side effects were noticed with the use of naloxone. Researchers found that naloxone infusions were consistently associated with a decrease in scratching activity in treated patients. Researchers concluded that increased opioid agonist activity contributes to scratching seen in patients with primary biliary cirrhosis. Moreover, they noted that naloxone infusions, although cumbersome in the number of infusions or injections needed, may be beneficial in the emergency treatment of itching related to this liver disease.

For more information see page 1351.

*Generic: **Naltrexone** (nal-TREKS-one)*
*Brands: **Naltrexone, ReVia***

Naltrexone is used to treat dependence on opiate drugs (narcotics) or alcohol. Naltrexone blocks the "high" that these substances produce. Unrelieved itching in primary biliary cirrhosis may be indicating the need for liver transplantation. In primary biliary cirrhosis, opiate antagonists such as naltrexone are considered by doctors to be a last-line effort to control itching before liver transplantation. Side effects associated with the drug include anxiety, difficulty sleeping, dizziness, headache, increased tiredness, nausea, nervousness, and vomiting.

Researchers in the Netherlands evaluated the use of naltrexone in a clinical trial in 16 patients with primary biliary cirrhosis. Patients with itching and primary biliary cirrhosis were randomly selected to receive a four-week course of naltrexone daily or placebo. Researchers then evaluated the patients' fatigue, quality of life, side effects of treatment, and liver function every two weeks. Results from this study showed that changes from the start of the study were significantly different and favored the naltrexone-treated group for daytime itching and nighttime itching. In four patients treated with naltrexone, side effects consistent with an opiate withdrawal syndrome were noted. Researchers concluded that oral naltrexone may be an effective and well-tolerated alternative drug for the itching associated with primary biliary cirrhosis.

For more information see page 1352.

*Generic: **Prednisolone** (pred-NISS-oh-lone)*
*Brands: **Predalone, Prelone***

Prednisolone belongs to a class of drugs known as corticosteroids. As a drug class, corticosteroids have strong anti-inflammatory properties and are used in a number of inflammatory diseases such as arthritis, asthma, and bronchitis, among others. Prednisolone helps to reduce swelling, redness, itching, and allergic reactions. Side effects include diarrhea, constipation, headache, increased or decreased appetite, increased sweating, nervousness, restlessness, and upset stomach, among others. Prednisolone can also impair the immune system's ability to fight infections.

In a three-year trial, researchers evaluated the use of prednisolone in people with primary biliary cirrhosis. Patients received prednisolone tablets given as a single morning dose. Placebo was given in the same manner as prednisolone. After three years, liver symptoms were improved in patients who received prednisolone treatment. Additionally, all liver function tests results favored treatment with prednisolone. There were no significant differences in bone loss between both treatment groups. Researchers concluded that three-year treatment of prednisolone was associated with better liver outcome and little evidence of bone loss in patients with primary biliary cirrhosis.

For more information see page 1428.

Therapy-resistant Hepatitis C

Hepatitis C is a disease caused by the hepatitis C virus (HCV) and results in liver swelling and liver dysfunction. This disease is transmitted by sharing drug needles, getting pricked by a contaminated needle, having a blood transfusion before 1992, having sex with an infected person, and being born to a mother who is infected with HCV. Symptoms include tiredness, stomach pains, fever, appetite loss, and diarrhea. Some patients are unresponsive to conventional treatment with interferons (immunomodulator drugs); hence these patients have a form of hepatitis that is resistant to these types of drugs and is called "therapy-resistant hepatitis C."

***Commonly Prescribed (On-Label) Drugs:** None*

OFF-LABEL PRESCRIPTION DRUGS
BREAKTHROUGH OPTIONS

*Generic: **Peginterferon Alfa-2a** (peg-in-ter-FEER-on AL-fa-2a)*
*Brand: **Pegasys***

Peginterferon alfa-2a (pegylated interferon), a man-made protein, is classified as an immunomodulator and an antiviral drug. In the body, natural interferons (proteins) help the immune system fight off viral infections and certain types of cancers. Peginterferon alfa-2a works in a way similar to natural interferons and is used to treat hepatitis C infection; however, it is not known if this drug can cure HCV infections, prevent liver failure or liver cancer, or prevent the spread of HCV to other persons. Side effects associated with peginterferon alfa-2a include diarrhea, dry skin, fever, chills, hair loss, headaches, and appetite loss, among others.

In general, treatment with interferon-based drug regimens has shown limited success in the treatment of hepatitis C. The safety and efficacy of peginterferon alpha alone or in combination with oral ribavirin (an antiviral drug) has not been entirely identified in previously treated patients who failed other alfa interferon therapies. However, among many doctors, peginterferon alfa-2a in combination with ribavirin is considered to be the treatment of choice in people with therapy-resistant hepatitis C.

In a recent study, use of peginterferon alpha-2a and ribavirin in people with advanced hepatic fibrosis and therapy-resistant hepatitis C resulted in an 18 % serologic response rate. Factors that positively influenced the response to this drug regimen included the type of virus and previous treatment with interferon alone. Retreatment in those with therapy-resistant hepatitis C depends on their previous type of response to treatment, the type of treatment previously used, disease severity, viral genotype, and other predictive factors for response. Interferons are also associated with the exacerbation of neuropsychiatric disorders including depression, suicide attempts, and drug dependence.

For more information see page 1398.

*Generic: **Peginterferon Alfa-2b*** *(peg-in-ter-FEER-on AL-fa-2b)*
*Brand: **PEG-intron***

Peginterferon alfa-2b (pegylated interferon), a man-made protein, is an immune modifier and an antiviral drug. In the body, natural interferons (proteins) help the immune system fight off viral infections and certain types of cancers. Peginterferon alfa-2b works similar to natural interferons and is used to treat hepatitis C infection; however, it is unknown if this drug can cure HCV infections, prevent liver failure or liver cancer, or prevent the spread of HCV to other persons. Peginterferon alfa-2b differs from standard interferons (immunomodulator drugs) in that it contains a substance called polyethylene glycol, which enhances its antiviral effects.

In general, treatment with interferon-based drug regimens has shown limited success in the treatment of hepatitis C. Combinations of pegylated interferons and ribavirin (an antiviral drug) are now the preferred treatments for most patients with chronic hepatitis C. In one study, a 48-week course of pegylated interferon in combination with ribavirin showed a sustained viral response rate of 55% in patients previously untreated for hepatitis C. Researchers with the University of Vermont evaluated the effects of peginterferon alfa-2b in 182 patients with therapy-resistant hepatitis C (who failed to respond to prior conventional interferon-based therapy). Ribavirin was given each day by mouth during the entire study. In patients who did not respond to previous therapy, the sustained viral response to peginterferon alfa-2b was 20%, and 55% in patients who previously relapsed. Results from this study suggest that combination peginterferon alfa-2b and ribavirin may be a treatment in people with therapy-resistant hepatitis C who have not responded to conventional therapy.

For more information see page 1399.

*Generic: **Ribavirin*** *(rye-ba-VYE-rin)*
*Brands: **Rebetol, Ribasphere, Virazole***

Ribavirin belongs to a class of drugs known as antivirals. Ribavirin is used to treat hepatitis C in combination with another antiviral known as peginterferon alfa. It is not known if treatment with ribavirin and interferon alfa (an immunomodulator drug) or peginterferon alfa therapies will prevent the spread of hepatitis

C to other persons, cure hepatitis C, or prevent complications associated with this liver disease. Side effects of ribavirin include headache, heartburn, itching, nausea, skin rash, and vomiting.

Spanish researchers noted the use of ribavirin alone for six months in four patients with therapy-resistant hepatitis C that did not respond to treatment with alfa interferon. In these patients, ribavirin was well tolerated and researchers concluded that this drug has a role, most likely in combination with interferon, in the treatment of therapy-resistant hepatitis C. Physicians recommend using oral ribavirin along with pegylated interferon alfa drugs for paients who have been treated with standard interferon alone or in combination with oral ribavirin but still have high levels of the virus in their blood. Study results have found that 15% to 20% of patients with therapy-resistant hepatitis C that did not respond to standard treatment improved and sustained low or undetectable levels of the virus after treatment with oral ribavirin and peginterferon alfa.

In another study, the combination of oral ribavirin and pegylated interferon sifnificantly reduced the level of the virus in the blood of 55% of the patients. In general, this treatment combination appears to be a well-recognized possible treatment option in people with therapy-resistant hepatitis C who do not respond to conventional therapy.

For more information see page 1446.

*Generic: **Ribavirin-interferon alfa-2b** (rye-ba-VYE-rin–in-ter-FEER-on AL-fa-2b)*
*Brands: **Copegus, Rebetron***

Ribavirin-interferon alfa-2b is a combination drug containing the antivirals ribavirin and interferon alfa-2b. Interferon alfa-2b is similar to natural interferons that are produced by the immune system to fight viral infections. Side effects associated with ribavirin-interferon alfa-2b include flu-like symptoms, thinning hair, headache, heartburn, itching, nausea, skin rash, and vomiting.

A review article published noted two trials involving patients who had hepatitis C relapse after treatment with interferon alfa-2b. In these instances, treatment with ribavirin plus interferon alfa-2b was found to be more effective than interferon alfa-2b alone in attaining undetectable blood virus levels and normalizing liver function for at least six months after the treatment was stopped. In a study conducted by researchers at Tufts University School of Medicine in Boston, Massachusetts, the combination of ribavirin and interferon alfa-2b was identified as a life-prolonging and cost-effective treatment in people with therapy-resistant hepatitis C. In comparison with interferon therapy alone, combination treatment with these two drugs was estimated to prolong life expectancy by two years with modest cost increases.

For more information see page 1448.

LUNG AND AIRWAY DISORDERS

ASTHMA

Asthma is a disorder that affects the lungs and is characterized by repeated wheezing, breathlessness, chest tightness, and early morning or nighttime coughing. During an asthma attack, the airways become swollen and inflamed, airway muscles tighten, and a reduced amount of air passes in and out of the lungs. Mucus may also block the airways. Attacks of asthma can be triggered by secondhand smoke, dust mites, air pollution, and pets, among other causes. Asthma can be subcategorized depending on symptoms, sensitivities, and triggers.

Acute Asthma

Acute asthma is a rapid onset, short and severe exacerbation of wheezing that is unresponsive to usually effective treatment and requires emergency room intervention. Acute asthma attacks are characterized by airway inflammation and narrowing, hyperinflation of the airways, pulmonary dysfunction, alterations in ventilation, and low levels of oxygen in the blood. Symptoms are those of an asthma attack such as wheezing, coughing, and shortness of breath; however, these sudden symptoms are persistent and can worsen.

Commonly Prescribed (On-Label) Drugs: *Betamethasone, Methylprednisolone*

OFF-LABEL PRESCRIPTION DRUGS
BREAKTHROUGH OPTIONS

*Generic: **Furosemide*** *(fyoor-OH-se-mide)*
*Brand: **Lasix***

Furosemide belongs to a class of drugs known as diuretics, or "water pills." Furosemide happens to be a strong diuretic, and is indicated to treat excess fluid and swelling in the body caused by conditions such as heart failure, kidney failure, and cirrhosis (a liver disease). Side effects associated with furosemide include low blood pressure, and water and electrolyte depletion.

Furosemide may be used in people with acute asthma since there is evidence that it blocks sodium-calcium pumps in the body and produces smooth muscle relaxation thereby preventing airway narrowing that is seen in asthma attacks. In a clinical study, Canadian researchers compared the effects of nebulized (administered in a fine spray) salbutamol (an adrenergic bronchodilator) and either nebulized furosemide or a saline solution in 42 patients with acute asthma. After 15 minutes and 30 minutes, there was no notable difference in the peak expiratory flow rate (PEFR) in patients treated with salbutamol and furosemide and salbutamol and saline treatment combinations. In patients who had short duration asthma exacerbations (for less than eight hours), PEFR improved significantly more in patients receiving furosemide. The respiratory rate, heart rate, and pulse rate also improved; however, there were no major differences between the treatment groups. The positive benefits of furosemide were not seen in patients with asthma symptoms greater than eight hours' duration. Researchers concluded that based on these findings, furosemide may provide added bronchodilator benefits in those patients with naturally occurring asthma symptoms of less than eight hours.

For more information see page 1204.

*Generic: **Ipratropium*** *(i-pra-TROE-pee-um)*
*Brands: **Atrovent, Atrovent HFA***

Ipratropium belongs to a class of drugs known as anticholinergic bronchodilators (drugs that open up narrowed airways), often used to treat symptoms of lung diseases such as asthma, chronic bronchitis, and emphysema. Ipratropium helps to decrease coughing, wheezing, shortness of breath, and difficult breathing by increasing airflow in the lungs. In severe asthma attacks, ipratropium is only used off-label in combination with other bronchodilators.

Canadian researchers highlighted the positive benefits of ipratropium combined with a beta2-agonist (a bronchodilator). Using the combination of ipratropium and a beta2-agonist was associated with a combined 7.3% improvement in forced expiratory flow in one second and a 22.1% improvement in peak expiratory flow rate (PEFR) compared with patients who received a beta2-agonist alone. In children with severe asthma, this drug combination improved lung function and decreased hospitalization rates. Researchers concluded that ipratropium, when used in combination with a beta2-agonist, offers modest improvements in airflow obstruction and appears to improve clinical outcomes in children.

For more information see page 1245.

Allergen-induced Asthma

Allergen-induced asthma, also referred to as allergic asthma, is characterized by airway obstruction associated with allergies and is triggered by substances called allergens. Allergen triggers that can induce allergic asthma include molds, animal dander, airborne pollens, house dust mites, and cockroach droppings. Exposure to the above-mentioned allergens, among others, can prompt an allergic reaction causing asthma symptoms such as wheezing, coughing, and airway obstruction. Investigators estimate that 90% of all asthma sufferers have allergic asthma as at least a portion of their disease.

Commonly Prescribed (On-Label) Drugs: *Montelukast*

OFF-LABEL PRESCRIPTION DRUGS
BREAKTHROUGH OPTIONS

Generic: **Cyclosporine** *(si-klo-SPOR-een)*
Brands: **Gengraf, Neoral, Sandimmune**

Cyclosporine belongs to a class of drugs known as immunosuppressives. Cyclosporine and other immunosuppressives are used to reduce the body's natural immunity in patients who received a transplanted kidney or liver. Cyclosporine is a strong drug; therefore, its use is associated with serious side effects such as high blood pressure, kidney and liver problems, and increased risk of infection. It is thought to influence immune cell activity in a number of inflammatory conditions including allergen-induced asthma; however, its activity in asthma is not fully understood.

In a study conducted at The London Chest Hospital, when cyclosporine was added to another drug and administered to people with chronic, severe steroid-dependent asthma during three months of treatment there was an improvement in lung function and a reduction in asthma exacerbations. In a nine-month follow-up study, low-dose oral cyclosporine substantially reduced the need for oral steroid therapy and significantly improved the morning peak expiratory flow rate (PEFR) when compared with placebo.

Additionally, other researchers studied the effects of cyclosporine on 12 patients with allergen-induced asthma. They were given two oral doses of either cyclosporine or placebo before inhaled allergen challenges (exposure to allergic-asthma triggers). In patients treated with cyclosporine, the drug reduced both the late asthmatic reaction and the late increase in inflammatory cells in the blood; however, the drug did not affect the early asthmatic reaction. Based on these results, researchers noted that cyclosporine provided anti-inflammatory properties in asthma, and may be useful in reducing the inflammatory aspect of asthma.

For more information see pages 1125 and 1127.

*Generic: **Furosemide** (fyoor-OH-se-mide)*
*Brand: **Lasix***

Furosemide is classified as a diuretic drug, commonly known as a "water pill," used to treat excess fluid and swelling in the body caused by conditions such as heart failure, kidney failure, and cirrhosis. Side effects associated with furosemide include low blood pressure, and water and electrolyte depletion. Close medical monitoring is necessary when using this drug because of the risk of these serious side effects.

The effect of furosemide on the airways in asthma is still uncertain. In allergen-induced asthma, researchers believe that furosemide affects electrolyte transport, prostaglandins (hormone-like substances), and inflammatory cell activity. In people with allergen-induced asthma, the use of furosemide has prevented or eased bronchospasm. Researchers in Spain evaluated the effects of furosemide in allergen-induced asthma. In this experiment, 56 blood samples from patients with allergen-induced asthma were stimulated with allergens like pollen. Blood samples that were treated with furosemide were also exposed to these same allergens. Results from this study showed that exposure to furosemide in the presence of allergen-induced asthma may block the release of histamine (a chemical in the body that is released during an allergic reaction) and other mediators responsible for the bronchial hyper-reactivity seen in this lung and airway disorder. Researchers concluded that furosemide may interfere with changes in the cells that store histamine. It should be noted that this drug is not commercially available as inhaled formulation.

For more information see page 1204.

Aspirin-sensitive Asthma

In about 3–5% of persons with asthma, aspirin use can cause asthma to worsen and prompt a severe and sudden asthma attack. In these people, aspirin can cause the body to produce excess amounts of chemicals known as leukotrienes; however, the complete mechanism by which aspirin induces an asthma attack is not fully known. Leukotrienes (a group of hormones that causes the symptoms of hayfever and asthma) makes the muscles around the bronchial tubes contract and results in shortness of breath and wheezing. Experiencing a negative reaction to aspirin is the only way to uncover if you have asthma sensitive to this drug. Most doctors recommend avoidance of aspirin for those with asthma.

Commonly Prescribed (On-Label) Drugs: *Montelukast, Zileuton*

OFF-LABEL PRESCRIPTION DRUG
BREAKTHROUGH OPTION

Generic: **Furosemide** *(fyoor-OH-se-mide)*
Brand: **Lasix**

Furosemide belongs to a class of drugs known as diuretics, or "water pills," used to treat excess fluid and swelling in the body caused by conditions such as heart failure, kidney failure, and cirrhosis. Side effects associated with furosemide include low blood pressure, and water and electrolyte depletion. You must be monitored when using this drug because of the risk of these serious side effects.

In clinical practice, furosemide has been used as an anti-asthma drug. In studies, furosemide stopped bronchoconstriction that was triggered by cold air, exercise, antigens, and metabisulfite (a preservative). In an article by a Polish researcher, in aspirin-sensitive asthma, furosemide provided a preventive effect on bronchoconstriction that was induced by aspirin. A clinical trial examined the effects of inhaled furosemide compared with placebo in six female patients with asthma and aspirin sensitivity. After inhaling furosemide or placebo, the six women inhaled increasing amounts of aspirin. Inhaling aspirin induced bronchoconstriction in all of the women who were pretreated with placebo. In this study, inhaled furosemide protected the women with asthma against bronchoconstriction induced by aspirin exposure. Researchers concluded that these results are compatible with the hypothesis that furosemide works by blocking neurotransmission (the passing of nerve signals from one cell to another through chemicals or electrical signals). It should be noted that this drug is not commercially available as inhaled formulation.

For more information see page 1204.

Chronic Asthma

Some people have occasional asthma attacks; however, a larger group of patients develops more long-lasting, recurrent symptoms of asthma such as coughing, shortness of breath, and wheezing on every day or most days. This syndrome is known as chronic asthma. In people with chronic asthma, several medications on a regular schedule are required daily. Continued exposure to antigens (substances that cause the immune system to produce antibodies) results in a chronic state of airway inflammation. Chronic asthma requires maintenance treatment to control asthma exacerbations.

Commonly Prescribed (On-Label) Drugs: *Montelukast, Pirbuterol*

OFF-LABEL PRESCRIPTION DRUGS
BREAKTHROUGH OPTIONS

Generic: **Furosemide** *(fyoor-OH-se-mide)*
Brand: **Lasix**

Furosemide is a diuretic drug, more commonly known as a "water pill," used to treat excess fluid and swelling in the body caused by conditions such as heart failure, kidney failure, and cirrhosis. Side effects associated with furosemide include low blood pressure, and water and electrolyte depletion. Close medical monitoring is necessary when using this drug because of the risk of these serious side effects.

Furosemide is also used to treat chronic asthma by increasing airway and lung hormone levels, inducing airway smooth muscle relaxation, and inhibiting the release of immune cells that result in airway inflammation.

In a review article by a researcher in Poland, furosemide was noted to be an anti-asthmatic drug. This researcher mentioned the efficacy of furosemide in premature infants with lung disease who were dependent on a ventilator. Aerolized furosemide given in saline solution increased tidal volume and respiratory lung compliance and improved lung resistance significantly after one to two hours after inhalation. Additionally, there were no adverse effects related to furosemide such as urine output difference or urinary electrolyte losses. The positive effect of furosemide was seen in as little as 30 minutes after the dose was given, and persisted for at least four hours. However, increasing the dose did not further improve lung function. Despite the positive benefits exerted by furosemide on lung function in a number of studies involving infants and children with lung disease, routine use of this drug in infants three weeks and older has not been recommended in the medical literature.

For more information see page 1204.

Generic: **Ipratropium** *(i-pra-TROE-pee-um)*
Brands: **Atrovent, Atrovent HFA**

Ipratropium belongs to a class of drugs known as anticholinergic bronchodilators (drugs that open up narrowed airways), often used to treat symptoms of lung diseases such as asthma, chronic bronchitis, and emphysema. It helps to decrease coughing, wheezing, shortness of breath, and difficult breathing by increasing airflow in the lungs. When ipratropium is given for acute, severe attacks of asthma, it is only used with other bronchodilators. Side effects associated with ipratropium include dry mouth, cough, and unpleasant taste.

Physicians have used effectively orally inhaled ipratropium for the treatment of chronic asthma. Some doctors recommend a trial of ipratropium as second-line treatment in those with moderate to severe asthma exacerbations who do not respond to other drugs. Researchers believe that the benefits of using ipratropium as a maintenance treatment (to prevent and control exacerbations) in chronic asthma remains to be seen. It has been suggested that this drug may serve as an alternate option in those having adverse events with beta-adrenergic agonists. Medical experts believe orally inhaled anticholinergics, such as ipratropium, have a limited role in managing asthma in children.

For more information see page 1245.

Exercise-induced Asthma

See Exercise-induced Bronchospasm, Prevention

Exercise-induced Bronchoconstriction

See Exercise-induced Bronchospasm, Prevention

Exercise-induced Bronchospasm, Prevention

Exercise-induced bronchospasm (EIB) occurs when the airways shrink during or after exercise. In people with EIB, exercising for more than 30 minutes can be challenging. Symptoms of EIB typically occur after five to 20 minutes of nonstop exercise, and include wheezing, difficulty breathing, coughing, chest tightness, or chest pain. EIB may be triggered by breathing in air that is cooler and drier compared with the air in the lungs. Your doctor may prescribe certain medications called "controllers" to prevent EIB.

Commonly Prescribed (On-Label) Drugs: *Albuterol, Formoterol, Salmeterol*

OFF-LABEL PRESCRIPTION DRUGS
BREAKTHROUGH OPTIONS

Generic: **Furosemide** *(fyoor-OH-se-mide)*
Brand: ***Lasix***

Furosemide is classified as a diuretic, or "water pill," used to treat excess fluid and swelling in the body caused by conditions such as heart failure, kidney failure, and cirrhosis. Side effects associated with furosemide include low blood pressure, and water and electrolyte depletion. Close medical monitoring is necessary when using this drug because of the risk of these serious side effects.

Inhaled formulations of furosemide have been used with success in people to prevent EIB. Furosemide was as effective as sodium cromoglycate (an anti-inflammatory drug) in children with EIB in a clinical study, as mentioned in a review article by researchers in Italy. It was also significantly more effective when compared with placebo and amiloride (a diuretic drug) in patients with asthma. These researchers also noted that furosemide was effective in preventing bronchoconstriction that was induced by the inhalation of dry air in patients with asthma compared with amiloride. Also highlighted by researchers were the beneficial effects of furosemide in patients with asthma sensitive to cold air.

However, it should be noted that this drug is not commercially available as an inhaled formulation.

For more information see page 1204.

Generic: **Ipratropium** *(i-pra-TROE-pee-um)*
Brands: **Atrovent, Atrovent HFA**

Ipratropium belongs to a class of drugs often used to treat symptoms of lung diseases such as chronic asthma, chronic bronchitis, and emphysema. This drug is used off-label for those suffering from exercise-induced asthma. Ipratropium helps to decrease coughing, wheezing, shortness of breath, and difficult breathing by increasing airflow in the lungs. The most common side effects associated with ipratropium include cough, dry mouth, and unpleasant taste.

The American Journal of Medicine reviewed the use of ipratropium to prevent EIB in patients with asthma. It was noted that ipratropium primarily affects the central airways compared with other drugs that act on the small, peripheral airways. The researchers reviewed a number of small studies evaluating the variable effects of ipratropium in people with EIB. In these studies, the time before exercise challenge after the drug was given ranged from 30 minutes to 90 minutes. Some of the studies in this review showed that bronchoconstrictor response was not altered by ipratropium use. Other studies showed that use of this drug resulted in a partial response in some patients. Among those that had a response to ipratropium, it was found that these patients had less severe asthma, milder exercise-induced bronchoconstriction, and mostly central airways responses to exercise. The researcher emphasized that a recurring theme among the studies reviewed was that ipratropium was more effective when the obstruction involved the central airways. Lastly, in the studies involving cold weather, pretreatment with ipratropium did not affect the change in airway measurements when compared with no pretreatment.

For more information see page 1245.

*Generic: **Nedocromil** (ne-doe-KROE-mil)*
*Brand: **Tilade***

Nedocromil is used to prevent the symptoms of asthma. If used on a regular basis, nedocromil can lessen the number and severity of asthma attacks by reducing lung inflammation. A side effect associated with nedocromil is unpleasant taste; other effects include cough, headache, nausea and vomiting, runny or stuffy nose, and throat irritation, among others.

Italian researchers evaluated the effects of nedocromil in the prevention of EIB in 13 athletes. In nine of the 13 athletes, nedocromil provided a good protective effect. In the remaining four athletes, the protective effect was not satisfactory. In these athletes with less than optimal response, a larger dose was found to be effective. In two instances, the drug resulted in prolonged bronchodilation. These researchers concluded that prevention of EIB with nedocromil may be based on the dose used and may be related to the degree of bronchial hyper-reactivity or other factors.

For more information see page 1355.

Steroid-dependent Asthma

Steroids help to regulate a number of body functions, including inflammation. In patients with asthma, the use of steroids helps open up the airways by reducing inflammation in airway walls. With the positive benefits of steroids there are also some negative effects. If steroids are taken for a long time, the body may stop making its own supply, and in turn, steroid drugs become necessary. In instances of severe asthma, some patients may become steroid-dependent if they take steroids for an extended period of time.

***Commonly Prescribed (On-Label) Drugs:** None*

OFF-LABEL PRESCRIPTION DRUGS
BREAKTHROUGH OPTIONS

*Generic: **Cyclosporine** (si-klo-SPOR-een)*
*Brands: **Gengraf, Neoral, Sandimmune***

Cyclosporine belongs to a class of drugs known as immunosuppressives that are used to reduce the body's natural immunity and prevent rejection of a transplanted organ. It is associated with serious side effects such as high blood pressure, kidney and liver problems, and increased risk of infection.

In asthma, cyclosporine is thought to block the activity of inflammatory cells and thereby reduce inflammation, although its exact action in asthma is not fully understood. The drug is also thought to reduce the need for steroids. Several researchers have noted the "steroid-sparing" effects that cyclosporine offers in people with asthma. In a trial, researchers in Poland sought to examine the effects of cyclosporine in patients with severe, corticosteroid-dependent asthma. In this study, 34 patients with steroid-dependent asthma were selected to receive: 1) cyclosporine or placebo for 12 weeks; 2) cyclosporine or placebo and oral prednisone (a steroid) reduction for 22 weeks; and 3) follow-up observation at eight weeks. In those who received cyclosporine, researchers noted only a slightly positive effect on asthma severity; however, no positive effects on lung function were seen. Cyclosporine appeared to be slightly better than placebo in reducing the amount of steroid needed, although a reduction in steroids was associated with some impairment in lung function. Researchers concluded that cyclosporine has a limited role in people with steroid-dependent asthma.

For more information see pages 1125 and 1127.

*Generic: **Furosemide** (fyoor-OH-se-mide)*
*Brand: **Lasix***

Furosemide belongs to a class of drugs known as diuretics, or "water pills," used to treat excess fluid and swelling in the body caused by conditions such as heart failure, kidney failure, and cirrhosis. Side effects associated with furosemide include low blood pressure and water and electrolyte depletion.

In studies, furosemide stops bronchoconstriction that is triggered by cold air, exercise, antigens, and metabisulfite (a preservative). The action of this drug in steroid-dependent asthma is not fully clear. In the medical literature, furosemide has documented use as an anti-asthma drug. In patients with steroid-dependent asthma, aspirin and furosemide offered a combined beneficial antiasthmatic effect. The combination of both of these drugs resulted in a reduction in the amount of steroids needed. In a study conducted in Italy of nine patients with chronic asthma requiring a high dose of inhaled steroids, researchers examined the effects of inhaled furosemide combined with a form of aspirin. Patients were treated with this drug combination or placebo and inhaled steroids twice daily. In those who received combined furosemide and a form of aspirin, two patients stopped steroids and seven patients reduced their steroid intake. It was concluded that the combination of inhaled furosemide and a form of aspirin reduced the need for steroids without major side effects in those with steroid-dependent asthma.

For more information see page 1204.

Generic: **Methotrexate** *(meth-oh-TREKS-ate)*
Brands: **Rheumatrex, Trexall**

Methotrexate belongs to a class of drugs that slow the growth of certain cells in the body. High doses of this drug are used to control certain cancers; at low doses, the drug is less toxic and still retains its anti-inflammatory properties. Use of methotrexate is associated with nausea and vomiting, liver dysfunction, thinned or brittle hair, blistering skin or acne, and appetite or weight loss. Additionally, methotrexate may induce asthma symptoms and cause lung disease itself.

How methotrexate works in steroid-dependent asthma is not fully known; however, it is thought to block histamine (a chemical produced by the body) release from immune cells and interfere with the way the body breaks down steroids. In a study of 14 patients with steroid-dependent asthma, methotrexate provided a 36.5% reduction in prednisone (steroid) use compared with placebo. In a follow-up study of 25 patients receiving methotrexate for at least 18 months, a reduction in daily prednisone use was reported. Fifteen patients in this study tapered off the dose of prednisone and another nine patients reduced their steroid dose by more than

50%. In another study involving 60 patients, use of methotrexate resulted in a 50% reduction in prednisolone (a steroid) dose, compared with 14% of those receiving placebo. Once methotrexate was stopped, the amount of steroid that was needed returned to levels seen at the beginning of the study. A combined review of several studies has indicated that methotrexate given for three to six months provides about a 20% reduction in steroid needs, although only 60% of patients show a dramatic response.

For more information see page 1312.

BACTERIAL LUNG DISEASE

Atypical Pneumonia

Atypical pneumonia, or "walking pneumonia" is caused by *Legionella pneumophila*, *Mycoplasma pneumoniae*, and *Chlamydia pneumoniae* bacteria. Usually, atypical pneumonias are associated with milder forms of pneumonia; however, pneumonia caused by *Legionella* can be severe and result in death. Those at risk for atypical pneumonias include the elderly, smokers, and those with weakened immune systems. Also, infected air conditioning systems have been linked to pneumonia caused by *Legionella*. Symptoms of atypical pneumonia include chills, fever, cough, muscle stiffness, and rapid breathing, among others.

Eaton Agent

See Mycoplasma Pneumonia

Legionellosis

See Legionnaire's Disease

Legionnaire's Disease

Legionnaire's disease is a lung disease caused by *Legionella pneumophila* bacteria, which are found in bodies of water and in soil. In water or water systems, *Legionella* will attach, colonize, and form a biofilm (a protective adhesive excreted by microorganism). Since Legionnaire's disease is a water-borne illness and is mainly acquired through drinking water, it is not contagious. Between two and 10 days after exposure to the bacteria, symptoms appear and can include tiredness, weakness, high fever, cough, diarrhea, nausea, vomiting, headache, muscle aches, and shortness of breath, among others.

Commonly Prescribed (On-Label) Drugs: *Cyclosporine, Erythromycin*

OFF-LABEL PRESCRIPTION DRUGS
BREAKTHROUGH OPTIONS

Generic: **Ciprofloxacin** *(sip-roe-FLOKS-a-sin)*
Brands: **Ciloxan, Cipro, Cipro XR**

Ciprofloxacin is used to treat a wide variety of infections including pneumonia, bronchitis, bacterial diarrhea, and urinary tract infections. This antibiotic is also used to treat Legionnaire's disease; however, it does not show activity against bacteria that can function without oxygen. Side effects associated with the use of ciprofloxacin include upset stomach, vomiting, stomach pain, indigestion, headache, nervousness, and agitation, among others.

Most of the data supporting the use of antibiotics, such as ciprofloxacin, come from review articles, lab studies, and patient case study reports. Lab studies have shown that quinolone antibiotics have a high intracellular activity against *Legionella*. In a patient case study, researchers from Japan noted the effects of ciprofloxacin in a 69-year-old man with cough and fever. Tests revealed that he had Legionnaire's disease, and he was subsequently treated with IV ciprofloxacin. After treatment, his symptoms rapidly improved. Researchers concluded that IV ciprofloxacin should be the first treatment choice for this disease.

For more information see page 1093.

Generic: **Clarithromycin** *(kla-RITH-roe-mye-sin)*
Brands: **Biaxin, Biaxin XL**

Clarithromycin is often used in a wide variety of infections such as pneumonia, bronchitis, and infections of the lungs, ears, sinuses, skin, and throat. Therapy with antibiotics, such as clarithromycin, should last for two weeks in mild forms of disease. In individuals with decreased immunity or more severe Legionnaire's disease, antibiotic treatment should be taken for three weeks. Clarithromycin may cause side effects such as diarrhea, upset stomach, abnormal taste, stomach pain, and headache.

In a review article by a researcher with The Clinical Pharmacology Research Center in Cooperstown, New York, clarithromycin is among the list of recommended antibiotics for Legionnaire's disease. In a clinical study conducted by researchers in the United Kingdom, oral azithromycin (an antibiotic) given once daily was more effective than clarithromycin in preventing fever and reducing the number of bacteria and lung lesions in guinea pigs. Researchers found that an eight-fold higher dose of clarithromycin was needed to gain the same effect as low-dose azithromycin in this study. Finally, in a clinical study conducted by researchers in Pakistan, use of clarithromycin was associated with a 98% clinical cure rate in 34 patients with Legionnaire's disease. Researchers concluded that clarithromycin is a safe and effective treatment in patients with severe Legionnaire's disease that may be used in those who do not respond to azithromycin.

For more information see page 1098.

Generic: **Gemifloxacin** *(je-mi-FLOKS-a-sin)*
Brand: **Factive**

Gemifloxacin is approved to treat a number of infections including pneumonia and bronchitis. Among many doctors, this type of antibiotic is considered one of the preferred drugs for the treatment of Legionnaire's disease. Side effects associated with gemifloxacin include diarrhea, stomach pain, vomiting, lightheadedness, and confusion, among others.

Researchers with the University of Pennsylvania School of Medicine documented the activity of gemifloxacin in guinea pigs with Legionnaire's disease. In this study, guinea pigs treated with gemifloxacin were compared with guinea pigs treated with azithromycin and others treated with levofloxacin. All 15 treated with gemifloxacin for two days survived for nine days, and 13 of the 14 guinea pigs given this same drug for five days survived. All 12 azithromycin-treated guinea pigs survived, and 11 of the 12 guinea pigs given levofloxacin survived. Researchers concluded that gemifloxacin is effective in Legionnaire's disease, even when the drug regimen is shortened.

For more information see page 1210.

*Generic: **Minocycline** (min-OH-sik-leen)*
*Brands: **Dynacin, Minocin***

Minocycline is used to treat a number of bacterial infections. For Legionnaire's disease, certain antibiotics, such as minocycline, are recommended since they have high concentrations and are active against *Legionella* bacteria. Therapy with antibiotics, in general, should last for two weeks in mild disease, and three weeks in severe disease and in persons with decreased immunity. Side effects associated with minocycline include upset stomach, diarrhea, dizziness, unsteadiness, drowsiness, headache, and vomiting, among others.

In a study conducted at the Department of Health in Pennsylvania, five antibiotics, including minocycline, were tested in guinea pigs with Legionnaire's disease. In this study, the most effective antibiotic was minocycline; use of this drug resulted in a 50% survival rate in infected guinea pigs. The other antibiotics, rifampin, amikacin, tobramycin, and gentamycin, were less effective. In this study, surviving guinea pigs remained healthy and were able to produce antibodies (molecules in body fluids that destroy or neutralize bacteria and toxins) to the *Legionella* bacteria. In another laboratory study, minocycline was found to be the most effective drug in guinea pigs infected with Legionnaire's disease. Minocycline was as effective as doxycycline (an antibiotic) in blocking the growth of *Legionella* bacteria, and prolonged the animals' survival. Overall, minocycline is recognized as having antibiotic activity against this type of bacteria.

For more information see page 1331.

Generic: **Moxifloxacin** *(moxs-i-FLOKS-a-sin)*
Brands: **Avelox, Vigamox**

Moxifloxacin is used to treat a number of bacterial infections, and stops bacterial growth in diseases such as Legionnaire's. Among many doctors, fluoroquinolone antibiotics such as moxifloxacin are considered the preferred drugs for the treatment of Legionnaire's disease. In the treatment of respiratory infections, moxifloxacin has been reported to be effective. Moreover, this drug has activity against atypical pneumonias, such as *Legionella pneumophila*. Despite the fact that fluoroquinolone antibiotics are not recommended in those under age 18 with Legionnaire's disease, these types of antibiotics may be used in certain instances in children. Side effects include dizziness, nausea, and diarrhea.

Researchers in Germany evaluated the newer fluoroquinolones, including moxifloxacin for the treatment of Legionnaire's disease. In this study, six strains of *Legionella* were tested and proven to be highly susceptible to the fluoroquinolones, including moxifloxacin, which was found to prevent the overall growth of *Legionella pneumophila*. Researchers concluded that moxifloxacin could be very valuable in the treatment of Legionnaire's disease.

In another study, researchers at the University of Pittsburgh, in Pennsylvania, compared the activity of different classes of antibiotics (quinolones, macrolides, and ketolides) on 112 strains of *Legionella*. Quinolone-type antibiotics such as moxifloxacin were found to have the greatest degree of intracellular activity against *Legionella pneumophila*. Ketolide- and macrolide-type antibiotics, respectively, showed less activity.

For more information see page 1342.

Generic: **Rifampin** *(ri-FAM-pin)*
Brand: **Rifadin**

Rifampin is used to prevent and treat tuberculosis and other infections. In people who are severely ill or have decreased immunity, IV rifampin may be added at the start of treatment. Additionally, if *Legionella pneumophila* is identified in patients with community-acquired pneumonia, experts recommend the use of a macrolide or fluoroquinolone antibiotic with or without IV rifampin. Alternatively, the antibiotic, doxycyline, may be given in these instances with or without IV rifampin.

In a study by researchers at Stratton Veterans Affairs Medical Center in Albany, New York, evaluating various antibiotics and rifampin on Legionnaire's disease, only levofloxacin and rifampin worked against *Legionella pneumophila* when used in combination. Rifampin dosing was mentioned in a review article by researchers in Spain, which recommended that persons with severe illness or decreased immunity with Legionnaire's disease, IV or oral rifampin every 12 hours should be added to the erythromycin (an antibiotic) dose. In another analysis, researchers in France reviewed cases of Legionnaire's disease and concluded that combined therapy with erythromycin, rifampin, or perfloxacin (an antibiotic) is superior to erythromycin alone.

For more information see page 1450.

Generic: **Tetracycline** *(tet-ra-SYE-kleen)*
Brands: **Sumycin, Wesmycin**

Tetracycline is an antibiotic used in a wide variety of infections including pneumonia and bladder infections. In Legionnaire's disease, tetracycline is considered to be an alternate drug treatment. In some instances, IV rifampin may be added on to tetracycline to treat infected persons. In general, treatment of Legionnaire's disease with an antibiotic should last for two weeks in mild disease and up to three weeks in those with severe disease or decreased immunity. Side effects associated with tetracycline are uncommon but possible, and include upset stomach, diarrhea, and sore mouth.

Journal of Antimicrobial Chemotherapy reported the activities of tetracycline and two other antibiotics (minocycline and doxycycline) in guinea pigs infected with *Legionella pneumophilia*. In this analysis, minocycline and doxycycline were equally effective against these bacteria; however, tetracycline was the least effective of all three antibiotics. Minocycline was the only antibiotic to have statistically significant effects, although doxycycline increased survival rates. The researchers concluded that tetracycline-derived antibiotics (minocycline and doxycycline) are effective treatments in the management of Legionnaire's disease.

For more information see page 1503.

Generic: **Trimethoprim-sulfamethoxazole**
(try-METH-oh-prim sul-fah-meth-OX-ahzole)
Brands: **Bactrim, Septra**

Trimethoprim-sulfamethoxazole is an antibiotic that contains a combination of two drugs: trimethoprim and sulfamethoxazole. It is used in several different types of infections including pneumonia, bronchitis, ear infections, and urinary tract infections. In Legionnaire's disease, trimethoprim-sulfamethoxazole is considered to be a treatment alternative to other antibiotics. Side effects associated with trimethoprim-sulfamethoxazole include diarrhea, dizziness, appetite loss, mouth sores, nausea, and vomiting, among others. In general, therapy with antibiotics should last for two weeks in mild Legionnaire's disease, and up to three weeks in those with severe disease or immune system dysfunction.

Although macrolide antibiotics are the treatment of choice according to a pediatric infectious disease and immunology specialist with the University of Florida Health Science Center, trimethoprim-sulfamethoxazole is an effective alternative for Legionnaire's disease. Evidence of the use, efficacy, and safety of trimethoprim-sulfamethoxazole is limited to a few review articles and patient case studies in the medical literature. In one review article by researchers with the Winthrop-University Hospital in Mineola, New York, trimethoprim-sulfamethoxazole was reported to be active against *Legionella pneumophilia.*

For more information see page 1530.

Mycoplasma Pneumonia

Mycoplasma pneumonia, an atypical pneumonia, is a lung infection caused by a type of bacteria known as *Mycoplasma pneumoniae*. People at highest risk for mycoplasma pneumonia are those who work or reside in crowded areas. About 15 to 50% of pneumonia in adults is mycoplasma pneumonia. Symptoms occur within one to three weeks after infection and include headache, fever, chills, excessive sweating, chest pain, sore throat, and cough.

Commonly Prescribed (On-Label) Drugs: *Clarithromycin, Erythromycin, Tetracycline*

OFF-LABEL PRESCRIPTION DRUGS
BREAKTHROUGH OPTIONS

Generic: **Ciprofloxacin** *(sip-roe-FLOKS-a-sin)*
Brands: **Ciloxan, Cipro, Cipro XR**

Ciprofloxacin is used to treat lung infections including pneumonia and bronchitis as well as a number of other bacterial infections such as urinary tract, sinus, and sexually transmitted diseases. In mycoplasma pneumonia, ciprofloxacin appears to relieve most of the infection-related symptoms. Ciprofloxacin is generally used for 10 to 14 days and may cause side effects such as upset stomach, vomiting, stomach pain, indigestion, headache, nervousness, and agitation, among others.

A researcher from Denmark reviewed a number of studies to summarize the efficacy of ciprofloxacin in respiratory infections. In these studies, ciprofloxacin was dosed from seven to 16 days, and in up to 103 patients with a variety of lung infections. Additionally, based on the findings from a number of experiments with animals infected with *Mycoplasma pneumoniae*, this researcher suggested that ciprofloxacin has a role in the treatment of human mycoplasma pneumonia.

Researchers in Japan compared the efficacy of ciprofloxacin with other quinolone-type antibiotics, temafloxacin and ofloxacin, in mycoplasma pneumoniae-infected hamsters. In this study, both temafloxacin and ofloxacin, but not ciprofloxacin, were active when the oral formulations given once daily for five days were started 24 hours after infection. Additionally, continuous administration of ciprofloxacin or ofloxacin for 15 days did not significantly reduce the amount of *Mycoplasma pneumoniae* in the lungs. Use of ciprofloxacin must be considered in conjunction with a physician.

For more information see page 1093.

Generic: **Minocycline** *(min-OH-sik-leen)*
Brands: **Dynacin, Minocin**

Minocycline is used to treat a number of bacterial infections. According to a clinical microbiologist at the University of Alabama at Birmingham, erythromycin has been the long-standing drug of choice for mycoplasma pneumonia infections, but these bacteria are also susceptible to tetracycline-type antibiotics such as minocycline. Side effects can include allergic reactions, dark-colored urine or pale stools, headache, blurred vision, nausea, vomiting, and appetite loss, among others.

In a review of patient case studies, researchers in Austria reviewed 58 reports of children with mycoplasma pneumonia. Researchers found that in the 44 children treated with antibiotics (primarily minocycline or erythromycin) only one patient was cured as a direct result of the drugs (in this case the antibiotic was chloramphenicol). In a patient case study in Japan, minocycline treatment alone or in combination with levofloxacin (an antibiotic) was ineffective in a patient with mycoplasma pneumonia. This 16-year-old patient experienced gradual improvement once minocycline was stopped and after erythromycin (an antibiotic) was given. In a laboratory study evaluating the activity of antibiotics against *Mycoplasma pneumoniae*, Japanese researchers found that grepafloxacin had stronger antibacterial activity than ofloxacin and minocycline.

For more information see page 1331.

Pneumocystis Jiroveci Pneumonia

Pneumocystis jiroveci, which was formerly known as pneumocystis carinii, is caused by the microorganism *Pneumocystis jiroveci*. This form of pneumonia is rare among healthy persons, but more common and possibly fatal in those with decreased immunity such as people with the human immunodeficiency virus (HIV). Symptoms of pneumocystis jiroveci pneumonia (PCP) include high fever, nonproductive cough, weight loss, shortness of breath, and night sweats. Investigators believe that PCP is spread by breathing in *Pneumocystis jiroveci* cysts that colonize in the respiratory tract.

Commonly Prescribed (On-Label) Drugs: *None*

OFF-LABEL PRESCRIPTION DRUGS
BREAKTHROUGH OPTIONS

*Generic: **Clindamycin** (klin-da-MYE-sin)*
*Brands: **Cleocin, Clindamycin***

Clindamycin is usually reserved for use in more serious infections because it is associated with colitis (inflammation of the large intestine). Although trimethoprim-sulfamethoxazole is considered to be the treatment of choice for PCP, other treatments for mild, moderate, and severe disease include IV clindamycin with oral primaquine (an antimalarial drug). In general, clindamycin is given with primaquine for PCP. Clindamycin works by blocking bacterial protein production and stopping bacterial growth. Possible side effects include colitis, diarrhea, stomach cramps, fever, and increased thirst.

Results from clinical studies have shown that IV clindamycin or oral clindamycin used with oral primaquine for 21 days was effective treatment for PCP in adults with HIV. In these studies, most patients demonstrated clinical improvement within two to seven days with this regimen, and the combination was well tolerated. Moreover, the FDA recognizes the use of clindamycin for the treatment of PCP in patients with HIV. When compared with trimethoprim and sulfamethoxazole-type antibiotic drugs, clindamycin was shown to be just as effective. Therefore, clindamycin may be used in people who fail to respond to, who are contraindicated for, or have an inadequate response to trimethoprim-sulfamethoxazole. In a study of 497 patients with PCP conducted by researchers in South Africa, the combination of clindamycin and primaquine was the most effective alternative treatment in patients who failed to respond to other drugs.

For more information see pages 1099 and 1101.

*Generic: **Dapsone** (DAP-zone)*
*Brand: **None***

Dapsone is an antibiotic used to treat leprosy and skin infections. It is considered an alternative drug for the treatment of mild to moderate PCP, and is given in combination with another antibiotic drug, trimethoprim.

In PCP, dapsone can be used with trimethoprim as initial treatment in adults with acquired immune deficiency syndrome (AIDS). Dapsone once daily along with trimethoprim in four divided doses for 21 days has been proven to be effective for the initial treatment of PCP in this population. In one study conducted in Belgium, the use of this drug regimen resulted in a 93% response rate in patients with mild to moderate PCP. In general, researchers note that most patients show clinical improvement with dapsone and trimethoprim after six days of treatment, and both of these drugs are well tolerated. Furthermore, the FDA recognizes the use of dapsone in patients with AIDS.

The combination of dapsone and trimethoprim appears to be just as effective as trimethoprim and sulfamethoxazole-type antibiotic drugs for mild to moderately severe PCP. However, dapsone and trimethoprim are better tolerated in patients with AIDS versus trimethoprim-sulfamethoxazole. Therefore, dapsone and trimethoprim in combination may serve as an alternative treatment in patients who are intolerant to trimethoprim-sulfamethoxazole.

For more information see page 1131.

Generic: **Prednisone** *(pred-NIS-zone)*
Brands: **Deltasone, Liquid Pred, Meticorten, Orasone, Sterapred**

Prednisone is frequently used to treat inflammation and to prevent rejection of transplanted organs and to treat certain types of cancer. In PCP, prednisone can blunt inflammatory lung responses and reduce deterioration of oxygenation and respiratory failure. Prednisone is indicated to treat moderate to severe PCP in people with HIV who have low blood oxygen levels. Side effects associated with prednisone include upset stomach, vomiting, headache, dizziness, insomnia, and depression, among others. Additionally, the use of prednisone increases the risk for infection.

In a review conducted at the Thomas Jefferson University Hospital in Philadelphia, researchers found that early therapy with corticosteroids can help people with moderate to severe AIDS-related PCP. Use of corticosteroids in patients with AIDS-related PCP was associated with decreased mortality, respiratory failure, and deterioration of oxygenation. Steroid therapy was found to be most beneficial when given within 72 hours of the start of PCP treatment. A small, increased rate of infection was associated with the use of corticosteroids in this review article.

For more information see page 1429.

Generic: **Trimethoprim** (try-METH-oh-prim)
Brands: **Primsol, Proloprim**

Trimethoprim is used in a number of bacterial infections, particularly urinary tract infections. It is also combined with other drugs to treat PCP. Although side effects are generally uncommon, upset stomach, vomiting, anemia, and diarrhea can occur with use of this drug.

In people with AIDS and PCP who received trimethoprim and dapsone, improvement is generally seen within six days, and this drug combination is well tolerated. Based on evidence in clinical studies of animals with induced PCP, trimethoprim alone appears to be ineffective in the treatment of this type of pneumonia. The combination of trimethoprim and sulfamethoxazole is considered the drug of choice for the initial treatment of mild, moderate, and severe PCP infections. In the treatment of PCP, higher doses of trimethoprim are usually necessary compared with other infections. In PCP, trimethoprim and dapsone can be used as initial treatment in adults with AIDS. Trimethoprim along with dapsone for 21 days has been proven effective for the initial treatment of PCP in this population. In one study, the use of this drug regimen resulted in a 93% response rate in patients with mild to moderate PCP.

For more information see page 1529.

Pneumocystis, Prevention

Prevention of pneumocystis, a potentially fatal respiratory infection caused by the microorganism *Pneumocystis jiroveci*, is necessary in persons with a very low CD4 immune cell (a type of white blood cell that fights infections) count. Preventive Pneumocystitis jiroveci pneumonia (PCP) medication has shown to have a positive impact on patients with HIV disease. People who should receive preventive PCP drugs include those infected with HIV, and possibly those with decreased immune system function that is not attributed to HIV.

Commonly Prescribed (On-Label) Drugs: Atovaquone, Cotrimoxazole (Trimethoprim-Sulfamethoxazole), Trimetrexate

---

OFF-LABEL PRESCRIPTION DRUGS
BREAKTHROUGH OPTIONS

Generic: **Dapsone** *(DAP-zone)*
Brand: **None**

Dapsone is an antibiotic used to treat leprosy and skin infections. In PCP, dapsone blocks the growth of bacteria. Although trimethoprim-sulfamethoxazole is considered the preferred treatment for the prevention of PCP, dapsone is considered the next alternative, and is often combined with pyrimethamine (an antimalarial drug). Side effects associated with the use of dapsone include fever, rash, nausea, anemia (decreased number of red blood cells), vomiting, headache, insomnia, and upset stomach.

Dapsone is recognized as a drug used in the prevention of PCP in persons with HIV. A trial conducted in Australia demonstrated that dapsone was effective for PCP in persons with HIV and low immune cell counts. Additionally, a small study showed that dapsone was effective in both the primary and secondary prevention of PCP. Finally, in a study conducted in Belgium, dapsone and a combination of pyrimethamine and sulfadoxine (an antibiotic) appeared to be similarly effective at preventing PCP in 193 patients with HIV.

For more information see page 1131.

Pneumocystosis Interstitial

See Pneumocystis Jiroveci Pneumonia

AIRWAY DISORDERS

More than 30 million Americans have lung disease, which may cause intermittent or chronic symptoms. Airway diseases include seasonal allergic rhinitis, Cheyne-Stokes respiration, chronic obstructive pulmonary disease (COPD), cystic fibrosis, and laryngitis, among others. Common symptoms of lung disease include difficulty breathing, shortness of breath, chronic cough, coughing up blood, or pain when breathing in or out. Lung diseases can result from smoking; exposure to gases, asbestos (a natural fiber), chemicals, or other irritants; and air or environmental pollution, among many other causes.

Besnier-Boeck-Schaumann Syndrome

See Sarcoidosis

Boeck Disease

See Sarcoidosis

Boeck Sarcoid

See Sarcoidosis

Chronic Obstructive Pulmonary Disease

Chronic obstructive pulmonary disease, or COPD, is a slow, progressive airways disease that results in gradual loss of lung function. It also encompasses the lung condition called emphysema, which is when the walls between many of the air sacs in the lungs are destroyed. The number one risk factor for COPD is cigarette smoking. Other forms of tobacco smoking, exposure to second-hand smoke, and work-related dusts or chemicals also increase a person's risk of COPD. Signs and symptoms include productive cough; bluish tinge to the skin, lips, and nailbeds; shortness of breath; barrel chest; pursed-lips breathing; wheezing, weight loss, and swelling of feet and ankles.

Commonly Prescribed (On-Label) Drugs: *Acetylcysteine, Azithromycin, Doxapram, Dyphylline, Formoterol,*

Ipratropium, Ipratropium/Albuterol, Isoetharine,
Metaproterenol, Salmeterol, Salmeterol/Fluticasone,
Theophylline, Tiotropium

OFF-LABEL PRESCRIPTION DRUG
BREAKTHROUGH OPTION

Generic: **Methylprednisolone** *(meth-il-pred-NIS-oh-lone)*
Brands: **Depo-Medrol, Medrol, Solu-Medrol**

Methylprednisolone belongs to a class of drugs known as corticosteroids and is used in a number of conditions such as asthma and arthritis, and in severe allergies. For the treatment of COPD, corticosteroids have been shown to be effective in speeding up recovery from acute exacerbations of this disease.

Methylprednisolone may be given in IV form in the emergency room for people experiencing acute COPD exacerbations. The oral formulation of this corticosteroid appears to be just as effective as IV. Side effects are generally uncommon with methylprednisolone use, but can include upset stomach, stomach irritation, vomiting, headache, dizziness, and insomnia. Also, this drug can increase your risk of infections.

Clinical Pharmacy reported the use of methylprednisolone and bronchodilator therapy in patients with COPD undergoing upper abdominal surgery. In an effort to combat the post-operative deterioration of lung function that is a result of abdominal surgery, methylprednisolone was used. Patients showed a significant improvement in the post-operative lung recovery compared with the placebo group. Results from this study also suggested that methylprednisolone improved diaphragm function. Investigators concluded that immediate post-operative administration of methylprednisolone improves lung function.

For more information see page 1316.

Clarke-Hadfield Syndrome

See Cystic Fibrosis

Cystic Fibrosis

Cystic fibrosis is a life-threatening lung disorder and can cause severe lung damage and nutritional deficiencies. It affects the cells that produce saliva, mucus, sweat, and digestive fluids in the body; in persons with cystic fibrosis, these secretions become thick and sticky. Cystic fibrosis is an inherited disorder caused by gene defects; the number one risk factor is a family history of the disease. Signs and symptoms of cystic fibrosis include a salty taste to the skin, bowel obstruction, delayed growth, thick sputum, and coughing and wheezing, among others. Respiratory failure is the most dangerous result of cystic fibrosis. For information on off-label drugs for children with cystic fibrosis, see Children's Health Disorders chapter on page 192.

Commonly Prescribed (On-Label) Drugs: *Acetylcysteine, Aztreonam, Ceftazidime, Chloramphenicol, Dornase Alfa, Fusidic Acid, Medium Chain Triglycerides, Pancrelipase, Ticarcillin/Clavulanic Acid, Tobramycin, Ursodiol*

OFF-LABEL PRESCRIPTION DRUGS
BREAKTHROUGH OPTIONS

Generic: **Ipratropium** *(i-pra-TROE-pee-um)*
Brands: **Atrovent, Atrovent HFA**

Ipratropium belongs to a class of drugs known as anticholinergic bronchodilators that are often used to treat symptoms of lung diseases such as asthma, chronic bronchitis, and emphysema. Ipratropium helps to decrease coughing, wheezing, shortness of breath, and difficult breathing by increasing airflow to the lungs. Oral ipratropium has been used in cystic fibrosis for bronchodilation in a limited number of patients in clinical studies. Side effects include cough, dry mouth, and unpleasant taste.

In a small study in Canada, the effect of large doses of ipratropium and another drug were studied in nine patients with cystic fibrosis. After inhalation of each drug, and at four and eight hours after inhalation, the FEV1 and airway resistance improved on both days. Researchers concluded that single and sequential treatment of large doses of bronchodilating drugs provide similar bronchodilator effects in persons with cystic fibrosis.

For more information see page 1245.

*Generic: **Omeprazole*** *(oh-ME-pray-zol)*
*Brands: **Prilosec, Zegerid***

Omeprazole, a proton pump inhibitor which stops the production and release of gastric acid in the stomach, belongs to a class of drugs that block the production of acid by the stomach and are used in gastroesophageal reflux disease (GERD) and other diseases where the stomach overproduces acid. Most people with cystic fibrosis suffer from excess fat in their stools. Use of omeprazole may produce side effects such as stomach pain, diarrhea, dizziness, mild rash, constipation, and dry cough.

Researchers in the Netherlands examined the effect of adding omeprazole to treatment with pancreatin (an enzyme-type drug) in nine adults with cystic fibrosis with lung and pancreas involvement. It was concluded that omeprazole added on to high-dose pancreatin treatment reduced fat excretion in cystic fibrosis.

For more information see page 1386.

Fibrocystic Disease of the Pancreas

See Cystic Fibrosis

Hydrothorax

See Pleural Effusion

Laryngitis

Inflammation of the larynx (voice box) as a result of irritation, overuse, or infection is called laryngitis. When vocal cords become irritated or inflamed, swelling occurs and results in distortion of sounds. Hoarseness and faintness of voice can result along with tickling sensations in the back of the throat, sore throat, and cough. Laryngitis can be acute or chronic; chronic laryngitis may be a sign of a more serious disorder. Causes of laryngitis include viral infections, bacterial infections, heavy smoking or alcohol consumption, and gastroesophageal reflux disease (GERD).

Commonly Prescribed (On-Label) Drugs: *Omeprazole*

OFF-LABEL PRESCRIPTION DRUGS
BREAKTHROUGH OPTIONS

Generic: **Lansoprazole** *(lan-SOE-pra-zole)*
Brands: **Prevacid, Prevacid IV, Prevacid Solutabs**

Lansoprazole, a proton pump inhibitor that stops the production and release of gastric acid in the stomach, belongs to a class of drugs that block the production of acid by the stomach and are used in GERD and other diseases where the stomach overproduces acid. It is used to treat ulcers, heartburn, and gastroesophageal reflux disease (GERD). Possible side effects of lansoprazole include stomach pain and diarrhea. In some patients, GERD results in laryngeal and lung symptoms such as coughing, hoarseness, and sore throat. Lansoprazole may help treat GERD-associated laryngitis.

In a clinical trial, 22 patients with chronic laryngitis with or without esophageal symptoms were given lansoprazole for three months and had a significantly higher rate of complete symptom response compared with placebo (50% versus 10%, respectively). Researchers concluded that lansoprazole is a promising drug for chronic laryngitis. In another trial, a researcher with Baylor University in Texas along with researchers from other U.S. universities examined the effects of lansoprazole and placebo for three months in 20 people with chronic laryngitis. Results from this study demonstrated that six patients (50%) in the lansoprazole group and one patient in the placebo group had a complete response to treatment. These researchers reasoned that lansoprazole should be considered as a first-line treatment for chronic laryngitis.

For more information see page 1269.

Generic: **Pantoprazole** *(pant-OH-pray-zoll)*
Brands: **Protonix, Protonix IV**

Pantoprazole is a proton pump inhibitor that stops the production and release of gastric acid in the stomach, thereby decreasing acid production and allowing the stomach and esophagus to heal. Side effects include diarrhea, headache, stomach pain, and gas or bloating.

Pantoprazole has been studied for the treatment of laryngitis in two clinical trials involving 51 adults. In these studies, pantoprazole alone was administered and then given in combination with cisapride (a prokinetic drug). In the study using a high-dose of pantoprazole with cisapride in 22 patients with gastroesophageal reflux disease (GERD)-related laryngitis, patients had significant reductions in all laryngitis symptoms. In another study of 29 patients with persistent hoarseness and voice disorders, pantoprazole was given once daily for six weeks. After six weeks of treatment, significant reductions in hoarseness, heartburn, sore throat, and indigestion were noticed. Moreover, after three months of treatment, these effects remained.

For more information see page 1393.

Mucoviscidosis

See Cystic Fibrosis

Pleural Effusion

An abnormal accumulation of fluid between the layers of the membrane that line the lungs and chest cavity (pleura) is known as pleural effusion. The two types of pleural effusions are transudative pleural effusions and exudative pleural effusions. Transudative effusions are normally caused by abnormal lung pressure (such as in congestive heart failure). Exudative effusions occur from pleural inflammation (such as in instances of lung disease). Symptoms of pleural effusion include shortness of breath, chest pain, cough, hiccups, and rapid breathing; however, there may be no symptoms in some cases.

Commonly Prescribed (On-Label) Drugs: *Bleomycin, Talc*

OFF-LABEL PRESCRIPTION DRUGS
BREAKTHROUGH OPTIONS

Generic: ***Alteplase*** *(AL-te-plase)*
Brands: ***Activase, Cathflo Activase***

Alteplase, a thrombolytic drug, is used to dissolve blood clots that form in the blood vessels, heart, or lungs after a heart attack. It may also be used to prevent blood clots in other diseases. In pleural effusion, it has been suggested that the use of alteplase may help to increase the drainage of fluid in people with complicated pleural effusions.

Investigators at Kansas University Medical Center found that use of alteplase was more effective than thoracostomy tube (inserting a chest tube) alone in pleural drainage in 53 children with complicated pleural effusions. Moreover, the amount of time chest tube placement was required was significantly less in the early alteplase group (84 hours) compared with the late or thoracostomy group (209 hours versus 130 hours). Adverse events reported in clinical studies with this drug included minor bleeding , pain, and coughing. Early data from studies involving alteplase suggest that this drug may be effective in promoting drainage and maintaining pleural tube patency (preventing blockage) for patients with complicated pleural effusions.

For more information see page 1000.

*Generic: **Streptokinase** (strep-toe-KYE-nace)*
*Brand: **Streptase***

Streptokinase, a thrombolytic drug, is used to dissolve blood clots that form in the blood vessels, heart, or lungs after a heart attack. It may also prevent blood clots in other diseases. In pleural effusion, its use may help to increase the drainage of fluid. Side effects associated with streptokinase include dizziness, lightheadedness, and fever.

Experts say that pleural drainage is recommended for persons with moderate or high risk for a poor outcome with pleural effusion. Additionally, in clinical studies, the use of streptokinase has been shown to be effective in adults with pleural effusion. In one study, the use of streptokinase in 24 people with pleural effusions resulted in more drainage and smaller pleural effusions at hospital discharge. Researchers in Turkey evaluated the use of streptokinase in children with complicated pleural effusion and concluded that daily use of streptokinase was effective and safe in both the early and late phases of pleural effusion.

For more information see page 1480.

Pulmonary Edema

Pulmonary edema is a condition where increased pressure in the blood vessels of the lungs forces fluid into the air sacs and prevents absorption of oxygen. Usually, heart problems are the main cause of pulmonary edema; other causes include pneumonia, exercise, or the use of certain drugs. Signs and symptoms of pulmonary edema include extreme shortness of breath, difficulty breathing, wheezing, anxiety or restlessness, a cough that produces frothy sputum and that may contain blood, excessive sweating, pale skin, and chest pain.

Commonly Prescribed (On-Label) Drugs: *Ethacrynic Acid, Furosemide, Trimethaphan*

OFF-LABEL PRESCRIPTION DRUGS
BREAKTHROUGH OPTIONS

Generic: **Captopril** *(KAP-toe-pril)*
Brand: **Capoten**

Captopril, an antihypertensive drug, is used to control high blood pressure and has been used to treat heart failure; it works by relaxing blood vessels. "Afterload reducers" such as captopril reduce systemic vascular resistance, increase cardiac output (total amount of blood being pumped by the heart over a particular period of time), and allow for water loss in pulmonary edema. Captopril is associated with the following side effects: cough, taste loss, fatigue, and increased sensitivity to the sun.

Clinical studies have shown that captopril improves afterload (tension produced by a chamber of the heart in order to contract) and cardiac output, and decreases breathing difficulty within 10 minutes to 15 minutes in pulmonary edema. In a case study, Polish researchers documented the effects of captopril in a 59-year-old patient presenting with diabetes, renal insufficiency, uremic toxicity, and pulmonary edema. Use of captopril resulted in a gradual decrease of pulmonary edema between two and eight days of treatment, decreased heart rate, and reduced blood pressure. After 14 days, the patient's condition remained stable and the captopril dose went unchanged. Researchers concluded that treatment with captopril can reverse pulmonary edema and is life-saving.

For more information see page 1066.

Generic: **Dobutamine** *(doe-BYOO-ta-meen)*
Brand: **Dobutrex**

Dobutamine is used to regulate the pumping of the heart. It is often used in instances of shock or in heart failure. In pulmonary edema, dobutamine provides vasodilation and increases the force with which the heart muscle contracts. At increased doses, these types of drugs may increase heart rate. In pulmonary edema, dobutamine provides a combination of beneficial blood circulation effects such as increased cardiac output. Side effects associated with the use of dobutamine include headache and nausea.

In a case study of a 58-year-old woman with cerebral hemorrhage and pulmonary edema, the effects of dobutamine were reported by a study group from Denmark. In this instance, an IV of dobutamine was given for a few minutes and then decreased. Within 20 minutes, secretions from the tracheal tube stopped. Additionally, her blood pressure was reduced. Researchers concluded that dobutamine helped to restore blood pressure and an adequate cerebral perfusion pressure.

For more information see page 1149.

Generic: **Dopamine** *(DOE-pa-meen)*
Brand: **None**

Dopamine, a naturally occurring catecholamine, is used to make the heart pump more effectively; it is often used in instances of heart failure and shock. In pulmonary edema, catecholamine-type drugs provide vasodilation and increase the force with which the heart muscle contracts. At increased doses, these drugs may increase heart rate. In pulmonary edema, dopamine stimulates both adrenergic and dopaminergic receptors. Side effects associated with the use of dopamine include nausea and headache.

The use of dopamine for pulmonary edema in the medical literature is primarily restricted to laboratory experiments involving animals. In a study at the University of Illinois at Chicago, researchers noted that results of an animal experiment showed that dopamine restored the lungs' ability to clear edema by increasing recruitment of sodium pumps from the plasma membrane of lung cells.

For more information see page 1151.

Generic: **Enalapril** (e-NAL-a-pril)
Brands: **Vasotec, Vasotec I.V.**

Enalapril, an antihypertensive, increases cardiac output (total amount of blood being pumped by the heart over a particular period of time) and allows for water loss in pulmonary edema. In pulmonary edema, enalapril decreases aldosterone (a hormone that controls sodium and potassium in the blood) secretion. Side effects of enalapril include cough and tiredness.

The use of enalapril in people with severe heart failure improved in preload, afterload, and cardiac output. In a study in France of 20 patients with acute pulmonary edema, the use of enalapril showed improvements in cardiac preload and afterload; however, no significant effect on cardiac output was noticed. Enalapril significantly decreased blood pressure by 21% at eight hours. Enalapril was shown to have an excellent safety profile in both studies. According to recommendations from a Canadian joint medical conference, enalapril should be given to all patients with adequate blood pressure who have acute pulmonary edema.

For more information see page 1166.

Generic: **Ipratropium** (i-pra-TROE-pee-um)
Brands: **Atrovent, Atrovent HFA**

Ipratropium belongs to a class of drugs known as bronchodilators, used to help facilitate breathing by opening up airways. This class of drugs is often used to treat symptoms of lung diseases such as asthma, chronic bronchitis, and emphysema. Ipratropium helps to decrease coughing, wheezing, shortness of breath, and difficult breathing by increasing airflow in the lungs.

A small study documented the use of ipratropium in smoking and nonsmoking persons with congestive heart failure to improve lung function. After four puffs of ipratropium, breathing improved in all patients.

For more information see page 1245.

Generic: **Milrinone** *(MIL-ri-none)*
Brand: **Primacor**

Milrinone is used to make the heart beat stronger. It can dilate blood vessels, thereby increasing the amount of blood pumped by the heart and improving heart rate. Additionally, this drug is thought to block clumping of blood platelets and block harmful immune cells. Side effects associated with milrinone include blurred vision, diarrhea, and headache.

Several studies compare milrinone with dobutamine in patients with congestive heart failure and fluid retention due to pulmonary edema. Investigators feel that results from these studies show that milrinone offered greater improvements in heart function without significant increases in heart muscle oxygen consumption. Researchers in Taiwan studied the effects of milrinone in patients with pulmonary edema resulting from hand, foot, and mouth disease in another analysis. Medical records from 24 children with pulmonary edema resulting from severe hand, foot, and mouth disease from 1998 to 2003 were evaluated. Researchers found that mortality was lower in children treated with milrinone compared with those that did not receive this drug (36.4% versus 92.3%). Rapid heart rate was also reduced in children treated with milrinone compared with those who did not receive this drug. Milrinone also reduced white blood cell counts and blood platelets in this study. Researchers concluded that this drug can help patients with hand, foot, and mouth disease, pulmonary edema, and survival of heart and lung collapse.

For more information see page 1330.

Generic: **Morphine** *(MOR-feen)*
Brands: **DepoDur, Duramorph, Kadian, MS Contin, Oramorph SR**

Morphine, a narcotic, is used to relieve severe pain following childbirth, surgery, and other medical procedures. It has been shown to relieve shortness of breath and anxiety. For many years, morphine has been the mainstay drug to treat cardiac lung edema since there is evidence from clinical studies that it causes blood vessels to widen by releasing of histamine (a chemical produced by the body). However, the mechanism of morphine-induced histamine release is not fully clear. In instances of pulmonary edema, morphine decreases heart rate, blood pressure, blood flow output, and heart oxygen consumption. Side effects of morphine include itching, blurred vision, clumsiness, constipation, dizziness, drowsiness, dry mouth, breathing difficulties, and nervousness, among others.

In a study published in *Circulation*, 13 patients with mild pulmonary edema received morphine, after which congestive heart symptoms improved and venodilation was induced. Researchers speculated that the positive benefits of morphine in pulmonary edema may be attributed to afterload reduction and reduced breathing effort. The use of morphine for pulmonary edema has declined during the past few years. Although morphine produces calming effects on the body, its use is associated with significant respiratory depression. Some doctors believe that the risk of morphine use outweighs the benefits, and they may tend to use other, more effective drugs.

For more information see page 1341.

Generic: **Nitroglycerin IV** *(nye-troe-GLI-ser-in)*
Brand: **Nitro-Bid IV**

Nitroglycerin IV belongs to a class of drugs known as vasodilators and is used to relax blood vessels and increase the oxygen and blood supply to the heart. Infusions of nitroglycerin are used to relieve pain associated with angina (chest pain), to control blood pressure, and to treat congestive heart failure. In pulmonary edema, "preload reducers," such as nitroglycerine IV, decrease lung capillary pressure and reduce fluid in the lungs. This drug is considered to be the drug of choice in patients who do not have low blood pressure. Nitroglycerine also has a rapid onset and offset (within minutes) and allows for the rapid effects and stopping of adverse reactions when this drug is given. Side effects associated with nitroglycerine IV include dizziness, fainting, flushing of the face or neck, headache, irregular heartbeat, nausea, and vomiting.

In a study of nitroglycerin IV in patients with acute pulmonary edema, 16 of the 24 (66.7%) patients showed significant improvement after 20 minutes of this drug. In a study evaluating different routes of administration of nitroglycerine, researchers found that the best blood pressure reduction was seen in 68% of patients treated with IV nitroglycerin compared with 41% of patients receiving nitroglycerin sublingually.

For more information see page 1364.

Generic: *Norepinephrine* (nor-ep-i-NEF-rin)
Brand: *Levophed*

Norepinephrine, a naturally occurring catecholamine, is used to treat several serious heart problems. In pulmonary edema, catecholamine-type drugs provide vasodilation and increase the force with which the heart muscle contracts. At increased doses, these types of drugs may increase heart rate. Norepinephrine is generally reserved for patients with severe hypotension or patients with severe hypotension who are unresponsive to other medications. Side effects of norepinephrine include anxiety, nervousness, difficulty sleeping, headache, increased sweating, nausea, vomiting, and weakness.

In a review article by researchers at Duke University Medical Center in North Carolina, dogs with induced pulmonary edema were treated with norepinephrine, which improved blood circulation. The dogs' condition remained stable during one hour of continuous infusion while all other treatment groups circulation worsened and some died. In another study of pulmonary edema induced in dogs, researchers noted that norepinephrine improved ventricular function over a wide range of blood pressures and afterloads.

For more information see page 1369.

Generic: *Nitroprusside* (nye-troe-PRUS-ide)
Brand: *Nitropress*

Sodium nitroprusside IV belongs to a class of drugs known as hypotensive drugs and is used to neutralize or reduce acids in the blood or urine. Sodium nitroprusside IV is often used during emergency situations such as heart attacks or lung problems to restore the normal acid-base balance in the blood. "Afterload reducers" like sodium nitroprusside IV reduce systemic vascular resistance, increase cardiac output (total amount of blood being pumped by the heart over a particular period of time), and allow for water loss in pulmonary edema. Specifically, in pulmonary edema, sodium nitroprusside IV offers strong direct smooth muscle relaxation and improved cardiac output. Sodium nitroprusside IV can also cause sharp decreases in blood pressure.

According to an emergency medicine specialist with the University of Maryland School of Medicine, sodium nitroprusside IV is an excellent drug to use in critically ill patients because of its rapid onset and offset of action (within one to two minutes). Also, sodium nitroprusside IV is a highly effective drug for use in pulmonary edema associated with severe high blood pressure that is not responsive to other drugs. In a study conducted in China, sodium nitroprusside was given to 39 patients with acute high-altitude pulmonary edema (HAPE). In this study, 33 patients (84%) fully recovered and six patients (15%) improved in 72 hours. The total efficacy of the drug was 100%, and improvements in heart pumping and function were also realized.

For more information see page 1367.

Pulmonary Hypertension

See Cardiovascular Disease Chapter

Sarcoid

See Sarcoidosis

Sarcoidosis

Sarcoidosis is a systemic disease involving inflammation that produces microscopic lumps of cells in body organs. Granulomas can grow and come together to form large and small groups of these lumps, and can affect the lungs, lymph nodes, skin, eyes, and liver function. In some instances, sarcoidosis may scar the tissues in certain body organs and affect the way they work.

Commonly Prescribed (On-Label) Drugs: *Betamethasone, Cortisone, Dexamethasone, Methylprednisolone, Prednisolone, Prednisone, Triamcinolone*

OFF-LABEL PRESCRIPTION DRUGS
BREAKTHROUGH OPTIONS

*Generic: **Azathioprine** (ay-za-THYE-oh-preen)*
*Brand: **Imuran***

Azathioprine is used to reduce the body's natural immunity in patients who receive organ transplants and also to treat rheumatoid arthritis and the inflammation that is characteristic of sarcoidosis. Use of azathioprine may result in cough or hoarseness, nausea, fever, chills, lower back pain, painful or difficult urination, and tiredness. It can also reduce the number of white blood cells in the body and may increase your risk of cancer.

Azathioprine has been shown to reduce the need for steroids in people with sarcoidosis, and was mentioned to be an effective steroid-sparing agent in the long-term management of this disease according to an Italian researcher. Researchers in Germany evaluated the use of azathioprine in patients with sarcoidosis to evaluate its steroid-sparing effects, and concluded that results from this study showed that all patients had dramatic symptomatic relief and disease improvements without any serious adverse effects.

For more information see page 1033.

*Generic: **Budesonide** (byoo-DES-oh-nide)*
*Brands: **Entocort EC, Pulmicort Respules, Pulmicort Turbohaler, Rhinocort Aqua***

Budesonide is used for treating asthma and has strong anti-inflammatory properties that reduce inflammation in the airways. Side effects include nose irritation or burning, bleeding or sores in the nose, upset stomach, lightheadedness, cough, and hoarseness, among others.

Inhaled budesonide for eight weeks has been found to significantly reduce the ratio of immune cells in the lung fluid in patients with sarcoidosis. In a study conducted by a Swedish researcher, 20 patients with sarcoidosis were treated with inhaled budesonide. Four were symptom-free during the entire study. Sixteen complained of breathing difficulty at rest or during exercise. Chest lesions were reduced with the use of budesonide, respiratory function improved, and the treatment was well tolerated. Researchers noted that although more studies are needed, inhaled budesonide is beneficial for sarcoidosis. In another study in Finland, researchers discovered that early treatment of sarcoidosis with prednisolone (a steroid) and inhaled budesonide improved lung function.

For more information see page 1055.

Generic: **Chloroquine** (klor-OH-kwin)
Brand: **Aralen**

Chloroquine belongs to a class of drugs known as antimalarials, which also have been used to treat other inflammatory disorders such as rheumatoid arthritis. In the treatment of sarcoidosis, antimalarial drugs are more likely to be effective if there is skin or neurologic involvement, or a high level of calcium in the blood. Side effects associated with chloroquine include diarrhea, difficulty seeing, headache, itching, appetite loss, nausea, vomiting, and stomach cramps, among others. Physicians recommend that patients taking this drug have eye exams every six months.

Chloroquine is well recognized in review articles for the treatment of sarcoidosis and is considered to be a treatment alternative to the disease's mainstay treatment, corticosteroids, when the disease is steroid-resistant or when the use of steroids is contraindicated. Canadian researchers found chloroquine to be effective for lung sarcoidosis. Prolonged treatment with chloroquine in 23 patients with sarcoidosis resulted in significant improvements in pulmonary function. Patients who received maintenance chloroquine treatment had fewer relapses and a slower decline in lung function. Researchers concluded that chloroquine should be considered for the treatment and maintenance of chronic pulmonary sarcoidosis.

For more information see page 1082.

Generic: **Cyclophosphamide** (sye-kloe-FOS-fa-mide)
Brands: **Cytoxan, Neosar**

Cyclophosphamide, an immunosuppressant, is used to treat certain cancers, kidney diseases, and others. In sarcoidosis, this drug acts similar to corticosteroids—it suppresses inflammation and the immune system. Cyclophosphamide is often reserved for severe cases of sarcoidosis, because of its side effects, low white blood cell counts, nausea, bladder irritation, increased risk of cancer, darkening of the skin and fingernails, appetite loss, hair loss, nausea, and vomiting, among others.

In an Italian review article the researcher reported cyclophosphamide to be a steroid-sparing drug in sarcoidosis. Also, in a small study conducted by researchers with the Medical University of South Carolina, patients with neurosarcoidosis who were resistant to or unable to tolerate corticosteroid drugs were treated with IV cyclophosphamide. Of the seven patients treated, four patients reported symptom improvement, but all treated patients demonstrated clinical improvement based on the results from medical tests. Researchers concluded that a short-term course of cyclophosphamide may be a viable steroid-sparing treatment for people with neurosarcoidosis.

For more information see page 1123.

Generic: *Hydroxychloroquine* (hye-droks-ee-KLOR-oh-kwin)
Brand: *Plaquenil*

Hydroxychloroquine, an immunosuppressant, is an antimalarial drug used to treat rheumatoid arthritis. In people with systemic disease, hydrochloroquine has been found to relieve skin inflammation, hair loss, mouth sores, fatigue, and joint pains. It is also helpful in preventing relapses of active disease.

Antimalarial drugs, such as hydroxychloroquine, have been shown to be particularly effective in sarcoidosis with skin involvement and high levels of calcium in the blood. In instances where corticosteroids are not indicated, or the patient is resistant to or experiences adverse reactions with steroid treatment, hydroxychloroquine may be an effective second-line treatment for sarcoidosis. Side effects associated with hydroxychloroquine include visual disturbances, color blindness, hair loss, irritability, weakness, nausea, itching, and headache, among others. If hydroxychloroquine is used for an extended time period, regular eye exams (once every six months) are required.

In a case study by researchers at the University of Southern California, researchers evaluated the efficacy of chloroquine and hydroxychloroquine for neurosarcoidosis. Results showed that both chloroquine and hydroxychloroquine either stabilized symptoms or controlled neurological symptoms in 10 of 12 patients. Researchers concluded that both of these drugs were effective in controlling neurological sarcoidosis in those who failed to respond to corticosteroids or developed severe side effects.

For more information see page 1225.

*Generic: **Infliximab** (in-FLIKS-e-mab)*
*Brand: **Remicade***

Infliximab, an immunosuppressant, is used to treat Crohn's disease (an inflammatory disease of the intestines); it has also been used in rheumatoid arthritis and other inflammatory conditions. In instances of sarcoidosis where corticosteroids are contraindicated, infliximab has been used as an alternative treatment. Use of infliximab may result in fevers, night sweats, pale skin, swollen lymph nodes, cough, abdominal pain, fainting, headache, muscle pain, nasal congestion, tiredness, and nausea, among others.

Clinical studies and case reports emphasize the use of infliximab for the treatment of sarcoidosis. Infliximab is recognized by investigators as a promising and upcoming treatment for sarcoidosis, and a treatment alternative to steroids. In one study by researchers in Germany, a 59-year-old woman with granulomas (microscopic lumps seen in sarcoidosis) who was unable to take steroids because of her history of uncontrolled diabetes was given infliximab. Within four to six months, most of the granulomas resolved leaving behind lesions. New lesions that arose disappeared within two weeks. Moreover, no new lesions were seen after 16 months of follow-up. Researchers deduced that infliximab may be a treatment for people with sarcoidosis or other chronic diseases involving granulomas.

For more information see page 1239.

*Generic: **Methotrexate** (meth-oh-TREKS-ate)*
*Brands: **Rheumatrex, Trexall***

Methotrexate slows the growth of certain cells in the body. High doses of this drug are used to control certain cancers; at low doses, the drug is less toxic and still retains its anti-inflammatory properties. Methotrexate is associated with nausea and vomiting, decreased white blood cells, liver dysfunction, thinned or brittle hair, blistering skin or acne, and appetite or weight loss. It may also induce asthma symptoms. Methotrexate is used in various types of cancers and in rheumatoid arthritis. Physicians recommend that blood tests be performed from time to time to monitor the effects of this drug on the body. Combining methotrexate with folic acid may reduce the incidence of side effects.

In sarcoidosis, methotrexate acts similar to corticosteroids; reducing inflammation and suppressing the immune system. Methotrexate has been used as a second-line alternative in patients who cannot take steroids or do not achieve a significant response with these types of drugs. In a study in Denmark, 16 patients with sarcoidosis with skin involvement (15 of these patients also had other body organs affected) were treated with methotrexate. In 12 patients, the skin lesions resolved; in three of four patients, eye inflammation also cleared. However, 10 patients experienced side effects, which primarily involved nausea. Researchers concluded that a low dose of methotrexate is an effective treatment alternative to steroid treatment in sarcoidosis with skin and eye involvement.

For more information see page 1312.

*Generic: **Pentoxifylline** (pen-TOKS-i-fi-leen)*
*Brands: **Pentoxil, Trental***

Pentoxifylline belongs to a class of drugs known as hemorrheologic agents and is used to improve blood flow through blood vessels. In sarcoidosis with lung involvement, pentoxifylline used alone or in combination with low doses of corticosteroids significantly improves respiratory function. This drug works by blocking tumor necrosis factor (proteins that activate immune cells). Its side effects include dizziness, nausea, vomiting, headache, and stomach discomfort.

In a study German researchers compared dexamethasone (a corticosteroid), with pentoxifylline, which improved the treatment regimens. Results showed that pentoxifylline suppressed tumor-necrosis alpha release from immune cells, and blocked interleukin-10 (a product of immune cells in the body) production. In another study, patients with sarcoidosis received pentoxifylline. Of 18 patients, 11 improved, seven remained stable, and none worsened. Use of pentoxyfylline improved lung function, and researchers concluded that this drug may help to replace or reduce the need for corticosteroids for the treatment of sarcoidosis.

For more information see page 1405.

Generic: **Thalidomide** *(tha-LI-doe-mide)*
Brand: **Thalomid**

Thalidomide is used to treat and prevent a painful skin disease associated with leprosy known as erythema nodosum leprosum. It may be beneficial for sarcoidosis since it works by blocking tumor necrosis factor; this effect may be important in the early and chronic phases of inflammation and the associated granulomas. When used in low doses, thalidomide has been shown to be effective in selected instances of sarcoidosis with skin or lung involvement. Its side effects include constipation, diarrhea, dizziness, drowsiness, nausea, and stomach pain, among others.

Thalidomide has demonstrated efficacy in skin symptoms of sarcoidosis, according to a review article by a researcher at the University of California. In a clinical trial by researchers in France, thalidomide for patients with skin symptoms of sarcoidosis regressed skin legions within one to five months. Four patients in this study achieved complete response to treatment; six patients had partial response; and two patients' skin lesions did not regress. Overall, treatment with thalidomide was well tolerated, but researchers concluded that further examination of this drug is needed. In a study at University of Cincinnati Medical Center in Ohio, thalidomide was effective to some degree for 14 patients with sarcoidosis with skin involvement who received the drug.

For more information see page 1505.

Schaumann Syndrome

See Sarcoidosis

Seasonal Allergic Rhinitis

Seasonal allergic rhinitis, or hay fever, happens when the body's immune system overreacts to particles such as ragweed, plant pollens, and mold spores. During an allergic attack, a chemical called histamine is released from cells in the body. This chemical release opens blood vessels in the body and results in symptoms such as runny and/or itchy nose, nasal congestion, and sneezing. Seasonal allergic rhinitis is very common; affected individuals have symptoms during the spring and fall. This condition may often coexist with asthma in some individuals.

Commonly Prescribed (On-Label) Drugs: Acrivastine, Cyproheptadine, Desloratadine, Desloratadine/ Pseudoephedrine, Dexchlorpheniramine, Fexofenadine, Flunisolide, Loratadine/Pseudoephedrine, Mometasone, Pheniramine, Tetrahydrozoline

---

OFF-LABEL PRESCRIPTION DRUG
BREAKTHROUGH OPTION

Generic: **Zafirlukast** *(za-FIR-loo-kast)*
Brand: **Accolate**

Zafirlukast is used to prevent and manage asthma. It has also been used to treat seasonal allergic rhinitis. In one trial, patients with seasonal allergic rhinitis who received zafirlukast before exposure to ragweed pollen had less nasal congestion, sneezing, and runny nose compared with patients who received placebo.

In a study in Italy, 35 patients with allergic rhinitis and asthma who tested positive for allergy to grass pollen were given zafirlukast twice daily for two weeks. Researchers noted that zafirlukast significantly reduced asthma and allergic rhinitis symptoms. Nasal resistance decreased after treatment with zafirlukast and the number of certain inflammatory cells in nasal fluid decreased, and the drug was well tolerated. Researchers concluded that zafirlukast may be useful for patients affected with asthma and allergic rhinitis. In another study evaluating four different doses of zafirlukast, researchers noted that the use of this drug resulted in a decrease in sneezing and runny nose.

For more information see page 1548.

Viscidosis

See Cystic Fibrosis

MENTAL HEALTH DISORDERS

ANXIETY DISORDERS

Anxiety disorders are among the most common and most treatable mental disorders. About 25 million Americans are affected. Anxiety disorders range in severity from feelings of uneasiness to immobilizing bouts of terror. You may suffer from depression, and may use or abuse alcohol or drugs to try to relieve your symptoms. Performance on the job or in school and personal relationships may suffer.

Anxiety

See Generalized Anxiety Disorder

Generalized Anxiety Disorder

People with general or generalized anxiety disorder (GAD) have ongoing, severe tension that interferes with their everyday lives. You worry constantly about jobs, school, health, and more minor issues such as chores and appointments and feel helpless about overcoming these worries. You may have trouble sleeping, muscle aches and pains, headaches, and feelings of weakness or shakiness. Those with GAD are often irritable and may have trouble concentrating.

Commonly Prescribed (On-Label) Drugs: *Escitalopram, Paroxetine, Venlafaxine*

OFF-LABEL PRESCRIPTION DRUGS
BREAKTHROUGH OPTIONS

*Generic: **Fluvoxamine** (floo-VOKS-a-meen)*
*Brand: **Luvox***

Fluvoxamine is a selective serotonin reuptake inhibitor (SSRI) used for treating obsessive-compulsive disorder in children and adolescents. It is also used for GAD in adults, children, and adolescents. A study published in the *New England Journal of Medicine* reported that fluvoxamine administered to 128 pediatric patients with anxiety disorders was effective in reducing anxiety. The investigators of this study recommended using a lower dose in children ages 6–11, relative to doses used in adolescents and adults. They felt that fluvoxamine was well tolerated by the pediatric patients in this study. The most common side effect was abdominal pain.

Fluvoxamine has also helped depressed patients with coexisting anxiety, a condition that may also be controlled by many commonly used antidepressants. Fluvoxamine was studied at the Depression Clinical and Research Program at Massachusetts General Hospital and Harvard Medical School. In this study, a small group of 30 outpatients with major depression with coexisting anxiety received fluvoxamine. Fluvoxamine significantly reduced both depression and anxiety in these patients. The investigators were encouraged by these results and suggested that fluvoxamine be tested in a larger group of patients. In a study, 19 of these patients more than 50 years old were treated with fluvoxamine for 21 weeks, and researchers observed that most were helped.

For more information see page 1199.

*Generics: Selective Serotonin Reuptake Inhibitors such as **Gabapentin** (GA-ba-pen-tin) and **Pregabalin** (pre-GAB-a-lin)*
*Brands: **Neurontin (gabapentin), Lyrica (pregabalin)***

Pregabalin and gabapentin are selective serotonin reuptake inhibitors (SSRIs). Studies of pregabalin have focused on dosage, adverse effects, onset of action, and withdrawal. Gabapentin was developed to treat epileptic seizures and has also been used in the treatment of neuropathic pain, depression, and anxiety and is chemically related to the neurotransmitter GABA (a brain chemical) and to pregabalin. It works at GABA receptors to facilitate the movement of calcium across the cell membrane.

In several studies, pregabalin was administered at 150, 300, 400, 450, or 600 mg/day, and all doses except 150 mg/day were effective in controlling anxiety. In these studies, pregabalin was well tolerated. Its most common side effects were sleepiness and dizziness, and these were mild to moderate and, sometimes, transitory.

In other studies, pregabalin was compared to alprazolam and venlafaxine used to treat anxiety. Researchers found that pregabalin was effective after one week of treatment, earlier than the other drugs. Also, they found that sexual dysfunction, a common side effect of SSRIs, was not evident with pregabalin. Discontinuation of pregabalin did not cause withdrawal symptoms, a significant problem with benzodiazepine treatment. Based on these results, researchers concluded that pregabalin is promising as a treatment for GAD.

For more information see pages 1206 and 1431.

Generic: *Tiagabine* (tie-GA-been)
Brand: *Gabatril*

Tiagabine was developed to treat epilepsy and works as a selective GABA reuptake inhibitor (SGRI), just as the SSRI drugs act as selective serotonin reuptake inhibitors. Doses used to treat anxiety are much lower than those used to treat epilepsy. In one study, people who were not helped by other drugs, including benzodiazepines and SSRIs, experienced relief from anxiety when treated with tiagabine. In another study published in the *Journal of Clinical Psychiatry*, tiagabine was compared with paroxetine in 40 patients with GAD. Researchers found that the two drugs were equally effective in reducing anxiety and depression and in improving sleep and overall functioning.

Tiagabine was also studied in 48 patients who had partial improvement with SSRI treatment for six weeks. These patients were given tiagabine in addition to an SSRI. The patients were treated for eight weeks, and then their anxiety was assessed. Researchers found that about half of these patients were helped by this therapy. About one third of them achieved complete remission by the end of the study. In addition to the positive effect on their anxiety, the patients reported increased quality of sleep and improvement in their overall functioning. Researchers concluded that tiagabine was generally well tolerated. The most commonly reported adverse effects were sleepiness and dizziness. Several researchers agreed that tiagabine may be helpful in treating anxiety, alone or with other drugs, in doses much lower than those used to treat epilepsy.

For more information see page 1510.

Obsessive-compulsive Disorder (OCD)

Obsessive-compulsive disorder (OCD) is an anxiety disorder characterized by recurrent, unwanted thoughts (obsessions) and/or repetitive behaviors (compulsions). For example, if you have OCD you may be obsessed with germs or dirt and wash your hands compulsively over and over. With OCD you may be aware that your behavior is senseless but are unable to stop it, but some adults and many children with OCD aren't even aware that their behavior is abnormal.

Commonly Prescribed (On-Label) Drugs: *Clomipramine, Fluoxetine, Fluvoxamine, Paroxetine, Sertraline*

OFF-LABEL PRESCRIPTION DRUGS
BREAKTHROUGH OPTIONS

*Generic: **Citalopram** (sye-TAL-oh-pram)*
*Brand: **Celexa***

Citalopram is a selective serotonin reuptake inhibitor (SSRI) that increases the amount of serotonin available in the brain. It is approved for use in treating depression. Researchers from the Imperial College of Science, Technology and Medicine in London conducted a trial involving 401 patients who were given a low, medium, or high dose of citalopram or placebo for 12 weeks. All three doses of citalopram were more effective than placebo. The patients' work situation, family life, and home responsibilities also improved.

Success treating OCD in adults was demonstrated in another study. Twenty-nine people were treated with citalopram for 24 weeks, and the drug was effective in 76% of them. The effects of citalopram in long-term treatment of OCD have also been reported. Thirty-eight patients were treated with citalopram for one to two years and their OCD improved for up to one year. Additionally, intravenous administration of citalopram was given to 39 patients who had tried taking citalopram or similar drugs with no improvement in their OCD. After 21 days of intravenous administration of citalopram, 59% of the patients had significant improvement in their OCD. Patients were then given citalopram orally, and all of them had substantial further improvement in their OCD by day 84.

For more information see page 1096.

Generic: **Mirtazapine** *(mir-TAZ-a-peen)*
Brands: **Remeron, Remeron SolTab**

Mirtazapine increases the activity of the neurotransmitters (brain chemicals) norepinephrine and serotonin. It is approved for use in the treatment of major depressive disorder.

Mirtazapine was tested by researchers at Stanford University School of Medicine for the treatment of OCD. The study involved 30 patients. Researchers found that those who continued taking mirtazapine had additional improvement in their OCD, but those who took placebo had a worsening of their condition.

For more information see page 1332.

Generic: **Pindolol** *(PIN-doe-lole)*
Brand: **Visken**

Pindolol is a beta-blocker approved for use in the treatment of high blood pressure and angina (chest pain). The effect of pindolol as an add-on treatment was studied by researchers in Israel. Fourteen patients were given paroxetine for 17 weeks. Those who did not improve on paroxetine were then given either pindolol or a placebo in addition to paroxetine. Researchers found that those who received pindolol in addition to paroxetine had a significantly greater improvement in their OCD than those taking placebo and paroxetine.

For more information see page 1418.

Generic: **Risperidone** *(RIS-peer-i-dohn)*
Brands: **Risperdal, Risperdal M-TAB**

Risperidone blocks the access of the neurotransmitters (brain chemicals) dopamine and serotonin. It is approved for use in the treatment of schizophrenia, bipolar mania, and psychotic disorders.

Researchers with the Department of Psychiatry and Behavioral Neurobiology at the University of Alabama at Birmingham examined 16 OCD patients; the patients received risperidone, haloperidol, or placebo in addition to another drug. Both risperidone and haloperidol decreased the patients' obsessive symptoms, while placebo had no effect. Risperidone was also studied in 45 OCD patients who took fluvoxamine for 12 weeks. Then all patients, regardless of how well they did on fluvoxamine, were given risperidone in addition to fluvoxamine for another six weeks. Patients who were not helped by fluvoxamine experienced improvement on risperidone plus fluvoxamine. However, patients who were helped by fluvoxamine did not derive any additional benefit from adding risperidone to fluvoxamine. Risperidone has also been studied in patients who had OCD in addition to other psychiatric disorders. In one such study, 20 people were treated for two months with risperidone in addition to other drugs, and all of these patients had improvement in their OCD.

For more information see page 1456.

Generic: **Venlafaxine** *(ven-la-FAX-een)*
Brands: **Effexor, Effexor XR**

Venlafaxine is an antidepressant and antianxiety drug. The approved uses of venlafaxine are for the treatment of depression, generalized anxiety disorder, and social anxiety disorder. It is used off-label in the treatment of OCD.

Venlafaxine was compared with clomipramine, a drug approved for treating OCD. The patients in this study were given clomipramine or venlafaxine for 12 weeks. The percentage of patients whose symptoms improved was about equal in the two treatment groups. Venlafaxine has also been compared with paroxetine, another drug approved for use in the treatment of OCD. In this study, 150 patients were given either paroxetine or venlafaxine for 12 weeks, after which approximately 40% of the patients' OCD in each treatment group improved. The incidence of adverse effects was also similar in the two groups. In another study, venlafaxine was prescribed to 39 patients, some of whom were being treated for other conditions in addition to OCD and were taking more than one medication. According to researchers, in this study, 69% of the patients taking venlafaxine showed improvement in their OCD.

For more information see page 1542.

Obsessive-compulsive Personality Disorder

See Obsessive-compulsive Disorder

Panic Disorder

Panic disorder is a serious condition and quite different from fear and anxiety in everyday life. If you have panic disorder you may have panic attacks, in which you experience a sudden surge of overwhelming fear that comes without warning and without any obvious reason. Although panic attacks are not dangerous, the persistent fear of panic attacks can dominate and disrupt your life because you may avoid situations in which you believe a panic attack will occur.

Commonly Prescribed (On-Label) Drugs: *Alprazolam, Clonazepam, Fluoxetine, Paroxetine, Sertraline*

OFF-LABEL PRESCRIPTION DRUGS
BREAKTHROUGH OPTIONS

Generic: Tricyclic Antidepressants such as **Amitriptyline**
(a-mee-TRIP-ti-leen), **Clomipramine** *(kloe-MI-pra-meen)*,
Desipramine *(des-IP-ra-meen)*, **Imipramine**
(im-IP-ra-meen), **Nortriptyline** *(nor-TRIP-ti-leen)*, and
Trimipramine *(trye-MI-pra-meen)*
Brands: **Elavil (amitriptyline), Anafranil (clomipramine),
Norpramin (desipramine), Tofranil, Tofranil-PM
(imipramine), Aventyl, Pamelor (nortriptyline),
Surmontil (trimipramine)**

Amitriptyline, clomipramine, desipramine, imipramine, nortriptyline, and trimipramine are tricyclic antidepressants that treat panic attacks by altering receptor sensitivity in the brain. Tricyclic antidepressants can treat panic attacks and elevate depressed moods and are usually administered in a single daily dose. Tricyclic antidepressants are generally now used to treat panic disorder in either of two situations: (1) when other medications have been tried but are not effective or (2) in addition to another medication which is partially effective. The tricyclic antidepressant imipramine has proven effectiveness in preventing panic attacks in approximately 70% of people. It is a non-addicting drug and you will not develop a tolerance to it, although it may take several weeks for you to notice an improvement of your symptoms.

Desipramine may be prescribed to you if you suffer from depression as well as panic attacks. You will not develop a tolerance to this drug. Also it causes little or no drowsiness. However, desipramine may cause increased sensitivity to the sun and is not helpful for anticipatory anxiety, which you may experience before starting a difficult activity.

Nortriptyline works much like desipramine in that it treats panic attacks and depression. Researchers note that you will see improvement in your symptoms within a few weeks or months, and will often need blood tests during the first few weeks to establish the correct dosage.

Clomipramine eases obsessive-compulsive disorders by affecting the duration and intensity of your symptoms. It also affects the anxiety that obsessive-compulsive sufferers may experience. This drug also treats symptoms of depression.

Amitriptyline treats panic attacks and depression and has less incidence of causing insomnia. This drug may be prescribed to you if you have difficulty sleeping because of amitriptyline's sedating effects. However, researchers state it is not helpful to you once an attack begins and may cause problems with concentration.

For more information see pages 1009, 1105, 1132, 1230, 1378, and 1532.

Generic: Serotonin Specific Reuptake Inhibitors such as **Citalopram** *(sye-TAL-oh-pram),* **Fluvoxamine** *(floo-VOKS-a-meen),* and **Venlafaxine** *(ven-la-FAX-een)* **Brands: *Celexa (citalopram), Luvox (fluvoxamine), Effexor, Effexor XR (venlafaxine)***

Citalopram, fluvoxamine, and venlafaxine are SSRIs that work by balancing brain chemicals called neurotransmitters and enabling more serotonin to be available, which process reduces the frequency and severity of attacks. You may not respond to SSRIs for three to six weeks but clinical trials have shown that this drug reduces frequency of panic attacks by 75 to 80%.

In a study in Scotland, researchers examined the efficacy of citalopram versus clomipramine in patients with panic attacks. A total of 475 patients received citalopram, clomipramine, or placebo and were evaluated for eight weeks. Researchers concluded that citalopram significantly reduced the frequency of panic attacks.

Fluvoxamine has been frequently studied in clinical trials for its efficacy in treating patients with panic disorder. Researchers at the Albert Einstein College of Medicine compared fluvoxamine versus placebo in treating panic attacks. The study consisted of 188 people with panic disorder. Researchers observed that fluvoxamine significantly reduced the frequency and severity of panic disorder as well as easement of discomfort and distress caused by attacks. Results were seen in patients as early as the first week of treatment with fluvoxamine.

Venlafaxine affects the brain chemicals norepinephrine and serotonin. The *Journal of Clinical Psychiatry* documented a case report at the University of Cincinnati Medical Center of four patients with panic disorder who received low doses of venlafaxine.

Panic disorder was eliminated in all four patients treated with a low dosage of venlafaxine. Three of the four patients experienced no further panic attacks. According to researchers, these results suggest that venlafaxine may have a high onset of action in treating panic disorders.

For more information see pages 1096, 1199, and 1542.

Generic: **Gabapentin** *(GA-ba-pen-tin)*
Brand: **Neurontin**

Gabapentin, originally approved as an anticonvulsant and later as a treatment for post-herpetic pain, has been used to treat a wide variety of illnesses including panic disorder. There are case reports involving a small number of patients that show the effectiveness of gabapentin in treating panic disorder. Its effectiveness has also been demonstrated in a group of 103 patients who received gabapentin or placebo for an eight-week period. The study was published in the *Journal of Clinical Psychopharmacology*. When all patients receiving gabapentin were compared with all patients receiving placebo, researchers observed significant difference in the drug's effectiveness in alleviating the symptoms of panic disorder. However, when the researchers considered only those patients who were severely ill with panic disorder, they found different results. In these patients, those treated with gabapentin had significantly greater improvement than those receiving placebo. Additionally, researchers found that women showed a greater response than men to the drug treatment. The researchers concluded that gabapentin may be useful for the treatment of panic disorder in severely ill patients.

For more information see page 1206.

Generic: **Mirtazapine** *(mir-TAZ-a-peen)*
Brands: **Remeron, Remeron SolTab**

Mirtazapine is an antidepressant drug that affects the chemicals noradrenaline and serotonin. It is sometimes effective in the treatment of panic disorder. A study conducted in the Netherlands examined the efficacy of mirtazapine in the treatment of panic disorder, involving 28 people for 15 weeks. Researchers studied the reduction of panic attacks and the number of patients completely free of panic attacks. They found that 74% of patients had significant improvements in their panic disorder while being administered mirtazapine. Results were seen within the first two weeks of active treatment. These researchers concluded that mirtazapine is a fast and effective treatment as an alternative therapy for people with panic disorder.

For more information see page 1332.

Generic: **Phenelzine** (FEN-el-zeen)
Brand: **Nardil**

Phenelzine is an antidepressant that belongs to the class of drugs called monoamine oxidase inhibitors (MAOIs). Of the MAOIs, phenelzine is among the most commonly prescribed drug for treating panic disorders. Physicians administer relatively low dosages of phenelzine at the beginning of treatment for panic disorder and gradually increase it until panic attacks cease. Treatment with phenelzine normally lasts for six months to a year, and is tapered at the end of the specified period of time.

For more information see page 1408.

Generic: **Pindolol** (PIN-doe-lole)
Brand: **Visken**

Pindolol is a beta-blocker used for the treatment of high blood pressure. Researchers at Tel Aviv University in Israel reported on the drug's use in the treatment of panic disorder. They used pindolol in addition to fluoxetine. In this way, they learned that pindolol has an augmenting effect on fluoxetine treatment. This is important because fluoxetine and other SRRIs, which are commonly used as the first line of defense in treating panic disorder, do not give good results consistently. In fact, about 30% of people either cannot tolerate the side effects or do not get adequate relief of their panic symptoms. The subjects in this study were 25 outpatients with panic disorder, some of whom also had agoraphobia (fear of being in open spaces or in public and feeling helpless). They all had previously been treated with antidepressants and fluoxetine with little benefit on their panic disorder symptoms. During this study, patients continued taking fluoxetine and also received pindolol or placebo for four weeks. Those who received pindolol plus fluoxetine had greater reductions in their panic symptoms than those receiving fluoxetine and placebo alone. The researchers concluded that these results show that pindolol increases the beneficial effects of fluoxetine in patients with treatment-resistant panic disorder.

For more information see page 1418.

Generic: *Tiagabine* (tie-GA-been)
Brand: *Gabitril*

Tiagabine was originally developed for the treatment of seizures. Later, investigators found it to have therapeutic benefits for the treatment of mental health disorders, too. It acts by inhibiting the reuptake of the neurotransmitter GABA in the brain. In a trial, people with panic disorder were treated successfully with tiagabine. This drug was also studied in healthy subjects by investigators from the Department of Psychiatry at the University of Munich in Munich, Germany. When the patients were given tiagabine, the effects of the chemicals that cause panic attacks were greatly reduced. According to researchers, this study adds weight to the findings of tiagabine's therapeutic effects in people with anxiety disorder.

For more information see page 1510.

Generic: *Valproic Acid* (val-PRO-ick AS-id)
Brands: *Depacon, Depakene, Depakote Delayed Release, Depakote ER, Depakote Sprinkle*

Valproic acid was originally developed as an anticonvulsant. Like many neurological drugs, it was subsequently used to treat mental health conditions. There have been case reports that it is effective in people who have panic disorder in addition to other disorders, including alcoholism, substance abuse, withdrawal from benzodiazepines, and multiple sclerosis. Case reports show that valproic acid can be effective when other medications are not. A physician at the University of Michigan Medical School has recommended that it be used in addition to another effective treatment, if the other drug is only partially effective. In a study conducted at the Royal Victoria Hospital in Canada, researchers examined 10 patients with panic disorder. The researchers noted significant reduction of panic disorder symptoms. In another study, 12 patients with panic disorder were treated with valproic acid. Again, the drug was found to be successful in treating panic disorder. The researchers followed the progress of the patients for 18 months, during which valproic acid was effective the whole period of time.

For more information see page 1534.

Post-traumatic Stress Disorder

Post-traumatic Stress Disorder (PTSD) is a type of anxiety disorder that is triggered by memories of a traumatic event that affected you directly or that you witnessed. The disorder affects survivors of traumatic events such as sexual or physical assault, war, torture, a natural disaster, a car accident, a hostage situation, or a death camp. It affects more than five million adults per year in the United States. PTSD often resists drug treatment.

Commonly Prescribed (On-Label) Drugs: *None*

OFF-LABEL PRESCRIPTION DRUGS
BREAKTHROUGH OPTIONS

Generic: **Amitriptyline** *(a-mee-TRIP-ti-leen)*
Brand: **Elavil**

Amitriptyline is a tricyclic antidepressant that increases the concentrations of norepinephrine and serotonin, two important neurotransmitters (chemicals) in your brain for regulating moods. Like many other drugs for PTSD, amitriptyline has been studied in combat veterans. In one study, 46 combat veterans were treated with amitriptyline and studied for eight weeks. The dose of amitriptyline was tailored to the needs of each individual. Amitriptyline was found to reduce PTSD symptoms. Also, the researchers found that the amitriptyline reduced depression and anxiety in the combat veterans.

For more information see page 1009.

Generic: **Carbamazepine** *(kar-ba-MAZ-e-peen)*
Brands: **Carbatrol, Epitol, Tegretol, Tegretol XR**

Carbamazepine is used to prevent and control seizures that occur in epilepsy by reducing excessive nerve signals in your brain. In a study of veterans, researchers reported that carbamazepine is effective in decreasing PTSD symptoms. The beneficial effects of carbamazepine were seen shortly after drug treatment began. Most veterans started to experience therapeutic effects three to five days after starting to take the drug. However, a small proportion of people taking carbamazepine have a serious decrease in the number of white blood cells. Other possible side effects include liver damage and adverse interactions with other drugs.

For more information see page 1068.

Generic: **Citalopram** *(sye-TAL-oh-pram)*
Brand: **Celexa**

Citalopram, a selective serotonin uptake inhibitor (SSRI), affects the brain in ways similar to other SSRIs. Citalopram has been recommended for treatment of PTSD by investigators. This drug is believed to function in the same way as fluoxetine. Two other drugs, sertraline and paroxetine, have been approved by the FDA for treating PTSD, because of which, researchers feel that citalopram would also be useful in its treatment.

For more information see page 1096.

Generic: Tricyclic Antidepressants such as **Clomipramine** *(kloe-MI-pra-meen)*, **Desipramine** *(des-IP-ra-meen)*, **Imipramine** *(im-IP-ra-meen)*, **Nortriptyline** *(nor-TRIP-ti-leen)*, and **Trimipramine** *(trye-MI-pra-meen)*
Brands: **Anafranil (clomipramine), Norpramine (desipramine), Tofranil, Tofranil-PM (imipramine), Aventyl, Pamelor (nortriptyline), Surmontil (trimipramine)**

Clomipramine, desipramine, imipramine, nortriptyline, and trimipramine are all tricyclic antidepressants. All of these drugs work in similar ways in your brain: They increase the concentrations of the neurotransmitters (brain chemicals) dopamine, norepinephrine, and serotonin. Researchers feel that the useful-ness of tricyclic antidepressants is limited by their side effects, which include sedation, constipation, and dry mouth, and the possibilities of more serious side effects.

Researchers state that a few studies of clomipramine, de-sipramine, imipramine, nortriptyline, and trimipramine have been reported. In one of these studies conducted by the Depart-ment of Psychiatry at the VA Medical Center in California, 18 combat veterans with PTSD were given desipramine or placebo for four weeks and their PTSD symptoms assessed. In this study, desipramine was no more effective than placebo. The investiga-tors suggested that the lack of efficacy was due to the relatively short duration of the treatment. In another study, 60 combat veterans were given imipramine, phenelzine, or placebo. Both imipramine and phenelzine were found to be more effective than placebo at controlling symptoms of PTSD. Several case reports and small studies on clomipramine, desipramine, imipramine, nortriptyline, and trimipramine found mixed re-sults, and improvement in PTSD symptoms, when present, was modest. One group of researchers combined the results of 15 such studies and analyzed the results. They concluded that 45% of patients receiving a tricyclic antidepressant had moderate to good improvement in their symptoms.

For more information see pages 1105, 1132, 1230, 1378, and 1532.

Generic: **Cyproheptadine** *(si-proe-HEP-ta-deen)*
Brand: **Periactin**

Cyproheptadine is an antihistamine drug that also induces drowsiness and sleep. It is of special interest to researchers and pa-tients with PTSD because nightmares are common and very dis-turbing in patients with PTSD.

One case reported on a nine-year-old boy with PTSD and several other mental disorders. He was particularly troubled by night-mares, and tried several sleep-promoting drugs with no success. He was then given cyproheptadine in addition to a drug that he was taking for an attention deficit disorder. Researchers observed that cyproheptadine had a dramatic effect on him: He had a com-plete remission of his nightmares within four weeks of starting the drug. His remission continued for the entire follow-up period of six months. This study concluded that cyproheptadine may be an alternative therapy in children with PTSD who do not respond well to more commonly used drugs, and that more research on the effects of cyproheptadine on children with PTSD is needed.

For more information see page 1128.

Generic: **Fluoxetine** *(floo-OKS-e-teen)*
Brands: **Prozac, Prozac Weekly, Sarafem**

Fluoxetine, an SSRI (serotonin specific reuptake inhibitor), is similar to sertraline and paroxetine, which are also SSRIs. This is important because sertraline and paroxetine have been approved by the FDA for the treatment of PTSD. Since fluoxetine is closely related to the other two drugs, it may also be effective in treating PTSD.

In a study by researchers from Duke University Medical Center, 12 combat veterans were given fluoxetine or placebo. They found that fluoxetine was no more effective than placebo in alleviating the symptoms of PTSD. In another small study, 20 Vietnam veterans with PTSD were all given fluoxetine. Of the 20 men, 13 had a decrease in their PTSD symptoms after taking fluoxetine.

A larger study has also been published by researchers at Massachusetts General Hospital, involving 64 men and women with civilian or combat-related PTSD. In this study, fluoxetine was more effective than placebo in reducing the symptoms of PTSD. The researchers found the civilian patients appeared to benefit from fluoxetine more than combat veterans. Another study by researchers at Duke University Medical Center involved 53 civilians with PTSD who were given fluoxetine or placebo for 12 weeks. At the end of the 12-week period, they were evaluated on several different scales of mental health and well-being. Fluoxetine was superior to placebo in several ways, notably in treating PTSD. In fact, 59% of fluoxetine-treated patients were rated as very much improved, as compared to 19% of placebo-treated patients. Fluoxetine was also superior to placebo in other tests of mental functioning assessed by the researchers and the patients themselves.

For more information see page 1192.

Generic: **Gabapentin** *(GA-ba-pen-tin)*
Brand: **Neurontin**

Gabapentin has been used to treat many mental health conditions. In a case report, one man with PTSD was treated with gabapentin and had a significant decrease in anxiety symptoms and nightmares, which were among his PTSD symptoms. In another study, researchers from Ralph H. Johnson Veterans Affairs Medical Center reviewed the records of 30 patients with PTSD. The majority of these patients had moderate or marked improvement in their duration of sleep, and most also experienced a decrease in the frequency of their nightmares. The researchers were encouraged by these results and suggested that further studies were needed to clarify the effects of gabapentin on sleep difficulties and other symptoms associated with PTSD.

For more information see page 1206.

Generic: **Lamotrigine** *(la-MOE-tri-jeen)*
Brand: **Lamictal**

Lamotrigine is a drug originally developed and approved for the treatment of epilepsy and later approved for the treatment of bipolar disorder. Researchers are unsure of how it works, but they have proposed that it acts on the brain by affecting the chemicals in the brain that pass into and out of the cells. Lamotrigine is available as tablets that can be chewed, swallowed whole, or dispersed in water, and it can be given to infants, children, adults, and the elderly. The side effect of greatest concern is the development of rashes, which, in rare cases, can be fatal. These adverse effects are slightly more common in children than in adults.

Ten patients with PTSD were treated with lamotrigine or placebo for 12 weeks. Fifty percent of those receiving lamotrigine improved compared with 25% of those receiving placebo. The researchers suggested that lamotrigine be studied again in larger groups of patients.

For more information see page 1268.

Generic: **Mirtazapine** *(mir-TAZ-a-peen)*
Brands: **Remeron, Remeron SolTab**

Mirtazapine is an antidepressant drug that affects two neuro-transmitters (brain chemicals), norepinephrine and serotonin. The outcome of these effects is an increase in the release of both norepinephrine and serotonin.

Since the most troubling symptom of PTSD is chronic, recurrent nightmares, scientists have hypothesized that mirtazapine would also be effective in treating PTSD and have tested it in patients with PTSD. In a study conducted at the Duke University Medical Center, patients were treated with mirtazapine or placebo for eight weeks. Researchers found that mirtazapine caused improvements in some patients. The effects of mirtazapine were also studied in more than 300 people treated at several community clinics serving people in the Chicago metropolitan area. Approximately 75% of the patients experienced a reduction of nightmares and sleeplessness when they were treated with mirtazapine, and a few of the patients reported a total absence of trauma-related nightmares when they were treated with mirtazapine.

For more information see page 1332.

Generic: **Prazosin** *(PRA-zoe-sin)*
Brand: **Minipress**

Prazosin is approved for the treatment of high blood pressure. It affects the activity of the nervous system outside the brain, like a traffic controller at a central station. The nervous system, in turn, regulates the constricting and dilating of the blood vessels. Prazosin therefore dilates the blood vessels and thereby decreases blood pressure.

Prazosin has been investigated for treating mental health conditions, including PTSD. In a case study, an outpatient with persistent nightmares who had been exposed to civilian trauma was studied. He had not been helped by any of several drug treatments, but when he started taking prazosin, his sleep improved and he had fewer nightmares. His positive response prompted investigators to study the effects of prazosin in five additional outpatients with PTSD that was not related to combat. The patients were started on a low dose of prazosin, which was gradually increased until there were positive results. The total time of the drug treatment was six weeks. All six patients showed moderate to marked reduction in nightmares.

Additionally, ten male Vietnam combat veterans with frequent, severe nightmares related to combat trauma were treated with prazosin or placebo. The results were published in the *American Journal of Psychiatry*. After treatment with prazosin or placebo, the patients were evaluated for the effects on nightmares and other symptoms of PTSD. Researchers found that the patients had greater improvement while on prazosin than on placebo.

For more information see page 1427.

Generic: **Propranolol** *(proe-PRAN-oh-lole)*
Brands: **Inderal, Inderal LA, InnoPran XL, Propranolol Intensol**

Propranolol is a beta-blocker approved for the treatment of high blood pressure. It lowers blood pressure by its effects on the heart, the liver, and the brain and nervous system. When propranolol treatment is started shortly after the traumatic event, it may prevent you from developing PTSD. This effect has not been proven, but it has been explored in several studies.

A case published in the *Journal of Traumatic Stress* reported on a 44-year-old woman who was in five traffic accidents. After the last three, she developed severe PTSD episodes that lasted over six months each. After she had recovered from the PTSD, she was in a sixth accident and again began to develop PTSD. This time, however, she started taking propranolol 48 hours after the accident. Her PTSD symptoms were reduced quickly and markedly. These findings prompted a group of investigators to design a study to see whether propranolol could prevent PTSD if it was given shortly after the trauma. The study involved 19 people taken to emergency rooms after physical assaults or automobile accidents and offered treatment with propranolol. Two months after the traumatic event, almost all the patients showed some degree of symptoms associated with PTSD. However, the severity of the symptoms was twice as high in the patients who had not taken propranolol as in those who had.

The effects of propranolol have also been studied in children who were subjected to trauma, usually physical and/or sexual abuse.

There were three phases to the study: no drug, then propranolol, then no drug again. The children exhibited significantly fewer PTSD symptoms while receiving propranolol than either before or after they received the drug.

For more information see page 1438.

*Generic: **Tiagabine** (TIE-ga-been)*
*Brand: **Gabitril***

Tiagabine is approved for the treatment of epilepsy as it affects nerve activity by interacting with the neurotransmitter GABA, a chemical in the brain. One case report on tiagabine and PTSD concerned a 43-year-old man who developed PTSD and depression after the terrorist attacks on September 11, 2001. He started with a low dose of tiagabine, and the dose was gradually increased until it was effective. Then he had a major and dramatic improvement in his PTSD.

Tiagabine was also studied in seven women with PTSD who were started on a low dose of tiagabine and the dose was increased gradually until it became effective. After two weeks, six of the seven patients' PTSD symptoms markedly improved. Researchers rated the patients as much improved or very much improved. Another study involved six patients with PTSD and other mood disorders who were taking various medications. They were given tiagabine and evaluated after one and six weeks. At both times, their anxiety (one of several symptoms of PTSD) was significantly reduced.

For more information see page 1510.

*Generic: **Topiramate** (TOE-pie-rah-mate)*
*Brand: **Topamax***

Topiramate is approved for treating epilepsy. It affects receptors for two neurotransmitters (brain chemicals), GABA and glutamate. Its overall effect is to increase the activity of GABA and to decrease the activity of glutamate.

The use of topiramate for the treatment of PTSD has been studied by researchers at the University of Washington in Seattle. It had a marked effect on these patients, reducing or eliminating their nightmares and flashbacks. The researchers later published a study on 35 civilian outpatients, including nine men and 26 women. All were given topiramate, and some also took other medications. Topiramate reduced nightmares in 79% of the patients and reduced flashbacks in 86% of the patients. In a third study, researchers examined the effects of topiramate in 33 civilian outpatients with PTSD. After four weeks of treatment with topiramate, total symptoms decreased by 49%.

For more information see page 1516.

Generic: **Trazodone** *(TRAZ-oh-done)*
Brand: **Desyrel**

Trazodone is an antidepressant thought to affect the serotonin in the brain. In one study, six people with combat-related PTSD were given trazodone. Four patients were reported as much improved, and two patients were rated as minimally improved. Lack of sleep was the first symptom to decrease, and this happened after two to three months of treatment. Another study involved 74 patients who were admitted to a Veterans Affairs hospital for PTSD. Of the 60 patients who maintained their trazodone treatment, 72% found the drug helped decrease their nightmares. In addition, 92% found that the drug helped them fall asleep, and 78% said that it helped them stay asleep. The researchers concluded that trazodone was effective for the treatment of nightmares and insomnia, which are particularly troubling and disruptive symptoms of PTSD.

For more information see page 1521.

Generic: **Valproic Acid** *(val-PRO-ick AS-id)*
Brands: **Depacon, Depakene, Depakote Delayed Release, Depakote ER, Depakote Sprinkle**

Valproic acid is an anticonvulsant drug approved to treat epilepsy. In two case reports, researchers have shown that valproic acid caused significant reduction of PTSD symptoms. The symptom that most improved was irritability. Valproic acid was also studied in 16 Vietnam veterans with combat-related PTSD, and the results were published in *The Journal of Clinical Psychiatry*. Ten of the 16 patients showed significant improvement and particularly reduced their heightened states of arousal and reactivity. In another study, of 16 outpatients receiving treatment for PTSD at a Veterans Administration hospital, three of the patients dropped out of the study because they experienced unacceptable side effects of the drug. The 13 patients who completed the drug trial of eight weeks had significant decreases in their anxiety, heightened states of arousal, and flashbacks about their trauma. Researchers noted that an unexpected benefit of valproate was a decrease in the patients' depression.

For more information see page 1534.

Social Phobia

Social phobia, or social anxiety disorder, is a condition in which you have a marked and persistent fear of one or more social or performance situations. You may fear that you will act in a way (or show anxiety symptoms) that will be humiliating or embarrassing. You may recognize that the fear is excessive or unreasonable. Exposure to the feared social situation almost invariably provokes anxiety, which may take the form of panic attacks. In children, the anxiety may be expressed as crying, tantrums, freezing, or shrinking from social situations with unfamiliar people.

Commonly Prescribed (On-Label) Drugs: *Paroxetine, Sertraline, Venlafaxine*

OFF-LABEL PRESCRIPTION DRUGS
BREAKTHROUGH OPTIONS

Generic: ***Buspirone*** *(byoo-SPYE-rone)*
Brand: ***BuSpar***

Buspirone is approved for the treatment of short-term relief of anxiety in people with generalized anxiety disorder. It differs from other drugs used to treat anxiety disorders in two important ways. First, it causes little or no sedation. Second, it usually takes one to two weeks of treatment to be effective, while many other anxiety drugs start producing effects after one dose.

Researchers in the Netherlands studied buspirone in 30 people with social phobia. The patients received buspirone or placebo for 12 weeks. Researchers observed that neither buspirone nor placebo was particularly effective. Only one patient on buspirone and one on placebo had improvement in their symptoms. Another study had different results. Seventeen patients were treated with buspirone for 12 weeks, at the end of which period, 47% of the patients' social phobia symptoms were much or very much improved. Among the 12 patients who took a high dose of buspirone, 67% were improved or much improved in their symptoms.

For more information see page 1061.

Generic: **Citalopram** *(sye-TAL-oh-pram)*
Brand: *Celexa*

Citalopram is a member of a class of drugs called selective serotonin reuptake inhibitors (SSRIs) which block the uptake of the brain chemical serotonin. Most SSRIs also block the uptake of two other brain chemicals, dopamine and norepinephrine. It is different from the other SSRIs because it affects serotonin but has almost no effect on dopamine or norepinephrine. It is approved for use in the treatment of depression.

Citalopram was administered to 22 people with social phobia for 12 weeks. A total of 86% of the patients had improved symptoms. In another study, citalopram was compared with meclobemide in the treatment of social phobia. Researchers felt that the two drugs were equally effective. Seventy-five percent of patients were much improved or very much improved in both treatment groups.

For more information see page 1096.

Generics: Anticonvulsants such as **Gabapentin** *(GA-ba-pen-tin)* and **Pregabalin** *(pre-GAB-a-lin)*
Brands: **Neurontin (gabapentin), Lyrica (pregabalin)**

The chemical structure of gabapentin is similar to the structure of the neurotransmitter (brain chemical) GABA. Gabapentin and pregabalin act similarly. Gabapentin is approved for treatment of epilepsy and post-herpetic neuralgia, but it has been used off-label for many other medical conditions. One of the reasons that it is used so widely is that it is relatively safe. Pregabalin is approved for use in neuropathic pain associated with diabetic peripheral neuropathy and post-herpetic neuralgia.

The effects of gabapentin on 69 patients were published in the *Journal of Clinical Psychopharmacology*. They received either gabapentin or placebo for 14 weeks. Researchers observed a significant reduction in the symptoms of social phobia in patients on gabapentin compared with those on placebo.

Additionally, pregabalin was evaluated in a trial of 135 patients. The patients were given either a high dose of pregabalin, a low dose of pregabalin, or placebo for 10 weeks. Social phobia symptoms were significantly reduced by the high dose of pregabalin relative to placebo. However, the response of the patients on low dose of pregabalin was not significantly different from placebo.

For more information see pages 1206 and 1431.

Generic: **Clonazepam** *(kloe-NA-ze-pam)*
Brand: **Klonopin**

Clonazepam is a drug that enhances the activity of the neurotransmitter (brain chemical) GABA (gamma-aminobutyric acid) in the brain. It is approved for the treatment of seizure disorders and panic disorder.

In a study with 23 patients, clonazepam was compared to no treatment for eight weeks. Researchers observed that clonazepam had a significant effect on the patients. Although 70% of the patients experienced sedation when they started taking the drug, this effect wore off with time or when the dosage was reduced. The effectiveness of clonazepam was also studied in a larger group of 75 patients who were given clonazepam or placebo for up to 10 weeks. Clonazepam treatment was successful in 78% of the patients, while only 20% of those on placebo had positive results. Significant differences in the two groups were evident in the first week of treatment.

Clonazepam was also studied as an add-on treatment in patients who were taking another drug, paroxetine. Patients were divided into two groups and given paroxetine plus clonazepam or paroxetine plus placebo. The addition of clonazepam to paroxetine made little or no difference. The percentage of patients who experienced relief from their symptoms was approximately the same in both treatment groups. In another study, 75 patients received either clonazepam or paroxetine for a brief period and then were reevaluated after two years. Researchers noted that even after two years, the patients who had taken clonazepam experienced relief from their social phobia.

For more information see page 1107.

Generic: **Fluoxetine** *(floo-OKS-e-teen)*
Brands: **Prozac, Prozac Weekly, Sarafem**

Fluoxetine is a selective serotonin reuptake inhibitor (SSRI). It has numerous effects in the brain, all of which derive from its effects on the neurotransmitter serotonin, a brain chemical. Fluoxetine has little or no effect on neurotransmitters other than serotonin. It is approved for the treatment of depression, bulimia nervosa (an eating disorder), and obsessive-compulsive disorder. The effects of fluoxetine were studied in 16 patients with social phobia who took the drug for 12 weeks. After 12 weeks of treatment, 81% had significant reduction in their symptoms. In another study conducted by the Dean Foundation for Health, Research and Education in Middleton, Wisconsin, 60 patients were given fluoxetine or placebo for 14 weeks. All the patients' social phobia improved, whether taking fluoxetine or placebo. The success rates were similar for both drug and placebo.

Additionally, fluoxetine was also compared to psychotherapy (cognitive therapy) in two studies. In the first study by researchers from the Department of Psychology at the Institute of Psychiatry in London, 60 patients were treated with drug or psychotherapy for 16 weeks. At all evaluation times, cognitive therapy was more successful than drug therapy. In the second study, 295 patients were treated for 14 weeks with fluoxetine, psychotherapy (comprehensive cognitive behavioral group therapy), or a combination of the two. Researchers found that both drug therapy and psychotherapy were more successful than placebo, and both treatments had similar response rates. It suggests that fluoxetine may be beneficial to people suffering social phobia; however, further study is necessary.

For more information see page 1192.

*Generic: **Fluvoxamine** (floo-VOKS-a-meen)*
*Brand: **Luvox***

Fluvoxamine is a selective serotonin reuptake inhibitor (SSRI). It increases the amount of serotonin that is available to interact with neurons and changes their electrical activity. Fluvoxamine has been approved for the treatment of depressive illness and obsessive-compulsive disorder. The effect of fluvoxamine on social phobia was studied in 30 people who were given drug or placebo for 12 weeks. A substantial improvement was observed in 46% of the patients who took fluvoxamine and only 7% of those who took placebo. The findings of this study served as the basis for another study comparing the short-term and long-term effects of fluvoxamine, involving 35 centers in Europe, South Africa, and the United States. The results were published in the *International Journal of Neuropsychopharmacology*. In the short-term phase, patients received fluvoxamine for 12 weeks. In the long-term phase, the patients who had some improvement in their social phobia symptoms were given the chance to continue taking the drug for another 12 weeks. At the end of the second 12-week period, the patients who had taken the drug tended to have a decrease in their social phobia symptoms, and a significant decrease in the severity of the disorder.

Another study was a "real life" test in which 15 patients were given a five-minute performance task of simulated public speaking. They performed this task before and after taking fluvoxamine for six weeks. Social phobia was significantly reduced by drug treatment. One week after the drug trial ended, the patients had a follow-up session and they still had beneficial effects of the drug. In all of these studies, some patients were helped by fluvoxamine (responders) and some were not (nonresponders). A group of researchers compared the characteristics of responders and nonresponders in the hope that they could make more informed decisions about who would be helped by the drug. Thirty patients were treated for 12 weeks with fluvoxamine or a similar drug and 72% of the patients were responders. The researchers found that the nonresponders had higher heart rates, higher blood pressure, and more severe forms of social phobia than the responders.

For more information see page 1199.

*Generic: **Nefazodone*** *(nef-AY-zoe-done)*
*Brand: **Serzone***

Nefazodone works by interfering with the uptake of serotonin and norepinephrine, two important brain chemicals. In very rare cases, nefazodone may cause life-threatening liver disease. The effects of nefazodone on social phobia were studied in 23 patients who took the drug for 12 weeks. At the end of the 12-week trial, 70% of the patients were considered responders (moderate or marked improvement) and 30% were nonresponders (minimal or no improvement). Nefazodone was also studied in a series of five clinical cases. Three of the patients showed significant improvement in their social phobia symptoms.

For more information see page 1356.

DEPRESSIVE DISORDERS

Depressive disorders involve your body, mood, and thoughts. Your eating and sleeping patterns, feeling of self-worth, and mental outlook are affected by depressive disorders. These disorders are not to be mistaken with a passing blue mood. If you have a depressive illness you cannot merely "pull yourself together" and get better. Without treatment, symptoms can last for weeks, months, or years. The longer they last, the more difficult they are to treat.

Bipolar Disorder

Bipolar disorder, also known as manic-depressive illness, is a brain illness that causes unusual shifts in mood, energy, and ability to function. Bipolar disorder is much more severe than the ups and downs of mood that most people experience. A concern in the treatment of depression in patients with bipolar disease is the possibility that the patients will switch into mania. It is estimated that more than two million American adults have bipolar disorder.

Commonly Prescribed (On-Label) Drugs: *Aripiprazole, Carbamazepine, Lamotrigine, Lithium, Olanzapine, Olanzapine/Fluoxetine, Valproic Acid, Ziprasidone*

OFF-LABEL PRESCRIPTION DRUGS
BREAKTHROUGH OPTIONS

Generic: **Bupropion** *(byoo-PROE-pee-on)*
Brands: **Wellbutrin, Wellbutrin SR, Wellbutrin XL, Zyban**

Bupropion alters the electrical activity of neurons in the brain. It was originally approved for use as an antidepressant and marketed under the name Wellbutrin. It has since been approved as an aid for smoking cessation and marketed as Zyban.

Bupropion has been studied as a treatment for bipolar disorder when taken in addition to other medications. In one study conducted by the Department of Psychiatry at the University of Toronto in Canada, bupropion was compared with the anticonvulsant drug topiramate in 36 patients. The patients continued their other medications and added either bupropion or topiramate. The percentage of patients who experienced a 50% decrease in their symptoms was similar for bupropion (59%) and topiramate (56%). In another study published in the *Journal of Affective Disorders* bupropion was compared to idazoxan in bipolar depressed patients. The two drugs had similar effects. Both caused a 50% decrease in symptoms over a six-week period. In a third study, bupropion was compared with the tricyclic antidepressant desipramine. Bipolar patients who were taking lithium or an anticonvulsant drug were given either bupropion or desipramine in addition to their other medications and monitored for a year. Both drugs were similar in their antidepressant effects, but patients were less likely to switch to mania with bupropion than with desipramine.

For more information see page 1058.

Generic: **Citalopram** *(sye-TAL-oh-pram)*
Brand: **Celexa**

Citalopram is a selective serotonin reuptake inhibitor (SSRI) that increases the amount of serotonin available in the brain. It is approved for use in treating depression. Citalopram was tested as an add-on therapy in bipolar depressed patients. The patients were given citalopram in addition to their other medications for eight weeks. Twenty-one patients responded favorably to citalopram, and they continued taking the drug for another 16 weeks. During the 16-week treatment period, 14 of the 21 patients had remission of their symptoms and stayed in remission. Two other patients experienced remission followed by relapse. Several studies have shown that SSRIs are effective in treating bipolar disorder but you must take these drugs for at least two weeks before you experience relief of your symptoms.

For more information see page 1096.

Generic: *Fluoxetine* (floo-OKS-e-teen)
Brands: *Prozac, Prozac Weekly, Sarafem*

Fluoxetine is a selective serotonin reuptake inhibitor (SSRI) approved for use in treating depression, bulimia nervosa (an eating disorder), and obsessive-compulsive disorder. The efficacy of fluoxetine treatment was compared in people with bipolar disorder and people with major depressive disorder. In the short-term treatment phase of the study, patients were given fluoxetine for twelve weeks. In the next phase of the study, all patients who were in remission were treated with fluoxetine, placebo, or fluoxetine and then placebo. This phase was long-term treatment, and it lasted for 52 weeks. Relapse rates were similar in the two groups of patients.

Researchers from the Department of Psychiatry at the University of California, Los Angeles compared the effects of fluoxetine, imipramine (a tricyclic antidepressant), and placebo in 89 patients with bipolar disorder. After six weeks of treatment, 86% of the patients receiving fluoxetine, 57% of those receiving imipramine, and 38% of those receiving placebo experienced an improvement of 50% or more in their depressive symptoms. Fluoxetine was associated with significantly fewer adverse effects than imipramine. Only 7% of fluoxetine-treated patients dropped out of the study because of adverse drug effects, compared to 30% of those treated with imipramine.

For more information see page 1192.

Generic: *Gabapentin* (GA-ba-pen-tin)
Brand: *Neurontin*

The chemical structure of gabapentin is similar to the structure of the neurotransmitter (brain chemical) GABA (gamma-aminobutyric acid). Gabapentin is approved for treatment of epilepsy and post-herpetic neuralgia, but it has been used off-label for many other medical conditions.

Gabapentin has been studied in bipolar patients in various mood states: mania, hypomania, depression, and rapid cycling (switching from depression to mania and back rapidly). In one study, 28 bipolar patients experiencing mania, depression, or rapid cycling were given gabapentin in addition to their other medications. Only 18 patients completed the study. Among these, 14 treated for mania or hypomania had a positive response to gabapentin. Patients with hypomania responded the fastest. All five patients treated for depression had a positive response to gabapentin. Only one of the five patients cycling rapidly had a positive response. Overall, researchers found that gabapentin was effective in treating mania and hypomania but not effective in treating rapid cycling. A similar study involved patients who were suffering from mania, hypomania, or a mixed state. They were taking lithium, valproate, or both, but not experiencing relief from their symptoms. They were given gabapentin or placebo in addition to their other medications. There was a significant difference between the gabapentin group and the placebo group; the antimanic response was significantly greater in the placebo group than in the gabapentin group. Researchers observed that gabapentin and placebo were equally effective in relieving depression.

Two additional studies involved bipolar patients who were depressed. In the first study, the effect of gabapentin was assessed in patients with chronic illness. Of the 22 patients in the study, 12 had moderate to marked improvement; eight had complete remission. In the second study, gabapentin was given to patients who had taken other medications and experienced relief followed by frequent relapses. After gabapentin treatment, 50% of the patients had significant improvement in their depression.

For more information see page 1206.

*Generic: **Levetiracetam** (lee-va-tye-RA-se-tam)*
*Brand: **Keppra***

Levetiracetam is an anti-seizure drug approved for add-on use in the treatment of partial seizures in adults and children four years of age and older with epilepsy. Researchers at the National Institutes of Health (NIH) evaluated levetiracetam in 34 patients with bipolar disorder who had not experienced relief of their symptoms with other drugs. Some were depressed; some were manic; and some were cycling rapidly between depression and mania. Patients who were severely depressed at the beginning of the study did not go into remission, while those who were less severely depressed did. Researchers observed that a majority of the manic patients showed improvement of their symptoms, and 44% of them went into remission.

A case report described a man with rapid cycling bipolar disorder whose disease was extremely resistant to medications. He had tried 15 different medications, individually or in various combinations (maximum of six) unsuccessfully. He was then given levetiracetam with no other medications, and this treatment worked for him.

For more information see page 1276.

Generic: **Methylphenidate** *(meth-il-FEN-i-date)*
Brands: **Concerta, Metadate CD, Metadate ER, Methylin, Methylin ER, Ritalin, Ritalin LA, Ritalin-SR**

Methylphenidate is a central nervous system stimulant that increases the amounts of neurotransmitters norepinephrine and dopamine into the brain. It is approved for the treatment of attention deficit hyperactivity disorder (ADHD). Researchers from the University of Louisville School of Medicine in Kentucky studied the safety and efficacy of methylphenidate in the treatment of 14 depressed patients with bipolar disorder. When the patients took methylphenidate in addition to their other medications, their depression and other psychiatric symptoms decreased. However, they felt significant adverse effects from the drug. Three of the patients dropped out of the study because they experienced anxiety. Another study involved the use of methylphenidate and amphetamine, another central nervous system stimulant, in treating bipolar disease. Eight patients were given methylphenidate or amphetamine in addition to their other medications. The patients' bipolar illness substantially improved overall and their depression and medication-induced sedation moderately improved. None of the patients switched from depression into mania, and none of them abused methylphenidate or amphetamine.

For more information see page 1315.

Major Depression

See Major Depressive Disorder

Major Depressive Disorder

Major depressive disorder (also called clinical depression and unipolar depression) is a condition in which you feel consistently sad for long periods of time. You do not take pleasure in activities you used to enjoy. You often have changes in your sleep pattern, loss of appetite, inability to concentrate, and forgetfulness. You feel worthless, helpless, and hopeless. Major depressive disorder is quite common. It has been estimated that 15% of the population experiences major depression at least once in their life.

Commonly Prescribed (On-Label) Drugs: None

OFF-LABEL PRESCRIPTION DRUGS
BREAKTHROUGH OPTIONS

Generic: Alprazolam (al-PRAY-zoe-lam)
Brands: Alprazolam Intensol, Xanax, Xanax XR

Alprazolam is approved for use in the treatment of panic disorder. It affects the electrical activity of key neurons in the brain. The effectiveness of alprazolam in treating major depressive disorder has been studied in comparison with drugs of the tricyclic antidepressant class, since the latter are known to be effective. Alprazolam was compared with desipramine, a tricyclic antidepressant, in three studies with varying results. In one study, 52 depressed patients took alprazolam or desipramine for six weeks. The two drugs were equally effective in treating their depression, and neither drug gave troublesome side effects.

In the second study, patients were given alprazolam, desipramine, or a combination of alprazolam and desipramine for six weeks. All three treatments gave similar degrees of improvement in symptoms of depression. However, there was a difference in the time course of antidepressant effects among the treatment groups. Patients taking alprazolam experienced relief of their depressive symptoms earlier than those not taking alprazolam, with significant improvement often occurring within the first week of treatment. In the third study, 54 patients were given either alprazolam or desipramine for six weeks, but the results were different from those in the other two studies. Neither alprazolam nor desipramine was particularly effective in treating depression. Researchers believe the variation in results could be due to differences in the severity of depression among the patients.

For more information see page 997.

Generic: *Clonazepam* (kloe-NA-ze-pam)
Brand: *Klonopin*

Clonazepam is a member of the benzodiazepam class of drugs. It works within the brain to enhance the effects of the neurotransmitter GABA (gamma-aminobutyric acid). It is approved for the treatment of seizure disorders and panic disorder.

The antidepressant effect of clonazepam was studied in 27 people with major depressive disorder or bipolar disorder. A marked or moderate improvement of depression was observed in 84% of these patients. In most cases, the reduction in depression occurred during the first week of drug treatment. In another study designed to determine whether clonazepam could enhance the antidepressant effect of the drug fluoxetine, patients taking fluoxetine were also given clonazepam or placebo in addition to fluoxetine. Clonazepam caused a modest decrease in depression compared to fluoxetine alone. The patients who received clonazepam in addition to fluoxetine had improvement of their depression more quickly than those who received fluoxetine and placebo. In another study, the effect of clonazepam as an add-on therapy to a variety of other drugs was assessed. Sixty-nine patients with chronic depression were given clonazepam at different doses in addition to their other medications during a four-week period. Clonazepam enhanced the antidepressant effects of the other medications, particularly when the dose of clonazepam was greater than 1.5 mg per day. The improvement in depression occurred within two weeks of starting clonazepam.

For more information see page 1107.

*Generic: **Selegiline** (se-LE-ji-leen)*
*Brand: **Eldepryl***

Selegiline is a MAOI (monoamine oxidase inhibitor) approved for use in the treatment of Parkinson's disease and is administered in capsule form. Recently, selegiline has also been incorporated into a patch that you can apply to the skin.

Selegiline in patch form was compared to a placebo patch in 365 outpatients with major depressive disorder. Selegiline had a modest but statistically significant antidepressant effect. In a similar study, selegiline in patch form was compared to a placebo patch in 177 outpatients. A significant difference in antidepressant effect was seen in patients receiving selegiline compared to those receiving placebo, and the difference occurred as early as the first week of treatment.

For more information see page 1466

Manic-depressive Psychosis

See Bipolar Disorder

Seasonal Affective Disorder

Seasonal affective disorder, or SAD, is a type of major depressive disorder or the depressive part of bipolar disorder in which the depressive episodes occur at certain times of the year. SAD typically appears as winter depression, and you may experience depressive episodes starting in the fall and occurring through the winter; symptoms usually resolve by the spring and summer. Symptoms of SAD include depressed mood, lack of energy, increased sleep, and weight gain. As the hours of daylight decrease, SAD symptoms increase. Treatments for SAD include phototherapy (therapy with artificial light) and drugs.

Commonly Prescribed (On-Label) Drugs: *None*

OFF-LABEL PRESCRIPTION DRUGS
BREAKTHROUGH OPTIONS

Generic: **Modafinil** *(moe-DAF-i-nil)*
Brand: **Provigil**

Modafinil is a drug used to treat excessive sleepiness caused by narcolepsy (a condition that causes excessive daytime sleepiness) or shift work sleep disorder (sleepiness during scheduled waking hours and difficulty falling asleep or staying asleep during scheduled sleeping hours in people who work at night or on rotating shifts). Modafinil is also used along with breathing devices or other treatments to prevent excessive sleepiness caused by obstructive sleep apnea/hypopnea syndrome (OSAHS) a sleep disorder in which the patient briefly stops breathing or breathes shallowly many times during sleep and therefore does not have enough restful sleep. Modafinil belongs to a class of drugs known as central nervous system (CNS) stimulants. Based on studies involving animals, this drug is thought to work by changing the amounts of certain natural substances in the area of the brain that controls sleep and wakefulness.

A researcher at Foothills Psychiatry in Boise, Idaho, evaluated the efficacy and safety of modafinil in 13 patients with SAD/winter depression. In this study, modafinil significantly decreased winter depression at week one through week eight. Moreover, modafinil significantly improved overall clinical condition at all time points, reduced fatigue, and improved wakefulness from weeks two through eight. The researcher concluded that modafinil may be an effective and well-tolerated drug for patients with SAD/winter depression.

For more information see page 1338.

Generic: **Sertraline** *(SER-tra-leen)*
Brand: **Zoloft**

Sertraline belongs to a class of antidepressants known as selective serotonin reuptake inhibitors (SSRIs) and is used to treat depression, obsessive-compulsive disorder (OCD), panic disorder, premenstrual dysphoric disorder (PMDD), post-traumatic stress disorder (PSTD), and social anxiety disorder. It is thought to work by increasing the activity of a chemical in the brain known as serotonin; this SSRI-type antidepressant has been shown to be effective and well tolerated if you are affected with seasonal affective disorder.

The International Collaborative Group on Sertraline in the Treatment of Outpatients With Seasonal Affective Disorder conducted a study evaluating this drug in 187 outpatients with seasonal pattern recurrent winter depression. Results from this study showed that sertraline produced a significantly greater response than placebo. Additionally, more sertraline-treated patients achieved a response greater than those in the placebo-treated group. Sertraline was well tolerated; the most frequent adverse events were nausea, diarrhea, insomnia, and dry mouth. Researchers concluded that sertraline offers an important treatment option in the management of seasonal affective disorder. This drug may be particularly useful if you do not tolerate, cannot comply with, or are unresponsive to phototherapy.

For more information see page 1468.

EATING DISORDERS

Eating disorders include extreme emotions, attitudes, and behaviors that surround weight and food issues. These types of disorders include anorexia, bulima, and binge eating. They affect girls and boys, men and women, and cause serious emotional and physical problems that may be life threatening.

Anorexia Nervosa

Anorexia nervosa is an illness in which you refuse to maintain a reasonable body weight, defined as at least 85% of the weight expected for your height and age. You have an intense fear of gaining weight or becoming overweight, even though you are underweight. You also have disturbances in your perception of your own body weight and deny the seriousness of your own low body weight.

Commonly Prescribed (On-Label) Drugs: Megestrol

OFF-LABEL PRESCRIPTION DRUG
BREAKTHROUGH OPTION

Generic: **Fluoxetine** *(floo-OKS-e-teen)*
Brands: **Prozac, Prozac Weekly, Sarafem**

Fluoxetine is a selective serotonin reuptake inhibitor (SSRI) that increases the amount of serotonin available in the brain. It is approved for use in treating depression, bulimia nervosa, and obsessive-compulsive disorder. Fluoxetine has been studied for the treatment of anorexia nervosa several times, and the results were mixed. One study was designed to determine whether fluoxetine would improve clinical outcome and reduce relapse after normal weight was restored. The 35 patients participating in this study were given fluoxetine or placebo during treatment as inpatients and as outpatients for one year.

The patients who continued taking fluoxetine for one year had a reduced relapse rate as determined by a significant increase in weight and reduction in symptoms.

For more information see page 1192.

Binge Eating

People with serious binge eating problems eat an unusually large amount of food and feel that their eating is out of control. You may eat much more quickly than usual; eat unusually large amounts of food; eat alone because you're embarrassed about your eating; and feel disgusted, depressed, or guilty about your overeating. Binge eating differs from bulimia nervosa in that bulimics purge (vomit or take diuretics or laxatives), fast, or exercise excessively to keep from gaining weight.

Commonly Prescribed (On-Label) Drugs: *None*

OFF-LABEL PRESCRIPTION DRUGS
BREAKTHROUGH OPTIONS

*Generic: **Naltrexone** (nal-TREKS-one)*
*Brands: **Naltrexone, ReVia***

Naltrexone is approved for use in the treatment of dependence on opiates and alcohol. A preliminary study investigated the effect of naltrexone in one patient with binge eating disorder. The patient was given naltrexone, then placebo, and then naltrexone at twice the dose used earlier. The patient also received psychotherapy during the study. Researchers found that binge symptoms were reduced by drug treatment.

For more information see page 1352.

*Generic: **Sibutramine** (si-BYOO-tra-meen)*
*Brand: **Meridia***

Sibutramine is approved for use in the management of obesity, including weight loss and maintenance of weight loss. It is to be used in conjunction with a low-calorie diet.

The effect of sibutramine was studied in 20 patients with binge eating disorder who were given the drug or placebo for 12 weeks. Researchers found that binge frequency was significantly lower on sibutramine than on placebo. In addition, sibutramine was effective in promoting and maintaining weight loss in these patients. In a similar study conducted in Brazil, 60 obese outpatients received sibutramine or placebo for 12 weeks. The researchers noted a significant reduction in the number of days with binge eating episodes in the sibutramine group compared with the placebo group. Sibutramine was also associated with weight loss and a decrease in depressive symptoms.

For more information see page 1470.

*Generic: **Topiramate** (TOE-pie-rah-mate)*
*Brand: **Topamax***

Topiramate, approved for the treatment of epilepsy, works by affecting brain chemicals. Since topiramate is associated with weight loss in the treatment of epileptics, it has been studied for possible use in the treatment of binge eating disorder. In one study by researchers at the University of Cincinnati College of Medicine, 61 outpatients were given topiramate or placebo for 14 weeks. Topiramate was associated with a significantly greater reduction in binge frequency than placebo (94% and 46% respectively). In another study, 13 outpatients were treated with topiramate. Nine of the 13 patients had a moderate or better improvement in their binge eating disorder during drug treatment, and their improvement was maintained for three to 30 months. In addition, their weight loss was significantly correlated with their topiramate dose.

For more information see page 1516.

Bulimia Nervosa

Bulimia nervosa (BN) is a disorder with recurrent episodes of binge eating. Binge eating lasts for a longer period of time than normal eating and is characterized by a sense of lack of control over eating. With BN, you also have recurring episodes of inappropriate behaviors to prevent gaining weight, such as self-induced vomiting; inappropriate use of laxatives, enemas, diuretics, or other medications; fasting; or excessive exercise.

Commonly Prescribed (On-Label) Drugs: *Fluoxetine*

OFF-LABEL PRESCRIPTION DRUGS
BREAKTHROUGH OPTIONS

Generic: **Desipramine** *(des-IP-ra-meen)*
Brand: **Norpramin**

Desipramine is an antidepressant drug of the tricyclic type. Like other tricyclic antidepressants, it blocks the reuptake of the neurotransmitters norepinephrine and serotonin, brain chemicals. The effect of desipramine on bulimia nervosa has been studied several times with mixed results—effective, somewhat effective, and ineffective. In the first study, 12 patients were given desipramine or placebo for six weeks. Then their treatments were reversed, so that those who had taken desipramine received placebo and those who had taken placebo received desipramine for another six weeks. Desipramine was effective in reducing bingeing and vomiting frequency.

In the second study, short-term and long-term effects of desipramine were evaluated in 80 bulimic patients. In the short-term phase of the study, the patients were given either desipramine or placebo for eight weeks. Patients who were helped by desipramine enrolled in the long-term phase of the study, in which they were given desipramine or placebo for six months. In the short-term phase, desipramine was superior to placebo. Patients who received desipramine had an average reduction of 47% in their binge frequency, while those on placebo had an average increase of 7% in their binge frequency. The results of the long-term phase of the study were different; 29% of the patients who participated in the long-term phase relapsed in the following four months.

In the third study, psychotherapy was compared with drug treatment. Patients were given cognitive-behavioral therapy (CBT), desipramine, or a combination of CBT and desipramine. Some of the patients treated with desipramine dropped out of the study because of adverse effects of the drug, and those who continued taking treatment were not helped by the drug.

For more information see page 1132.

*Generic: **Imipramine** (im-IP-ra-meen)*
*Brands: **Tofranil, Tofranil-PM***

Imipramine is a tricyclic antidepressant approved for use in the treatment of depression and enuresis (bed-wetting) in children. A report published in the *American Journal of Psychiatry* documented the effects of imipramine in 22 chronically bulimic women. The women received imipramine or placebo. In this study, imipramine was associated with a significantly reduced frequency of binge eating. The effect of phenelzine has also been studied in patients with both bulimia and atypical depression. The patients were given phenelzine, imipramine, or placebo. Researchers found that phenelzine was more effective than either imipramine or placebo. In fact, imipramine was only minimally effective.

In another study, imipramine treatment was compared with group psychotherapy. Patients were treated with imipramine, placebo, imipramine plus intensive group therapy, or placebo plus intensive group therapy for 12 weeks. All patients except those taking placebo alone had significant reductions in their bulimic behaviors.

For more information see page 1230.

Generic: **Phenelzine** *(FEN-el-zeen)*
Brand: **Nardil**

Phenelzine belongs to the class of drugs called monoamine oxidase inhibitors (MAOIs), which increases the amount of these neurotransmitters and affects the electrical activity of neurons in the brain. Because of their toxicity, MAOIs are not widely used today. They are generally used when other medications fail to work. Phenelzine is approved for use in the treatment of some types of depression.

Phenelzine has been shown to be effective in treating bulimia in several studies. In one study, 20 bulimic women were divided into two groups; one group took phenelzine and the other, placebo. The women on phenelzine had significantly fewer binges per week than those on placebo. Five of the phenelzine-treated patients ceased bingeing entirely, but none of the placebo-treated patients did. Four of the phenelzine-treated patients reduced their binge frequency by at least 50%, compared to 22% in the placebo group.

The effect of phenelzine has also been studied in patients with both bulimia and atypical depression. The patients were given phenelzine, imipramine, or placebo. Reseachers found that phenelzine was more effective than either imipramine or placebo. In fact, imipramine was only minimally effective. At the New York State Psychiatric Institute researchers studied 50 patients with both bulimia and atypical depression. They were treated with phenelzine or placebo. Phenelzine was significantly superior to placebo in the reduction of binge frequency (64% vs. 5%) and in the fraction of patients who had ceased bingeing.

For more information see page 1408.

Generic: **Sertraline** *(SER-tra-leen)*
Brand: **Zoloft**

Sertraline is a selective serotonin reuptake inhibitor (SSRI) approved for use in the treatment of major depressive disorder, obsessive-compulsive disorder, panic disorder, post-traumatic stress disorder, premenstrual dysphoric disorder, and social anxiety disorder. The effects of sertraline were studied by researchers in Italy in 20 women. They were divided into two groups and were given sertraline or placebo for 12 weeks. The group treated with sertraline had a statistically significant reduction in the number of bingeing and purging episodes compared with the placebo group. No one discontinued drug treatment because of adverse effects.

In another study, 18 women were treated with sertraline for eight weeks. There was no placebo group in this study. The treated women had significant reductions in the number of binges and purges per week as well as reductions in their depressive symptoms. None of the women experienced adverse effects of sertraline.

For more information see page 1468.

SUBSTANCE ABUSE AND ADDICTIVE BEHAVIORS

Symptoms of substance abuse include fatigue, poor health, personality changes, social withdrawal, and decreased interest in work, school, or social activities, among others. Effects of substance abuse include increased heart rate and blood pressure; AIDS; hepatitis; behavioral changes; hallucinations; clinical depression; sleeplessness; tremors; liver, lung, and kidney impairment; and death. The hallmark traits of addictive behaviors include: obsession on the object, activity, or substance; seeking out and engaging in the behavior despite awareness of the negative consequences; compulsive behavior; withdrawal symptoms after stopping the addictive behavior; loss of control; denial; concealing the behavior from others; episodic blackout; depression; and low self-esteem.

Alcoholism (Cravings and Dependence)

Alcoholism is a common, serious, and expensive disease. Alcohol affects practically every organ in the body; it affects many neurotransmitter systems in the brain including opiates, gamma-aminobutyric acid (GABA), glutamate, serotonin, and dopamine. Elevated opiate levels explain the euphoric effect of alcohol while its effects on GABA result in anxiolytic and sedative effects. When alcohol is withdrawn, the central nervous system (CNS) experiences excitability. Those who abuse alcohol are more prone to alcohol withdrawal. Long-term abuse can result in cell death and brain degeneration. Signs of alcoholism include accidents, anxiety, depression, breakdown of relationships, and insomnia, among others. In the reviewed studies, the use of drug therapy was typically part of a larger overall program, including behavioral therapy, which was all targeted toward improvement in alcohol abuse.

Commonly Prescribed (On-Label) Drugs: Disulfiram, Naltrexone

OFF-LABEL PRESCRIPTION DRUGS
BREAKTHROUGH OPTIONS

Generic: **Baclofen** (BAK-low-fen)
Brands: **Kemstro, Lioresal**

Baclofen belongs to a class of drugs known as muscle relaxants; it is used to relieve muscle spasms and contractions in conditions such as multiple sclerosis.

Researchers in Italy evaluated the effects of baclofen on the alcohol craving, ethanol intake, and abstinence from alcohol in 10 alcoholic men. Nine subjects finished the study; two of these nine still drank alcohol, but substantially less. Seven of the nine subjects did not drink throughout the study. With baclofen, craving was significantly reduced from the first week until the end of the study. Moreover, it was noted that their obsessional thinking about alcohol disappeared. Drug side effects included headache, vertigo, nausea, and constipation, among others. Researchers concluded that this drug may have a role for alcohol cravings.

In another study, researchers in Italy evaluated the use of baclofen plus naltrexone (a drug used for alcoholism) in a rat model of alcohol drinking. Although either drug alone did not affect alcohol drinking, when used together, the combination offered significant reduction in daily alcohol intake and retardation in the alcohol drinking behavior in rats. Based on these findings, researchers suggested that the combination may have benefits.

For more information see page 1037.

Generic: **Buspirone** *(byoo-SPYE-rone)*
Brand: **BuSpar**

Buspirone belongs to a class of drugs known as anxiolytics. This class of drugs is used to relieve certain kinds of anxiety. Buspirone is different from other drugs used to treat anxiety in that it has little effect on mental alertness.

Clinical studies evaluating the use of buspirone have proven that this drug is safe and has some efficacy for the treatment of alcoholism, although researchers noted that high doses may be needed for best results. Buspirone may work indirectly by treating the underlying anxiety rather than by affecting drinking behavior. Researchers in Korea and the United States evaluated the use of buspirone in 33 men. Researchers found that cortisol response to buspirone was significantly decreased in alcoholic subjects versus normal subjects. This effect demonstrated decreased receptor selectivity. Although more understanding is needed with regard to receptor sensitivity changes, researchers noted that these results improve their knowledge about the role of receptors and alcoholism.

For more information see page 1061.

Generic: **Citalopram** *(sye-TAL-oh-pram)*
Brand: **Celexa**

Citalopram belongs to a class of antidepressant drugs known as selective serotonin reuptake inhibitors (SSRIs). This drug treats depression by increasing the amount of serotonin, a natural substance in the brain that maintains mental balance. Citalopram is sometimes used to treat alcoholism, eating disorders, panic disorder, premenstrual dysphoric disorder, and social phobia.

Some researchers suggest that the use of SSRIs, such as citalopram, may decrease alcohol intake and cravings in certain subtypes of alcoholics. In one study, researchers in Germany compared the effects of a number of SSRIs, including citalopram, in an animal model of alcoholism. In this study, each SSRI reduced alcohol consumption; however, the degree of selectivity and specificity of the effect varied between the drugs. With regard to selectivity, fluoxetine and citalopram affected alcohol intake. Fluvoxamine and paroxetine affected food intake somewhat more markedly than alcohol.

Researchers in Toronto, Canada, examined the different effects of citalopram on alcohol intake in nondepressed men and women with mild to moderate alcohol dependence. The patients received up to 12 weeks of citalopram or placebo. Men receiving citalopram reduced average drinks per day by 44%, whereas women had a 27% decrease in average drinks per day. Researchers concluded that men may benefit more than women from citalopram in the treatment of alcohol dependence.

For more information see page 1096.

Generic: *Fluoxetine* (floo-OKS-e-teen)
Brands: *Prozac, Prozac Weekly, Sarafem*

Fluoxetine belongs to a class of antidepressant drugs known as selective serotonin reuptake inhibitors (SSRIs). This drug is used to improve mood, and can also help treat anxiety, obsessive-compulsive disorder, eating disorders, panic disorder, premenstrual dysphoric disorder (PMDD), and post-traumatic stress. Fluoxetine is used to treat a number of other disorders including alcoholism, attention-deficit disorder, borderline personality disorder, sleep disorders, headaches, mental illness, and obesity.

Some study researchers suggest that the use of SSRIs, such as fluoxetine, may decrease alcohol intake and cravings in certain subtypes of alcoholics. Across the SSRIs, reductions in alcohol intake ranging from 10% to 70% have been observed, as noted in a review article by Canadian researchers.

In one study, researchers in Germany compared the effects of a number of SSRIs, including fluoxetine, in an animal model of alcoholism. In this study, each SSRI reduced alcohol consumption; however, the degree of selectivity and specificity of the effect varied across the compounds. With regard to selectivity, fluoxetine affected alcohol intake; citalopram affected this similarly. Fluvoxamine and paroxetine affected food intake somewhat more markedly than alcohol. Therefore, fluoxetine is considered to be the most selective, followed by citalopram, fluvoxamine, and paroxetine, which was nonspecific.

For more information see page 1192.

Generic: *Fluvoxamine* (floo-VOKS-a-meen)
Brand: *Luvox*

Fluvoxamine belongs to a class of antidepressant drugs known as SSRIs, and is used to treat obsessive-compulsive disorder. This drug is sometimes used to treat depression. SSRI-type drugs, such as fluvoxamine, may be helpful in treating later-onset alcoholism and alcoholism that is complicated by major depression.

In one review article, a researcher noted that SSRIs may indirectly work in alcoholism by treating underlying depression rather than affecting alcohol intake. Some researchers suggest that the use of SSRIs, such as fluvoxamine, may decrease alcohol intake and cravings in certain subtypes of alcoholics. A number of factors, such as gender, alcoholic subtype, and extent of drinking appear to affect the treatment efficacy of the SSRI-type drugs. With the use of SSRIs, reductions in alcohol intake ranging from 10% to 70% have been observed, as noted in a review article by Canadian researchers.

Researchers in Italy performed a 16-week study to test the efficacy of two SSRIs drugs (fluvoxamine and citalopram) in decreasing relapse and craving in alcoholics. Researchers concluded that the study proved that SSRI-type drugs are effective in combination with psychotherapy to prevent relapse in alcoholics.

For more information see page 1199.

Generic: *Ondansetron* (on-DAN-se-tron)
Brands: *Zofran, Zofran ODT*

Ondansetron belongs to a class of drugs known as anti-emetics. These types of drugs are used to prevent nausea and vomiting that may occur after treatment with chemotherapy, radiation, or surgery.

Since anxiety often accompanies drinking, researchers have proposed that ondansetron may reduce alcohol intake by reducing anxiety. The effects of ondansetron (short-term use) on alcohol consumption was evaluated in two studies involving 400 alcoholics. In the first study, 71 alcoholics were given low-dose ondansetron or high-dose ondansetron. At the end of the study, 39% of the low-dose group and 16% of the high-dose group had reduced drinking. However, in this study, low-dose ondansetron seemed to be more effective in light drinkers than heavy drinkers. Mild constipation was the only adverse event noted in this study.

In a study conducted at the University of Texas in San Antonio, 321 patients with alcoholism received ondansetron for 11 weeks. Those who received ondansetron had fewer drinks per day than those receiving placebo. Based on these results, researchers concluded that ondansetron is an effective treatment for patients with early-onset alcoholism.

For more information see page 1387.

Generic: *Paroxetine* (pa-ROKS-e-teen)
Brands: *Paxil, Paxil CR*

Paroxetine belongs to a class of antidepressant drugs known as SSRIs, and is used to improve mood by treating depressive symptoms. This drug may be used to treat social anxiety disorder, obsessive-compulsive disorder, panic attacks, post-traumatic stress disorder, or premenstrual dysphoric disorder.

Researchers in Germany compared the effects of a number of SSRIs, including paroxetine, in an animal model of alcoholism. In this study, each SSRI reduced alcohol consumption; however, the degree of selectivity and specificity of the effect varied across the compounds. With regard to selectivity, fluoxetine affected alcohol intake; citalopram affected these parameters in a similar fashion. Fluvoxamine and paroxetine affected food intake somewhat more markedly than alcohol. Therefore, fluoxetine is considered to be the most selective, followed by citalopram, fluvoxamine, and paroxetine, which was nonspecific. Overall, SSRI-type drugs are considered to be important drugs for the treatment of alcoholism, and they may be particularly effective in treating late-onset alcoholism and alcoholism complicated by coexisting major depression.

For more information see page 1395.

Generic: **Sertraline** *(SER-tra-leen)*
Brand: **Zoloft**

Sertraline belongs to a class of antidepressants known as SSRIs, and is used to treat depression, obsessive-compulsive disorder, panic disorder, premenstrual dysphoric disorder, post-traumatic stress disorder, and social anxiety disorder. Sertraline is thought to work by increasing the activity of a chemical in the brain known as serotonin; in alcoholism, this drug may decrease other central nervous system-related factors associated with craving and/or motivation to drink.

Researchers at the Medical University in South Carolina in Charleston evaluated the use of sertraline and cognitive behavioral therapy (CBT) in depressed alcoholics. In this 12-week trial, 82 depressed and actively drinking alcohol-dependent individuals were given sertraline or placebo. Researchers noted that sertraline was well tolerated and all patients had decreases in both depression and alcohol use. Those who received sertraline had fewer drinks per drinking day than those who received placebo; however, other drinking outcomes were not different between the two treatment groups. Treatment with sertraline was associated with less depression at the end of treatment in female subjects compared with female subjects who received placebo. Overall, less drinking was associated with improved depression outcome. Findings indicate that sertraline may provide modest benefit in terms of drinking outcome and may lead to improved depression in female alcohol-dependent subjects. Additionally, alcohol relapse prevention CBT appeared to be of benefit to subjects.

For more information see page 1468.

Generic: **Topiramate** *(TOE-pie-rah-mate)*
Brand: **Topamax**

Topiramate belongs to a class of drugs known as anti-epileptic drugs and is used to prevent epileptic seizures, and may be used to prevent migraine headaches.

In a study, 150 adults diagnosed with alcohol dependence were given topiramate at increasing dosages for 12 weeks. By week 12 of the study, drinking was significantly reduced in both treatment groups; however, topiramate was significantly more effective compared with placebo in reducing cravings and drinking. In an article reviewing this study, it was suggested that topiramate has a greater effect on drinking compared with other drugs used in the treatment of alcoholism (naltrexone and acamprosate).

Topiramate also has been proved effective in individual patients. In a case study report, two middle-aged patients with bipolar disorder, post-traumatic stress disorder, and alcohol dependence resistant to other drugs experienced significant decreases in alcohol craving and use with topiramate. In both instances, the patients remained completely alcohol-free at two-year follow-up.

For more information see page 1516.

Alcohol Withdrawal

Alcohol withdrawal syndrome is characterized by early symptoms of hypertension, abnormally rapid heart rate, overstimulation of the nervous system, anxiety, and irritability. Neurologic symptoms include tremor, hallucinations, and a reduced seizure threshold. Alcohol withdrawal symptoms start within six to 24 hours after the last alcoholic drink in chronic drinkers. In some instances, alcohol withdrawal syndrome can be life threatening. Clinical management of alcohol withdrawal entails symptom relief, prevention of seizures and delirium, and a transition to a treatment program to maintain abstinence from alcohol. In the reviewed studies, the use of drug therapy was typically part of a larger overall program, including behavioral therapy, which was all targeted toward improvement in alcohol abuse.

Commonly Prescribed (On-Label) Drugs: *Chlordiazepoxide, Clorazepate, Diazepam, Hydroxyzine, Oxazepam*

OFF-LABEL PRESCRIPTION DRUGS
BREAKTHROUGH OPTIONS

*Generic: **Alprazolam** (al-PRAY-zoe-lam)*
*Brands: **Alprazolam Intensol, Xanax, Xanax XR***

Alprazolam belongs to a class of drugs known as benzodiazepines. As a drug class, benzodiazepines slow down the central nervous system. This drug is used to relieve anxiety and nervousness and helps to treat panic attacks. Long-term use of benzodiazepine drugs, such as alprazolam, can lead to dependence; withdrawal symptoms can occur with sudden cessation of the drug.

Benzodiazepines are the treatment of choice for alcohol withdrawal. They work to eliminate the clinical symptoms of this disorder, and to prevent seizures and delirium. Patients with alcohol dependence commonly experience symptoms of anxiety, depression, and insomnia. Benzodiazepines can be used to prevent and treat withdrawal seizures and delirium tremens.

Researchers at the University of North Texas Health Science Center in Fort Worth examined the effects of alprazolam and abecarnil on ethanol withdrawal-induced anxiety-like behaviors in rats. Male rats received an ethanol-containing liquid diet for seven to 10 days and were tested for withdrawal symptoms 12 hours after stopping the diet. Researchers found that alprazolam was more potent than abecarnil in reversing ethanol withdrawal-induced anxieties. Results from this study suggest that alprazolam may have therapeutic potential for treatment of ethanol withdrawal-induced anxiety-like symptoms.

For more information see page 997.

Generic: **Atenolol** *(a-TEN-oh-lole)*
Brand: **Tenormin**

Atenolol belongs to a class of drugs known as beta-blockers, and is used alone or in combination with other drugs to treat high blood pressure. It also is used to prevent angina (chest pain) and to treat heart attacks. Atenolol works by slowing the heart rate and relaxing blood vessels so the heart does not have to pump as hard. This drug may be used to treat alcohol withdrawal, heart failure, or irregular heartbeat, and to prevent migraine headaches.

There are a number of studies that have demonstrated that beta-blockers, such as atenolol, are effective at reducing heart rate, blood pressure, and tremor associated with alcohol withdrawal syndrome. Atenolol has been used along with a benzodiazepine drug in the management of acute alcohol withdrawal. However, beta-blockers alone are not effective in preventing delirium or seizures; therefore, these drugs should be used in addition to benzodiazepines for alcohol withdrawal.

In a study, 61 patients received atenolol, and 59 patients received placebo. Compared with placebo-treated patients, atenolol-treated patients had a significant reduction in the length of hospital stay. On each treatment day, significantly fewer patients receiving atenolol required related treatment with benzodiazepines, and patients receiving placebo required a significantly higher daily dose of benzodiazepines. Among patients who had withdrawal symptoms at the start of the study, vital signs became normal more rapidly in the patients receiving atenolol, and their abnormal behavior and clinical characteristics also resolved more rapidly. None of the 120 patients in this study developed delirium tremens. Researchers deduced that atenolol is helpful in the treatment of patients with alcohol withdrawal syndrome.

For more information see page 1027.

Generic: **Baclofen** (BAK-loe-fen)
Brands: **Kemstro, Lioresal**

Baclofen belongs to a class of drugs known as muscle relaxants and is used to relieve muscle spasms and contractions in people who have conditions such as multiple sclerosis.

Baclofen has been used in a number of instances to reduce alcohol cravings. In animal studies, this drug has suppressed the severity of alcohol withdrawal. It suppressed the intensity of alcohol withdrawal syndrome in rats physically dependent on alcohol. Also, researchers in Italy examined the effects of this drug in humans in a small case study series for 30 days. With the use of baclofen, all patients experienced a rapid reduction in symptoms as shown by reduced withdrawal scores and reductions in blood pressure and pulse rates. After 30 days, all patients were without withdrawal symptoms and alcohol-free. Baclofen was well tolerated; three patients experienced transient drowsiness within 30 to 60 minutes after baclofen administration during the first week of treatment. Researchers concluded that baclofen, in a dose lower than that for the treatment of muscle spasms, produced a rapid disappearance of alcohol withdrawal in all five people in this study.

For more information see page 1037.

Generic: **Buspirone** *(byoo-SPYE-rone)*
Brand: **BuSpar**

Buspirone belongs to a class of drugs known as anxiolytics, which are used to relieve certain kinds of anxiety. It is different from other drugs used to treat anxiety in that it has little effect on mental alertness. In general, this drug takes about two to four weeks for benefits to be seen. Side effects associated with buspirone include disturbed dreams, nightmares, dizziness, drowsiness, headache, nasal congestion, nausea, restlessness, nervousness, and stomach upset.

Researchers at the Benjamin Rush Center in Syracuse, New York examined the role of buspirone in the management of alcohol withdrawal. They evaluated the efficacy of buspirone as treatment to eliminate or reduce the complications of alcohol withdrawal during the detoxification process. One hundred patients were considered for the study, which consisted of buspirone every four hours. All but one patient given buspirone completed the treatment within six days in a manner that effectively controlled their withdrawal symptoms. Hospital staff and patients alike offered favorable comments regarding treatment effects. Staff noted that patients were more alert and were able to participate in support group meetings; patients remarked that they did not feel lethargic or addicted to buspirone. Researchers concluded that buspirone was effective in managing withdrawal symptoms in 100 hospitalized alcohol-dependent patients; yet, larger studies are needed to fully examine the advantages and disadvantages to treatment.

For more information see page 1061.

Generic: **Carbamazepine** *(kar-ba-MAZ-e-peen)*
Brands: **Carbatrol, Epitol, Tegretol, Tegretol XR**

Carbamazepine belongs to a class of drugs known as mood stabilizers. Depending on its use, this drug also may be classified as an antineuralgic, antidiuretic, or an anticonvulsant drug. It is used to control some types of seizures in the treatment of a neurologic condition known as epilepsy; also it may be used to relieve neurogenic pain, to prevent bipolar disorder symptoms, and used to treat a certain type of diabetes, alcohol withdrawal, or some mental illnesses.

Your doctor may use carbamazepine in an off-label manner to treat alcohol withdrawal psychosis. In a study conducted in Turkey, 83 men classified as alcoholics with severe alcohol withdrawal symptoms received either carbamazepine or diazepam (another benzodiazepine drug) for seven days. In this study, 33 men in the carbamazepine group and 34 men in the diazepam group finished the trial. Overall, both drugs were found to be equally effective in treating the withdrawal symptoms. Additionally, there were not significant differences with regard to side effects between the drugs. Researchers concluded that based on these findings, carbamazepine is as effective as diazepam in the treatment of alcohol withdrawal.

In a study published in a Scandinavian psychiatry journal, 72 hospitalized patients with alcohol withdrawal symptoms were treated with either carbamazepine or barbital (a barbiturate drug). Researchers found no statistically significant differences in effectiveneess between the two treatments, and both drugs were well tolerated. They concluded that carbamazepine is a valuable alternative drug in the treatment of mild and moderate alcohol withdrawal symptoms.

Additionally, researchers from the Department of Psychiatry and Behavioral Sciences at the Medical University of South Carolina conducted a study of 86 alcoholic men with severe alcohol withdrawal. They received carbamazepine or oxazepam. The researchers found that the drugs were equally effective in treating the withdrawal syndrome and the side effects were not significantly different. However, the people who received carbamazepine had a decline in physiological distress. Based on these results, researchers suggest that carbamazepine may be effective to treat psychosis associated with alcohol withdrawal.

For more information see page 1068.

Generic: **Clonidine** *(KLON-i-deen)*
Brands: **Catapres, Catapres-TTS, Duraclon**

Clonidine is classified as an antihypertensive drug, and is used to treat high blood pressure. It works by stimulating certain brain receptors, which relaxes blood vessels in other parts of the body, causing them to widen. This drug may also be used to ease withdrawal symptoms associated with the long-term use of alcohol, narcotics, and nicotine. Your doctor may prescribe clonidine for alcohol withdrawal delirium.

Doctors have used clonidine to relieve opiate withdrawal symptoms for more than 20 years. Researchers at Orebro University in Sweden evaluated the effect of intrathecal (administered directly into the spinal fluid) and oral clonidine as supplements to spinal anesthesia with lidocaine in patients at risk of postoperative alcohol withdrawal syndrome. Forty-five alcohol-dependent patients undergoing prostate surgery were divided into three groups. The diazepam group was premedicated with diazepam orally; the intrathecal clonidine group received a placebo (saline) tablet and clonidine intrathecally; and the oral clonidine group received clonidine orally. Twelve patients in the diazepam group had symptoms of alcohol withdrawal syndrome, compared with two in the intrathecal clonidine group and one in the oral clonidine group. Two patients in the diazepam group had severe delirium. Researchers found that patients receiving oral clonidine had a slightly decreased arterial blood pressure six hours to 12 hours after spinal anesthesia; patients in the diazepam group had a circulatory reaction 24 hours to 72 hours after surgery. Overall, preoperative clonidine (intrathecally or orally) prevented significant postoperative alcohol withdrawal syndromes in alcohol-dependent patients.

For more information see page 1108.

*Generic: **Divalproex** (DI-val-proe-ix)*
*Brands: **Depakote Delayed Release, Depakote ER,***
Depakote Sprinkle

Divalproex sodium belongs to a class of drugs known as mood stabilizers, and is used to control seizures in certain types of epilepsy. Divalproex sodium is used in other conditions such as bipolar disorder, mania, migraine prevention, and control of behavioral problems associated with dementia (the loss of thinking, remembering, and reasoning abilities). There are a number of side effects associated with divalproex sodium including breast enlargement, changes in menstrual periods, clumsiness, diarrhea or constipation, difficulty speaking, dizziness or drowsiness, loss of bladder control, nausea or vomiting, and headache, among others.

A researcher at the University of Maryland in Baltimore conducted a medical chart review of psychiatric outpatients with alcohol or substance abuse and mood disorders. It was found that some patients treated with divalproex sodium diminished their substance abuse during the period of treatment for their disorders. Of the 46 patients, 24 showed a reduction in alcohol or other substance abuse, two showed a change in their usage, and none of the patients increased usage.

Researchers from the University of Washington School of Medicine evaluated 36 patients undergoing alcohol withdrawal. The patients received divalproex sodium or placebo. Also, all patients had access to oxazepam as a rescue medication in case alcohol withdrawal symptoms became unmanageable. Researchers observed that those patients on divalproex sodium had less use of oxazepam as an escape medication. They concluded that divalproex sodium significantly affects the course of alcohol withdrawal and reduces the need for treatment with a benzodiazepine.

For more information see page 1147.

Generic: *Gabapentin* (GA-ba-pen-tin)
Brand: *Neurontin*

Gabapentin is in a class of drugs known as anticonvulsants, and is used to help control some types of seizures in the treatment of a neurologic condition known as epilepsy. This drug is also used to control pain associated with shingles. In studies, gabapentin has been shown to have a positive effect in the treatment of moderate alcohol withdrawal in four inpatients when added to clomethiazole (a drug known as a hypnotic).

In case study reports, the use of this drug has been associated with a reduction in alcohol cravings and/or withdrawal scores. In a trial, 15 adult alcoholics with persistent insomnia received gabapentin within a two-week period. In this study, most patients had some relief of insomnia with gabapentin 600 mg each night. Seven patients in this study needed higher doses (900 mg/day to 1200 mg/day) and three patients required 1500 mg/day. One patient in this study responded to 200 mg at night. Reported reactions in this study include dizziness, fatigue, and/or sedation. Since gabapentin has few interactions with drugs or alcohol, and has minimal abuse or dependency potential, its role in alcohol and substance abuse disorders is being explored.

For more information see page 1206.

*Generic: **Lorazepam** (lore-AZ-ee-pam)*
*Brands: **Ativan, Lorazepam Intensol***

Lorazepam, a benzodiazepine drug, is an anti-anxiety drug primarily used to relieve anxiety in affected persons, although your doctor may prescribe this drug for other reasons, such as alcohol withdrawal psychosis or delirium. Side effects of lorazepam include drowsiness, dizziness, tiredness, weakness, memory loss, diarrhea, upset stomach, and appetite changes.

Benzodiazepine-type drugs are fast acting and offer a sedative effect; they are considered to be the mainstay treatment for mild-to-moderate alcohol withdrawal. However, long-term use of benzodiapines is associated with dependence and may result in withdrawal when the drug is stopped.

A clinical trial comparing patient responses to the benzodiazepine drugs lorazepam and carbamazepine was conducted by researchers at the substance abuse clinic at the Medical University of South Carolina. Patients with moderate alcohol withdrawal syndrome received carbamazepine or lorazepam on day one, and then reduced dosages of carbamazepine or lorazepam. In this study, both drugs were equally effective at decreasing the symptoms of alcohol withdrawal. In the post-treatment period, 89 patients drank on at least one day. Carbamazepine-treated patients drank less than one drink per drinking day (on average) and lorazepam patients drank almost three drinks per drinking day.

In those patients with multiple previous detoxifications, the carbamazepine group drank less than one drink per day (on average) and the lorazepam group drank about five drinks per day (on average). Lorazepam-treated patients had a significant rebound of alcohol withdrawal symptoms post-treatment, and the risk of having a first drink was three times greater compared with the carbamazepine-treated patients. Researchers concluded that carbamazepine was superior to lorazapam in preventing rebound withdrawal symptoms and decreasing post-treatment drinking.

For more information see page 1287.

Generic: **Midazolam** *(MID-aye-zoe-lam)*
Brand: **Versed**

Midazolam belongs to a class of drugs known as benzodiazepines, which slow down the central nervous system. It is a sedative hypnotic that causes relaxation and sleep. In anesthesia, it provides loss of awareness and memory for short diagnostic tests and surgical procedures; produces sleep at the start of surgery; or supplements other types of general anesthetics. Midazolam does not reduce pain or cause loss of consciousness.

In an article by researchers at Stanford University Medical Center in California, it was noted that treatment with newer benzodiazepines, such as lorazepam and midazolam, has become more widespread, and death from severe alcohol withdrawal has decreased in recent years. In another article, researchers at the Michael Reese Hospital and Medical Center in Chicago, Illinois, reported their results of midazolam and its effects on alcohol withdrawal in rats. In this study, researchers tested the ability of midazolam to modify alcohol-induced changes: blood flow and cerebral oxygen consumption after alcohol withdrawal in alcohol-dependent rats. Results from this study showed that midazolam may be effective in lowering blood pressure and brain metabolism and reversing the blood flow changes produced by alcohol withdrawal, demonstrating that midazolam may be of benefit in alcoholics, particularly those receiving anesthesia for surgical procedures. The drug may help treat alcohol withdrawal and improve anesthesia levels for surgery.

For more information see page 1325.

Benzodiazepine Withdrawal

Long-term use of benzodiazepines can lead to dependency on the drug. Abrupt cessation of benzodiazepine drug use can produce withdrawal symptoms. These symptoms include anxiety, panic, hypersensitivity to sensory stimuli, depersonalization and derealization, abnormal perception of movement, appetite and weight loss, and depressed mood. Less common symptoms also include epileptic seizures and psychotic or neuropsychiatric symptoms. Even with conservative and gradual benzodiazepine dose reductions, symptoms of withdrawal have been observed in some persons. In the reviewed studies, the use of drug therapy was typically part of a larger overall program, including behavioral therapy, which was all targeted toward improvement in substance abuse.

Commonly Prescribed (On-Label) Drugs: None

OFF-LABEL PRESCRIPTION DRUG
BREAKTHROUGH OPTION

Generic: ***Carbamazepine*** *(kar-ba-MAZ-e-peen)*
Brands: ***Carbatrol, Epitol, Tegretol, Tegretol XR***

Carbamazepine belongs to a class of drugs known as mood stabilizers. Depending on its use, this drug also may be classified as an antineuralgic, antimanic, antipsychotic, antidiuretic, or anticonvulsant drug. It is used to control some types of seizures in the treatment of epilepsy; also it may be used to relieve neurogenic pain, to prevent bipolar disorder symptoms, and to treat a certain type of diabetes, alcohol withdrawal, or some mental illnesses.

Researchers in Germany evaluated the efficacy of carbamazepine for benzodiazepine withdrawal. In 18 patients, a benzodiazepine drug was withdrawn. The dose was gradually reduced in nine patients; the other nine patients were given carbamazepine syrup for 15 days after the benzodiazepine drug was stopped. In those patients treated with carbamazepine, there was a trend toward less severe benzodiazepine withdrawal symptoms. Researchers concluded that carbamazepine offers a therapeutic benefit for those at risk for benzodiazepine withdrawal.

In another study, researchers in Poland found that carbamazepine was found to be comparable with another drug used for benzodiazepine withdrawal, tianeptine, and was safe and effective in treating withdrawal symptoms. These two studies provide some evidence that carbamazepine may be helpful for benzodiazepine withdrawal but more evidence is needed.

For more information see page 1068.

Cocaine Addiction

The effects of cocaine are immediate, pleasurable, and brief; the drug produces strong yet short-lived euphoria. Similar to caffeine, cocaine produces wakefulness and reduces hunger. Once the drug wears off, intense depression, anxiety, lethargy, and excessive sleeping occur. Addiction to cocaine can happen quickly and is challenging to break. Individuals who are addicted to cocaine will go to great lengths to obtain cocaine and will continue using the drug despite the negative consequences. Addicted people may have difficulty quitting cocaine because the resulting depression can be overwhelming, and will cause them to use more drug to overcome their depressed mood. In the reviewed studies, the use of drug therapy was typically part of a larger overall program, including behavioral therapy, which was all targeted toward improvement in substance abuse.

Commonly Prescribed (On-Label) Drugs: None

OFF-LABEL PRESCRIPTION DRUGS
BREAKTHROUGH OPTIONS

*Generic: **Amantadine** (a-MAN-to-deen)*
*Brand: **Symmetrel***

Amantadine belongs to a class of drugs known as antivirals, although depending on how its used, it might be classified as an antifatigue or antishaking drug. This drug is used to prevent or treat certain influenza infections (type A infections). Amantadine may be given alone or in combination with flu shots.

There have been a number of studies evaluating the use of amantadine for cocaine addiction, all with variable results. In one study, 42 people were chosen to receive amantadine or placebo for 10.5 days. Through one month, more amantadine-treated patients had urine samples that tested negative for cocaine. In another study, patients were chosen to receive a higher dose of amantadine or placebo for four weeks, in addition to psychosocial care. Results from this study showed no significant differences between conditions for urine drug testing, self-report of drug use, retention, craving, or global improvement.

Researchers at the Friends Research Institute in Los Angeles, California, evaluated amantadine twice daily for cocaine dependence. In this 16-week trial with group counseling included, patients were chosen to receive amantadine or placebo. Researchers found that amantadine-treated patients were more likely to not use cocaine on the last day of the eight-week study compared with those patients who received placebo. These findings were similar at the end of the study (at week 16).

For more information see page 1001.

Generic: **Baclofen** (BAK-loe-fen)
Brands: **Kemstro, Lioresal**

Baclofen belongs to a class of drugs known as muscle relaxants; it is used to relieve muscle spasms and contractions in conditions such as multiple sclerosis. It is also used to treat trigeminal neuralgia, which is severe burning or stabbing pain along the nerves in the face.

There are a number of studies and patient case studies indicating that baclofen may be useful in the treatment of cocaine, heroin, nicotine, and alcohol dependence; however, more research is needed. Animal studies involving baclofen have shown that this drug reduces self-administration of cocaine, but the effects depend on the amount of cocaine used. At low doses of cocaine, baclofen reduced cocaine use; however, at higher doses, baclofen did not affect cocaine self-administration in rats. In a human study, researchers at the UCLA Integrated Substance Abuse Program in Los Angeles, California, compared baclofen three times daily plus counseling sessions with placebo in those with cocaine dependence. Results from this study showed that people who received baclofen showed significant and stepwise increases in the probability of having urine samples that tested negative for cocaine. It was concluded that baclofen effects were apparent for those individuals with chronic levels of cocaine use.

For more information see page 1037.

Generic: **Carbamazepine** (kar-ba-MAZ-e-peen)
Brands: **Carbatrol, Epitol, Tegretol, Tegretol XR**

Carbamazepine belongs to a class of drugs known as mood stabilizers. Depending on its use, this drug also may be classified as an antineuralgic, antimanic, antipsychotic, antidiuretic, or anticonvulsant drug. Carbamazepine is used to control some types of seizures in the treatment of a neurologic condition known as epilepsy; it may be used to relieve neurogenic pain, to prevent bipolar disorder symptoms, and to treat a certain type of diabetes, alcohol withdrawal, or some mental illnesses.

Carbamazepine may be a useful drug in the treatment of cocaine addiction since it has a low potential for addiction, and may also treat co-existing disorders. Researchers at the National Institute on Drug Abuse, Addiction Research Center in Baltimore, Maryland, reported that carbamazepine is an effective treatment for cocaine dependence based on findings from studies. A large decrease in cocaine use during eight weeks in 12 cocaine-dependent men was observed. Patients received carbamazepine for four weeks, then decreased doses of the study drug during the next four weeks in addition to counseling. Throughout the study, five men remained cocaine-free. During treatment with carbamazepine, six men reported that they achieved their longest abstinence of cocaine. Researchers concluded that these results support the utility of carbamazepine for cocaine dependence.

For more information see page 1068.

Generic: *Desipramine* (des-IP-ra-meen)
Brand: *Norpramin*

Desipramine belongs to a class of drugs known as antidepressants, and is used to treat depression. This drug is also used to treat cocaine withdrawal and eating disorders. Side effects associated with desipramine include upset stomach, drowsiness, weakness or tiredness, excitement, anxiety, insomnia, nightmares, dry mouth, skin sensitivity to sunlight, and appetite or weight changes.

Researchers at the University of Kansas Medical Center in Kansas City, Kansas compared the effects of desipramine or carbamazepine with placebo in an outpatient program for cocaine abuse. Patients received desipramine, carbamazepine, or placebo for eight weeks. The patients improved over time on all self-ratings related to cocaine use, mood, and craving. Those in the two treatment groups reported significantly more improvement on self-ratings of depression and irritability. No treatment differences were noted for sustained abstinence or for the number of positive urine drug tests. Based on these findings, researchers concluded that there may be a possible role for desipramine in cocaine abuse treatment.

In a 26-week study, researchers at Yale University School of Medicine in Connecticut evaluated the efficacy of desipramine in 109 male and female cocaine- and opiate-dependent patients treated with buprenorphine or methadone. Once stabilized on buprenorphine or methadone (during the first two weeks), half of the patients received desipramine for the first half of the trial and placebo for the second, with the order of drugs reversed for the second half of the trial. Results from this study showed that desipramine reduced the use of opiates only when administered at the beginning rather than in the middle of the trial, whereas cocaine use was reduced when desipramine was introduced at either time.

For more information see page 1132.

Generic: **Divalproex** *(DI-val-proe-ix)*
Brands: **Depakote Delayed Release, Depakote ER, Depakote Sprinkle**

Divalproex sodium belongs to a class of drugs known as mood stabilizers, and is used to control seizures in certain types of epilepsy. It is used in other conditions such as bipolar disorder, mania, migraine prevention, and control of behavioral problems associated with dementia (the loss of thinking, remembering, and reasoning abilities). There are a number of side effects associated with divalproex sodium including breast enlargement, changes in menstrual periods, clumsiness, diarrhea or constipation, difficulty speaking, dizziness or drowsiness, loss of bladder control, nausea or vomiting, and headache, among others.

Researchers at the University of Minnesota in Minneapolis examined the effectiveness of increasing levels of valproic acid (a drug related to divalproex sodium) on cocaine abstinence in 55 patients. With valproic acid treatment, the total number of days of cocaine use decreased significantly and improved levels of subject functioning were noticed. Researchers concluded that based on these results, the divalproex sodium form of valproic acid may be an effective add-on drug in the management and treatment of cocaine dependency.

Researchers at the Medical University of South Carolina found that anticonvulsant drugs, particularly valproate, are a class of drugs with potential utility in the treatment of addictive disorders. Finally, in a study conducted at the Department of Mental Health at Tewksbury Hospital in Massachusetts, divalproex sodium was found to be safe and effective when used alone or in combination with other psychiatric drugs in patients with substance abuse and mood disorders.

For more information see page 1147.

*Generic: **Gabapentin** (GA-ba-pen-tin)*
*Brand: **Neurontin***

Gabapentin is a member in a class of drugs known as anticonvulsants, and is used to help control some types of seizures in the treatment of epilepsy. This drug is also used to control pain associated with shingles. Side effects associated with the use of gabapentin include blurred or double vision; cold or flu-like symptoms; delusions; dementia; drowsiness; hoarseness; lack or loss of strength; lower back or side pain; swelling of the hands, feet, or lower legs; and trembling and shaking; among others.

Across the medical literature, gabapentin has been noted to be a potential treatment for cocaine dependence. Gabapentin is thought to work in dependence disorders through dopaminergic actions. In clinical studies, gabapentin has been used for up to nine months. In a study, 30 cocaine-dependent patients were selected to receive gabapentin twice daily for eight weeks. Six patients completed the entire study. At eight weeks, the extent and frequency of cocaine cravings were significantly reduced from the start of the study. Reductions in depression, anxiety, and the percentage of patients with a positive urine screen were also seen. Researchers concluded that gabapentin is well tolerated and effective in reducing cocaine cravings in patients with cocaine dependence; however, more studies are needed to validate findings from smaller studies.

For more information see page 1206.

*Generic: **Modafinil** (moe-DAF-i-nil)*
*Brand: **Provigil***

Modafinil is a central nervous system stimulant that is prescribed for narcolepsy (sudden and uncontrollable attacks of drowsiness and sleep), obstructive sleep apnea (periodic cessation of breathing at night), and shift work sleep-related disorders. It is used to promote wakefulness and alertness.

Because the primary symptoms of cocaine withdrawal are increased sleep, low energy, and depression, modafinil may have utility since it decreases sleepiness, improves mood, and increases energy, sense of well being, and concentration. In a study conducted by researchers at the University of Pennsylvania, patients were pretreated with modafinil and then given an IV infusion of cocaine. No toxic reactions were seen with the drug combination, and modafinil blocked a number of cocaine effects including euphoria and vital sign elevations (heart rate).

An eight-week study of modafinil treatment in 17 cocaine-dependent patients was conducted by the same group of researchers at the University of Pennsylvania. In addition to treatment, all patients received cognitive behavioral therapy twice weekly. Patients in the modafinil-treated group had 47% cocaine-free urines; subjects in this group also reported decreased depression, increased sense of well being, and decreased craving. Moreover, there were no serious adverse events. Researchers concluded that modafinil appears to be a promising drug for the treatment of cocaine dependence.

For more information see page 1138.

Generic: *Topiramate* (TOE-pie-rah-mate)
Brand: *Topamax*

Topiramate belongs to a class of drugs known as anti-epileptic drugs. This drug is used to prevent epileptic seizures, and may be used to prevent migraine headaches. Side effects associated with topiramate include headache, nausea, tremor, fatigue, back pain, chest pain, gastrointestinal upset, visual disturbances, sleepiness, and weight loss, among others.

Researchers affiliated with the University of Pennsylvania School of Medicine evaluated the effects of this drug on subjects with cocaine addiction in a 13-week study. Forty patients in this study received placebo or an increasing daily dose of topiramate for eight weeks. At the end of the study, subjects' doses were gradually decreased. In addition, patients received twice-weekly cognitive behavioral therapy. Results from this study demonstrate that those who received topiramate were more likely than those who received placebo to abstain from cocaine after the eighth week of the study. Additionally, those who received counseling and topiramate were more likely to achieve three or more weeks of continuous cocaine abstinence compared with the placebo and counseling group (59% versus 26%, respectively). Researchers concluded that topiramate can successfully produce a stable period of cocaine abstinence.

For more information see page 1516.

Pathological Gambling

Pathological gambling is classified as a major psychological disorder. Criteria for this disorder involves at least five of the following traits: a preoccupation with gambling; a need to gamble with increasing amounts to achieve desired excitement; repeated and unsuccessful attempts to control or stop gambling, restlessness and/or irritability when trying to stop gambling; gambling to escape problems and/or mood; lying to family members about gambling; committing illegal acts to support gambling monies; jeopardizing or losing important relationships and/or jobs; and relying on others to relieve the debts incurred by gambling. Treatment for this addictive disorder involves therapy and drug treatment.

Commonly Prescribed (On-Label) Drugs: *None*

OFF-LABEL PRESCRIPTION DRUGS
BREAKTHROUGH OPTIONS

Generic: **Citalopram** *(sye-TAL-oh-pram)*
Brand: **Celexa**

Citalopram belongs to a class of drugs known as SSRI-type antidepressants. This drug is used to treat depression or other related problems. Clinical studies have indicated that SSRI-type drugs may be effective for pathological gambling, although a few subjects in these studies had problems with machine gambling.

SSRI-type drugs, such as citalopram, are considered to be the treatment of choice for obsessive-compulsive disorder (OCD) and related conditions. Since pathological gambling and OCD may be related, researchers have studied the effects of SSRI-type drugs, such as citalopram, for this addictive disorder. In a study conducted by researchers at Brown University School of Medicine in Providence, Rhode Island, 15 adult pathological gamblers were given citalopram for up to 12 weeks. After treatment with citalopram, patients reported significant reductions on all gambling measures including the number of days gambled, amount of money lost gambling, preoccupation with gambling, and urges to gamble. Thirteen patients (86.7%) were rated as "much improved" or "very much improved." Moreover, patients with major depression improved to about the same degree as patients without depression. For the majority of patients, improvement was seen during the first two weeks of treatment. Researchers concluded that citalopram seems to be an effective drug for the treatment of pathological gambling, and benefits seen were separate from the drug's antidepressant effects.

For more information see page 1096.

*Generic: **Naltrexone** (nal-TREKS-one)*
*Brands: **Naltrexone, ReVia***

Naltrexone alleviates dependence on opiate drugs (narcotics) or alcohol. This drug works by blocking the elevated mood (high) that these substances produce. Naltrexone therapy is often combined with counseling and support groups. It is generally used after an initial detoxification period. If naltrexone is used while a person is still taking opiate drugs, withdrawal symptoms may occur.

Support for the use of naltrexone for pathological gambling stems from evidence of its efficacy in the treatment of alcoholism, bulimia, drug abuse, borderline personality disorder, and other psychiatric disorders in which urges are the main symptom. Since one of the primary symptoms of pathological gambling is an uncontrolled urge triggered by potential reward, researchers at the University of Minnesota Medical School in Minneapolis evaluated naltrexone for the treatment of this addictive disorder. In this study, 83 subjects with pathological gambling disorders were enrolled in a 12-week study. Patients received placebo or naltrexone. Researchers evaluated data from 45 subjects in this study and found that significant improvement was seen in all gambling symptom measures. At the end of the study, 75% of subjects treated with naltrexone were "much" or "very much improved" compared with 24% of subjects who received placebo. Nausea was the most common side effect seen during the first week of the study in the naltrexone group. Based on these findings, researchers concluded that naltrexone is effective in reducing symptoms of pathological gambling.

For more information see page 1352.

Smoking Cessation

Despite the known risks, numerous awareness campaigns, and publication of research studies that show the health hazards of cigarette smoking, smoking continues to be a major health problem. Although most cigarette smokers who have quit have done so without treatment, the success rate per quit attempt is low—less than 5% of unassisted quit attempts lead to successful long-term abstinence from cigarette smoking. A number of therapies have been directed toward smoking cessation. These include behavioral therapies (counseling) and drug treatments. Drug treatments include nicotine replacement therapies (nicotine gum and patches) and blockade treatments. In the reviewed studies, the use of drug therapy was typically part of a larger overall program, including behavioral therapy, which was all targeted toward improvement in substance abuse.

Commonly Prescribed (On-Label) Drugs: None

OFF-LABEL PRESCRIPTION DRUGS
BREAKTHROUGH OPTIONS

---

*Generic: **Clonidine** (KLON-i-deen)*
*Brands: **Catapres, Catapres-TTS, Duraclon***

Clonidine is classified as an antihypertensive drug, and is used to treat high blood pressure by stimulating certain brain receptors (of the alpha adrenergic type), which relaxes blood vessels in other parts of the body, causing them to widen. It may also be used to ease withdrawal symptoms associated with the long-term use of alcohol, narcotics, and nicotine. Your doctor may prescribe clonidine for delirium related to alcohol withdrawal.

Clonidine should be used three to four days before a person's quit date, to build up enough drug in the body. The patch is changed weekly; and treatment with the patch formulation can last up to 10 weeks. This drug was one of the first non-nicotine drugs studied for its smoking cessation effects. Since this drug has been effective in treating opiate and alcohol withdrawal, researchers have investigated its utility in reducing nicotine craving and withdrawal. It is thought that this drug blocks anxiety, irritability, and cravings that characterize nicotine withdrawal. In studies, recipients of clonidine were more likely to quit smoking compared with placebo-treated subjects. Additionally, clonidine was found to be more effective when given by a skin patch rather than by mouth, and when given with behavioral therapy.

A group of three researchers sought to determine the efficacy of clonidine in smoking cessation. Researchers employed the Cochrane Tobacco Addiction Group trials registry in search of relevant clinical studies. Out of the six trials reviewed by the group, it was found that clonidine is effective in promoting smoking cessation; however, side effects, such as dry mouth, sedation, dizziness, and postural hypotension, may limit the use of this drug.

For more information see page 1108.

Generic: **Mecamylamine** *(meh-CAM-el-ah-mean)*
Brand: **Inversine**

Mecamylamine is a drug that belongs to a class of drugs known as antihypertensives, which are used to lower high blood pressure. Mecamylamine is also classified as a nicotine antagonist, or a drug that blocks the effects of nicotine. It was discovered that mecamylamine can block the rewarding effects of nicotine, thereby reducing the urge to smoke. At high doses, mecamylamine may produce significant adverse effects such as drowsiness, hypotension, and constipation. Lower doses along with nicotine replacement therapy (gum or patches) may negate adverse effects.

Two researchers evaluated the efficacy of mecamylamine in smoking cessation through a review of existing medical literature. They found two studies that demonstrated the efficacy of mecamylamine with nicotine replacement therapy. In the first study, 48 people received mecamylamine plus nicotine replacement therapy; combination treatment was found to be more effective than nicotine patch alone. The abstinence rate at one year was 37.5% versus 4.2% for the patch alone.

In the second study, 80 patients were treated for four weeks before quitting with one of four treatments: nicotine patch plus mecamylamine capsules; 2) nicotine alone; 3) mecamylamine alone; or 4) no active drug. In this study, up to 40% of subjects who received the patch plus mecamylamine abstained from smoking, compared with 20%, 25%, and 15% of the other groups, respectively. It is important to note that up to 40% of subjects who received mecamylamine required dose reductions because of constipation.

For more information see page 1293.

Generic: **Naltrexone** *(nal-TREKS-one)*
Brands: **Naltrexone, ReVia**

Naltrexone alleviates dependence on opiate drugs (narcotics) or alcohol. This drug works by blocking the elevated mood (high) that these substances produce. Naltrexone therapy is often combined with counseling and support groups and is generally used after an initial detoxification period. If naltrexone is used while a person is still taking opiate drugs, withdrawal symptoms may occur.

Naltrexone may help block the rewarding effects of smoking. In a study conducted by researchers at the University of Chicago in Illinois, naltrexone significantly reduced cigarette craving and desire to smoke. Reductions in craving persisted in a subsequent one-hour nonsmoking period. Use of naltrexone also significantly reduced the total number of cigarettes smoked.

For more information see page 1352.

Generic: **Nortriptyline** *(nor-TRIP-ti-leen)*
Brands: **Aventyl, Pamelor**

Nortriptyline belongs to a class of drugs known as tricyclic antidepressants, or TCAs. This drug is used to elevate mood and treat depression. Your doctor may prescribe nortriptyline for other conditions, such as smoking cessation and attention-deficit disorder. Side effects associated with nortriptyline include anxiety, constipation, diarrhea, dry mouth, drowsiness, dizziness, headache, increased sensitivity to sunlight, appetite loss, nausea, vomiting, skin rash, or weight loss or gain.

In clinical studies, nortriptyline was found to be comparable with the smoking cessation and antidepressant drug bupropion. In a clinical trial, 158 smokers (age range from 18 years to 65 years) were given placebo or nortriptyline up to 12 weeks after their designated smoking quit day. The nicotine patch was started on the quit day and continued for eight weeks. In addition to nortriptyline and the patch, subjects received behavioral intervention. Researchers found that nortriptyline along with the nicotine patch resulted in an increased smoking cessation rate with minimal effect on withdrawal symptoms. At six months, the smoking cessation rates were 23% for the bupropion and nortriptyline group and 10% for the placebo group. In this study, nortriptyline use resulted in frequent side effects such as dry mouth (38%) and sedation (20%). In 13% of patients, nortriptyline was stopped due to adverse events.

According to researchers in the Netherlands, nortriptyline should be considered a first-line drug for smoking cessation, based on their review of the medical literature. Compared with placebo treatment in five studies, nortriptyline use provided higher smoking abstinence rates after at least six months of treatment.

For more information see page 1378.

Generic: **Selegiline** (se-LE-ji-leen)
Brand: **Eldepryl**

Selegiline helps to increase or extend the effects of drugs used to treat Parkinson's disease (i.e., levodopa or carbidopa), and slow the progression of the disease. This drug may promote smoking cessation in central dopamine systems by blocking dopamine metabolism.

Researchers at the Program for Research in Smokers with Mental Illness in New Haven, Connecticut, examined the safety and efficacy of selegiline versus placebo for smoking cessation in nicotine-dependent cigarette smokers. In this study, 40 people were chosen to receive either selegiline hydrochloride or placebo during an eight-week trial. Results from this study showed that selegiline increased smoking cessation rates during the last four weeks of the trial versus placebo. Selegiline was well tolerated in cigarette smokers. Researchers suggested that selegiline is safe for use and enhances smoking cessation rates compared with placebo in nicotine-dependent cigarette smokers.

In another study by researchers at Johns Hopkins University School of Medicine in Baltimore, Maryland, selegiline decreased cigarette craving, particularly during abstinence, and it reduced the number of cigarettes smoked and smoking satisfaction ratings. Results from this study prove that early treatment with selegiline during a quit attempt may promote smoking cessation.

For more information see page 1466.

MEN'S HEALTH DISORDERS

EJACULATORY DISORDERS

The most common problems of sexual dysfunction in men are ejaculation disorders, which include premature ejaculation, retrograde ejaculation, partial retrograde ejaculation, and post-spinal injury ejaculation. These and other sexual dysfunctions in men can result from physical causes such as diabetes, heart and vascular disease, hormonal imbalances, side effects from certain drugs, drug or alcohol abuse, and surgery, or psychological causes such as work-related stress and anxiety, concerns about sexual performance, marital or relationship problems, and sexual trauma.

Premature Ejaculation

Premature ejaculation is the occurrence of ejaculation before a man wishes it to happen or too quickly to satisfy his sexual partner. A common condition, premature ejaculation is rarely the result of a physical problem. It can occur before penetration or just after penetration, and may leave the couple feeling sexually unfulfilled. Treatments for premature ejaculation include behavioral methods, exercise methods, condom use, and drug treatments.

Commonly Prescribed (On-Label) Drugs: *Bumetanide*

OFF-LABEL PRESCRIPTION DRUGS
BREAKTHROUGH OPTIONS

Generic: **Clomipramine** *(kloe-MI-pra-meen)*
Brand: **Anafranil**

Clomipramine belongs to the class of drugs known as tricyclic antidepressants, or TCAs, and is the most widely studied drug for premature ejaculation. Antidepressants, such as clomipramine, may be effective in premature ejaculation since a common side effect is delayed sexual climax.

The use of clomipramine for premature ejaculation is well documented in the medical literature. A clinical study conducted by researchers at the Johns Hopkins School of Health & Hygiene wanted to determine if men with premature ejaculation who fail to respond to 25 mg clomipramine would respond to an increase in the dosage of up to 30 mg of clomipramine. During this study, four men kept daily logs of their sexual activities and ejaculations while increasing the daily doses of clomipramine (10 mg, 20 mg, and 30 mg). Results from this study showed that there was a dose-response effect on ejaculation with increasing levels of clomipramine. Moreover, 30 mg of clomipramine was significantly more effective than the 25-mg dose in men who failed to respond to 25 mg of clomipramine.

In a study of life-long premature ejaculation conducted by researchers in the Netherlands, clomipramine provided clinically meaningful delays in ejaculation whereas paroxetine, a selective serotonin reuptake inhibitor (SSRI), did not.

For more information see page 1105.

Generic: **Fluoxetine** *(floo-OKS-e-teen)*
Brands: **Prozac, Prozac Weekly, Sarafem**

Drugs with selective serotonin reuptake inhibitors (SSRI)-type side effects, such as fluoxetine, have been shown to be safe and effective to treat premature ejaculation. In fact, many doctors use SSRIs since they have been noted to be the most successful drugs to delay early ejaculation. The mechanism of action of SSRIs, such as fluoxetine, increases the availability of a chemical in the body known as serotonin in the central nervous system.

Delayed ejaculation was noted in a study in 51 men with premature ejaculation. Among other SSRIs, fluoxetine was found to increase the amount of time before intravaginal ejaculation. In another study by Korean researchers, the efficacy and safety of fluoxetine, sertraline (an SSRI), clomipramine (a TCA), and placebo were compared in 36 men who ejaculated in less than two minutes. Men took each of the three drugs and the placebo consecutively during a four-week period per medication. After four weeks of treatment, time before ejaculation increased significantly for placebo, fluoxetine, sertraline, and clomipramine. However, researchers noted that in this study clomipramine and sertraline treatments resulted in a greater increase in time before ejaculation compared with fluoxetine or placebo.

For more information see page 1192.

Generic: *Paroxetine* (pa-ROKS-e-teen)
Brands: *Paxil, Paxil CR*

Several clinical studies have shown that the use of selective serotonin reuptake inhibitors (SSRIs) are safe and effective to treat premature ejaculation. Paroxetine, which is a strong SSRI often used to treat premature ejaculation, works by increasing serotonin, a chemical in the body, in the central nervous system. Studies have shown that SSRIs, such as paroxetine, have fewer adverse effects compared with tricyclic antidepressants (TCAs).

With paroxetine, improvements in premature ejaculation may not be seen until at least three weeks after the start of treatment. The drug should be stopped if no improvements are seen after six weeks of therapy or if adverse events become troublesome. Besides sexual side effects, other adverse effects associated with paroxetine include sour stomach, decreased appetite, gas, heartburn, nervousness, and sleepiness.

In clinical studies, paroxetine has been shown to be effective for premature ejaculation, and according to *American Family Physician*, it should be considered as a first-line treatment for this disorder. In a study conducted in the Netherlands, 34 men with premature ejaculation were given 20 mg or 40 mg daily of paroxetine for seven weeks. At the end of the study, 27 men completed treatment, and both treatment groups showed an improvement in ejaculation time. Based on these results, researchers concluded that 20 mg of paroxetine may be an adequate treatment for primary premature ejaculation.

For more information see page 1395.

Generic: **Sertraline** *(SER-tra-leen)*
Brand: **Zoloft**

Several studies indicate that selective serotonin reuptake inhibitors (SSRIs), such as sertraline, are safe and effective to treat premature ejaculation. Many doctors use SSRIs precisely for premature ejaculation. Overall, according to research at the Cleveland Clinic Foundation in Ohio, SSRIs have shown the most success in delaying premature ejaculation.

Sertraline, a potent SSRI, is often used to treat premature ejaculation. It works by increasing the available serotonin in the central nervous system. The use of these antidepressants results in fewer side effects compared with tricyclic antidepressants. One of the most common side effects of SSRIs, such as sertraline, is delayed sexual climax; hence, doctors may prescribe this drug for premature ejaculation. With sertraline, improvement in premature ejaculation may not occur until at least three weeks after the treatment is started. If no improvement is noticed after six weeks of treatment, or if adverse effects become troublesome, sertraline should be discontinued. Besides sexual side effects, use of sertraline may result in sour stomach, belching, decreased appetite or weight loss, diarrhea, dizziness, drowsiness, and dry mouth, among others.

In a clinical study of 46 men with premature ejaculation, sertraline daily delayed ejaculation with the fewest side effects. With a higher dose of sertraline daily, ejaculation was delayed even further, but at the higher dose, two men experienced side effects such as drowsiness, appetite loss, and upset stomach. Researchers found that increasing the dose of sertraline increased the drug's efficacy in delaying ejaculation. Other study results suggest that sertraline can be taken on an "as-needed basis" and within a few hours before sexual contact.

For more information see page 1468.

Retrograde Ejaculation

Retrograde ejaculation occurs when the semen enters the bladder instead of emerging from the penis during an orgasm. During retrograde ejaculation, a tiny muscle (a sphincter) at the opening of the bladder does not work properly, and semen travels backward into the bladder. Causes of retrograde ejaculation include injury to the bladder neck muscle or bladder neck nerves during surgery, nerve damage from diabetes or other illnesses, or side effects from certain medications. Retrograde ejaculation can impair fertility, but otherwise is not harmful.

Commonly Prescribed (On-Label) Drugs: Bethanidine

OFF-LABEL PRESCRIPTION DRUG
BREAKTHROUGH OPTION

Generic: ***Imipramine*** *(im-IP-ra-meen)*
Brands: ***Tofranil, Tofranil-PM***

Imipramine belongs to the class of antidepressants known as tricyclic antidepressants, or TCAs, and may be used to treat retrograde ejaculation. As a drug class, TCAs decrease desire, decrease ability to gain and sustain erection, and inhibit orgasm and ejaculation, as noted by two U.S. researchers at Albert Einstein College of Medicine and at the Department of Psychiatry & Behavioral Sciences in Galveston, Texas, respectively. Imipramine affects sexual function as well, although this has been noted to a lesser extent than clomipramine (another TCA).

In a German review of 36 clinical studies, imipramine was more effective than pseudoephedrine (a central nervous system stimulant) for retrograde ejaculation. Similar to pseudoephedrine, imipramine provides muscle contraction and helps ejaculation in affected patients. When compared with ephedrine, imipramine demonstrated a significantly higher reversal rate in patients with retrograde ejaculation. Based on this review, researchers concluded that medical treatment with imipramine to reverse retrograde ejaculation provides a real opportunity in natural conception of offspring and should be the treatment of choice in affected men.

For more information see page 1230.

Partial Retrograde Ejaculation

Retrograde ejaculation refers to the entry of semen into the bladder instead of it exiting through the urethra during ejaculation. Partial retrograde ejaculation may be caused by prior prostate or urethral surgery, illness such as diabetes, or certain drugs like high blood pressure drugs. Although this disorder is relatively uncommon, it may result in infertility in some men.

Commonly Prescribed (On-Label) Drugs: *None*

OFF-LABEL PRESCRIPTION DRUG
BREAKTHROUGH OPTION

Generic: **Midodrine** *(MI-doe-dreen)*
Brand: **ProAmatine**

Midodrine is indicated to treat severe cases of low blood pressure. This drug increases blood pressure and is therefore called an antihypotensive. Midodrine works by stimulating nerve endings in blood vessels resulting in constriction of smooth muscles that surround blood vessels. By constricting these muscles, the width of the blood vessels narrows, thereby elevating blood pressure. Midodrine as an injection helps to transform a retrograde ejaculation into an anteretrograde ejaculation by reinforcement of the blood vessels surrounding the sphincter. Side effects associated with midodrine use include rapid or irregular heart rate, itching, headache, numbness or tingling in the hands and feet, goose bumps, chills, and urinary difficulties.

There are a few reports of midodrine use for ejaculatory disorders. Even fewer are reports of midodrine used specifically in patients with partial retrograde ejaculation. In a study conducted by researchers in Chile, the semen of two patients with partial retrograde ejaculation was collected and frozen after injection of midodrine. The frozen/thawed semen samples were mixed with fresh semen recently ejaculated to evaluate the number of motile sperm, and for subsequent artificial insemination. In both instances, pregnancies occurred. In a study in *European Urology*, midodrine use in six patients with partial ejaculatory incompetence resulted in a significant increase in orgasmic sensation and a statistically significant improvement in ejaculatory function. In another study published in a European urology journal, normal ejaculation was induced in seven out of 12 patients with the use of oral midodrine. Additionally, emission of normal sperm into the urethra was restored in three out of 12 patients with a single intravenous (IV) injection of midodrine.

For more information see page 1327.

Post-Spinal Injury Ejaculation

The inability to ejaculate as a result of damage to the spinal cord affects approximately 90% of men with spinal cord injuries, and is referred to as post–spinal injury ejaculation. Another problem that may affect men with spinal cord injuries is retrograde ejaculation, or the entry of semen into the bladder instead of exiting through the urethra during ejaculation. Additionally, the motility of sperm in men with spinal cord injuries is considerably lower than for men without injury to the spine.

Commonly Prescribed (On-Label) Drugs: None

OFF-LABEL PRESCRIPTION DRUG
BREAKTHROUGH OPTION

---

*Generic: **Midodrine** (MI-doe-dreen)*
*Brand: **ProAmatine***

Midodrine is typically used to treat severe cases of low blood pressure. It increases blood pressure and stimulates nerve endings in blood vessels, resulting in constriction of smooth muscles that surround blood vessels. By constricting these muscles, the width of the blood vessels narrows and elevates blood pressure. In injectable form, midodrine helps to transform a retrograde ejaculation into an anteretrograde ejaculation by reinforcement of the blood vessels surrounding the sphincter. Side effects associated with midodrine use include rapid or irregular heart rate, itching, headache, numbness or tingling in the hands and feet, goose bumps, chills, and urinary difficulties.

Clinical evidence of midodrine use in men with spinal cord injury in the medical literature is limited to a few international studies. In one study conducted by French researchers, midodrine was used to induce ejaculation in 10 patients (mean age of 28.5 years) with spinal cord injury who wanted to father a child. Fourteen trials of drug-induced ejaculation were performed.

Midodrine was given through slow IV infusion, and sperm was collected. In 10 cases (71.4%), ejaculation was obtained. Results from this trial demonstrated that midodrine offered good results with regard to ejaculation in patients with spinal cord injury, although the quality of the sperm collected was often poor. Researchers concluded that after antibiotic treatment, use of midodrine can serve an alternative to other treatments such as vibromassage and electrostimulated ejaculation to induce ejaculation in men with spinal cord injury. In another study of men with spinal cord injury conducted by French researchers, midodrine was effective in treating absence of ejaculation. In this study, it was concluded that midodrine helped achieve ejaculation in men with spinal cord injury.

For more information see page 1327.

ERECTILE DISORDERS

The symptoms of erectile disorders include a persistent or recurrent inability to attain or maintain an adequate erection until completion of sexual activity. Erectile disorders are characterized by marked distress or interpersonal difficulty and can be caused by psychological or physiological factors at different times in a man's life or may be lifelong in duration. Types of erectile disorders include erectile dysfunction, Peyronie's disease, and priapism.

Erectile Dysfunction

Erectile dysfunction can be a total inability to achieve erection, an inconsistent ability to achieve erection, or a tendency to sustain erections only for a brief time. Physiological causes of erectile dysfunction include damage to the nerves, arteries, smooth muscles, and tissues by diseases such as diabetes. Other causes include surgeries such as radical prostate surgery for cancer, certain drugs (blood pressure drugs), psychological factors like stress, as well as smoking and hormone imbalances.

Commonly Prescribed (On-Label) Drugs: *Alprostadil, Sildenafil, Tadalafil, Vardenafil*

OFF-LABEL PRESCRIPTION DRUGS
BREAKTHROUGH OPTIONS

Generic: **Apomorphine** *(a-poe-MOR-feen)*
Brand: **Apokyn**

Apomorphine is often used to treat Parkinson's disease and was previously used to induce vomiting in people who ingested poisonous chemicals. It is thought to act on areas of the central nervous system that control male erection, although the precise involvement of dopamine in sexual motivation and arousal is not fully known. Investigators believe that dopamine can trigger erection by acting on specific neurons in the brain and areas of the spinal cord.

In a study in 849 men with erectile dysfunction conducted at Loyola University Medical Center, after apomorphine was given, 39.4% of men had erections firm enough for sexual intercourse compared with 13.1% before the drug. Attempts at erection that resulted in sexual intercourse also increased 38.3% from 12.7% before the drug was given. In this study, the most common side effect was nausea (11.7% of patients), which was dose-related and decreased with continued use of the drug. Researchers concluded that it was safe and effective for mild, moderate, and severe erectile dysfunction.

In a small German study examining the effects of apomorphine on brain activity in 12 patients with erectile dysfunction, apomorphine appeared to induce brain activity in the prefrontal cortex—an area associated with male sexual arousal during orgasm. Increased brain activity associated with apomorphine was associated with penile rigidity, which supports this drug's use.

For more information see page 1022.

Generic: **Papaverine** *(pa-PAV-er-een)*
Brand: **Para-Time S.R.**

Papaverine hydrochloride belongs to a class of drugs known as vasodilators, which expand blood vessels thereby increasing blood flow, and are generally used to treat poor blood circulation. Self-injection of papaverine hydrochloride into the penis combined with small doses of phentolamine mesylate has been effective for erectile dysfunction, increasing swelling of the penis and resulting in an erection. Many investigators conclude that papaverine hydrochloride injection is one of the most effective, well-studied drugs for erectile disorders.

Injection of papaverine hydrochloride with or without other drugs is generally reserved for patients who do not respond to other treatments such as other drugs, psychotherapy/behavioral therapy, and vacuum constriction devices, and in instances where altering any drug-related or medical cause of erectile dysfunction has not helped.

In a Brazilian study of 168 men ranging in age from 43 years to 78 years with erectile dysfunction due to prostate cancer surgery, self-injection of papaverine hydrochloride, phentolamine mesylate, and prostaglandin E1 (a hormone-like substance) was evaluated. This drug combination resulted in a 94.6% success rate and no life-threatening complications. Moreover, use of these drugs for erectile dysfunction resulted in a 13.1% cure rate. Researchers concluded that self-injection of papaverine hydrochloride, phentolamine mesylate, and prostaglandin E1 is a safe, effective treatment in men with erectile dysfunction due to radical prostate surgery.

For more information see page 1394.

Generic: **Phentolamine** *(fen-TOLE-a-meen)*
Brands: **Regitine, Rogitine**

Phentolamine mesylate is given by injection and results in expansion of blood vessels and increases in blood flow. When injected into the penis, phentolamine mesylate increases blood, thereby resulting in an erection.

Sexual intercourse should be attempted within two hours after injection of phentolamine mesylate. Side effects associated with phentolamine mesylate injection include tingling at the tip of the penis, prolonged or painful erection, dizziness, lumps in the penis, bruising or bleeding at the injection site, ejaculation difficulties, and burning along the penis.

A low-dose injectable drug combination consisting of phentolamine mesylate, papaverine hydrochloride, and alprostadil are often used to treat erectile dysfunction. Self-injection of phentolamine mesylate and papaverine hydrochloride has been shown to increase penile swelling and produce an erection. In general, injection of phentolamine mesylate with or without papaverine hydrochloride or other drugs into the penis are considered after other drug therapies have failed or caused side effects, and before moving on to surgery to treat the erectile disorder.

In an Israeli study of men with erectile dysfunction and cardiovascular disease, a variety of penile injections consisting of phentolamine mesylate, papaverine hydrochloride, prostaglandin (a hormone-like substance), and atropine sulfate (an anticholinergic) resulted in a success rate of 94.3%. Researchers concluded that penile injections of vasoactive drugs may be viable for patients with erectile dysfunction and cardiovascular disease.

For more information see page 1411.

Impotence

See Erectile Dysfunction

Penile Fibromatosis

See Peyronie's Disease

Peyronie's Disease

Peyronie's disease is an inflammatory condition that is characterized by the formation of plaque or hardened scar tissue beneath the skin of the penis. The scarring is noncancerous, but often results in painful erections and curvature of an erect penis. The exact causes of Peyronie's disease are not fully understood, although researchers have speculated that penile trauma such as from sports injuries and vigorous sexual activity results in short-term instances of this condition. Genetic factors and connective tissue disorders are also thought to contribute to the development of this disease.

Commonly Prescribed (On-Label) Drugs: *None*

OFF-LABEL PRESCRIPTION DRUG
BREAKTHROUGH OPTION

Generic: **Interferon Alfa-2b** *(in-ter-FEER-on AL-fa-2b)*
Brand: **Intron A**

Interferon alfa-2b contains interferons, which are naturally occurring proteins produced by the immune system. Interferon alfa-2b works by directing the immune system to attack foreign substances such as bacteria, viruses, and tumors that invade the body. Once the drug detects a foreign substance, it alters the substance by slowing, blocking, or changing its growth or function. Dosing for interferon alfa-2b depends on the disease being treated and is generally tailored to the individual patient. Side effects associated with interferon alfa-2b include flu-like symptoms such as fever, chills, and headache, increased heart rate, confusion, and low white blood cell count, among others.

In clinical studies, use of interferon alfa-2b for Peyronie's disease has had variable results. In a study at Tulane University Health Science Center during 12 weeks in 120 men with Peyronie's disease, both placebo and interferon alfa-2b showed significant benefit, but the patients treated with interferon alfa-2b had greater improvement than placebo-treated patients (68% versus 40%, respectively). In a German study of 30 affected men, interferon alfa-2b was not useful for early Peyronie's disease. Researchers concluded that this treatment is ineffective since the disease progress often continues at different sites in about 25% of patients. In 26 patients, treated plaques remained unchanged in this study. Moreover, use of interferon alfa-2b resulted in considerable side effects (in 74 of the 90 injections administered) including fever and muscle aches.

For more information see page 1243.

Priapism

Priapism is the occurrence of any persistent erection for more than four hours in the absence of sexual stimulation. Priapism is not associated with sexual excitement, and the erection does not stop after ejaculation occurs. This condition is a genuine urologic emergency, and medical intervention is necessary to avoid complications such as infection and loss of penis. Causes of priapism include diseases including sickle-cell disease, cancer, and certain psychiatric drugs.

Commonly Prescribed (On-Label) Drugs: Etilefrine

OFF-LABEL PRESCRIPTION DRUGS
BREAKTHROUGH OPTIONS

Generic: **Phenylephrine** *(fen-ill-EPH-rhine)*
Brand: **Neo-Synephrine**

Phenylephrine is a decongestant typically used to maintain blood pressure in instances of low blood pressure such as during shock or anesthesia. It may also be used to treat priapism and is often given as an injection in a vein or muscle, or under the skin. Side effects associated with phenylephrine include headache, nausea, or vomiting.

In general, for people with priapism of four to six hours, use of decongestants is the first-line recommendation. In clinical studies, use of phenylephrine has been shown to be safe and effective for priapism. In a study at the University of Manitoba, nine patients with priapism were injected with phenylephrine diluted with saline into the penis. After the injection, eight of the nine patients experienced a loss of erection, no changes in blood pressure or heart rate, and no side effects. Additionally, in a Spanish review of medical records involving 67 men with priapism in one hospital from 1978 through 1994, researchers found that injection of phenylephrine into the penis was the initial treatment for priapism. Of the men treated, 64 patients also received surgery whereas three patients were successfully treated with medication. Additionally, medical complication rates were low for patients receiving phenylephrine injection. The use of this drug should be discussed with your doctor before treatment.

For more information see page 1412.

Generic: **Terbutaline** *(ter-BYOO-ta-leen)*
Brand: **Brethine**

Terbutaline is a bronchodilator that is used to relieve and prevent asthma attacks by relaxing breathing muscles. It also relaxes some other types of muscles in the body, hence its potential use in priapism. Side effects associated with the use of terbutaline include rapid or irregular heart rate, elevated blood pressure, tremor, nausea, nervousness, dizziness, and heartburn, among others. The use of terbutaline for priapism may act to decrease blood flow to the penis and eliminate erection.

According to a published commentary by two doctors at Memorial Hospital in Houston, Texas, and Tulane Medical School, oral terbutaline can be given if a person has a sustained erection of more than two hours. This regimen can be repeated every 15 minutes until the erection is eliminated, or if the patient has taken a total of three tablets. According to these doctors, terbutaline is effective in 20–30% of patients with priapism.

In a study in India, oral terbutaline resulted in elimination of erection in 42% of patients who had a drug-induced priapism that had been previously treated with a vasoactive drug. The researcher concluded that an initial trial with terbutaline for drug-induced priapism may be successful. In another study at George Baptist Medical Center, researchers noted the successful use of terbutaline in patients with priapism when another medical procedure including a shunt procedure had not worked. Terbutaline has also been used to manage priapism in patients under general and local anesthesia.

For more information see page 1499.

Van Buren Disease

See Peyronie's Disease

PROSTATE DISORDERS

The prostate is a small organ located below the bladder that produces a fluid substance that becomes part of the semen. Prostate disorders are quite common in men, and include benign prostatic hypertrophy (BPH), nonbacterial prostatitis, and prostate cancer. The most common prostate problem in men under age 50 is prostatitis, an inflammatory condition. In men over the age of 50, the most common prostate disorder is BPH. Older men are also at risk for prostate cancer; however, this disease is much less common than BPH.

Abacterial Thrombotic Endocarditis

See Nonbacterial Prostatitis

Benign Prostatic Hypertrophy

Also referred to as benign prostatic hyperplasia, BPH is a non-cancerous enlargement of the prostate and is a common occurrence in older men. Many men over 40 have a slight enlargement of the prostate; more than 90% of men over 80 have enlarged prostates. Less than half of men may experience symptoms associated with BHP which include a weak urine stream, dribbling after urinating, straining to urinate, incomplete emptying of the bladder, and the need to urinate more than two times per night, among others. Treatments for BPH include "watchful waiting," lifestyle changes, drugs, and surgery.

Commonly Prescribed (On-Label) Drugs: *Doxazosin, Finasteride, Terazosin*

OFF-LABEL PRESCRIPTION DRUGS
BREAKTHROUGH OPTIONS

---

*Generic: **Prazosin** (PRA-zoe-sin)*
*Brand: **Minipress***

Prazosin, typically prescribed for high blood pressure, also improves urine flow rates by relaxing smooth muscle in BPH. The advantage of prazosin compared with nonselective alpha-adrenergic blockers is its lower risk of causing adverse events.

In BPH, prazosin has been recognized to improve urinary flow rate and frequency of urination. According to early clinical trials in England, prazosin offered convincing evidence of its efficacy in BPH. In these trials, prazosin relieved obstructive and irritative BPH symptoms and also improved urinary flow rates and decreased urethral pressure. The researcher concluded that between 60% and 70% of patients receiving prazosin can expect benefits. Conversely, in a comparison study in India of prazosin versus transurethral resection of the prostate (a surgical procedure) in 62 patients with BPH, surgery was more effective than prazosin treatment in alleviating BPH symptoms.

According to clinical guidelines issued by the American Urological Association, prazosin data are insufficient to recommend its use for BPH symptoms.

For more information see page 1426.

Generic: *Phenoxybenzamine* (fen-oks-ee-BEN-za-meen)
Brand: *Dibenzyline*

Phenoxybenzamine is classified as a nonselective alpha-adrenergic receptor blocker. Use of phenoxybenzamine can worsen the symptoms of respiratory infections, fatigue, dizziness, impaired ejaculation, and nasal stuffiness; visual problems may also occur. Moreover, there are cancer concerns associated with the use of phenoxybenzamine, although in a review of published medical literature from 1966 until 2002 conducted at Cornell University, despite cancer concerns associated with phenoxybenzamine, a researcher found no reports of drug-related tumors since its introduction.

In clinical studies, when compared with placebo, phenoxybenzamine use resulted in urinary flow rate improvements as reported by the patients themselves. Up to 75% BPH symptom improvement has been reported in the medical literature. Off-label use of phenoxybenzamine for symptoms of urinary retention was well recognized in the Cornell study, which also noted significant urinary symptom relief with the use of phenoxybenzamine in men with BPH. The most common side effects of phenoxybenzamine in the literature review were dizziness, impotence and ejaculatory problems, and nasal stuffiness. According to clinical guidelines issued by the American Urological Association, however, phenoxybenzamine data are insufficient to recommend its use for BPH symptoms.

For more information see page 1410.

Nonbacterial Prostatitis

Nonbacterial prostatitis is the most common type of prostatitis and involves inflammation of the prostate gland (male sex gland) without known causes. Researchers have several theories regarding the causes of nonbacterial prostatitis including the presence of certain fungi, viruses, and bacteria (even though tests for bacteria come back negative). It has been suggested that irritation caused by the reflux of urine into the prostate may result in nonbacterial prostatitis. Up to 65% of men with chronic prostatitis have this nonbacterial form. Symptoms include pain, frequent urination, and pain or burning on urination, among others. Complications of nonbacterial prostatitis involve sexual and urinary problems. Overall, researchers feel that treatment of nonbacterial prostatitis is challenging, drug failures are quite common, and there is very little evidence to support any type of treatment.

Commonly Prescribed (On-Label) Drugs: Allopurinol, Pentosan Polysulfate Sodium

---

OFF-LABEL PRESCRIPTION DRUGS
BREAKTHROUGH OPTIONS

Generic: **Ciprofloxacin** *(sip-roe-FLOKS-a-sin)*
Brands: **Ciloxan, Cipro, Cipro XR**

Ciprofloxacin is classified as a fluoroquinoline, which is a type of antibiotic that kills certain types of bacteria. Ciprofloxacin does not kill anaerobic bacteria (bacteria that does not need oxygen). In nonbacterial prostatitis, ciprofloxacin diffuses into prostate fluid and inhibits the synthesis and growth of bacteria. Ciprofloxacin is not indicated in persons under the age of 18. Its most common side effects include nausea, vomiting, diarrhea, and abdominal pain, among others.

Patients with nonbacterial prostatitis may be treated with antibiotics, such as ciprofloxacin, to assure that bacteria is not the cause of their prostatitis-like symptoms. According to *Canadian Journal of Urology*, ciprofloxacin has shown efficacy in the treatment of chronic bacterial prostatitis caused by *E. coli.* as well as in patients with nonbacterial prostatitis; however, prolonged use in the absence of proven infection or symptom improvement is not recommended. Researchers believe that clinical studies in the published medical literature reporting the safety and efficacy of ciprofloxacin for nonbacterial prostatitis are lacking.

For more information see page 1093.

Generic: **Doxazosin** *(doks-AY-zoe-sin)*
Brand: **Cardura**

Doxazosin is an antihypertensive drug (used to lower high blood pressure), which results in vasodilation (widening of veins and arterioles) and decrease in blood pressure. In prostatitis, doxazosin has been found to be quite effective in improving urine flow and decreasing urinary obstruction and symptoms of irritation.

Symptoms of nonbacterial prostatitis should then be reassessed, and the dose should be maintained if treatment has worked. If no effect has been seen, an increase in the dose should be considered. If a patient is already taking blood pressure medications, blood pressure should be monitored when doses of doxazosin are increased. Common side effects associated with doxazosin include dizziness, drowsiness, headaches, constipation, and appetite loss, among others.

In a Turkish study, doxazosin or a placebo was given to 60 men with chronic nonbacterial prostatitis for three months. Patients completed a survey regarding their pain-related symptoms during treatment. Patients receiving doxazosin reported overall improvements in disease symptoms (32.9% of patients), pain (36.6% of patients), and quality of life (36.8% of patients).

For more information see page 1152.

Generic: **Levofloxacin** *(lee-voe-FLOKS-a-sin)*
Brands: **Levaquin, Quixin**

Levofloxacin is an antibiotic used in nonbacterial prostatitis because it penetrates the prostate (male sex gland). Levofloxacin has broad-spectrum antibiotic effects. Common side effects include upset stomach, appetite loss, diarrhea, nausea, and headache, among others.

Although prostatitis may be nonbacterial, oftentimes doctors will treat it with antibiotics, such as levofloxacin, to assure that bacteria is not the underlying cause of symptoms. Some patients with nonbacterial prostatitis may actually improve with the use of antibiotics; however, prolonged use of these types of drugs in the absence of proven infection or symptom improvement is not recommended by doctors.

Researchers believe that data in the medical literature on the use of levofloxacin for nonbacterial prostatitis is quite limited. It remains to be seen how effective certain types of antibiotics, such as levofloxacin, are in the treatment of this prostate disorder. In *Urology*, levofloxacin was reported to be one of the more popular antibiotics used for nonbacterial prostatitis. Overall, treatment of nonbacterial prostatitis is challenging and treatment failures are very common.

For more information see page 1278.

*Generic: **Terazosin** (ter-AY-zoe-sin)*
*Brand: **Hytrin***

Terazosin is used to lower high blood pressure. In general, antihypertensives like terazosin are very effective in people with nonbacterial prostatitis because they improve urine flow and reduce disease-associated irritation. A selective alpha1-receptor blocker, terazosin relaxes smooth muscles of the arteries, the prostate, and the bladder neck.

In a study at the University of Texas, use of terazosin was evaluated in 25 patients with nonbacterial prostatitis and prostate pain. Of the 25 patients, 19 patients (76%) responded to terazosin given during one month. Eleven patients (58%) continued to have no symptoms of nonbacterial prostatitis and prostate pain three months later. Researchers concluded that terazosin is an effective treatment in patients affected with this prostate disorder. Notably, terazosin has been identified among other drugs to effectively treat urinary obstruction associated with nonbacterial prostatitis.

For more information see page 1048.

*Generic: **Trimethoprim-sulfamethoxazole***
(try-METH-oh-prim sul-fah-meth-OX-ah-zole)
*Brands: **Bactrim, Septra***

Trimethoprim-sulfamethoxazole is an antibiotic drug; trimethoprim acts to block an enzyme and sulfamethoxazole blocks bacterial production in the body. Antibiotics as a drug class are often used in nonbacterial prostatitis to check for improvement in symptoms and to rule out infection with an organism. Adverse effects associated with trimethoprim-sulfamethoxazole include upset stomach, diarrhea, nausea, vomiting, and headache.

Researchers believe that evidence of the efficacy and safety of trimethoprim-sulfamethoxazole is lacking in the medical literature. In most patients, a trial of antibiotics is initially used and may include trimethoprim-sulfamethoxazole. Most medical experts recommend three to four weeks of treatment with an antibiotic.

For more information see page 1530.

Terminal Endocarditis

See Nonbacterial Prostatitis

Thromboendocarditis

See Nonbacterial Prostatitis

MISCELLANEOUS DISORDERS

In addition to ejaculatory, erectile, and prostate disorders, and urogenital cancers, a number of other conditions affect certain populations of men. Two important miscellaneous men's health disorders are gynecomastia (enlarged breasts) and infertility (inability to impregnate naturally).

Gynecomastia

Gynecomastia is abnormally enlarged male breasts. In adolescent boys, this condition is fairly common and in 90% of cases gynecomastia disappears within a matter of months. Possible causes of gynecomastia include puberty, steroid use, obesity, tumors, aging, drug side effects, and genetic disorders, among others. Psychologically, gynecomastia can be emotionally devastating and feelings of shame, embarrassment, and self-hate may arise. Treatment of gynecomastia may involve weight loss, drug treatment, or surgery.

Commonly Prescribed (On-Label) Drugs: *None*

OFF-LABEL PRESCRIPTION DRUGS
BREAKTHROUGH OPTIONS

Generic: **Danazol** *(DA-na-zole)*
Brand: **Danocrine**

Danazol is typically used for a variety of medical problems such as endometriosis, breast cysts, and abnormal swelling of the body tissues. Danazol may also be used to treat gynecomastia since one of the more common side effects associated with its use is decreased breast size. Other side effects include flushing or redness of skin, mood or mental changes, and nervousness.

In a Korean review of medical records, the efficacy of danazol was compared with another drug, tamoxifen. In this analysis, researchers reviewed 68 men with gynecomastia. Twenty-three patients were treated with tamoxifen and 20 were treated with danazol. Complete resolution of gynecomastia was noted in 18 patients (78.2%) treated with tamoxifen and eight patients (40%) treated with danazol. In the tamoxifen group, five patients experienced gynecomastia recurrence. Researchers noted that although tamoxifen was more effective in reducing gynecomastia, it also resulted in a higher relapse rate.

British researchers at the Princess of Wales Royal Air Force Hospital examined the efficacy of danazol for gynecomastia in a comparison with placebo. In this study of 52 men, danazol reduced breast tenderness significantly more than placebo and was associated with a significant improvement in the degree of gynecomastia and breast size. A notable side effect with danazol treatment was weight gain. Researchers concluded that danazol provided effective control of gynecomastia and may eliminate the need for surgical breast reduction.

For more information see page 1129.

Generic: **Tamoxifen** *(ta-MOKS-i-fen)*
Brand: **Nolvadex**

Tamoxifen blocks the effect of estrogen (a hormone) on tissue. Tamoxifen is typically prescribed for the treatment of invasive breast cancers following surgery and/or radiation and in the prevention of breast cancer in both women and men. Common side effects associated with tamoxifen include cataracts or other eye problems, liver problems, bone pain, headache, nausea, vomiting, skin rash or dryness, inability to maintain erection, and loss of sexual desire, among others.

A recent study at the Department of Urology, National Tumor Institute, suggested that the use of tamoxifen may reduce breast pain and gynecomastia associated with the use of bicalutamide (a hormone drug given for prostate cancer). In a study of 151 men with prostate cancer, 51 patients received bicalutamide, 50 patients bicalutamide and tamoxifen for 24 weeks, and 50 patients received bicalutamide and radiotherapy. Of the 51 patients who only received bicalutamide, 35 of these patients developed gynecomastia or breast pain. In men treated with bicalutamide and tamoxifen, only four out of 50 patients developed gynecomastia. Seventeen out of the 50 patients treated with bicalutamide and radiotherapy developed gynecomastia. Researchers commented that tamoxifen use in patients with prostate cancer may treat the gynecomastia side effect of bicalutamide treatment. Furthermore, the drug combination of tamoxifen and bicalutamide did not increase adverse events or quality of life.

Additionally, in a British study, use of tamoxifen in men with painful gynecomastia was shown to be safe and effective. Thirteen men were given tamoxifen, and 10 patients responded well to treatment. One patient stopped drug treatment because of calf tenderness; no other adverse effects were reported.

For more information see page 1493.

Infertility

The National Institutes of Health have reported that male infertility affects approximately 40% of the 2.6 million infertile married couples in the U.S. Infertility is defined as the inability to conceive after at least one year of unprotected intercourse. In men, hormone disorders, illness, trauma or obstruction to reproductive body organs, or sexual dysfunction can permanently or temporarily affect sperm and prevent conception. The main causes of male infertility are impairments in sperm production, sperm delivery, and testosterone (a male hormone) deficiency.

Commonly Prescribed (On-Label) Drugs: *Balsalazide, Clomiphene*

OFF-LABEL PRESCRIPTION DRUGS
BREAKTHROUGH OPTIONS

*Generic: **Anastrozole** (an-AS-troe-zole)*
*Brand: **Arimidex***

Anastrozole belongs to a class of drugs known as aromatase inhibitors; these drugs block aromastase (an enzyme) that is a major source of estrogen (a female hormone) in body. Anastrozole is typically given in patients with breast cancer to reduce hormone blood levels that contribute to tumor growth, but it may be particularly helpful for men whose infertility is associated with abnormal levels of hormones (testosterone and estrogen). Common side effects associated with the use of anastrozole include headache, diarrhea, nausea, back pain, weakness, and reduced energy.

Overall, researchers have noted that hormonal drugs for male infertility have had minimal success with the exception of aromatase inhibitors like anastrozole. In clinical trials, the testosterone-to-estradiol (a female hormone also present in men) ratio levels in infertile men improve with anastrozole. Use of anastrozole also causes semen changes that improve fertility. Two researchers with Cornell University Medical School studied 140 infertile men with abnormal hormone levels, and evaluated the effects of testolactone (an anticancer drug) daily or anastrozole daily. Men who received testolactone had increases in testosterone-to-estradiol ratios, sperm concentration, sperm motility, and improved in sperm structure. Treatment with anastrozole resulted in similar improvements in male-to-female hormone ratios, semen volume, sperm concentration, and sperm motility. Researchers concluded that anastrozole provides similar effects on hormones and semen as testolactone, and can help men who are infertile due to abnormal hormone ratios.

For more information see page 1020.

*Generic: **Bromocriptine** (broe-moe-KRIP-teen)*
*Brand: **Parlodel***

In infertile men, bromocriptine has been used to restore fertility since it has been found to increase sperm count during and after treatment. Its use is associated with nausea, headaches, dizziness, and fatigue.

The use of bromocriptine for male infertility has been documented in case reports and clinical studies. In one study in *Journal of Andrology*, nine men with benign growths that were secreting increased levels of prolactin (a hormone that prompts milk production) and decreased sperm counts were treated for 90 days with bromocriptine. After treatment, all nine had significant decreases in prolactin levels; sperm counts increased in five of the nine patients. In four men, testosterone levels increased. Researchers concluded that bromocriptine appears to be useful. In a case report of a man with a benign pituitary growth, high levels of prolactin, absence of sperm, impotence, underactivity of the testes, and decreased sexual desire, researchers tested the effects of high doses of bromocriptine for five months and noted significant improvement in sexual desire, sperm concentration, and reduction in the size of the benign growth.

For more information see page 1054.

Generic: *Clomiphene* (KLOE-mi-feen)
Brands: *Clomid, Serophene*

Clomiphene is an estrogen receptor-blocker that increases the secretion of a certain hormone, known as gonadotropin-releasing hormone, which blocks estrogen. Typically, clomiphene is used to induce ovulation in women who do not produce eggs but desire to become pregnant. Low doses of clomiphene for male infertility may help increase sperm production, and it has been used to treat this condition. Side effects associated with the use of clomiphene include upset stomach, vomiting, and headache.

In a study by a Japanese researcher of 59 men with abnormal sperm, 36 men received a gonadotropin-releasing hormone analogue and 23 patients received oral clomiphene for three months. Sperm density increased in men treated with the hormone analogue, but no significant change in sperm density occurred in men treated with clomiphene. Similarly, sperm motility improved with the hormone analogue but there were no statistically significant increases in men treated with clomiphene. Overall, no adverse events were noted in either treatment group. Alternatively, in a Saudi Arabian study, clomiphene used for abnormal sperm was associated with a significant increase in total sperm count and total motile sperm count. The researchers concluded that clomiphene may be more effective in certain men with abnormal sperm and high levels of prolactin.

For more information see page 1103.

Generic: **Human Chorionic Gonadotropin** *(kor-ee-ON-ik goe-NAD-oh-troe-pin)*
Brand: **Novarel**

Human chorionic gonadotropin belongs to a class of drugs known as gonadotropins, which stimulate the production of gonadal steroid hormones, and is produced by the human placenta. Use of this hormone in male infertility stimulates certain cells to produce testosterone. Adverse effects associated with the use of human chorionic gonadotropin include headache, irritability, restlessness, and enlarged breasts (gynecomastia) in males.

Hormone therapy has had limited success in infertile men with the exception of human chorionic gonadotropin, which is often helpful in restoring male fertility in men with abnormal levels of gonadotropin. This hormone has been found to be effective in restoring sperm production after chemotherapy treatments.

In a Japanese review of medical charts of 36 males between the ages of 11 and 42 years with hypogonadism (abnormally decreased functioning of the testicles and/or retardation of growth or sexual development) treated at various fertility centers, the long-term administration of human chorionic gonadotropin resulted in sperm production in 36% of men with small testicular volume and in 71% of males with large testicular volume. In general, treatment with this drug for three months results in semen improvements. Human chorionic gonadotropin is often accompanied with increased sexual desire and improved sexual performance. On the average, gynecomastia occurs in less than 5% of patients toward the end of treatment.

For more information see page 1502.

*Generic: **Letrozole*** *(LET-roe-zole)*
*Brand: **Femara***

The anticancer therapy letrozole belongs to a class of drugs known as aromastase inhibitors, which block aromastase (an enzyme) that is a major source of estrogen (a female hormone) in the body. Use of letrozole prevents almost all estrogen production. Typically, letrozole is used to treat certain forms of breast cancer. Side effects associated with this drug include back, bone, joint, and muscle pain.

This drug may be helpful in men who are infertile because of abnormal hormone levels. Clinical studies specifically evaluating the use of letrozole in infertile males are limited. In a study in the Netherlands, the use of letrozole normalized testosterone in severely obese men with hypogonadism (abnormally decreased functioning of the testicles and/or retardation of growth or sexual development). In this study, 10 severely obese men were given letrozole for six weeks, after which estradiol levels decreased and testosterone levels increased. Researchers concluded that short-term use of letrozole, as dosed in this study, normalized testosterone levels.

For more information see page 1273.

MUSCULOSKELETAL DISORDERS

ARTHRITIDES DISORDERS

Arthritides is the plural of arthritis, which literally means inflammation ("itis") of a joint ("arrhro"). This disease includes any disorders, acute or chronic, whether caused by a bacterial, viral, or fungal infection, or an autoimmune disease, or whether it is idiopathic, meaning due to unknown causes.

Ankylosing Spondylitis

Ankylosing spondylitis (AS) is a chronic disease that mainly affects the spine, although the hips, shoulders, knees, or ankles also may become involved. Symptoms initially are stiffness and pain in the lower back, but inflammation of the joints and ligaments that enable the back to move may eventually cause the joints and bones to fuse together and inhibit movement. Genetics, particularly a gene called HLA-B-27, seems to play a major role in causing AS, usually in men.

Commonly Prescribed (On-Label) Drugs: *Betamethasone, Cortisone, Dexamethasone, Diclofenac, Etanercept, Indomethacin, Infliximab, Methylprednisolone, Naproxen, Phenylbutazone, Prednisolone, Prednisone, Sulindac, Triamcinolone*

OFF-LABEL PRESCRIPTION DRUGS
BREAKTHROUGH OPTIONS

Generic: **Flurbiprofen** *(flure-BI-proe-fen)*
Brand: **Ansaid**

Flurbiprofen belongs to a class of drugs called non-steroidal anti-inflammatory drugs (NSAIDs). They help reduce pain and inflammation and are widely prescribed for rheumatoid arthritis and osteoarthritis, and also widely used off-label in other arthritides. However, not everyone can take them because of their side effects on the gastrointestinal (GI) tract.

British Medical Journal reported a study conducted at the Research Institute for Rheumatic Diseases in the Slovak Republic. Two hundred patients with various arthritides, including 20 with AS, were given sustained-release flurbiprofen for six months and monitored monthly. A total of 75.5% completed the study. Most who withdrew did so in the first month or so, half due to mild to moderate GI side effects. The investigators of the study concluded that flurbiprofen was effective, well tolerated, and suitable for long-term treatment of most patients with chronic arthritic conditions.

Another *British Medical Journal* article compared flurbiprofen to phenylbutazone, an older NSAID, in treating AS in 35 patients over a four-week period. Halfway through, patients were switched from one drug to the other. Results showed little difference between the two on most criteria, but the researchers concluded flurbiprofen is likely to have an important role in the management of AS.

For more information see page 1194.

Generic: **Ketoprofen** *(kee-toe-PROE-fen)*
Brand: **Oruvail**

Ketoprofen is a non-steroidal anti-inflammatory drug (NSAID), which is widely prescribed to reduce inflammation and pain in various types of arthritis. Unfortunately, their main side effect is gastrointestinal (GI) tract upset.

A recent trial reported in *Arthritis & Rheumatism* showed that treatment with celecoxib (a selective COX inhibitor) reduced the progression of AS as shown on x-rays, and this was grounds for gaining U.S. FDA approval for celecoxib for AS. However, it has since been shown that celecoxib has little GI benefits over other selective COX inhibitors, that it may have greater cardiac risks, and it is much more expensive. Therefore, some physicians are turning to other selective COX inhibitors, particularly to ketoprofen, which was part of the original study out of which the celecoxib trial grew.

For comparative purposes a recent review of the therapy of AS in *Arthritis Research* looking at the newer therapies noted, "There is evidence that the new, more COX-2 selective drugs [such as] . . . celecoxib are no less effective in treating back pain of AS patients than conventional NSAIDs such as ketoprofen."

For more information see page 1261.

*Generic: **Meloxicam** (mel-OKS-i-kam)*
*Brand: **Mobic***

Meloxicam is part of a group of therapeutic drugs called COX-2 selective drugs, which is a new sub-group of the larger class of non-steroidal anti-inflammatory drugs (NSAIDs). It is used to ease inflammation and pain in osteoarthritis and rheumatoid arthritis. Another COX-2 selective drug, celecoxib, was recently shown to reduce progression of AS as documented on x-rays, reported in *Arthritis & Rheumatism.* However, because of the publicity surrounding the possible greater cardiac risks of NSAIDs, particularly COX-2 inhibitors, as well as its significant costs, some physicians have looked for other options for their patients.

A recent review of the therapy of AS in *Arthritis Research* looking at the newer therapies noted, "There is evidence that the new, more COX-2 selective drugs [such as] . . . meloxicam are no less effective in treating back pain of AS patients than conventional NSAIDs," which had long been the accepted mainstay of treatment, according to researchers.

A study at Guangzhou General Hospital in China explored the efficacy of combining meloxicam with either of two different doses of methotrexate (a powerful immunosuppressive drug) in the treatment of AS. The researchers of the study concluded that this combination yielded satisfactory results.

For more information see page 1303.

Generic: **Methotrexate** *(meth-oh-TREKS-ate)*
Brands: **Rheumatrex, Trexall**

Methotrexate is a powerful suppressor of key factors in the immune system. It is approved for the treatment of certain cancers as well as rheumatoid arthritis and juvenile rheumatoid arthritis, because it also suppresses inflammation.

According to a report from the Center for Sports Medicine and Orthopedics, in Chattanooga, Tennessee, suppressing inflammation is probably methotrexate's main action in AS, leading to a reduction in pain, swelling, and stiffness, but it may have other actions on the immune system. However, there is no evidence that it actually induces remission. Methotrexate takes time to work, and you may not see a benefit for three to six or eight weeks. Further, if improvement is not seen in five or six weeks, your doctor may gradually increase the dose.

A study at Guangzhou General Hospital in China evaluated use of two different doses of methotrexate combined with meloxicam in the treatment of AS and concluded that both yielded satisfactory results. Because methotrexate poses toxic risks to the liver, it should not be taken by people with liver damage, patients should not drink alcohol while taking it, and patients must have regular liver function tests. It is unsafe during pregnancy.

For more information see page 1312.

Generic: **Pamidronate** *(pa-mi-DROE-nate)*
Brand: **Aredia**

Pamidronate belongs to a class of drugs known as bisphosphonates. It is given intravenously to treat Paget's diseases, hypercalcemia of malignancy, and low bone-density problems related to cancer or its treatment.

A recent article in *Indian Journal of Medical Sciences* reviewed the potential anti-arthritic and anti-inflammatory effects of bisphosphonates in general and pamidronate in particular, noting that animal studies have shown that bisphosphonates prevent erosive arthritis and chronic inflammation. *Journal of Rheumatology* reported a study of 16 patients with AS who had not responded to NSAID treatment. Half received six intravenous infusions per month for six months, while the other group received only monthly infusions. Both groups improved, but the first group significantly more so. The improvements developed three to six months after treatment and persisted for at least three months after treatment. A second study of nine patients, reported in *Rheumatology*, assessed an intensive regimen—with infusions on day 1, 2, 14, 28, and 56—and followed patients for 84 days. Benefits were seen not only in the spine, but also in peripheral joints with a decrease in the average number of tender and swollen joints of 98.2%. According to researchers, although benefits were seen even in those with long duration of disease, greater benefits were seen in those with shorter duration of disease.

For more information see page 1391.

Generic: *Sulfasalazine* (sul-fa-SAL-a-zeen)
Brands: *Azulfidine, Azulfidine EN-tabs*

Sulfasalazine is used to treat ulcerative colitis, an inflammatory bowel disease frequently associated with AS. It is also U.S. FDA-approved for rheumatoid arthritis. *Arthritis Research* called sulfasalazine the best-investigated disease-modifying antirheumatic drug for the treatment of AS.

The Cochrane Central Register of Controlled Trials evaluated clinical trials examining the efficacy of sulfasalazine on AS and found 11 studies meeting their criteria. Researchers looked at both laboratory measures of inflammation and patients' subjective experience of pain and stiffness. They concluded that sulfasalazine demonstrated some benefit in reducing measures of inflammation and easing morning stiffness, but no evidence of benefit in physical function, pain, spinal mobility, enthesitis (a traumatic disease that affects the attachment point of skeletal muscle to bone), and patient and physical global assessment. They concluded that patients at an early disease stage, those with higher levels of inflammation, and those with peripheral arthritis would most likely benefit. An article in *Drugs* defined sulfasalazine as a second-line treatment that has been used in severe AS with positive results.

For more information see page 1483.

*Generic: **Thalidomide** (tha-LI-doe-mide)*
*Brand: **Thalomid***

The benefits of thalidomide seem to be related to immunosuppressive effects and/or effects on neural tissue. In 1998, U.S. FDA approved thalidomide for use in treating leprosy symptoms. According to the National Institutes of Health, studies are also being conducted to determine its effectiveness in treating symptoms associated with AIDS, some cancers, and rheumatic diseases, including AS.

Journal of Rheumatology reported on a study at several Chinese university hospitals of thalidomide for severe AS in 13 patients who had not responded to conventional therapies. Four had a 50% improvement, and four had a 20% improvement. The investigators concluded that thalidomide is a promising treatment.

For more information see page 1505.

Arthritis Deformans

See Rheumatoid Arthritis

Arthropathia Psoriatic

See Psoriatic Arthritis

Arthritis

See Osteoarthritis

Degenerative Arthritis

See Osteoarthritis

Degenerative Joint Disease

See Osteoarthritis

Fibromyalgia

Fibromyalgia (FM), also called fibromyalgia syndrome, is a chronic illness characterized by musculoskeletal aches, pain, and stiffness, tenderness in soft tissue, general fatigue, and sleep disturbances. The areas that are painful to the touch tend to occur in specific areas of the body known as "tender points." These points aid in diagnosis of this illness, which is difficult to diagnose. The most common sites of pain include the neck, back, shoulders, pelvic area, and hands, but any part of the body can be involved. Symptoms tend to ebb and flow over time.

Commonly Prescribed (On-Label) Drugs: None

OFF-LABEL PRESCRIPTION DRUGS
BREAKTHROUGH OPTIONS

Generics: Antidepressants such as **Amitriptyline**
(*a-mee-TRIP-ti-leen*) and **Cyclobenzaprine**
(*sye-kloe-BEN-za-preen*)
Brands: **Elavil (amitriptyline), Flexeril
(cyclobenzaprine)**

Amitriptyline and cyclobenzaprine are older types of antidepressants. Cyclobenzaprine is approved for treatment of muscle spasms. While depression may also affect people with fibromyalgia, these drugs' primary effects on the illness appear not to be psychological but rather are related to their ability to interfere with certain chemical messengers in the brain and thereby change the way the brain perceives pain messages.

The American College of Rheumatology reports that antidepressants have emerged as "the mainstay in the pharmacologic approach to patients with fibromyalgia," and early studies emphasized the use of tricyclic antidepressants. In three of four trials, amitriptyline compared favorably with placebo, although the benefit appeared to be relatively small and side effects such as dry mouth and drowsiness were troublesome. These studies were reported in *Arthritis & Rheumatism* and *Journal of Rheumatology*, but according to a recent review article on fibromyalgia in *Journal of the American Medical Association*, studies demonstrate that amytriptyline often helps with sleep (a major problem for people with fibromyalgia) and overall well-being and there is strong evidence for its efficacy.

Experts note that cyclobenzaprine, similar in chemical structure to amitriptyline, was evaluated for fibromyalgia because it was thought to offer some of amitriptyline's benefits without its side effects. In fact, only modest benefits have been found in short-term clinical trials. One trial compared the two drugs as well as placebo in 208 patients. After one month, 21%, 12%, and none of the amitriptyline, cyclobenzaprine, and placebo patients, respectively, had significant clinical improvement. These percentages increased to 36%, 33%, and 19%, respectively, at the six-month assessment. According to researchers, promising recent data suggest that combining amitriptyline with another type of antidepressant, a selective serotonin reuptake inhibitor such as fluoxetine, may yield even better results, according to *Arthritis & Rheumatism*.

For more information see pages 1009 and 1121.

Generic: Selective Serotonin Reuptake Inhibitors such as **Citalopram** (sye-TAL-oh-pram), **Fluoxetine** (floo-OKS-e-teen), and **Paroxetine** (pa-ROKS-e-teen)
Brands: **Celexa (citalopram), Prozac, Prozac Weekly, Sarafem (fluoxetine), Paxil, Paxil CR (paroxetine)**

Citalopram, fluoxetine, and paroxetine belong to the first generation of a class of drugs called selective serotonin reuptake inhibitors (SSRIs), approved for the treatment of depression. The best known is fluoxetine. Although people with fibromyalgia often also suffer with depression and SSRIs may alleviate that, the beneficial impact on fibromyalgia itself has nothing to do with depression. Rather, the SSRIs increase a neurotransmitter in the brain, called serotonin, which affects the way the brain perceives the pain message.

Studies demonstrating modest evidence for the efficacy of fluoxetine in fibromyalgia were cited in a review article in *Journal of the American Medical Association (JAMA)*, including one showing improvement in pain but no change in mood. Another showed the combination of amitriptyline and fluoxetine better than either alone, and another showed the same in combination with cyclobenzaprine. These drugs sometimes need two to three months to see full benefit.

Additionally, a four-month study of citalopram was reported in *European Journal of Pain*. Among those who completed the trial, 52.9% improved compared to 22.2% of the placebo group, with significant effects on pain, after two months of therapy, but the effect diminished after four months, although the alleviation of depression was increasing at the end.

For more information see pages 1096, 1192, and 1395.

Generic: Selective Serotonin and Norepinephrine Reuptake Inhibitors such as **Duloxetine** *(doo-LOX-e-teen)*, **Mirtazapine** *(mir-TAZ-a-peen)*, and **Venlafaxine** *(ven-la-FAX-een)*
Brands: **Cymbalta (duloxetine), Remeron, Remeron SolTab (mirtazapine), Effexor, Effexor XR (venlafaxine)**

Duloxetine, mirtazapine, and venlafaxine belong to a class of drugs called selective serotonin and norepinephrine reuptake inhibitors (SNRIs). In contrast to the SSRIs discussed above, these block the reuptake of two chemical messengers, both serotonin and norepinephrine, and therefore are proposed to be potentially more effective in their basic roles. They are all approved as antidepressants.

Arthritis & Rheumatism reported on a study comparing duloxetine to placebo in 207 people with fibromyalgia. After 12 weeks, duloxetine-treated patients improved significantly more on the Fibromyalgia Impact Questionnaire and the Brief Pain Inventory average pain severity score and had significantly greater improvement in mean tender point pain threshold. A trial of 90 patients reported in *Arthritis & Rheumatism* found that venlafaxine was not significantly different from placebo, although two small trials using high doses, reported in *Psychosomatics* and *Annals of Pharmacotherapy,* found it useful.

The University of Medical Sciences in Poznan, Poland, conducted a study of mirtazapine in 29 fibromyalgia patients for six weeks. The majority had a 40% or greater reduction in the intensity of fibromyalgia symptoms (pain, sleep disturbance, and fatigue). The researchers concluded mirtazapine is an effective, promising therapy in fibromyalgia.

For more information see pages 1164, 1332, and 1542.

Generic: Anti-epileptic drugs such as **Gabapentin**
(GA-ba-pen-tin), **Pregabalin** *(pre-GAB-a-lin),* **Tiagabine**
(tie-GA-been), and **Topiramate** *(TOE-pie-rah-mate)*
Brands: **Neurontin (gabapentin), Lyrica (pregabalin),**
Gabitril (tiagabine), Topamax (topiramate)

Gabapentin, pregabalin, tiagabine, and topiramate are all anti-epileptic drugs approved to treat seizures. Pregabalin is a derivative of gabapentin, which is also approved for treating diabetic neuropathy and post-herpetic neuralgia. Topiramate is approved to treat migraines. These drugs are prescribed for people with fibromyalgia because they inhibit certain chemical messengers in the brain and therefore lower sensitivity to pain. Further, they may help with disturbed sleep and depression. The addition of anti-epileptic drugs to medication regimens may be particularly valuable for fibromyalgia patients with increased pain sensitivity, especially marked pain that results from a non-injurious touch to the skin.

A clinical trial compared various doses of pregabalin in 529 patients with fibromyalgia and found that 450 mg per day significantly reduced the average severity of pain compared with placebo, according to *Arthritis & Rheumatism*. There also were significant improvements in sleep, fatigue, and health-related quality of life.

Arthritis Today notes that topiramate "may be useful for treating specific symptoms or conditions, such as cluster headaches, mood disturbances and eating disorders, which may occur in people with fibromyalgia."

Tiagabine increases sleep efficiency and maintenance and decreases whole-body pain in fibromyalgia patients, according to the Department of Internal Medicine at the Baptist Medical Center.

With all anti-epileptic drugs, doses should be increased slowly to avoid dizziness and excess sleepiness, as well as dullness of thought that some users characterize as "dopey brain."

For more information see pages 1206, 1431, 1510, and 1516.

Generic: **Modafinil** *(moe-DAF-i-nil)*
Brand: **Provigil**

Modafinil is a central nervous system stimulant. It changes the amounts of certain natural substances in the brain that control sleep and wakefulness. It also enhances wakefulness, mood, and memory, but, in contrast to traditional stimulants such as amphetamines or caffeine, is not likely to cause jitteriness and anxiety. Modafinil is approved to treat the excessive sleepiness caused by narcolepsy, which causes severe daytime sleepiness, and shift work sleep disorder (sleepiness during scheduled waking hours). It is also used to prevent excessive daytime sleepiness in people with obstructive sleep apnea, a disorder in which people briefly stop breathing frequently during sleep and therefore don't get enough restful sleep.

Journal of Neuropsychiatry and Clinical Neuroscience reported on the successful use of modafinil in four patients with fibromyalgia. All patients reported improvements in daily function, alertness, and fatigue within three weeks. Recurrences were immediate if doses were missed, and improvements returned the same day when dosing was restored. The researchers concluded that modafinil is a good potential treatment option.

For more information see page 1338.

Generic: **Tramadol** *(TRAM-a-dole)*
Brand: **Ultram**

Tramadol is an analgesic that is generally considered effective for moderate to severe pain, including neuropathic pain. It not only acts on opioid receptors in the brain, it also acts similar to the SSRIs and SNRI antidepressants by increasing the availability of the two chemicals in the brain—serotonin and noradrenaline—involved in communicating pain messages. It also can have an antidepressant effect.

Three studies demonstrating modest evidence for efficacy for tramadol in fibromyalgia were cited in *Journal of the American Medical Association.* Two were trials of tramadol alone and showed tramadol to be effective and well tolerated, with improvements in pain relief and decreased pain threshold. The third was also a trial but used a tramadol-acetaminophen combination, and researchers also noted it yielded better pain scores in the active drug group compared to placebo.

For more information see page 1518.

Fibromyalgia Syndrome

See Fibromyalgia

Fiessinger-Leroy-Reiter Syndrome

See Reiter's Syndrome

Gout

Gout is one of the most painful forms of inflammatory arthritis. It develops when too much uric acid builds up in the body. This leads to the deposition of uric acid crystals in joints, often in the big toes or other small joints. Lumpy deposits of uric acid, called tophi, may occur and kidney stones from uric acid crystals develop. The immediate goal of treatment is to alleviate inflammation and pain, but long-term therapy is aimed at reducing uric acid levels.

Commonly Prescribed (On-Label) Drugs: *Allopurinol, Betamethasone, Colchicine, Cortisone, Dexamethasone, Indomethacin, Methylprednisolone, Naproxen, Phenylbutazone, Prednisolone, Prednisone, Sodium Thiosalicylate, Sulfinpyrazone, Sulindac, Triamcinolone*

OFF-LABEL PRESCRIPTION DRUGS
BREAKTHROUGH OPTIONS

Generic: Non-steroidal Anti-inflammatory Drugs such as **Diclofenac Sodium** *(dye-KLO-fen-ak),* **Etodolac** *(ee-toe-DOE-lak),* and **Ketoprofen** *(kee-toe-PROE-fen)* **Brands: Voltaren, Voltaren-XR *(diclofenac sodium),* Lodine, Lodine XL *(etodolac),* Oruvail *(ketoprofen)***

Diclofenac sodium, etodolac, and ketoprofen belong to a group of drugs known as non-steroidal anti-inflammatory drugs

(NSAIDs), commonly prescribed to reduce inflammation and pain in arthritis. Unfortunately, their main side effect is gastro-intestinal (GI) tract upset, but this can be almost eliminated with the addition of a proton pump inhibitor. These three are variously approved for rheumatoid and osteoarthritis and ankylosing spondylitis and painful menstruation, or pain in general. Arthritis-Symptom.com notes that NSAIDs are considered the best treatment available and preferred over any other medication in acute gout. They block the production of prostaglandins, the substance that dilates blood vessels and causes inflammation and the pain of gout.

A report from the General Hospital of Mexico in the *Clinical Investigations Review* on a survey of physicians indicated that diclofenac was the drug most frequently used to acute gout attacks. *Drugs for the Aging* noted that caution is necessary when prescribing NSAIDs for arthritis in the elderly and that diclofenac and ketoprofen are preferred.

Journal of Rheumatology reported that a study of gout patients who received either ketoprofen or an older NSAID, indomethacen, found that more than 90 in both groups reported pain relief starting the first day of treatment. By day seven, most patients in both groups improved markedly. Hence, researchers stated that ketoprofen was rated favorably for safety and efficacy. The early responders possibly benefited from the analgesic effects of NSAIDs, not the anti-inflammatory effects.

Bandolier, the website providing evidence-based clinical information to physicians, reported that in two small studies etodolac was as effective as naproxen in the treatment of acute gout.

For more information see pages 1143, 1179, and 1256.

Generic: *Fenofibrate* (fen-oh-FYE-brate)
Brands: *Antara, Lofibra, TriCor*

Fenofibrate is normally used (with dietary changes to restrict cholesterol and fat intake) to reduce the amount of cholesterol and triglycerides (fatty substances) in patients' blood. Accumulation of cholesterol and fats inside arterial walls (atherosclerosis) decreases blood flow and oxygen supply to the heart, brain, and other parts of the body. Lowering levels of cholesterol and fats may help to prevent heart disease, angina, strokes, and heart attacks. For this reason, fenofibrate is FDA-approved for treating high cholesterol and triglyceride levels and certain other abnormal lipid (blood fat) fat conditions.

In a study, three adult patients with recurrent gout attacks experienced decreases in uric acid ranging from 29% to 39% after the addition of fenofibrate for three weeks. Two were also on allopurinol. Two stopped fenofibrate for short periods, with subsequent increases in uric acid. Once fenofibrate therapy was reinstated, uric acid levels dropped. In all three patients, no further gout attacks occurred during the follow-up period. However, researchers state that fenofibrate addresses the underlying problem of elevated uric acid, not the immediate inflammation that causes pain.

For more information see page 1184.

Generic: **Ketorolac** *(KEE-toe-role-ak)*
Brand: **Toradol**

Ketorolac is a non-steroidal anti-inflammatory (NSAID) used to alleviate pain. Unlike other NSAIDs, ketorolac is usually reserved for moderately severe pain, the pain that occurs after an operation or other procedure. It can be given by pill or, unlike other NSAIDs, by injection or intravenous infusion. Because it is very potent, its side effects can be much more severe and sudden, even dangerous. Therefore, ketorolac should not be used for more than five days. This can make it valuable for acute attacks that only need a brief course of an NSAID but one that will be a very powerful painkiller and rapid anti-inflammatory.

The Arthritis Society of Canada reported on a series of studies with NSAIDs and found that 80 out of 100 patients who received intravenous ketorolac had their pain reduced by half within two hours. *Annals of Emergency Medicine* reported on a study in two Texas emergency rooms comparing the effects of intramuscular injections of ketorolac with oral indomethacin, an older NSAID. Twenty patients with acute gout received one of the two treatments. After two hours, pain scores had decreased from 4.5 to 1.4 in the ketorolac group and from 4.4 to 1.5 in the indomethacin group. After six hours, there was some rebound in the ketorolac group. The researchers concluded that pain relief was similar with the two drugs.

For more information see page 1263.

*Generic: **Meloxicam** (mel-OKS-i-kam)*
*Brand: **Mobic***

Meloxicam is one of a group of drugs called COX-2 selective drugs, a new sub-group of the larger class of non-steroidal anti-inflammatory drugs (NSAIDs). Meloxicam is approved to ease inflammation and pain in osteoarthritis and rheumatoid arthritis. A Chinese study reported in *Clinical Therapeutics* compared meloxicam, diclofenac and rofecoxib (recently removed from the U.S. market) in the treatment of acute gout attacks. Sixty-two patients received one of the three drugs. On day three, pain relief was obtained in 84.2% of those on rofecoxib vs. 40% of those on meloxicam; on day eight, pain relief for rofecoxib was 94.7% vs. 60% respectively. No significant differences for diclofenac were found. The investigators concluded that rofecoxib provided better, more effective therapy than meloxicam but, as noted above, rofecoxib is no longer on the market.

For more information see page 1303.

Lyme Arthritis

Lyme disease is the most common illness transmitted by ticks in the United States. Its first symptoms are usually a rash at the site of the tick bite, fever, chills, muscle and joint aches, headache, and fatigue. However, one of the complications may be Lyme arthritis that may develop quickly or weeks to months after the tick bite, most commonly in the knee. The disease is named after Lyme, Connecticut, where the first outbreak in the United States was first observed in the 1970s.

Commonly Prescribed (On-Label) Drugs: *None*

OFF-LABEL PRESCRIPTION DRUGS
BREAKTHROUGH OPTIONS

*Generic: **Doxycycline** (doks-i-SYE-kleen)*
*Brands: **Adoxa, Doryx, Doxy 100, Monodox, Periostat, Vibra-Tabs, Vibramycin***

Doxycycline is an antibiotic. According to a report from Children's Hospital of Boston, treatment for all stages of Lyme disease requires antibiotics, and the choice of antibiotic should be one that is comprehensive and will cover all likely pathogens—that is, including possible infectious causes other than Lyme. Doxycycline is first on their list for localized and early Lyme disease without evidence of central nervous system involvement. It can also be used for arthritis that is not persistent or recurrent. A report on Medscape recommends doxycycline for the treatment of Lyme arthritis for 28 days. A report from the Tufts University School of Medicine, in *Medical Clinics of North America*, from the physician who led the initial identification of Lyme, states that joint pain can usually be treated successfully with a one- or two-month course of oral doxycycline or amoxicillin, although if you have persistent or recurrent arthritis you may need anti-inflammatory drugs, too.

Physicians in Europe report that the most frequently used drug for Lyme arthritis is doxycycline, as noted in a German review, and a recommendation from the University of Genova, Italy. However, a report from Poland noted that relapses of Lyme arthritis happen despite prior effective antibiotic therapy. In a study of 64 patients, 25 were treated with oral doxycycline and 39 with intravenous ceftriaxone for 28 days. All experienced remission. Subsequently, relapse occurred in 36% of the doxycycline patients and 23% of the ceftriaxone patients. Researchers observed that relapse was more common among those older than 50 years.

For more information see page 1158.

Generic: **Hydroxychloroquine** *(hye-droks-ee-KLOR-oh-kwin)*
Brand: **Plaquenil**

Hydroxychloroquine was originally developed to treat malaria but has since been discovered to act as an anti-inflammatory drug and to modulate the immune system in ways that are not fully understood. It has been approved to treat autoimmune disorders such as lupus and rheumatoid arthritis.

A report from the Tufts University School of Medicine in Boston, in *Medical Clinics of North America*, from the physician who led the initial identification of Lyme, states that patients with certain genetic and immune markers may have persistent arthritis despite treatment with oral or intravenous antibiotics. For these cases doctors may prescribe anti-inflammatory drugs.

A colleague at Tufts further reported in *Medical Clinics of North America* on the specific genetic marker that can trigger this treatment-resistant arthritis in which antibiotic therapy is ineffective and wrote that in these instances drugs such as hydroxychloroquine and methotrexate can induce remission.

For more information see page 1225.

*Generic: **Methotrexate** (meth-oh-TREKS-ate)*
*Brands: **Rheumatrex, Trexall***

Methotrexate is a potent immunosuppressant drug that also suppresses inflammation. It is approved to treat certain cancers as well as rheumatoid and juvenile rheumatoid arthritis.

In an article in *Medical Clinics of North America*, the physician who led the initial identification of Lyme reports that patients with certain genetic and immune markers may have persistent arthritis despite oral or intravenous antibiotic therapy and may need anti-inflammatory drugs. In another article in *Medical Clinics of North America*, a researcher discussed the specific genetic marker that can trigger such antibiotic-resistant arthritis and wrote that drugs such as methotrexate or hydroxychloroquine are needed to induce remission in such cases.

Methotrexate can be severely toxic to the liver. Therefore, it should not be taken by people with liver damage. Also, you should not drink alcohol while taking it, and you must have regular liver function tests. Do not take methotrexate if you are pregnant.

For more information see page 1312.

Marie-Strümpell Disease

See Ankylosing Spondylitis

Nodose Rheumatism

See Rheumatoid Arthritis

Osteoarthritis

Osteoarthritis (OA), the most common joint disease affecting older adults, involves progressive damage to cartilage—the rubbery material at the end of long bones—and structures around the joint. OA may cause fluid accumulation, bony overgrowth, and weakness of muscles and tendons, limiting movement and causing pain and swelling. Any joint may be affected but most common are the knees, hips, spine, and hands.

Commonly Prescribed (On-Label) Drugs: *Betamethasone, Capsaicin, Celecoxib, Choline Salicylate, Cortisone, Dexamethasone, Diclofenac, Diclofenac/Misoprostol, Diflunisal, Estrogens, Etodolac, Fenoprofen, Flurbiprofen, Ibuprofen, Indomethacin, Ketoprofen, Meclofenamate, Meloxicam, Methylprednisolone, Nabumetone, Naproxen, Oxaprozin, Oxycodone, Phenylbutazone, Piroxicam, Prednisolone, Prednisone, Salsalate, Sodium Hyaluronate, Sulindac, Tolmetin, Triamcinolone, Trolamine Salicylate, Valdecoxib*

OFF-LABEL PRESCRIPTION DRUG
BREAKTHROUGH OPTION

Generic: **Doxycycline** *(doks-i-SYE-kleen)*
Brands: **Adoxa, Doryx, Doxy 100, Monodox, Periostat, Vibra-Tabs, Vibramycin**

Doxycycline is one of a class of antibiotics known as tetracyclines, which are approved for treating various bacterial infections. Such infections have never been shown to cause OA, but antibiotics have other effects in the body. They inactivate several enzymes that play a role in inflammation and decrease the production of substances that modulate immune system activity.

Arthritis & Rheumatism reported a clinical trial in which 431 patients with moderately advanced OA in one knee received either doxycycline or placebo for 30 months. X-rays were taken every six months, and 71% of the patients completed the study, at which time the mean loss of joint space width in the diseased knee (a measure of disease progression) in the doxycycline group was 33% less than in the placebo group. Yet, despite significantly slowing disease progression, researchers observed that doxycycline did not reduce the severity of joint pain. However, mean pain scores at baseline were low in both treatment groups, leaving only limited opportunity to demonstrate improvement in joint pain.

On the other hand, the drug significantly reduced the frequency with which subjects reported increases in knee pain 20% or greater than the level of pain they had at their previous semi-annual visit. Fewer than 5% of all subjects reported side effects. The researchers concluded that doxycycline showed benefits in slowing the rate of joint space narrowing in knees with established OA but its value in the early treatment and symptomatic management of OA will require further investigation.

For more information see page 1158.

Osteoarthrosis

See Osteoarthritis

Psoriatic Arthritis

Psoriatic arthritis (PsA) is a unique combination of destructive, disabling arthritis in three or more joints in an asymmetrical pattern (that is, not the same joints on both sides of the body), and a tendency to finger deformities and spine problems, all of which may precede the development of the skin disease psoriasis by months or years. The psoriasis is characterized by raised scales and plaques ranging from red to grey or silvery-white covering large areas.

Commonly Prescribed (On-Label) Drugs: *Betamethasone, Cortisone, Dexamethasone, Etanercept, Infliximab, Interferon Gamma, Methylprednisolone, Prednisolone, Prednisone, Triamcinolone*

OFF-LABEL PRESCRIPTION DRUGS
BREAKTHROUGH OPTIONS

Generic: ***Auranofin*** *(au-RANE-oh-fin)*
Brand: ***Ridaura***

Auranofin is a salt made from gold that is approved for use in treating rheumatoid arthritis. It is not clear how it works to treat inflammation, but according to MedicineNet.com, gold salts can decrease the inflammation of the joint lining in people with inflammatory arthritis, such as adult and juvenile rheumatoid arthritis. This can prevent destruction of bone and cartilage. Such benefits have led doctors to consider its use in PsA.

In *Annals of Rheumatic Diseases*, experts in PsA reviewing traditional disease modifying anti-rheumatic drugs (DMARDs) reported a beneficial response in some assessment measures with gold. In a six-month study of auranofin in 238 patients, the treated group showed a modest but significant improvement compared to the placebo group in occupational/daily function, but no significant difference in morning stiffness or joint tenderness/swelling scores.

British Journal of Rheumatology reported on a study comparing auranofin, gold thiomalate (an injected version of gold), and placebo. After 24 weeks, based on pain scores and indicators of inflammation and joint swelling, significant improvement was seen only in the group receiving the injected gold.

For more information see page 1032.

Generic: Purine Analogues such as ***Azathioprine***
(ay-za-THYE-oh-preen) and ***Mercaptopurine***
(mer-kap-toe-PYOOR-een)
Brands: ***Imuran (azathioprine), Purinethol***
(mercaptopurine)

These drugs are purine analogues—that is, related to uric acid. Azathioprine is a prodrug of mercaptopurine. (A prodrug is a compound that breaks down into the active drug once in the body.) These drugs are also known as antimetabolites. They prevent cells (including those in the immune system) from dividing. Azathioprine is classified as an immunosuppressant medication for the prevention of organ transplant rejection and treatment of rheumatoid arthritis. Although its exact mechanism of action in rheumatoid arthritis is not known, its suppressing of the immune system appears to decrease the activity of this illness. Mercaptopurine is approved to treat certain types of leukemia.

In *Annals of Rheumatic Diseases*, experts in PsA reviewed traditional disease modifying anti-rheumatic drugs and wrote that, although favorable results have been reported with azathioprine and mercaptopurine, the studies have been small and no placebo-controlled data are available. But in one report, 11 of 13 people treated with mercaptopurine showed improvement in both their skin and joint symptoms within three weeks of starting therapy. And a report on six patients showed marked improvement in skin symptoms in six patients on azathioprine.

For more information see pages 1033 and 1305.

Generic: **Bromocriptine** *(broe-moe-KRIP-teen)*
Brand: **Parlodel**

Bromocriptine blocks the release of a hormone called prolactin that affects the menstrual cycle and breast milk production. Bromocriptine is approved for treating amenorrhea (absence of menstruation), female infertility, hyperprolactinemia, acromegaly (excessive growth hormone), and Parkinson's disease.

Seminars in Arthritis and Rheumatism suggests that evidence supports the idea that the hormone prolactin may play a causative role in some rheumatic diseases, including PsA. This would support the use of bromocriptine in its treatment, if not as the primary therapy then as an add-on. Researchers reviewed the literature and found clinical trials showing efficacy with bromocriptine in various rheumatic diseases. For PsA, only case reports were found, and further investigation was urged. Bromocriptine may be a relatively safe, efficacious alternative therapy.

A skin clinic in Germany presented four cases in the *Journal of the American Academy of Dermatology* demonstrating the therapeutic effectiveness of bromocriptine in PsA. Subsequently, a study group of 35 patients suffering from PsA, in whom long-term treatment with commonly used drugs had not led to recovery nor significant benefits, was given bromocriptine. According to researchers, 77% achieved significant improvement in joint symptoms.

For more information see page 1054.

Generic: Antimalarials such as **Chloroquine** *(klor-OH-kwin)* and **Hydroxychloroquine** *(hye-droks-ee-KLOR-oh-kwin)*
Brands: **Aralen (chloroquine), Plaquenil (hydroxychloroquine)**

Chloroquine and hydroxychloroquine are anti-malarials and were originally developed to treat malaria. Subsequently, it was discovered that they modulate the immune system in ways that are not fully understood and can have anti-inflammatory effects. Hydroxychloroquine has also been approved to treat certain autoimmune disorders such as rheumatoid arthritis and lupus.

Studies reporting a favorable response to these drugs in about 75% of PsA patients treated have been offset by concerns that they may have an adverse effect on their psoriasis, according to an article in *Annals of Rheumatic Diseases* by experts in PsA. While improvements in joint problems were observed by researchers, a wide spectrum of psoriasis as well as photosensitivity, dermatitis, and other skin problems have been reported in participants in these trials.

Journal of Rheumatology reported on 32 patients given chloroquine in the University of Toronto Psoriatic Arthritis Clinic, of whom only six subsequently had an exacerbation of psoriasis, and only one discontinued therapy. Six of their control patients who were not given chloroquine also had an exacerbation of psoriasis. Therefore, researchers concluded that chloroquine may be an effective PsA treatment, does not exacerbate psoriasis, and warrants more study. However, another article in the *Journal of Rheumatology* from Ohio State University reported on a single patient with PsA whose psoriasis was markedly exacerbated by hydroxychloroquine.

Nonetheless, a report from the South Nassau Communities Hospital on *eMedicine* recommended hydroxychloroquine, while acknowledging that how it works on PsA remains unknown.

For more information see pages 1082 and 1225.

Generic: *Cyclosporine* (si-klo-SPOR-een)
Brands: *Gengraf, Neoral, Sandimmune*

Cyclosporine is a very potent immunosuppressant medication that is considered a disease modifying anti-rheumatic drug (DMARD) because it not only decreases the pain and swelling of arthritis but may also prevent joint damage and reduce the risk of long-term disability. It is approved to prevent the rejection of transplanted kidneys, hearts, and livers, but it is used off-label by people with rheumatoid arthritis, psoriatic arthritis, and some other rheumatic conditions that have not responded well to conventional therapies.

Rheumatology International reported on a study at University Hospital in Milan, Italy in which 60 PsA patients were given cyclosporine. After 12 months inflammation lessened. At two years, skin symptoms improved. The researchers concluded that cyclosporine is a helpful second choice treatment for patients with active PsA, although they state that careful follow-up of patients is needed. Additionally, *International Journal of Clinical Pharmacology Research* reported on a study from the Research Institute of Rheumatic Diseases in the Slovak Republic of cyclosporine given to PsA patients for 18 weeks. As early as two weeks, skin symptoms improved by 65.5%. The most intense arthritis benefits were seen by 18 weeks. The average time to improvement was 10 weeks.

An Italian study in the *Journal of Rheumatology* compared cyclosporine with sulfasalazine in a study that assigned 99 patients to one of the two drugs. After six months, cyclosporine was shown to lessen the pain, swollen and tender joints, arthritis impact, and psoriasis area and its severity.

For more information see pages 1125 and 1127.

Generic: *Leflunomide* (le-FLOO-noh-mide)
Brand: *Arava*

Leflunomide is an anti-inflammatory drug known as a disease modifying anti-rheumatic drug (DMARD) because it not only reduces arthritis pain and joint swelling but may also decrease damage to the joints and long-term disability. It is approved for the treatment of rheumatoid arthritis. Although rheumatoid arthritis is an autoimmune disease—one in which the body attacks part of itself as if it were a foreign invader—it is not completely clear how this drug works in rheumatoid arthritis. However, leflunomide interferes with the formation of DNA, which is important for developing cells, such as those in the immune system. The drug decreases white blood cells that play an important role in the immune system.

Arthritis & Rheumatism reported on a clinical trial in which 190 PsA patients received either leflunomide or placebo. After 24 weeks, 58.9% of the leflunomide patients and 29.7% of the placebo patients responded well with decreased joint and skin symptoms, pain, and other indicators of disease. Based on these results, researchers stated that treatment was relatively well tolerated with no unusual toxic side effects. The researchers concluded that leflunomide is safe and effective.

Expert Opinions in Pharmacotherapy reported from a German rheumatology clinic that leflunomide has not only demonstrated significant efficacy in PsA but these benefits are maintained with long-term use.

For more information see page 1270.

Generic: *Meclofenamate* (meh-clo-PHEN-a-mate)
Brand: *Meclomen*

Meclofenamate belongs to a class of medications called non-steroidal anti-inflammatory drugs (NSAIDs), originally developed to reduce the inflammation and pain of arthritis. They have also been found useful in other painful conditions. Meclofenamate is approved for the treatment of rheumatoid and osteoarthritis, painful menstruation, and other pain.

NSAIDs act by inhibiting cyclooxygenase enzymes that lead to the formation of inflammatory substances. Based on anecdotal reports that meclofenamate did a better job than other NSAIDs in dealing with the inflammation of PsA, a clinical study conducted in Ann Arbor, Michigan and Chicago, Illinois was reported in the *Journal of the American Academy of Dermatology*. In the first four weeks, 103 patients were divided to receive either meclofenamate or placebo. Most meclofenamate-treated patients had no change in their psoriasis. Then 89 patients continued in a four-week study of meclofenamate and one-third of the patients showed improvement.

An article from South Nassau Communities Hospital on *eMedicine* notes that, despite the possibility of worsening psoriasis, NSAIDs are used widely to alleviate joint inflammation. About two-thirds of patients who use them find relief without an increase in symptoms. Meclofenamate was among the NSAIDs recommended.

For more information see page 1296.

Generic: **Methotrexate** *(meth-oh-TREKS-ate)*
Brands: **Rheumatrex, Trexall**

Methotrexate is a powerful immunosuppressant drug. By blocking an enzyme in the body called dihydrofolate reductase, it interferes with the production of a form of folic acid that is important for actively growing cells of the skin, blood, gastrointestinal tissues, and immune system. In this way, it can help suppress cancer as well as diseases that involve the immune system.

In *Annals of Rheumatic Diseases*, experts in PsA reviewing traditional disease modifying anti-rheumatic drugs reported that the efficacy of methotrexate in PsA was first demonstrated in 1964 in a study of 21 patients in which those on the active drug experienced significant improvement in their arthritis and skin rash, but had recurrence of both within one to four months of cessation of therapy. In this trial methotrexate was given by injection.

The current method of giving methotrexate is orally once a week. There have been no controlled trials using this dosing, but several reviews of PsA patients on such regimens, reported in *Journal of Rheumatology* and *Clinical Rheumatology*, found good joint improvement and resolution of skin rashes. It may take four to eight weeks to see a benefit.

For more information see page 1312.

Generic: **Sulfasalazine** *(sul-fa-SAL-a-zeen)*
Brands: **Azulfidine, Azulfidine EN-tabs**

Sulfasalazine is an anti-inflammatory medication that belongs to a class of drugs called sulfa drugs and is called a disease modifying anti-rheumatic drug (DMARD) because it may change the course of the disease, prevent damage to the joints, and reduce the risk of long-term disability, although it is not entirely clear why it is effective. It is approved to treat rheumatoid arthritis as well as ulcerative colitis, which is also an inflammatory disease. Sulfasalazine is also used to treat other forms of arthritis such as juvenile rheumatoid arthritis, ankylosing spondylitis, and psoriatic arthritis, often in combination with other drugs.

In a supplement to the *Annals of Rheumatic Diseases*, experts in PsA reviewing traditional DMARDs reported that sulfasalazine was tried for PsA based on its success in rheumatoid arthritis.

The trial was a 24-week study of 30 patients in which those on sulfasalazine showed significant improvement in joint pain compared to those on placebo, as reported in the *Journal of Rheumatology*. Similar results continued to be reported in larger studies. However, researchers feel that the benefits of sulfasalazine appear to be limited to peripheral joints and does not benefit spinal disease nor skin rash.

For more information see page 1483.

Reiter Disease

See Reiter's Syndrome

Reiter's Syndrome

Reiter's syndrome is named for the physician who first described it in 1916 and defined it as a cluster of three problems: arthritis, nongonococcal urethritis (infection of the urethra caused by pathogens other than gonorrhea), and conjunctivitis. It is called a reactive arthritis because it complicates an infection (often minor) elsewhere in the body. The arthritis lasts longer than a month and is associated with inflammation of the urethra or cervix with diarrhea.

Commonly Prescribed (On-Label) Drugs: *None*

OFF-LABEL PRESCRIPTION DRUG
BREAKTHROUGH OPTION

*Generic: **Bromocriptine** (broe-moe-KRIP-teen)*
*Brand: **Parlodel***

Bromocriptine blocks the release of prolactin (a hormone that affects the menstrual cycle and breast milk production). It is approved for treatment of the cessation of menstruation, female infertility, excess prolactin, Parkinson's disease, and excessive growth hormone.

Physicians from the Montgomery Veterans' Affairs Hospital in Missouri indicated in an article in *Seminars in Arthritis and Rheumatism* that prolactin may play a causative role in some rheumatic diseases, including Reiter's syndrome. If so, then bromocriptine would be useful in its treatment. The investigators reviewed the literature and found a number of clinical trials showing efficacy with bromocriptine in various rheumatic diseases. For Reiter's syndrome enthesopathy, only case reports were found, and further investigation was urged. (Enthesopathy is an abnormality involving an attachment of a tendon or ligament to bone.) The investigators suggested that bromocriptine may be a relatively safe and efficacious alternative therapy.

In an article in the *Journal of Rheumatology*, researchers from the Specialty Hospital in Mexico City reported on four patients with Reiter's syndrome treated with bromocriptine. All had infectious gastroenteritis and enthesopathy that persisted despite treatment with three anti-inflammatory drugs and one with sulfasalazine for long periods. Such treatment was discontinued eight days before bromocriptine therapy was initiated. In two, dramatic improvement began 24 hours after bromocriptine treatment began, and the other two improved after four days of therapy.

For more information see page 1054.

Rheumatoid Arthritis

Rheumatoid arthritis (RA) is an autoimmune disease that causes chronic inflammation of the tissue around the joints, as well as other organs in the body. In autoimmune diseases, the immune system mistakenly attacks the body's own tissues as if they were foreign invaders. Although RA is usually a progressive illness, leading to joint destruction and disability, there may be quiet periods where there are few or no symptoms. However, because it is a chronic disease, RA continues indefinitely and may not go away.

Commonly Prescribed (On-Label) Drugs: *Adalimumab, Anakinra, Aspirin, Auranofin, Aurothioglucose, Azathioprine, Betamethasone, Celecoxib, Choline Salicylate, Corticotropin, Cortisone, Cyclosporine, Dexamethasone, Diclofenac, Diclofenac/Misoprostol, Diflunisal, Etanercept, Etodolac, Fenoprofen, Flurbiprofen, Gold Sodium Thiomalate, Hydroxychloroquine, Ibuprofen, Indomethacin, Infliximab, Ketoprofen, Leflunomide, Magnesium Salicylate, Meclofenamate, Meloxicam, Methotrexate, Methylprednisolone, Nabumetone, Naproxen, Oxaprozin, Penicillamine,*

Phenylbutazone, Piroxicam, Prednisolone, Prednisone,
Salsalate, Sodium Salicylate, Sulfasalazine, Sulindac, Tolmetin,
Triamcinolone, Valdecoxib

OFF-LABEL PRESCRIPTION DRUGS
BREAKTHROUGH OPTIONS

Generic: **Bromocriptine** *(broe-moe-KRIP-teen)*
Brand: **Parlodel**

Bromocriptine inhibits the release of the hormone prolactin, which affects the menstrual cycle and production of breast milk and is approved for treating hyperprolactinemia (an excess of prolactin), amenorrhea (absence of menstruation), female infertility, acromegaly (excessive growth hormone), and Parkinson's disease.

An article in *Seminars in Arthritis and Rheumatism* from the Montgomery Veterans' Affairs Hospital in Missouri suggests that evidence supports the idea that the hormone prolactin would play a causative role in some rheumatic diseases, including RA. This would support the use of bromocriptine in treating of RA, at the very least as an add-on therapy. Clinical trials showed it to be effective in various rheumatic diseases, but for RA, only a few studies with relatively few patients were found. In these, bromocriptine was associated with improvements in morning stiffness, grip strength, numbers of swollen and painful joints, and disability. The researchers suggested bromocriptine may be a relatively safe and efficacious alternative therapy.

For more information see page 1054.

Generic: **Captopril** *(KAP-toe-pril)*
Brand: **Capoten**

Captopril belongs to a class of drugs called angiotensin converting enzyme (ACE) inhibitors. It inhibits an enzyme needed to produce a substance that causes blood vessels to tighten. Therefore, blood vessels relax, lowering blood pressure. Captopril is approved for the treatment of hypertension as well as heart failure and post–heart attack left ventricular dysfunction, because it helps lower the workload of the heart. However, captopril also has immunosuppressant activity and therefore researchers consider it a potential slow-acting drug for the treatment of RA. Its molecular structure is similar to another immunosuppressant approved for RA called penicillamine (unrelated to the antibiotic penicillin).

A Hungarian study compared captopril and penicillamine in animals with rheumatoid arthritis. Researchers concluded that captopril would be valuable to evaluate in humans. *The Lancet* described a study in which 15 patients with RA were given captopril for 48 weeks. Two-thirds reported benefits, and lab tests showed improvements in important indicators of inflammation. Side effects were mild, although two patients withdrew because of them.

For more information see page 1066.

Generic: **Chlorambucil** (khlor-AM-byoo-sil)
Brand: *Leukeran*

Chlorambucil belongs to a class of drugs called alkylating drugs that work by binding DNA strands so that cell division is not possible. They also bind other important biochemicals, thereby impairing their function so that cancer cells and other cells that rapidly divide cannot reproduce. Chlorambucil is approved for treating a type of leukemia and malignant lymphomas. Lymphocytes, white blood cells whose normal function involves antibody production and other immune activities, are also very sensitive to the effects of alkylating drugs. This makes alkylating drugs helpful in treating autoimmune diseases such as RA.

Studies experimenting with chlorambucil for RA started as long as 35 years ago with an early report in *Reviews in Rheumatology.* In the *Medical Journal of Australia*, a five-year follow-up of 22 patients treated at Rachel Forster Hospital in Sydney reported a total of 12 in full remission, seven in partial remission, and three had died due to malignancies not related to RA.

For more information see page 1079.

Generic: **Cyclophosphamide** *(sye-kloe-FOS-fa-mide)*
Brands: **Cytoxan, Neosar**

Cyclophosphamide belongs to a class of drugs known as alkylating drugs, which were originally developed and are still used to treat some types of cancer. It is approved for treating various leukemias and cancers. Because of its immunosuppressant benefits, it is also used off-label to treat a number of autoimmune diseases such as lupus, scleroderma, and some of the complications of rheumatoid arthritis, such as vasculitis or blood vessel inflammation.

The Cochrane Library reported on a series of trials comparing oral cyclophosphamide against placebo or an active drug at a dose considered to be ineffective in patients with RA. Of 70 patients, 31 were receiving cyclophosphamide. A significant benefit was observed for cyclophosphamide compared to placebo for tender and swollen joints. The researchers found benefits similar to DMARDs such as antimalarials or sulfasalazine but lower than methotrexate, but concluded that toxicity was severe.

In a review on the Johns Hopkins Hospital arthritis website, serious toxicities such as bone marrow depression, hemorrhagic cystitis, premature ovarian failure, infection, and secondary malignancy were also mentioned.

For more information see page 1123.

Generic: **Doxycycline** *(doks-i-SYE-kleen)*
Brands: **Adoxa, Doryx, Doxy-100, Monodox, Periostat, Vibra-Tabs, Vibramycin**

Doxycycline is part of the tetracycline group of antibiotics and is approved for treatment of a variety of bacterial infections. It has never been shown that infections cause RA, but that may not be why doxycycline helps RA. Antibiotics have other effects in the body. Tetracyclines inactivate several enzymes that play a role in inflammation. They also decrease the production of substances that modulate immune system activity. However it works, doxycycline may slow the progression of joint damage in arthritis and prevent disability, like other drugs in the class known as disease modifying antirheumatic drugs (DMARDs). Therefore, it is sometimes prescribed for patients with symptoms of mild rheumatoid arthritis and Lyme arthritis.

Journal of the Association of Physicians in India reported on a small clinical trial comparing doxycycline with methotrexate in 35 patients with RA for six months. Both therapies produced clinically significant improvements in tender and swollen joints, pain, and inflammation. Researchers observed that there were no differences in improvement between the groups. *Rheumatology International* reported on a small study of 12 patients for three months, yielding significant improvement of all symptoms.

For more information see page 1158.

*Generic: **Minocycline** (min-OH-sik-leen)*
*Brands: **Dynacin, Minocin***

Minocycline is one of the tetracycline group of antibiotics, which help kill bacteria that cause infections. It is approved to treat a variety of bacterial infections. Minocycline is sometimes prescribed for patients with symptoms of mild rheumatoid arthritis. It may take two to three months before improvement begins and a year before maximum benefits occurs.

Arthritis & Rheumatism reported on a study in 46 patients in their first year of RA who received either minocycline or placebo. After six months, those on minocycline significantly improved compared to those on placebo. In a follow-up study of 38 of these patients for an average of four years, those who had received minocycline initially were most likely to be in remission (40% vs. 17%) and less likely to require a DMARD (50% vs. 90%). Based on these results, researchers strongly suggest that minocycline in early RA is beneficial.

A trial, also published in *Arthritis & Rheumatism*, involved 219 people with mild-to-moderate RA who received placebo or minocycline for 48 weeks. Minocycline patients experienced a greater than 50% improvement in joint swelling and tenderness, and all improvements were significant compared to the placebo group.

For more information see page 1331.

Rheumatoid Spondylitis

See Ankylosing Spondylitis

BONE DISEASE

While bone seems hard as a rock it is constantly renewing itself. Old bone is removed (bone resorption) and replaced by new bone (bone formation). When it's in balance, humans maintain normal bone density. Abnormal bone density may be due to aging or drugs.

Osteoporosis

When bone loss exceeds formation to the degree that bone density drops and patients are at significant risks for fractures, osteoporosis (OP) is present. This may be due to aging, most commonly in women after menopause due to their loss of estrogen. Also, it is common among elderly men, especially in those who smoke or use alcohol excessively. Or OP may be caused by taking steroid medications such as prednisone, prednisolone, or cortisone. Steroids slow bone formation, interfere with the body's handling of calcium, and affect levels of sex hormones, leading to increased bone loss. The same drugs may be used to prevent or treat OP.

Commonly Prescribed (On-Label) Drugs: *Alendronate, Calcitonins, Estrogens, Ibandronate, Risedronate, Teriparatide*

OFF-LABEL PRESCRIPTION DRUGS
BREAKTHROUGH OPTIONS

Generic: ***Chlorthalidone*** *(klor-THAL-i-done)*
Brand: ***Thalitone***

Chlorthalidone is a thiazide-like diuretic. Thiazides are the most commonly used and oldest type of antihypertensive drugs used. They accomplish that goal by reducing the volume of fluid in the body. However, it has been observed that people taking thiazide diuretics have hypocalciuria—decreased calcium in their urine—which might be useful in preventing OPs in elderly women who do not exercise adequately.

An article in *Osteoporosis International* from the Hawaii Osteoporosis Center reported on a trial monitoring 113 postmenopausal women assigned to take chlorthalidone or placebo.

According to investigators, after an average of 2.6 years, use of the active drug was associated with significant reductions in annual bone loss rates and an average increment of 0.9% per year, whereas use of placebo was associated with bone loss at two sites and borderline bone gain at one site. The investigators concluded that the data support a causal relationship between chlorthalidone use and reduced bone loss.

For more information see page 1083.

Generic: **Etidronate** *(e-ti-DROE-nate)*
Brand: **Didronel**

Etidronate is one of a group of drugs known as bisphosphonates. They help slow bone loss. While some are approved for treatment of OP, etidronate is not. Rather, it is approved for the treatment of symptomatic Paget's disease of bone and in the prevention and treatment of heterotopic ossification following total hip replacement or due to spinal cord injury. Nonetheless, it is sometimes used for OP.

An article in *Thorax* from Llandough Hospital, Penarth, UK, reported on a five-year study of etidronate and/or calcium as prevention and treatment of OP in patients with asthma receiving long-term oral and/or inhaled glucocorticoids. Those receiving etidronate had significantly increased bone mineral density at the lumbar spine but not at the hip, although there was little if any protective effect against fractures, except possibly in postmenopausal women.

An article in the *Journal of Rheumatology* analyzed different therapeutic regimens for the prevention of vertebral fractures in women treated with steroids. Researchers concluded that calcium, vitamin D, and a low-cost bisphosphonate such as cyclic etidronate decrease vertebral fracture risk at acceptable cost and should be started when initiating corticosteroid treatment in women who do not already have OP.

For more information see page 1177.

Generic: **Pamidronate** *(pa-mi-DROE-nate)*
Brand: **Aredia**

Pamidronate belongs to a class of drugs, called bisphosphonates, that help slow bone loss. It is approved for the treatment of Paget's disease, osteolytic lesions, and certain malignancies. Unlike the bisphosphonates approved for treatment of osteoporosis that are given as pills taken daily or weekly, pamidronate may be given orally or as an intravenous infusion given every three months.

An article in the *Journal of Bone and Mineral Research* reported on a study from Belgium comparing the benefits of a single intravenous infusion of pamidronate at the start of steroid therapy versus such infusions every three months over the course of a year in the prevention of OP in 32 patients. At the end of the year, either method achieved primary prevention as measured by bone mineral density. However, lab tests of evolving bone turnover showed a sustained decrease of bone resorption over time only in the group that received the frequent infusions.

An article in *Calcification Tissue International* reported a study from Mont-Godinne University Hospital in Belgium in which 27 patients starting on corticosteroid therapy were divided to receive either intravenous pamidronate (every three months) and calcium or calcium alone. After one year, the pamidronate group showed a significant increase in spinal and hipbone mineral density compared to the calcium alone group. Researchers observed that in the calcium group, bone density had dropped.

An article in the *Journal of Clinical Pharmacological Therapy* reported a study from Wilhelmininspital, in Vienna, Austria, that enrolled 86 women with postmenopausal (69) or glucocorticoid-induced (17) OP. All received intravenous pamidronate every three months. The researchers concluded that this cyclic treatment increases spinal bone mineral density in postmenopausal OP.

An article in the *Journal of Clinical Endocrinology and Metabolism* from the University of Auckland, New Zealand, reported that the researchers used oral pamidronate in their study of 48 women with postmenopausal osteoporosis. After two years, bone mineral density increased in the total body, spine, and hip in those receiving pamidronate but decreased significantly in those receiving placebo. Vertebral fracture rates were almost twice as high in those receiving placebo.

For more information see page 1391.
For more information see page 1391.

*Generic: **Simvastatin** (SIM-va-stat-in)*
*Brand: **Zocor***

Simvastatin belongs to a class of drugs called statins. It is approved to treat hyperlipidemia and hypercholesterolemia—that is, to lower blood fats and reduce the risk of heart disease and cardiovascular events in high-risk patients. Statins block the liver's synthesis of cholesterol by blocking a pathway involved in the process.

A study in *Bone* from the University of Siena, Italy reported that 30 postmenopausal hypercholesterolemic women were treated with simvastatin for 12 months and 30 normocholesterolemic postmenopausal women provided control data. The difference between the two groups was significant for bone mineral density at the spine and hip, with the treated women showing increases at both sites, and a positive effect shown for simvastatin.

An article in *Pharmacoepidemiological Drug Safety* reported on a study from Brigham and Women's Hospital in Boston that examined the relationship between statin use and bone density among postmenopausal women. They did a survey of postmenopausal women who had bone densitometry and agreed to a telephone interview about their OP risk factors, use of hormone replacement therapy, and osteoporosis medications and statin exposure. Of 339 women studied, 162 were current or past users of statins. Statin users has significantly higher body mass index and rates of thiazide use and were more likely to abstain from alcohol. Researchers found that statin use was associated with significantly higher bone mineral density at the hip compared to non-users.

For more information see page 1474.

*Generic: **Zoledronic Acid** (zoe-lyn-DRAN-ic AS-id)*
*Brand: **Zometa***

Zoledronic acid belongs to a class of drugs known as bisphosphonates that increase bone density and reduce the rate of fracture in OP. It is given by intravenous infusion and is only approved for the treatment of certain malignancies. Oral bisphosphonates are widely used for treating osteoporosis, but many women have difficulty sticking to the regimen because of gastrointestinal side effects, and the drugs are not absorbed well in some patients.

According to researchers, receiving an intravenous infusion every six months might solve these problems.

As reported in an article in the *New England Journal of Medicine*, zoledronic acid is one of the most potent bisphosphonates that has been studied in clinical trials to date. It is superior to pamidronate in the treatment of cancer-related hypercalcemia. Because it has high potency, only small doses are required for the inhibition of bone resorption, and long dosing intervals may be used. An international trial was undertaken to examine the effect of intravenous zoledronic acid on bone density and bone turnover in postmenopausal women with low bone density and to assess the effects of varying the total dose administered and the dosing interval. Researchers studied five regimens in 351 women (different doses at three- or six-month intervals or a single dose) with low bone mineral density in a one-year trial. There were similar increases in bone mineral density in all the zoledronic acid groups for the spine and hip that were 3% to 5% higher than the placebo group. The researchers concluded that an annual infusion might be an effective treatment for postmenopausal osteoporosis.

For more information see page 1553.

CONNECTIVE TISSUE DISEASES

Connective tissue is the "cellular glue" that holds the body together. It is between the cells giving tissues form and strength. It also helps deliver nutrients and is involved in special tissue functions. Connective tissue is constructed of dozens of proteins including collagens, proteoglycans, and glycoproteins. If any of the genes that encode these proteins have defects or mutations, the result may be a susceptibility to a connective tissue disorder. It is currently believed that patients need such genetic risk(s) plus interaction with one or more environmental factors to trigger a heritable connective tissue disorder.

Arteritis Nodosa

See Polyarteritis Nodosa

Dermatomyositis/Polymyositis

Since dermatomyositis and polymyositis are similar in signs, symptoms, and treatment, both conditions are often mentioned together. Both dermatomyositis and polymyositis are categorized in the family of inflammatory muscle diseases. Dermatomyositis is characterized by muscle weakness and a patchy, bluish-purple rash on the face, neck, shoulders, upper chest, elbows, knees, knuckles, and back. The most common symptom of polymyositis is gradual onset of muscle weakness that may begin in the trunk muscles and progress to more distant body muscles.

OFF-LABEL PRESCRIPTION DRUGS
BREAKTHROUGH OPTIONS

*Generic: **Azathioprine** (ay-za-THYE-oh-preen)*
*Brand: **Imuran***

Azathioprine belongs to the class of drugs known as immunosuppressive drugs. The use of azathioprine may decrease proliferation of immune cells, thus reducing autoimmune activity. In patients with dermatomyositis/polymyositis, azathioprine has become an increasingly popular alternative to corticosteroids since it is well tolerated and its use results in fewer adverse effects. Prednisone is the drug of choice for this type of immune disorder; however, doctors may decide to give azathioprine for dermatomyositis/polymyositis in patients who have serious complications with steroids, repeated disease relapses when the steroid dose was lowered, no improvement in muscle strength with steroids, or in progressive disease with severe weakness and breathing failure.

In a study of 70 patients with diffuse lung disease and polymyositis or dermatomyositis, treatment generally consisted of prednisone for initial control followed by lower doses of prednisone plus azathioprine or another immunosuppressive drug, methotrexate, for disease suppression. According to researchers, survival in this study was significantly better than that observed for historical control subjects. In another study, 19 patients with juvenile dermatomyositis were examined. All except one patient was treated with prednisolone, 13 patients received methotrexate, and three patients received azathioprine. Eight patients achieved complete remission, eight patients experienced partial remission, and two patients had no response. According to some researchers, azathioprine may not work as fast or be as effective as methotrexate.

For more information see page 1033.

Generic: *Chloroquine* (klor-OH-kwin)
Brand: *Aralen*

Chloroquine belongs to the class of drugs known as antimalarials, and may be used as a steroid-sparing drug to treat skin diseases. Chloroquine is a second-line therapy for the treatment of dermatomyositis/polymyositis. In a study of 17 adult patients with signs and symptoms of dermatomyositis who did not respond to antimalarial therapy alone, researchers examined a variety of treatments including antimalarials, prednisone (a corticosteroid), and methotrexate (an antineoplastic drug), among other medications. Seven out of 17 patients had at least near resolution of skin symptoms with antimalarial therapy alone. Of these seven patients, four patients required combination antimalarial therapy consisting of chloroquine and quinacrine or hydroxychloroquine and quinacrine hydrochloride, and three patients responded well to antimalarial therapy alone. Based on these results, researchers concluded that there may be a subgroup of patients whose skin lesions respond well to combination therapy of antimalarials, such as chloroquine and quinacrine.

Chloroquine is one of the most common antimalarial drugs and is often used in a number of autoimmune diseases. Chloroquine is recognized for its benefits in skin conditions, and its efficacy and safety profile makes it a practical treatment option for the symptoms of dermatomyositis/polymyositis.

For more information see page 1082.

Generic: *Cyclophosphamide* (sye-kloe-FOS-fa-mide).
Brands: *Cytoxan, Neosar*

Cyclophosphamide inhibits cell growth and proliferation, and it appears to interfere with the growth and proliferation of immune cells in dermatomyositis/polymyositis. When steroids fail, cyclophosphamide is the next treatment option for affected patients.

Use of cyclophosphamide carries the risk of abnormal or uncontrolled cell growth called neoplasia, therefore regular blood monitoring is required. In clinical studies, cyclophosphamide has shown promising results for the treatment of dermatomyositis/polymyositis, and may be particularly useful in those with interstitial lung disease. Interstitial lung disease can occur before muscle or skin symptoms of dermatomyositis/polymyositis are present. Patients with dermatomyositis/polymyositis and progressive lung disease benefit from cyclophosphamide given as daily oral or IV therapy in combination with steroids. A study conducted at the Juvenile Dermatomyositis Research Centre, Institute of Child Health in London highlighted the efficacy of IV cyclophosphamide in children with severe dermatomyositis. Ten out of 12 children showed a significant improvement in muscle function, muscle strength, and skin disease severity with cyclophosphamide pulse therapy, and improvement lasted until the most recent follow-up, which was between six months to seven years. Additionally, no side effects associated with cyclophosphamide were reported. Also, according to researchers, there is accumulating evidence that cyclophosphamide is effective in patients with nonspecific interstitial pneumonia and dermatomyositis.

For more information see page 1123.

Generic: *Cyclosporine* *(si-klo-SPOR-een)*
Brands: *Gengraf, Neoral, Sandimmune*

Cyclosporine is a strong immunosuppressant drug that blocks important immune cells known as T-cells, which are activated in autoimmune diseases such as dermatomyositis/polymyositis. Serious side effects associated with cyclosporine include high blood pressure and kidney problems. Other side effects include headache, nausea, vomiting, abdominal pain or dyspepsia, and swelling of the hands or feet.

In patients who are resistant to steroids, cyclosporine has been reported to be just as effective as methotrexate, an antineoplastic drug and first-line treatment for dermatomyositis/polymyositis. Moreover, researchers feel that there are more recent data that mention IV cyclosporine is effective in patients with dermatomyositis/polymyositis and lung diseases such as interstitial pneumonitis or pulmonary fibrosis. In an analysis of 28 patients with interstitial lung disease comparing polymyositis with dermato-myositis, researchers found that giving cyclosporine early on bene-fited four steroid-resistant patients with dermatomyositis and interstitial lung disease. Results from this study also showed that patients with dermatomyositis and interstitial lung disease are more resistant to steroids than those with polymyositis and inter-stitial lung disease, and that aggressive therapy with cyclosporine should be considered in these patients. Interstitial pneumonia in polymyositis and dermatomyositis is recognized to be a major complication of both of these autoimmune disorders, and cy-closporine may also reduce the amount of steroids required. Some researchers have suggested that cyclosporine may be more effective in children rather than adults.

For more information see pages 1125 and 1127.

Generic: **Diltiazem** *(dil-TYE-a-zem)*
Brands: **Cartia XT, Cardizem, Dilacor XR, Diltia XT, Taztia XT, Tiazac**

Diltiazem is a calcium channel blocker, and may be helpful in treating calcinosis (calcium deposits) associated with dermato-myositis/polymyositis. In high blood pressure and chest pain, dil-tiazem inhibits calcium ions from entering the slow channels and voltage-sensitive areas of vascular smooth muscle and heart mus-cle; however, its action is not fully understood in other diseases. Researchers believe that diltiazem works by preventing new layers of calcium from forming.

Calcinosis is a complication in autoimmune disorders such as dermatomyositis, and it may cause severe disability. These de-posits appear as hard bumps under the skin. Several patient case studies have recognized the efficacy of diltiazem on calcium de-posits in patients with dermatomyositis. In one report, a three-year-old girl in Japan with dermatomyositis since age one was unsuccessfully treated with a steroid for multiple calcium deposits under the skin. Despite therapy with steroids and aluminum hy-droxide, these deposits grew larger. Only treatment with diltiazem completely stopped the development of calcinosis. Finally, an eight-year-old girl in Argentina with dermatomyositis developed calcinosis 26 months after her diagnosis. In this case, the patient also experienced bone loss as a result of steroid use. Treatment with immunosuppressive drugs and steroids did not affect the calcium deposits. After treatment with oral diltiazem and oral pamidronate, in addition to calcium and vitamin D supplements for 21 months, there was significant regression of the calcinosis, and her bone mass returned to normal.

For more information see page 1146.

Generic: **Hydroxychloroquine** *(hye-droks-ee-KLOR-oh-kwin)*
Brand: **Plaquenil**

Hydroxychloroquine belongs to the drug class known as antimalarials, which are used in a number of autoimmune disorders, especially in skin conditions. Hydroxychloroquine is the preferred antimalarial to be used to treat dermatomyositis/polymyositis, and may promote partial or complete control of the disease. It acts to inhibit movement of immune cells and impairs antigen-antibody reactions.

Several small studies involving the use of hydroxychloroquine for dermatomyositis have been conducted. In one study, nine patients with childhood dermatomyositis and incomplete response to corticosteroid therapy or exacerbation of disease when corticosteroids were tapered received hydroxychloroquine and corticosteroids. After three months, researchers observed significant reduction in rash and proximal and abdominal muscle strength. After six months of therapy, the prednisone dose was reduced. Researchers in this study suggested that use of hydroxychloroquine may be helpful in certain patients with dermatomyositis, especially those with major skin disease or significant steroid toxicity.

Overall, researchers concluded that hydroxychloroquine has a favorable safety and efficacy profile, is the preferred antiviral drug for dermatomyositis/polymyositis, and may be a treatment alternative for those patients who are resistant or intolerant to steroids.

For more information see page 1225.

Generic: **Immune globulin IV** *(eh-mune GLOB-ewe-lyn)*
Brands: **Gamimune N, Gamunex, Octagam, Polygam S/D, Venoglobulin S**

Immune globulin IV belongs to the family of immunoglobulins, and may be a third drug option in patients in whom steroids and immunosuppressive drugs have failed to treat dermatomyositis/polymyositis. Immune globulin improves the clinical and immunologic parts of the disease, and may decrease autoantibody production and increase removal of immune complexes.

Immune globulin IV has been shown to be effective in dermatomyositis, and improvement is generally noted after the first infusion and evident by the second monthly infusion. After the second or third dose, if no improvement is seen, then immune globulin is unlikely to be successful. Several clinical studies have shown that at high doses, immune globulin is a promising and safe choice, although it is expensive and may have to be repeated to maintain benefit. A study showed that in patients with dermatomyositis resistant or partially responsive to conventional therapies, immune globulin IV was very effective in improving skin rash and muscle strength. Up to 20% of patients experienced improvements in daily living activities, and specific muscles in the body (such as those used in swallowing), showed improvements with immune globulin when compared with placebo. In polymyositis, small studies have shown muscle strength improvements in up to 70% of patients receiving immune globulin IV.

For more information see page 1235.

Generic: **Methotrexate** *(meth-oh-TREKS-ate)*
Brands: **Rheumatrex, Trexall**

Methotrexate, which belongs to a class of drugs known as antineoplastic drugs, inhibits cell growth and proliferation. In inflammatory conditions, methotrexate has been demonstrated to relieve symptoms of pain, swelling, and stiffness; it also offers benefits in muscle and skin disease.

Methotrexate may be offered as a second-line drug when patients with dermatomyositis/polymyositis do not respond to steroids, and it may be more effective than azathioprine, another antineoplastic drug. Researchers feel that methotrexate is well recognized as an alternative drug for the treatment of dermatomyositis/ polymyositis. In 19 patients with juvenile dermatomyositis, all patients received prednisolone, a steroid, and 13 patients received methotrexate. Eight patients achieved complete remission of their disease, eight patients experienced partial remission, and two patients had no response. In a study comparing the efficacy and safety of methotrexate and cyclosporine added to corticosteroids in patients with severe polymyositis or dermatomyositis, both treatment groups had significant improvements in muscle function, clinical assessment, and patient's assessment of symptoms. However, researchers observed that patients treated with methotrexate showed a better response than patients treated with cyclosporine. Overall, methotrexate has been shown to be effective in the treatment of dermatomyositis/polymyositis.

For more information see page 1312.

Generic: *Mycophenolate mofetil*
(my-koe-FEN-oh-late MOE-feh-till)
Brands: *CellCept, Myfortic*

Mycophenolate mofetil, an immunosuppressive drug, is useful for both skin and muscle diseases since it inhibits the proliferation of inflammatory cells known as lymphocytes. Mycophenolate mofetil has been used to treat psoriasis, a common skin condition.

It has demonstrated promising results in patient case studies, and is recognized in medical literature as an effective treatment alternative in patients who are not responsive to other therapies. In four patient cases exhibiting evidence of severe dermatomyositis, conventional therapy with corticosteroids, hydroxychloroquine (an antimalarial), and/or methotrexate (an antineoplastic drug) were limited by side effects or insufficient response. Mycophenolate mofetil was then given to these patients and was found to be effective at controlling skin disease activity and reducing the dose of steroids. The mean duration of treatment was 13 months.

If mycophenolate mofetil is given for an extended time, there may be an increased risk of lymphoma. At high doses, there is an increased risk for gastrointestinal intolerance. With the use of mycophenolate mofetil, there is increased risk of infection, increased toxicity in those with renal impairment, and caution should be used in patients with active peptic ulcer disease. Researchers state that mycophenolate mofetil has a well-tolerated side effect profile, and its use in dermatomyositis/polymyositis continues to be studied.

For more information see page 1344.

Generic: **Tacrolimus** *(ta-KROE-li-mus)*
Brands: **Prograf, Protopic**

Tacrolimus is a drug that suppresses the immune system and is commonly used to prevent rejection of transplanted body organs. Dermatomyositic skin lesions can be quite resistant to systemic and topical drugs, and tacrolimus has been used in these instances with documented improvement. In a study published in *Dermatology* of six patients (five adults and one child) with resistant dermatomyositic skin lesions, topical tacrolimus (0.1%) ointment was applied. All patients in this study experienced improvement of skin lesions after six to eight weeks of tacrolimus treatment. Two of the patients had dramatic responses. In another study conducted in Japan, topical tacrolimus was applied to 11 patients with facial skin lesions from cutaneous lupus erythematosus and dermatomyositis. Of the 11 patients, six patients (three with systemic lupus erythematosus and two with dermatomyositis) showed a marked regression of skin lesions. Four patients (three with lupus erythematosus and one with dermatomyositis) were resistant to therapy.

Based on these results, researchers suggested that topical tacrolimus may be another drug for managing skin lesions in dermatomyositis/polymyositis. Tacrolimus has also been documented to be effective in patients with interstitial lung disease and dermatomyositis/polymyositis. Common side effects of tacrolimus are burning and itching during the first or second applications. Other side effects include severe and blurred vision, liver and kidney problems, seizures, tremors, hypertension, diabetes mellitus, insomnia, loss of appetite, weakness, and depression, among others.

For more information see page 1489.

Disseminated Lupus Erythematosus

See Systemic Lupus Erythematosus

Kussmaul Disease

See Polyarteritis Nodosa

Periarteritis Nodosa

See Polyarteritis Nodosa

Polyarteritis Nodosa

Polyarteritis nodosa (PAN) is a rare autoimmune disease. It causes inflammation of arteries and can therefore affect any part of the body, but the muscles, joints, intestines, bowels, nerves, kidneys, and skin are most commonly involved. Damaged function of any of these organs can be uncomfortable, but impaired blood supply to the bowel can be painful and life threatening when arteries supplying the intestines die (necrotize). The underlying immunological cause of the disease or what causes the subsequent vascular injuries remains poorly understood.

Commonly Prescribed (On-Label) Drugs: *None*

OFF-LABEL PRESCRIPTION DRUGS
BREAKTHROUGH OPTIONS

Generic: **Cyclophosphamide** *(sye-kloe-FOS-fa-mide)*
Brands: **Cytoxan, Neosar**

Cyclophosphamide is one of a group of medications called alkylating drugs. They were originally developed as cancer therapies and work by binding DNA strands to prevent cell division, thus slowing or halting the cancer. Cyclophosphamide's impact on cells in the immune system makes it a drug that can tamp down the immune response. As a result, although cyclophosphamide is approved for treating various leukemias and cancers, it is used off-label to treat a number of autoimmune diseases such as lupus, scleroderma, and polyarteritis nodosa.

An article in the *American Journal of Medicine* from the National Institute of Allergy and Infectious Diseases reported on two patients with far advanced PAN involving multiple organ systems with extensive aneurysms (arteries with weak patches about to burst) who were treated with oral cyclophosphamide and alternate-day prednisone therapy. Patients experienced dramatic remissions within weeks, and angiograms a year later revealed that the aneurysms had been healed. The prednisone was withdrawn and the patients were then maintained on cyclophosphamide alone at the time of the report when each was 18 and 27 months from the original start of therapy, respectively. The researchers concluded that cyclophosphamide could be considered highly effective even in far advanced PAN.

An article from the University of California at Irvine on *eMedicine* includes cyclophosphamide on the list of alkylating drugs recommended for polyarteritis nodosa.

For more information see page 1123.

Generic: **Famciclovir** *(fam-SYE-kloe-veer)*
Brand: **Famvir**

Famciclovir is a prodrug—that is, a drug that is broken down in the body into another drug that is the active drug. It is converted in the body into the antiviral drug penciclovir. This drug helps block the duplication of the DNA that viruses need in order to reproduce and survive.

Physicians have observed that 20% to 30% of patients with PAN also are infected with hepatitis B virus (HBV), while less than 1% overall of those with HBV develop PAN. Conventional regimens for those with both include steroids and immunosuppressive drugs such as cyclophosphamide, methotrexate, and antiviral drugs such as interferon alfa.

An article in the *Journal of Hepatology* from physicians in Hanover, Germany reported on the case of a man with HBV and PAN who did not respond to prednisolone or interferon alfa, and therefore famciclovir was added. With this regimen, there was a 79% reduction in the DNA of HBV after the first week and 88% after the second week, with a corresponding decline in PAN symptoms. After a year of therapy with famciclovir, physicians were able to reduce the dose and the patient has been taking the drug for three years with no PAN symptoms. The investigators of this study recommend the drug as an effective, well-tolerated long-term therapy in PAN patients with HBV associated disease.

For more information see page 1180.

*Generic: **Interferon Alfa-2b** (in-ter-FEER-on AL-fa-2b)*
*Brand: **Intron A***

Interferon exists naturally in the human body and helps protect the body from viruses. Interferon alfa-2b is a protein produced in the laboratory. It is approved for treatment of hepatitis B and C, and cancer.

According to researchers, the relationship between PAN and hepatitis B virus (HBV) is interesting and well established: 20% to 30% of those with PAN are infected with HBV, while less than 1% of those with HBV develop PAN. Conventional regimens for those with both include steroids and immunosuppressive drugs such as cyclophosphamide, methotrexate, and antiviral drugs such as interferon alfa.

An article in *Hepatogastroenterology* from Keystone Digestive Disease Consultants in Pittsburgh, PA, reported on a patient with PAN and HBV resistant to multiple therapies. He was treated with famciclovir, interferon, and granulocyte macrophage colony stimulating factor (GM-CSF). Artery inflammation but not the HBV responded to therapy with the cyclophosphamide and corticosteroids. The HBV also did not respond to a year of interferon. However, when famciclovir and GM-CSF were added, the HBV infection quickly resolved and the PAN did not recur with continued antiviral treatment.

In an article on *Dermatology Journal Online* from New York University of a case of PAN, an investigator noted that for the most severe and life-threatening forms of HBV-associated disease concomitant antiviral drugs such as interferon alfa-2b enhance survival.

For more information see page 1243.

*Generic: **Methotrexate** (meth-o-TREKS-ate)*
*Brands: **Rheumatrex, Trexall***

Methotrexate is a drug that suppresses the immune system by affecting the metabolism of cells. It is approved for the treatment of a number of cancers, psoriasis, rheumatoid and juvenile rheumatoid arthritis. However, it is used off-label in a number of related autoimmune diseases.

In a report from the University of California at Irvine on *eMedicine*, researchers noted that immunosuppressive has been the standard therapy for PAN, and that a combination of two or more different such drugs can improve the outcome. Methotrexate is one of their recommended alkylating drugs, although its mechanism of action in treatment is unknown. Researchers believe that methotrexate ameliorates symptoms of inflammation, but they advise that the dose should be adjusted gradually to achieve the best response.

An article in the *Canadian Medical Association Journal* from a physician at Montreal General Hospital reported on a man with severe PAN who had not responded to six months of prednisone therapy. After 18 weeks of weekly infusions of methotrexate, the patient's condition resolved: the PAN-caused diabetes disappeared, the blood pressure dropped, and he was able to return to work for the first time in a year. Additionally, the physician had been able to lower the dose of prednisone.

An article in *Dermatology* from the Institut Gustave-Roussy in France provided information on two patients with cutaneous PAN who responded well to treatment with methotrexate. The skin lesions started to heal within three weeks. One patient reported full recovery, which lasted for two years after stopping methotrexate.

For more information see page 1312.

Generic: **Prednisone** (pred-NIS-zone)
Brands: **Deltasone, Liquid Pred, Meticorten, Orasone, Sterapred**

Prednisone is a corticosteroid drug related to the hormone that the adrenal glands make. It is approved to treat a wide range of autoimmune, inflammatory, and allergic diseases, as well as certain malignancies. In low to moderate doses, these drugs suppress inflammation, perhaps by suppressing the activity of certain blood cells involved in inflammation. In higher doses, prednisone more potently suppresses the underlying immune responses that cause the inflammation, albeit then putting you at higher risk of side effects including a greater risk of infections.

A report on *eMedicine* from the Department of Neurology at the University of California at Irvine notes that corticosteroids yield profound and diverse effects, including modifying immune responses to various stimuli and helping to suppress the inflammation of PAN. Prednisone is first on its list of corticosteroids. Prednisone may block certain enzymes, which in turn inhibit prostaglandins, hormone-like substances that contribute to inflammations. According to investigators, the result of these processes will be reduced disease activity throughout the body and, of course, reduced pain.

For more information see page 1429.

Polymyalgia Rheumatica

Polymyalgia rheumatica (PMR) is an inflammatory disorder that causes widespread muscle aching and stiffness, especially in the neck, shoulders, upper arms, thighs, and hips. Symptoms usually start over a period of several days or weeks, and occasionally even overnight, are worse in the morning and after staying in one position for long periods, especially after sleep. Morning stiffness after sleep can be so severe that getting dressed can be painful. But, most importantly, patients should report any severe headaches to their doctor immediately in case they are converting to temporal arteritis (see below). Vision might be at risk without immediate stepped-up treatment.

Commonly Prescribed (On-Label) Drugs: *Methotrexate, Methylprednisolone, Prednisolone, Simvastatin*

OFF-LABEL PRESCRIPTION DRUG
BREAKTHROUGH OPTION

Generic: ***Prednisone*** *(pred-NIS-zone)*
Brands: ***Deltasone, Liquid Pred, Meticorten, Orasone, Sterapred***

Prednisone is a steroid drug related to the hormone made by the adrenal glands. It is approved to treat a wide range of autoimmune, inflammatory, and allergic diseases, as well as some cancers.

In the *Manual of Rheumatology and Outpatient Orthopedic Disorders* prepared by physicians of the Hospital for Special Surgery in New York City, one of the leading rheumatic disease centers, prednisone is recommended as the initial therapy for PMR. Most symptoms should ease within 72 hours, after which the dose will be reduced to the lowest possible to keep you symptom free long term. In an article on *eMedicine* from the emergency medicine department of Sentara Careplex Hospital, researchers state that patients may require treatment for several months to several years.

An article in the *Annals of Internal Medicine* from the Systemic Vasculitis Study Group of the Italian Society for Rheumatology presents a study in 72 newly diagnosed PMR patients comparing prednisone alone to prednisone plus methotrexate (an immunosuppressive drug) to discern whether those taking methotrexate were able to more effectively taper prednisone without flare-ups. The result was positive—enabling patients to get off prednisone sooner and yielding fewer PMR flares—suggesting that this immune suppressant may be useful in patients who are at high risk for steroid-related toxic problems.

For more information see page 1429.

Scleroderma

Scleroderma, an autoimmune disorder, occurs in two variations, each with its own subtypes. Localized scleroderma (linear and morphea) affects the skin or possibly underlying muscles and bones, but does not affect internal organs and is relatively mild. Systemic scleroderma (limited, and diffuse), also known as systemic sclerosis (SSc) may affect the skin, blood vessels, and/or internal organs. When it affects the internal organs, it may cause disability or even death.

Commonly Prescribed (On-Label) Drugs: *Cyclofenil, Epoprostenol*

OFF-LABEL PRESCRIPTION DRUGS
BREAKTHROUGH OPTIONS

Generic: **Colchicine** *(KOL-chi-seen)*
Brand: **None**

Colchicine is a drug that modulates the immune system by arresting cell division, and in this way it helps suppress inflammation. It is used to prevent and treat attacks of gouty arthritis by reducing inflammation.

In a letter to the editor of *The Lancet* from 30 years ago, physicians in Mexico suggested that until the causative mechanisms of scleroderma were better understood, a rational approach to its treatment would be modification of collagen metabolism. Their group had attempted to do so in a clinical trial with colchicine vs. placebo in 14 patients. After six months, it was converted to an open study of colchicine alone for another six months, although the patients were assessed with photographs and other objective measures at baseline, six months, and 12 months. Researchers concluded that colchicine had a significant impact on skin markers of improvement variously on six to nine patients at different stages of the trial, and the researchers recommended it for further study.

Nonetheless, some 25 years later, a Johns Hopkins University researcher writing in *Expert Opinions on Investigative Drugs* wrote that traditional medications such as colchicine have proved disappointing in clinical practice despite anecdotal evidence of benefit, an opinion shared by a Paris University researcher writing then as well. This is contradicted by a report from New York University in the *Dermatology Online Journal* at about the same time. Researchers stated that colchicine has shown some promise in the treatment of aggressive disease.

Researchers believe that these varying views confirm that in complex diseases such as scleroderma, treatment must be tailored exquisitely to the individual and to each stage of the disease.

For more information see page 1115.

Generic: *Cyclophosphamide* (sye-kloe-FOS-fa-mide)
Brands: *Cytoxan, Neosar*

Cyclophosphamide belongs to a group of drugs known as alkylating drugs. It is approved for various leukemias, lymphomas, cardinomas, and other cancers.

Because cells involved in the immune system are also very sensitive to the effects of alkylating drugs and their function can be blocked, cyclophosphamide is called an immunosuppressant—a medicine that can inhibit the immune response. It has long been used to treat a number of autoimmune diseases such as some of the complications of rheumatoid arthritis, lupus, and scleroderma.

In a review of the American College of Rheumatology scientific sessions from the Johns Hopkins University, physicians discussed the effects of cyclophosphamide/prednisolone therapy on the clinical findings and endothelial functions of patients with early diffuse SSc. Turkish researchers found improvements in skin scores, ability to open the mouth, flex the fingers, decreased joint tenderness, and improved lung function. In addition, there was improvement in lab measures of disease. The Johns Hopkins researchers commented that the clinical improvement was very interesting but noted that kidney function must be closely monitored if corticosteroids are used in early diffuse scleroderma.

A report from New York University in the *Dermatology Online Journal* notes that cyclophosphamide may be useful in the treatment of lung fibrosis, in which researchers at the University of California at Los Angeles and the University of Paris agree. A survey found that more than 92% of members of the American College of Rheumatology would use cyclophosphamide for interstitial lung disease, and that rose to 97% if they were SSc experts.

For more information see page 1123.

Generic: **Cyclosporine** *(si-klo-SPOR-een)*
Brands: *Gengraf, Neoral, Sandimmune*

Cyclosporine is a biochemically powerful immunosuppressant drug. It is approved to prevent the rejection of transplanted kidneys, hearts, and livers. However, it is used off-label to treat people with various arthritides and connective tissue diseases, such as scleroderma, that have not responded well to traditional treatments. It is believed to help because cyclosporine inhibits a sub-group of white blood cells, called T-lymphocytes; these lymphocytes are critical in the immune system and contribute to the development of autoimmune diseases, such as rheumatoid arthritis, lupus, and scleroderma.

Johns Hopkins University physicians offered an abstract from an Italian study of cyclosporine in the treatment of SSc made at the American College of Rheumatology 2000 scientific sessions. Patients were divided to receive isradipine (a calcium channel blocker) plus cyclosporine or isradipine alone. Researchers observed that only in the cyclosporine group did the skin score improve and only in this group was there stabilization of lung function. The study was small but patients were followed for two years. Two patients in this trial developed renal impairment despite the fact that all patients were on a calcium channel blocker. While several studies suggest that cyclosporine may be helpful in scleroderma, the researchers of this study felt its use is limited by the renal toxicity that can be life threatening.

For more information see pages 1125 and 1127.

*Generic: **Methotrexate** (meth-o-TREKS-ate)*
*Brands: **Rheumatrex, Trexall***

Methotrexate belongs to a class of drugs known as antimetabolites, which means they can block the metabolism of cells and help control the immune system. This makes them useful in treating diseases associated with abnormally rapid cell growth, such as cancer and psoriasis. Methotrexate is also a potent immunosuppressive and anti-inflammatory drug and is approved for treatment of a variety of cancers, psoriasis, and rheumatoid arthritis and juvenile rheumatoid arthritis, because it also suppresses inflammation. It seems to work, in part, by altering aspects of immune function, which may play a role in causing rheumatoid arthritis.

According to The Arthritis Society of Canada, two studies showed that more people receiving methotrexate injections had improved skin thickness by 30% and could breathe better by 15% than people receiving a placebo or sugar pill. By the society's standards, they considered this "silver level" evidence that methotrexate decreases skin thickness and such symptoms and breathing problems (the only higher level being gold.)

For more information see page 1312.

*Generic: **Mycophenolate Mofetil***
(my-koe-FEN-oh-late MOE-feh-till)
*Brands: **CellCept, Myfortic***

Mycophenolate mofetil, originally created to prevent the rejection of transplanted organs, is approved for patients receiving kidney and heart transplants. However, many drugs that inhibit the immune system to prevent organ rejection also come to the attention of physicians who take care of people with autoimmune diseases such as scleroderma. Mycophenolate mofetil prevents the proliferation of certain white blood cells, suppresses the synthesis of antibodies, and decreases the recruitment of other white blood cells to sites of inflammation, thus suppressing inflammation overall, all of which can be of use in autoimmune diseases, and it is now also used off-label in several of them, including lupus and scleroderma.

An article in *Rheumatology* reported on a study of 13 patients at the Royal Free Hospital in London to assess the safety and efficacy of antithymocyte globulin, given intravenously for five days, followed by oral mycophenolate mofetil for 12 months. Improvements were seen in skin scores, but hand contractures worsened. Average systemic disease remained stable. One patient died after a scleroderma kidney crisis. However, five patients developed serum sickness early on after the antithymocyte globulin treatment, although this was controlled by corticosteroids. Researchers concluded that the mycophenolate was well tolerated.

For more information see page 1344.

Generic: *Penicillamine* (pen-ah-SILL-amine)
Brands: *Cuprimine, Depen*

Penicillamine is used in the treatment of the genetic disorder Wilson's disease, which causes copper to build up in the body tissues, and it is approved for that disease.

An article in the *Archives of Dermatology* reports on its use in *localized* scleroderma, which has no recognized internal organ involvement and for which there is no proven treatment. They discuss case reports of 11 patients with severe disease, in which penicillamine was judged to have a favorable effect in seven (64%). Improvement began within three to six months, the typical delayed benefit seen with DMARDs. It yielded skin softening and more normal growth in the affected limb in two of the three children. It caused mild, reversible kidney problems in three patients. The researchers concluded that penicillamine may be effective in severe cases of localized scleroderma.

In a survey of physicians on the use of drugs for systemic sclerosis (SSc) reported in the Scleroderma Clinical Trials Consortium, it was found that experts in SSc versus generalist rheumatologists were less likely to use penicillamine for skin, joint, or lung manifestations where a negative trial exists in early diffuse scleroderma.

An article in *Expert Opinions and Investigatory Drugs* from the Johns Hopkins University School of Medicine noted that penicillamine has been disappointing in clinical practice for systemic scleroderma despite anecdotal benefit.

For more information see page 1401.

Generic: **Thalidomide** *(tha-LI-doe-mide)*
Brand: **Thalomid**

Thalidomide is being researched for its immunomodulatory aspects. Studies are under way to assess thalidomide's efficacy in AIDS, some cancers, and a number of arthritides and connective tissue diseases, including scleroderma.

In a review of the American College of Rheumatology 2000 scientific sessions on the Johns Hopkins University website, physicians reported that Thalomid may be potentially helpful in scleroderma. Eleven patients had participated in a study where clinical benefit was reported.

An expert from New York University in *Dermatology Online Journal* wrote that thalidomide is one of the drugs that has shown some promise in the treatment of aggressive disease. In 2005 an article from the University Medicine and Dentistry of New Jersey-New Jersey Medical School, noted thalidomide as one of the possible immunosuppressants to be used.

It is absolutely essential that women avoid pregnancy while taking thalidomide because it definitely causes birth defects. Therefore the government mandates that women register with a special program, use two forms of birth control, and take monthly pregnancy tests.

For more information see page 1505.

Systemic Lupus Erythematosus

Systemic lupus erythematosus (SLE) is a chronic autoimmune disease. It causes inflammation that can affect the joints, skin, kidneys, lungs, heart, nervous system, and other organs of the body. The most common symptoms are fatigue, skin rashes (varying from a marked facial blush to a butterfly shaped blush across the face), and arthritis (usually in the same joints on both sides of the body, often accompanied by a low fever). Symptoms wax (called flares) and wane over time.

Commonly Prescribed (On-Label) Drugs: *Aspirin, Betamethasone, Cortisone, Dexamethasone, Hydroxychloroquine, Methylprednisolone, Prednisolone, Prednisone, Triamcinolone*

OFF-LABEL PRESCRIPTION DRUGS
BREAKTHROUGH OPTIONS

Generic: ***Azathioprine*** *(ay-za-THYE-oh-preen)*
Brand: ***Imuran***

Azathioprine is a drug that prevents certain cells (including those in the immune system) from dividing. It is an immunosuppressant medication approved for the prevention of organ transplant rejection and treatment of rheumatoid arthritis. Although its exact mechanism of action in rheumatoid arthritis is not known, its effect in suppressing the immune system appears to decrease the activity of this illness.

In an article from the University of Texas Health Science Center at San Antonio on *eMedicine*, it was reported that immunosuppressives including azathioprine are used for disease control and that this drug may decrease proliferation of immune cells and result in lower autoimmune activity.

An article in *Lupus* from Ben-Gurion University in Israel noted that azathioprine is widely used for SLE management in patients who need high doses of prednisone, who experience recurrent flares, and those who develop lupus nephritis (kidney disease). An article in *Arthritis & Rheumatism* reported that although a majority of patients with lupus nephritis, given a choice, switched to cyclophosphamide to increase their odds of kidney survival, 31%

refused to do so because of the toxicity risks of cyclophosphamide and remained on azathioprine.

For more information see page 1033.

Generic: **Bromocriptine** *(broe-moe-KRIP-teen)*
Brand: **Parlodel**

Bromocriptine inhibits the release of a hormone called prolactin. A woman's menstrual cycle and breast milk production are affected by such hormone inhibition. Bromocriptine is approved for treating an excess of prolactin called hyperprolactinemia, an excess of growth hormone called acromegaly, certain types of infertility in women, amenorrhea (the absence of menses), and Parkinson's disease.

An article in *Seminars in Arthritis and Rheumatism* from the Montgomery Veterans' Affairs Hospital in Missouri suggests that prolactin may play a causative role in some rheumatic diseases, including lupus. This supports the idea that bromocriptine would therefore be useful in therapy, at least in an add-on role. The investigators reviewed the literature and found two clinical trials showing benefits for lupus, one showing it reduced the number of flares and the other showing it to be as effective as hydroxychloroquine (the most commonly used background drug for treating lupus) in reducing lupus disease activity indices. Researchers concluded that bromocriptine was a relatively safe and effective alternative therapy.

An article in *Lupus* from the Specialty Hospital in Mexico City reported on a study in which 66 people were divided to receive either bromocriptine or placebo and followed for two to 17 months. The SLE Disease Activity Index on the fifth visit decreased significantly in the bromocriptine group compared to controls, as did the average number of flares per patient per month. Researchers concluded that long-term treatment with a low dose of bromocriptine was a safe and effective means of decreasing lupus flares.

For more information see page 1054.

Generic: **Chlorambucil** *(khlor-AM-byoo-sil)*
Brand: **Leukeran**

Chlorambucil is approved for treating a type of leukemia and malignant lymphomas. Further, lymphocytes, white blood cells that are involved in such immune system activities as antibody production, are also sensitive to the impact of alkylating drugs such as chlorambucil. This makes them potentially useful in the treatment of autoimmune diseases such as lupus.

An article on lupus and kidney diseases from the Lupus Foundation of America reports that cytotoxic or immunosuppressive drugs are considered standard treatment for those with serious lupus nephritis. These medications inhibit the immune system, which in turn prevents further kidney damage. Although the most commonly used drug is cyclophosphamide, the article notes that chlorambucil is one of the less frequently used immunosuppressives.

In an article in the *American Heart Journal*, physicians from the Radcliffe Infirmary in Oxford, England treated six lupus patients with deteriorating kidney function who were suffering with severe side effects due to high prednisone doses. With chlorambucil therapy, kidney function improved and prednisone was able to be withdrawn or doses lowered. At the time of the report, the patients remained well at one and one-half to six years after beginning chlorambucil treatment.

In another study reported in the *American Journal of Kidney Disease* from the Maggiore Hospital in Milan, Italy, a small trial comparing methylprednisolone alone to methylprednisolone with chlorambucil concluded that the combination may induce a more stable remission of nephrotic syndrome and better protect long-term kidney function.

For more information see page 1079.

Generic: **Cyclophosphamide** *(sye-kloe-FOS-fa-mide)*
Brands: **Cytoxan, Neosar**

Cyclophosphamide is approved for treating various leukemias and cancers. In addition, alkylating drugs such as cyclophosphamide also affect some cells in the immune system, so cyclophosphamide is also referred to as an immunosuppressant.

Because of its immunosuppressant benefits, cyclophosphamide is also used off-label as a therapy for autoimmune diseases including lupus.

In an article from the University of Texas Health Science Center at San Antonio on *eMedicine*, it was noted that immunosuppressives are important for disease control and that cyclophosphamide may act by interfering with the growth of normal cells.

In an article in *Transplantation Proceedings*, researchers from the Military Medical Academy in Belgrade, Yugoslavia, discussed the use of high doses of cyclophosphamide in the treatment of severe SLE. They noted that the protocol of the National Institute of Health (NIH) for use of this drug, in cases where the kidneys or central nervous system are affected, is used around the world. They reported on their 10-year experience with high monthly "pulse" doses of intravenous cyclophosphamide over six months (and then at a maximum of six more times at three-month intervals) in their treatment of the most severe forms of lupus in 178 patients. Complete remission was achieved in 75% and incomplete remission in 10%, with a positive effect usually observed after a third pulse.

For more information see page 1123.

*Generic: **Cyclosporine** (si-klo-SPOR-een)*
*Brands: **Gengraf, Neoral, Sandimmune***

Cyclosporine is a powerful immunosuppressive drug that prolongs the survival of multiple organ transplants. It is approved for the prevention of cardiac, kidney, and liver transplant rejection. Cyclosporine also has been shown to suppress certain aspects of the immune system that also may be helpful in autoimmune diseases such as lupus. It inhibits a group of white blood cells, known as T-lymphocytes, which contribute to the development and maintenance of lupus and other autoimmune diseases. Therefore it is sometimes used to treat lupus, rheumatoid arthritis, and other autoimmune diseases that have not responded to conventional therapies. In this regard, it is considered a disease modifying antirheumatic drug (DMARD) because it not only decreases the pain and swelling of arthritis but it may also prevent joint damage and reduce the risk of long term disability.

The Lupus Foundation of America reports that cytotoxic or immunosuppressive drugs are deemed standard treatment for patients with serious lupus nephritis. These drugs inhibit the immune system, which in turn prevents further kidney damage. Although the most commonly used medication cited is cyclophosphamide, researchers note that cyclosporine is one of the less frequently used immunosuppressives.

An article in *Clinical Nephrology* from physicians at the Columbia University College of Physicians and Surgeons reports that although cyclosporine has long been used to treat patients with systemic lupus, only a few of these patients have had lupus membranous nephropathy. They did a pilot study to assess cyclosporine in 10 nephrotic patients with the problem, using the medication alone in two patients or in conjunction in the rest, for up to 43 months. All experienced symptomatic improvement, and serum creatinine was not significantly increased at the end of the study period. Only three had systemic lupus flares requiring additional immunosuppressive therapy. Researchers observed that repeat kidney biopsies in five showed a decrease in the lupus activity index.

For more information see pages 1125 and 1127.

*Generic: **Methotrexate** (meth-o-TREKS-ate)*
*Brands: **Rheumatrex, Trexall***

Methotrexate belongs to a class of drugs known as antimetabolites that prevent certain cells (including those in the immune system) from dividing. This helps slow or halt the progression of cancer, which is why methotrexate is approved for the treatment of leukemia and certain other cancers. Because it also is a powerful suppressor of key factors in the immune system and therefore inhibits inflammation, methotrexate is also approved to treat rheumatoid arthritis and juvenile rheumatoid arthritis. Drugs that have worked for rheumatoid arthritis have often been tried for other rheumatic diseases. According to the American College of Rheumatology (ACR), "methotrexate is one of the most effective and commonly used medicines to treat various forms of arthritis and other rheumatic conditions." Further, it notes that since 1988, when methotrexate gained FDA approval for rheumatoid arthritis, lupus has been among these diseases so treated.

In an update on the treatment of SLE in the *American Family Physician*, an expert in lupus care reported that when patients need prednisone doses greater than 10 mg per day, immunosuppressive drugs should be added to help lower the steroid dose. The researcher recommended low dosages of methotrexate once a week as extremely effective in this regard. Further, it was pointed out that it is now standard practice to prescribe folic acid to counter some of the minor side effects of methotrexate.

Because methotrexate can be toxic to the liver, it should not be taken if you have liver disease. Further, you should not drink alcohol while taking methotrexate in order to reduce the risk of cirrhosis.

For more information see page 1312.

Generic: *Mycophenolate Mofetil*
(my-koe-FEN-oh-late MOE-feh-till)
Brands: *CellCept, Myfortic*

Mycophenolate mofetil was developed to prevent the rejection of transplanted organs. It modulates the immune system through multiple mechanisms. Among them, it prevents the proliferation of certain white blood cells, suppresses the synthesis of antibodies, and decreases the recruitment of other white blood cells to the sites of inflammation, thus suppressing inflammation overall. Because of these mechanisms, it is now also used off-label in the treatment of certain autoimmune and inflammatory diseases such as lupus.

According to a patient education report on lupus therapy from the American College of Rheumatology, aggressive therapy is needed for the more serious and potentially life-threatening complications of lupus. Recently, mycophenolate mofetil has been used to treat severe lupus kidney disease.

For inducing remission in severe lupus nephritis and systemic necrotizing vasculitis, as defined by the National Institutes of Health, the combination of cyclophosphamide and steroids may be used. After such induction, maintenance of remission with cyclophosphamide long term is limited because of toxicity. Ongoing studies are comparing the benefits of mycophenolate mofetil in maintaining remission.

However, researchers at the Mayo Clinic have already shown that mycophenolate mofetil is effective for managing symptoms of systemic lupus in patients whose condition does not affect the kidneys. Researchers report that the drug is well tolerated and has fewer side effects than many other medications used to treat lupus.

For more information see page 1344.

Generic: **Rituximab** *(ri-TUK-si-mab)*
Brand: **Rituxan**

Rituximab is a genetically engineered antibody that targets B cells and eliminates them from the blood. Rituximab is approved for the treatment of non-Hodgkin's lymphoma. However, B cells are a type of white blood cell that plays a central role in the development of lupus.

An article in *Arthritis & Rheumatism* reported on research with rituximab at the University of Rochester in New York. Seventeen patients were divided into low-, intermediate-, and high-dose groups and received one or four infusions over the course of a month at one of two different doses. The primary clinical measurement was the SLAM index—a global lupus activity index that evaluates how patients feel and all the organ systems. In addition, laboratory measures of B cell depletion were done. A majority of participants—11 of 17—had profound B cell depletion, and their SLAM score was significantly improved by two to three months. At the end of a year, those who had gotten better continued to stay well with no difference in how they felt. After the end of the study, three of the 17 went into remission and remain on no medications whatsoever.

According to an article in the Alliance for Lupus Research newsletter *Lupus Research Update*, researchers believe that rituximab appears to be a promising drug that is a safe and effective treatment, at least for the majority of people who experience profound B cell depletion. In some people it may produce permanent remission. In others, it may only induce a remission that must be sustained with other drugs, albeit much milder drugs than would otherwise be needed. However, researchers feel that large clinical trials are needed to prove that it works and learn how to best use it.

For more information see page 1457.

Generic: **Thalidomide** *(tha-LI-doe-mide)*
Brand: **Thalomid**

Research into thalidomide's immunomodulatory effects has led it to be FDA approved for use in treating leprosy symptoms. According to the National Institute of Health (NIH), studies are also being conducted to determine the effectiveness of thalidomide in treating symptoms associated with AIDS, some cancers, and a number of rheumatic diseases, including lupus.

An article from the University of Texas Health Science Center at San Antonio on *eMedicine* includes thalidomide in its list of recommended immunosuppressive drugs for lupus.

An article in the *American Journal of Medicine* from St. Thomas' Hospital in London reported the use of thalidomide for resistant cutaneous lupus unresponsive to antimalarials, prednisolone, methotrexate, azathioprine, and cyclosporine. A group of 48 patients were variously given one of three different doses. They had an excellent response rate, including 60% with complete remission, 21% with partial remission, and 19% who did not respond.

For more information see page 1505.

Systemic Scleroderma

See Scleroderma

Systemic Sclerosis

See Scleroderma

Temporal Arteritis

Temporal arteritis (TA), also known as giant cell arteritis, is an inflammatory disease of the arteries (blood vessels) in the scalp and head, especially right around the temples. Some people who have TA also have symptoms of polymyalgia rheumatica (PMR). Five to 15% of those with PMR at some point are diagnosed with TA. Both diseases may occur together, separately, or one following the other. Treatment is similar, but the threat in temporal arteritis is vision loss without rapid treatment.

Commonly Prescribed (On-Label) Drugs: Infliximab

OFF-LABEL PRESCRIPTION DRUG
BREAKTHROUGH OPTION

Brand: **Methotrexate** *(meth-o-TREKS-ate)*
Brands: **Rheumatrex, Trexall**

Methotrexate is one of a group of drugs called antimetabolites that block the metabolism of cells and help control the immune system, which makes them helpful in the therapy of cancer and psoriasis and other illnesses associated with abnormally rapid cell growth. It's also a powerful anti-inflammatory drug.

An article in the *Annals of Internal Medicine* from the Systemic Vasculitis Study Group of the Italian Society for Rheumatology presented a study in 72 newly diagnosed PMR patients. They divided the patients to receive prednisone and placebo or prednisone plus methotrexate (an immunosuppressive drug) and subsequently lowered the prednisone doses on a regular schedule until it was fully withdrawn quickly. Methotrexate or placebo was given weekly until the end of the 24-month follow-up. Participants were monitored for number of flares (which were treated), cumulative dose of steroid, and adverse events, to discern whether those taking methotrexate were able to more effectively taper prednisone without flare-ups. Researchers observed that the methotrexate group experienced significantly fewer relapses (45% vs. 85%) and received a significantly smaller total dose of prednisone.

An article in *Arthritis & Rheumatism* reported on a study from the United States that had essentially the opposite result. Researchers enrolled 80 TA patients, found no difference in relapse rates between those treated with prednisone alone or prednisone plus methotrexate. However, according to researchers, the design varied somewhat in that the American study called for prednisone to be tapered to an every-other-day dose, which could explain the conflicting results.

For more information see page 1312.

MUSCULAR DISORDERS

Dystrophia Myotonica

See Myotonic Dystrophy

Muscular Dystrophy

Muscular dystrophy (MD) is a general term for a group of genetic diseases characterized by progressive weakness and degeneration of the skeletal muscles that control movement. The most common is Duchenne, which primarily affects male children, progresses rapidly, and leads to an inability to walk by early adolescence and need for a respirator by age 20.

Commonly Prescribed (On-Label) Drugs: None

OFF-LABEL PRESCRIPTION DRUGS
BREAKTHROUGH OPTIONS

*Generic: **Albuterol** (al-BYOO-ter-ole)*
*Brands: **Proventil, Ventolin, Volmax***

Albuterol is a drug normally given by inhaler for the prevention and treatment of asthma, and for the treatment of bronchitis, emphysema, and obstructive pulmonary disease. It is a drug that belongs to a class known as "beta-2 agonists" and it has long been thought to have positive effects on muscle. Evidence suggests it may increase muscle protein synthesis and slow muscle protein breakdown.

When given by inhaler as done for asthma, albuterol has no effect on skeletal muscle. However, as reported in *Neurology*, a slow-release oral preparation of albuterol has been shown to improve symptoms of MD in children in a small pilot study over three months. The children taking albuterol showed improvements in muscle strength, mostly in their thigh, compared to those taking placebo. Other studies have shown that albuterol may lead to growth of muscle tissue. However, no benefit was found in muscle function tests. The researchers recommended longer-term studies.

For more information see page 991.

Generic: **Prednisolone** *(pred-NISS-oh-lone)*
Brands: **Prelone, Predalone**

Prednisolone is a corticosteroid drug approved to treat numerous cancers and autoimmune, inflammatory, and allergic diseases.

According to an article in *Neuromuscular Disorders*, the potential benefits of corticosteroids in the treatment of MD was first demonstrated in 1974, and the usefulness of prednisolone was subsequently shown to improve muscle function in a study in 1987. Two years later they showed improvement in muscle strength. Over the years, efforts have been made to find the right dose to obtain maximum benefits with minimum side effects. In an article in the journal from a group at Hammersmith Hospital in London, an effective, low-dosage, intermittent dosage was recommended.

According to an article in *Postgraduate Medicine*, most clinicians in the United States prescribe prednisone, which in many instances is effective. However, in many European countries, prednisolone is the most widely used corticosteroid. Patients with liver disease are sometimes unable to metabolize prednisone (which is technically a prohormone, a precursor to a hormone) and may be given prednisolone instead (in the same dose as prednisone).

For more information see page 1428.

Generic: **Prednisone** *(pred-NIS-zone)*
Brands: **Deltasone, Liquid Pred, Meticorten, Orasone, Sterapred**

Prednisone is one of a group of drugs variously known as corticosteroids, or steroids. They are related to the hormone cortisol made by the adrenal glands, and are approved for treatment of a number of malignancies as well as various allergic, autoimmune, and inflammatory diseases.

An article in *Neuromuscular Disorders* discusses the history of steroid use in MD. Their benefits were first shown more than 30 years ago, and they have been in use ever since as doctors have investigated various dosages to achieve maximum benefit with the least toxicity.

Another article in *Neuromuscular Disorders* discusses causative elements of MD and how they relate to treatments. They conclude that the work suggests that prednisone exerts a direct effect on muscle survival.

An article in the *Archives of Neurology* presents a study from the Netherlands comparing placebo with prednisone on the theory that the adverse effects of prednisone outweigh its benefits. The investigators concluded that the prednisone group did better because, although adverse effects were present, they did not impair quality of life and motor functions were preserved.

For more information see page 1429.

Myodystrophy

See Muscular Dystrophy

Myotonia Atrophica

See Myotonic Dystrophy

Myotonia Dystrophica

See Myotonic Dystrophy

Myotonic Dystrophy

Myotonic dystrophy (MMD) is one of a group of genetic diseases involving progressive weakness and degeneration of the skeletal muscles that control movement. People with MMD have a better prognosis than those with muscular dystrophy. However, they have prolonged muscle spasms in the fingers and facial muscles; a floppy-footed, high-stepping gait; cataracts; cardiac abnormalities; and endocrine disturbances.

Commonly Prescribed (On-Label) Drugs: *None*

OFF-LABEL PRESCRIPTION DRUGS
BREAKTHROUGH OPTIONS

Generic: **Mexiletine** *(MEKS-i-le-teen)*
Brand: **Mexitil**

Mexiletine is approved to treat a kind of abnormal heart rhythm called ventricular arrhythmia. It does this by slowing nerve impulses in the heart and making the tissue of the heart less sensitive. Its antiarrhythmic affect has to do with its ability to inhibit the inward sodium current, and that relates to its role in MMD, one type of which is called a "sodium channelopathy" because these patients have a genetic mutation in their sodium channel. According to an article in *Neurological Science*, in these patients, during rest after a period of exercise, there is an inactivation in their sodium channels with a loss of electrical excitability, leading to a paralytic attack.

An article in *Acta Neurologica of Scandinavia* from the Warsaw Medical Academy of Poland reported that disopyramide, phenytoin, tocainide, and mexiletine were compared in 30 patients with MMD. Mexiletine and tocainide were found to be the most potent anti-MMD drugs. Their efficacy was explained by their fast-blocking effect on the sodium channels in the muscle membrane. However, researchers state that their benefits must be weighed against the risk of blood problems.

For more information see page 1324.

Generic: **Nifedipine** *(nye-FED-i-peen)*
Brands: **Adalat CC, Apo-Nifed (PA), Novo-Nifedin, Nu-Nifed, Procardia**

Nifedipine belongs to a class of drugs called calcium channel blockers. It is approved for hypertension. While it is not clear how it dilates blood vessels to lower blood pressure, it is believed to have something to do with the way it regulates calcium transport into and out of cells.

According to an article in the *Journal of Neurology, Neurosurgery and Psychiatry* from Southern General Hospital in Glasgow, UK, abnormal calcium transport may be implicated in the membrane defect in MMD. A clinical trial comparing two different doses of nifedipine and placebo was performed in 10 patients with MMD and assessed by measuring finger extension. Researchers observed significant improvement using the drug.

For more information see page 1360.

Steinert Disease

See Myotonic Dystrophy

MISCELLANEOUS CONDITIONS

A variety of other conditions can affect the musculoskeletal system. Among those that are most common and troublesome are chronic fatigue syndrome, bursitis, and tendinitis.

Chronic Fatigue Syndrome

Chronic fatigue syndrome (CFS) is persistent fatigue, not due to exertion nor eased by rest, that results in substantial cuts in occupational, educational, social, or personal activities. Further, the syndrome occurs simultaneously with four or more of the following that do not predate the fatigue and have lasted six months or longer: substantial impairment in short-term memory or concentration; sore throat; tender lymph nodes; muscle pain; multi-joint pain without swelling or redness; headaches of a new type, pattern, or severity; unrefreshing sleep; and post-exertional malaise lasting more than 24 hours.

Commonly Prescribed (On-Label) Drugs: *None*

OFF-LABEL PRESCRIPTION DRUGS
BREAKTHROUGH OPTIONS

Generic: Tricyclic Antidepressants such as ***Amitriptyline*** *(a-mee-TRIP-ti-leen),* ***Clomipramine*** *(kloe-MI-pra-meen),* ***Desipramine*** *(des-IP-ra-meen),* ***Doxepin*** *(DOKS-e-pin),* ***Imipramine*** *(im-IP-ra-meen),* and ***Nortriptyline*** *(nor-TRIP-ti-leen)*
Brands: ***Elavil (amitriptyline), Anafranil (clomipramine), Norpramin (desipramine), Prudoxin, Sinequan (doxepin), Tofranil, Tofranil-PM (imipramine), Aventyl, Pamelor (nortriptyline)***

Low doses of tricyclic antidepressants have been prescribed for chronic fatigue syndrome patients to improve sleep and to relieve mild, generalized pain. The doses used are generally much lower than those used to treat depression. Some adverse reactions include dry mouth, drowsiness, weight gain, and elevated heart rate. *Health-cares.net* reports they may provide benefits by promoting deep sleep and inhibiting pain pathways in the nervous system.

An article in the *American Family Physician* reported that tricyclic antidepressants offer various benefits, including antidepressant effects, anti-inflammatory properties, effects on central skeletal muscle relaxation, and enhancement of pain-inhibiting factors through various brain pathways. Its major action seems to be that last one, that is, affecting how the brain perceives certain messages. The article reported on several studies using amitriptyline in CFS. In one study, after eight weeks, it yielded significant improvement in local pain, stiffness, and sleep pattern, but had little effect on tenderness.

In another study reported in the article, an amitriptyline/naproxen combination was compared with either alone. Those on amitriptyline alone or in combination had improvement in pain, sleep difficulties, fatigue on awakening, and tender point scores. Researchers noted that patients receiving combination therapy had no significant improvement in pain, compared with patients taking amitriptyline alone. Naproxen was not effective as a single drug.

An article by the National Library Society reported that the most widely used treatment for CFS is tricyclic antidepressants in low doses, and they specifically cite amitriptyline or doxepin. For unusually low doses, liquid forms may be necessary. An article from the Mayo Clinic reported the benefits of tricyclic antidepressants, again noting amitriptyline, desipramine, and nortriptyline. An article in *Biological Psychiatry* reported the benefits of nortriptyline in chronic fatigue syndrome based on a double blind, placebo-controlled study.

For more information see pages 1009, 1105, 1132, 1154, 1230, and 1178.

Generic: *Atenolol* (a-TEN-oh-lole)
Brand: *Tenormin*

Atenolol belongs to a class of drugs called beta-blockers and is used to reduce blood pressure, abnormal heart rhythms, and the workload of the heart. It is approved for people who have had heart attacks to reduce cardiovascular mortality.

Reports from Johns Hopkins University that have been published in the *Journal of the American Medical Association* and *The Lancet* suggest that some patients with chronic fatigue syndrome (CFS) may have neurally mediated hypotension (low blood pressure). This was based on a test in which patients were placed on a table that is suddenly tilted and their reactions measured. Abnormal responses of CFS patients have ranged from 25% to 96%.

According to the U.S. Centers for Disease Control, all CFS patients do not respond to treatment with antihypotensive medications, and the general use of such drugs may be harmful. However, they may be useful in specific circumstances, such as in patients who have orthostatic hypotension—a condition in which blood pressure drops suddenly when you stand up—and atenolol has benefitted such patients.

For more information see page 1027.

Generic: Corticosteroids such as ***Fludrocortisone***
(floo-droe-KOR-ti-sone) and ***Hydrocortisone***
(hi-dro-KOR-ti-sone)
Brands: ***Florinef (fludrocortisone), Cortef***
(hydrocortisone)

Hydrocortisone and fludrocortisone both belong to a class of drugs called corticosteroids. Steroids are typically used to treat malignancies and autoimmune, anti-inflammatory, and allergic diseases, as is commonly the case with hydrocortisone. Fludrocortisone is used specifically to treat Addison's disease and adreno-genital syndromes where excessive amounts of sodium are lost in the urine.

Studies from Johns Hopkins University, published in the *Journal of the American Medical Association* and *The Lancet*, suggest that some patients with chronic fatigue syndrome (CFS) may have neurally mediated hypotension (low blood pressure). Researchers based this on a test in which patients were placed on a table that is suddenly tilted and their reactions measured. Abnormal responses of CFS patients have ranged from 25% to 96%. Hypotension often responds to increasing salt retention in the body.

According to a report from the U.S. Centers for Disease Control (CDC), fludrocortisone has been prescribed for CFS patients who have had a positive tilt table test. However, in a study reported in the *Journal of the American Medical Association*, fludrocortisone alone was not effective in the general treatment of CFS patients. Nonetheless, the investigators believe that further studies are needed to determine whether other medications or combination therapy are more effective in treating orthostatic intolerance in CFS patients.

Given the overlap between the symptoms of Addison's disease and CFS, some researchers theorized that low cortisol levels may be an issue for CFS patients and a cause of their symptoms. An article in *The Lancet* from researchers in London and Cambridge, UK, reports on a study with 32 patients treated with low doses of hydrocortisone for one month and placebo in another month, the order of treatment randomly assigned. Fatigue levels dropped by 7.2 points for those on hydrocortisone and by 3.3 points for those on placebo.

For more information see pages 1189 and 1222.

Generic: Selective Serotonin Reuptake Inhibitors such as **Fluoxetine** *(floo-OKS-e-teen)*, **Paroxetine** *(pa-ROKS-e-teen)*, and **Sertraline** *(SER-tra-leen)*
Brands: **Prozac, Prozac Weekly, Sarafem (fluoxetine), Paxil, Paxil CR (paroxetine), Zoloft (sertraline)**

Fluoxetine, sertraline, and paroxetine belong to a class of drugs called selective serotonin reuptake inhibitors (SSRIs). They are approved to treat depression. The impact of SSRIs on CFS seems to derive from their ability to interfere with the reabsorption of a neurotransmitter called serotonin, so as to make it more available. This affects the way the brain perceives pain because the pain message simply does not get through the network. However, this does not appear to be the only method of action, although how it fully works remains unknown.

These antidepressants have been used to treat depression in CFS patients, although non-depressed CFS patients receiving treatment with SSRIs have also been found by some health care providers to benefit from this treatment as well as or better than depressed patients, according to the U.S. Centers for Disease Control (CDC). A number of adverse reactions, varying with the specific drug, may be experienced, but include agitation, sleep disturbances, increased fatigue, weight gain, and sexual dysfunction. A report from the Mayo Clinic indicates the benefits of SSRIs, and specifically mentioned fluoxetine, paroxetine, and sertraline.

For more information see pages 1192, 1395, and 1468.

Generic: **Midrodine** *(MI-doe-dreen)*
Brand: **ProAmatine**

Midrodine belongs to a class of drugs called alpha agonists that treat low blood pressure. However, midrodine also treats a special type of problem blood pressure called orthostatic hypotension in which the blood pressure drops suddenly when you stand up, leading to dizziness or fainting.

The U.S. Centers for Disease Control (CDC) does not recommend general use of antihypotensive drugs. However, it recognizes that such medications may be useful in specific circumstances, such as those who have been identified by an abnormal tilt test, and the CDC identifies midodrine as one drug that may be useful in selected patients that have been identified by this test. The test (involving reclining on a table, and the position is changed suddenly) identifies people with a rare disorder of the autonomic nervous system. According to researchers, articles in support of the theory have been recently published widely.

Midodrine, a drug that directly increases blood pressure, may be useful in selected patients identified by an abnormal tilt test, according to the CDC. Increased salt and water intake is also recommended for these patients but should be done only under supervision of a health care provider. The drug is also mentioned as beneficial for CFS in an article from the Mayo Clinic on cnn.com.

For more information see page 1327.

*Generic: **Modafinil** (moe-DAF-i-nil)*
*Brand: **Provigil***

Modafinil is a central nervous system stimulant that alters the amounts of some natural substances in the brain that control sleep and wakefulness. It also enhances wakefulness, mood, and memory, but, in contrast to traditional stimulants such as amphetamines or caffeine, modafinil is not apt to cause jitteriness and anxiety. Modafinil is approved to treat the excessive sleepiness caused by narcolepsy, which causes severe daytime sleepiness, and shift work sleep disorder. The drug is also used to prevent excessive daytime sleepiness in people with obstructive sleep apnea.

When fatigue represents lethargy or daytime sleepiness in people with CFS, treatment with modafinil may be useful. An article in *Human Psychopharmacology* reported a case of a man with CFS who suffered with severe fatigue, general malaise, generalized aches and pains, and poor sleep. He had suffered for 13 years and eventually sought psychiatric help. He was prescribed various antidepressants to no avail. A course of modafinil was then prescribed and was successful in treating the debilitating fatigue with energy levels improved from 20% to 60% of optimum within a few months. Researchers observed that he was able to return to part-time work and, at last, to enjoy a good quality of life.

For more information see page 1338.

Tendinitis/Bursitis

Bursa are small bags of fluid throughout our bodies at points where muscles and tendons glide over bone. They are designed to decrease friction between surfaces that move in opposite directions. Bursitis is inflammation of bursa that occurs when repetitive movement has been prolonged, caused too much pressure, or a bruise or traumatic injury has occurred. A tendon is a flexible band of tissue that connects muscle to bone, thus enabling movement. When a tendon is inflamed, the action of pulling the muscle becomes irritating and painful, yielding tendinitis.

Commonly Prescribed (On-Label) Drugs: *Betamethasone, Cortisone, Dexamethasone, Methylprednisolone, Naproxen, Prednisolone, Prednisone, Sulindac, Triamcinolone*

OFF-LABEL PRESCRIPTION DRUG
BREAKTHROUGH OPTION

Generic: **Diclofenac Sodium** *(dye-KLOE-fen-ak)*
Brands: **Voltaren, Voltaren-XR**

Diclofenac sodium is one of a class of drugs known as non-steroidal anti-inflammatory drugs (NSAIDs). They are commonly prescribed to reduce inflammation and pain in various types of arthritis. It is approved for rheumatoid and osteoarthritis, and synovitis (inflammation of the synovium inside a joint). NSAIDs work by interfering with enzymes that promote inflammation and, therefore, they are often prescribed for other types of inflammation.

An article in the *International Journal of Clinical Practice* from physicians in Germany and Switzerland assigned 1,222 patients with shoulder bursitis/tendinitis to receive either diclofenac or another NSAID, nimesulide (not available in the United States), for two weeks. Researchers found that the two drugs were therapeutically equivalent, with a slight superiority for nimesulide.

The primary problem with NSAIDs is their gastrointestinal (GI) side effects placing the patient at risk for ulcers. Therefore, it is sometimes prescribed together with misoprostol, which can prevent such toxicity. An article in *Drugs* from the Center of Medicine and Sport Trauma in Charleroi, Belgium, reported on a study of tendinitis/bursitis patients in which 185 were given misoprostol/diclofenac while 187 were given diclofenac alone for 14 days. While similar improvements were seen with both patients, abdominal pain, nausea, and vomiting occurred somewhat more frequently with the combination therapy.

For more information see page 1143.

NEUROPATHIC PAIN DISORDERS

CHRONIC PAIN DISORDERS

Pain, such as from stubbing your toe, has a physical cause. However, pain can also be generated by your body's nerves without a physical source. This type of pain is called neuropathic pain, and appears to have no cause, making treatment difficult. For some people neuropathic pain is unresponsive to traditional forms of therapy and may lead to serious disability.

Chronic Neuropathic Pain

Neuropathic pain is associated with abnormal functioning of the nervous system. The nerves that affect the perception of pain behave in abnormal ways in patients with neuropathic pain. Neuropathic pain often seems to have no cause. For example, you may feel pain in a limb that has been amputated (phantom limb pain). Stimuli that cause little or no pain in healthy people can cause very intense, long lasting neuropathic pain, which is very difficult to treat. Many painkillers, including some very powerful drugs such as morphine, have little effect on neuropathic pain. For this reason, there is a great deal of interest by researchers in using drugs not approved as painkillers to treat neuropathic pain.

Commonly Prescribed (On-Label) Drugs: *None*

OFF-LABEL PRESCRIPTION DRUGS
BREAKTHROUGH OPTIONS

Generic: Tricylic antidepressants such as ***Amitriptyline***
(a-mee-TRIP-ti-leen), ***Clomipramine*** *(kloe-MI-pra-meen)*,
Desipramine *(des-IP-ra-meen)*, and ***Nortriptyline***
(nor-TRIP-ti-leen)
Brands: ***Elavil (amitriptyline), Anafranil (clomipramine),***
Norpramin (desipramine), Aventyl, Pamelor
(nortriptyline)

Tricyclic antidepressants function by increasing the amount of the
neurotransmitters (chemicals in the brain) norepinephrine,
dopamine, and serotonin. Amitriptyline has been studied in
women recovering from breast cancer surgery. These women had
postmastectomy syndrome, a group of symptoms including pain
in the breast scar and the arm nearby. This pain was neuropathic,
caused by the cutting of nerves and subsequent changes in the remaining nerve cells after breast cancer surgery. Twenty women
started in this study, but four dropped out before study completion. Four withdrew from the study because of adverse effects of
the drug, mainly severe fatigue, but they had experienced pain relief while taking the drug. Fifteen of the 20 women who completed
the study had a major reduction (at least 50%) in the intensity of
their pain. According to researchers, the drug treatment was effective in reducing both the scar pain and arm pain. In spite of the effectiveness of amitriptyline in reducing pain, only three of the 15
women who finished the study wanted to continue taking the
drug. The other 12 cited the adverse effects of the drug (tiredness,
dry mouth, and constipation) as reasons for discontinuing.

Two other tricyclic antidepressants, clomipramine and nortriptyline, were studied in a group of 39 patients with severe neuropathic pain. Researchers concluded that both drugs were significantly better than placebo for reducing pain, and clomipramine
was more effective than nortriptyline. Additionally, researchers
noted that both drugs have fewer and milder side effects than
amitriptyline and work essentially as well.

For more information see pages 1009, 1105, 1132, and 1378.

Generic: **Bupropion** *(byoo-PROE-pee-on)*
Brands: **Wellbutrin, Wellbutrin SR, Wellbutrin XL, Zyban**

Bupropion is an antidepressant that is chemically different from other antidepressants. It has fewer side effects than the tricyclic antidepressants such as amitriptyline and imipramine and is tolerated well by most patients.

At the University of Arizona Neurology Clinic and Pain Clinic in Tucson, Arizona, the effect of bupropion was studied in 41 outpatients with chronic neuropathic pain. They had all experienced pain for at least three months, and some for more than 10 years. Bupropion caused a significant decrease in their pain, starting after only two weeks of treatment. Many other medications take six to eight weeks to be effective. Pain continued to decrease from week two to week six. Approximately 75% of the patients reported that their pain was improved or much improved with bupropion. The average reduction in pain scores was 30%. The patients also assessed their quality of life while taking the drug and reported better overall health, functioning, and enjoyment of life. When the patients discontinued bupropion, their pain recurred after two weeks. The researchers observed that the patients rated the drug's side effects as mild, and the side effects tended to decrease with time.

For more information see page 1058.

Generic: **Carbamazepine** *(kar-ba-MAZ-e-peen)*
Brands: **Carbatrol, Epitol, Tegretol, Tegretol XR**

Carbamazepine was originally developed as an anticonvulsant drug for epilepsy. It is now approved for the treatment of trigeminal neuralgia as well. According to researchers, although it is not known with certainty how it works, it probably affects the electrical activity of brain nerve cells, which are critical for seizures and for pain. Although it is safe for most people, a very small number of those who take it develop aplastic anemia, which is potentially life threatening. For this reason, physicians recommend that patients taking carbamazepine need to have their complete blood cell (CBC) counts monitored.

The effects of carbamazepine have been studied in 43 patients who had severe neuropathic pain for years. Conventional medications, including morphine, had little effect on their pain. Before the study, their pain was relieved by electric stimulation of their spinal cord (spinal cord stimulation, SCS). During the study, the SCS was turned off temporarily and their pain returned. Then they received carbamazepine, morphine, or a placebo for eight days. Researchers allowed them to resume SCS at any time if they could not tolerate the pain. The amount of time after discontinuation of SCS before severe pain returned was compared for treatment with carbamazepine, morphine, and placebo. The researchers observed that there was a significant delay in return of the pain when the patients took carbamazepine, but not morphine or placebo. The researchers concluded that carbamazepine can be useful for severe neuropathic pain, even when treatment with morphine is not successful.

For more information see page 1068.

*Generic: **Gabapentin** (GA-ba-pen-tin)*
*Brand: **Neurontin***

The chemical structure of gabapentin is similar to the structure of the neurotransmitter (brain chemical) GABA (gamma-aminobutyric acid). Gabapentin is approved for treatment of epilepsy and post-herpetic neuralgia, but has been used off-label by physicians for many other medical conditions.

Spine documented a trial in which gabapentin was used to treat severe neuropathic pain after a spinal cord injury. The study involved 20 paraplegic patients (age range 20 and 65 years), seven women and 13 men, all of whom had complete spinal cord injury at the thoracic or lumbar level and had had neuropathic pain for more than six months. Gabapentin decreased the intensity and frequency of pain; relieved all neuropathic pain symptoms except for the itchy, sensitive, dull and cold types; and improved the overall quality of life. Researchers concluded that gabapentin is an effective treatment for patients experiencing neuropathic pain following a spinal cord injury. Additionally, they recommend that doses be administered at low levels and gradually increased.

An Italian study tested the effects of gabapentin when used in addition to opioids (morphine, codeine, and related drugs) to treat severe neuropathic pain caused by cancer. The study included 121 cancer patients taking opioid drugs, which only partially relieved their pain. They continued taking these drugs and were given gabapentin or placebo in addition. Gabapentin was significantly more effective than placebo in reducing the cancer patients' pain.

For more information see page 1206.

Generic: *Lamotrigine* (la-MOE-tri-jeen)
Brand: *Lamictal*

Lamictal is an anticonvulsant drug typically used to treat epilepsy. In a study, two patients with chronic neuropathy were given lamotrigine. Researchers observed that lamotrigine reduced their pain to the extent that they were able to discontinue or reduce the dose of their other painkillers.

Neuropathic pain occurs commonly in HIV patients. At Mount Sinai Medical Center in New York, a study of 42 patients with HIV was conducted. The patients received lamotrigine or placebo for 14 weeks. Of 42 enrolled patients, 13 did not complete the study—five of whom dropped out due to rash. In the remaining 29, 20 patients received placebo and nine received lamotrigine. The pain scores between the placebo and lamotrigine groups at the start of the study were not significantly different. However, at the end of the trial, the lamotrigine group had a significant reduction of pain compared to the placebo group. Researchers concluded that the drug effectively decreased the patients' average pain, but did not change their peak worst pain.

Chronic neuropathic pain is also observed commonly after a nerve is cut. Lamotrigine was studied in six such patients after attempts to control their pain with surgery or medication failed. Lamotrigine decreased the patients' burning or shooting pains and also decreased the frequency of their pain attacks.

Pain is a significant problem in patients with spinal cord injury (SCI). About two thirds of these patients develop neuropathic pain, and the pain is severe in about one third of them. Lamotrigine was tested on 30 patients with SCI, and the results were mixed. The drug had no significant effect in patients with complete SCI. However, researchers noted that in patients with incomplete SCI, the drug caused a significant decrease in pain at or below the level of the SCI.

Twenty patients whose neuropathic pain was not successfully controlled by other drugs were treated with lamotrigine alone or with a combination of lamotrigine and morphine. Overall, researchers observed that the patients tended to be helped by lamotrigine alone or in combination with morphine.

For more information see page 1268.

Generic: *Lidocaine* (LYE-doe-kane)
Brands: *Anestacon, Xylocaine*

Lidocaine is an anesthetic (numbing) drug available as a cream and solution for intravenous use. When given intravenously, it acts on receptors in the brain to affect the passage of sodium ions into and out of neurons.

At the Department of Neurology and Danish Pain Research Center in Denmark, 24 patients with spinal cord injury received either lidocaine or placebo intravenously for a period of 30 minutes. Lidocaine, but not placebo, significantly reduced pain both at and below the level of the spinal cord injury. Additionally, 82 patients received intravenous lidocaine one time for 30 minutes at the time they were admitted to a hospice. The overwhelming majority of patients (90%) reported reduction in their pain. Of these patients, 82% had a major pain reduction, and 8% had a partial pain reduction. In both groups, pain relief was rapid (30 minutes), and there were no adverse reactions to the drug.

In a third study, lidocaine was administered through the skin using a patch that was changed every 24 hours. The 82 patients in this study had severe lower back pain and significantly reduced all four kinds of pain: sharp, hot, dull, and deep.

For more information see page 1283.

Generic: *Mexiletine* (MEKS-i-le-teen)
Brand: *Mexitil*

Mexiletine is an anesthetic that affects the passage of sodium ions into and out of neurons, and is approved for the treatment of heart arrhythmias (abnormal heartbeats). It works similarly to lidocaine but, unlike lidocaine, is effective when taken orally as a capsule.

Eleven men came to a pain clinic because other medications had failed to reduce their pain. They were given mexiletine or placebo for at least one month. Mexiletine caused a significant decrease in their pain. The men were then given the opportunity to continue taking the drug, and those who did so continued to experience relief from their pain.

Spinal cord injury pain is difficult to treat and occurs in 5–30% of patients with this injury. In a study by the Department of Physical Medicine and Rehabilitation at Baylor College of Medicine in Texas, researchers examined the effects of mexiletine in the treatment of spinal cord pain. The study involved 15 patients, of whom 11 completed, who received either mexiletine or placebo over four weeks. Researchers assessed the patients' pain using a variety of scales. According to the researchers, mexiletine did not appear to decrease spinal cord injury-related pain.

For more information see page 1324.

Generic: **Oxcarbazepine** *(ox-car-BAZ-e-peen)*
Brand: **Trileptal**

Oxcarbazepine is an antiseizure drug approved for the treatment of epilepsy. It alters the pattern of neuronal firing and transmission of nerve impulses to prevent seizures.

Researchers in Spain sought to examine the efficacy of oxcarbazepine in patients diagnosed with chronic neuropathic pain. Forty people with a long history of neuropathic pain that was resistant to treatment with other medications such as other anticonvulsants, non-steroidal anti-inflammatory drugs (NSAID), and opiates received oxcarbazepine and then were evaluated by researchers. According to researchers, treatment with oxcarbazepine reduces symptomatic variations of neuropathic pain, especially in the case of lancinating discharges (a sensation of cutting, piercing, or stabbing) and burning pain, although the allodynia (pain from a source that is not normally painful) also improved with treatment. In 50% of cases the opinion of the patients themselves in response to treatment was good or very good. Researchers noted that the side effects included dizziness, drowsiness, and abdominal upsets, but they concluded that oxcarbazepine has a good benefit-risk ratio and is a form of treatment that is well accepted by patients.

In another study, oxcarbazepine was tested in 36 people with neuropathic pain who were being treated with gabapentin, which did not give them relief from their pain. They were then given oxcarbazepine in addition to gabapentin, and the results were excellent. Almost two thirds of the patients experienced pain relief, and their pain symptoms improved by more than 70%.

Another study involved 18 patients with neuropathic pain who had tried gabapentin but had not gotten relief. They were given oxcarbazepine, which caused a marked reduction in their pain. Pain reduction was rated as good in 33% of the patients and excellent in 39% of the patients. In a similar study, oxcarbazepine was tested in 18 people whose pain was not relieved by gabapentin. In this study, 15 (83%) of the patients had good or excellent responses to oxcarbazepine, according to researchers.

Oxcarbazepine was also tested in 12 patients with neuropathic pain resulting from spinal cord injury. When they were treated with oxcarbazepine, 58% had moderate pain relief.

For more information see page 1390.

Generic: **Phenytoin** *(FEN-i-toyn)*
Brand: **Dilantin**

Phenytoin is one of the drugs used to treat epilepsy. It acts in the motor cortex (part of the brain that controls movement) to promote the passage of sodium ions out of neurons, which affects the electrical activity of neurons to inhibit epileptic seizures. Phenytoin was the first oral anticonvulsant drug used to treat neuropathic pain. It has also been administered intravenously to treat acute flare-ups of pain.

Journal of Pain Symptom Management documented a case where physicians administered intravenous phenytoin to a patient who had cancer and crescendo pain (pain that rapidly increases in severity) due to pelvic disease. The patient's pain was significantly reduced as a result of the intravenous phenytoin.

In an Irish study, 20 people who were experiencing acute flare-ups of neuropathic pain were given phenytoin or placebo intravenously for two hours. The researchers observed that, in the phenytoin group, the patients experienced a significant reduction in burning pain, shooting pain, sensitivity to pain, and overall pain. The reduction in overall pain persisted for one day, in sensitivity for two days, and in shooting pain for four days after infusion. Researchers concluded that IV phenytoin can be used to treat flare-ups of chronic neuropathic pain.

For more information see page 1413.

Generic: **Rituximab** *(ri-TUX-si-mab)*
Brand: **Rituxan**

Rituximab is a synthetic antibody made up of part of a human antibody and part of a mouse antibody. It works by interacting with human B lymphocytes, cells that are an important part of the immune system. Rituximab recognizes and binds to a specific protein on the surface of the B lymphocytes. Through a chain of reactions, the B lymphocytes are broken up and destroyed. The drug is approved for use in Hodgkin's and other lymphomas and cancers in which B lymphocytes multiply excessively and out of control. It is administered intravenously. In very rare cases, rituximab triggers adverse reactions that may be fatal.

In some cases, neuropathic pain is associated with abnormalities of the immune system, so researchers hypothesized that rituximab might be helpful in these cases. Rituximab was tested on one woman with neuropathic pain associated with immune system abnormalities. She had chronic neuropathic pain that worsened over time and had tried several pain medications—gabapentin, oxcarbazepine, bupropion, topiramate, and tricyclic antidepressants—that failed to relieve her pain and/or had intolerable adverse effects. Doctors then treated her with intravenous rituximab once a week for four weeks and her pain and other symptoms associated with neuropathy were reduced. The beneficial effects lasted for at least 23 months after the drug treatment.

For more information see page 1457.

Generic: **Tiagabine** *(tie-GA-been)*
Brand: **Gabitril**

Tiagabine binds to receptors for the neurotransmitter (a brain chemical) GABA and blocks the uptake of GABA into neurons. It has been approved for use in addition to other drugs for epilepsy.

The Department of Neurology at The Ohio State University examined the painkilling effect of tiagabine on 17 patients (10 men, seven women) with chronic neuropathic pain. The patients discontinued use of all their other pain medications for one week before receiving tiagabine. Eight of the patients developed such severe pain that they dropped out of the study. The remaining nine patients were given a low dose of tiagabine once a day, and the dose was increased over a four-week period. Tiagabine caused significant decreases in all qualities of pain: sharp, burning, dull, cold, sensitive, itchy, unpleasant, deep, and superficial. Higher doses of the drug were no more effective than the lower dose, but there was a greater incidence of adverse effects at the higher doses. Tiagabine may have potential benefits for treatment of painful neuropathy, but assessment of its efficacy in a larger study is needed.

For more information see page 1510.

*Generic: **Venlafaxine** (ven-la-FAX-een)*
*Brands: **Effexor, Effexor XR***

Venlafaxine is an antidepressant and anti-anxiety drug that increases the amount of the neurotransmitters norepinephrine and serotonin (chemicals in the brain). It has a similar but less potent effect on the neurotransmitter dopamine. The approved uses of venlafaxine are for the treatment of depression, generalized anxiety disorder, and social anxiety disorder.

At the Department of Anaesthesia and Intensive Care Medicine, Helsinki University Central Hospital in Finland, venlafaxine was tested for effectiveness in reducing neuropathic pain following the treatment of breast cancer in 13 patients. The study lasted 10 weeks, and the number of tablets taken daily was increased by one at a one-week interval. Researchers found that the average pain relief and the maximum pain intensity were significantly lower with venlafaxine compared with placebo. Anxiety and depression were not affected. Adverse effects did not show significant differences between treatments. They concluded that the higher doses of venlafaxine could be used in order to improve pain relief.

For more information see page 1542.

Epileptiform Neuralgia

See Trigeminal Neuralgia

Facial Neuralgia

See Trigeminal Neuralgia

Fothergill Disease

See Trigeminal Neuralgia

Neuritis

See Chronic Neuropathic Pain

Neuropathia

See Chronic Neuropathic Pain

Post-herpetic Neuralgia

Post-herpetic neuralgia is triggered by the virus that causes chickenpox. A small amount of this virus can remain in the body for many years after the initial chickenpox illness. When the virus is reactivated by stress, age, or other unknown factors, it travels along nerve cells and causes pain. When the virus reaches the skin, it produces a rash and blisters. This condition is known as shingles or herpes zoster. You may continue to feel pain long after the rash and blisters disappear, which is called post-herpetic neuralgia.

Commonly Prescribed (On-Label) Drugs: Lidocaine

OFF-LABEL PRESCRIPTION DRUGS
BREAKTHROUGH OPTIONS

Generic: Tricyclic antidepressants such as **Amitriptyline** *(a-mee-TRIP-ti-leen)* and **Nortriptyline** *(nor-TRIP-ti-leen)* *Brands:* **Elavil (amitriptyline), Aventyl, Pamelor (nortriptyline)**

Tricyclic antidepressants function by increasing the amount of the neurotransmitters (chemicals in the brain) norepinephrine, dopamine, and serotonin. Tricyclic antidepressants are generally used to treat people who have not responded to other drugs or in combination with other medications.

Several studies have demonstrated the effectiveness of amitriptyline in treating post-herpetic neuralgia. In one study in *Neurology*, 24 patients with post-herpetic neuralgia were given amitriptyline or placebo. Sixteen of the 24 people experienced good to excellent pain relief when they took amitriptyline. The drug did not have an antidepressant effect in most of these patients; researchers believe that is due to the low dose of the drug being administered.

In another study by the Neurobiology and Anesthesiology Branch at the National Institute of Dental Research, 58 patients with post-herpetic neuralgia were given amitriptyline, lorazepam, or placebo for six weeks. The patients were asked to rate their level of pain in a diary. At the conclusion of the study, 47% of the patients had moderate or greater relief of their pain when they took amitriptyline. In contrast, only 15% of those treated with lorazepam and 16% of those taking placebo had the same degree of relief from their pain. Researchers concluded that the patients who took higher doses of amitriptyline had more pain relief than those who took lower doses. They also noted that in four patients lorazepam did not relieve pain and was associated with severe depressive reactions.

Researchers at the UCLA Pain Management Center conducted a study to evaluate if fluphenazine enhances the effects of amitriptyline for the treatment of post-herpetic neuralgia. The researchers divided 49 patients into four treatment groups: Group 1, amitriptyline; Group 2, amitriptyline plus fluphenazine; Group 3, fluphenazine; and Group 4, placebo. Patients taking amitriptyline or a combination of amitriptyline and fluphenazine had a significant reduction in their pain, but patients taking fluphenazine or placebo did not. There was no significant difference in pain relief between amitriptyline and the combination of amitriptyline and fluphenazine. Based on these results, researchers concluded that this study showed that (1) amitriptyline, but not fluphenazine, was effective in treating post-herpetic neuralgia and (2) there was no advantage to adding fluphenazine to amitriptyline.

Additionally, researchers at the University of Rochester School of Medicine and Dentistry stated that nortriptyline and amitriptyline provide equivalent therapeutic benefits for people with post-herpetic neuralgia but that nortriptyline is better tolerated.

Researchers at the University of Toronto support this finding, confirming that first-line therapy for neuropathic pain may be either an antidepressant such as amitriptyline or nortriptyline.

For more information see pages 1009 and 1378.

Generic: **Carbidopa-levodopa**
(kar-bi-DOE-pa lee-voe-DOE-pa)
Brands: **Sinemet, Sinemet CR**

Carbidopa-levodopa is approved for treating Parkinson's disease. Levodopa is converted to the neurotransmitter dopamine (a brain chemical). Carbidopa inhibits the breakdown of levodopa. The combination of these two drugs increases the amount of dopamine in the brain.

Journal of American Medicine Association reported on the effects of carbidopa-levodopa on 47 people with post-herpetic neuralgia. The patients started taking carbidopa-levodopa or placebo within five days of the onset of rash and blisters. Vomiting was the only side effect observed in both groups. The group receiving carbidopa-levodopa had significant decrease in pain intensity from the third day. Complete cessation of both pain and sleep disturbances was more frequent in all patients. Two months later, post-herpetic neuralgia was also less frequent in the group that received carbidopa-levodopa. Based on these results, researchers concluded that pain disappeared completely in more patients taking the drug than in patients taking placebo.

For more information see page 1070.

Generic: **Clonidine** *(KLON-i-deen)*
Brands: **Catapres, Catapres-TTS, Duraclon**

Clonidine is approved for the treatment of high blood pressure. It binds to the brain chemical norepinephrine within the brain and increases the electrical activity of neurons, which affects the electrical activity of another group of nerve cells important in the regulation of blood pressure. The net effect is a reduction of blood pressure.

National Institute of Dental Research evaluated the effects of clonidine compared to the effects of other painkillers in 40 patients with post-herpetic neuralgia. Patients received clonidine in tablet form. Patients reported significantly more pain relief from clonidine than from placebo. Codeine and ibuprofen were ineffective in reducing pain. Sedation, dizziness, and other side effects were more frequent after clonidine (74%) or codeine (69%) than after placebo (36%) or ibuprofen (28%). According to researchers, the incidence of side effects from clonidine was about the same as that from codeine, even though the former was more effective as a painkiller.

Additionally, clonidine in ointment form (not commercially available in this form in the United States) was also tested for the treatment of post-herpetic neuralgia in 10 patients, who applied the ointment directly to the painful area. Clonidine ointment produced a satisfactory effect in nine of the 10 patients within a few minutes, and there were no side effects.

For more information see page 1108.

Generic: **Desipramine** *(des-IP-ra-meen)*
Brand: **Norpramin**

Desipramine is a tricyclic antidepressant. It works by increasing the amount of the neurotransmitters (chemicals in the brain) norepinephrine, dopamine, and serotonin. Tricyclic antidepressants are generally used to treat people who have not had adequate relief with other drugs or as add on with other medications.

A study in *Clinical Pharmacology Therapy* showed that desipramine has the least reduction of smooth muscle spasms and sedative effects, as well as pain-relieving potential. Other antidepressant drugs—notably amitriptyline—are known to relieve post-herpetic neuralgia, but are often toxic. Twenty-six post-herpetic neuralgia patients received desipramine and placebo for six weeks of treatment.

Nineteen patients completed both treatments; 12 reported at least moderate relief with desipramine and two reported relief with placebo. Pain relief with desipramine was significantly reduced from weeks 3 to 6. Psychiatric interview at entry into the study produced a diagnosis of depression for four patients, although pain relief was similar in depressed and non-depressed patients. The researchers concluded that desipramine relieves post-herpetic neuralgia and that pain relief is not determined by mood elevation.

For more information see page 1132.

Tic Douloureux

See Trigeminal Neuralgia

Trigeminal Neuralgia

Trigeminal neuralgia is an extremely painful condition that usually affects people over age 50, most often women. In involves the fifth cranial nerve, which leads to the head. The trigeminal nerve can be compressed by a blood vessel, the pressure wearing away the nerve's myelin sheath. The intense, stabbing pain occurs in the jaw, gums, forehead or elsewhere on the face.

Commonly Prescribed (On-Label) Drugs: Carbamazepine

OFF-LABEL PRESCRIPTION DRUGS
BREAKTHROUGH OPTIONS

---

*Generic: **Botulinum Toxin Type A***
(BOT-yoo-lin-num TOKS-in type aye)
*Brands: **Botox, Botox Cosmetic***

Botulinum toxin A is approved for the treatment of moderate to severe facial lines and severe underarm sweating. Off-label, it has also been used to treat migraines, post-surgical pain, and trigeminal neuralgia. Botulinum toxin A works by blocking the release of certain chemicals in the brain, and researchers believe this action inhibits pain messages.

An article published in *Neurology* reported a study of 13 people with trigeminal neuralgia who were treated with botulinum toxin A injection. During the study, the patients remained on their other medications while undergoing injections. Their medication use and pain intensity scores were evaluated at 10, 20, 30, and 60 days after an injection. By day 20, researchers observed that the patients had a significant reduction in pain scores. By 60 days, four of 13 patients were medicine free and had markedly reduced pain levels. The remaining patients experienced less pain and a decrease in their medicine use by 50%. Researchers found that botulinum toxin A may be an effective and well-tolerated treatment for trigeminal neuralgia, especially in those who are unresponsive to conventional therapies.

For more information see page 1051.

Generic: **Gabapentin** (GA-ba-pen-tin)
Brand: **Neurontin**

Gabapentin is an anticonvulsant approved for use against partial seizures. It is not clear how it works, though it may help multiple sclerosis patients by modulating central pain pathways.

A study in *Southern Medical Journal* by a neurologist who gave gabapentin to 59 patients suffering from a variety of neurological complaints, including trigeminal neuralgia. Seeking an alternative to traditional treatments that many patients did not tolerate well, he turned to gabapentin as an alternative and found that more than half of the patients reported moderate-to-excellent pain control from the drug. Seven patients had trigeminal neuralgia and did particularly well with gabapentin.

In another published report, gabapentin was used for multiple sclerosis patients whose pain could not be controlled with the conventional therapy. In *Neurology,* neurologists at the Baltimore veterans hospital reported that seven people with multiple sclerosis received gabapentin and six had a complete elimination of symptoms, and a third partial. Patients maintained pain relief from gabapentin a year later.

For more information see page 1206.

Generic: **Lamotrigine** (la-MOE-tri-jeen)
Brand: **Lamictal**

Lamotrigine is an anti-epilepsy drug with chemical characteristics different from other epilepsy drugs. It works by suppressing the excessive release of amino acids that cause excess neurological firing.

Some clinicians have turned to lamotrigine for their patients who cannot tolerate the side effects of carbamazepine, the standard,

FDA-approved treatment for trigeminal neuralgia. British researchers related their study in the journal *Pain* of 14 patients whose symptoms were resistant to their current treatment with carbamazepine or phenytoin. One half received lamotrigine and the other placebo, in addition to their previous drug regimen. The first phase of the trial lasted for two weeks, then the groups' therapies were reversed. The people on lamotrigine did better than those on placebo.

Italian researchers reported in *Neurology* about their trial involving 20 trigeminal neuralgia patients who had gone off carbamazepine because of side effects. Soon thereafter, patients received lamotrigine in slowly increasing doses until dose was effective. Researchers noted that 16 patients had complete pain relief, with minimal side effects, that lasted at least three to eight months past the end of the study period.

For more information see page 1268.

Generic: **Oxcarbazepine** (ox-car-BAZ-e-peen)
Brand: **Trileptal**

Oxcarbazepine is traditionally used for epilepsy. It is closely related to carbamazepine. Because some patients experience negative side effects from carbamazepine, clinicians have tried oxcarbazepine, which has a relatively low side effects profile.

In a London study published in the *Journal of Neurology, Neurosurgery, and Psychiatry* involving six people with trigeminal neuralgia, researchers found that oxcarbazepine gave good pain control with no significant side effects.

Another study in *Pain* followed a small group whose pain from trigeminal neuralgia did not respond to the traditional drug treatment, such as carbamazepine. The study compared oxcarbazepine with surgery and found that the drug was effective for a time, but not over months or years. All of the patients eventually required surgery after 13 years.

For more information see page 1390.

ORAL HEALTH DISORDERS

Aphthae

See Canker Sores

Burning Mouth Syndrome

Patients with burning mouth syndrome have a tingling, burning, or numb sensation on the lips, tongue, and/or inside of the mouth. No visual signs, such as redness or swelling, accompany these sensations. You may experience symptoms that come and go or that increase steadily throughout the day. Others may have some symptom-free days. Possible causes of burning mouth syndrome include nutritional deficiencies, anxiety or depression, or nerve problems (such as damage to certain craniofacial nerves), although none of these causes has been proven.

Commonly Prescribed (On-Label) Drugs: None

OFF-LABEL PRESCRIPTION DRUG
BREAKTHROUGH OPTION

---

*Generic: **Clonazepam** (kloe-NA-ze-pam)*
*Brand: **Klonopin***

Clonazepam belongs to the class of drugs known as benzodiazepines. This drug is thought to exert its effects by acting on certain types of receptors in nerve cells. Benzodiazepines are used as muscle relaxants, to relieve anxiety, and as anti-epileptic drugs. Because they may produce dependence with long-term use, these drugs should be used for limited or defined periods.

A study conducted at Case Western Reserve University reported on 30 patients who experienced symptoms of burning mouth syndrome from one month to 12 years. Many of the patients felt the burning sensation starting in late morning, with intensity increasing throughout the day and peaking in the evening. The patients received clonazepam daily before bedtime. They were instructed to increase their dosage weekly until they experienced significant pain reduction or had adverse effects. Researchers found that 43% of patients had partial to complete relief and continued with the drug. Twenty-seven percent reported that the drug was beneficial but stopped due to side effects. For 30%, there was no pain reduction.

From these results, researchers compared the patient's age, history of burning mouth syndrome, and final dosage amounts between the three groups. They found that patients who had less pain were significantly younger than those who had relief accompanied by side effects. Based on this, researchers suggest that clonazepam may be an effective treatment for burning mouth syndrome.

For more information see page 1107.

Cancer Treatment-induced Mucositis/Stomatitis

The soft tissues within the mouth and the rest of the digestive tract contain some of the most rapidly dividing cells in the body. Treatments for cancer, such as chemotherapy and radiation, aim to stop or slow the rate at which abnormal cancer cells divide and reproduce. Because normal cells in the digestive tract also divide and reproduce rapidly, cancer treatments can slow the normal growth and repair of these tissues often leading to stomatitis (tissues lining the oral cavity are inflamed and painful) and/or mucositis (a painful inflammation of the cells that line the entire digestive tract, occurring from mouth to anus). These conditions are a common side effect of cancer treatments, especially with the anti-cancer drug 5-fluorouracil.

Commonly Prescribed (On-Label) Drugs: *None*

OFF-LABEL PRESCRIPTION DRUGS
BREAKTHROUGH OPTIONS

Generic: **Allopurinol** *(al-oh-PURE-i-nole)*
Brands: **Aloprim, Zyloprim**

Allopurinol is in a class of medications called xanthine oxidase inhibitors. It works by reducing the production of uric acid (a byproduct of metabolism) in the body. Allopurinol mouthwash has been shown to be effective in preventing and treating mucositis and stomatitis. This drug is often delivered in a mouthwash or spray that is rinsed out of the mouth after use. In studies of allopurinol to prevent stomatitis, the drug has been used in a variety of formulations and strengths, administered several times a day after 5-fluorouracil treatment. Patients are usually instructed not to swallow the mouthwash.

For more information see page 995.

Generic: **Amifostine** *(am-i-FOS-teen)*
Brand: **Ethyol**

Amifostine protects the salivary glands and is approved to treat dry mouth caused by radiation treatment. It is a type of drug known as a chemoprotectant, meaning that it protects the body against harmful effects of cisplatin and radiation treatment. Amifostine works by neutralizing the metabolites of cancer treatment and radiation in normal, noncancerous tissues so that DNA and RNA are not damaged. It has also showed promise in preventing mouth ulcers caused by cancer treatment, but another study conducted at the University of Dundee Dental Hospital seemed to contradict this use.

For more information see page 1002.

Generic: Symptom management with **Dicyclomine**
(dye-SYE-kloe-meen), **Sucralfate** *(soo-KRAL-fate),* and
Lidocaine *(LYE-doe-kane)*
**Brands: Bentyl, Bentylol, Di-Spaz (dicyclomine), Carafate
(sucralfate), Anestacon, Xylocaine (lidocaine)**

Drugs such as dicyclomine, sucralfate, and lidocaine lessen the
symptoms of mucositis and/or stomatitis but do not treat the underlying cause of the condition. Usually given as a mouthwash or
spray, they are used to help relieve the discomfort. Lidocaine in an
oral solution has helped relieve the symptoms of mucositis, although toxic reactions have occurred in children and in adults in
higher doses. Sucralfate has been shown to lessen the occurrence
of mucositis and stomatitis in patients receiving high-dose
chemotherapy for bone marrow transplantation.

For more information see pages 1145, 1283, and 1482.

Canker Sores

Canker sores, or aphthous stomatitis, are shallow ulcers that form
in the soft tissues of the mouth—usually on the insides of the
cheeks, on the tongue, or on the base of the gums. The cause of
canker sores is unknown in most cases, but they are sometimes related to stress, other illnesses, or certain medications. They are
painful and can make it uncomfortable to talk or eat. They are not
contagious and are not related to the cold sores caused by herpes
simplex virus. Canker sores usually go away without treatment
within 7–10 days, although treatment may be needed in more severe cases.

Commonly Prescribed (On-Label) Drugs: *None*

OFF-LABEL PRESCRIPTION DRUGS
BREAKTHROUGH OPTIONS

Generic: **Colchicine** *(KOHL-chi-seen)*
Brand: None

Colchicine is used to treat acute gout. It is useful in suppressing
the body's inflammation response. This drug has also been used
off-label with some success in people with severe canker sores. Re-

searchers in France studied use of colchicine on 54 patients with severe cases of recurrent canker sores. In this study, colchicine was given for a minimum of three months. Of 54 patients, 12 no longer had outbreaks of canker sores and were in complete remission. In 22 patients, lesions were significantly improved and no longer painful. In the remaining 20 patients, treatment failed or was poorly tolerated.

For more information see page 1115.

Generic: **Prednisone** *(pred-NIS-zone)*
Brands: **Deltasone, Liquid Pred, Meticorten, Orasone, Sterapred**

Steroid drugs such as prednisone work by turning off certain chemicals in cells that produce inflammation. A corticosteroid that reduces swelling, redness, itching, and allergic reactions, prednisone has been used off-label in the treatment of severe recurrent canker sores, although it can have many troubling side effects, such as hyptertension, hyperglycemia, and osteoporosis, when taken in large doses for extended periods.

For more information see page 1429.

Generic: Corticosteroids such as **Betamethasone** *(bay-ta-METH-a-sone)*, **Clobetasol** *(kloe-BAY-ta-sol)*, **Dexamethasone** *(deks-a-METH-a-sone)*, and **Fluocinonide** *(floo-oh-SIN-oh-nide)*
Brands: **Bet-Val, Diprosone, Luxiq, Maxivate, Teladar (betamethasone), Clobex, Cormax, Embeline, Olux, Temovate (clobetasol), Decadron, Dexone, Dexameth, Hexadrol (dexamethasone), Fluonex, Lidex, Lidex-E (fluocinonide)**

Topical treatments for canker sores are applied directly onto the affected area in the mouth. Betamethasone, clobetasol, dexamethasone, and fluocinonide are corticosteroids. Used to treat some skin conditions, topical steroids are absorbed through the skin or mucous membranes to reduce local inflammation. Although topical steroids for oral sores come in creams, lotions, gels, ointments, or solutions, the most effective are typically ointments or gels. When you have multiple canker sores in the mouth, or lesions far back in the mouth, steroid rinses are recommended. Topical steroids work by entering the nucleus of a cell and turning off the production of the chemicals that produce inflammation. Topical steroids also constrict the tiny vessels that supply blood to an inflamed area, thus reducing pain and swelling. These drugs do not eliminate the cause of canker sores, but they can reduce the discomfort of them and shorten the time to their disappearance.

For more information see pages 1042, 1102, 1138, and 1191.

Drug-induced Gingival Enlargement

Gingival enlargement, also known as gingival hyperplasia or enlargement of the gums, can be caused by certain drugs—most commonly, phenytoin, cyclosporin, or nifedipine, which are often used to prevent organ rejection in transplant recipients. These drugs may interfere in the normal breakdown of types of cells in gum tissue. Because these cells are not sloughed off normally, the gums become enlarged, appear puffy and red, are tender to the touch, and may bleed easily. In very severe cases, your teeth may be partially or even completely obscured.

Commonly Prescribed (On-Label) Drugs: *None*

OFF-LABEL PRESCRIPTION DRUGS
BREAKTHROUGH OPTIONS

*Generic: **Azithromycin** (az-ith-roe-MYE-sin)*
*Brands: **Tri-Pak, Zithromax Z-Pak, Zithromax***

Azithromycin is in a class of medications called macrolide antibiotics. It works by inhibiting the ability of bacterial cells to synthesize protein, which is needed for many cell functions and growth. Studies have found azithromycin to be effective for cyclosporine-induced gingival enlargement in transplant patients. In one Turkish study, the drug reduced gum swelling in all 18 patients who had developed gingival enlargement as a result of cyclosporine therapy for kidney transplants.

For more information see page 1035.

Generic: **Chlorhexidine Gluconate**
(klor-HEX-i-deen GLOO-koe-nate)
Brands: **Peridex, PerioChip, PerioGard**

Chlorhexidine Gluconate is an antiseptic and disinfectant medication that is effective against various bacteria, viruses, bacterial spores, and fungi. This drug kills the organisms that cause mouth and throat infections, and other common conditions in the mouth such as *Candida albicans* fungi that cause thrush infection in the mouth, and bacteria that may infect mouth ulcers or other sore areas in the mouth, especially after dental surgery. Infection of these areas increases discomfort and delays healing. Few studies have evaluated the use of mouth rinses in the treatment of gingival enlargement. However your dentist may prescribe it to treat redness, swelling, and bleeding of inflamed gums. It may be useful in the treatment of gingival enlargement.

For more information see page 1081.

Gingivitis

Gingivitis is an inflammation of the gums (gingiva) that produces soreness, redness, and swelling. It is most commonly caused by a buildup of tartar and plaque, a sticky substance produced by bacteria that forms on teeth surfaces. When teeth are not cleaned regularly, plaque hardens into tartar, which builds up on the base of the teeth and can irritate the gums. If this tartar buildup is not removed, the gums may become increasingly inflamed and infected with the many strains of bacteria that the mouth normally harbors. Gingivitis can also be caused by injury or trauma to the gums, such as that caused by brushing or flossing too forcefully, or by poorly fitting dentures or crowns. Allergic reactions may also cause gingivitis.

Commonly Prescribed (On-Label) Drugs: *Chlorhexidine*

OFF-LABEL PRESCRIPTION DRUGS
BREAKTHROUGH OPTIONS

Generic: Antibiotics such as ***Ciprofloxacin***
(sip-roe-FLOKS-a-sin), ***Clindamycin*** *(klin-da-MYE-sin)*,
Doxycycline *(doks-i-SYE-kleen)*, ***Erythromycin***
(er-ith-roe-MYE-sin), and ***Metronidazole***
(me-troe-NI-da-zole)
Brands: ***Ciloxan, Cipro, Cipro XR (ciprofloxacin),***
Cleocin, Clindamycin (clindamycin), Adoxa, Doryx,
Doxy-100, Monodox, Periostat, Vibramycin, Vibra-Tabs
(doxycycline), Akne-Mycin, E.E.S., Eryc, Ery-Tab,
Erythrocin (erythromycin), Flagyl, Flagyl ER, Metro-
Cream, MetroGel, MetroLotion, MetroGel Vaginal
(metronidazole)

Antibiotics are part of a larger group of drugs known as anti-microbials, which kill or slow the growth of microorganisms that cause disease. Ciprofloxacin, clindamycin, doxycycline, erythromycin, and metronidazole are not the only ones in the family of antibiotics but are the ones used off-label specifically to treat gingivitis.

Antibiotics work in a variety of ways. Some interfere with the bacteria's ability to synthesize protein, thereby inhibiting their growth. Others block DNA replication or nucleic acid synthesis. Antibiotics are broadly classified into Gram-positive and Gram-negative species based on their reactions in a test known as Gram staining, which differentiates these two classes of bacteria by how the organisms appear under a microscope after being stained with a special dye. The results of Gram staining can help clinicians choose the antibiotics that will act against the bacteria causing the infection.

Of the antibiotics listed here, both clindamycin and erythromycin are often used as alternatives to penicillin in penicillin-allergic patients. Clindamycin, a narrow spectrum antibiotic, was found in one study to be particularly effective in treating gingivitis with few side effects. Other antibiotics, such as ciprofloxacin, are broad-spectrum antibiotics, meaning that they are effective against a wide variety of both Gram-positive and Gram-negative bacterial species.

For more information see pages 1093, 1101, 1158, 1170, and 1322.

Oral Leukoplakia

Oral leukoplakia is a clinical term for a white lesion on the tongue or on the inside of the mouth whose cause is unknown. Only when a biopsy or sample of the lesion is taken can a doctor determine if the lesion is dysplastic or pre-cancerous. If it is dysplastic, the cells of the lesion have early signs of cancer and may eventually develop into cancer, though this is rare.

An oral leukoplakia that is dysplastic may appear as a white or gray, thick, and slightly raised patch, forming over weeks or months. The lesions are usually painless, but may become sensitive to heat, spicy foods, or other irritation. Often, oral leukoplakias are attributed to rough teeth or dentures that irritate the tissues of the tongue or mouth. Smoking also appears to increase the risk of dysplastic oral leukoplakia.

Commonly Prescribed (On-Label) Drugs: *Aminolevulinic Acid, Deflazacort, Dexamethasone, Hydrocortisone, Methyl-prednisolone*

OFF-LABEL PRESCRIPTION DRUGS
BREAKTHROUGH OPTIONS

Generic: ***Bleomycin*** *(BLEE-o-mice-in)*
Brand: ***Blenoxane***

Bleomycin belongs to the drug class of anti-neoplastic drugs, which are used to treat cancer. The drug works by interfering with DNA production inside cells.

One study conducted in Finland evaluated bleomycin in the treatment of oral leukoplakia in 10 patients. The drug was dissolved in a solution and applied to the lesion once a day for five days and again for another five days after a two-day break. At two weeks after treatment, the lesions appeared unchanged, but after three months most of the lesions had grown noticeably smaller. By five months after treatment, the lesions had disappeared completely in five patients and had improved in three patients. No improvement at all was seen in the remaining two patients.

For more information see page 1050.

Generic: Retinoids such as **Isotretinoin**
(eye-soe-TRET-i-noyn) and **Tretinoin** *(TRET-i-noyn)*
Brands: **Avita, Retin-A, Renova** *(tretinoin),* **Accutane, Claravis** *(isotretinoin)*

Isotretinoin belongs to a class of drugs called retinoids, which are synthetic derivatives of vitamin A. They are used to treat severe acne and other skin conditions. Because isotretinoin is derived from vitamin A, users of this drug should be careful to avoid vitamin A supplements, as they can cause dangerous side effects.

One Italian study showed isotretinoin to be effective in treating oral leukoplakia. Applied as a topical gel, the drug produced treatment responses in nine of 10 patients with oral leukoplakia. No side effects of the drug were observed.

For more information see pages 1242 and 1523.

Oral Lichen Planus

Lichen planus is a skin disease that causes reddish or purplish bumps on the skin. Lichen planus can also affect the oral cavity, causing white or mixed red and white lesions inside the mouth, on the gums, or under the tongue. In the most common form of oral lichen planus, lesions are typically painless and in many cases go away on their own. However, in severe cases, they can be painful and persistent, and may interfere with eating, swallowing, speaking, or toothbrushing. The cause of oral lichen planus is not known but researchers believe it is related to an immune or allergic-type reaction.

Commonly Prescribed (On-Label) Drugs: Dexamethasone

OFF-LABEL PRESCRIPTION DRUGS
BREAKTHROUGH OPTIONS

Generic: Corticosteroids such as **Betamethasone**
(bay-ta-METH-a-sone), **Clobetasol** *(kloe-BAY-ta-sol)*, and
Dexamethasone *(deks-a-METH-a-sone)*
Brands: **Bet-Val, Diprosone, Luxiq, Maxivate, Teladar
(betamethasone), Clobex, Cormax, Embeline, Olux,
Temovate (clobetasol), Decadron, Dexameth, Dexone,
Hexadrol (dexamethasone)**

Topical drugs to treat oral lichen planus include corticosteroids.
Betamethasone, clobetasol, and dexamethasone are corticosteroids. Absorbed through the skin or mucous membranes to reduce inflammation locally, these topical steroids are used to treat
various skin conditions. Topical steroids enter the nucleus of a cell
and turn off the production of the chemicals that produce inflammation. They also constrict the tiny vessels that supply blood to an
inflamed area, thus reducing pain and swelling.

Betamethasone as a mouth rinse to treat oral lichen planus significantly reduced painful symptoms of these lesions, as well as their
size.

For more information see pages 1042, 1044, 1102, and 1138.

Generic: Immunosuppressives such as **Azathioprine**
(ay-za-THYE-oh-preen), **Mycophenolate Mofetil**
(my-koe-FEN-oh-late MOE-feh-till), and **Tacrolimus**
(ta-KROE-li-mus)
Brands: **Imuran (azathioprine), CellCept, Myfortic
(mycophenolate mofetil), Prograf, Protopic (tacrolimus)**

Systemic treatments are usually drugs taken by mouth. The drugs
listed here are taken orally to treat oral lichen planus, in contrast
to topical treatments, which are applied directly to the lesions.
These systemic medications are used when there is little or no response to topical treatments. Since researchers believe that lichen
planus is caused by some type of immune reaction, many of the
systemic drugs used to treat the condition work by interfering
with the body's immune response.

Azathioprine, mycophenolate mofetil, and tacrolimus are immunosuppressive drugs used to suppress the immune system. They work by inhibiting the production of cells called T lymphocytes, which play a crucial role in the body's immune response. They are most often used to suppress a patient's immune system in organ transplantation to reduce the likelihood of rejection. A few studies have shown it to be effective in treating oral lichen planus. Azathioprine was evaluated in a small study of nine patients with lichen planus, seven of whom had oral lesions. The drug produced a good to excellent response in six people.

Mycophenolate mofetil targets an enzyme that helps form DNA and impairs the production of DNA by cells that become overactive in autoimmune diseases. In a case report published in Germany, mycophenolate mofetil was used to treat very severe cases of oral lichen planus in two people, with excellent results.

Tacrolimus has been shown to be an effective alternative therapy of more severe forms of oral lichen planus. *Journal of American Academy of Dermatology* reported that a group of patients with oral lichen planus treated with topical tacrolimus demonstrated a significant improvement within one week of beginning therapy. Thirteen of the 17 patients enrolled in the study suffered a relapse of oral lichen planus within two to 15 weeks of cessation of tacrolimus therapy.

For more information see pages 1033, 1344, and 1489.

Generic: ***Isotretinoin*** *(eye-soe-TRET-i-noyn)*
Brands: ***Accutane, Claravis***

Isotretinoin belongs to a class of drugs called retinoids, which are synthetic derivatives of vitamin A. These drugs are used to treat severe acne and other skin conditions. Topical isotretinoin has been shown to be effective as a treatment in combination with other medications for oral lichen planus. Because isotretinoin is derived from vitamin A, users of this drug should be careful to avoid vitamin A supplements, as this can cause dangerous side effects.

For more information see page 1252.

Periodontitis

Periodontitis is a deep infection in the gums around the base of the tooth. Unlike gingivitis, which is marked by relatively minor redness and swelling of the gums, periodontitis is a more severe bacterial infection. In periodontitis, the gums begin to pull away from the teeth, forming pockets that harbor the growth of bacteria. Left untreated, the infection in these pockets can spread into the tissue beneath the gum line and into the underlying bone and connective tissue. Alveolar bone, a thin layer of compact bone that forms the tooth socket surrounding the roots of teeth, may be lost and the teeth may need to be removed as a result.

Commonly Prescribed (On-Label) Drugs: *Chlorhexidine, Doxycycline, Tetracycline*

OFF-LABEL PRESCRIPTION DRUGS
BREAKTHROUGH OPTIONS

Generic: Antibiotics such as **Ciprofloxacin** *(sip-roe-FLOKS-a-sin)*, **Clindamycin** *(klin-da-MYE-sin)*, **Erythromycin** *(er-ith-roe-MYE-sin)*, and **Metronidazole** *(me-troe-NI-da-zole)*

Brands: **Ciloxan, Cipro, Cipro XR** *(ciprofloxacin),* **Cleocin, Clindamycin** *(clindamycin),* **Akne-Mycin, E.E.S., Eryc, Ery-Tab, Erythrocin** *(erythromycin),* **Flagyl, Flagyl ER, MetroCream, MetroGel, MetroLotion, MetroGel Vaginal** *(metronidazole)*

Antibiotics are part of a larger group of drugs known as antimicrobials, which kill or slow the growth of microorganisms that cause disease. The drugs listed here are just those used off-label specifically to treat periodontitis. They are drugs used to treat bacterial infections; they will not work against infections caused by viruses or other types of microorganisms.

Antibiotics work in a variety of ways. Some interfere with the bacteria's ability to synthesize protein, thereby inhibiting their growth. Others block DNA replication or nucleic acid synthesis. Antibiotics are broadly classified into Gram-positive and Gram-negative species based on their reactions in a test known as Gram staining, which differentiates these two classes of bacteria by how the organisms appear under a microscope after being stained with a special dye. The results of Gram staining help clinicians choose the antibiotics that will act against the bacteria causing the infection.

Of the antibiotics listed here, both clindamycin and erythromycin are often used as alternatives to penicillin in penicillin-allergic patients. Clindamycin in particular was effective in treating periodontitis with few side effects. Other antibiotics, such as ciprofloxacin, are broad-spectrum antibiotics, meaning that they are effective against a wide variety of both Gram-positive and Gram-negative bacterial species. For periodontitis, antibiotics may be taken orally or, in the case of doxycycline and minocycline, applied directly into infected pockets of the gums.

For more information see pages 1093, 1099, 1170, and 1322.

Generic: Nonsteroidal anti-inflammatory drugs (NSAIDs) such as ***Flurbiprofen*** *(flure-BI-proe-fen)*, ***Ibuprofen*** *(eye-byoo-PROE-fen)*, ***Ketoprofen*** *(kee-toe-PROE-fen)*, ***Meloxicam*** *(mel-OKS-i-kam)*, and ***Naproxen*** *(na-PROKS-en)*
Brands: ***Ansaid (flurbiprofen), Motrin, Ultraprin (ibuprofen), Oruvail (ketoprofen), Mobic (meloxicam), Anaprox (DS), EC-Naprosyn, Naprelan, Naprosyn (naproxen)***

NSAIDs are drugs that reduce pain, fever, and inflammation. They are distinguished from steroidal anti-inflammatory drugs, which have similar action but also suppress the immune system. These drugs also inhibit the production of prostaglandin, a hormone produced in the body that creates inflammation and pain.

NSAIDs show promise in their ability to slow the progression of periodontal disease. They appear not only to reduce pain and swelling but also, in the case of meloxicam, to reduce the rate at which bone is lost in advanced disease. The reduction of pain and swelling by the use of NSAIDs is important not only for overall comfort but also allows toothbrushing and flossing, both of which are critical to preventing advancement of disease.

NSAIDs also inhibit substances produced by inflamed gums in periodontitis, which appear to contribute to the loss of bone in advanced periodontitis. Flurbiprofen, ibuprofen, and naproxen in particular have been shown to reduce these substances in animal studies.

For more information see pages 1194, 1228, 1261, 1303, and 1354.

Recurrent Aphthous Stomatitis

See Canker Sores

SKIN DISORDERS

Acne

Acne results from the action of hormones on the skin's oil glands, which leads to plugged pores and outbreaks of lesions commonly called pimples. Acne lesions usually occur on the face, neck, back, chest, and shoulders. Nearly 17 million people in the United States have acne, making it the most common skin disease. Although acne is not a serious health threat, severe acne can lead to disfiguring, permanent scarring, which can be upsetting to the affected people.

Commonly Prescribed (On-Label) Drugs: *Adapalene, Azelaic Acid, Benzoyl Peroxide, Clindamycin, Dexamethasone, Doxycycline, Erythromycin (topical), Fusidic Acid, Gentamicin, Isotretinoin, Minocycline, Oxytetracycline, Salicylic Acid, Sodium Thiosulfate, Sulfacetamide, Sulfur, Tazarotene, Tetracycline, Tretinoin*

OFF-LABEL PRESCRIPTION DRUGS
BREAKTHROUGH OPTIONS

Generic: **Desogestrel-Ethinyl Estradiol**
(des-oh-JES-trel ETH-in-il es-tra-DYE-ole)
Brands: **Apri, Cyclessa, Desogen, Kariva, Mircette, Ortho-Cept**

Desogestrel ethinyl estradiol is used most commonly to prevent pregnancy or regulate the menstrual cycle. It may also be used for treating acne.

Acne and facial oiliness are related and affect a high proportion of women after their first menstrual bleeding. One of the treatment options is hormonal therapy, especially for women who require contraception. The effect of combined oral contraceptives in skin disorders depends on their estrogen-progestogen balance. The choice of product should be tailored as much as possible to the individual. Several combined oral contraceptives containing new-generation progestogens such as desogestrel have demonstrated efficacy in treating women with acne. Facial oil has been less well studied, but the few available studies show an improvement in women using combined oral contraceptives.

For more information see page 1136.

---

*Generic: **Erythromycin** (er-ith-roe-MYE-sin)*
*Brands: **Akne-Mycin, E.E.S., Eryc, Ery-Tab, Erythrocin***

Erythromycin is an antibiotic used to treat a wide variety of bacterial infections, such as respiratory tract infections, middle ear infections, and skin infections. It is also widely used off-label in the treatment of acne.

Antibiotic therapy has been integral to the management of inflammatory acne for many years. Commonly prescribed antibiotics include tetracyclines, erythromycin, and trimethoprim, with or without sulfamethoxazole. In selecting the appropriate antibiotic, you should ask your doctor to take into account the severity of the acne, cost-effectiveness, the safety profile of the drug, and the potential for your developing of resistance. The widespread, long-term use of antibiotics over the years has unfortunately led to the emergence of resistant bacteria. The global increase in the antibiotic resistance of *Propionibacterium acnes* contribute significantly to treatment failures. Clinicians prescribing antibiotics for acne must adopt strategies to minimize further development of resistant bacteria. Use combination therapies, avoid prolonged antibiotic treatment, and avoid concomitant topical and oral antibiotics with chemically dissimilar antibiotics and make sure you comply with instructions.

For more information see page 1170.

---

*Generic: **Finasteride** (fi-NAS-teer-ide)*
*Brands: **Propecia, Proscar***

Finasteride is typically used in men to treat urinary problems caused by an enlarged prostate but may be used to treat acne in women. It blocks an enzyme that is instrumental in converting testosterone to another hormone that causes the growth of the prostate. The prostate decreases as a result. This effect only lasts as long as treatment with finasteride continues. Since the enzyme that produces an enlarged prostate also is responsible for acne, finasteride may be prescribed by your doctor for acne.

An Italian study at the University of Palermo compared the relative effectiveness of flutamide and finasteride with cyproterone acetate, at both low and high doses in the treatment of moderate to severe acne in 48 women who produce elevated amounts of the androgen hormone. The women received the following treatments for one year: cyproterone acetate with ethinylestradiol; flutamide; and finasteride. Researchers observed that the hormone levels decreased with flutamide and both low and high doses of cyproterone acetate. Therefore, researchers concluded that women with moderate to severe acne can be helped by low doses of certain antiandrogen medications, such as finasteride.

For more information see page 1187.

Generic: *Flutamide* (FLOO-ta-mide)
Brand: *Eulexin*

Flutamide is a nonsteroidal antiandrogen drug. A study in China examined 52 women with acne, including 42 with oligomenorrhea (less menstrual blood flow than usual) or amenorrhea (the absence of menstrual cycles) (Group 1) and 10 with regular menstrual cycles (Group 2). As a control, another 15 oligomenorrheic women without acne were also studied (Group 3). Patients in Group 1 received flutamide combined with estrogen-progestogen preparations. Group 2 received flutamide alone, Group 3 was treated with estrogen-progestogen.

Groups 1 and 2 showed a significant decrease in inflammatory lesions at the end of three and six months of treatment and even after discontinuation of therapy for six months. Three and six months after treatment, Group 1's hormones, testosterone and androstenedione, decreased. Group 2 showed improvement of acne by flutamide alone without alteration in androgens. Researchers concluded that low dose of flutamide, with or without estrogen-progestogen, is effective for the improvement of acne in women with or without oligomenorrhea or amenorrhea.

For more information see page 1196.

*Generic: **Levonorgestrel-Ethinyl Estradiol***
(LEE-voe-nor-jes-trel ETH-in-il ess-tra-DYE-ole)
*Brands: **Alesse, Aviane, Enpresse, Lessina, Levlen, Levlite, Levora, Lutera, Nordette, Portia, PREVEN, Seasonale, Tri-Levlen, Triphasil, Trivora***

Levonorgestrel-ethinyl estradiol is used to prevent pregnancy or regulate the menstrual cycle. Acne is a disorder in which androgens appear to play an important role. A low-dose oral contraceptive containing ethinyl estradiol and levonorgestrel (EE/LNG) has been shown to improve hormone levels. A study at the University of Pennsylvania Hospital evaluated the efficacy and safety of a low-dose oral contraceptive containing this drug for the treatment of moderate acne. In the trial, healthy women with regular menstrual cycles and moderate facial acne received either EE/LNG or placebo for six cycles of 28 days. At the end of the study, researchers found that the number of inflammatory and total lesions was significantly lower with EE/LNG compared with placebo. A low-dose oral contraceptive containing EE/LNG appears effective and safe for treating moderate acne.

For more information see page 1279.

*Generic: **Norgestimate-Ethinyl Estradiol***
(nor-JES-ti-mate ETH-in-il es-tra-DYE-ole)
*Brands: **MonoNessa, Ortho-Cyclen, Ortho Tri-Cyclen, Ortho Tri-Cyclen Lo, Sprintec***

Norgestimate ethyinyl estradiol is used to prevent pregnancy or regulate the menstrual cycle. Certain brands of birth control pills may also be used for treating acne or as a "morning after" pill for emergency contraception.

A study in *Dermatology* compared the efficacy of a combination oral contraceptive (OC) containing norgestimate and ethinyl estradiol for treating of 12 women with acne.

According to researchers, after six months of therapy, the number of acne counts improved. The success of treatment was rated positively both by the researchers and by all women except one who did not report any changes. Therefore, researchers concluded that norgestimate and ethinyl estradiol is a good therapeutic option for women of fertile age suffering from mild to moderate acne.

For more information see page 1374.

*Generic: **Spironolactone*** *(speer-on-oh-LAK-tone)*
*Brand: **Aldactone***

Spironolactone is used to treat high blood pressure. Lowering high blood pressure helps prevent strokes, heart attacks, and kidney problems. It is also used to treat swelling (edema) caused by conditions such as congestive heart failure by removing excess fluid and improving symptoms such as breathing problems.

Androgen hormones play an important role in acne, yet despite the demonstrated effects, spironolactone, an androgen receptor blocker, is not commonly used to treat acne. A study in Turkey evaluated the effects and side effects of spironolactone in women with acne. Thirty-five women were treated with spironolactone for three months. Lesion numbers and hormone levels before and after treatment were compared. Researchers noted clinically significant improvement in 24 women (85.71%). No response was seen in four women. Spironolactone is a safe, effective medication for women with acne. Although its side effects seem to be high, researchers state that in the majority of cases this is not a reason to stop treatment.

For more information see page 1478.

*Generic: **Trimethoprim-sulfamethoxazole***
(try-METH-oh-prim suhl-fah-meth-OX-ah-zole)
*Brands: **Bactrim, Septra***

Trimethoprim-sulfamethoxazole is a combination of two antibiotics used to treat a wide variety of bacterial infections and to prevent and treat a certain type of pneumonia.

Antibacterial medications have been used off-label to treat acne for many years, and several commonly used antibacterials have established efficacy and safety records, including tetracycline, doxycycline, minocycline, erythromycin (and other macrolide antibiotics), and trimethoprim/sulfamethoxazole (cotrimoxazole). Your choice of antibacterial should take into account efficacy, cost-effectiveness, benefit-risk ratios, and the potential for developing resistance. To help prevent the development of resistance, physicians typically prescribe antibacterials for an average of six months. Generally, antibacterials should be taken for at least two months before considering switching because you're not responding to it.

For more information see page 1530.

Acne Rosacea

See Rosacea

Acne Vulgaris

See Acne

Acquired Leukoderma

See Vitiligo

Alopecia Areata

Alopecia areata is a highly unpredictable, autoimmune skin disease resulting in the loss of hair on the scalp and elsewhere on the body. In alopecia areata, the affected hair follicles are mistakenly attacked by your immune system (white blood cells), resulting in the arrest of hair growth. Alopecia areata usually starts with one or more small, round, smooth bald patches on the scalp and can progress to total scalp hair loss (alopecia totalis) or complete body hair loss (alopecia universalis).

Commonly Prescribed (On-Label) Drugs: *Betamethasone, Clobetasol, Dexamethasone, Fluocinolone Acetonide, Fluocinonide*

OFF-LABEL PRESCRIPTION DRUGS
BREAKTHROUGH OPTIONS

*Generic: **Cyclosporine** (si-klo-SPOR-een)*
*Brands: **Gengraf, Neoral, Sandimmune***

Cyclosporine is used to prevent or treat organ rejection in transplant patients. Eight patients with alopecia areata (AA) affecting at least 95% of the scalp were enrolled in a study at the University of British Columbia. The average duration of their disease was 7.5 years. All were started on a regimen of cyclosporine and prednisone, and then the dosage of cyclosporine was decreased after 10 weeks if the scalp response was good and there were no significant side effects. Every six weeks thereafter cyclosporine was reduced if the response showed more than 75% regrowth of cosmetically acceptable hairs. At week 24, cyclosporine was stopped and prednisone was continued for one month. Two of eight patients had cosmetically acceptable results.

For more information see pages 1125 and 1127.

*Generic: **Pimecrolimus** (pie-meh-CROW-lie-mus)*
*Brand: **Elidel***

Pimecrolimus is used to treat certain skin conditions such as eczema (atopic dermatitis), in people who have not responded well to or who should not use other eczema medications such as topical steroids. Pimecrolimus belongs to a new class of topical immunomodulators (TIMS). These drugs inhibit inflammatory skin reactions while producing fewer side effects than topical steroids. This medication penetrates the top layer of the skin to alter the immune response in skin diseases, but since it only reaches the upper layers of the skin, researchers are unsure whether it can have an effect on alopecia areata. Currently, studies are ongoing to develop this topical cream into an oral treatment.

For more information see page 1415.

Generic: **Prednisone** *(pred-NIS-zone)*
Brands: **Deltasone, Liquid Pred, Meticorten, Orasone, Sterapred**

Prednisone is a corticosteroid hormone (glucocorticoid) that decreases the body's immune system's response to various diseases in order to reduce symptoms such as swelling and allergic-type reactions. It is used to treat arthritis, blood disorders, breathing problems, certain cancers, eye problems, immune system diseases, and skin diseases. Systemic corticosteroids such as prednisone have been demonstrated to be effective in treating severe alopecia areata. Eighteen people with alopecia areata were treated with systemic corticosteroids during a study conducted in Saudi Arabia. Satisfactory hair regrowth was achieved in seven patients (38.9%). Hair fall subsequently occurred in all patients when they discontinued or tapered off corticosteroid therapy. Therefore, researchers concluded that corticosteroid therapy does not prevent the spread or relapse of severe alopecia areata.

For more information see page 1429.

Generic: **Tacrolimus** *(ta-KROE-li-mus)*
Brands: **Prograf, Protopic**

Topical tacrolimus is used to treat a skin condition called eczema (atopic dermatitis) in patients who have not responded well to, or who should not use, other eczema medications such as topical steroids. A study at the University of California at San Francisco Hair Research Center examined 11 people with alopecia areata affecting 10% to 75% of the scalp. People who had alopecia areata for an average duration of six years had no hair growth response to tacrolimus ointment applied twice daily for 24 weeks. Researchers concluded that this treatment failure may reflect insufficient depth of penetration of the ointment, but may be more beneficial in those who have less duration of this disorder.

For more information see page 1489.

Alopecia Areata Totalis

See Alopecia Areata

Alopecia Areata Universalis

See Alopecia Areata

Bullous Pemphigoid

Bullous pemphigoid (BP) is an autoimmune disorder that causes chronic blistering of the skin. It ranges from mildly itchy welts to severe blisters and infection and may affect a small area of the body or be widespread. The vast majority of those affected are elderly, but it has been seen at all ages.

Commonly Prescribed (On-Label) Drugs: None

OFF-LABEL PRESCRIPTION DRUGS
BREAKTHROUGH OPTIONS

*Generic: **Azathioprine** (ay-za-THYE-oh-preen)*
*Brand: **Imuran***

Azathioprine is used to prevent rejection of transplanted organs and for cases of severe arthritis that do not respond to other therapies. In a report in *British Journal of Dermatology* a 59-year-old man developed lesions during the course of a long-lasting severe psoriasis, which had been treated for years with different topical treatments as well as with PUVA and UV-B radiations. The man was successfully treated with a combination of acitretin and azathioprine.

Azathioprine has an important role in treating many inflammatory skin diseases. In view of this, researchers in the United Kingdom performed a questionnaire-based survey to establish current practice in the use of azathioprine by dermatologists and associate specialists. They found that the response rate was 68%. These data provided evidence that azathioprine is useful in the treating a wide variety of dermatological diseases. The most common conditions treated were pemphigoid, pemphigus, and atopic eczema. In addition, most dermatologists felt that azathioprine was well tolerated.

For more information see page 1033.

*Generic: **Clobetasol** (kloe-BAY-ta-sol)*
*Brands: **Clobex, Cormax, Embeline, Olux, Temovate***

Clobetasol is a corticosteroid used to treat swelling, redness, and itching in certain scalp conditions. BP is the most common autoimmune blistering skin disease, which until recently, was treated with oral corticosteroids. However, high-dose corticosteroids are poorly tolerated in the elderly, and their use has probably contributed to high death rates. Accordingly, physicians have directed considerable effort at identifying corticosteroid-sparing drugs, such as immunosuppressant drugs, intravenous immunoglobulins, and tetracyclines. Many options have appeared to be useful, but then found to be ineffective or only marginally effective when tested in trials. An important breakthrough occurred with the use of clobetasol propionate. It was not only associated with a significant decrease in severe complications of BP patients but was also more effective than oral prednisone. Based on this evidence, researchers suggest that new strategies for BP should include topical clobetasol propionate as a possible therapy option, especially in those who are resistant to conventional forms of treatment.

For more information see page 1102.

*Generic: **Cyclophosphamide** (sye-kloe-FOS-fa-mide)*
*Brands: **Cytoxan, Neosar***

Cyclophosphamide, used to treat various types of cancer, works by slowing or stopping cell growth. The mainstay treatment of BP is systemic steroids and other immunosuppressive therapies. Researchers in India at Bangalore Medical College enrolled 50 people with autoimmune vesiculobullous disorders (a group of disorders characterized by fluid-filled vesicles on the skin) for dexamethasone-cyclophosphamide pulse therapy (DCP). Researchers state that this therapy is very effective in the treatment of vesiculobullous disorders.

For more information see page 1123.

Generic: **Dapsone** *(DAP-zone)*
Brand: **None**

As an anti-infective drug, dapsone has been used to treat leprosy, malaria, and *Pneumocystic carinii* in AIDS patients. However, it has also been prescribed for a variety of non-infectious diseases as well, such as bullous pemphigoid.

Dermatologica reported that three people with BP successfully responded to dapsone within two weeks of treatment, which supports findings by other physicians and researchers. *British Journal of Dermatology* reported that in a study with 18 patients with bullous pemphigoid, eight patients (44%) had a complete response and six (66%) had a partial response.

Another study tested the use of dapsone in combination to treat people who had severe or recurrent BP and who initially responded to prednisone and azathioprine but experienced flare-ups, even while on high doses of the drug. Researchers added dapsone to the treatment and 12 patients (92%) had complete remission, which enabled prednisone to be tapered. This suggests that dapsone may be effective in people with BP who are resistant to systemic steroids, can't take them, or are intolerant of side effects caused by other treatment options.

For more information see page 1131.

Generic: **Mycophenolate Mofetil**
(my-koe-FEN-oh-late MOE-feh-till)
Brands: **CellCept, Myfortic**

Mycophenolate mofetil, which is used in organ transplants to prevent rejection of the new organ, has recently been shown to help in autoimmune blistering disorders. In a study at the University of Ulm in Germany a case of BP that was difficult to control with systemic steroids was successfully treated with mycophenolate mofetil as additional therapy.

Mycophenolate mofetil seems also to help in the treatment of psoriasis and rheumatic arthritis. Recently, there have been six reported cases of successful treatment of blistering autoimmune diseases with mycophenolate mofetil in combination with high dose prednisone therapy. On the basis of these reports, researchers in Germany examined mycophenolate mofetil treatment in several patients with blistering autoimmune diseases. Besides using a combination of mycophenolate mofetil and high-dose prednisone, evaluation of mycophenolate mofetil monotherapy was evaluated for its effect in treating blistering autoimmune diseases. Five patients who had severe pemphigus vulgaris or BP were treated with mycophenolate mofetil. Two patients received mycophenolate mofetil in combination with high-dose prednisone therapy and three patients received mycophenolate mofetil monotherapy. According to researchers, all patients were completely free of symptoms within eight to 11 weeks of therapy.

For more information see page 1344.

Generic: **Prednisone** *(pred-NIS-zone)*
Brands: **Deltasone, Liquid Pred, Meticorten, Orasone, Sterapred**

Prednisone is a corticosteroid hormone that decreases the immune system's response to various diseases to reduce symptoms such as swelling and allergic-type reactions. It is used to treat arthritis, blood disorders, breathing problems, certain cancers, eye problems, immune system diseases, and skin diseases.

BP is the most common autoimmune blistering skin disease. Until recently the condition was treated with oral corticosteroids such as prednisone. However, high-dose corticosteroids are poorly tolerated in the elderly, and can even lead to death. According to researchers, prednisone should be considered only in the very rare cases that are either resistant or intolerant to other treatments.

For more information see page 1429.

Generic: **Tetracycline** *(tet-ra-SYE-kleen)*
Brands: **Sumycin, Wesmycin**

Tetracycline, an antibiotic that works by stopping the growth of bacteria, is used to treat a wide variety of infections, including acne. According to investigators at the University of Toronto, tetracycline with or without nicotinamide may benefit people with mild BP.

For more information see page 1503.

*Generic: **Immune Globulin IVIG***
(EH-mune GLOB-ewe-lyn)
*Brands: **Gamimune N, Gamunex, Octagam, Polygam S/D, Venoglobulin S***

In a study conducted at the New England Baptist Hospital fifteen people with recurrent BP who had experienced several significant side effects resulting from conventional therapy were treated with intravenous immunoglobulin (IVIG) therapy. While receiving IVIG, all people achieved a sustained clinical remission. IVIG improved quality of life and did not produce any serious side effects. IVIG appears to be an effective alternative in treating patients with severe BP who do not respond to conventional therapy. IVIG may be particularly useful, if treatment is begun early, in those who are at risk of experiencing serious or potentially fatal side effects from conventional immunosuppressive therapy.

For more information see page 1235.

Cheloid

See Keloids

Climatic Keratopathy

See Dermatitis (Chronic Actinic)

Dermatitis (Atopic)

Atopic dermatitis, also known as eczema and atopic eczema, is a chronic, itchy skin condition that is very common in children but may occur at any age. It is the most common form of dermatitis and usually occurs in people who have an "atopic tendency." That is, they have a tendency to develop any or all of three closely linked conditions: atopic dermatitis, asthma, and hay fever (allergic rhinitis). Often these conditions run within families with a parent, child, or sibling also affected. A family history of asthma, eczema, or hay fever is particularly useful in diagnosing atopic dermatitis in infants.

Atopic dermatitis is not contagious. It arises because of a complex interaction of genetic and environmental factors. These include skin irritants, the weather, temperature, and nonspecific triggers.

Commonly Prescribed (On-Label) Drugs: Methdilazine

OFF-LABEL PRESCRIPTION DRUGS
BREAKTHROUGH OPTIONS

Generic: **Azathioprine** *(ay-za-THYE-oh-preen)*
Brand: **Imuran**

Azathioprine is used to prevent rejection of transplanted organs and for cases of severe arthritis that do not respond to other therapies. There is a limited range of treatments for severe atopic dermatitis. Azathioprine has often been used but researchers note that there has been no clinical trial of this drug to confirm its efficacy in atopic dermatitis. A study of azathioprine was conducted in the United Kingdom with 37 adult patients with severe atopic dermatitis. Each treatment period lasted three months.

During the study, the disease decreased 26% during treatment with azathioprine vs. 3% on placebo. Pruritus, sleep disturbance, and disruption of work/daytime activity all improved significantly on active treatment but not on placebo. Gastrointestinal disturbances were reported by 14 patients during azathioprine treatment and four were withdrawn as a result of severe nausea and vomiting. Researchers concluded that azathioprine is an effective and useful drug in severe atopic dermatitis.

For more information see page 1033.

Generic: **Cyclosporine** *(si-klo-SPOR-een)*
Brands: **Gengraf, Neoral, Sandimmune**

Cyclosporine is an immunosuppressive drug used in the treatment of arthritis. It is used in adults with atopic dermatitis that has not responded to other treatments. Cydosporine is effective in blocking inflammation. In a study in *British Journal of Dermatology*, researchers evaluated the effects on quality of life of people with atopic dermatitis. Thirty-three patients with severe atopic dermatitis that did not respond to other treatments received either placebo for eight weeks followed by cyclosporine or the reverse (cyclosporine followed by placebo).

Cyclosporine significantly improved quality of life, especially with regard to psychosocial activities, sleep, home management, work, and recreation. Sleep improved and itching decreased. Additionally, the group that had received cyclosprine before placebo had a sustained quality of life after treatment was stopped. Researchers also noted that there was no correlation between disease activity and quality of life score.

For more information see pages 1125 and 1127.

Generic: ***Mycophenolate Mofetil***
(mye-koe-FEN-oh-late MOE-feh-till)
Brands: ***CellCept, Myfortic***

Mycophenolate mofetil is a medication that suppresses the body's immune system. A study in Germany evaluated whether mycophenolate mofetil is effective for treating moderate-severe atopic dermatitis that is not responsive to standard therapy.

Then patients received mycophenolate mofetil twice daily for four weeks. At week 5, the dosage was reduced until study end (week 8). Researchers observed that treatment with mycophenolate mofetil notably reduced the severity of atopic dermatitis within four weeks in all patients. Mycophenolate mofetil was well tolerated in most patients. Six of seven people who had responded to mycophenolate mofetil had no relapse of disease during 20-week follow-up. Therefore, researchers concluded that mycophenolate is a highly effective drug for treating moderate-severe atopic dermatitis, with no serious adverse effects occurring in any patients.

For more information see page 1344.

Dermatitis (Chronic Actinic)

Dermatitis, also called eczema, is an inflammation of the skin. It can have many causes and occur in many forms, but generally describes swollen, reddened, and itchy skin. Dermatitis is a common condition that is not life threatening or contagious, but it can make you uncomfortable and self-conscious. Every year, more than 12 million people in the United States visit a doctor because of a skin rash, such as dermatitis.

Commonly Prescribed (On-Label) Drugs: *Coal Tar, Methdilazine, Pimecrolimus, Tacrolimus*

OFF-LABEL PRESCRIPTION DRUGS
BREAKTHROUGH OPTIONS

Generic: **Acitretin** *(a-si-TRE-tin)*
Brand: **Soriatane**

Acitretin is a retinoid medication used in the treatment of severe psoriasis and other skin disorders in adults. Hand eczema is a common skin disease that tends to become chronic and may interfere with many types of work. Emollients have been shown to help reduce eczema and prevent hand eczema. Researchers in Denmark conducted a study of 29 patients who were diagnosed with dermatitis on their palms. Fourteen of the patients received acitretin while the remaining 15 received placebo.

After four weeks of treatment, patients receiving acitretin had a 51% reduction of symptoms compared with a 9% reduction in the placebo group. No further improvement was seen over another 4 weeks of treatment. Additionally, there were no changes in blood biochemistry, and no patients discontinued therapy because of side effects. Researchers concluded that acitretin is efficacious and safe to use in patients with dermatitis of the palms.

For more information see page 988.

Generic: **Cyclosporine** *(si-klo-SPOR-een)*
Brands: **Gengraf, Neoral, Sandimmune**

Cyclosporine is an immunosuppressive drug that treats chronic actinic by blocking the body's immune system. In a report in *European Journal of Dermatology,* doctors at the Institute of Dermatology in Italy treated a 69-year-old man with chronic atopic dermatitis. Initially, he was treated with oral steroids that resolved the dermatitis; however, once the dosage was lowered, he relapsed. Doctors then prescribed cyclosporine, which resulted in significant improvement, but symptoms again reappeared when the dosage was lowered so doctors administered the original dosage

(1.5 mg). He is still being treated with cyclosporine, and has no visible symptoms and no side effects.

For more information see pages 1125 and 1127.

Generic: **Danazol** *(DA-na-zole)*
Brand: **Danocrine**

Danazol is a synthetic derivative of ethisterone (a hormone). Researchers in Israel used danazol as a preventive treatment for recurrent episodes of autoimmune progesterone dermatitis, a rare condition appearing during the perimenstrual period or following progesterone treatment, in two young women. Other treatments have been ineffective. The treatment regimen consisted of danazol twice daily, starting one to two days before the expected date of each menses and continuing for three days thereafter. Researchers found this regimen to be highly effective in preventing the eruptions in these two women and concluded that people with autoimmune progesterone dermatitis may benefit from preventive treatment with danazol.

For more information see page 1129.

Erythema Solare

See Pruritus

Hives

See Urticaria

Impetigo

Impetigo is one of the most common skin infections. It usually appears on the face, especially around the nose and mouth. Although it commonly occurs when bacteria enter the skin through cuts or insect bites, it can also develop in skin that is perfectly healthy. Impetigo starts as a red sore that quickly ruptures, oozes for a few days, and then forms a yellowish-brown crust that looks like honey or brown sugar. This skin infection is highly contagious and scratching or touching the sores is likely to spread the infection to other parts of the body as well as to other people. Impetigo is seldom serious, and minor infections may clear without treatment in two to three weeks.

Commonly Prescribed (On-Label) Drugs: *Ammoniated Mercury, Cefditoren, Clioquinol, Gentamicin, Mupirocin, Nafcillin*

OFF-LABEL PRESCRIPTION DRUG
BREAKTHROUGH OPTION

Generic: **Erythromycin** *(er-ith-roe-MYE-sin)*
Brands: **Akne-Mycin, E.E.S., Eryc, Ery-Tab, Erythrocin**

Erythromycin is an antibiotic used to treat a wide variety of bacterial infections. *Staphylococcus aureus* remains one of the most common and troublesome of bacteria causing disease in humans. Skin and soft tissue infections that are predominantly caused by *S. aureus* include bullous and nonbullous impetigo.

Treatment of staphylococcal skin infections varies from topical antiseptics to prolonged intravenous antibacterials, depending on severity of the lesions and the health of the patient. According to investigators, the treatment of choice for oral antibacterials remains the penicillinase-resistant penicillins such as flucloxacillin. Cefalexin and erythromycin are suitable cost-effective alternatives with broader usage, although doctors should be careful to prescribe in ways that don't promote the development of resistance.

For more information see page 1170.

Impetigo Contagiosa

See Impetigo

Impetigo Vulgaris

See Impetigo

Itching

See Pruritus

Keloids

Keloids are raised overgrowths of scar tissue that occur at the site of a skin injury where trauma, surgery, blisters, vaccinations, acne, or body piercing have injured the skin. Less commonly, keloids may form in places where the skin has not had a visible injury. Keloids differ from normal mature scars in composition and size. Some people are prone to keloid formation and may develop them in several places.

Commonly Prescribed (On-Label) Drugs: *Betamethasone, Dexamethasone*

OFF-LABEL PRESCRIPTION DRUGS
BREAKTHROUGH OPTIONS

*Generic: **Bleomycin** (BLEE-o-mye-sin)*
*Brand: **Blenoxane***

Bleomycin is a medication used most commonly for treatment in cancer. Numerous treatments have been described for the treatment and prevention of scars, but researchers feel that the optimal management has yet to be defined. Researchers have studied the treatment and prevention of scars and keloids and found that a variety of new treatments exists with the potential to treat scars and keloids, including: interferon, imiquimod cream, tacrolimus, botulinum toxin, 5-fluorouracil, bleomycin, and verapamil. Several drugs have been effective in reducing scarring in vitro and in animal studies.

For more information see page 1050.

*Generic: **Interferon Alfa-2b** (in-ter-FEER-on AL-fa too-bee)*
*Brand: **Intron A***

Interferon alfa is a family of proteins with antiviral and immunomodulating activities. Researchers in the Department of Dermatology and Cutaneous Surgery at the University of Miami School of Medicine studied whether postsurgical treatment of keloids reduces the recurrence of keloids after they have been removed. The investigators administered either triamcinolone acetonide (TAC) or interferon alfa-2b (IFN-alpha 2b) in a postoperative injection.

Of keloids that were removed and then did not receive a postoperative injection 51.1% recurred. In comparison, 58.4% of TAC-treated lesions recurred and 18.7% of IFN-alpha 2b-treated lesions recurred. Researchers concluded that postoperative TAC injections do not reduce the number of keloid recurrences. However, injection of keloid excision sites with IFN-alpha 2b seems to have a therapeutic advantage over keloid surgery.

For more information see page 1243.

Generic: **Tretinoin** *(TRET-i-noyn)*
Brands: **Avita, Renova, Retin-A**

Tretinoin, a retinoid drug, is a medication used in the treatment of acne. It reduces the formation of pimples and promotes quick healing of pimples that do develop. Retinoids are potent inhibitors of MMPs (zinc-dependent enzymes that break down skin at the cellular level in both normal and diseased skin), especially in the treatment of aged skin and cancers. Researchers from the University of Tokyo also examined whether or not tretinoin affects MMPs that produce keloids, and found that tretinoin appeared to reverse the abnormal expression of keloids. The results suggest that tretinoin may be clinically useful to improve the chronic inflammation seen in keloids and prevent expansion of keloid tissues into normal skin.

For more information see page 1523.

Pruritus

Pruritus is a common manifestation of dermatologic diseases, including eczema, atopic dermatitis, and allergic contact dermatitis. Effective treatment of pruritus can prevent scratch-induced complications such as lichen simplex chronicus and impetigo. People, particularly elderly adults, with severe pruritus that does not respond to conservative therapy should be evaluated for an underlying systemic disease. Causes of systemic pruritus include uremia, cholestasis, polycythemia vera, Hodgkin's lymphoma, hyperthyroidism, and human immunodeficiency virus (HIV) infection. You may need skin scraping, biopsy, or culture if you have skin lesions.

Commonly Prescribed (On-Label) Drugs: Apomorphine, Cefazolin, Glutamine, Rifaximin

---

OFF-LABEL PRESCRIPTION DRUGS
BREAKTHROUGH OPTIONS

Generic: **Amitriptyline** *(a-mee-TRIP-ti-leen)*
Brand: **Elavil**

Amitriptyline is a tricyclic antidepressant medication used to treat depression, obsessive-compulsive disorders, and bed-wetting in children over six years of age. *Journal of the American Academy of Dermatology* reported an investigation into whether topically applied solutions of doxepin hydrochloride and amitriptyline hydrochloride affected pruritus in comparison to a solution of diphenhydramine alone. Researchers observed that doxepin, amitriptyline, and diphenhydramine all produced significantly higher relief. These researchers suggest that tricyclic antidepressants are effective topical antipruritic drugs.

For more information see page 1009.

Generic: **Nalmefene** *(NAL-me-feen)*
Brand: **Revex**

Nalmefene is used to reverse the effects of narcotic pain relievers used in medical procedures. Researchers at the National Institute of Diabetes and Digestive and Kidney Diseases evaluated the effects of naloxone on pruritus. The study involved 11 people with generalized pruritus complicating chronic liver disease. They were administered nalmefene or placebo for two months. At the end of the study, researchers concluded that nalmefene therapy was associated with a 75% reduction in the hourly scratching activity and a decrease in the visual perception of pruritus in all eight patients. Based on these results, researchers concluded that oral administration of nalmefene can relieve pruritus complicating chronic liver disease.

For more information see page 1350.

Generic: **Naltrexone** *(nal-TREKS-one)*
Brands: **Naltrexone, ReVia**

Naltrexone is used to maintain a drug-free state in people previously addicted to opiates. It is used in combination with behavior adjustment programs and only after you have completed a detoxification program.

Chloroquine induces a severe generalized pruritus, in predisposed African-American patients, during treatment of malaria fever, and also in some Caucasian patients treated for rheumatological diseases. A study in *International Journal of Dermatology* assessed and compared the antipruritic efficacy of naltrexone and the antihistamine, promethazine, in chloroquine-treated patients with malaria fever. The study compared the chloroquine-induced pruritus intensity and time profile in people with malaria fever who were pretreated with a single dose of either naltrexone or promethazine (six patients each). According to researchers, both naltrexone and promethazine reduced itching severity. One patient on naltrexone and two on promethazine never experienced any itching. Researchers concluded that naltrexone exerted an antipruritic action, at least to a similar extent to promethazine in people with chloroquine-induced itching in malaria fever.

For more information see page 1352.

Generic: **Ondansetron** *(on-DAN-se-tron)*
Brands: **Zofran, Zofran ODT**

Ondansetron is used to prevent nausea and vomiting caused by cancer chemotherapy or after surgery by blocking the hormone (serotonin) that causes vomiting.

Postoperative itching after intrathecal (the administration of medication into the spinal cord) delivery of narcotics may be a difficult problem for both the anesthesiologist and the person in the postanesthetic care unit. Since some studies have reported success in preventing itching with ondansetron, a study was conducted at the Departments of Medical Research and Anesthesiology in Taiwan tested whether preventive intravenous (IV) ondansetron effectively reduces the incidence of pruritus. Thirty-four patients underwent surgery after spinal anesthesia with intrathecal lidocaine and intrathecal sufentanil.

Ondansetron did not reduce the incidence of pruritus (77 vs. 81%) compared to placebo. The pruritus scores of the two groups were not significantly different. However, according to investigators, there are contradictory findings in the literature regarding the effectiveness of ondansetron in preventing narcotic-induced itching. Although some studies have indicated that ondansetron could prevent this side effect of intrathecal narcotics, researchers suggest that ondansetron is not effective in preventing narcotic-induced itching after a caesarean section.

For more information see page 1387.

Generic: **Paroxetine** *(pa-ROKS-e-teen)*
Brands: **Paxil, Paxil CR**

Paroxetine, a selective serotonin-reuptake inhibitor (SSRI), is an antidepressant drug used to treat depression, panic attacks, obsessive-compulsive disorder (OCD), social anxiety disorder (social phobia), posttraumatic stress disorder (PTSD), and generalized anxiety disorders (GAD).

Studies have suggested that, in people experiencing severe pruritus, paroxetine has a rapid anti-itching effect. One study in the Netherlands compared paroxetine and placebo. Twenty-six people were involved; 17 of them had solid tumors; four had blood disorders; and five had various nonmalignant conditions.

Patients were assigned to treatment with paroxetine or placebo. Two patients discontinued treatment because of adverse effects of paroxetine. Twenty-four patients treated with paroxetine had lower itching intensity over the seven treatment periods as compared to placebo. According to researchers, the outcome of this study indicates that paroxetine is effective in treating of severe itching of non-dermatological origin.

For more information see page 1395.

Generic: **Thalidomide** *(tha-LI-doe-mide)*
Brand: **Thalomid**

Thalidomide is an immunomodulatory drug with anti-inflammatory, sedative, and hypnotic activity. Researchers in the United Kingdom conducted a study of thalidomide's effects on pruritus with 11 patients with chronic pruritus caused by other skin disorders. Researchers noted that nocturnal scratch movement was decreased by thalidomide, and indicated that it may be an effective treatment for pruritus.

For more information see page 1505.

Psoriasis

Psoriasis is a common, chronic skin disorder. Plaque psoriasis is the most common type of psoriasis, characterized by red skin covered with silvery scales and inflammation. Patches of circular to oval shaped red plaques that itch or burn are typical of plaque psoriasis. The patches are usually found on the arms, legs, trunk, or scalp but maybe found on any part of the skin. The most typical areas are the knees and elbows.

Commonly Prescribed (On-Label) Drugs: *Acitretin, Alefacept, Amcinonide, Ammoniated Mercury, Anthralin, Betamethasone, Calcipotriene, Clobetasol Coal Tar, Cortisone, Cyclosporine, Desonide, Desoximetasone, Dexamethasone, Diflorasone, Efalizumab, Etanercept, Etretinate, Fluocinolone, Fluocinonide, Flurandrenolide, Fluticasone, Fusidic Acid, Gentamicin, Halcinonide, Juniper Tar, Methotrexate, Methoxsalen, Methylprednisolone, Mometasone, Prednicarbate, Prednisolone, Prednisone, Salicylic Acid, Tazarotene, Triamcinolone*

OFF-LABEL PRESCRIPTION DRUGS
BREAKTHROUGH OPTIONS

Generic: ***Infliximab*** *(in-FLIKS-e-mab)*
Brand: ***Remicade***

Infliximab is a monoclonal antibody that decreases swelling and decreases immune system function. According to researchers, encouraging results from clinical trials suggest that infliximab is effective for psoriasis. A study at The Johns Hopkins University School of Medicine evaluated the scientific evidence for the efficacy and safety of drugs for psoriasis, including data on alefacept, efalizumab, etanercept, and infliximab. Overall, researchers concluded that these drugs represent an important addition to psoriatic therapies and improve the disease course and life quality of those afflicted with psoriasis.

For more information see page 1239.

Generic: *Leflunomide* (le-FLOO-noh-mide)
Brand: *Arava*

Leflunomide has anti-inflammatory and immunosuppressive effects, used to treat arthritis (rheumatoid type). It works by suppressing the immune system, since rheumatoid arthritis is caused by damage from an overactive immune system.

Leflunomide is highly effective in treating rheumatoid arthritis, and small studies have suggested similar efficacy in psoriatic arthritis. In a German clinical trial, one hundred ninety patients with active psoriatic arthritis and psoriasis (at least 3% skin involvement) were divided to receive leflunomide or placebo for 24 weeks. At 24 weeks, 56 of 95 leflunomide-treated patients and 27 of 91 placebo-treated had responded. Researchers concluded that leflunomide is an effective treatment for psoriatic arthritis and psoriasis, providing a safe, convenient alternative to current therapies.

For more information see page 1270.

Generic: *Sirolimus* (sear-OH-le-mus)
Brand: *Rapamune*

Sirolimus is a potent immunosuppressive drug used to prevent the rejection of transplanted organs.

Sirolimus has also demonstrated efficacy in psoriasis when taken internally, so a study in *British Journal of Dermatology* sought to determine the efficacy and safety of sirolimus when applied topically. Researchers wanted to evaluate if sirolimus penetrates human skin. Twenty-four people with stable, chronic psoriasis received a small concentration of sirolimus for six weeks and then a greater concentration for an additional six weeks. There was a significant reduction in disease activity with topical sirolimus. When researchers evaluated the effects of sirolimus on psoriasis using a computerized imaging analysis of the biopsies, they also found a significant reduction in proliferating cells in the skin with sirolimus treatment. They concluded that topically applied sirolimus penetrates normal skin and has some antipsoriatic benefits.

For more information see page 1475.

Generic: **Topiramate** *(TOE-pie-rah-mate)*
Brand: **Topamax**

Topiramate is an anticonvulsant and antimigraine drug. Potomac Ridge Behavioural Health initiated a study following a finding in which a patient with both a mood disorder and psoriasis experienced significant improvement of her psoriasis following treatment with topiramate. Researchers evaluated the effectiveness of topiramate for the treatment of psoriasis. The patients were treated for a minimum of four months. For all patients, their psoriasis decreased after treatment. According to researchers, these results represent the first known report of the efficacy of topiramate in the treatment of psoriasis.

For more information see page 1516.

Rosacea

Rosacea is a chronic disease that affects the skin and sometimes the eyes. The disorder is characterized by redness, pimples, and in advanced stages thickened skin. Rosacea usually affects the face; other parts of the upper body are only rarely involved.

Commonly Prescribed (On-Label) Drugs: *Azelaic Acid, Dexamethasone, Metronidazole, Sulfacetamide, Sulfur*

OFF-LABEL PRESCRIPTION DRUGS
BREAKTHROUGH OPTIONS

Generic: **Clindamycin** *(klin-da-MYE-sin)*
Brands: **Cleocin T, Clindagel, ClindaMax, Clindets**

Clindamycin, used to treat a wide variety of serious bacterial infections, is an antibiotic that stops the growth of bacteria. In a study at Ohio State University, the topical antibiotic preparation, clindamycin in a lotion base, was compared with oral tetracycline in the treatment of rosacea in 43 people. Patients used topical clindamycin lotion applied twice daily or tetracycline. Patients' lesions were examined at three-week intervals over a period of 12 weeks. Topical clindamycin produced similar clinical results to oral tetracycline and was superior in the eradication of pustules, and researchers concluded that topical clindamycin in a lotion base is a safe, effective alternative to oral tetracycline therapy for treating rosacea.

For more information see page 1099.

Generic: Tetracycline antibiotics such as **Doxycycline** *(doks-i-SYE-kleen)*, **Minocycline** *(min-OH-sik-kleen)*, and **Tetracycline** *(tet-ra-SYE-kleen)*
Brands: **Adoxa, Doryx, Doxy-100, Monodox, Periostat, Vibramycin, Vibra-Tabs (doxycycline), Dynacin, Minocin (minocycline), Sumycin, Wesmycin (tetracycline)**

Doxycycline, minocycline, and tetracycline are antibiotics used to treat a wide variety of bacterial infections including acne.

The systemic treatment of erythrosis (a chronic state of capillary dilation in rosacea) is based on the association of *H. pylori* with rosacea, although researchers are still debating this association. Studies have shown the eradication of *H. pylori* using systemic treatments such as doxycycline and minocycline. Additionally, researchers are currently investigating a low-dose doxycycline. This treatment may provide greater safety than existing oral antibiotics.

Researchers are also examining the role of tetracycline in treating rosacea. Data pooled from three studies in the Netherlands of oral tetracycline versus placebo involving 152 patients showed that, according to physicians, tetracycline was effective, so there is some evidence that oral tetracycline is effective.

For more information see pages 1158, 1331, and 1503.

Scabies

Scabies is a common infestation of the skin with the microscopic mite *Sarcoptes scabei*. It is found worldwide, and affects people of all races and social classes. Scabies spreads rapidly under crowded conditions where there is frequent skin-to-skin contact between people, such as in schools and child-care facilities.

Commonly Prescribed (On-Label) Drugs: *Crotamiton, Lindane, Permethrin Cream*

OFF-LABEL PRESCRIPTION DRUG
BREAKTHROUGH OPTION

Generic: **Ivermectin** *(eye-ver-MEK-tin)*
Brand: **Stromectol**

Ivermectin is used to treat infections of certain parasites and has been used as an alternative drug for the treatment of scabies. Most clinicians consider topical permethrin to be the scabicide of choice because of its safety and efficacy relative to other available drugs, particularly lindane. Recommendations for alternative therapy differ among various clinicians. Experts recommend topical lindane or oral ivermectin as alternative scabicides, but some clinicians recommend oral ivermectin or topical crotamiton as alternatives. Oral ivermectin may be particularly useful in therapy-resistant infestations, for control of outbreaks in institutions, and when compliance with topical therapy is difficult.

Some clinicians consider ivermectin, alone or in combination with a topical scabicide, the regimen of choice for treatment of crusted scabies in immunocompromised people. Because substantial treatment failure might occur with topical scabicide or oral ivermectin treatment alone, some clinicians recommend simultaneous therapy with a topical scabicide and oral ivermectin or repeated treatments with oral ivermectin. Other clinicians recommend oral ivermectin for therapy-resistant infections or in people who cannot tolerate topical therapy.

For more information see page 1258.

Sunburn

Sunburn results from too much sun or sun-equivalent exposure. Almost everyone has been sunburned or will become sunburned at some time. Anyone who visits a beach, goes fishing, works in the yard, or simply is out in the sun can get sunburn. Improper use of tanning beds is also an increasing cause of sunburn. Although seldom fatal, sunburn can be disabling and cause quite a bit of discomfort. Severe sunburns increase the risk of developing skin cancer.

Ultraviolet B (UVB) radiation causes much of the damage after both acute and long-term exposure to the sun and is also the major cause of human skin cancer. UVB exposure initially induces an inflammatory response that has been linked to tumor formation.

Commonly Prescribed (On-Label) Drugs: Dibucaine

OFF-LABEL PRESCRIPTION DRUG
BREAKTHROUGH OPTION

Generic: **Indomethacin** *(in-doe-METH-a-sin)*
Brands: **Indocin, Indocin IV, Indocin SR**

Indomethacin treats the pain, swelling, and stiffness associated with arthritis, gout, bursitis, or tendonitis. An animal study by researchers in Japan studied the effects of indomethacin on sunburn and found that indomethacin was more effective as a preventive for sunburn, rather than a treatment for already existing sunburn. Its use as a preventive is still being studied.

For more information see page 1238.

Urticaria

Urticaria, or hives as it is commonly called, is an itchy rash consisting of localized swellings of the skin that usually lasts for a few hours before fading away. When urticaria develops around loose tissues of the eyes or lips, the affected area may swell excessively. Although frightening in appearance, the swelling (called angiooedema) goes away in 12 to 24 hours with treatment.

Commonly Prescribed (On-Label) Drugs: Astemizole, Brompheniramine, Cetirizine, Clemastine, Cyproheptadine, Desloratadine, Diphenhydramine, Fexofenadine, Loratadine, Methdilazine, Methylprednisolone, Tripelennamine

OFF-LABEL PRESCRIPTION DRUGS
BREAKTHROUGH OPTIONS

*Generic: **Amitriptyline*** *(a-mee-TRIP-ti-leen)*
*Brand: **Elavil***

Amitriptyline is a tricyclic antidepressant used to treat depression, obsessive-compulsive disorders, and bed-wetting in children over six years of age. Some of the psychiatric disorders that are usually associated with dermatological disorders and respond to antidepressants include major depressive disorder, obsessive-compulsive disorder, social phobia, and posttraumatic stress disorder. Skin disorder symptoms may be the feature of a primary psychiatric disorder, such as body image problems and dermatitis artefacta (self-induced skin lesions from itching or scratching).

The SSRI antidepressants such as amitriptyline are potentially beneficial in the management of all the major psychiatric syndromes that are encountered in dermatological disorders. The generally more favorable side effects of the SSRIs, such as lower toxicity to the heart in contrast to the tricyclic antidepressants, has made them the first-line treatment for the treatment of depression. Furthermore, some of the properties of the antidepressant drugs that are not related to their antidepressant activity, such as the histamine blocking effect of medications such as doxepin, amitriptyline, and trimipramine, are of benefit in dermatological conditions such as urticaria (hives) and itching.

For more information see page 1009.

*Generic: H_2 blockers such as **Cimetidine*** *(sye-MET-i-deen)*
and ***Ranitidine*** *(rah-nit-a-deen)*
*Brands: **Tagamet (cimetidine), Zantac, Zantac EFFER-dose (ranitidine)***

Cimetidine and ranitidine block secretion of acid from the stomach and are classified as antihistamines. Itch can originate as a disorder of the skin, neuropathic (multiple sclerosis), neurogenic (cholestasis), or psychogenic. Although itch of skin origin shares a common neural pathway with pain, the fiber involved in this type of itch are distinct. They respond to histamine and acetylcholine (a chemical in the brain) but are insensitive to mechanical stimuli. Histamine is the main component for itch in insect bite reactions and in most forms of hives, and in these circumstances the itch responds well to antihistamines. According to researchers, cimetidine and ranitidine may have a role in treating hives that are a symptom of an allergic reaction.

For more information see pages 1091 and 1443.

Generic: Cyclosporine (si-klo-SPOR-een)
Brands: Gengraf, Neoral, Sandimmune

Cyclosporine, an immunosuppressive drug, is used to prevent or treat organ rejection in transplant patients. An Italian study evaluated the effectiveness and safety of cyclosporine in the treatment of people with chronic hives (urticaria) who failed to respond to conventional therapy and who had to resort to long-term oral steroid treatment. In the study, 40 adults received either cyclosporine or cetirizine and then they were followed up for nine months.

All 40 patients completed the 16-week cyclosporine therapy without dropping out because of side effects. During cyclosporine treatment, 20 people had relapses resolving spontaneously or with antihistamines. During the nine-month follow-up period, 22 patients had relapses resolving spontaneously or with antihistamines. According to researchers, these results show the long-term efficacy and tolerability of cyclosporine in patients with severe chronic urticaria that is unresponsive to conventional treatments.

For more information see pages 1125 and 1127.

Generic: Doxepin (DOKS-e-pin)
Brands: Prudoxin, Sinequan

Doxepin is a tricyclic antidepressant used to treat depression, obsessive-compulsive disorders, and bed-wetting in children over 6 years of age.

The primary treatment of urticaria (hives) involves identification and discontinuation of the cause. Addition of an antihistaminic drug may be necessary to control itching. Because patients responded differently, several alternative drugs may need to be tried before the most effective one is found. Based on studies, low-dose doxepin seems effective and well tolerated by those who do not respond to conventional antihistamines. This success may be due in part to doxepin's more potent antihistamine-blocking properties. However, according to investigators, doxepin cream does not appear to be as effective as systemic therapy, and adverse effects (including sedation) and drug interactions are problematic. Researchers feel that topical use may be best suited to conditions involving intact skin that does not need treatment of large areas of the body, thereby reducing systemic absorption and adverse effects.

For more information see page 1154.

Generic: **Methotrexate** *(meth-oh-TREXS-ate)*
Brands: **Rheumatrex, Trexall**

Methotrexate is an immunosuppressant used to treat certain cancers and to control severe psoriasis or rheumatoid arthritis. It works by interfering with cell growth and suppressing the immune system.

In a Mexican study, researchers examined the role of methotrexate in seven people with autoimmune urticaria (hives). The patients were treated with methotrexate every 12 hours, two days a week. In cases where no toxicity was present in patients, doses increased to three days a week for a six-week period. Researchers observed a significant reduction in itching, the presence of spots, and the patient's ability to carry out daily activities. They concluded that methotrexate is effective treating autoimmune urticaria.

For more information see page 1312.

Generic: **Methylprednisolone** *(meth-il-pred-NIS-oh-lone)*
Brands: **Depo-Medrol, Medrol, Solu-Medrol**

Methylprednisolone, a systemic corticosteroid, is used principally as an anti-inflammatory or immunosuppressive drug. Although histamine blockers are known to alleviate the symptoms of urticaria effectively in most cases, more resistant patients may need systemic corticosteroids. A Canadian study examined the effects of a seven-day course of corticosteroids or placebo on histamine releasing factor (HRF) production in non-lesional skin of 19 chronic urticaria patients. Researchers observed no significant changes occurring in HRF production and histamine content after placebo treatment. In contrast with this, significant decrease of HRF activity was observed after one week of oral methyl-prednisolone. There was no change for histamine secretion. Researchers believe that these data suggest that corticosteroid therapy improves symptoms of chronic urticaria because of a decreased production of HRF in uninvolved skin.

For more information see page 1316.

Generic: **Montelukast** *(mon-te-LOO-kast)*
Brand: **Singulair**

Montelukast is an antiasthmatic drug used to control chronic asthma and help decrease the number of asthma attacks. It is also used to treat hay fever.

Many patients' chronic hives (urticaria) are not sufficiently controlled with histamine blockers. Researchers in Japan studied the effectiveness of montelukast for the treatment of chronic urticaria. Twenty-five patients were treated with montelukast for one week or more, without changing any treatment that they were using before the study, including histamine blockers. Twelve people, including six who had been treated with corticosteroids, were evaluated as "markedly improved" or "improved" following treatment with montelukast. Researchers concluded that montelukast may be worth trying for patients with chronic urticaria, when the condition is not sufficiently controlled with histamine blockers.

For more information see page 1340.

Generic: **Prednisolone** *(pred-NISS-oh-lone)*
Brands: **Predalone, Prelone**

Prednisolone reduces swelling and is used for many conditions, among them: allergic reactions, skin diseases (psoriasis, hives), breathing problems; cancers, blood disorders, and eye problems; arthritis, digestive problems, and for hormone replacement.

Researchers in Germany studied people with acute urticaria attending a department of dermatology and a rural dermatology office during the course of one year. Most patients suffered from moderate (42%) to severe (40%) disease. Patients received either loratadine or prednisolone. Both treatment regimens were effective in controlling itchy, raised patches of skin, but the corticosteroid-treated patients' symptoms ceased earlier, with complete remission occurring within three days of treatment in 93.8%, compared to 65.9% of patients treated with loratadine.

For more information see page 1428.

Generic: **Prednisone** (pred-NIS-zone)
Brands: **Deltasone, Liquid Pred, Meticorten, Orasone, Sterapred**

Prednisone is a synthetic glucocorticoid. To evaluate the efficacy of a four-day course of prednisone added to standard treatment with histamine blockers for the management of acute hives (urticaria), the emergency department of Maricopa Medical Center in Arizona conducted a trial. The study included adult patients with rash of no more than 24 hours' duration, regardless of cause. All patients were asked to evaluate the severity of itching and given diphenhydramine. When discharged, they were prescribed a regimen of hydroxyzine for itching, plus either prednisone or placebo for four days.

Forty-three patients were enrolled; 24 received prednisone and 19 received placebo. The two groups had similar severity of itching at enrollment, but at two- and five-day follow-up the prednisone group had significantly less itching and greater improvement of the rash. Researchers concluded that the addition of a prednisone burst improves the response of acute hives to antihistamines. Patients' conditions improved more quickly and more completely when prednisone was administered, without any apparent adverse effects.

For more information see page 1429.

Vitiligo

Vitiligo is a pigmentation disorder in which melanocytes (the cells that make pigment) in the skin, the mucous membranes (tissues that line the inside of the mouth and nose and genital and rectal areas) and the retina (inner layer of the eyeball) are destroyed. As a result, white patches of skin appear on different parts of the body. The hair that grows in areas affected by vitiligo usually turns white. The cause of vitiligo is not known, but doctors and researchers have several different theories.

Commonly Prescribed (On-Label) Drugs: Dihydroxyacetone, Methoxsalen, Monobenzone, Trioxsalen

---

OFF-LABEL PRESCRIPTION DRUG BREAKTHROUGH OPTION

Generic: **Tacrolimus** *(ta-KROE-li-mus)*
Brands: **Prograf, Protopic**

Tacrolimus is an immunosuppressant approved to treat eczema in people who have not responded well to, or who should not use, other eczema medications such as topical steroids. Since its introduction, researchers have found topical tacrolimus also to be effective and well tolerated in people with a variety of other skin disorders.

Tacrolimus is one of the newer immunosuppressants that act by inhibiting T-cell (a type of white blood cell involved in the body's immune system) activation and cytokine release (protein molecules that promote the communication between immune system cells). Tacrolimus appears to minimize the need for topical glucocorticoids and does not cause skin wasting. However, researchers feel that further studies are needed to clarify its effects on a variety of conditions.

For more information see page 1489.

Warts, Non-genital

Warts are a type of infection caused by viruses in the human papillomavirus (HPV) family. There are at least 60 types of HPV viruses. Warts can grow on all parts of your body. They can grow on the skin, on the inside of the mouth, on the genitals, and in the rectal area. Some varieties of HPV tend to cause warts on the skin, while other HPV types tend to cause warts on the genitals and rectal area. Some people are more naturally resistant to the HPV viruses and do not seem to get warts as easily as other people.

Commonly Prescribed (On-Label) Drugs: Interferon Alfa-N3, Podofilox

OFF-LABEL PRESCRIPTION DRUGS
BREAKTHROUGH OPTIONS

*Generic: **5-Fluorouracil** (flure-oh-YOOR-a-sil)*
*Brand: **Adrucil***

Fluorouracil is a medication that interferes with DNA synthesis. According to researchers, fluorouracil is effective in treating warts, but the method in which it is applied directly onto the affected tissue is not always been effective. Researchers in Turkey sought to evaluate the safety and efficacy of 5-fluorouracil in the treatment of verrucae (small skin lesion commonly found on the bottom of the foot). Seventy-six patients with a 315 total verrucae received a 5-fluorouracil, lidocaine, and epinephrine (5-FU + LE) mixture or placebo injection into the lesion. Complete response was noted in an average of 70% of the verrucae treated with the 5-FU + LE mixture and in 29% of those in the placebo group. No clinically significant systemic and local adverse effects occurred. Recurrence rates were evaluated and no statistically significant difference between the two groups was found. Researchers concluded that treatment of verrucae with 5-FU + LE mixture is safe and effective.

For more information see page 981.

*Generic: **Cimetidine** (sye-MET-i-deen)*
*Brand: **Tagamet***

Cimetidine blocks secretion of acid from the stomach. Several clinicians have reported successfully using cimetidine against warts but previous studies comparing cimetidine with placebo therapy have failed to statistically and scientifically corroborate those results. *Journal of American Podiatry Medical Association* reported that between 1995 and 2002, 216 people underwent treatment with oral cimetidine for plantar's wart. Physicians concluded that cimetidine may be used as a safe, effective, lone treatment for verrucae in all age groups.

For more information see page 1091.

Generic: **Imiquimod** *(i-mi-KWI-mod)*
Brand: **Aldara**

Imiquimod is used to treat a precancerous skin condition known as actinic keratosis and a cancerous skin condition called superficial basal cell carcinoma. It is also used to treat external genital and anal warts and is not recommended for use to remove human papilloma virus (HPV) growths.

Researchers at University of California at Irvine reported that infections with five of the herpes viruses (herpes simplex virus (HSV) 1, HSV-2, varicella zoster virus, Epstein-Barr virus, and cytomegalovirus) are treated with topical or systemic antiviral therapies. More than 100 types of HPVs may manifest as warts, skin cancers, cervical cancer, anogenital cancers, and upper digestive tract cancers and researchers suggest that immunomodulating medications, such as imiquimod, act on HPV indirectly by inducing immune responses, thereby reducing recurrences.

For more information see page 1233.

WOMEN'S HEALTH DISORDERS

GYNECOLOGIC CONDITIONS

Endometrial Implants

See Endometriosis

Endometriosis

Endometriosis is a chronic condition that affects the tissue that lines the uterus (endometrium). The abnormal tissue called endometrial implants grows outside of the uterus in other areas of the body, including ovaries, bowel, rectum, bladder, and the lining of the pelvis. When this occurs there may be: pain, irregular vaginal bleeding, and frequently infertility. Endometriosis affects five to 10% of women. The most common treatment is oral contraceptives; it is rare to find women who do not respond to oral contraceptives for the symptoms of endometriosis. Birth control pills help control the hormones responsible for the buildup of endometrial tissue each month and taking the pill long-term may reduce or eliminate the pain of endometriosis. Most women also have lighter and shorter menstrual flow when taking the pill.

Commonly Prescribed (On-Label) Drugs: *Danazol, Goserelin, Leuprolide, Nafarelin, Norethindrone*

OFF-LABEL PRESCRIPTION DRUGS
BREAKTHROUGH OPTIONS

Generic: **Levonorgestrel-Ethinyl Estradiol**
(LEE-voe-nor-jes-trel ETH-in-il es-tra-DYE-ole)
Brands: **Levlen, Levora, Nordette, Portia, Seasonale**

Levonorgestrel and ethinyl estradiol belong to the class of medication known as oral contraceptives (OCs) or birth control pills. This drug contains two types of hormones, estrogen and progestin. When these hormones are taken together they interfere with the normal hormonal fluctuations during the menstrual cycle and maintain hormone levels at a more constant level. Because the abnormal tissue in endometriosis is sensitive to menstrual cycle hormones, oral contraceptives are widely used to treat it and are often the first line of therapy for endometriosis. They can be given cyclically (three weeks on the pill and one week off) or continuously without interruption.

This medication inhibits hormones and suppresses ovarian estrogen production. The endometrial tissue is reduced, and swelling, bleeding and inflammation decrease. This combination oral contraceptive has reduced pelvic pain and abnormal menstruation in up to 89% of patients. As with other hormonal therapy, there is no documented improvement in fertility. Oral contraceptives have been widely used in the United States for the past 40 years, and current estimates show that about 10 million American women use them annually.

For more information see pages 1279.

Generic: **Medroxyprogesterone Contraceptive Injection**
(me-DROX-ee-proe-JES-te-rone)
Brand: **Depo-Provera**

Medroxyprogesterone acetate (MPA) is a commonly prescribed progestin hormone therapy for endometriosis that shrinks endometrial tissue. A long-acting injection is generally given every three months. Progestin therapy has been shown to limit estrogen-stimulated endometrial tissue growth. With this regimen, improvement has been reported in 57% to 96% of women and lesion regression observed in 40% to 60%.

A study examined the efficiency and side-effects of depot MPA (DMPA) in the treatment of moderate or severe endometriosis. Ninety-four women with moderate or severe endometriosis after surgery were divided into three groups: 34 cases in the group of DMPA received DMPA by injection every 28–30 days for six months; 30 cases in the group of gonadotropin releasing hormone agonists (GnRH-a) received leuprorelin acetate by injection every 28–30 days for six months; 30 cases in the control group did not receive any postoperative medical treatment. Patients' symptoms and signs, including pelvic pain, pelvic tenderness, menstrual and weight changes, were recorded before and after treatment, as well as liver and renal functions and sex hormone level. Both DMPA and GnRH-a treatment achieved similar significant relief of pelvic symptoms and signs (88% and 93%) compared with the control group. The recurrence rates in the DMPA and GnRH-a groups were 6% and 7%, significantly lower than the control group.

The researchers concluded that DMPA seems to be an effective, safe, and convenient treatment for endometriosis with low-cost, good compliance, and few side effects.

For more information see page 1299.

*Generic: **Medroxyprogesterone Acetate***
(me-DROX-ee-proe-JES-te-rone AS-eh-tate)
*Brand: **Provera***

Medroxyprogesterone acetate (MPA) oral is a progestin hormone medication. Oral progestins are the oldest drugs used for endometriosis. Progestins can prevent ovulation and reduce the risk for endometriosis in two ways. They reduce luteinizing hormone (LH), one of the reproductive hormones important in ovulation and they also change the lining of the uterus and eventually cause the lining to waste away. Some experts recommend progestins as the first choice for women with endometriosis who do not want to become pregnant. Progestins should not be taken during the luteal phase of the menstrual cycle (the premenstrual phase, which is 14 days before a period.)

MPA is typically administered orally for three months. Pain relief with progestin therapy has been reported as excellent. Clinical trials have shown a pain relief rate of up to 90% and improvement of pelvic density and tenderness in 80% of patients. Progestins have not been shown to improve fertility. Studies of women with early-stage endometriosis who were treated with MPA or expectant management had similar pregnancy rates over an 18-month period of time. Adverse effects include abnormal vaginal bleeding in about 20%, nausea, breast tenderness, fluid retention and depression. If effective, researchers have found that this medication can be used safely for long periods of time.

For more information see page 1297.

Generic: **Mifepristone** *(mi-FE-pris-tone)*
Brand: **Mifeprex**

Mifepristone triggers a miscarriage by blocking the actions of two hormones—the female sex hormones progesterone and glucocorticoids. Researchers at the University of California at San Diego spearheaded studies on mifepristone as a treatment for fibroids and endometriosis. Researchers concluded that the drug was "likely to be effective for both," reporting that a daily dose of mifepristone could shrink fibroids by 50% with few side effects. The drug also relieved pain and physical abnormalities associated with endometriosis. Moreover, mifepristone was shown to cause "less severe disruption of female hormones and fewer side effects" than some other hormonal treatments.

Case reports have shown that treatment with mifepristone can reduce pain and abnormal vaginal bleeding. Researchers believe that it might reduce abnormal endometrial tissue without dangerously lowering estrogen levels. Although use of antiprogestin reduced pain in all women, significant relief of symptoms occurred only when treatment lasted longer than six months.

For more information see page 1328.

Generic: **Norethindrone Acetate-Ethinyl Estradiol**
(NOR-eth-in-drone AS-eh-tate ETH-in-ill ess-tra-DYE-ole)
Brands: **Estrostep, Junel, Loestrin, Microgestin**

Norethindrone acetate-ethinyl estradiol is a combination of progesterone and estrogen drugs approved for use as oral contraceptives. The combination oral contraceptives combine natural or synthetic estrogens and progestins, similar to the natural sex hormones (estrogen and progesterone) produced in a woman's body. Ethinyl estradiol is an estrogen and norethindrone is a progestin. Together this combination can prevent ovulation and pregnancy. In general, a combination of estrogen and progestin works better than a single-ingredient product. Ethinyl estradiol/norethindrone tablets can also help regulate menstrual flow, treat acne, or may be used for other hormone related problems in women.

Combination oral contraceptives are often prescribed off-label to relieve pain with menses and other symptoms associated with endometriosis. They successfully reduced swelling, bleeding, inflammation and endometriotic lesions associated with endometriosis in 89% of patients. It does not improve fertility rates. Estrogen-progestin products are available as pills, skin patches, and vaginal rings; you can take them continuously without stopping treatment, or cyclically, with a week of no treatment (or placebo pills) between treatment cycles.

Although drug treatments will not cure endometriosis, they can provide significant symptom relief for many women. The treatment regimens for endometriosis with oral contraceptives are sometimes given continuously for several months (skipping the seven-day pill-free period). Taking the combination oral contraceptive pill continuously eliminates the incidence of period-related pain.

For more information see page 1370.

*Generic: **Norgestrel-Ethinyl Estradiol***
(nor-JES-trel ETH-in-il es-tra-DYE-ole)
*Brands: **Cryselle, Lo/Ovral, Low-Ogestrel, Ogestrel, Ovral***

Norgestrel-ethinyl estradiol is approved for use as a combination oral contraceptive medication. The combination oral contraceptive pill contains the hormones estrogen and progestogen. The oral contraceptives favored for treating endometriosis have a higher progestogen-to-estrogen ratio. The oral contraceptive pill may be useful off-label for women who have milder endometriosis symptoms, particularly adolescents and women who do not wish to take the other drugs available.

Continuously taking the combined oral contraceptive pill eliminates withdrawal bleeding and the incidence of period-related pain. It also reduces the amount of blood and the appearance of additional endometrial implants. Common side effects include fluid retention, nausea, breast tenderness, headaches, vaginal discharge and decreased sexual drive. Norgestrel-ethinyl estradiol is especially useful for minimizing the side effects of spotting and breakthrough bleeding.

For more information see page 1376.

Generic: *Norgestimate-Ethinyl Estradiol*
(nor-JES-ti-mate ETH-in-il es-tra-DYE-ole)
Brands: *MonoNessa, Ortho-Cyclen, Ortho Tri-Cyclen, Ortho Tri-Cyclen Lo, Sprintec*

Norgestimate-ethinyl estradiol is approved for use as a combination oral contraceptive containing both estrogen and progestin. The combination is used off-label for endometriosis and its symptoms. The progesterone in the drug breaks down the endometrium and endometriotic tissue. Treatment with this drug also decreases the likelihood of new lesions. These supplemental hormones reduce or eliminate the pain of endometriosis by interfering with the rise and fall of hormones during a menstrual cycle that cause endometrial implants to thicken, break down and bleed.

Researchers believe that the combination of estrogen and progestin in oral contraceptives alleviates cyclic pain by suppressing the cyclic growth of endometriotic implants. Norgestimate ethinyl estradiol is especially useful in avoiding side effects such as spotting, breakthrough bleeding, androgenic effects, and dyslipidemia.

For more information see page 1374.

Fibromyoma

See Uterine Fibroids

Leiomyomas

See Uterine Fibroids

Mastalgia

Mastalgia is defined as breast pain and tenderness. Women may experience mastalgia with their monthly ovulation, called cyclic, or mastalgia that does not follow any pattern, called noncyclic. Cyclic pain is the most common and may be caused by hormone changes. It is usually felt in both breasts or as sensations in the underarm region. Noncyclic breast pain is present at all times in a specific area and is not affected by a woman's menstrual cycle. Severe breast pain is a common symptom, affecting up to 70% of women at some time in their lives. It accounts for approximately 50% of referrals to a specialized breast clinic, two-thirds of women having cyclical and one-third experiencing noncyclical mastalgia. Most women require reassurance only, and the pain often subsides spontaneously after a few months. For the remainder, simple lifestyle changes are suggested initially, such as wearing a well-fitted sports bra, weight reduction, regular exercise and a reduction in caffeine intake. In only 15% of women is the pain severe enough to affect their lifestyle and warrant drug therapy.

Commonly Prescribed (On-Label) Drugs: None

OFF-LABEL PRESCRIPTION DRUGS
BREAKTHROUGH OPTIONS

Generic: **Bromocriptine** *(broe-moe-KRIP-teen)*
Brand: **Parlodel**

If you have moderate to severe mastalgia lasting more than seven days every month, persisting for longer than three months and interfering with everyday activities you should be considered for drug treatment. Bromocriptine is an effective treatment for mastalgia, as has been shown in trials with three and six month treatment groups. For cyclical mastalgia, response rates of 54% have been reported and for non-cyclical, 33%. Side effects such as headache and dizziness are reported in 35% of cases. Trials comparing the effectiveness of bromocriptine with danazol show a higher response rate with danazol. Bromocriptine may be used where danazol may interfere with other drugs or with other conditions, such as for women with a history of thromboembolism.

Researchers have found that using EF-12 (gammalinolenic acid; gamolenic acid) as first-line therapy with danazol and bromocriptine usually as second-line drugs, provides improvement in pain in 92% of women with cyclical mastalgia and in 64% of women with noncyclical mastalgia.

For more information see page 1054.

Generic: **Danazol** *(DA-na-zole)*
Brand: **Danocrine**

Danazol is a synthetic testosterone. Researchers have found that women with mastalgia who use danazol have reported significant relief: up to 70% in cyclical mastalgia and 31% in noncyclical mastalgia. In both groups, a relapse rate of 50% has been reported. Danazol use is limited by side effects including body hair growth, acne, and depression.

A recent study evaluated the effectiveness and side effects of danazol limited to use only during the luteal phase (days 14–28) of the menstrual cycle. Effective relief of cyclical mastalgia was demonstrated with only minimal side effects after a three-month trial. Further study is needed to determine optimal use with minimal side effects. If you are using oral contraceptives, you need adequate mechanical contraception while on danazol, as this drug will interfere with the effectiveness of the contraceptive pill. A response to danazol therapy is usually seen within three months.

For more information see page 1129.

Generic: **Tamoxifen** *(ta-MOX-I-fen)*
Brand: **Nolvadex**

Tamoxifen belongs to the class of drugs known as antineoplastics. A three-month low-dose of tamoxifen has been found to be the most effective drug for treating mastalgia. Studies have reported response rates as high as 90% in women with severe mastalgia. Treatment is effective in 78% of women with two to four months of treatment. However, the relapse rate is high too, at 50%. If there is a relapse, an extension of treatment by three months is often required.

For more information see page 1493.

Mastodynia

See Mastalgia

Myoma

See Uterine Fibroids

Pelvic Congestion

Sometimes chronic pelvic pain does not have an identifiable cause. When testing has ruled out endometriosis, fibroids, and uterine prolapse and there are no obvious signs of inflammation, pelvic congestion syndrome may be the source of debilitating pain. This is a common problem in women of reproductive age but the causes are poorly understood. There are several possible explanations, including: undetected irritable bowel syndrome or possible vascular problems. Because the underlying causes are poorly understood, treatment usually focuses on relieving the symptoms.

Commonly Prescribed (On-Label) Drugs: *None*

OFF-LABEL PRESCRIPTION DRUGS
BREAKTHROUGH OPTIONS

Generic: ***Goserelin*** *(GOE-se-rel-in)*
Brand: ***Zoladex***

Goserelin produces a reversible, low-estrogen condition. Researchers believe that lowering the amount of estrogen in the body can reduce pelvic pain. Improvement usually begins within four weeks of starting therapy. In studies, goserelin has been as effective as other medications commonly used to treat pelvic pain. Typically, within eight weeks of initiating therapy, absence of menstruation develops in 80–92% of women. Menses usually returns within eight weeks of discontinuation of this medication.

A study in *Human Reproduction* identified the proportion of pelvic congestion among women complaining of chronic pelvic pain and in a group of patients requesting tubal ligation. The efficiency of goserelin acetate versus medroxyprogesterone acetate (MPA) was also compared. Patients received either goserelin acetate for six months or MPA for six months. Among women with chronic pelvic pain, those with pure pelvic congestion were mostly birth mothers, had the most severe pelvic signs and symptoms, lowest rates of sexual functioning, and higher states of anxiety and depression compared with others. At one year after treatment, goserelin acetate remained superior to MPA. Goserelin acetate achieved a statistically significant advantage compared with MPA in alleviating signs and symptoms, improving sexual functioning, and reducing anxiety and depression.

For more information see page 1215.

Generic: **Leuprolide** *(loo-PROE-lide)*
Brands: ***Eligard, Lupron, Lupron Depot, Lupron Depot-Ped, Viadur***

Leuprolide acetate belongs to the group of medications called gonadotropin-releasing hormones (GnRH). In a study comparing leuprolide acetate (long-acting) and placebo administration every four weeks for six doses in women, leuprolide acetate was more effective than the placebo at reducing pelvic pain. When the treatment was discontinued, symptoms recurred within three to twelve months. Pain returned to its original severity within three months in 54% of patients.

One of the most common gynecological causes of chronic pelvic pain is endometriosis. As endometriotic lesions are affected by hormones, GnRH drugs cause shrinkage of the lesions and reduce the symptoms caused by them. One study conducted in St James's University Hospital in the United Kingdom examined the effect of leuprolide acetate on pelvic pain. Preliminary data showed a significant decrease in pain scores from before to after treatment. In addition, there was a general improvement in other symptoms. It was concluded that it is beneficial to treat women with chronic pelvic pain with GnRH drugs as first-line management to relieve painful symptoms. This approach could avoid the risks and discomforts of surgery.

For more information see page 1274.

*Generic: **Medroxyprogesterone Acetate***
(me-DROKS-ee-proe-JES-te-rone AS-eh-TATE)
*Brand: **Provera***

Medroxyprogesterone acetate (MPA) is a medication containing the female hormone progesterone. Studies have shown that medroxyprogesterone can reduce pain for women with pelvic congestion.

A study conducted in Turkey of women with pelvic pain looked at the efficiency of goserelin acetate versus MPA. The study measured symptom relief, improvement of psychological status, and sexual functioning. Patients received either goserelin acetate for six months or MPA for six months. Among patients with chronic pelvic pain, those with pure pelvic congestion were mostly women who had prior pregnancies, had the most severe pelvic signs and symptoms, lowest rates of sexual functioning, and higher states of anxiety and depression when compared to others.

At one year after treatment, goserelin acetate remained superior to MPA. Goserelin acetate achieved a statistically significant advantage compared with MPA in alleviating signs and symptoms, improving sexual functioning, and reducing anxiety and depression.

Researchers also identified treatments for chronic pelvic pain in women of reproductive age. The review included studies of women with a diagnosis of pelvic congestion syndrome or adhesions. MPA was consistently associated with a reduction of pain during treatment. Counseling supported by ultrasound scanning was also associated with reduced pain and improvement in mood.

For more information see page 1297.

Pelvic Pain, Chronic

Chronic pelvic pain is a common problem among women of reproductive age. Its cause is poorly understood. Chronic pelvic pain is diagnosed when: it has been present for six or more months, it is unresponsive to conventional therapy, and when the degree of pain seems greater than the identifiable tissue damage. Emotional and physical problems are usually present. Because chronic pelvic pain is poorly understood, treatment is often not satisfactory. Many people may have bladder or bowel dysfunction, sexual dysfunction or other systemic symptoms. Chronic pelvic pain is estimated to affect one in seven women in the United States.

Commonly Prescribed (On-Label) Drugs: *None*

OFF-LABEL PRESCRIPTION DRUGS
BREAKTHROUGH OPTIONS

Generic: **Goserelin** *(GOE-se-rel-in)*
Brand: **Zoladex**

Goserelin is a gonadotropin-releasing hormone (GnRH) that will stop ovulation and cause an artificial menopause. Side effects can include symptoms often experienced during menopause, including bone mineral loss, because of which use of goserelin is usually not long-term.

A study in *British Journal of Obstetrics and Gynaecology* was conducted to find out if preventing the function of the ovaries by taking GnRH could assist in the diagnosis of chronic pelvic pain in women. The study included eight women who were given goserelin every 28 days, followed by surgery to remove their ovaries. The women's response to goserelin and surgery (12 months or more post-operatively) was assessed. Goserelin resolved pelvic pain in six women. The only woman who did not respond to goserelin also failed to gain relief with surgery. One woman who responded to goserelin declined surgery. The investigators concluded that suppression of ovarian function by GnRH may relieve pelvic pain caused by certain ovary abnormalities. The investigators concluded that this approach may help doctors select cases likely to benefit from surgery, avoiding potentially difficult surgery in women who will gain little or no relief of symptoms from it.

For more information see page 1215.

Generic: **Leuprolide** *(loo-PROE-lide)*
Brands: **Eligard, Lupron, Lupron Depot, Lupron Depot-Ped, Viadur**

Leuprolide belongs to the group of medications called gonadotropin-releasing hormone (GnRH). One of the most common gynecological causes of chronic pelvic pain is endometriosis. As endometriotic lesions are under hormonal influence, the effects of GnRH cause shrinkage of the deposits, reducing symptoms caused by them.

In a study comparing leuprolide acetate and placebo administration every four weeks for six doses in women, leuprolide was more effective than the placebo at reducing pelvic pain. When the treatment was discontinued, symptoms recurred within three to twelve months. Pain returned within three months in 54% of women.

A study in *Journal of Obstetrics and Gynaecology* documented the effect of leuprorelin on pelvic pain. Preliminary data showed a decrease in pain scores from before to after treatment. In addition, there was a general improvement in other symptoms. Doctors found that symptom intensity was not always related to the severity of endometriosis and that patients with the worst symptoms were not necessarily the patients with the most physical findings. Therefore, if you have chronic pelvic pain, you can likely be treated beneficially with GnRH as first-line management to relieve painful symptoms and, hopefully, avoid surgical risks.

For more information see page 1274.

Generic: *Medroxyprogesterone Acetate*
(me-DROKS-ee-proe-JES-te-rone AS-eh-tate)
Brand: *Provera*

Medroxyprogesterone acetate is a progesterone hormone. Taking this medication for pelvic pain will stop ovulation and prevent over-production of estrogen, if present.

Clinical trials have clearly shown that laparoscopic surgery and medical treatment with medroxyprogesterone acetate, danazol, or nafarelin are effective. At six months, absolute decreases in pain scores were similar with surgical or medical treatment. Medical therapy after surgical treatment significantly reduced pain, but six months after it was stopped there was no difference between women treated and not treated post-operatively. The researchers concluded that although either surgical or medical treatment of endometriosis in women with chronic pelvic pain is clearly indicated, pain relief of six or more months' duration can be expected in only 40 to 70% of women with endometriosis-associated chronic pelvic pain.

For more information see page 1297.

Polycystic Ovary Syndrome

Polycystic ovary syndrome (PCOS) is characterized by enlarged ovaries with multiple small cysts, an abnormally high number of ovarian follicles at various stages of maturation, and a thick scarred capsule surrounding each ovary. The syndrome includes: absence of menses (amenorrhea), infertility, unwanted hair (hirsutism), and enlarged polycystic ovaries. Polycystic ovary syndrome occurs as a result of abnormal hormonal regulation.

Commonly Prescribed (On-Label) Drugs: None

OFF-LABEL PRESCRIPTION DRUGS
BREAKTHROUGH OPTIONS

Generic: ***Medroxyprogesterone Acetate***
(me-DROKS-ee-proe-JES-te-rone AS-eh-tate)
Brand: ***Provera***

Medroxyprogesterone acetate (MPA) is a progesterone hormone that can be used in polycystic ovary syndrome (PCOS) to treat abnormal uterine bleeding.

A study conducted in Turkey looked at the 10-day effects of MPA and progesterone administered either orally or vaginally, on women with PCOS to see if short-term progesterone treatment can stop abnormal uterine bleeding and control insulin abnormalities in patients with PCOS. Twenty-eight women with PCOS received 10-day MPA, oral, or vaginal progesterone. Hormone levels, insulin levels, oral glucose tolerance test, lipid profiles, and other blood values were studied in all groups before and after treatment.

Oral MPA and oral progesterone decreased luteinizing hormones and total testosterone levels. Hormonal levels did not change with vaginal progesterone. Basal insulin decreased significantly in the oral MPA group. Low-density lipoprotein cholesterol and lipoprotein (a) levels decreased only in the MPA group. Vaginal progesterone had no effect on glucose metabolism and lipid profiles. It was concluded that oral MPA could be considered for treatment of abnormal uterine bleeding symptoms in women with PCOS and also treat insulin abnormalities in women with PCOS.

For more information see page 1297.

Generic: **Metformin** *(met-FOR-min)*
Brands: **Glucophage, Glucophage XR, Riomet**

Metformin is a medication typically used in type-2 or non-insulin dependent diabetes. Preliminary studies have shown that metformin has been effective in restoring normal menstrual cycles in about 50% of women with polycystic ovary syndrome. Stimulation of ovulation may increase the likelihood of becoming pregnant while on this medication. A study at the University of Hull in the United Kingdom compared metformin therapy to another drug, orlistat in 21 women with PCOS. After an eight-week period of dietary change, the women were scheduled to receive either metformin three times daily or orlistat three times daily for three months.

Testosterone levels declined significantly in both groups. Levels of sex hormone-binding globulin did not change. Fasting insulin concentrations did not decrease significantly in either treatment group. Lipid levels failed to improve significantly in either group and did not differ substantially in the two groups. Women treated with orlistat had a 4.7% reduction in body weight, a more significant loss than metformin-treated women (1.0%). Researchers concluded that metformin and orlistat both decrease serum testosterone levels, but orlistat appears to reduce body weight more effectively in women with PCOS.

For more information see page 1308.

Generic: **Levonorgestrel-Ethinyl Estradiol**
(LEE-voe-nor-jes-trel ETH-in-il es-tra-DYE-ole)
Brands: **Levlen, Levora, Nordette, Portia, Seasonale**

Levonorgestrel and ethinyl estradiol are combination oral contraceptives (COC), usually containing two types of hormones, estrogens and progestins. When these hormones are taken together they interfere with the normal hormonal fluctuations during the menstrual cycle and maintain them at a more constant level. This medication can also help reduce excessive production of androgens, body hair growth, acne and painful menstruation in polycystic ovary syndrome (PCOS).

COCs are the most often used treatment for PCOS as they suppress androgen production, thus reducing skin androgenic symptoms and improving menstrual dysfunction. On the other hand, much still remains unknown about their metabolic effects. COCs could decrease insulin sensitivity and affect glucose tolerance, although the negative influence on insulin sensitivity is dependent on other factors (especially obesity) that may not be an issue if you are not obese. This impairment of glucose tolerance may be reversible, as the incidence of diabetes is not increased in past COC users.

A study looked at whether a multi-drug that combines oral contraceptives (COC) and metformin is beneficial compared to COC alone. Altogether, 30 women in the study were randomly assigned to two groups treated with either COC (COC group) or COC and metformin (METOC group) for six months. Two dropped out. Investigators concluded that adding metformin slightly modified the effect of COC, causing a more significant decrease in testosterone. Researchers concluded that the available data do not offer enough evidence to advocate the standard use of combined treatment in PCOS, but the combination might be beneficial for specific subgroups.

For more information see page 1279.

Generic: **Norethindrone Acetate-Ethinyl Estradiol**
(nor-eth-IN-drone AS-a-tate ETH-in-ill ess-tra-DYE-ole)
Brands: **Estrostep, Junel, Loestrin, Microgestin**

Norethindrone acetate-ethinyl estradiol is especially useful for minimizing side effects of polycystic ovary syndrome, such as carbohydrate changes, weight gain, acne, and body hair growth. This drug therapy also has less of an impact on glucose levels and plasma insulin concentrations. Researchers have concluded that these combination contraceptives are suitable if you have lipid disorders and diabetes.

For more information see page 1370.

Generic: **Norgestimate-Ethinyl Estradiol**
(nor-JES-ti-mate ETH-in-il es-tra-DYE-ole)
Brands: **MonoNessa, Ortho-Cyclen, Ortho Tri-Cyclen, Ortho Tri-Cyclen Lo, Sprintec**

Norgestimate-ethinyl estradiol is an estrogen and progestin combination medication that can be used for polycystic ovary syndrome (PCOS). This treatment often reduces symptoms related to PCOS, including body hair growth, acne, and slight or infrequent menstrual flow. New treatments such as norgestimate-ethinyl estradiol that increase insulin sensitivity as well as weight reduction in obese women with PCOS may be useful in modifying the complications of this common disorder among young adult women.

For more information see page 1374.

Generic: **Norgestrel-Ethinyl Estradiol**
(nor-JES-tril ETH-in-il es-tra-DYE-ole)
Brands: **Cryselle, Lo/Ovral, Low-Ogestrel, Ogestrel, Ovral**

Norgestrel-ethinyl estradiol is a combination oral contraceptive containing both estrogen and progestin. It is frequently used to treat menstrual irregularity and acne when they appear in women with polycystic ovary syndrome (PCOS). Oral contraceptives induce regular menstrual periods with a higher degree of reliability than any other form of treatment. In addition, they normalize hormone levels within 18 to 21 days.

Estrogen and progestin are more effective in combination than either one alone in suppressing excessive production of androgens. Low-dose oral contraceptive pills like ethinyl estradiol are usually effective in controlling excessive body hair growth and acne, which are commonly seen in PCOS.

For more information see page 1376.

Generic: **Spironolactone** *(speer-on-oh-LAK-tone)*
Brand: **Aldactone**

Spironolactone is commonly used to treat high blood pressure. It is also used to treat swelling caused by certain conditions such as congestive heart failure by removing excess fluid and improving symptoms such as breathing problems. For women with polycystic ovary syndrome (PCOS), the drug is prescribed off-label to reduce the male sex hormones that give rise to masculine characteristics. This medication has been useful in stopping body hair growth in women whose condition is not responsive to oral contraceptives. Spironolactone interferes with androgen activity and secretion, and the side effects are minimal.

A trial in Italy assessed the effects of long-term therapy with spironolactone on women with PCOS. Twenty-five patients received oral spironolactone for 12 months, which was effective in treating the androgenic aspects of PCOS. Long-term treatment with spironolactone had no negative effects on lipoprotein profile and glucose metabolism; there were also beneficial effects on glucose and lipid metabolism when the drug was given to overweight PCOS women who lost weight using this therapy.

For more information see page 1478.

Pudendal Neuralgia

See Vulvodynia

Sclerocystic Disease of the Ovary

See Polycystic Ovary Syndrome

Stein-Leventhal Syndrome

See Polycystic Ovary Syndrome

Uterine Fibroids (Leiomyomas)

Uterine fibroids are among the most common noncancerous tumors found in women of reproductive age. Also called fibromyomas, leiomyomas, and myomas, they are not associated with an increased risk of uterine cancer and almost never develop into cancer. Most of the time uterine fibroids are not harmful. As many as three out of four women have uterine fibroids. Typically, fibroids cause no problems so women are often unaware that they have them. When problems do occur (in about one out of four women), they are generally found during the 30- and 40-year age group.

Commonly Prescribed (On-Label) Drugs: Leuprolide

OFF-LABEL PRESCRIPTION DRUG
BREAKTHROUGH OPTION

Generic: **Mifepristone** *(mi-FE-pris-tone)*
Brand: **Mifeprex**

Mifepristone is a synthetic steroid that is effective in shrinking uterine fibroids and improving symptoms, such as heavy bleeding, pelvic pain, abnormally enlarged abdomen, and pain during sexual intercourse. One study at the University of Rochester, New York, compared the effect of two low doses of mifepristone on uterine fibroid size and symptoms, as well as their side effects. Forty women with large, symptomatic fibroids received the drug daily for six months. Uterine fibroids shrank by approximately 48%. Fibroid-related symptoms were reduced. Side effects included: reduced or absent menstruation (about 65%), hot flashes, and endometrial hyperplasia in about 28% of the participants. Researchers concluded that mifepristone should be considered for shrinking fibroids and relieving fibroid symptoms.

For more information see page 1328.

Vaginal Ulceration

Vaginal ulceration can occur as the primary or secondary event in a large variety of conditions. These include infections, autoimmune and/or inflammatory diseases and dermatoses, neoplasias, and conditions with unknown causes. Ulcerating lesions of the vagina may be solitary or multiple and painful or nontender. Solitary, nontender ulcers are characteristic of syphilis, lymphogranuloma venereum, and neoplasia. Multiple painful ulcers occur in herpes simplex virus, Behçet's syndrome, and Crohn's disease. Laboratory evaluation is often necessary to determine the causes of vulvar ulcers.

Commonly Prescribed (On-Label) Drugs: None

OFF-LABEL PRESCRIPTION DRUG
BREAKTHROUGH OPTION

Generic: **Sucralfate** *(soo-KRAL-fate)*
Brand: **Carafate**

Vaginal ulceration is at times resistant to traditional methods of treatment. Sucralfate binds to ulcerated areas and promotes healing. One report from Bowman Gray School of Medicine at Wake Forest University showed that vaginal ulceration treated with vaginal douches of sucralfate twice daily was successful in three cases, each with a different cause of vaginal ulcerations.

In another case, forty patients with Behçet's disease—a rare, chronic condition that affects the inner lining of the mouth and genitals—received either sucralfate or a placebo four times a day for three months. All patients were instructed to use sucralfate or placebo as an oral rinse for one to two minutes after routine mouth care and before sleep. Patients with genital ulcerations were also given sucralfate or placebo, to be applied as topical therapy or a vaginal douche. The sucralfate treatment significantly decreased frequency, healing time, and pain associated with oral ulcerations, and decreased healing time and pain associated with genital ulcerations. Patients in the placebo group showed no significant relief of symptoms, except for decreased pain of oral ulcerations. Researchers conclude that topical sucralfate suspension is effective and inexpensive in treating the oral and genital ulcerations characteristic of Behçet's disease.

For more information see page 1482.

Vulvodynia (Vulvar Dysesthesia)

Vulvodynia is characterized by widespread burning pain throughout the vulvar region (vilva and external genitalia) lasting a minimum of three months. This condition is considered by many to reflect a disease of the distal nerves of the affected areas because of the burning quality of the pain. Pain may be present in the labia, clitoris, vestibule, perineum, mons pubis, and inner thighs. The pain may be constant or unprovoked by touch or pressure to the vulva.

Commonly Prescribed (On-Label) Drugs: *None*

OFF-LABEL PRESCRIPTION DRUGS
BREAKTHROUGH OPTIONS

*Generic: **Amitriptyline** (a-mee-TRIP-ti-leen)*
*Brand: **Elavil***

There have been few clinical trials to determine effective treatment of vulvodynia. Tricyclic antidepressants are commonly prescribed off-label for treatment. Tricyclic antidepressants are thought to affect pain transmission in the spinal cord by increasing the levels of the brain chemicals norepinephrine and serotonin, both of which influence pain. Amitriptyline has this analgesic effect, reducing the symptoms of vulvodynia. It is also effective in treating the nerve pain of vulvodynia.

Patients are usually started on a low dose daily, taken at night to minimize side effects. The dose may be gradually increased, depending on the response and tolerability of side effects. Relief is not immediate, and it may take several weeks for the drug to become fully effective.

In a study of 104 women diagnosed with vulvodynia and treated over a period of six years, a follow-up questionnaire study found that a majority were doing well, reporting a sizable reduction in pain compared to when they first sought treatment. A small percentage (10.6%) reported cessation of pain. For most, over 89%, the condition was not cured but was under control. A majority of women reported improvements in their symptoms following pregnancy. Side effects are seen in up to 50% of women taking amitriptyline.

For more information see page 1009.

*Generic: **Desipramine** (des-IP-ra-meen)*
*Brand: **Norpramin***

Desipramine is an antidepressant. It works by increasing serotonin and norepinephrine levels in the brain and is sometimes prescribed off-label for neuropathic pain. Doctors recommend that after symptoms are controlled, dosage should be gradually reduced to the lowest level that will maintain relief. Tricyclic antidepressants also promote sleep and stabilize mood. The side effects include dry mouth, excessive sedation, urinary retention, orthostatic hypotension and cardiac arrhythmia. Desipramine can be used to manage the neuropathic pain of vulvodynia. It appears to be almost as effective as amitriptyline in most studies and has fewer side effects including less drowsiness. Successful treatment with desipramine for vulvodynia is well documented.

For more information see page 1132.

*Generic: **Carbamazepine** (kar-ba-MAZ-e-peen)*
*Brands: **Carbatrol, Epitol, Tegretol, Tegretol XR***

There are many approaches to the treatment for vulvodynia including general vulvar care, topical medications, oral medications, injectables, biofeedback and physical therapy, dietary changes with supplementations, acupuncture, hypnotherapy, and surgery. Carbamazepine is a drug typically used as an anticonvulsant, but it is also prescribed off-label for the relief of vulvodynia, as well as for various psychiatric disorders. There are minimal studies with limited data on using carbamazepine to treat vulvodynia. Anti-epileptic drugs such as carbamazepine act at several sites that may be relevant to pain, but the precise way they work remains unclear. These drugs are thought to limit excitement of the neurons in the brain. Side effects include dizziness, double vision, and nausea. Treatment with carbamazepine can cause aplastic anemia.

For more information see page 1068.

*Generic: **Nortriptyline** (nor-TRIP-ti-leen)*
*Brands: **Aventyl, Pamelor***

Nortriptyline is a tricyclic antidepressant that appears also to work as a pain killer. Most studies of antidepressant use in the symptomatic treatment of neuropathic pain have involved amitriptyline, but nortriptyline has been shown to reduce pain equally.

There is a complex relationship between depression and pain. Patients suffering from depression are known to be at a greater risk for developing a variety of chronic pain syndromes compared to individuals without depression. Vulvodynia is often associated with depression. The condition may respond favorably to antidepressant treatment, but to date only specific case reports, not controlled studies, support its use. The case reports consistently show that patients with major depression and vulvodynia dramatically improve with a tricyclic antidepressant such as nortriptyline.

For more information see page 1378.

HIRSUTISM

Hirsutism is a condition in which too much hair grows on the face or body. Although hirsutism can occur in both men and women, it is usually only a problem for women. Women with hirsutism have dark, thick hair on their face, chest, abdomen and back. This hair is different from the hair that some women have on their upper lip, chin, breasts or stomach, or the fine "baby" hair all over their body. Women from certain ethnic groups tend to have more body hair than others. This does not mean that they have hirsutism. It is generally caused by abnormally high levels of male hormones called androgens. Conditions such as polycystic ovary syndrome, Cushing's disease, and tumors in the ovaries or adrenal glands are common causes of hirsutism. Other causes may be from certain medications or hair follicles that are overly sensitive to male hormones. All combination oral contraceptives are beneficial for treating hirsutism.

Commonly Prescribed (On-Label) Drugs: Eflornithine

OFF-LABEL PRESCRIPTION DRUGS
BREAKTHROUGH OPTIONS

Generic: **Dexamethasone** *(deks-a-METH-a-sone)*
Brands: **Decadron, Dexameth, Dexone, Hexadrol**

Dexamethasone is a synthetic glucocorticoid. It affects almost all body systems but is used principally for its strong anti-inflammatory and immunosuppressant effects.

The College of Physicians and Surgeons of Columbia University studied whether the addition of dexamethasone to antiandrogen therapy prolongs remission in women with hirsutism. Fifty-four women with hirsutism were treated with one of four regimens:

spironolactone for one year, dexamethasone for one year, dexamethasone plus spironolactone for one year, or dexamethasone plus spironolactone for two years.

Androgen levels remained low one year after the withdrawal of dexamethasone treatment, either alone or in combination with spironolactone. In women who were treated with spironolactone alone, hirsutism scores had returned to pre-study values after one year. The researchers concluded that the addition of a drug that suppresses androgen levels may be useful to prolong the remission of hirsutism in women who are treated with antiandrogens.

For more information see page 1138.

Generic: *Finasteride* (fi-NAS-teer-ide)
Brands: *Propecia, Proscar*

Finasteride is an inhibitor of steroid 5-reductase, which appears to be the principal androgen responsible for stimulation of hair growth. A study at the Tehran University of Medical Sciences compared the clinical and hormonal effects of finasteride and a combination regimen of cyproterone acetate (CPA) plus ethinyl estradiol (EE2) in the treatment of hirsutism. Of forty hirsute women in the trial, twenty-nine had polycystic ovary syndrome (PCOS) and 11 had hirsutism. Patients were randomly treated with finasteride or CPA plus EE2 for nine months. Improvement of hirsutism induced by the two treatment methods was similar (47.6 % vs. 51.1%).The investigators concluded that finasteride and CPA plus EE2 are equally effective in decreasing hirsutism, despite significantly different effects on hormone levels.

For more information see page 1187.

Generic: *Flutamide* (FLOO-ta-mide)
Brand: *Eulexin*

Flutamide, a nonsteroidal antiandrogen, stops the growth of malignant cells. It has no other hormonal effects, except for a decrease in the secretion of adrenal androgens. The effectiveness of flutamide on hirsutism, used as single therapy or combined with oral contraceptives (OC), was studied by researchers in Chile. Women with hirsutism received flutamide alone or flutamide plus an oral contraceptive (ethynylestradiol and desogestrel). Hirsute women with polycystic ovary syndrome received flutamide plus an oral contraceptive. At three months, the reduction in hirsutism was 11.2% in women with hirsutism receiving flutamide alone; 15.9% for women receiving flutamide plus an oral contraceptive; and 24.7% in women with PCOS receiving flutamide plus an oral contraceptive. At twelve months, the figures were 57.2, 57.3, and 52.5% respectively. No side effects were observed. The researchers concluded that flutamide is effective for hirsutism in women with normal or elevated androgen levels. Adding oral contraceptives did not make the treatment more effective.

For more information see page 1196.

Generic: **Ketoconazole** *(kee-toe-KOE-na-zole)*
Brand: **Nizoral**

Ketoconazole is approved as an antifungal agent. In a report by researchers from the Institute of Obstetrics and Gynecology in Italy, 66 hirsute women were treated with: flutamide; finasteride; ketoconazole; and ethinyl estradiol (EE)-cyproterone acetate daily for the first week. Treatment continued with varying dosages for the next 12 months. All treatments produced a significant decrease in the hirsutism score, hair diameter, and daily hair growth rate.

Flutamide is the fastest in decreasing hair diameter; EE-CPA is the fastest in slowing down hair growth, even though at the end of the treatment there was a significant difference between flutamide and finasteride only. Flutamide, ketoconazole, and EE-CPA induced a significant decrease in total and free testosterone. Very few side effects were observed during treatment with low doses of flutamide, EE-CPA and particularly finasteride. Flutamide induced a decrease whereas EE-CPA induced an increase in triglycerides and cholesterol, showing higher values within the normal range. Ketoconazole induced several side effects and complications and several people dropped out of that part of the study. Despite different modes of action and significantly different effects on androgen levels, researchers concluded that low doses of flutamide, finasteride, and EE-CPA may constitute promising therapies in the treatment of hirsutism.

For more information see page 1259.

Generic: **Leuprolide** *(loo-PROE-lide)*
Brands: **Eligard, Lupron, Lupron Depot, Lupron Depot-Ped, Viadur**

Leuprolide is typically used as a drug to stop the growth of malignant cells and for its endocrine effects. A report by researchers at the University of Alabama evaluated the effects of treatment with leuprolide in hirsute women. Reseachers believed that leuprolide could improve hirsutism more rapidly compared to treatment with oral contraceptives (OC). Seventeen women were studied before and during six months of treatment with leuprolide with and without an oral contraceptive. Women who were not taking the leuprolide plus an OC noted a decrease in hair growth and improvement in texture. No significant difference between the two groups was found in facial hair density or outer hair diameter. Leuprolide plus cyclic estrogen/progestin appears to provide a more rapid and possibly greater improvement in hirsutism, compared to a standard OC regimen.

For more information see page 1274.

Generic: **Levonorgestrel-Ethinyl Estradiol**
(LEE-voe-nor-jes-trel ETH-in-il es-tra-DYE-ole)
Brands: **Levlen, Levora, Nordette, Portia, Seasonale**

Levonorgestrel-ethinyl estradiol is a combination oral contraceptive that contains both estrogen and progestin. A comparison of oral contraceptives (OCs) in the treatment of hirsutism was conducted by investigators at the University of Texas Medical Branch. Women with hirsutism received an OC containing either ethinyl estradiol/desogestrel or ethinyl estradiol/levonorgestrel for nine months of treatment. The sex hormone–binding globulin increased significantly in subjects using the desogestrel-containing OC compared with the levonorgestrel-containing OC. Ten subjects completed the nine months of treatment in the levonorgestrel group and 11 in the desogestrel group. Researchers concluded that treatment of hirsute women with OCs containing desogestrel results in a significant increase in sex hormone–binding globulin and decrease in free testosterone.

For more information see page 1279.

*Generic: **Medroxyprogesterone Acetate***
(me-DROKS-ee-proe-JES-te-rone AS-eh-tate)
*Brand: **Provera***

Medroxyprogesterone acetate is a synthetic progestin. A study in *British Journal of Dermatology* analyzed 26 hirsute women who were treated with medroxyprogesterone acetate (MPA). Treatments included: an ointment containing MPA in 13 patients; injection under the skin of MPA into the hairy areas of the face in five patients; and intramuscular injection of low doses of MPA in 13 patients. Each treatment was continued for an average duration of 16 weeks. The best clinical result was achieved by injection under the skin, the next most successful was the intramuscular injection, and the least successful was the topical application. Hair diameter measurements were reduced by 33% on average. Androgen levels, measured monthly, remained unaffected by topical treatment, but were decreased by the other treatments.

For more information see page 1297.

*Generic: **Norethindrone Acetate-Ethinyl Estradiol***
(nor-eth-IN-drone AS-a-tate ETH-in-ill ess-tra-DYE-ole)
*Brands: **Estrostep, Junel, Loestrin, Microgestin***

Norethindrone acetate-ethinyl estradiol is a combination oral contraceptive that contains estrogen and progestin. A study was conducted of 51 hirsute women, treated for nine months with either ethinyl estradiol plus norethindrone, or ethinyl estradiol plus norethindrone acetate if they needed contraception, or spironolactone daily if they did not. Ethinyl estradiol plus norethindrone and spironolactone were more effective in improving hirsutism.

For more information see page 1370.

*Generic: **Norgestimate-Ethinyl Estradiol***
(nor-JES-ti-mate ETH-in-il es-tra-DYE-ole)
*Brands: **MonoNessa, Ortho-Cyclen, Ortho Tri-Cyclen, Ortho Tri-Cyclen Lo, Sprintec***

Norgestimate-ethinyl estradiol is a combination oral contraceptive that contains estrogen and progestin. A study in the Netherlands evaluated changes in androgen metabolism and compared healthy women taking one of four low-dose modern oral contraceptives (OCs). One hundred women were divided into groups receiving: ethinyl estradiol (EE) plus norgestimate; EE plus desogestrel; or EE plus gestodene.

All three OC formulations may be beneficial in treating women with androgen-related syndromes such as acne and hirsutism.

For more information see page 1374.

*Generic: **Norgestrel-Ethinyl Estradiol** (nor-JES-tril ETH-in-il es-tra-DYE-ole)*
*Brands: **Cryselle, Lo/Ovral, Low-Ogestrel, Ogestrel, Ovral***

Norgestrel-ethinyl estradiol is a combination oral contraceptive (OC) that contains estrogen and progestin and is sometimes used off-label to treat hirsutism. Today's low-dose OC typically do not affect lipid levels. (Fats stored in the body and used for energy.) They also offer birth control when used in combination with other antiandrogen or gonadotropin-releasing hormone (GnRH) agonist therapy. Such combinations enhance effectiveness and prolong the amount of time the therapy is effective.

For more information see page 1376.

*Generic: **Spironolactone** (speer-on-oh-LAK-tone)*
*Brand: **Aldactone***

Spironolactone is typically used to treat high blood pressure and swelling (edema) caused by certain conditions such as congestive heart failure by removing excess fluid and improving symptoms such as breathing problems. Spironolactone has also been effective in treating hirsutism in women with polycystic ovary syndrome (PCOS) or hirsutism without a known cause. In the treatment of hirsutism, spironolactone appears to work by interfering with ovarian androgen secretion and androgen activity.

Hirsutism is often treated with oral contraceptive pills (OCs), topical medications, or antiandrogens such as spironolactone, flutamide and finasteride, as well as topical medications. Recent studies have shown that lower doses of antiandrogens are as effective as high doses and have the advantage of decreased cost and side-effects.

For more information see page 1478.

MENOPAUSAL SYMPTOMS

Menopause

The medical definition of menopause is the absence of menstruation for 12 months. In American women, the average age for menopause is 51. However, it can occur between a woman's late thirties and her late 50s. Menopause also occurs when a woman's uterus and ovaries are surgically removed. Menopause is the time in a woman's life when the function of the ovaries—production of eggs (ova) and female hormones such as estrogen and progesterone—ceases. Loss of ovarian function is associated with hot flashes and other menopausal symptoms.

Commonly Prescribed (On-Label) Drugs: *Levormeloxifene, Medroxyprogesterone*

OFF-LABEL PRESCRIPTION DRUGS
BREAKTHROUGH OPTIONS

Generic: ***Clonidine*** *(KLON-i-deen)*
Brands: ***Catapres, Catapres-TTS, Duraclon***

Clonidine is approved to treat high blood pressure. Lowering high blood pressure helps prevent strokes, heart attacks, and kidney problems. Clonidine has also been used off-label both orally and with transdermal patches for the management of symptoms such as hot flashes associated with menopause. Some clinicians recommend the use of clonidine for management of symptoms mainly in postmenopausal women in whom estrogen replacement therapy is not advised or in those with preexisting hypertension.

A study at Wayne State University School of Medicine examined the effects of clonidine on the sweating threshold in postmenopausal women with and without hot flashes. Twelve healthy postmenopausal women reporting frequent hot flashes and seven reporting none participated. In two separate sessions, participants received an intravenous injection of clonidine HCl or placebo, followed by body heating. The investigators collected data on core body temperature, skin temperature, sweat rate, and blood pressure. Women with hot flashes had significantly lower core body temperature sweating thresholds than women without hot flashes after receiving placebo. The investigators concluded that elevated brain norepinephrine levels reduce the sweating threshold in symptomatic women, thereby contributing to the start of menopausal hot flashes.

For more information see page 1108.

Generic: **Medroxyprogesterone Contraceptive Injection** (me-DROX-ee-proe-JES-te-rone)
Brand: **Depo-Provera**

Medroxyprogesterone is a synthetic progestin. Hot flashes are frequent in postmenopausal breast cancer patients, especially when treated with tamoxifen. Estrogen replacement therapy is the most effective treatment for hot flashes, but its use is controversial in breast cancer survivors. Progestins may offer a good alternative for the control of hot flashes for women who have had breast cancer.

A study comparing oral megestrol acetate with depot medroxyprogesterone acetate (MPA) for the control of hot flashes in postmenopausal patients with a history of breast cancer was conducted in Italy. Seventy-one postmenopausal women received either an injection of depot MPA or oral megestrol acetate. At week six, hot flashes were reduced by 86% on average in the whole group of patients, without significant differences between the two progestins. The investigators concluded that a short cycle of MPA injections provides significant, long-lasting relief from postmenopausal hot flashes in women with a history of breast cancer, offering an alternative to estrogen replacement therapy or prolonged administration of oral megestrol.

For more information see page 1299.

Generic: **Gabapentin** (GA-ba-pen-tin)
Brand: **Neurontin**

Gabapentin is approved to help control seizures in adults and children three years of age and older. It is also used to relieve nerve pain associated with shingles in adults.

In a report published by investigators at the University of Buffalo School of Medicine, a 32-year-old woman with surgically induced menopause experienced 20–30 severe hot flashes per day and failed to respond to various formulations of hormone replacement therapy and selective serotonin reuptake inhibitor (SSRI) therapy for 17 years. She markedly responded to gabapentin therapy. Researchers concluded that gabapentin should be considered another option in the treatment of menopausal symptoms.

For more information see page 1206.

Generic: *Levonorgestrel-Ethinyl Estradiol*
(LEE-voe-nor-jes-trel ETH-in-il es-tra-DYE-ole)
Brands: *Levlen, Levora, Nordette, Portia, Seasonale*

Levonorgestrel-ethinyl estradiol triphasic is a combination oral contraceptive (OC) that contains the two female hormones estrogen and progestin.

The once-weekly transdermal patch has been shown to be highly effective in rapidly reducing or significantly improving all categories in the quality of life in women with menopausal symptoms. In addition, this transdermal combination was not associated with any cases of increased growth of endometrial tissue or adverse effects on cholesterol or lipid values, but was associated with an increasing rate of amenorrhea (absence of periods) over time.

For more information see page 1279.

Generic: *Medroxyprogesterone Acetate*
(me-DROKS-ee-proe-JES-te-rone AS-eh-tate)
Brand: *Provera*

A study examined the effect of two continuous combined menopausal hormone therapies (MHTs) on the well-being of women starting treatment ("starters") and women switching from mainly sequential MHT ("switchers"). In a one-month trial, 249 postmenopausal women were treated with eitheran-estrogen plus medroxyprogesterone acetate or 17-beta-Estradiol plus norethisterone acetate continuously. Twelve items for measuring symptoms and well being were reported daily on a symptom scale. Women taking conjugated estrogen plus medroxyprogesterone acetate reported lower scores for breast tenderness, depression, irritability and tension, compared with women taking 17-beta-estradiol plus norethisterone acetate.

Compared with pretreatment, both groups developed side effects during the first week: breast tenderness, swelling and depression. Starters, but also switchers, reported less sweating. Compared with pretreatment ratings, switchers reported higher scores for breast tenderness, depression and negative effects on daily life, whereas starters reported only physical side-effects. A history of premenstrual syndrome (PMS) predicted high scores for swelling, depression, tension, irritability, headache and negative effects on daily life. The researchers concluded that conjugated estrogen plus medroxyprogesterone acetate is better tolerated than 17-beta-estradiol plus norethisterone acetate, and starters react differently from switchers. Side effects occur more frequently than benefits with MHT and are more frequent in women with previous PMS.

For more information see page 1297.

*Generic: **Megestrol Acetate** (mee-GES-trawl AS-eh-tate)*
*Brand: **Megace***

Megestrol acetate, a synthetic progestin, is typically used to treat certain cancers by limiting the growth of malignant cells. It also stimulates appetite in patients with certain types of significant weight loss.

A medical literature review conducted by researchers at the University of Oklahoma Health Sciences Center evaluated the effectiveness and safety of nonestrogen treatments for menopause symptoms not due to cancer or chemotherapy. Medications reviewed included clonidine hydrochloride, danazol, gabapentin, methyldopa, mirtazapine, progestins, propranolol hydrochloride, selective serotonin-reuptake inhibitors (SSRIs) and venlafaxine.

According to the review, postmenopausal symptom treatments with gabapentin, medroxyprogesterone acetate, and SSRIs such as paroxetine hydrochloride have been shown to be safe and effective in short-term use. Initial, small reports suggest that megestrol acetate and venlafaxine are effective in treating menopausal symptoms.

For more information see page 1302.

Generic: **Norethindrone Acetate-Ethinyl Estradiol Triphasic** *(nor-eth-IN-drone ASS-a-tate ETH-in-ill ess-tra-DYE-ole)*
Brands: **Estrostep, Junel, Loestrin, Microgestin**

Norethindrone acetate-ethinyl estradiol is a combination oral contraceptive containing both estrogen and progestin. A study of the CombiPatch transdermal system consisting of 17-beta-estradiol plus norethindrone acetate at Florida GYN Group evaluated improvements in menopausal quality of life. The 193 postmenopausal women between the ages of 45 and 65 years who participated in the study reported at least five daily moderate-to-severe hot flashes and episodes of nocturnal sweating for at least one month and applied one patch twice a week for 12 weeks.

Among women in study, transdermal 17-beta-estradiol plus norethindrone acetate significantly reduced the daily number of moderate-to-severe hot flashes from 4.1 at week 1 to 0.6 at week 12. The ratings of headache severity, insomnia, and vaginal irritation/dryness also improved significantly by week six and were maintained at week 12. At week 12, 92.4% of the subjects and 97.3% of the physicians reported that they were "satisfied" or "very satisfied" with the transdermal hormone delivery system. Researchers concluded that the results of this study compare favorably with previous placebo-controlled studies of transdermal hormone therapy in managing menopausal signs and symptoms. Patients reported that their quality of life significantly improved with the transdermal hormone therapy system.

Another study of postmenopausal women determined effects of five years of treatment with an oral continuous combined regimen of estradiol and norethisterone acetate on endometrial tissue. They found that long-term treatment (for up to five years) with continuous combined hormone replacement therapy was not associated with either endometrial hyperplasia or malignancy. In women who had complex hyperplasia during previous sequential (not continuous) treatments, the endometrium returned to normal during treatment with continuous combined hormone replacement therapy. These findings provide reassurance about the long-term safety of this continuous combined regimen for the endometrium.

For more information see page 1370.

Generic: **Norgestimate-Ethinyl Estradiol**
(nor-JES-ti-mate ETH-in-il es-tra-DYE-ole)
Brands: **MonoNessa, Ortho-Cyclen, Ortho Tri-Cyclen, Ortho Tri-Cyclen Lo, Sprintec**

Norgestimate-ethinyl estradiol is a combination oral contraceptive (OC) with estrogen and progestin, two female hormones. A review by researchers at Adis International Limited of menopausal hormone therapy (MHT) with continuous administration of estradiol, plus intermittent administration of oral norgestimate. A number of studies indicates that MHT with continuous estradiol plus intermittent norgestimate is effective in relieving menopausal symptoms and increasing bone mass density (BMD) in postmenopausal women. This MHT regimen is well tolerated. The norgestimate component of the treatment provides good endometrial protection and reduces bleeding. Investigators concluded that continuous oral estradiol plus intermittent oral norgestimate is an effective new option for MHT in postmenopausal women.

For more information see page 1374.

Generic: **Venlafaxine** *(ven-la-FAX-een)*
Brands: **Effexor, Effexor XR**

Venlafaxine is an antidepressant that restores the balance of natural chemicals (neurotransmitters) in the brain, thereby improving mood and feelings of well being.

Researchers from the University of California, San Francisco, studied the efficacy of extended-release venlafaxine for postmenopausal hot flashes. Eighty postmenopausal women with more than 14 hot flashes per week were treated with either extended-release venlafaxine or placebo for 12 weeks. Of the 80 women who enrolled in the study, 40 were in the treatment group and 40 in the placebo group. Hot flash symptoms and quality of daily living significantly improved in the treatment group. Hot flash severity was somewhat lower in the treatment group. Three side effects (dry mouth, sleeplessness, and decreased appetite) were significantly more frequent in the venlafaxine group, but others, including dizziness, tremors, anxiety, diarrhea, and rash, were significantly less frequent. Ninety-three percent of participants in the venlafaxine group chose to continue treatment at the end of the study. Researchers concluded that extended-release venlafaxine is an effective treatment for postmenopausal hot flashes in otherwise healthy women.

For more information see page 1542.

Perimenopause

Perimenopause is the 10- to 15-year period of natural physical changes that precede menopause (which is usually defined by a lack of periods for 12 months). The defining feature of perimenopause is hormone changes which can begin when a woman is in her mid to late 30s. Most women do not experience severe enough hormonal fluctuations until their forties to produce symptoms. The symptoms that are often reported are: hot flashes, night sweats, loss of sexual desire, vaginal dryness and itching, sleep disturbance, eating and weight issues, mood swings, anxiety, and skin changes.

Commonly Prescribed (On-Label) Drugs: None

OFF-LABEL PRESCRIPTION DRUGS
BREAKTHROUGH OPTIONS

Generic: **Norethindrone Acetate-Ethinyl Estradiol**
(nor-eth-IN-drone ASS-a-tate ETH-in-ill ess-tra-DYE-ole)
Brands: **Estrostep, Loestrin, Microgestin**

Norethindrone acetate ethinyl estradiol triphasic is a combination oral contraceptive (OC) containing estrogen and progestin female hormones. Two different regimens on perimenopausal and menopausal women with irregular bleeding episodes were studied to compare the incidence of women following nine months of treatment with a low dose continuous combined hormone replacement therapy consisting of estradiol and norethisterone acetate versus a sequential hormone replacement therapy consisting of equine estrogens and medrogestone. This study analyzed late peri- and postmenopausal women at 35 sites in Austria and Germany. A total of 446 women were allocated into two groups based on time since last bleeding and then divided to receive either a low-dose continuous combined therapy or a sequential therapy for nine months. Regarding the occurrence of irregular bleeding, the low-dose continuous combined therapy was superior to the sequential therapy. The low dose continuous combined norethindrone acetate ethinyl estradiol regimen is also suitable for late perimenopausal women since more than 80% of the women had no bleeding or spotting after nine months of treatment.

For more information see page 1370.

*Generic: **Norgestimate-Ethinyl Estradiol***
(nor-JES-ti-mate ETH-in-ill ess-tra-DYE-ole)
*Brands: **MonoNessa, Ortho-Cyclen, Ortho Tri-Cyclen, Ortho Tri-Cyclen Lo, Sprintec***

Norgestimate-ethinyl estradiol is a combination oral contraceptive (OC) that contains the two female hormones estrogen and progestin. Because progestin-related side effects are among the main reasons for discontinuation of menopausal hormone therapy (MHT), the selection of a formulation that contains the same well-tolerated progestin as in an oral contraceptive can be particularly important to the success of MHT. Available data suggest that the new, norgestimate hormone replacement therapy formulation may offer advantages over regimens that contain older progestins with more side effects.

For more information see page 1374.

MENSTRUAL DISORDERS

Abnormal Uterine Bleeding

Dysfunctional uterine bleeding (DUB) is irregular uterine bleeding that occurs without a known cause. It reflects a disruption in the normal cyclic pattern of hormonal stimulation of the endometrial lining at ovulation. The bleeding is unpredictable in many ways. It might be excessively heavy or light, prolonged, frequent, or random. This condition usually is associated with menstrual cycles not accompanied by ovulation, but also can occur in women with infrequent or irregular ovulation.

Commonly Prescribed (On-Label) Drugs: *Medroxyprogesterone Acetate, Norethindrone, Progesterone*

OFF-LABEL PRESCRIPTION DRUGS
BREAKTHROUGH OPTIONS

Generic: **Desmopressin** *(dez-moe-PREZ-in)*
Brands: **DDAVP, Minirin, Stimate**

Desmopressin is a drug that stimulates the release of blood components that are particularly important for women with bleeding disorders, especially von WilleBrand's disease. A study found that high doses of a nasal spray containing desmopressin acetate produced excellent results in treating abnormal uterine bleeding in women with bleeding disorders, including von WilleBrand's disease and mild hemophilia. It may even be useful if you do not have a bleeding disorder but you have abnormally slow blood clotting. Side effects were mild to moderate, and included headache, nausea, and weakness.

Women with von WilleBrand's disease and excessive menstrual blood loss may be misdiagnosed as having dysfunctional uterine bleeding (DUB); von WilleBrand's disease is the most common bleeding disorder and is present in approximately 1% of the population. It is much more common than previously recognized. There are improved diagnostic tests to identify this disorder and, most important, a high-concentration desmopressin acetate nasal spray is available as treatment.

For more information see page 1134.

Generic: **Leuprolide** *(loo-PROE-lide)*
Brands: **Eligard, Lupron, Lupron Depot, Lupron Depot-Ped, Viadur**

Leuprolide acetate may be used for cancer treatment or for its effects on hormones. Drugs like leuprolide, known as gonadotropin-releasing hormones (GnRH), are used under special circumstances for abnormal uterine bleeding, generally when no other medical treatment reduced uterine bleeding and a woman would like to avoid surgery.

Treatment with a GnRH-like leuprolide creates a menopausal-like condition. Cessation of menstruation usually occurs within three months of treatment. Menopausal symptoms, including hot flashes, night sweats, vaginal dryness, bone loss, joint pain, decreased concentration, and diminished libido, may occur. Compliance to therapy is generally good, despite these symptoms. Because osteoporosis is one of the risks of prolonged therapy, treatment is limited to six months unless additional estrogen is prescribed. GnRH is a good option for older women in late perimenopause who may have significant contraindications to other medical therapy. Halting menses is a relief to many of these patients, and after therapy many women spontaneously transition into menopause.

For more information see page 1274.

Generic: **Levonorgestrel-Ethinyl Estradiol**
(LEE-voe-nor-jes-trel ETH-in-il es-tra-DYE-ole)
Brands: **Levlen, Levora, Nordette, Portia, Seasonale**

Levonorgestrel-ethinyl estradiol is an estrogen-progestin combination contraceptive. Ethinyl estradiol and levonorgestrel are forms of estrogen and progesterone. Ethinyl estradiol and levonorgestrel prevent ovulation (the release of an egg from an ovary), disrupt fertilization (joining of the egg and sperm), and inhibit implantation (attachment of a fertilized egg to the uterus).

Short-term high-dose therapy can be used for excessive uterine bleeding. Any low-dose ethinyl estradiol product can be taken every six hours for five days to rapidly stop heavy menstrual bleeding. Once bleeding has stabilized, a single daily maintenance dose will provide a regular menstrual cycle as well as contraception. Oral contraceptives may help stop acute bleeding and decrease menstrual flow by approximately 50%.

Few studies demonstrate the benefits of low-dose oral contraceptives (OCs) on dysmenorrhea and menstrual flow. A clinical trial of patients with dysfunctional uterine bleeding (DUB) showed an 81–87% improvement in bleeding within three months compared to a 36–45% improvement reported in placebo treated patients.

The likelihood of iron-deficiency anemia appears to decrease in both current and past combination OC users. Several reports support the effectiveness of oral contraceptives for treating abnormal uterine bleeding.

For more information see page 1279.

Generic: **Norethindrone Acetate-Ethinyl Estradiol**
(nor-eth-IN-drone AS-a-tate ETH-in-ill ess-tra-DYE-ole)
Brands: Estrostep, Junel, Loestrin, Microgestin

Norethindrone acetate-ethinyl estradiol is an estrogen-progestin combination contraceptive containing estrogenic and progestinic steroids. In a study of continuous estrogen-progestin replacement therapy, 77 thin, nonsmoking white women, who were 12 to 60 months postmenopausal and had normal medical histories, were assigned to receive one of five dose combinations of daily ethinyl estradiol and norethindrone acetate or conjugated estrogens and medroxyprogesterone acetate. An additional 10 women meeting the same criteria served as a comparison group by taking calcium only. During 12 months of therapy, continuous users had significantly less vaginal bleeding and spotting than sequential users.

Another study confirmed the efficacy of norethindrone acetate-ethinyl estradiol and norethindrone ethinyl estradiol for abnormal uterine bleeding. At three months, norethindrone acetate ethinyl estradiol therapy significantly reduced the incidence of bleeding and spotting, compared with conjugated equine estrogens/medroxyprogesterone acetate therapy.

Norethindrone Acetate-Ethinyl Estradiol Fe is an estrogen-progestin combination contraceptive containing estrogenic and progestinic steroids, plus iron. This type of combination low-dose oral contraceptives has reduced the severity of dysfunctional uterine bleeding (DUB) in trials.

OC use decreases menstrual blood flow and seems to reduce prevalence of anemia and increased hemoglobin concentrations in anemic women. OCs are extremely effective for maintaining cycle control and alleviating cyclical symptoms. Many studies have shown that the days with moderate to heavy menstrual flow are consistently lower in women who use OCs compared to non-users. OC use has also been associated with a 60% reduction in menstrual flow, suggesting it can help women with abnormal uterine bleeding and the predisposition to anemia.

For more information see page 1370.

Generic: **Norgestimate-Ethinyl Estradiol**
(nor-JES-ti-mate ETH-in-il es-tra-DYE-ole)
Brands: **MonoNessa, Ortho-Cyclen, Ortho Tri-Cyclen, Ortho Tri-Cyclen Lo, Sprintec**

Norgestimate-ethinyl estradiol is an estrogen-progestin combination contraceptive containing estrogenic and progestinic steroids. A study at Beth Israel Deaconess Medical Center compared a triphasic combination oral contraceptive (OC) containing norgestimate and ethinyl estradiol (E2) with placebo in the treatment of dysfunctional uterine bleeding (DUB). Two hundred one women (15–50 years of age) with DUB received triphasic norgestimate-ethinyl E2 or placebo, for three consecutive 28-day treatment cycles. More than 80% of subjects who received triphasic norgestimate ethinyl estradiol had improvements in their abnormal bleeding patterns compared with fewer than 50% of subjects in the placebo treatment group. Abnormal bleeding patterns were reported by significantly fewer subjects receiving norgestimate-ethinyl estradiol than in the placebo treatment group. Physical functioning such as self-care, walking, lifting, exercising was significantly more improved in the triphasic norgestimate ethinyl estradiol group than in the placebo group. The investigators concluded that triphasic combination of norgestimate ethinyl estradiol is effective for DUB.

For more information see page 1374.

Generic: **Norgestrel-Ethinyl Estradiol**
(nor-JES-trel ETH-in-il es-tra-DYE-ole)
Brands: **Cryselle, Lo/Ovral, Low-Ogestrel, Ogestrel, Ovral**

Norgestrel-ethinyl estradiol is an estrogen-progestin combination contraceptive containing estrogenic and progestinic steroids. To determine the efficacy of oral contraceptives in the treatment of menstrual disorders, 44 patients received a norgestrel-ethinyl estradiol combination oral preparation. The drug was extremely well tolerated in all patients: only two reported minimum side effects. Oral contraceptive preparations are highly effective in the therapeutic manipulation of menstrual function.

Treatment with combination oral contraceptives helps women with persistent uterine bleeding. Correction of the cause of bleeding is the first consideration when providing treatment. Estrogen-progestin combinations, such as norgestrel-ethinyl estradiol helped stop bleeding and stabilize the uterine tissues. Once an acute bleeding episode is controlled, additional treatment may be needed for several months. The dose of the oral combination contraceptive will be different for the acute and the long-term management of abnormal uterine bleeding.

For more information see page 1376.

Amenorrhea

A woman normally menstruates every 23 to 35 days. Amenorrhea means not having menstrual periods. Primary amenorrhea is not having menstrual periods by the age of 16. Secondary amenorrhea is the absence of three or more periods in a row in a woman who has had regular menstrual periods. Menstruation requires that the uterus, cervix (opening to the uterus), vagina, and ovaries be normal and healthy. The pituitary gland and the hypothalamus, both located in the brain, must also be functioning properly. A problem with any of these parts of the body may keep a woman from having a period.

Commonly Prescribed (On-Label) Drugs: *Bromocriptine, Gonadorelin, Hydroxyprogesterone, Medroxyprogesterone, Norethindrone, Progesterone*

OFF-LABEL PRESCRIPTION DRUG
BREAKTHROUGH OPTION

Generic: **Norgestrel-Ethinyl Estradiol** *(nor-JES-trel ETH-in-il es-tra-DYE-ole)*
Brands: **Cryselle, Lo/Ovral, Low-Ogestrel, Ogestrel, Ovral**

Norgestrel-ethinyl estradiol is an estrogen-progestin contraceptive. Forty-four women with menstrual disorders that included spasmodic dysmenorrhea, dysfunctional uterine bleeding, and menorrhagia (heavy menstrual bleeding) were treated with a norgestrel-ethinyl estradiol combination. Those women who were bleeding heavily at the time of examination took one tablet of norgestrel and ethinyl estradiol 3–4 times daily until the bleeding stopped and then were maintained on one daily dose along with the other women with less serious bleeding episodes until day 21 of treatment. All 14 women with spasmodic dysmenorrhea had complete relief of symptoms and one case of infertility conceived after the therapy. The dysfunctional uterine bleeding group had similar results. Endometrial biopsies revealed a return to normal endometrial function. The drug was extremely well tolerated in all women with only two reporting minimum side effects. The oral contraceptive norgestrel-ethinyl estradiol is effective in the manipulation of the menstrual cycle functions.

For more information see page 1376.

Dysmenorrhea

Dysmenorrhea is simply the medical term for menstrual cramps, that dull or throbbing pain in the lower abdomen many women experience just before and during their menstrual periods. For some women, the discomfort is merely annoying. For others, it can be severe enough to interfere with everyday activities for a few days every month. Primary dysmenorrhea involves no physical abnormality and usually begins within three years after menstruation begins. Secondary dysmenorrhea involves an underlying physical cause, such as endometriosis or uterine fibroids.

Commonly Prescribed (On-Label) Drugs: *Acetaminophen, Aspirin, Belladonna, Celecoxib, Diclofenac, Ibuprofen, Ketoprofen, Meclofenamate, Mefenamic Acid, Naproxen, Valdecoxib*

OFF-LABEL PRESCRIPTION DRUGS
BREAKTHROUGH OPTIONS

Generic: ***Danazol*** *(DA-na-zole)*
Brand: ***Danocrine***

Danazol is a synthetic derivative of ethisterone (ethinyl testosterone). In a study in *Fertility and Sterility*, researchers examined the efficacy of an intrauterine device (IUD) containing danazol. The device was inserted for six months in a group of women who had been diagnosed with endometriosis and recurrent pelvic pain. Dysmenorrhea, dyspareunia, and pelvic pain significantly decreased after the first month, with a persistent effect during the six months of IUD insertion. According to investigators, a danazol-loaded IUD is an effective therapy for women with endometriosis-related pelvic pain.

Significant improvements in dysmenorrhea, deep dyspareunia, and nonmenstrual pain with low-dose danazol are well documented. Menstrual blood loss was also significantly reduced. Very low-dose danazol may be an alternative for temporary relief of endometriosis-associated pain. Ovulation is not always inhibited and barrier contraception is needed while taking low-dose danazol. Side effects occur but are rarely severe.

For more information see page 1129.

Generic: *Flurbiprofen* (flure-BI-proe-fen)
Brand: *Ansaid*

Flurbiprofen is a nonsteroidal anti-inflammatory drug (NSAID) that also reduces pain and fever. The efficacy of flurbiprofen and naproxen-sodium was studied in Sweden in women who complained of severe (23%) or very severe (77%) dysmenorrhea that interfered with their daily life. The severity of pain was significantly reduced during treatment with both flurbiprofen and naproxen-sodium. There was no significant difference in pain relief from the two drugs. More than 60% of the women reported no, or only mild, interference with daily activities during treatment. No serious side effects were reported, and none of the women stopped treatment because of side effects. Flurbiprofen and naproxen-sodium were both shown to be effective in relieving pain in women suffering from severe primary dysmenorrhea and markedly improved their capacity for normal activities during menstruation.

For more information see page 1194.

Generic: **Goserelin** *(GOE-se-rel-in)*
Brand: **Zoladex**

Goserelin is used for the treatment of endometriosis. Goserelin, like other GnRH analogs, reduces estrogen, which is thought to be principally responsible for endometriosis. A six-month course of goserelin can relieve pain and reduce endometriotic lesions; some degree of improvement has persisted in many patients for at least six months after completion of therapy. Substantial improvement of symptoms usually occurs within four weeks of starting goserelin.

In studies, goserelin was as effective as danazol in relieving symptoms such as dysmenorrhea, dyspareunia, pelvic pain, pelvic tenderness, and invasion of the pelvis by endometriosis; it also reduced the size of endometrial lesions. In two comparative studies, the extent of endometrial lesions was substantially reduced in 62–63% or 42–51% of women receiving goserelin or danazol, respectively. In these studies, amenorrhea, or absence of menstruation, developed in 80–92% of women receiving goserelin within eight weeks of initiation of drug therapy; menstruation usually returned within eight weeks after completion of therapy.

For more information see page 1215.

Generic: **Isoxsuprine** *(eye-SOKS-syoo-preen)*
Brand: **Vasodilan**

Isoxsuprine helps to widen blood vessels so blood flows better. Investigators in Mexico gave a drug combination including isoxsuprine, acetaminophen and caffeine to 80 women divided into two groups, 40 with premenstrual tension and 40 with primary dysmenorrhea. The results showed an excellent or very good response in 95% of cases of premenstrual tension and in 92.5% of cases of dysmenorrhea. Overall effectiveness of the compound in both conditions is 93.75%. Researchers concluded that the orally administered therapeutic combination is effective in both dysmenorrhea and premenstrual tension. However, another study of isoxsuprine used for the treatment of primary dysmenorrhea found no significant effect.

For more information see page 1254.

Generic: **Levonorgestrel-Ethinyl Estradiol**
(LEE-voe-nor-jes-trel ETH-in-il es-tra-DYE-ole)
Brands: **Levlen, Levora, Nordette, Portia, Seasonale**

Levonorgestrel-ethinyl estradiol is an estrogen-progestin contraceptive. A study evaluated whether a low-dose oral contraceptive (OC) is more effective than placebo for dysmenorrhea pain in adolescents. In a clinical trial, 76 healthy adolescents aged 19 years or younger with moderate or severe dysmenorrhea received either ethinyl estradiol and levonorgestrel or a matching placebo for three months. Participants used their usual pain medications as needed during the trial. The OC group had less pain than the placebo group. By cycle three, OC users rated their worst pain as less and used fewer pain medications than placebo users. By cycle three, OC users reported fewer days of any pain, fewer days of severe pain, and fewer hours of pain on the worst pain day than placebo users; however, these differences were not significant. The investigators concluded that among adolescents, a low-dose oral contraceptive relieved dysmenorrhea-associated pain more effectively than placebo.

In another study, the effectiveness of a 1-month course of OC was compared to that of a 3-month course for relief of primary dysmenorrhea in a study in 30 women who had been previously taking three-phase OCs. The study showed that for these women, the 1-month course was the better alternative. The fact that 19 of 23 women who continue treatment on the single-phase OC indicated that this type of pill may be chosen as the first alternative for women with primary dysmenorrhea.

For more information see page 1279.

Generic: **Nafarelin** *(NAF-a-re-lin)*
Brand: **Synarel**

Nafarelin, a synthetic gonadotropin-releasing hormone (GnRH), is used for its endocrine effects. Nafarelin, like other GnRH analogs, produces a low estrogen state. Since nafarelin in high dose is a potent inhibitor of ovarian function, most women stop menstruating while on therapy. Cessation of menstruation for any reason will result in improvement of dysmenorrhea, which is usually thought of as pain or cramps due to the menstrual flow. In women who received intranasal nafarelin for endometriosis, amenorrhea developed in 65, 80, and 90% of women within 60, 90, and 120 days of starting the drug, respectively. In women who did not become pregnant, menses returned within one, two, and three months of discontinuance of therapy in four, 82, and 100% of women, respectively.

A six-month course of nafarelin therapy can relieve pain and reduce endometriotic lesions, and some degree of improvement persists for at least six months following completion of therapy in many patients. In comparative studies, intranasal nafarelin was as effective as oral danazol in relieving pelvic pain, dysmenorrhea, dyspareunia of endometriosis and in reducing the size of endometrial lesions.

For more information see page 1349.

Generic: **Nifedipine** *(nye-FED-i-peen)*
Brands: **Adalat CC, Apo-Nifed (PA), Novo-Nifedin, Nu-Nifed, Procardia**

Nifedipine is a calcium channel blocker that treats menstrual contractions and pain in normal and dysmenorrhoeic women. In a Swedish study of nifedipine in women with primary dysmenorrhea caused by myometrial hyperactivity, twelve patients with severe primary dysmenorrhea received an oral dose of nifedipine on the first day of menstruation. Nine patients reported prompt relief of the menstrual cramps (within 15–60 min). Three patients had no pain relief. Researchers concluded that nifedipine can be used as a simple test to identify patients suffering from severe primary dysmenorrhea. In addition, it offers another treatment option for the pain.

For more information see page 1360.

Generic: **Norethindrone Acetate**
(NOR-eth-in-drone AS-eh-tate)
Brand: **Aygestin**

Norethindrone is a synthetic progestin, a female hormone used for the treatment of secondary amenorrhea and for the treatment of abnormal uterine bleeding caused by hormonal imbalance in women without underlying problems such as fibroids or uterine cancer.

In a study to evaluate the efficacy of norethindrone acetate, 52 women with dysmenorrhea, dyspareunia, and noncyclic pelvic pain with endometriosis were evaluated. Dysmenorrhea and noncyclic pelvic pain were relieved in 92.3% and 89.2% of patients, respectively. Overall pain relief was obtained in 94.2% of women. Breakthrough bleeding, of variable severity, was the most common side effect experienced by 30 women (57.6%); however, only four women (7.7%) dropped out from this side effect. One other woman dropped out for severe breast tenderness, and three for noncyclic pelvic pain. In general, treatment was successful in 44/52 (84.5%) of women with the above symptoms. Investigators concluded that norethindrone acetate is a cost-effective alternative with relatively mild side effects in the treatment.

For more information see page 1371.

Generic: *Norethindrone Acetate-Ethinyl Estradiol*
(nor-eth-IN-drone AS-a-tate ETH-in-ill ess-tra-DYE-ole)
Brands: *Estrostep, Junel, Loestrin, Microgestin*

Norethindrone acetate-ethinyl estradiol is a contraceptive containing estrogenic and progestinic steroids. Few studies have clearly documented the beneficial effects of low-dose oral contraceptives on menstrual flow and dysmenorrhea. In a clinical trial, it was demonstrated that women with dysfunctional uterine bleeding and pain using ethinyl estradiol tricyclic oral contraceptive experienced an 81–87% improvement in bleeding during three months, compared with a 36–45% improvement seen in the placebo group. Researchers hypothesize that the combination of estrogen and progestin in oral contraceptives essentially stabilizes the endometrium with time. A number of anecdotal reports document the effectiveness of oral contraceptives as treatment for primary dysmenorrhea. Oral contraceptives likely decrease the pain by reducing the prostaglandin content of menstrual fluid, leading to less local endometrial constriction of blood vessels. In addition, pain is reduced by decrease of uterine contracting.

Norethindrone ethinyl estradiol is a contraceptive containing estrogenic and progestinic steroids. In a clinical trial, women with dysfunctional uterine bleeding and pain used ethinyl estradiol tricyclic oral contraceptive and experienced an 81–87% improvement in bleeding and pain during three months compared with a 36–45% improvement in the placebo group. Researchers believe that the combination of estrogen and progestin in oral contraceptives essentially stabilize the endometrium over time.

For more information see page 1370.

*Generic: **Norgestrel-Ethinyl Estradiol***
(nor-JES-trel ETH-in-il es-tra-DYE-ole)
*Brands: **Cryselle, Lo/Ovral, Low-Ogestrel, Ogestrel, Ovral***

Norgestrel-ethinyl estradiol is a contraceptive containing estrogenic and progestinic steroids. In order to determine the efficacy of oral contraceptives in the treatment of menstrual dysfunction 44 women with spasmodic dysmenorrhea, dysfunctional uterine bleeding, and menorrhagia (heavy bleeding) were treated with a norgestrel-ethinyl estradiol combination oral preparation. Those patients who were bleeding heavily at the time of examination received norgestrel and ethinyl estradiol three to four times daily until the bleeding stopped and then were maintained on one daily dose along with the other patients with less serious bleeding episodes until day 21 of treatment.

All 14 women with spasmodic dysmenorrhea had complete relief of symptoms and one case of primary infertility conceived after the therapy. The dysfunctional uterine bleeding group had similar results. Endometrial biopsies in the metropathic and menorrhagic patients revealed a return to normal endometrial function. The drug was extremely well tolerated in all patients with only two patients reporting minimum side effects. Researchers concluded that oral contraceptive preparations such as norgestrel-ethinyl estradiol are highly effective in the treating of menstrual dysfunction.

For more information see page 1376.

*Generic: **Norgestimate-Ethinyl Estradiol***
(nor-JES-ti-mate ETH-in-il es-tra-DYE-ole)
*Brands: **MonoNessa, Ortho-Cyclen, Ortho Tri-Cyclen,
Ortho Tri-Cyclen Lo, Sprintec***

Norgestimate-ethinyl estradiol is a contraceptive containing estrogenic and progestinic steroids. Research has shown that oral contraceptives (OCs) protect women against dysmenorrhea and menorrhagia, menstrual cycle irregularities, iron deficiency anemia, and other disorders, as well as endometrial cancer and ovarian cancer. In addition to these noncontraceptive health benefits, OCs have proven valuable in managing gynecologic disorders, including dysfunctional uterine bleeding, persistent anovulation, premature ovarian failure, functional ovarian cysts, pelvic pain (including secondary dysmenorrhea), mittelschmerz (pain on ovulation), endometriosis, and the control of bleeding in women with blood dyscrasias.

In a trial assessing the safety and efficacy of norgestimate and ethinyl estradiol, a 12-month study of 661 women showed excellent contraceptive efficacy. Good cycle control was maintained. The incidence of dysmenorrhea and premenstrual syndrome was sharply reduced. Side effects were typical of those associated with use of low-dose OCs.

For more information see page 1374.

Generic: **Terbutaline** *(ter-BYOO-ta-leen)*
Brand: **Brethine**

Terbutaline relaxes the smooth muscle in the lungs and dilates airways to improve breathing. It is approved for the treatment of asthma, chronic bronchitis, or emphysema. Terbutaline also shows promise for treating dysmenorrhea, but further study is needed. In a report in *British Journal of Obstetrics & Gynaecology* on the effects of terbutaline on local uterine blood flow and lower abdominal pain, 11 women with severe primary dysmenorrhea were examined during the first day of menstruation. During uterine contractions, the local endometrial blood flow decreased markedly, and the women experienced the most intense pain.

For more information see page 1499.

Hypermenorrhea

See Menorrhagia

Late Luteal Phase Dysphoria

See Premenstrual Syndrome

Late Luteal Phase Dysphoric Disorder

See Premenstrual Syndrome

Menorrhagia

It is very common for women to experience heavy bleeding during a menstrual period. Some women have heavy periods almost every cycle. Menorrhagia is the medical term for excessive and/or prolonged menstrual bleeding. This condition is also known as hypermenorrhea. Although heavy menstrual bleeding is a common concern among premenopausal women, only a few women experience blood loss severe enough to be defined as menorrhagia.

Commonly Prescribed (On-Label) Drugs: *Meclofenamate*

OFF-LABEL PRESCRIPTION DRUGS
BREAKTHROUGH OPTIONS

Generic: **Danazol** *(DA-na-zole)*
Brand: **Danocrine**

Danazol is a synthetic derivative of ethisterone (ethinyl testosterone). In a report of 18 women with menorrhagia who were treated with danazol for 12 weeks, danazol was found to significantly reduce menstrual blood loss in the first month of treatment. A rapid increase in red blood cell counts and reduction in the number of days of bleeding were also observed. Three months after stopping treatment with danazol, blood loss remained significantly less than pretreatment levels.

Danazol treatment has consistently been effective in reducing menstrual blood loss. In some studies, reduction in blood loss is as high as 80% when compared to pretreatment blood loss. Following danazol therapy 20% of patients report amenorrhea and 70% report oligomenorrhea (infrequent or light menstruation). Approximately 50% of the patients report no side effects with danazol, while 20% reported minor but acceptable side effects. The most common complaint is weight gain, an increase of two to six pounds in 60% of patients. Danazol appears to be effective in treating for heavy menstrual bleeding compared to other medical treatments, though it is uncertain whether women will want to use it because of its frequent side effects.

For more information see page 1129.

Generic: **Leuprolide** (loo-PROE-lide)
Brands: **Eligard, Lupron, Lupron Depot, Lupron Depot-Ped, Viadur**

Leuprolide is used for its effects on hormones. In clinical trials, monthly intramuscular administration of leuprolide for a period of three or six months has been shown to decrease excess vaginal bleeding, resulting in improvement in blood counts. In one clinical trial leuprolide once monthly produced an increase in the percentage of red blood cells in a blood sample by six percent or greater and an increase in hemoglobin concentration in 77% of patients at three months. At three months, 80% of patients experienced relief from menorrhagia or menometrorrhagia, although some patients noted episodes of spotting or menstrual-like bleeding. A decrease of 25% or greater of blood flow occurred in 60% and 54% of patients treated, respectively. In addition, treatment relieved symptoms such as bloating, pelvic pain, and pressure.

For more information see page 1308.

Generic: **Levonorgestrel-Ethinyl Estradiol**
(LEE-voe-nor-jes-trel ETH-in-il es-tra-DYE-ole)
Brands: **Levlen, Levora, Nordette, Portia, Seasonale**

Levonorgestrel-ethinyl estradiol is an estrogen-progestin combination oral contraceptive (OCs). It is an extended-cycle OC, designed to reduce the number of menstrual periods from 13 to four per year. The 91-day regimen is taken daily as 84 active tablets containing the drug, followed by seven placebo tablets. Thus, users have their period once every season (once every three months).

Combination OCs help manage menstrual disorders, including dysmenorrhea, irregular cycles, mittelschmerz (pain on ovulation), and dysfunctional uterine bleeding. Suppression of ovulation with OCs effectively eliminates mid-cycle pain associated with rupture of the ovarian follicle. OCs decrease endometrial proliferation and thus the volume and duration of menstrual flow, which reduces many of the problems associated with menorrhagia. The OCs also reduce symptoms in women with endometriosis.

Administration of levonorgestrel daily can reduce bleeding by up to 96% after twelve months of use; 44% of patients treated with levonorgestrel develop amenorrhoea.

For more information see page 1279.

Generic: **Levonorgestrel-Releasing Intrauterine System**
(LEE-voe-nor-jes-trel)
Brand: **Mirena**

Levonorgestrel-releasing IU system is a progestin-releasing intrauterine device (IUD) that produces a dramatic decline in menstrual blood loss (65% to 98%) within 12 months of beginning treatment.

Researchers in Finland compared the long-term efficacy of the levonorgestrel intrauterine system and surgery (transcervical resection) on the endometrium in the treatment of menorrhagia in a three-year trial. Blood loss decreased for the levonorgestrel intrauterine system and somewhat less for surgery on the endometrium. Nineteen women out of 30 using the levonorgestrel intrauterine system completed the three-year follow-up compared with 22 out of 29 for surgery. Both treatments efficiently reduced menstrual bleeding. The high continuation rate suggests that the levonorgestrel intrauterine system is comparable with transcervical resection of the endometrium. Other studies have shown a reduction in blood loss by up to 90%.

For more information see page 1281.

Generic: **Medroxyprogesterone Contraceptive Injection**
(me-DROKS-ee-proe-JES-te-rone)
Brand: **Depo-Provera**

Medroxyprogesterone acetate is a synthetic progestin that can be used for the treatment of menorrhagia after an acute bleeding episode is controlled. It is most useful in women with adequate amounts of internal estrogen being produced for normal growth of the tissues in the uterus. These drugs usually do not stop excessive ongoing bleeding episodes.

The effectiveness of this drug on menorrhagia attributed to uterine fibroids has been studied by researchers in South Africa. In one study, twenty premenopausal women with menorrhagia attributed to uterine fibroids received medroxyprogesterone acetate for six months. Following a period of six months after the initiation of treatment, 30% became amenorrhoeic, 70% noticed improvement in their bleeding pattern and 15% had an increase in their blood hemoglobin levels.

For more information see page 1299.

Generic: **Naproxen** *(na-PROKS-en)*
Brands: ***Anaprox (DS), EC-Naprosyn, Naprelan,***
Naprosyn

Naproxen is an anti-inflammatory drug (NSAID) that also relieves pain and fever. It is used to relieve mild to moderately severe pain. NSAIDs reduce heavy menstrual bleeding when compared with placebo but are less effective than some of the other medications used for menorrhagia such as tranexamic acid or danazol. In the limited number of studies available, NSAIDs did not differ significantly in effectiveness compared to other treatments. However, there have been some reports of fewer side effects with NSAIDs.

In one study conducted in New Zealand, 45 ovulatory women with a complaint of menorrhagia were divided into three treatment groups. They received therapy with mefenamic acid in two cycles and one of three other agents in two cycles: naproxen, a low dose monophasic combined oral contraceptive, or low dose danazol. Mefenamic acid reduced measured blood loss by 20%; 38%; and 39% in groups one to three respectively. Naproxen reduced blood loss by 12%; the oral contraceptive by 43%; and danazol by 49%. There was no statistically significant difference in blood loss reduction between any of the treatments, although women on danazol experienced a dramatic, highly significant further reduction in blood loss after the first treatment cycle.

For more information see page 1354.

Generic: **Norethindrone Acetate**
(NOR-eth-in-drone AS-eh-tate)
Brand: **Aygestin**

Norethindrone acetate is a synthetic progestin used for the treatment of secondary amenorrhea and for the treatment of abnormal uterine bleeding caused by hormonal imbalance in women without other underlying conditions such as fibroids or uterine cancer. Oral luteal-phase (after ovulation) progestins may help regulate bleeding patterns in irregular bleeding but are ineffective in regular dysfunctional uterine bleeding and may actually increase menstrual bleeding.

Longer regimens (days five–25 of the menstrual cycle) have been found to have similar results when compared to the levonorgestrel intrauterine system for treatment of dysfunctional uterine bleeding. These longer treatment regimens have been studied in randomized controlled trials, but only 30% of women reported that they would have the treatment again.

For more information see page 1371.

Generic: **Norethindrone Acetate-Ethinyl Estradiol**
(NOR-eth-in-drone AS-eh-tate ETH-in-il es-tra-DYE-ole)
Brands: **Estrosep, Junel, Loestrin, Microgestin**

Norethindrone acetate-ethinyl estradiol is an estrogen-progestin combination contraceptive. A study of 350 postmenopausal women compared the effects on vaginal bleeding patterns of continuous combined hormone replacement therapy with norethindrone acetate and ethinyl estradiol versus conjugated equine estrogens and medroxyprogesterone acetate. At three months, norethindrone acetate/ethinyl estradiol therapy reduced the incidence of bleeding (12% vs. 23%) and bleeding and/or spotting (22% vs. 44%), compared with conjugated equine estrogens/medroxyprogesterone acetate therapy. The mean duration of bleeding and bleeding and/or spotting were also reduced with norethindrone acetate and ethinyl estradiol therapy versus conjugated equine estrogens/medroxyprogesterone acetate. The incidence of cumulative amenorrhea at every monthly interval was significantly better with norethindrone acetate and ethinyl estradiol therapy versus conjugated equine estrogens/medroxyprogesterone acetate therapy. The norethindrone acetate and ethinyl estradiol therapy provides significantly better control of vaginal bleeding than conjugated equine estrogens/medroxyprogesterone acetate therapy at all time points investigated in this 12-month study. Associated adverse side effects such as headache, breast pain incidence rates were similar in the two active treatment groups.

For more information see page 1370.

Generic: **Norgestimate-Ethinyl Estradiol**
(nor-JES-ti-mate ETH-in-il es-tra-DYE-ole)
Brands: **MonoNessa, Ortho-Cyclen, Ortho Tri-Cyclen, Ortho Tri-Cyclen Lo, Sprintec**

Norgestimate-ethinyl estradiol is an estrogen-progestin combination oral contraceptive containing estrogenic and progestinic steroids. A study compared the efficacy of a combination oral contraceptive (OC) containing norgestimate and ethinyl estradiol (E2) and placebo in the treatment of several menstrual disorders. Investigators at Beth Israel Deaconess Medical Center gave triphasic norgestimate-ethinyl E2 or placebo, for three consecutive 28-day treatment cycles to 201 women (15–50 years of age) with dysfunctional uterine bleeding (DUB). More than 80% of subjects receiving triphasic norgestimate-ethinyl E2 had significantly fewer abnormal bleeding patterns compared with fewer than 50% in the placebo treatment group. Physical functioning such as self-care, walking, lifting, and exercising was significantly more improved in the triphasic norgestimate-ethinyl E2 group than in the placebo group. Therefore, the triphasic combination of norgestimate and ethinyl E2 is an effective treatment for menstrual disorders.

For more information see page 1374.

Generic: **Norgestrel-Ethinyl Estradiol**
(nor-JES-trel ETH-in-il es-tra-DYE-ole)
Brand: **Cryselle, Lo/Ovral, Low-Ogestrel, Ogestrel, Ovral**

Norgestrel-ethinyl estradiol is an estrogen-progestin combination oral contraceptive. To determine the efficacy of oral contraceptives in the treatment of menstrual dysfunction, 44 women were treated with a norgestrel-ethinyl estradiol combination oral preparation. The women's major complaints included spasmodic dysmenorrhea, dysfunctional uterine bleeding, and menorrhagia. Those who were bleeding heavily at the time of examination received norgestrel and ethinyl estradiol three to four times daily until the bleeding stopped and then were maintained on one daily dose along with the other patients with less serious bleeding episodes until day 21 of treatment. All 14 patients who had reported spasmodic dysmenorrhea had complete relief of symptoms. The dysfunctional uterine bleeding group had similar results. Endometrial biopsies revealed a return to normal endometrial function. The medication was extremely well tolerated in all patients with only two patients reporting slight side effects. Oral contraceptive preparations are highly effective in the treatment of menstrual function.

For more information see page 1376.

Generic: **Tranexamic Acid IV** *(tran-eks-AM-ik AS-id)*
Brand: **Cyklokapron**

Tranexamic acid is used for short-term control of bleeding in hemophiliacs, including dental extraction procedures, and has been studied in a number of small clinical trials in women with menorrhagia. It reduced menstrual blood loss by 34–59% over two to three cycles, significantly more than placebo and other drug treatments.

In a large study, 81% of women were satisfied with tranexamic acid for three to four days/cycle for three cycles, and 94% judged their menstrual blood loss to be "decreased" or "strongly decreased" compared with untreated menstruations.

The oral drug tranexamic acid is an effective, well-tolerated treatment for menorrhagia and may be considered a first-line treatment for the initial management of menorrhagia, especially if you do not want hormonal treatment.

For more information see page 1520.

Menstrual Molimina

See Premenstrual Syndrome

Premenstrual Syndrome (PMS)

Premenstrual syndrome (PMS) is a group of symptoms related to the menstrual cycle, which may include fatigue, headache, gastro-intestinal problems, breast swelling and tenderness, changes in appetite, joint and muscle pain, tension, irritability, mood swings, crying spells, anxiety, depression, memory and concentration trouble. PMS symptoms occur in the week or two weeks before menses (menstruation or monthly bleeding). The symptoms usually go away after menses starts. PMS may interfere with normal activities at home, school, or work. Menopause, when monthly periods stop, brings an end to PMS.

Commonly Prescribed (On-Label) Drugs: Chlorotrianisene

OFF-LABEL PRESCRIPTION DRUGS
BREAKTHROUGH OPTIONS

Generic: **Alprazolam** (al-PRAY-zoe-lam)
Brands: **Alprazolam Intensol, Xanax, Xanax XR**

Alprazolam is a benzodiazepine tranquilizer that is typically used to treat anxiety disorders. Benzodiazepines like alprazolam enhance the actions of a natural brain chemical, GABA (gamma-aminobutyric acid), a neurotransmitter that carries messages between brain nerve cells. GABA inhibits the transmission of nerve signals, thereby reducing the perception of pain. Several studies have confirmed the effectiveness of short-term alprazolam use for premenstrual syndrome (PMS). Although short-term use (several weeks) are not problematic, larger doses for long-term daily use may be needed to achieve the same beneficial effects. Studies suggest that the risk of developing dependence for alprazolam appears to be greater in patients treated with doses greater than 4 mg/day and for long periods (more than 12 weeks). This is a risk common to all benzodiazepines. Because of these effects, suddenly discontinuing the use of a medication like alprazolam may result in hyperexcitability of the nervous system, which can cause serious withdrawal symptoms such as convulsions, depression, hallucinations, restlessness and sleeping difficulties, particularly when stopped abruptly. One study suggests that alprazolam is only effective for relieving the anxiety or mood changes associated with PMS, but not any of the other mood or physical symptoms. Therefore, although treatment with alprazolam is effective for some women with PMS, the side effects limit its use as a first-line approach.

For more information see page 997.

*Generic: **Bromocriptine** (broe-moe-KRIP-teen)*
*Brand: **Parlodel***

Bromocriptine inhibits the release of prolactin, the hormone that stimulates the breasts to produce milk, and is used primarily for treating breast tenderness or pain (mastalgia).

In one survey of women with premenstrual syndrome (PMS), 68% of women experienced breast symptoms associated with menstruation. Other studies have also reported that between 8% and 22% of women experience breast pain, described as moderate to severe, with menstruation. This condition is called cyclical mastalgia (or, cyclic mastopathy) and occurs after ovulation, increasing in intensity during the premenstrual phase and then receding at menstruation. There is no substantial support that bromocriptine is effective for PMS symptoms such as irritability, depression, and anxiety. Studies have not shown significant improvement with treatment of bromocriptine compared to placebo. Bromocriptine appears to be the treatment of choice in premenstrual mastalgia. Therefore researchers suggest that bromocriptine may have a place in selected cases of PMS with associated mastalgia.

For more information see page 1054.

*Generic: **Buspirone** (byoo-SPYE-rone)*
*Brand: **BuSpar***

Buspirone is a unique anti-anxiety medication known as an azapirone. Unlike the benzodiazepines, buspirone is not addictive. It also seems to have less pronounced side effects than benzodiazepines and no withdrawal effects, even when the drug is discontinued abruptly. Buspirone is typically used for managing anxiety disorders and for short-term relief of the symptoms of anxiety. The effectiveness of buspirone for long-term use (longer than 3–4 weeks) has not been established by controlled studies, but it has been used in some patients for substantially longer periods (6–12 months) with continuing good results. If it is used for extended periods, the need for continued therapy should be reassessed periodically.

Buspirone has only a modest effect on premenstrual syndrome (PMS). One study at Institute of Clinical Neuroscience in Sweden reported that buspirone reduced premenstrual irritability. It has a lower incidence of adverse sexual side effects than some other drugs, such as often reported with selective serotonin-reuptake inhibitor (SSRI). In patients experiencing sexual dysfunction with other treatments, buspirone may be a useful alternative.

For more information see page 1061.

*Generic: **Citalopram** (sye-TAL-oh-pram)*
*Brand: **Celexa***

Citalopram hydrobromide, a selective serotonin-reuptake inhibitor (SSRI), is typically prescribed as an antidepressant. It increases levels of serotonin, a neurotransmitter chemical that transmits messages between brain nerve cells and regulates pain, pleasure, anxiety, panic, arousal, and sleep behavior. Like other SSRIs, citalopram specifically acts on serotonin, and has a minimal effect on the other neurotransmitters, norepinephrine and dopamine. Because SSRI antidepressants like citalopram selectively block serotonin reuptake, they produce fewer side effects than earlier medications for depression.

Evidence shows that the selective serotonin reuptake inhibitors (SSRIs) effectively reduce the symptoms of severe premenstrual syndrome (PMS). According to investigators, results from a small number of subjects suggest that citalopram treatment is effective for PMS patients even in those who have failed previous SSRI treatment. You may only need to take SSRIs during the 14-day premenstrual period; this is called "intermittent treatment." This approach is also associated with fewer adverse effects than other standard regimens.

For more information see page 1096.

*Generic: **Clomipramine*** *(kloe-MI-pra-meen)*
*Brand: **Anafranil***

Clomipramine is typically prescribed as an antidepressant, but it has been also used to manage premenstrual syndrome (PMS). In a limited number of women with severe premenstrual irritability and depressed mood, clomipramine has been shown to be more effective than placebo in reducing these symptoms.

Researchers in Sweden demonstrated the effectiveness of clomipramine by comparing a treatment group with a placebo. Twenty-nine nondepressed women displaying severe premenstrual irritability and/or depressed mood were treated daily from the day of ovulation until the onset of the menstruation either with clomipramine or placebo for three consecutive menstrual cycles; another nine women (seven on clomipramine, two on placebo) dropped out during treatment. In both treatment groups, premenstrual irritability and depressed mood were significantly reduced during treatment; in the placebo group, this symptom reduction was about 45%, whereas in the clomipramine group it was greater than 70%. The premenstrual ratings of irritability and depressed mood during the three treatment cycles were significantly lower in the clomipramine group than in the placebo group. Global improvement with clomipramine was significantly better than with placebo. Researchers believe that this study confirms the effectiveness of low doses of clomipramine in the treatment of premenstrual syndrome.

For more information see page 1105.

*Generic: **Danazol*** *(DA-na-zole)*
*Brand: **Danocrine***

Danazol is a synthetic substance that resembles male hormones. It suppresses estrogen and menstruation and is used in low doses for severe premenstrual syndrome (PMS). It is particularly useful for premenstrual migraines. Taking it only during the luteal phase (after ovulation) relieves cyclical mastalgia (severe breast pain) and avoids potential side effects, but this intermittent regimen has no effect on the other PMS symptoms.

One study compared the effectiveness and safety of danazol with placebo in the treatment of severe premenstrual syndrome. Nineteen patients received danazol for three months followed by placebo, and 18 received treatment in the reverse order. Improvement was significantly more likely with danazol than with placebo after three months. Significant improvements were reported for breast discomfort, irritability, depression, anxiety, mood swings, crying, depressed libido, and abdominal swelling. Therefore, researchers concluded that danazol provides effective and generally well tolerated treatment for severe PMS. However, continuous therapy is not recommended because of side effects.

For more information see page 1129.

*Generic: **Drospirenone-Ethinyl Estradiol***
(droh-SPYE-re-none ETH-in-il Es-tra-DYE-ole)
*Brand: **Yasmin***

Drospirenone-ethinyl estradiol is a combination oral contraceptive containing estrogenic and progestinic steroids. This medication is a low-dose oral contraceptive (OC) birth control pill that contains estrogen and drospirenone. Drospirenone influences the regulation of water retention and electrolyte balance in the body, as well as having antiandrogenic (anti–male hormone) properties. An oral contraceptive containing drospirenone should ease water retention, bloating, weight gain, and breast tenderness. Furthermore, the anti-androgenic properties of drospirenone are believed to decrease irritability and tension. A study at University of Tennessee Health Science Center evaluated the effectiveness, safety, and cycle control of a low-dose combination OC containing drospirenone and ethinyl estradiol. Three hundred twenty-six women with menstrual symptoms showed a statistically significant decrease of water retention. The OC containing ethinyl estradiol and drospirenone was well tolerated and reduced the severity of menstrual cycle symptoms.

For more information see page 1162.

*Generic: **Fluvoxamine** (floo-VOKS-a-meen)*
*Brand: **Luvox***

Fluvoxamine, a selective serotonin-reuptake inhibitor (SSRI), is an antidepressant. A number of small trials shows this drug appears to be an effective treatment for premenstrual symptoms. In one such trial at the University of Pennsylvania fluvoxamine was taken daily for two menstrual cycles. Symptoms that most improved were irritability, anxiety, feeling out of control, and decreased interest in usual activity. Sixty percent of the subjects reported at least a 50% reduction in unwanted symptoms.

Other reports show improvement in symptoms such as tension and irritability. In a small study, fluvoxamine was taken for 14 days premenstrually for only three menstrual cycles. Seventy-five percent of the women reported significant improvement in premenstrual symptoms. Thus, noncontinuous use of fluvoxamine for premenstrual syndrome may be an effective option.

For more information see page 1199.

*Generic: **Goserelin** (GOE-se-rel-in)*
*Brand: **Zoladex***

Goserelin is used for its effect on hormones. Gonadotropin-releasing hormone (GnRH) medications like goserelin have been used to treat women with premenstrual syndrome (PMS). Depending on the dosages, menstrual cycling can be eliminated completely or ovulation alone can be suppressed. GnRH agonists lead to a "chemical menopause" and thus cause clinical concerns about low levels of estrogen and the development of osteoporosis and other symptoms associated with menopause. To compensate for the low level of female hormones when GnRH drugs are used, several types of steroid "add-back" regimens have been developed to create an artificial hormonal environment to minimize unwanted side effects. Add-back therapy refers to regimens that provide doses of estrogen and progestin that are high enough to maintain bone density, but are too low to offset the beneficial effects of the GnRH drug.

Treatment of PMS with such regimens has produced mixed results. Some studies have found no clinical improvement when women take a GnRH-like goserelin when compared to no treatment at all. Other studies suggest that women with severe mood symptoms may not benefit from this therapeutic approach. There are, however, studies showing a clear benefit with GnRH drugs plus add-back therapy for women with PMS.

For more information see page 1215.

*Generic: **Leuprolide*** *(loo-PROE-lide)*
*Brands: **Eligard, Lupron, Lupron Depot, Lupron Depot-Ped, Viadur***

Leuprolide is used for its effects on hormones. The Department of Clinical Pharmacy at the University of Tennessee studied the effect of leuprolide on 25 women with PMS. Leuprolide depot or saline was administered by injection for three consecutive treatment cycles. Leuprolide depot treatment was significantly more effective than placebo on all assessments. Irritability, neurologic symptoms, breast tenderness, and fatigue were most responsive to treatment. Symptoms were reduced only in women without premenstrual depression. Women with moderate premenstrual depression improved but remained symptomatic, whereas the group with severe premenstrual depression showed no improvement. Adverse side effects were lowest in those without premenstrual depression and highest in those with severe depression.

Leuprolide reduced both behavioral and physical symptoms and was well tolerated in the absence of severe PMS. You should be evaluated for depression before receiving a GnRH agonist. According to researchers, the different responses to leuprolide suggest that it may be helpful in diagnosing distinct subtypes of PMS.

For more information see page 1274.

*Generic: **Medroxyprogesterone Acetate***
(me-DROKS-ee-proe-JES-te-rone AS-eh-tate)
*Brand: **Provera***

Medroxyprogesterone acetate is a synthetic progestin, which is far more powerful than the body's own natural progesterone.

Studies have not consistently demonstrated that injectable hormone treatment compared to placebo improves PMS when progesterone was administered during the last week to 10 days before menses. On the other hand, progesterone treatment that is used as a contraceptive, such as norethisterone enantate, may be effective because it blocks ovulation. This medication causes irregular menstrual bleeding patterns but with continued use may result in an absence of menstrual bleeding altogether.

For more information see page 1297.

*Generic: **Mefenamic Acid** (me-fe-NAM-ik AS-id)*
*Brand: **Ponstel***

Mefenamic acid is a nonsteroidal anti-inflammatory drug (NSAID) used to treat inflammation, mild to moderate pain, and fever. Non-steroidal anti-inflammatory medication prevents the body from producing prostaglandins hormone-like substances that trigger pain and inflammation, and which may stimulate the symptoms associated with premenstrual syndrome (PMS). Therefore, reducing the amount of prostaglandins in the body may help to eliminate many of the inflammatory symptoms of PMS such as menstrual cramps, breast pain, headache, swelling, and other discomforts.

Steroids work by suppressing the immune system, whereas NSAIDs work mainly by preventing the formation of prostaglandins which are produced within the body's cells by the enzyme cyclooxygenase (COX). There are two varieties of the COX enzyme, COX-1 and COX-2. COX-1 is continuously secreted within the stomach and small bowel, and is important for maintaining a healthy stomach lining, normal kidney function, and the clotting action of blood platelets. In contrast, the COX-2 enzyme is primarily found at sites of inflammation. First-generation NSAIDs like mefenamic acid work by inhibiting both COX-1 and COX-2 enzymes and are considered non-selective COX-2 inhibitors.

Mefenamic acid therapy given during the luteal phase (after ovulation) is effective in relieving symptoms of PMS, but gastrointestinal toxicity prohibits its use. Overall, NSAIDs may alleviate a wide range of symptoms of PMS, but they do not appear to improve all symptoms such as mastalgia.

For more information see page 1300.

*Generic: **Nafarelin** (NAF-a-re-lin)*
*Brand: **Synarel***

Nafarelin prevents the release of eggs (ovulation) and menses. In a study, injections of an early GnRH agonist resulted in a 75% reduction in PMS symptoms. The beneficial effects began with the second month of treatment. Several other studies using different GnRH agonists have confirmed these results.

Various GnRH agonists are effective for PMS: most patients report complete resolution of their symptoms during therapy. However, because of their cost and associated adverse side effects, these drugs are usually reserved for patients with severe PMS who are unresponsive to other therapies. Adverse effects include hot flashes, headaches, muscle aches, vaginal dryness, and emotional lability, some of which (such as hot flashes) may decrease in severity over several weeks or months. The adverse side effects from low estrogenic associated with GnRH agonists, such as loss of bone mineral density (osteoporosis), make them impractical for long-term use and GnRH agonist therapy is not recommended for longer than six months. More recently, there have been reports that an estrogen/progestin combination can be added to GnRH agonist therapy to maintain the beneficial effects on PMS symptoms. These findings suggest that such modified GnRH agonist therapy may be safe and effective for long-term treatment of PMS.

For more information see page 1349.

Generic: **Naproxen** *(na-PROKS-en)*
Brands: **Anaprox (DS), EC-Naprosyn, Naprelan, Naprosyn**

Naproxen is a non-steroidal anti-inflammatory drug (NSAID) that reduces inflammation and pain as well as fever. Non-steroidal anti-inflammatory drugs (NSAIDs) are worth considering if PMS is associated with dysmenorrhea, headaches or musculoskeletal symptoms. Several early studies showed that naproxen is effective for treating PMS. In one study of naproxen sodium in Italy, both menstrual and premenstrual pain decreased during active drug treatment, while placebo was ineffective. In addition, a significant improvement was observed in premenstrual behavioral changes (likely related to the relief of pain). Improvements in symptoms including headache, fatigue, aches and pains, and mood are well documented. NSAIDs block prostaglandins, hormone-like substances that dilate blood vessels and cause inflammation. NSAIDs are usually the first drugs tried for almost any kind of minor pain. For PMS pain studies indicate that NSAIDs are most helpful when started seven days from menstruation and continued for four days into the cycle.

For more information see page 1354.

Generic: **Norethindrone Acetate** *(NOR-eth-in-drone AS-eh-tate)*
Brand: **Aygestin**

Norethindrone acetate is a synthetic progestin that inhibits ovulation. Progesterone is a natural hormone produced by the ovary during the second half of the menstrual cycle. Its biological function is to change the lining of the uterus so that the cells that line the uterus can provide nutrition to the developing embryo during the earliest phases of development after conception. If conception fails to occur, the drop in progesterone and estrogen levels in the blood lead to menstruation, a shedding of the lining of the uterus, which is an important preventive mechanism for the development of uterine cancer. Women who lack progesterone and who produce or are exposed to persistent levels of estrogen are at greater risk for this form of cancer. Other biological effects of progesterone include assisting in the final development of the female breast during puberty. Progesterone is also known to have mild sedative effects. Many clinicians feel that premenstrual syndrome (PMS) is related to levels of progesterone, although how it is related is poorly understood.

For more information see page 1371.

Generic: **Nortriptyline** *(nor-TRIP-ti-leen)*
Brands: **Aventyl, Pamelor**

Nortriptyline is a tricyclic antidepressant drug, which increases the levels of neurotransmitters in the brain. It has been shown to be very effective in the treatment of premenstrual syndrome (PMS) when given during the luteal phase (after ovulation) as well as with treatment continuously throughout the cycle. It also decreases the symptoms of depressed mood, irritability, and mood swings. However, the clinical use of this class of medication for the treatment of PMS is limited by its adverse side effects which include drowsiness, dizziness, increased sun sensitivity, and blurred vision. Because of the overlap of premenstrual mood symptoms with depression or anxiety, recent studies have enlisted antidepressants in the treatment of mood symptoms—anxiety, irritability, and mood swings—that are the most frequent symptoms in women with PMS.

For more information see page 1378.

Generic: **Spironolactone** *(speer-on-oh-LAK-tone)*
Brand: **Aldactone**

Spironolactone functions as a potassium-sparing diuretic. It increases urination to help eliminate water and sodium from the body. Diuretics reduce bloating in women with PMS and also have a beneficial effect on mood, breast tenderness, and food craving. Spironolactone is the only diuretic that is effective in relieving PMS symptoms.

A study in Sweden reported on the effectiveness of spironolactone for PMS. Thirty-five women with PMS were given spironolactone or placebo daily from day 14 of the menstrual cycle until the first day of the following menstruation. Spironolactone improved PMS symptoms compared to placebo; negative mood symptoms and somatic symptoms significantly decreased. Spironolactone significantly improved irritability, depression, feeling of swelling, breast tenderness, and food craving compared to placebo. Spironolactone appears to be an effective therapy for the negative mood changes and somatic symptoms of PMS.

For more information see page 1478.

Premenstrual Dysphoric Disorder

Premenstrual dysphoric disorder (PMDD) is a severe form of premenstrual syndrome (PMS). According to the Committee on Gynecologic Practice of the American College of Obstetricians and Gynecologists, up to 80% of women of reproductive age have physical changes with menstruation; 20 to 40% of them experience symptoms of PMS, while 2 to 10% report severe disruption of their daily activities, which is called premenstrual dysphoric disorder (PMDD). Key symptoms are severe depression, irritability, and tension before menstruation.

Commonly Prescribed (On-Label) Drugs: *Fluoxetine, Paroxetine, Sertraline*

OFF-LABEL PRESCRIPTION DRUGS
BREAKTHROUGH OPTIONS

*Generic: **Alprazolam** (al-PRAY-zoe-lam)*
*Brands: **Alprazolam Intensol, Xanax, Xanax XR***

Alprazolam is used to manage anxiety disorders or for the short-term relief of symptoms of anxiety or anxiety associated with depressive symptoms. It has been shown to reduce premenstrual symptoms, in particular premenstrual anxiety.

Alprazolam has also been shown to be superior in reducing symptoms of PMDD when compared to progesterone and placebo. A 50% improvement of symptoms is reported in 37% of the group treated with alprazolam, compared with 29% on progesterone, and 30% with placebo. The alprazolam tended to work better on the symptoms associated with mood disturbances (irritability, sadness) than the physical symptoms.

In another study, 30 women took alprazolam or placebo. Alprazolam was found to be superior to placebo in reducing symptoms. Low-dose alprazolam, administered intermittently during the luteal (after ovulation) phase, has been shown to be effective and is considered a good second-line treatment. Because of the addiction potential of this medication, use is generally limited. Long-term use is discouraged.

For more information see page 997.

*Generic: **Citalopram** (sye-TAL-oh-pram)*
*Brand: **Celexa***

Citalopram, a selective serotonin-reuptake inhibitor (SSRI), is an antidepressant. It has been used in a limited number of women with PMDD. Clinical experience suggests that the onset of action of SRRIs in women with PMDD is more rapid than when used for other psychiatric conditions; therefore, administration only during the luteal phase (after ovulation, the last two weeks of the menstrual cycle) may be effective in treating PMDD.

In a trial, intermittent administration of citalopram (10–30 mg daily during the luteal phase) for three menstrual cycles appeared to be more effective than continuous (10–30 mg daily throughout the menstrual cycle) or semi-intermittent administration (5 mg daily during the follicular—the period during menstrual bleeding—phase and 10–30 mg daily during the luteal phase of the drug and substantially more effective than placebo. Citalopram was well tolerated in all three regimens, and adverse side effects generally were mild. Researchers believe additional controlled studies are needed to determine whether the drug's effectiveness is sustained during longer-term, maintenance therapy in women with PMDD.

For more information see page 1096.

Generic: *Clomipramine* (kloe-MI-pra-meen)
Brand: *Anafranil*

Clomipramine is a tricyclic antidepressant. A Swedish study reported on 40 non-depressed women who had severe premenstrual irritability and/or dysphoria and late luteal phase (after ovulation) dysphoric disorder. Women with PMDD were treated daily for three menstrual cycles with either clomipramine or placebo. In both treatment groups premenstrual irritability and dysphoria were significantly reduced. In the placebo group, this reduction was only about 40%, whereas, in the clomipramine group, the symptom decrease was greater than 80%. For all three treatment cycles, women on clomipramine had significantly lower symptoms than placebo patients. Global improvement was considerably and significantly better with clomipramine than with placebo. Therefore, researchers concluded that low doses of clomipramine effectively reduce premenstrual irritability and dysphoria with a response rate close to 100%. Clomipramine given either continuously or intermittently is effective in reducing premenstrual irritability and depressed mood. However, preliminary data suggest that if you have premenstrual syndrome you may be particularly sensitive to the adverse side effects associated with the drug.

For more information see page 1105.

Generic: **Drospirenone** *(droh-SPYE-re-none) and* **Ethinyl Estradiol** *(ETH-in-il Es-tra-DYE-ole)*
Brand: **Yasmin**

Drospirenone is an estrogen-progestin combination contraceptive. Although oral contraceptives are used to treat mild-to-moderate symptoms associated with premenstrual syndrome, few trials support the efficacy of an oral contraceptive combined with drospirenone for moderate-to-severe symptoms associated with PMDD. A study of drospirenone in women with PMDD by researchers at the University of Pennsylvania showed a consistently greater reduction of symptoms for all 22 premenstrual symptoms compared to the placebo group. In addition, acne and food craving was significantly improved in the treatment group.

Another study confirms that drospirenone is beneficial for treating PMDD. Sixty-four patients with PMDD received either the 24/4 (four-day pill-free interval) regimen or placebo for three cycles. The 24/4 low-dose oral contraceptive was significantly more effective than placebo in treating emotional symptoms of PMDD including depression, anxiety, mood swings, anger, irritability and feeling overwhelmed.

For more information see page 1162.

Generic: **Escitalopram** *(es-sye-TAL-oh-pram)*
Brand: **Lexapro**

Escitalopram is a selective serotonin-reuptake inhibitor (SSRI) that is typically prescribed as an antidepressant. A study published in *Journal of Clinical Psychiatry* compared the efficacy and tolerability of escitalopram for premenstrual dysphoric disorder (PMDD) at symptom onset or given throughout the luteal phase (after ovulation). Twenty-seven women with PMDD were given escitalopram for three consecutive menstrual cycles. Premenstrual symptoms significantly improved; the luteal (after ovulation) phase group had 57% decrease and the symptom-onset group a 51% decrease. Clinical improvement was reported by 11 of 13 women in the luteal phase group and nine of 14 women in the symptom-onset group. Escitalopram was well tolerated, its adverse side effects mild and transient, with only two patients discontinuing due to side effects. PMDD improved significantly with either luteal phase or symptom-onset dosing of escitalopram. Women with more severe PMDD may respond better to luteal phase dosing than symptom-onset dosing.

For more information see page 1172.

Generic: *Fluvoxamine* *(floo-VOKS-a-meen)*
Brand: *Luvox*

Fluvoxamine, a selective serotonin-reuptake inhibitor (SSRI), is an antidepressant. It increases the amount of the neurotransmitter (brain chemical) serotonin in the brain. PMDD experts recommend an SSRI for PMDD when the main symptoms are depression, sudden mood shifts, anxiety, anger, irritability or fatigue. If PMDD symptoms are severe or if PMDD is associated with another condition requiring an SSRI, treatment is usually continuous (medication is taken every day). For less severe symptoms, intermittent dosing (about two weeks before menses) may be all that is necessary.

A large number of studies have evaluated SSRIs for treating women with PMDD. In a review of 12 trials with continuous dose administration of SSRIs and eight trials with luteal phase dose administration (from ovulation to menses), SSRIs were found to enhance mood, improve premenstrual irritability and dysphoria with a rapid onset of action. These studies demonstrate the successful treatment of symptoms overall and from the onset of the treatment cycle, which is significant because some SSRIs can take 2 to 3 weeks to work.

For more information see page 1105.

Generic: *Goserelin* *(GOE-se-rel-in)*
Brand: *Zoladex*

Goserelin may be used as a cancer-fighting medication and for its effects on hormones. Gonadotropin-releasing hormone (GnRH) agonists such as goserelin work by preventing ovulation and treatments are usually reserved for women who have severe PMDD that has not responded to better established and tolerated treatments. Because these drugs cause a premature menopause, they are often used together with supplemental estrogen and progestin to prevent the symptoms and long-term effects of the loss of estrogen at menopause.

In a study, goserelin was given to 27 women diagnosed with premenstrual tension. Over the course of three months, goserelin significantly reduced physical symptoms, such as breast discomfort and swelling. According to researchers, goserelin reduced cyclical fluctuations of anxiety and irritability, but any improvement in depressive symptoms was not consistent.

For more information see page 1215.

Generic: Leuprolide (loo-PROE-lide)
Brands: Eligard, Lupron, Lupron Depot, Lupron Depot-Ped, Viadur

Leuprolide is used for its effects on hormones. GnRH agonists like leuprolide are reserved mainly for women with severe symptoms of PMDD, primarily physical symptoms, that do not respond to other treatments. GnRH agonists such as leuprolide cause the ovary to temporarily stop making estrogen and progesterone, creating what some refer to as "artificial menopause." Side effects primarily result from the reduced amount of estrogen and include hot flashes, bone loss, and a risk of osteoporosis. To prevent bone loss, doctors often prescribe estrogen or the drug alendronate for women being treated with a GnRH agonist.

In a study at the University of Tennessee, leuprolide depot was given by injection for three consecutive cycles in 25 women with late luteal (after ovulation) PMDD. This treatment was ineffective for women with severe premenstrual depression and associated with adverse side effects. Leuprolide depot was well tolerated and effective in reducing less severe symptoms.

In a study at University of Pennsylvania Medical Center, women with PMS, and women with dysphoric symptoms were compared. Leuprolide depot was significantly more effective than placebo for women with PMS but not for women with premenstrual exacerbations of PMDD. Dysphoric symptoms for women with PMS did not decrease until the third cycle. The researchers concluded that the different responses to the drug may indicate that premenstrual depression has different causes from those of other dysphoric mood disorders.

For more information see page 1274.

*Generic: **Mefenamic Acid** (me-fe-NAM-ik AS-id)*
*Brand: **Ponstel***

Mefenamic acid is a nonsteroidal anti-inflammatory drug (NSAID) that also relieves pain and fever. Nonsteroidal anti-inflammatory drugs (NSAIDs) block prostaglandins, substances that dilate blood vessels and cause inflammation. NSAIDs are usually the first drugs tried for almost any kind of minor pain. There are dozens of NSAIDs. Mefenamic acid is among the most effective for menstrual disorders.

Mefenamic acid relieved dysmenorrhea in one study more effectively than placebo. In a study of women with menorrhagia, mefenamic acid resulted in a reduction in blood loss of up to 80% and was accompanied by a reduction in duration of dysmenorrhea and menstrual-related headache.

Mefenamic acid given during the luteal phase (after ovulation) relieves symptoms, but for some women gastrointestinal toxicity may limit its use. Overall, NSAIDs have been found to alleviate a wide range of premenstrual symptoms, but they do not appear to improve breast pain. In addition, the effects of mefenamic acid on mood are inconsistent when compared to its effects on pain.

For more information see page 1300.

*Generic: **Metolazone** (me-TOLE-a-zone)*
*Brands: **Mykrox, Zaroxolyn***

Metolazone is a diuretic and antihypertensive drug. Commonly called water pills, diuretics help the body shed excess water and sodium from the body through urination. They reduce bloating in women with PMS and also improve mood, decrease breast tenderness and food craving. These medicines significantly help reduce the weight gain, breast swelling, and bloating associated with premenstrual syndrome.

Metolazone has been effective for women with premenstrual weight gain for symptoms that include irritability, tension, depression, headache and water retention. Excessive urination and weakness occurred occasionally with larger doses. The efficacy of this treatment, however, may be limited as the data suggest that only women who gain weight premenstrually may benefit from diuretic treatment for PMDD.

For more information see page 1319.

Generic: **Mirtazapine** *(mir-TAZ-a-peen)*
Brands: **Remeron, Remeron SolTab**

Mirtazapine is an antidepressant unrelated to the selective serotonin reuptake inhibitors (SSRIs). It is unique in its action, stimulating the release of neurotransmitters (chemicals that permit communication among nerve cells) norepinephrine and serotonin in the brain.

In studies, SSRIs have helped treat PMDD. Mirtazapine is an option if you are unresponsive to, or intolerant of, SSRIs. People taking mirtazapine do not experience the side effects typical of other antidepressants: reduced sex drive, nervousness, and insomnia. Current evidence suggests that mirtazapine is effective in the treatment of depressive illness at all levels of severity. In addition, analyses of trials in moderate and severe depression show mirtazapine is effective in subgroups of depressed patients, particularly those with anxiety, sleep disturbance, and agitation.

The proportion of responders who improved from week one was twice as great with mirtazapine (13% versus 6%) as with SSRIs.

For more information see page 1332.

Generic: **Nafarelin** *(NAF-a-re-lin)*
Brand: **Synarel**

Nafarelin is used for its effects on hormones. Gonadotropin-releasing hormone (GnRH) agonists like nafarelin are synthetic hormones that suppress ovulation. They have been shown to be more effective than placebo in treating behavioral and physical symptoms of PMDD. Because they suppress ovulation, they end the hormonal fluctuations that produce PMS and so are sometimes used for very severe PMS symptoms and to improve breast tenderness, fatigue, and irritability. GnRH analogs, however, appear to have little effect on depression. Some experts believe that they may be useful as first-line therapy in some women with menstrual pain and irregular periods.

For more information see page 1349.

Generic: **Naproxen** *(na-PROKS-en)*
Brands: **Anaprox (DS), EC-Naprosyn, Naprelan, Naprosyn**

Naproxen is an anti-inflammatory drug (NSAIDs) that also relieves pain and fever. Naproxen relieves common pain symptoms of premenstrual syndrome (PMS), with the exception of breast pain. NSAIDs are commonly given for menstrual cramps, headaches, and pelvic discomfort and reduce the severity of these symptoms in women with PMDD. Women who experience severe cramping may take naproxen 1 to 2 days before cramps begin. Naproxen improves physical symptoms and headache in women with PMS. Overall, NSAIDs may alleviate a wide range of symptoms except for breast pain.

For more information see page 1354.

Generic: **Nortriptyline** *(nor-TRIP-ti-leen)*
Brands: **Aventyl, Pamelor**

Nortriptyline is a "tricyclic" antidepressant (TCA) drug. Many physicians do not find them to be as effective as SSRIs for treating depression-related illness. Nonetheless, tricyclic drugs are still frequently used as antidepressant medication. Some believe that they work better in patients with severe depression or melancholic symptoms.

Tricyclic antidepressants are more effective than placebo for PMDD in studies involving continuous administration as well as in studies using an intermittent luteal phase (after ovulation) treatment. In one report of 11 women who met criteria for late luteal-phase PMDD, eight had a good therapeutic response, but the efficacy of TCA antidepressants for premenstrual depression needs confirmation with more studies.

For more information see page 1378.

*Generic: **Spironolactone** (speer-on-oh-LAK-tone)*
*Brand: **Aldactone***

Spironolactone is a diuretic. It increases urination and helps eliminate water and sodium from the body. It is most commonly used to reduce bloating in women with PMDD, improves mood, and decreases breast tenderness and food craving. Other common diuretics include hydrochlorothiazide and furosemide. Many diuretics deplete the body's supply of potassium, possibly leading to heart rhythm disturbances, unless potassium is replaced through diet or supplementation. Spironolactone, however, is a potassium-sparing drug and does not have this problem, although women should be sure not to take additional potassium if they take spironolactone.

Spironolactone was more effective than placebo in reducing irritability, depression, somatic symptoms, feelings of swelling, breast tenderness, and craving for sweets. Therefore, diuretics relieve some of the physical symptoms of PMDD, such as bloating.

For more information see page 1478.

*Generic: **Venlafaxine** (ven-la-FAX-een)*
*Brands: **Effexor, Effexor XR***

Venlafaxine is commonly prescribed as an antidepressant. A study at the University of Pennsylvania examined the efficacy and safety of venlafaxine in the treatment of PMDD. One hundred sixty-four women received venlafaxine or placebo for four menstrual cycles. Venlafaxine was significantly more effective than placebo in reducing PMDD symptoms. Sixty percent of venlafaxine versus 35% of placebo subjects improved. Forty-three percent of venlafaxine subjects versus 25% of placebo subjects experienced significant remission of mood, pain, and physical symptoms. Improvement was relatively swift, with approximately 80% symptom reduction in the first treatment cycle. Adverse side effects such as nausea, insomnia, and dizziness were mild and transient. Venlafaxine is significantly more effective than placebo for PMDD treatment. Response to treatment can occur in the first treatment cycle, and venlafaxine is well tolerated. Further studies are needed to evaluate the potential of intermittent (luteal phase—after ovulation) dosing for this cyclic disorder and the efficacy of long-term maintenance treatment with venlafaxine.

For more information see page 1482.

Premenstrual Tension Syndrome

See Premenstrual Syndrome

MISCARRIAGE

Miscarriage is defined by the absence of fetal breathing, heartbeats, pulsation of the umbilical cord, or definite movements of voluntary muscles. Early miscarriage occurs at less than 20 weeks of gestation. Intermediate miscarriage occurs at 20–27 weeks of gestation. Late miscarriage occurs at greater than 28 weeks of gestation.

Abortion

An abortion is the expulsion or removal of an embryo or fetus from the mother prematurely. This can be done as an artificial procedure, but it often happens naturally when the mother's body expels the fetus because of problems with the pregnancy. Medically induced abortions can be completed by a surgical procedure or treatment with special medications.

Commonly Prescribed (On-Label) Drugs: Carboprost, Dinoprost, Dinoprostone, Mifepristone, Oxytocin, Rho(D) Immune Globulin, Sodium Chloride

OFF-LABEL PRESCRIPTION DRUGS
BREAKTHROUGH OPTIONS

Generic: **Mifepristone** *(mi-FE-pris-tone)*
Brand: **Mifeprex**

Mifepristone blocks the hormone progesterone, which is needed for pregnancy to continue.

A study of misoprostol and sulprostone, two prostaglandins used for the termination of second and third trimester pregnancy, compared the effectiveness for the termination of second and third trimester pregnancy in cases of congenital or genetic abnormalities and for the induction of labor in cases of fetal death within a woman's uterus. In cases where the fetus was alive, misoprostol was usually (77%) combined with mifepristone.

In 94 patients whose fetuses had died in the womb, there was no significant difference between misoprostol and sulprostone in time to delivery, blood loss, operative removal of the placenta, and need for pain relief. In cases of intra-uterine death, the effectiveness of misoprostol for termination of the pregnancy is comparable to that of sulprostone. When the fetus is viable, combination of mifepristone-misoprostol is more effective than sulprostone alone.

For more information see page 1328.

*Generic: **Misoprostol** (mye-soe-PROST-ole)*
*Brand: **Cytotec***

Misoprostol is used to prevent stomach ulcers while you take NSAIDs such as aspirin, ibuprofen, and naproxen, especially if you are at risk for developing ulcers or have a history of ulcers.

A study of 39 trials compared different medical methods for first-trimester abortion. Combined regimen mifepristone/prostaglandin: mifepristone 600 mg compared to 200 mg shows similar effectiveness in achieving complete abortion (four trials). Misoprostol administered orally is less effective (more failures) than the vaginal route and may be associated with more frequent side effects such as nausea and diarrhea. Mifepristone alone is less effective compared to the combined regimen mifepristone/prostaglandin. In one trial comparing gemeprost with misoprostol, misoprostol was more effective. The reviewers concluded that these medical abortion methods are safe and effective. Combined regimens are more effective than single drug treatments. In the combined regimen, the dose of mifepristone can be lowered to 200 mg without significantly decreasing its effectiveness.

For more information see page 1334.

Generic: **Methotrexate** *(meth-o-TREX-ate)*
Brands: **Rheumatrex, Trexall**

Methotrexate is used to limit growth of malignant cells. Surgical abortion has been the method of choice for termination of pregnancy up to 63 days' gestation since the 1960s, but over the last three decades many studies have explored the use of medical methods for inducing abortion at these gestations. Earlier regimens assessed the systemic and intrauterine injection of prostaglandins.

Since the introduction of mifepristone, medical abortion has been steadily increasing in countries where mifepristone has been available for routine use. Most current clinical protocols require the use of prostaglandins such as misoprostol in combination with anti-progesterones such as methotrexate. The safety, efficacy, and acceptability of the medical regimen are now well established at all gestations of pregnancy.

For more information see page 1312.

Abortion, Incomplete

An incomplete abortion is the clinical situation where part of the fetus or placental material is retained within the uterus. This can happen after a natural or medical abortion. Typical symptoms include vaginal bleeding and lower abdominal cramping. In most cases, a surgical intervention called curettage is performed to remove the remaining material from the uterus. The goal of this treatment is to prevent prolonged bleeding or infection.

Commonly Prescribed (On-Label) Drugs: *Dinoprost*

OFF-LABEL PRESCRIPTION DRUGS
BREAKTHROUGH OPTIONS

Generic: **Carboprost** *(KAR-boe-prost)*
Brand: **Hemabate**

Carboprost causes the uterus to contract and is used for the termination of a pregnancy. It is also used to help control severe bleeding after giving birth.

A study in *Contraception* analyzed treatment with vaginal suppositories containing carboprost that were administered to 40 women to induce an early abortion. All subjects were 49 days or less from their last menstrual period. Twenty-four women (60%) had a successful termination of their pregnancy using two vaginal prostaglandin suppositories. Sixteen women (40%) did not abort. One of the women who failed treatment refused the second suppository due to gastrointestinal side effects and uterine cramping following the insertion of the suppository. A second woman had an incomplete abortion and developed mild endometritis. Sixteen women reported side effects that included nausea, emesis, diarrhea, uterine cramping requiring analgesia, restlessness, shakiness, and dizziness.

For more information see page 1072.

Generic: *Methylergonovine* (meth-il-er-goe-NOE-veen)
Brand: *Methergine*

Methylergonovine directly stimulates contractions of uterine smooth muscle. Investigators in Mozambique studied the capacity of vaginal misoprostol in combination with methylergometrine to achieve complete evacuation of the uterus without the need for subsequent surgical evacuation of the uterus. This study included 228 women seeking abortion. Vaginal misoprostol was given in the early second trimester. All women received related treatment with methylergometrine from the moment of misoprostol application every eight hours until uterine evacuation. Follow-up was continued until the first menstruation after interruption.

Complete uterine evacuation was achieved in 173/228 cases (76%). The remaining 55 women underwent manual evacuation of placenta remnants trapped in the cervix. In seven of these women a scraping of the uterus was carried out due either to ultrasound evidence of placental remnants or due to uterine bleeding. The interval between misoprostol application and fetal expulsion averaged 14.9 hours in group one and 21.0 hours in group two. The investigators concluded that misoprostol, in combination with methylergometrine, is efficient in achieving uterine evacuation without surgical intervention.

For more information see page 1315.

Generic: **Misoprostol** *(mye-soe-PROST-ole)*
Brand: **Cytotec**

Misoprostol is used to prevent stomach ulcers while you take NSAIDs such as aspirin, ibuprofen, and naproxen, especially if you are at risk for developing ulcers or have a history of ulcers.

A study of the efficiency of misoprostol in the termination of missed abortion (fetus stops developing but miscarriage does not take place spontaneously) in a group of 66 women aged 19–37, who received 400 microg of vaginal misoprostol for termination of missed abortion. The overall success rate for a complete abortion was 30.3% and for incomplete abortion 25.8%. Another 16.7% cases failed with the procedures used. The investigators concluded that vaginal misoprostol can induce the termination of missed abortion or dilation of the cervical canal.

Another study in Thailand evaluated the effectiveness and side effects of two regimens of oral misoprostol, single dose (600 microg) and repeated dose (1200 microg), in the treatment of incomplete abortion. One hundred women who had incomplete abortion (gestational age less than 20 weeks) were given a single oral 600-microg dose or repeated oral dose after four hours (total 1200 microg). The overall incidence of complete abortion was 86.9%, which was not statistically different between the single-dose and repeated-dose groups. Overall rate of acceptability and tolerability of side effects were 88.9% and 97.9%, respectively. Oral misoprostol may be a practical alternative in the management of incomplete abortion.

For more information see page 1334.

Abortion, Late

Late abortion is defined as the termination of a pregnancy after the first trimester.

Commonly Prescribed (On-Label) Drugs: *None*

OFF-LABEL PRESCRIPTION DRUGS
BREAKTHROUGH OPTIONS

*Generic: **Mifepristone** (mi-FE-pris-tone)*
*Brand: **Mifeprex***

Mifepristone is used for the medical termination of pregnancy and enables women as outpatients to have successful terminations of pregnancy up to 63 days gestation in 92–99%. In the inpatient setting, studies have shown that mifepristone in combination with prostaglandin is effective as a drug for abortion in the late first trimester. In the second trimester, the addition of mifepristone to a prostaglandin regimen can expedite the speed of the abortion. At all stages of pregnancy, the use of mifepristone facilitates and improves prostaglandins' expulsive effects on the uterine contents.

A study assessed the use of medication and the outcome of medical abortion in the late first trimester of pregnancy. The investigators reviewed 483 women who underwent medical abortion at 64 to 91 days of gestation and who used mifepristone that was followed 36 to 48 hours later by repeated doses of misoprostol. A total of 891 abortions were carried out at 64 to 91 days of gestation; of these, 483 cases (54.2%) were undertaken medically. Complete abortion occurred in 458 cases (94.8%). The older the fetus, however, the less efficient the drugs become from the beginning of the abortion. The researchers concluded that medical abortion between 64 and 91 days of gestation is effective and has a high success rate.

For more information see page 1328.

*Generic: **Misoprostol** (mye-soe-PROST-ole)*
*Brand: **Cytotec***

Misoprostol increases the magnitude and frequency of uterine contractions and stimulates uterine bleeding and total or partial expulsion of uterine contents in pregnant women. A review of 26 studies assessed the effects of vaginal misoprostol for third trimester cervical ripening (softening of the cervix) or induction of labor. Compared to placebo, misoprostol was associated with increased cervical ripening. It was also associated with a reduced need for treatment with oxytocin (a type of hormone). Misoprostol was more effective than prostaglandin for labor induction. The researchers concluded that vaginal misoprostol appears to be more effective in inducing labor than conventional methods of cervical ripening and labor induction.

For more information see page 1334.

Abortion, Missed

A missed abortion refers to a miscarriage where the fetus has died prior to 20 weeks of pregnancy, but neither the fetus nor the placenta has been expelled from the uterus and is retained in utero for two months or longer.

Commonly Prescribed (On-Label) Drugs: *Dinoprostone Vaginal Suppositories*

OFF-LABEL PRESCRIPTION DRUG
BREAKTHROUGH OPTION

Generic: **Misoprostol** *(mye-soe-PROST-ole)*
Brand: **Cytotec**

Misoprostol may be used to assist with childbirth and for the treatment of severe bleeding after delivery. When misoprostol is used vaginally for these purposes, it causes the womb muscles to contract.

Evaluation of the efficacy and tolerance of a high dose of vaginal misoprostol for outpatient medical management of missed abortion was conducted by researchers in Greece. Three doses of 400 mg misoprostol were administered intravaginally every four hours daily, for a maximum period of three days, to 108 women with uneventful first trimester pregnancy failure. A total of 98 women (90.7%) were managed successfully, with 74 (68.5%) of them within the first 24 hours. Only six of 108 women (9.3%) required surgical intervention.

For more information see page 1334.

PREGNANCY

Amnioreduction

Amnioreduction refers to the removal of excess amniotic fluid. Under ultrasound guidance and after numbing of the mother's abdominal wall, a long, very fine needle is introduced into the uterus and into the amniotic cavity. While the fetus is being monitored with ultrasound, excess fluid from the amniotic cavity is withdrawn. It is similar to amniocentesis, where a small amount of amniotic fluid is removed for diagnostic reasons. Amnioreduction is performed for the purpose of reducing large amounts of fluid, in order to correct too much amniotic fluid.

Commonly Prescribed (On-Label) Drugs: *None*

OFF-LABEL PRESCRIPTION DRUG
BREAKTHROUGH OPTION

Generic: **Sulindac** *(sul-IN-dak)*
Brand: **Clinoril**

Sulindac is an anti-inflammatory drug (NSAID) used to reduce pain and swelling. Cord entanglement is a common complication of twins who share a single amniotic sac, and it is associated with high perinatal death. Apart from preterm delivery, no treatment has previously been used to reduce the risks of this complication. A study tested to find out if reducing amniotic fluid volume would reduce the risk of cord accidents. Cord entanglement was documented in three cases of twins and sulindac administered to their mothers. Sulindac was associated with a reduction in amniotic fluid. All six twins were delivered without complications. The investigators concluded that medical amnioreduction with sulindac is a new way to reduce cord complications in twins sharing a single amniotic sac.

Another study examined newly developed methods for diagnosing twins sharing a single amniotic sac and reducing mortality. In the past two decades, technologies have enabled early diagnosis of this condition and its complications. As a result, the majority of cases can be diagnosed reliably at an early gestational age. Treatment with medical amnioreduction, surgical amnioreduction, or fetal reduction (removing one fetus so that the other's chances of normal development and delivery increases) in selected cases may be offered before 24 weeks' gestation. Later, intensive fetal surveillance should be offered until 32 weeks, at which point elective preterm delivery may be considered to prevent possible fetal death.

For more information see page 1486.

Cervical Ripening

In pregnancy, the uterine cervix serves two major functions. First, it maintains its firmness during pregnancy as the uterus dramatically enlarges. This physical integrity is critical so that the developing fetus can remain in the uterus until the appropriate time for delivery. Second, in preparation for labor and delivery, the cervix softens and becomes more distensible, a process called cervical ripening. These chemical and physical changes are required for cervical dilatation, labor, and delivery of a fetus. In women with a medical or obstetrical need for induction of labor, certain agents can "ripen" the cervix to facilitate the induction process.

Commonly Prescribed (On-Label) Drugs: *None*

OFF-LABEL PRESCRIPTION DRUG
BREAKTHROUGH OPTION

Generic: **Misoprostol** *(mye-so-PROST-ole)*
Brand: **Cytotec**

Misoprostol is used to prevent stomach ulcers while you are taking NSAIDs such as aspirin, ibuprofen, and naproxen, especially if you are at risk for developing ulcers or have a history of ulcers. Misoprostol helps to decrease risk of serious ulcer complications such as bleeding. It protects the stomach lining by lowering the amount of acid that comes in contact with it.

The American College of Obstetrics and Gynecology (ACOG) states that misoprostol has been used effectively (intravaginally using tablets formulated for oral administration) to improve cervical "ripening" in pregnant women with a medical or obstetric need for labor induction. A study at Stanford University School of Medicine examined the efficacy and safety of oral misoprostol versus vaginal misoprostol in 204 women between 32 to 42 weeks of gestation with an unfavorable cervix and an indication for labor induction. They received either oral or vaginal misoprostol every four hours up to four doses. Investigators found that oral misoprostol was as effective as vaginal misoprostol for cervical ripening and had a low incidence of uterine hyperstimulation (an inability to tolerate labor), no increase in side effects, a high rate of patient satisfaction. It is also associated with a lower cesarean section rate.

For more information see page 1334.

Cephalic Version

See External Cephalic Version

Eccyesis

See Ectopic Pregnancy

Ectopic Pregnancy

An ectopic pregnancy is a condition where a fertilized egg settles and grows in a location other than the inner lining of the uterus. The vast majority of ectopic pregnancies occurs in the fallopian tube (95%), but they can occur elsewhere, such as the ovary, cervix, and abdominal cavity. In the United States an ectopic pregnancy occurs in about one in 60 pregnancies. The major health risk of this condition is internal bleeding.

Commonly Prescribed (On-Label) Drugs: *None*

OFF-LABEL PRESCRIPTION DRUG
BREAKTHROUGH OPTION

Generic: **Methotrexate** *(meth-oh-TREKS-ate)*
Brands: **Rheumatrex, Trexall**

Methotrexate is an immunosuppressant used to limit growth of malignant cells. A study at the University of Tennessee Health Science Center compared success rates of 643 patients who had ectopic pregnancy and received multiple or single doses.

The success rates were comparable between patients with multi-dose and single-dose therapy (95% vs. 90%, respectively) as hormone levels, history of ectopic pregnancy (21.4% vs. 21.7%, respectively), number of treatment days, gestational age, ectopic size, ectopic volume and ectopic mass volume. Patients who received single-dose therapy were significantly heavier (146 vs. 159 pounds), had greater ectopic cardiac activity (3.1% vs. 10.3%), and received fewer methotrexate doses. The investigators concluded that single-dose methotrexate therapy is as effective as multidose therapy for the treatment of ectopic pregnancy.

For more information see page 1312.

External Cephalic Version

External cephalic version is the changing of a baby's position in the uterus by manipulation of the mother's abdomen. Usually it is done to turn a breech baby to a vertex (headfirst) position. A breech baby's bottom or feet are in a position to come out before the head during delivery through the birth canal. Such a delivery may be hazardous because for example, the baby's head may become trapped in the mother's cervix. If the baby is moved to a headfirst position, you may avoid having a vaginal breech delivery or cesarean section.

Commonly Prescribed (On-Label) Drugs: *Nitroglycerin*

OFF-LABEL PRESCRIPTION DRUGS
BREAKTHROUGH OPTIONS

Generic: **Terbutaline** *(ter-BYOO-ta-leen)*
Brand: **Brethine**

Terbutaline is used to relax the smooth muscle in the lungs and dilate airways to improve breathing. It is typically used in the treatment of asthma, chronic bronchitis, or emphysema.

The efficacy and safety of intravenous nitroglycerin was compared with that of subcutaneous terbutaline administered under the skin as a treatment for arresting uterine contractions for external cephalic version at terms as studied by researchers in the Department of Obstetrics and Gynecology at Stanford University. In a clinical trial, patients between 37 and 42 weeks of gestation received either nitroglycerin therapy or terbutaline therapy to stop contractions during external cephalic version.

Of 59 patients, 30 women received nitroglycerin, and 29 women received terbutaline. The overall success rate of external cephalic version was 39%. The rate of successful external cephalic version was significantly higher in the terbutaline group. Compared with nitroglycerin, terbutaline was associated with a significantly higher rate of successful external cephalic version at term.

For more information see page 1499.

Extrauterine Pregnancy

See Ectopic Pregnancy

Fetal Distress

Fetal distress refers to a difficulty the fetus encounters before labor or during the birth process. The term "fetal distress" is commonly used to describe low oxygen levels in the fetus (hypoxia). Fetal hypoxia may result in fetal damage or death if not reversed promptly. Fetal distress can be detected when the following signs are observed: abnormal slowing of labor, the presence of meconium (dark green fecal material from the fetus), other abnormal substances in the amniotic fluid, or abnormal indications on fetal electronic monitoring.

Commonly Prescribed (On-Label) Drugs: None

OFF-LABEL PRESCRIPTION DRUGS
BREAKTHROUGH OPTIONS

Generic: **Dexamethasone** *(deks-a-METH-a-sone)*
Brands: **Decadron, Dexameth, Dexone, Hexadrol**

Dexamethasone is a corticosteroid that reduces swelling and inflammation and is used to treat a variety of disorders. A study at Nuffield Department of Obstetrics and Gynaecology at Oxford looked at the effect of dexamethasone on fetal heart rate. Twenty-eight pregnant women, at 27 to 32 weeks of gestation, received dexamethasone to accelerate pulmonary maturation (in the fetus) in the expectation of preterm delivery. Dexamethasone was given on 51 occasions at weekly intervals (one to four occasions per patient). In 10 pregnancies without fetal distress there was a highly significant brief rise in short-term fetal heart rate variation after dexamethasone administration.

In 18 pregnancies with subsequent delivery for fetal distress (abnormal fetal heart rate pattern) the rise in short-term fetal heart rate variation was less. The investigators concluded that dexamethasone administration normally causes a rise in fetal heart rate variation for up to a day.

For more information see page 1138.

Generic: **Terbutaline** *(ter-BYOO-ta-leen)*
Brand: **Brethine**

Terbutaline relaxes the smooth muscle in the lungs and dilates airways to improve breathing. It is used in the treatment of asthma, chronic bronchitis, or emphysema. A study looked at the maternal impact of terbutaline versus magnesium sulfate in the treatment of fetal distress prior to cesarean delivery. Forty-six women received either subcutaneous terbutaline (administered under the skin) or intravenous magnesium sulfate for in utero fetal resuscitation before cesarean delivery. There were no significant differences between groups in arterial pressure, arterial pressure before and after induction of anesthesia, maternal heart rate, maternal oxygen saturation, and estimated blood loss. Magnesium sulfate-treated women received significantly more intraoperative intravenous fluids than the terbutaline group.

For more information see page 1499.

Heterotopic Pregnancy

See Ectopic Pregnancy

Hyperemesis Gravidarum

Nausea and vomiting during pregnancy, more widely known as morning sickness, is a common condition. Hyperemesis gravidarum is a rare disorder characterized by severe and persistent nausea and vomiting during pregnancy that may cause dehydration, vitamin and mineral deficit, and the loss of greater than five percent of their original body weight, and may necessitate hospitalization. Do not use any drug while pregnant without first consulting a physician.

Commonly Prescribed (On-Label) Drugs: None

OFF-LABEL PRESCRIPTION DRUGS
BREAKTHROUGH OPTIONS

Generic: Chlorpromazine (klor-PROE-ma-zeen)
Brand: Thorazine

Chlorpromazine is an antipsychotic used to treat symptoms of mental or emotional conditions. It is also used to control hiccups, reduce anxiety, and treat nausea and vomiting. Phenothiazines like chlorpromazine are used for preventing and controlling severe nausea and vomiting associated with various illnesses. This class of drugs has been effective when used in the management of postoperative nausea and vomiting. In general, phenothiazines are not effective in preventing vertigo or motion sickness, or for the management of vomiting. Chlorpromazine has been shown to reduce nausea and vomiting of pregnancy when compared with placebo.

Safe use of phenothiazines for the prevention and treatment of nausea and vomiting of pregnancy has not been established, and the manufacturers recommend that the drugs be used during pregnancy only when the potential benefits justify the possible risks to the fetus. Some phenothiazines are not recommended at all for use during pregnancy.

For more information see page 1086.

Generic: **Droperidol** *(droe-PER-i-dole)*
Brand: **Inapsine**

Droperidol is used to reduce the incidence of nausea and vomiting during surgical and diagnostic procedures. However, because of the risk of serious, sometimes fatal effects on heart rhythms, the manufacturer states that use of droperidol should be reserved only for those women who have failed to respond adequately to other drugs in the treatment of nausea and vomiting.

Researchers at University of California, Irvine, compared continuous droperidol infusion and single dose intravenous diphenhydramine for treatment of morning sickness. Women treated with droperidol-diphenhydramine had significantly shorter hospitalizations, fewer days per pregnancy hospitalized for excessive vomiting, and fewer re-admissions with this diagnosis. It was concluded that droperidol is a beneficial, cost-effective therapy for the treatment of morning sickness.

For more information see page 1161.

Generic: **Metoclopramide** *(met-oh-kloe-PRA-mide)*
Brand: **Reglan**

Metoclopramide is used in a variety of gastrointestinal (GI) disorders but principally for the management of gastroesophageal reflux, for the prevention of chemotherapy-induced nausea and vomiting, as well as postoperative nausea and vomiting.

Researchers at Tufts University School of Medicine compared pyridoxine-metoclopramide combination therapy to prochlorperazine and promethazine in the outpatient treatment of nausea and vomiting in pregnancy. In total, 174 first-trimester patients were divided into three treatment groups: pyridoxine-metoclopramide, prochlorperazine, or promethazine. Prior to and on the third day, women recorded their responses to the given treatment and their number of nausea episodes. There were no differences in the number of nausea episodes prior to treatment. Combination therapy with pyridoxine and metoclopramide appears to be superior to either monotherapy in the treatment of nausea and vomiting in pregnancy.

For more information see page 1318.

*Generic: **Prochlorperazine** (proe-klor-PER-a-zeen)*
*Brands: **Compazine, Compro***

Prochlorperazine is used to control severe nausea and vomiting of various causes. It is effective for postoperative nausea and vomiting, and for that caused by toxins, radiation, or cell-damaging drugs.

Pyridoxine-metoclopramide combination therapy has been compared to prochlorperazine and promethazine monotherapies in the treatment of 174 pregnant outpatients. Investigators at Tufts University School of Medicine divided women into three treatment groups: pyridoxine-metoclopramide, prochlorperazine, or promethazine. There were no differences in the number of nausea episodes prior to treatment, but combination therapy with pyridoxine and metoclopramide appears to be superior to either monotherapy in the treatment of nausea and vomiting in pregnancy.

For more information see page 1434.

*Generic: **Promethazine** (proe-METH-a-zeen)*
*Brands: **Phenadoz, Phenergan, Promethegan***

Promethazine is used to treat and manage motion sickness. It has been compared with methylprednisolone for the treatment of morning sickness. Women with a normal-appearing pregnancy of less than or equal to 16 weeks' gestation with morning sickness received either oral methylprednisolone, or oral promethazine. After three days, methylprednisolone was tapered over the course of two weeks, whereas the promethazine was continued without change for two weeks. For women who continued to vomit after two days, the medication was discontinued. Women receiving either medication at discharge continued to take the remainder of the assigned medication from the packaged pill dispensers. They were followed up weekly.

There were no significant differences between the groups with respect to maternal age, gestational age at entry, number of previous admissions, or greater than five percent body weight loss. Three women in the methylprednisolone group and two in the promethazine group failed to stop vomiting within two days. One woman from the promethazine group was unavailable for follow-up. No women from the methylprednisolone group was readmitted but five of the 17 women receiving promethazine were readmitted for excessive nausea within two weeks of discharge. No adverse effects were noted for either drug and it was concluded that a short course of methylprednisolone is more effective than promethazine for the treatment of morning sickness.

For more information see page 1435.

Generic: **Trimethobenzamide** *(trye-meth-oh-BEN-za-mide)*
Brand: **Tigan**

Trimethobenzamide is used for the control of nausea and vomiting, including the treatment of postoperative nausea and vomiting. It is also used for nausea associated with gastroenteritis. The drug is less effective as an anti-nausea medication than phenothiazine, but may have fewer adverse side effects than phenothiazine therapy. When vomiting is severe, potentially hazardous, and likely to be of short duration, phenothiazine antiemetics may be preferred. When long-term therapy is anticipated, non-phenothiazine antiemetics such as trimethobenzamide hydrochloride should be considered. If treatment with prochlorperazine or promethazine is unsuccessful, some physicians try other antiemetics, such as trimethobenzamide.

For more information see page 1528.

Infertility

Infertility is usually defined as not being able to get pregnant despite trying for one year. A broader view of infertility includes not being able to carry a pregnancy to term and have a baby. Infertility affects about 6.1 million Americans, or 10% of the reproductive age population, according to the American Society for Reproductive Medicine. It may be due to a single cause in either partner in a couple, or a combination of factors that prevents a pregnancy from occurring or continuing. The therapies in this section are for women.

Commonly Prescribed (On-Label) Drugs: Balsalazide, Bromocriptine, Clomiphene

---

OFF-LABEL PRESCRIPTION DRUGS
BREAKTHROUGH OPTIONS

---

*Generic: **Anastrozole** (an-AS-troh-zole)*
*Brand: **Arimidex***

Anastrozole prevents the growth of malignant cells by lowering estrogen hormone levels to help shrink tumors and slow their growth. During infertility treatment, ovarian stimulation with drugs is used either alone or in conjunction with intrauterine insemination and reproductive technologies. At present, the two main medications for ovarian stimulation include clomiphene citrate, and injectable gonadotropins. In spite of the high ovulation rate with the use of clomiphene citrate, the pregnancy rate is much lower. In clomiphene citrate failures, gonadotropin injections have generally been used as the next treatment option. Treatment with gonadotropins is difficult to control and characteristically associated with increased risk of multiple pregnancies. Therefore, it would be preferable to use an effective oral treatment without risk of multiple pregnancies and with minimal monitoring.

Aromastase inhibitors, such as anastrozole, can be administered early in the follicular phase (time during menstrual bleeding) to induce ovulation. Success of aromastase inhibitors like anastrozole in induction and augmentation of ovulation in addition to improving ovarian response to gonadotropin stimulation has been reported. There are other potential applications for aromastase inhibitors in infertility management, including improving implantation in assisted reproduction and in vitro maturation.

For more information see page 1020.

Generic: **Letrozole** *(LET-roe-zole)*
Brand: **Femara**

Letrozole prevents growth of malignant cells. It is typically used to treat advanced breast cancer in women after menopause. The effects of letrozole and clomiphene citrate were studied in women undergoing superovulation (stimulating the ovaries to develop multiple eggs) and intrauterine insemination (IUI) have been compared. There were a total of 238 cycles of superovulation and IUI in women with infertility. Women received either letrozole daily or clomiphene citrate daily.

There was no significant difference between the total number of developing follicles in the letrozole and in the clomiphene citrate groups. No difference was found in the endometrial thickness between the two groups. The pregnancy rate per cycle was 11.5% in the letrozole group and 8.9% in the clomiphene citrate group. Four of the 11 pregnancies in the clomiphene citrate group resulted in a miscarriage (36.6%). The investigators concluded that superovulation and IUI with letrozole and clomiphene citrate are associated with similar pregnancy rates, but the miscarriage rate is higher with clomiphene citrate. The ideal dose of letrozole remains unknown and further study is needed.

For more information see page 1273.

Generic: **Tamoxifen** *(ta-MOKS-I-fen)*
Brand: **Nolvadex**

Tamoxifen prevents growth of malignant cells. Tamoxifen and clomiphene have both been used for ovulation induction in women with infertility. Researchers reviewed studies in various professional medical journals to compare the effectiveness of tamoxifen versus clomiphene for the induction of ovulation and conception. Researchers at the Women's and Children's Hospital looked at clinical trials that compared tamoxifen and clomiphene for ovulation induction in women whose bodies do not ovulate. The main outcome measures were ovulation rate and clinical pregnancy rate. The use of tamoxifen and clomiphene citrate resulted in similar ovulation rates. There was no benefit of tamoxifen over clomiphene citrate in achievement of pregnancy per cycle or per ovulatory cycle. Clomiphene citrate and tamoxifen are equally effective in inducing ovulation.

For more information see page 1493.

Labor Induction

Sometimes, if labor does not start on its own, doctors use medicines to help labor begin. This is called "labor induction." The most common reason for labor induction is that the pregnancy has gone two weeks or more past the due date. The baby may get too big if you carry it this far past your due date and may not get enough nourishment from your body. Labor induction may also be recommended if there are concerns for you or your pregnancy for other reasons, such as, high blood pressure, infection, and diabetes.

Commonly Prescribed (On-Label) Drugs: Dinoprostone, Oxytocin

OFF-LABEL PRESCRIPTION DRUGS
BREAKTHROUGH OPTIONS

Generic: **Carboprost** (KAR-boe-prost)
Brand: **Hemabate**

Carboprost tromethamine causes the uterus to contract and is used for the termination of a pregnancy. It is also used to help control severe bleeding after giving birth. A study conducted in China examined the most effective dose of carboprost suppository for induction of labor. A total of 150 pregnant women were divided into three groups, each being administered different doses of carboprost: group one received 0.100 mg; group two 0.125 mg; and group three 0.200 mg. The success rates of induction were 90.0%, 94.0% and 100.0% for group one, two and three, respectively. There were three cases of precipitate delivery in group two and three. No uterine hyperstimulation (the uterine's inability to handle labor) occurred in group one and two, while three cases of uterine hyperstimulation were reported in group three. The researchers concluded that a single maximum dose of carboprost for term labor induction should be less than 0.200 mg.

For more information see page 1072.

Generic: **Mifepristone** *(mi-FE-pris-tone)*
Brand: **Mifeprex**

Mifepristone blocks a hormone called progesterone that inhibits contractions of the uterus. In a study involving 594 women taking mifepristone for labor induction, results show that patients have a favorable cervix within 48 to 96 hours and are less likely to need a cesarean.

For more information see page 1328.

Generic: **Misoprostol** *(mye-so-PROST-ole)*
Brand: **Cytotec**

Misoprostol is used to prevent stomach ulcers while you take NSAIDs such as aspirin, ibuprofen, and naproxen, especially if you are at risk for developing ulcers or have a history of ulcers. Misoprostol decreases risks of serious ulcer complications such as bleeding.

The American College of Obstetrics and Gynecology (ACOG) states that misoprostol has improved cervical "ripening" in pregnant women with a need for labor induction. A study at the University of Vermont looked at whether a single outpatient dose of intravaginal misoprostol reduces the synthetic oxytocin (a hormone that facilitates the birth process) use for induction, as synthetic oxytocin may overstimulate the uterus and harm the mother and fetus. Women received misoprostol or dinoprostone gel the evening before oxytocin induction. A single dose of misoprostol significantly decreased the cumulative dose of oxytocin, the cumulative time of oxytocin administration, and the dose intensity of oxytocin. There was no difference in cesarean delivery and there was no difference in short-term neonatal outcome. No women had hyperstimulation or required cesarean. The investigators concluded that a single dose of misoprostol administered in the outpatient setting significantly decreases oxytocin use.

For more information see page 1334.

Nonreassuring Fetal Status

See Fetal Distress

Ovulation Induction

Ovulation induction for in vitro fertilization, (IVF) uses medication to stimulate development of one or more mature follicles (where eggs develop) in the ovaries of infertile women who may not regularly develop mature follicles without the help. Ovulation induction may be necessary in women who do not ovulate consistently, but want to have a child. There are many reasons why women do not ovulate regularly.

Commonly Prescribed (On-Label) Drugs: Chorionic Gonadotropin, Follitropin Alfa, Follitropin Beta, Menotropins

---

OFF-LABEL PRESCRIPTION DRUGS
BREAKTHROUGH OPTIONS

---

*Generic: **Leuprolide** (loo-PROE-lide)*
*Brands: **Eligard, Lupron, Lupron Depot, Lupron Depot-Ped, Viadur***

Leuprolide, a synthetic analog of naturally occurring gonadatropin-releasing hormone (GnRH), is used to prevent growth of malignant cells and for its effects on hormones.

The use of two GnRHs, leuprolide and triptorelin, were compared in which 52 women underwent controlled ovarian hyperstimulation and in vitro fertilization (IVF). Patients received either leuprolide or triptorelin on days 21–23 of the menstrual cycle. Twenty-six women were included in each group. Significantly higher clinical implantation and pregnancy rates were found in the leuprolide group than the triptorelin group. The investigators concluded that leuprolide is associated with higher implantation and pregnancy rates than triptorelin when used in the midluteal phase.

For more information see page 1274.

*Generic: **Nafarelin** (NAF-a-re-lin)*
*Brand: **Synarel***

Nafarelin, a synthetic analog of gonadotropin-releasing hormone (GnRH), is used to affect hormones. In an in vitro fertilization (IVF) program, researchers studied the effect of the gonadotropin-releasing hormone agonist (GnRH-a) nafarelin on thirty women who had exhibited low ovarian response in at least two previous IVF cycles. They received nafarelin daily for seven to 10 days from the mid-luteal phase (days 21–23) of the previous cycle until the first day of menstruation. Menotropin was commenced on cycle day three (with no additional nafarelin). A significantly higher number of eggs were retrieved and a higher number of embryos transferred in the study cycles than in the control cycles. Pregnancy rates per embryo transfer and per cycle were 10.4% and 7.7% for the study cycles and 2.8% and 1.6% for the control cycles, respectively. Treatment with the GnRH-a nafarelin should be an additional option for ovulation induction for infertile patients in IVF programs.

For more information see page 1349.

Paracyesis

See Ectopic Pregnancy

POSTPARTUM DEPRESSION

Postpartum depression (PPD) may develop a few days or even months after childbirth. PPD can happen after the birth of any child, not just the first child. Feelings similar to the baby blues— sadness, despair, anxiety, irritability—are present but felt much more strongly. PPD may interfere with normal daily activities. If this is the case, help is needed for treatment and/or support. While PPD is a serious condition, it can be treated with medication and counseling.

Postpartum Psychosis and Lactation

Postpartum psychosis is a very serious mental illness that can affect a new mother. The episode of psychosis usually begins within one to three months after delivery. The mother with postpartum psychosis may lose touch with reality and have auditory hallucinations (hearing things that are not actually happening, like a person talking) and delusions (perceiving things differently from the way they are). Visual hallucinations (seeing things that are not there) are less common. Other symptoms may include insomnia, agitation, anger, and irrational guilt about somehow having done something wrong. Women who have postpartum psychosis need prompt evaluation and treatment and almost always need medication. If they are at risk for hurting themselves or someone else, women with postpartum psychosis need to be in a hospital. Postpartum psychosis is very rare, affecting 1 in 3 women/1000 births. Currently, it is thought to be a separate condition from postpartum depression.

Commonly Prescribed (On-Label) Drugs: Bromocriptine, Cabergoline, Chlormezanone, Chlorotrianisene, Clomiphene, Cyclofenil, Diethylstilbestrol, Dinoprostone, Lisuride, Metergoline, Quinagolide

---

OFF-LABEL PRESCRIPTION DRUGS
BREAKTHROUGH OPTION

---

*Generic: **Carbamazepine** (kar-ba-MAZ-e-peen)*
*Brands: **Carbatrol, Epitol, Tegretol, Tegretol XR***

Carbamazepine is an anticonvulsant. It is also used to relieve pain associated with trigeminal neuralgia (tic douloureux) as well as for psychiatric disorders.

Researchers at Prince of Wales Hospital in Australia examined the preventive usefulness of medications in women at risk of postpartum relapse of mental disorders. The postnatal period is a time of increased onset and relapse of mental illness, which poses a clinical dilemma, as many mothers require medication and will also choose to breast-feed.

Researchers reviewed the safety of psychotropes in breast-fed infants and the usefulness of preventive drugs for women at risk of postpartum relapse and, secondly, provided guidelines for the use of psychotropic drugs in breast-feeding women. Both tricyclic antidepressants (TCA) and specific serotonin re-uptake inhibitors (SSRIs) appear to be relatively safe in breast feeding. Antidepressants commenced in the early postpartum period may reduce depressive relapse. However, high-dose antipsychotics should be avoided, as they may be associated with long-term adverse side effects in the infant. Researchers concluded that on the basis of current knowledge, the use of SSRIs, TCA, carbamazepine, sodium valproate, and short-acting benzodiazepines are relatively safe.

For more information see page 1068.

Premature Labor

Premature or pre-term labor is labor that begins more than three weeks before you are expected to deliver your baby (but after the 20th week of pregnancy). Contractions (tightening of the muscles in the uterus) cause the cervix (lower end of the uterus) to open earlier than normal. Pre-term labor may result in the birth of a premature baby. However, labor often can be stopped to allow the baby more time to grow and develop in the uterus.

Commonly Prescribed (On-Label) Drugs: *Bretylium, Moxalactam, Quinestrol, Ritodrine, Tocainide*

OFF-LABEL PRESCRIPTION DRUGS
BREAKTHROUGH OPTIONS

Generic: ***Albuterol*** *(al-BYOO-ter-ole)*
Brands: ***Proventil, Ventolin, Volmax***

Albuterol is used as a bronchodilator for the treatment of asthma and as a uterine relaxant for the suspension of premature labor. A study conducted in Thailand examined the value of oral albuterol for the inhibition of preterm labor by review of medical records. Of 132 pregnancies reviewed, 81.1% were prolonged for more than 24 hours, 59.8% for more than two days, 32.6% for more than one week, and 8.3% for more than four weeks. The pregnancy outcome was significantly better in the group that had a prolongation time of at least 48 hours. The researchers concluded that oral albuterol is another effective method for inhibiting preterm labor and prolonging pregnancy. Because it requires no intensive medical nursing care and observations and no discomfort of an intravenous line, researchers suggest that oral albuterol may be an alternative drug for managing preterm labor.

For more information see page 991.

Generic: **Betamethasone** *(bay-ta-METH-a-sone)*
Brand: **Celestone**

Betamethasone is used principally as an anti-inflammatory treatment. It may also be used to enhance fetal lung maturity in the event of premature labor. The use of drugs to stop uterine contractions can be used for a few days to allow the betamethasone time to enhance lung maturity. A single course of corticosteroid treatment in two doses of 12 mg betamethasone or 6 mg of dexamethasone is important for the prevention of fetal respiratory distress in premature births between the 24th and 34th weeks of pregnancy. Multiple doses may be harmful and should be avoided. In these cases, medical decisions depend on fetal maturity.

For more information see page 1044.

Generic: **Dexamethasone** *(deks-a-METH-a-sone)*
Brands: **Decadron, Dexameth, Dexone, Hexadrol**

Dexamethasone is used principally as an anti-inflammatory or immunosuppressant drug. A review of the medical literature was conducted to determine the effects of corticosteroids administered to pregnant women to accelerate fetal lung maturity prior to preterm delivery. Eighteen trials including data on over 3,700 babies were included. Benefits extended to a broad range of gestational ages and were not limited by sex or race. No adverse consequences of preventive use of corticosteroids for preterm birth were identified. The reviewers concluded the corticosteroids given prior to preterm birth (as a result of either preterm labor or elective preterm delivery) are effective in preventing respiratory distress syndrome and neonatal mortality.

For more information see page 1138.

Generic: **Diltiazem** *(dil-TYE-a-zem)*
Brands: **Cardizem, Cartia XT, Dilacor XR, Diltia XT, Taztia XT, Tiazac**

Diltiazem is a calcium channel blocking drug. The safety and efficacy of maintenance control of contractions with oral diltiazem compared to oral nifedipine in achieving 37 weeks gestation was studied at Stanford University. After successful stoppage of contractions with magnesium sulfate, 69 women with preterm labor at less than 35 weeks gestation received either nifedipine or diltiazem. The primary outcome was the percentage of women achieving 37 weeks gestation. All sixty-nine women were available for final analysis. Fewer patients on diltiazem compared to nifedipine achieved 37 weeks. Gestational age at delivery was also less for women receiving diltiazem. There were fewer days gained in utero from beginning of treatment to delivery with diltiazem as compared to nifedipine; however, this difference was not statistically significant.

Maternal blood pressure and pulse during stoppage of contractions did not differ significantly between groups. Despite the theoretical advantages of diltiazem, maintenance with diltiazem offered no benefit over nifedipine in achieving 37 weeks gestation. The cardiovascular alterations with either drug in pregnant women appear minimal.

For more information see page 1146.

Generic: **Indomethacin** *(in-doe-METH-a-sin)*
Brands: **Indocin, Indocin IV, Indocin SR**

Indomethacin is a nonsteroidal anti-inflammatory drug (NSAID) that also reduces pain and fever. It is a type of tocolytic, meaning that it inhibits uterine contractions that stop labor. Tocolytics decrease the risk of pre-term delivery within seven days. Indomethacin was associated with significant prolongations in pregnancy. Maternal side effects significantly associated with tocolytic use were palpitations, nausea, tremor, chorioamnionitis, hyperglycemia, hypokalemia, and the need to discontinue treatment. The investigators concluded that although tocolytics may prolong pregnancy, they did not improve perinatal or neonatal outcomes in this study and may be risky to the mother.

For more information see page 1238.

Generic: **Isoxsuprine** *(eye-SOKS-syoo-preen)*
Brand: **Vasodilan**

Isoxsuprine widens blood vessels so blood flows better. Twenty pregnant women received 10 mg isoxsuprine hydrochloride orally every eight hours until the uterine contractions were abolished, followed by 10 mg 12 hourly up to 38 weeks of gestation. Successful tocolysis, or stoppage of contractions, was observed in 85% of cases receiving nifedipine in contrast to 40% of women receiving isoxsuprine hydrochloride.

For more information see page 1254.

Generic: *Ketorolac* (KEE-toe-role-ak)
Brand: *Toradol*

Ketorolac is a nonsteroidal anti-inflammatory drug (NSAID) that also reduces pain and fever with proven efficacy and safety. In a trial at the University of Mississippi Medical Center, 88 women in confirmed pre-term labor at less than or equal to 32 weeks' gestation received magnesium sulfate.

The study groups were similar with respect to age, number of prior pregnancies, cervical status, and gestational age on admission. Ketorolac was more rapid in the arrest of pre-term labor than magnesium sulfate. No women discontinued either drug due to adverse effects. There was no difference in the incidence of neonatal complications between the two groups. Researchers concluded that in pregnancies with pre-term labor at less than 32 weeks, ketorolac appears to be appropriate.

For more information see page 1263.

Generic: *Magnesium Sulfate* (mag-NEE-zhum SUL-fate)
Brand: *Magnesium Sulfate*

Magnesium sulfate is commonly used as an anticonvulsant. It has also been used in selected patients to inhibit uterine contractions in pre-term labor (tocolysis) and thus prolong gestation when such prolongation of intrauterine life would be expected to benefit the pregnancy's outcome. Previously, the American College of Obstetricians and Gynecologists (ACOG) considered drugs such as ritodrine (no longer commercially available in the United States), terbutaline, and magnesium sulfate the first-line tocolytic agents of choice. However, current ACOG guidelines for management of pre-term labor state that there is no clearly preferred first-line tocolytic drug because of conflicting results regarding efficacy in trials.

While use of magnesium sulfate may effectively delay delivery for at least 24–48 hours, the principal goal of prolongation of gestation is to reduce the incidence of neonatal death, respiratory distress syndrome, and long-term morbidity and mortality associated with prematurity. There is limited evidence substantiating the efficacy of magnesium sulfate in this regard. The main benefit currently derived from tocolytic therapy appears to be short-term to forestall labor prior to 34 weeks of gestation and prolong gestation (for 2–7 days), thus providing time for patients to receive other drugs such as corticosteroids to increase fetal maturation and/or to be transferred to other facilities. Whether pre-term use of magnesium sulfate also can reduce the risk of certain neuro-developmental defects needs to be more fully examined.

For more information see page 1292.

Generic: **Nicardipine** *(nye-KAR-de-peen)*
Brands: **Cardene, Cardene IV, Cardene SR**

Nicardipine is a calcium channel blocking drug. The efficacy and safety of oral nicardipine for preterm labor has been compared to magnesium sulfate. Women between 24 and 34 weeks' gestation with documented preterm labor received either oral nicardipine or intravenous magnesium sulfate as initial to-colytic therapy to arrest uterine contractions. The main outcome variables examined were time to uterine stillness, time gained in utero, recurrence of preterm labor, failure of tocolysis, and pertinent maternal and neonatal outcomes.

There were no significant differences in maternal demographic characteristics between the groups. Among patients who responded with uterine stillness within six hours, there was a significant decrease in the time to uterine stillness in the nicardipine group. Women in the magnesium sulfate group were more likely to have preterm labor recur. The women in the magnesium sulfate group had more adverse side effects, mainly nausea and vomiting. There were no differences in birth weight, estimated gestational age at delivery, or neonatal complications between the two groups. Investigators concluded that oral nicardipine is an effective, safe, and well-tolerated tocolytic drug.

For more information see page 1358.

Generic: **Nifedipine** *(nye-FED-i-peen)*
Brands: **Adalat CC, Apo-Nifed (PA), Novo-Nifedin, Nu-Nifed, Procardia**

Nifedipine is a calcium channel blocking drug that has been used in selected patients to inhibit uterine contractions in preterm labor (tocolysis) and thus prolong gestation when it was expected to benefit the fetus and birth. While the American College of Obstetricians and Gynecologists (ACOG) and many clinicians previously considered nifedipine a second-line tocolytic drug to be used only when first-line drugs had failed, current ACOG guidelines state that there is no clear first-line tocolytic agent because of conflicting results in trials. However, a recent analysis of data from a number of studies suggests that calcium channel blockers (principally nifedipine) may be more effective than, and preferable to, other drugs such as magnesium sulfate when inhibiting preterm labor is deemed necessary.

Calcium channel blockers are more effective in reducing births within seven days of initiation of tocolytic treatment and before 34 weeks' gestation and are associated with improved neonatal outcomes and a reduced frequency of adverse side effects in the mother that lead to discontinued treatment compared with other tocolytic drugs. Different dosages and dosage forms of nifedipine were used in these studies, and an optimal dosage regimen for the drug as a tocolytic has not been determined.

For more information see page 1360.

Generic: **Sulindac** *(sul-IN-dak)*
Brand: **Clinoril**

Sulindac is a nonsteroidal anti-inflammatory drug (NSAID) that also reduces pain and fever. A study to determine whether nimesulide causes fewer fetal side effects than indomethacin or sulindac was undertaken after short-term attempts to stop contractions (tocolysis). The study had three drug treatment groups comprised of women who were at 28 to 32 weeks of gestation with preterm contractions. The women were treated in the delivery suites of two busy inner-city teaching hospitals; the intervention consisted of 48 hours of treatment and with 72 hours of follow-up observation with indomethacin, sulindac, or nimesulide. There were no significant differences among drugs for any of these effects. The investigators concluded that nimesulide causes similar short-term fetal side effects to indomethacin and sulindac.

For more information see page 1486.

Generic: **Terbutaline** *(ter-BYOO-ta-leen)*
Brand: **Brethine**

Terbutaline relaxes the smooth muscle in the lungs and dilates airways to improve breathing. It is used in the treatment of asthma, chronic bronchitis, or emphysema.

Acute fetal distress is usually diagnosed by characteristic features in the fetal heart rate pattern. Intrauterine resuscitation consists of increasing oxygen delivery to the placenta and umbilical blood flow, in order to reverse hypoxia and acidosis. These measures include inhibition of uterine contractions usually with subcutaneous or intravenous terbutaline.

In a study to determine the impact of terbutaline versus magnesium sulfate in the treatment of fetal distress prior to cesarean delivery forty-six women received either subcutaneous (under the skin administration) terbutaline or intravenous magnesium sulfate for in-utero fetal resuscitation before cesarean delivery. There were no significant differences between groups in arterial pressure, arterial pressure before and after induction of anesthesia, maternal heart rate, maternal oxygen saturation, estimated blood loss, and pre- and postoperative hematocrits (red blood cell measure).

For more information see page 1499.

Puerperal Psychosis

See Postpartum Psychosis and Lactation

SEXUAL DISORDERS

Dyspareunia

Pain during or after sexual intercourse is known as dyspareunia. Although this problem can affect men, it is more common in women. Women with dyspareunia may have pain in the vagina, clitoris, or labia. There are numerous causes of dyspareunia, many of which are treatable. Women with dyspareunia may feel superficial pain at the entrance of the vagina, or deeper pain during penetration or thrusting of the penis. Some women also may experience severe tightening of the vaginal muscles during penetration, a condition called vaginismus. A common type of dyspareunia is female sexual arousal disorder, which is a condition described as a woman's inability to complete sexual activity due to inadequate lubrication.

Commonly Prescribed (On-Label) Drugs: *Goserelin, Histrelin, Nafarelin, Tamoxifen*

OFF-LABEL PRESCRIPTION DRUGS
BREAKTHROUGH OPTIONS

Generic: **Alprostadil** *(al-PROS-ta-dill)*
Brands: **Caverject, Caverject Impulse, Edex, Muse**

Alprostadil is a vasodilating drug that increases blood flow by expanding blood vessels. A report in *Journal of Sex & Marital Therapy* discussed the efficacy and safety of three doses of alprostadil cream in a study of 94 women who had female sexual arousal disorder of at least six month's duration. The women applied different, 10 premeasured doses of alprostadil or a placebo cream to the vulvar area prior to vaginal intercourse over a period of six weeks.

The primary measure, the arousal success rate, was highest in the highest alprostadil dose group and lowest in the lowest-dose group, but the responses were not different from that of the placebo cream, for any of the three doses. However, satisfaction with arousal during sexual activity improved. Adverse side effects were generally mild or moderate in intensity and mainly involved localized reactions in the genital area.

For more information see page 998.

Generic: **Phentolamine** *(fen-TOLE-a-meen)*
Brands: **Regitine, Rogitine**

Phentolamine is a drug known as an adrenergic blocking agent. Female sexual arousal disorder is a highly prevalent problem, although little is known about pathophysiology or treatment of the disorder. Given the potential role of blood vessels and circulation, a study was conducted on the effects of oral phentolamine in menopausal women with female sexual arousal disorder. Six postmenopausal women with a lack of lubrication and with sexual arousal difficulties of at least six months' duration participated. All received a single dose of oral phentolamine and placebo. Results indicated a mild, positive effect of phentolamine across all measures of arousal, with significant changes in self-reported lubrication and pleasurable sensations in the vagina. The drug was well tolerated, overall, with few reports of adverse side effects.

For more information see page 1411.

Generic: **Sildenafil** *(sil-DEN-a-fil)*
Brand: **Viagra**

Sildenafil increases blood flow to the penis for male sexual dysfunction. But sexual dysfunction also affects 30–50% of American women. Aside from hormone replacement therapy, there are no current FDA-approved medical treatments for female sexual disorders.

A study was conducted at Boston Medical Center to determine safety and efficacy of sildenafil for use in women with sexual arousal disorder. Evaluations were completed on 48 women with complaints of sexual arousal disorder. Physiologic measurements, including genital blood flow, vaginal lubrication, intravaginal pressure-volume changes and genital sensation were recorded pre- and post-sexual stimulation at the start of the study and following sildenafil.

At the end of the study the women also completed a report on the drug's effectiveness. Following sildenafil, physiologic measurements improved significantly. Low arousal, low desire, low sexual satisfaction, difficulty achieving orgasm, decreased vaginal lubrication and dyspareunia also improved following six weeks of sildenafil. Sildenafil appears to significantly improve both subjective and physiologic parameters of the female sexual response. Studies are currently in progress to further determine efficacy of this medication for treatment of female sexual dysfunction in different populations of women.

For more information see page 1472.

Female Orgasmic Disorder, Secondary to SSRI Use

Female orgasmic disorder, secondary to selective serotonin reuptake inhibitor (SSRI) use is a persistent or recurrent difficulty. It means delay in orgasm, or absence of orgasm following sufficient sexual stimulation and arousal, as a result of treatment with SSRI medication.

Commonly Prescribed (On-Label) Drugs: None

OFF-LABEL PRESCRIPTION DRUGS
BREAKTHROUGH OPTIONS

*Generic: **Bupropion** (byoo-PROE-pee-on)*
*Brands: **Wellbutrin, Wellbutrin SR, Wellbutrin XL, Zyban***

Bupropion is an antidepressant. A study at the University of Virginia compared the use of bupropion sustained release (SR) as a treatment for sexual dysfunction versus placebo in 42 patients with selective serotonin reuptake inhibitor (SSRI)-induced sexual dysfunction. An analysis of the association of testosterone and sexual functioning in the participants was also performed. Patients with major depression who experienced a therapeutic response to any SSRI and were experiencing medication-induced sexual dysfunction received either bupropion SR or placebo for four weeks, in addition to the SSRI.

There was a significant difference between the two groups at week four in desire as measured by self-report of feelings of desire and frequency of sexual activity. Desire/frequency showed a significantly greater improvement among those receiving bupropion SR compared with placebo. The investigators concluded that bupropion SR, as an effective antidote to SSRI-induced sexual dysfunction, produced an increase in desire to engage in sexual activity and frequency of engaging in sexual activity compared with placebo. However, researchers concluded that a larger study is needed to further investigate this finding.

For more information see page 1058.

Generic: **Sildenafil** *(sil-DEN-a-fil)*
Brand: **Viagra**

Sildenafil is used to treat male sexual function problems (impotence or erectile dysfunction) by blocking a certain enzyme in the body. Researchers reviewed the medical literature describing female orgasmic disorder and impaired sexual desire disorder (SSRIs) and their treatment, including the use of sildenafil. In addition, a sample case of a 38-year old woman who suffered from fluoxetine-induced arousal and orgasmic disturbance was included. Researchers concluded that in some case reports, sildenafil has been shown to be beneficial in reversing female sexual dysfunction induced by SSRIs.

For more information see page 1472.

Hypoactive Sexual Desire Disorder

Hypoactive sexual desire disorder is a lack of sexual desire that causes a woman personal distress. This includes a persistent or recurring deficiency or absence of sexual fantasies or thoughts, or a lack of interest in sex or being sexual. Often women suffering with this complaint will report they feel "flat" sexually or sexually "dead." This disorder occurs in approximately 20% of the population and occurs in both sexes, though more commonly in women.

Commonly Prescribed (On-Label) Drugs: *Alprostadil, Sildenafil*

OFF-LABEL PRESCRIPTION DRUGS
BREAKTHROUGH OPTIONS

*Generic: **Apomorphine** (a-poe-MOR-feen)*
*Brand: **Apokyn***

A study was conducted in Italy to verify whether apomorphine SL is effective in premenopausal women affected by hypoactive sexual desire disorder. Sixty-two women, aged 26 to 45 years, affected by arousal disorders and hypoactive sexual desire disorder participated in the study, which consisted of two parts. The first was four weeks of a taken-as-needed regimen of apomorphine SL. The second part of the study was for the nonresponders, who received treatment in one of six possible sequences of three study periods with apomorphine at different dosages, washout, and placebo.

Efficacy was assessed with a questionnaire. The questionnaire measured arousal, desire, orgasm, enjoyment, and frequency of sexual relationships. Fifty women completed the four-week drug regimen, and six of them benefited from this treatment regimen. The 44 women who reported no change with respect to baseline participated in the second part of the study.

The daily intake of the drug was effective with both dosages compared with placebo for arousal and desire. The effects of the larger dose of apomorphine were better than those obtained with the lower dose. The orgasm, enjoyment, and "satisfied by frequency" scores improved during treatment with daily apomorphine compared with baseline and placebo. The investigators concluded that daily apomorphine SL may improve the sexual life of women with sexual difficulties.

For more information see page 1022.

*Generic: **Bupropion** (byoo-PROE-pee-on)*
*Brands: **Wellbutrin, Wellbutrin SR, Wellbutrin XL, Zyban***

Bupropion is an antidepressant. A report describes the results of the first evaluation of bupropion sustained release (SR) in nondepressed females with hypoactive sexual desire disorder. Women entered a four-week trial. None responded to placebo, but continued in an active treatment phase where they received bupropion SR for up to eight additional weeks. Researchers at Case Western

Reserve University assessed hypoactive sexual desire disorder by rating sexual desire and sexual functioning. Of the 51 women who entered the active treatment phase, 29% responded to treatment with bupropion SR, which was generally well tolerated. Pending the results of further study, researchers concluded that bupropion SR may offer a treatment option.

Additionally, efficacy, tolerability, and effects on sexual functioning of bupropion SR and the selective serotonin reuptake inhibitor (SSRI) fluoxetine were compared. In a study, patients with recurrent major depression were treated with bupropion SR, fluoxetine, or placebo for up to 8 weeks. Depression and sexual-functioning status were assessed at weekly clinic visits; tolerability was assessed primarily by monitoring adverse side effects. The investigators concluded that bupropion SR and fluoxetine were similarly effective and well tolerated in the treatment of depression. Fluoxetine, however, was more frequently associated with sexual dysfunction compared with bupropion SR. Bupropion SR may be an appropriate initial choice for the treatment of depression if you are concerned about sexual functioning.

For more information see page 1058.

Generic: *Phentolamine* (fen-TOLE-a-meen)
Brands: *Regitine, Rogitine*

Researchers in Mexico assessed the potential of phentolamine as a treatment of postmenopausal women with female arousal disorder. The study consisted of forty-one women who received one of four treatments: low-dose and higher-dose vaginal solutions, an oral tablet of phentolamine, and placebo. Researchers found that in women who received placebo versus women who received hormone replacement therapy (HRT) with higher-dose phentolamine in vaginal solution had significantly different readings. Subjective reports also were significantly different from placebo with the vaginal solution 40 mg and the oral tablet of 40 mg of phentolamine among hormone replacement users. However, researchers found no significant differences between women not receiving HRT. The investigators concluded that results indicate that phentolamine may show promise as treatment for female sexual arousal disorder in estrogenized postmenopausal women.

For more information see page 1411.

Generic: **Testosterone** *(tes-TOS-ter-one)*
Brands: **Androderm, AndroGel, Delatestryl, Depo-Testosterone, Striant, Testim, Testoderm, Testoderm with Adhesive, Testopel**

Testosterone is a naturally occurring androgen, commonly referred to as the male hormone. Androgens also play an important role in healthy female sexual function, especially in stimulating sexual interest and in maintaining desire. Female sexual dysfunction is a complex problem, and women can have low androgen levels for many reasons including age, ovary removal, and the use of oral estrogens.

A review of clinical trials by researchers at Cedars-Sinai Medical Center found that most clinical trials in postmenopausal women with loss of libido have demonstrated that the addition of testosterone to estrogen significantly improved multiple facets of sexual functioning including libido and sexual desire, arousal, frequency and satisfaction. In clinical trials of up to two years' duration of testosterone therapy, women tolerated it well and demonstrated no serious side effects. The results of these trials suggest that testosterone therapy in low doses is effective for the treatment of women's sexual interest and desire disorder in postmenopausal women who do not have estrogen deficiency.

For more information see page 1502.

PART II

DRUG PROFILES

GUIDE TO PRESCRIPTION DRUG INFORMATION

Using This Guide

This guide is meant to be a quick reference only and is not intended to substitute for your doctor or pharmacist's instructions. In general, it covers only the most pertinent details on drugs described in Part I of this book. The side effects listed are the most common ones and are not necessarily all-inclusive, so if you experience unusual or bothersome symptoms that are not listed here, call your doctor for advice. Important: Most medications are not recommended for children. Consult your doctor if you have any questions on medication for your child or for yourself.

Pregnancy Risk Categories

While it is best to avoid drugs during pregnancy unless medically necessary, some medications can be more harmful to a developing fetus than others. The FDA assigns a Pregnancy Risk Category to each drug based on its potential to cause birth defects. The categories are determined using available clinical and pre-clinical information. Following are brief explanations of the categories:

A   Adequate studies in pregnant women have not demonstrated a risk to the fetus.

B   Animal studies have not demonstrated a risk to the fetus, but there are no adequate studies in pregnant women; or animal studies have shown an adverse effect, but adequate studies in pregnant women have not demonstrated a risk to the fetus.

C   Animal studies have shown an adverse effect on the fetus, but there are no adequate studies in humans; or there are no animal reproduction studies and no adequate studies in humans. Drugs should be taken only if benefits justify potential risks to the fetus.

D   There is evidence of human fetal risk, but the potential benefits from the use in pregnant women may be acceptable despite its potential risks.

X   Studies in animals or humans demonstrate fetal abnormalities or adverse reaction; reports indicated evidence of fetal risk. The risk of use in a pregnant woman clearly outweighs any possible benefit.

NR   Not rated.

5-FLUOROURACIL
(flure-oh-YOOR-a-sil)

Injectable

NEWLY DISCOVERED USES (OFF-LABEL)
Warts, non-genital

ORIGINAL USES (ON-LABEL)
To treat various cancers, including breast, colon, head and neck, pancreas, rectum, or stomach

BRAND NAME
Adrucil

DRUG CLASS
Antineoplastic

DESCRIPTION
5-Fluorouracil is used to treat cancers by interfering with the production of DNA and inhibiting an enzyme that is incorporated into RNA.

POTENTIAL SIDE EFFECTS
Mouth ulcers, diarrhea, changes in blood parameters such as decreased white blood cells, decreased red blood cells and platelets, chest pain, hair loss, skin reactions, rash, skin pigmentation, anorexia, nausea, vomiting, gastric ulcers, increased tearing, vision changes, fever.

CAUTIONS
- Notify your doctor if you have impaired kidney or liver function or if you recently received high-dose pelvic radiation.
- Immediately contact your doctor if you develop vomiting or diarrhea, mouth ulcers, numbness in the hands or feet, or chest pain.
- May require combination therapy with pyridoxine (Vitamin B-6).
- Contraceptive measures are recommended for both men and women during therapy.

DRUG INTERACTIONS
Rotavirus Vaccine, Live (established), warfarin. Consult your doctor prior to immunizations or vaccinations, or starting any other medications.

FOOD INTERACTIONS
Unknown

HERBAL INTERACTIONS
Avoid black cohosh, dong quai in estrogen-dependent tumors.

PREGNANCY AND BREAST-FEEDING CAUTIONS
FDA Pregnancy Risk Category D. Excretion into breast milk unknown. Breast-feeding is not recommended during therapy with this drug.

SPECIAL INFORMATION
Blood monitoring is required during therapy to assess for complications.

ACARBOSE
(AY-car-bose)

NEWLY DISCOVERED USES (OFF-LABEL)
Prevention of type 2 diabetes

ORIGINAL USES (ON-LABEL)
Diabetes Mellitus Type 2

BRAND NAME
Precose

DRUG CLASS
Anti-diabetic (alpha-glucosidase inhibitor)

DESCRIPTION
This drug delays the breakdown of ingested complex carbohydrates and the absorption of glucose (sugar). Also inhibits the conversion of sugar to other forms.

POTENTIAL SIDE EFFECTS
Abdominal pain, diarrhea, flatulence, increases in tests used to monitor for liver function.

CAUTIONS
- Not for use in severe liver disease (cirrhosis), inflammatory bowel disease, ulcerations of the colon, intestinal obstruction, or diseases where there is marked problems in digestion or absorption.
- Not for use if kidney function is reduced.

- Requires periodic blood glucose (sugar) monitoring.
- Acarbose may increase the risk of developing low blood glucose levels when taken with other diabetic drugs.

DRUG INTERACTIONS
Digoxin, digestive enzymes (pancreatic enzymes), charcoal

FOOD INTERACTIONS
Unknown

HERBAL INTERACTIONS
Guar gum, psyllium, bitter melon, St. John's wort, ginseng, eucalyptus, gymnema sylvestre, licorice, thioctic acid, glucosamine

PREGNANCY AND BREAST-FEEDING CAUTIONS
FDA Pregnancy Risk Category B. Excretion in breast milk unknown. Consult with your doctor.

SPECIAL INFORMATION
You should take this medication with the first bite of each main meal. Continue dietary instructions, a regular exercise program, and regular testing of urine and/or blood glucose. Stomach side effects tend to improve in frequency and intensity with continued therapy.

ACEBUTOLOL
(a-se-BYOO-toe-lole)

NEWLY DISCOVERED USES (OFF-LABEL)
Myocardial infarction post-incident, stable angina.

ORIGINAL USES (ON-LABEL)
Abnormal heart rhythm (ventricular arrhythmias), angina, high blood pressure

BRAND NAME
Sectral

DRUG CLASS
Antiarrhythmic, antihypertensive (beta-blocker)

DESCRIPTION
This drug blocks a type of cell membrane, called beta-adrenergic receptors, in the heart to stabilize heart rate and reduce blood pressure.

POTENTIAL SIDE EFFECTS

Fatigue, headache, dizziness, insomnia, depression, chest pain, edema (swelling related to fluid retention), abnormal dreams, rash, constipation, diarrhea, upset stomach, nausea, muscle aches, impotence, abnormal vision, shortness of breath.

CAUTIONS

- Do not use if you have a certain type of heart condition, such as congestive heart failure, cardiogenic shock, too low heart rate, or second- and third-degree heart block, sinus node dysfunction. Also, do not use during pregnancy.
- Do not stop this medication suddenly; instead, taper over a gradual period.
- May result in an exaggerated response such as increased heart rate, increased blood pressure, or chest pain. Consult with your doctor about possible effects on the heart.
- May cause or mask the symptoms of low blood glucose levels in diabetics.
- Notify your doctor if you have lung disease or problems with kidney function.
- Avoid this type of drug if you have congestive heart failure.

DRUG INTERACTIONS

Clonidine, reserpine, disopyramide, theophylline, aluminum salts, barbiturates, calcium salts, cholestyramine, colestipol, non-steroidal anti-inflammatory drugs (e.g., indomethacin, etc.), penicillins, rifampin, haloperidol, ergot alkaloids, prazosin, salicylates, some sulfonylureas

FOOD INTERACTIONS

Unknown

HERBAL INTERACTIONS

Dong quai, yohimbe, ginseng

PREGNANCY AND BREAST-FEEDING CAUTIONS

FDA Pregnancy Risk Category B (manufacturer), Category D (2nd and 3rd trimesters). Excreted in breast milk, consult your doctor prior to use.

SPECIAL INFORMATION

Notify your doctor of any chest pain, sensations of unusual heart rate, unresolved swelling of extremities, unusual weight gain, breathing difficulty, new cough, skin rash, unresolved fatigue, unresolved constipation or diarrhea, unusual muscle weakness.

ACETAZOLAMIDE
(a-set-a-ZOLE-a-mide)

NEWLY DISCOVERED USES (OFF-LABEL)
Ménière's disease

ORIGINAL USES (ON-LABEL)
Glaucoma (chronic simple open-angle, secondary glaucoma, pre-operatively in acute angle-closure), drug-induced edema (swelling related to fluid retention) or edema due to congestive heart failure, some types of seizures (immediate release dosage form), prevention or amelioration of symptoms associated with acute mountain sickness.

BRAND NAMES
Diamox, Diamox Sequels

DRUG CLASS
Anticonvulsant, diuretic (carbonic anhydrase inhibitor)

DESCRIPTION
This drug inhibits the activity of a certain enzyme in the central nervous system, which slows abnormal and excessive discharge from central nervous system neurons. This action also results in a decreased pressure.

POTENTIAL SIDE EFFECTS
Flushing, incoordination of muscles, confusion, depression, allergic skin reaction, photosensitivity (skin reaction related to sun exposure), electrolyte imbalance, increased blood or urine glucose, appetite decreased, diarrhea, nausea, frequent urination, blood disorders, liver disorders, numbness, hearing disturbance, ringing in the ears.

CAUTIONS
- Notify your doctor if you have an allergy to sulfonamides (antibacterials or diuretics) prior to therapy with this drug, as this drug should not be taken in patients with sulfonamide allergies.
- Not for use in liver disease or insufficiency (may result in coma), with decreased sodium and or potassium levels, adrenal gland insufficiency, severe kidney disease or dysfunction, severe lung obstruction.
- Not for long-term use if you have noncongestive angle-closure glaucoma.

- Requires blood monitoring during therapy to screen for blood disorders.
- Use with caution if you are diabetic.
- Impaired mental alertness and/or physical coordination may occur.

DRUG INTERACTIONS
Diflunisal, cyclosporine, salicylates, lithium, amphetamines, quinidine, primidone

FOOD INTERACTIONS
Unknown

HERBAL INTERACTIONS
Unknown

PREGNANCY AND BREAST-FEEDING CAUTIONS
FDA Pregnancy Risk Category C. Excreted in breast milk; breast-feeding not recommended during therapy.

SPECIAL INFORMATION
If you experience stomach upset when using this drug, take with food. Capsules may be opened and sprinkled over soft food. Avoid prolonged exposure to sunlight, and wear sunscreen during therapy. This drug may cause drowsiness, so use caution while performing tasks that require alertness. Notify your doctor if you develop a sore throat, fever, unusual bruising or tingling in the hands and feet during therapy.

ACETYLCYSTEINE
(a-se-teel-SIS-teen)

NEWLY DISCOVERED USES (OFF-LABEL)
Blepharitis, keratoconjunctivitis sicca (dry eye), prevention of nephrotoxicity due to contrast media in coronary procedures and CT scan

ORIGINAL USES (ON-LABEL)
Mucolytic therapy in patients with abnormal or viscous mucous secretions in acute and chronic lung disease, in lung complications related to surgery and in cystic fibrosis. Also used in diagnostic bronchial studies and as antidote for acute acetaminophen toxicity.

BRAND NAMES
Acetadote, Mucomyst

DRUG CLASS
Antidote, mucolytic (reduce secretion thickness)

DESCRIPTION
Acetylcysteine is used to reduce the degree of organ damage by lowering mucus viscosity.

POTENTIAL SIDE EFFECTS
Antidote use (large doses): nausea, vomiting, rash, itching, increased heart rate, low or high blood pressure.

Other uses: mouth ulcers, nausea, vomiting, fever, drowsiness, tightness in chest, increased heart rate.

CAUTIONS
- Use may result in an increased volume of liquefied lung secretions, which may require mechanical suction or the use of an drug that prevents constriction in the lung.
- When used as an antidote, hives have occurred rarely, indicating a possible allergic reaction. Stop medication immediately if this occurs.
- Administration of this drug may result in a temporary body odor.

DRUG INTERACTIONS
Activated charcoal

FOOD INTERACTIONS
Unknown

HERBAL INTERACTIONS
Unknown

PREGNANCY AND BREAST-FEEDING CAUTIONS
FDA Pregnancy Risk Category B. Use caution in breast-feeding, as it is unknown if this drug is excreted in breast milk.

SPECIAL INFORMATION
When used to treat acetaminophen overdose, you may dilute the 5% solution of this drug in cola, orange juice, or other soft drink.

ACITRETIN
(a-si-TRE-tin)

NEWLY DISCOVERED USES (OFF-LABEL)
Dermatitis (chronic actinic)

ORIGINAL USES (ON-LABEL)
Treatment of severe psoriasis

BRAND NAMES
Soriatane

DRUG CLASS
Retinoid-like compound (vitamin A derivative)

DESCRIPTION
The mechanism of action in psoriasis is unclear.

POTENTIAL SIDE EFFECTS
Night blindness, shaking, headache, pain, hair loss, skin peeling, dry skin, nail disorder, itching, numbness, cold/clammy skin, increased sweating, skin ulcers, sunburn, abnormal vision, eye irritation, abdominal pain, diarrhea, nausea, dry mouth, nosebleeds, gum bleeding or inflammation, mouth ulcers, joint aches, arthritis, back pain, muscle aches, and depression.

CAUTIONS
- You could become pregnant for at least 3 years after discontinuation of medication. An informed consent form must be signed prior to the initiation of therapy.
- Abstain from alcohol or alcohol containing products during therapy and for 2 months after discontinuation.
- Do not donate blood during or after 3 years following completion of therapy.
- Requires monitoring of lipids and liver function before and during therapy.
- Inform your doctor if decreased night vision or decreased tolerance to contact lenses develops. Also notify your doctor if you develop aggressive feelings or thoughts of self-harm.
- Inform your doctor if you have kidney or liver function.

DRUG INTERACTIONS
Vitamin A, oral retinoids, methotrexate, tetracycline, etretinate, sulfonylureas, oral contraceptives, phenytoin, and progestin "mini-pill"

FOOD INTERACTIONS
Do not drink alcohol during therapy.

HERBAL INTERACTIONS
Unknown

PREGNANCY AND BREAST-FEEDING CAUTIONS
FDA Pregnancy Risk Category X. Excreted in the breast milk. Do not breast-feed during therapy.

SPECIAL INFORMATION
This drug has a black box warning regarding contraindications of use during pregnancy. A pregnancy test is required within one week prior to therapy. Discuss risks of fetal defects and pregnancy during therapy.

Worsening of psoriasis may occur during initial therapy. The full benefits of therapy may not be observed for 2 to 3 months in the treatment of psoriasis. Wear sunscreen and protective clothing to avoid photosensitivity reaction. Read the Medication Guide prior to the initiation of therapy.

ACYCLOVIR
(ay-SYE-kloe-veer)

NEWLY DISCOVERED USES (OFF-LABEL)

Complicated mononucleosis/Epstein-Barr, outer retinal necrosis

ORIGINAL USES (ON-LABEL)
Treatment and prevention of mucosal and skin herpes simplex infections. Treats herpes simplex encephalitis, herpes zoster, genital herpes, varicella-zoster infections in healthy non-pregnant persons older than 13 years of age, and children older than 12 months old who have a chronic skin or lung disorder or are receiving long-term aspirin therapy and are immunocompromised.

BRAND NAME
Zovirax

DRUG CLASS
Antiviral

DESCRIPTION
This drug inhibits viral reproduction by interfering with the production of DNA in the virus.

POTENTIAL SIDE EFFECTS
Lightheadedness, headache, nausea/vomiting, stomach pain, diarrhea, malaise, mild pain/burning (topical).

CAUTIONS
- Use with caution if pre-existing kidney disease is present or if the drug is taken with other drugs, which can potentially harm the kidneys.
- This drug is not a cure for genital herpes and it is not known if this drug could prevent transfer of the virus. Avoid contact with lesions.
- Begin therapy within 72 hours of onset of symptoms for shingles (herpes zoster). Treatment is most effective when started within 48 hours after onset of rash.
- Severe kidney failure has occurred with this drug.
- Photosensitivity (skin reaction related to sun exposure) has occurred with this drug. Wear sunscreen and wear protective clothing to minimize exposure to sunlight.

DRUG INTERACTIONS
Zidovudine, probenecid, valproic acid, phenytoin, theophylline

FOOD INTERACTIONS
Unknown

HERBAL INTERACTIONS
Unknown

PREGNANCY AND BREAST-FEEDING CAUTIONS
FDA Pregnancy Risk Category B. Breast-feeding is compatible with this drug.

SPECIAL INFORMATION
Avoid sexual intercourse when visible lesions are present. Do not exceed recommended dosage. This drug may cause photosensitivity reaction (skin reaction related to sun exposure). Avoid prolonged exposure to sunlight and wear sunscreen during therapy. When using ointment, apply using a finger cot or glove.

ALBUTEROL
(al-BYOO-ter-ole)

NEWLY DISCOVERED USES (OFF-LABEL)
Bronchopulmonary dysplasia (in infants), muscular dystrophy, premature labor (preterm)

ORIGINAL USES (ON-LABEL)
Asthma, chronic obstructive pulmonary disease (COPD), exercise-induced bronchospasms

BRAND NAMES
Proventil, Ventolin, Volmax

DRUG CLASS
Bronchodilator (beta2-adrenergic agonist)

DESCRIPTION
This drug relaxes smooth muscle by acting on beta-2 receptors found in the lungs to prevent constriction, enabling easier breathing with little effect on heart rate.

POTENTIAL SIDE EFFECTS
Chest pain (angina), irregular heart rhythm (atrial fibrillation), flushing, dizziness, low potassium levels, headache, lightheadedness, rash, serum blood levels increased, dry mouth, unusual taste, muscle cramps/weakness, cough.

CAUTIONS
- Contact your doctor if initial symptoms do not improve upon treatment with this drug. Do not exceed the dose recommended by your doctor.
- Notify you doctor if you have cardiac disease, diabetes, glaucoma, or low potassium levels.

DRUG INTERACTIONS
Ipratropium, MAO inhibitors, tricyclic antidepressants, inhaled anesthetics, propranolol

FOOD INTERACTIONS
Limit caffeine intake.

HERBAL INTERACTIONS
Ephedra, ma huang, yohimbe

PREGNANCY AND BREAST-FEEDING CAUTIONS
FDA Pregnancy Risk Category C. It is not known if this drug is excreted in breast milk. Consult with your doctor prior to use during breast-feeding.

SPECIAL INFORMATION
Read the enclosed patient brochure that accompanies your prescription. Shake metered dose inhaler well before use and to prime prior to first use and whenever inhaler has not been used in the previous two weeks. Prime the inhaler by releasing four sprays into the air away from your face. Oral forms should be administered with water one hour before or two hours after a meal.

Metered dose inhalers are under pressure. Do not puncture or store near open heat or flame. Storage in temperatures greater than 120° F may result in bursting. If you detect an unusual taste or smell, contact your pharmacist.

ALEMTUZUMAB
(ay-lem-TU-zoo-mab)

NEWLY DISCOVERED USES (OFF-LABEL)
Multiple sclerosis

ORIGINAL USES (ON-LABEL)
B-cell chronic lymphocytic leukemia

BRAND NAME
Campath

DRUG CLASS
Antineoplastic (monoclonal antibody)

DESCRIPTION
This drug binds to the surface of the leukemic (cancerous site) cell and stimulates a breakdown of the cell.

POTENTIAL SIDE EFFECTS
Low or high blood pressure, swelling in legs or ankles, increased heart rate, fever, fatigue, headache, hives, rash, nausea, vomiting, anorexia, diarrhea, itching, various blood abnormalities (decrease in the number of white blood and red blood cells, anemia), shaking, skeletal muscle pain, weakness, shortness of breath, cough,

bronchitis, infection, chest pain, insomnia, malaise, depression, constipation

CAUTIONS

- Because this drug may suppress the immune system, the risk of serious infections is increased. Preventive therapy to prevent certain bacterial and viral infections is recommended if you decide to take this drug.
- Infusion site reactions may occur, including sudden low blood pressure, shaking, fever, shortness of breath, chills or rash. To prevent or reduce the risk of such reactions, an antihistamine or acetaminophen should be taken prior to dosing.
- Therapy should be stopped during serious infection, serious blood disorders, or other serious toxicity until the problem resolves.
- Live viral vaccines should not be taken during or recently after treatment.
- Effective contraceptive methods must be used during and six months following treatment.
- Do not use this drug if you have an infection.

DRUG INTERACTIONS
Live virus vaccines

FOOD INTERACTIONS
Unknown

HERBAL INTERACTIONS
Unknown

PREGNANCY AND BREAST-FEEDING CAUTIONS
FDA Pregnancy Risk Category C. It is not known if this drug is excreted in the breast milk. Stop breast-feeding during therapy and for at least three months after the last dose is given.

SPECIAL INFORMATION
A black box warning for this drug will alert you to the possibility of severe infusion reactions and serious abnormalities in the blood as a result of therapy. In addition, information regarding serious infections is discussed.

ALENDRONATE
(a-LEN-droe-nate)

NEWLY DISCOVERED USES (OFF-LABEL)
Bone loss reduction in spinal cord injury

ORIGINAL USES (ON-LABEL)
Osteoporosis in postmenopausal females, osteoporosis in males, osteoporosis caused by steroid drugs in males and females with low bone mineral density who are receiving a daily dosage of prednisone, Paget's disease

BRAND NAME
Fosamax

DRUG CLASS
Bisphosphonate derivative

DESCRIPTION
This drug reduces bone breakdown via actions on osteoblasts (cells that produce protein in the bone), which indirectly increases bone mineral density.

POTENTIAL SIDE EFFECTS
Low levels of calcium and phosphate, abdominal pain, gastric acid reflux, headache, stomach upset, nausea and flatulence.

CAUTIONS
- Do not use this drug if you have low levels of calcium.
- Do not use this drug if you have abnormalities of the esophagus which delay esophageal emptying.
- Do not use this drug if you are unable to sit upright or stand for at least 30 minutes.
- Do not use this drug if you have decreased kidney function.
- Low levels of calcium must be corrected before therapy is started; ensure that you have adequate calcium and vitamin D intake.
- This drug is irritating to the gastric tissue and should be used with caution if you have swallowing difficulties, esophageal disease, gastritis, or ulcers.

DRUG INTERACTIONS
Ranitidine (intravenous), aspirin-containing products. All oral medications may interfere with the absorption of this drug. Wait at least 30 minutes after taking alendronate before taking any oral medications.

FOOD INTERACTIONS
All foods and beverages interfere with the absorption of this drug.
Do not eat or drink anything but water within 30 minutes of taking this medication; if you fail to follow these directions, it can decrease your body's absorption of the drug up to 60%.

HERBAL INTERACTIONS
Unknown, except as stated above with absorption problems.

PREGNANCY AND BREAST-FEEDING CAUTIONS
FDA Pregnancy Risk Category C. Excretion into breast milk is unknown; use with caution in breast-feeding.

SPECIAL INFORMATION
Take this medication first thing in *the morning* with a full glass of plain water, at least 30 minutes before your first intake of food, beverage, or medication of the day. Do not take at night. Do not suck or chew the tablet. You should remain standing or sitting for at least 30 minutes and until first meal of the day to prevent esophageal erosion. Contact your doctor if you develop difficulty swallowing, pain on swallowing, chest pain, or new or worsening heartburn. You may need to take supplemental vitamin D and calcium while taking this medication.

ALLOPURINOL
(al-oh-PURE-i-nole)

NEWLY DISCOVERED USES (OFF-LABEL)
Prevention of mucositis/stomatitis induced by cancer treatment

ORIGINAL USES (ON-LABEL)
Hyperuricemia (gout), renal stone formation

BRAND NAMES
Aloprim, Zyloprim

DRUG CLASS
Anti-gout (xanthine oxidase inhibitor)

DESCRIPTION
This drug inhibits the activity of the enzyme responsible for the conversion of uric acid. Uric acid is responsible for accumulating in joints, creating inflammation and damage in gout.

POTENTIAL SIDE EFFECTS

Skin rash, headache, diarrhea, change in taste sensation, abdominal pain, numbness, upset stomach, Stevens-Johnson syndrome, nausea, drowsiness, various blood disorders.

CAUTIONS

- You should not use this drug to treat asymptomatic gout.
- A dosage adjustment will be required if you have reduced kidney function.
- Discontinue use of this drug at first sign of rash or allergic reaction.
- Use of this drug requires periodic monitoring during therapy (kidney and liver function).
- You should drink sufficient fluid to promote sufficient urine output to avoid problems. Drink greater than 10 to 12 glasses of fluid daily.
- Risk of rash may be increased if you are receiving ampicillin or amoxicillin.
- The risk of allergic reactions may be increased if you are taking thiazide diuretics.
- An increased risk of bone marrow suppression may occur when taken with myelosuppressive (suppress bone marrow function) drugs.

DRUG INTERACTIONS

Azathioprine, chlopropamide, mercaptopurine, theophylline, and oral anticoagulants, amoxicillin, ampicillin, ACE inhibitors, and thiazide diuretics. Iron supplements and vitamin C may increase kidney stone formation.

FOOD INTERACTIONS

Alcohol. This drug is better tolerated if taken with food or milk.

HERBAL INTERACTIONS

Unknown

PREGNANCY AND BREAST-FEEDING CAUTIONS

FDA Pregnancy Risk Category C. Excreted in breast milk. The American Academy of Pediatrics considers this drug compatible with breast-feeding. Consult your doctor if you have questions.

SPECIAL INFORMATION

Take this medication after meals with plenty of fluids. Notify your doctor if skin rash, painful urination, blood in the urine, swelling of the eyes, lips, or mouth occurs. This drug may produce drowsiness, so use caution when performing tasks that require alertness.

ALPRAZOLAM
(al-PRAY-zoe-lam)

NEWLY DISCOVERED USES (OFF-LABEL)

Alcohol withdrawal, irritable bowel syndrome (IBS), major depressive disorder, premenstrual dysphoric disorder (PMDD), premenstrual syndrome (PMS), therapy-resistant PMDD

ORIGINAL USES (ON-LABEL)
Anxiety associated with depression, general anxiety disorder (GAD), panic disorder

BRAND NAMES
Alprazolam Intensol, Xanax, Xanax XR

DRUG CLASS
Antianxiety

DESCRIPTION
Decreases excitability in the neurons by binding to receptors in the central nervous system and brain.

POTENTIAL SIDE EFFECTS
Lightheadedness, changes in libido, menstrual disorders, dry mouth, appetite increase or decrease, weight gain/loss, low blood pressure, confusion, derealization, dizziness, disinhibition, dermatitis, rash, difficulty urinating, salivation increased, upset stomach, sexual dysfunction, rigidity, tremor, muscle cramps, nasal congestion, muscle aches, shortness of breath, drowsiness, fatigue, difficulty walking, sweating.

CAUTIONS
- Do not suddenly stop therapy; if you stop using this drug, your use should be tapered gradually. Withdrawal symptoms, including seizures, have been reported 18 hours to three days after abrupt discontinuation or after large decreases in doses.
- Paradoxical reactions have been reported with use (excitability, anger, hostility).
- Elderly people should use this drug with caution (may require smaller doses). Cautions should also be used by debilitated patients, those with reduced liver or kidney function, obese patients, patients with history of dependence or depression.

- May cause anterograde amnesia (memory loss of recent actions, events).
- Use with caution if you are receiving concurrent CYP3A4 inhibitors (see drug interactions).
- May cause sedation and impair physical or mental capabilities. Concurrent use with other sedatives may increase the risk of severe sedation.

DRUG INTERACTIONS
Narcotic analgesics, barbiturates, phenothiazines, antihistamines, MAO inhibitors, sedative-hypnotics, cyclic antidepressants, imipramine and desipramine. This drug is cleared from the body by a specific set of liver enzymes (cytochrome P3A4). Concurrent use of alprazolam with other drugs that block this enzyme may result in increased levels of alprazolam. The list of drugs that inhibit this enzyme, increasing the potential for side effects, is large. Please check with your pharmacist before starting any new medication while taking alprazolam.

FOOD INTERACTIONS
Alcohol

HERBAL INTERACTIONS
Valerian, St. John's wort, kava kava, gotu kola, gingko biloba

PREGNANCY AND BREAST-FEEDING CAUTIONS
FDA Pregnancy Risk Category D. Excreted in breast milk, not recommended during breast-feeding.

ALPROSTADIL
(al-PROS-ta-dill)

NEWLY DISCOVERED USES (OFF-LABEL)
Dyspareunia

ORIGINAL USES (ON-LABEL)
Erectile dysfunction

BRAND NAMES
Caverject, Caverject Impulse, Edex, Muse

DRUG CLASS
Prostaglandin E-1

DESCRIPTION
Causes relaxation of blood vessels by direct effect on smooth muscle containing blood vessels. When injected along the penile shaft, allows blood flow into the penis.

POTENTIAL SIDE EFFECTS
Penile pain, urethral burning, increased heart rate, low blood pressure, headache, prolonged erection, injection site reaction, flushing, fever, apnea, dizziness, testicular pain, pelvic pain, back pain, urethral bleeding, penile fibrosis.

CAUTIONS
- You should not use this drug if you are predisposed to priapism (e.g., sickle cell anemia, multiple myeloma, leukemia).
- Inform your doctor if you have anatomical deformations of the penis, penile implants, or if sexual activity is inadvisable or contraindicated.
- Do not use this drug if you are pregnant.

DRUG INTERACTIONS
Antihypertensives, anticoagulants (e.g., warfarin)

FOOD INTERACTIONS
Alcohol

HERBAL INTERACTION
Saw palmetto

PREGNANCY AND BREAST-FEEDING CAUTIONS
FDA Pregnancy Risk Category X. This drug is not indicated for use in women, so breast-feeding is not recommended.

SPECIAL INFORMATION
When used for erectile dysfunction, persistent and painful erections may occur. It is important to seek medical attention and treat immediately to avoid penile tissue damage and permanent loss of potency.

ALTEPLASE
(AL-te-plase)

NEWLY DISCOVERED USES (OFF-LABEL)
Pleural effusion

ORIGINAL USES (ON-LABEL)
Acute stroke, acute heart attack, clots in the lung, blocked central, venous catheter

BRAND NAMES
Activase, Cathoflo

DRUG CLASS
Fibrinolytic

DESCRIPTION
Breaks down fibrin (a type of protein) by binding to fibrin in a clot.

POTENTIAL SIDE EFFECTS
Bleeding (particularly gastric or urinary but may occur anywhere), low blood pressure, fever, and allergic reactions.

CAUTIONS
- Do not use this drug if you have an increased risk for bleeding (recent surgery, stroke, aneurysm, brain tumor, active internal bleeding, severe uncontrolled high blood pressure.). Discuss these risks with your doctor.
- Requires blood testing for bleeding tendencies before administration (e.g., International normalized ratio, Prothrombin time, etc.).

DRUG INTERACTIONS
Warfarin, heparins, aspirin, aminocaproic acid, nitroglycerin, dipyridamole, abciximab, vitamin K antagonist, drugs that affect clotting and bleeding

FOOD INTERACTIONS
Unknown

HERBAL INTERACTIONS
Cat's claw, dong quai, evening primrose, feverfew, red clover, horse chestnut, garlic, green tea, ginseng, and gingko

PREGNANCY AND BREAST-FEEDING CAUTIONS
FDA Pregnancy Risk Category C. Excretion into breast milk is unknown, do not breast-feed while using this drug.

SPECIAL INFORMATION
Watch for signs of bleeding and bruising, and report findings to your doctor.

AMANTADINE
(a-MAN–to-deen)

NEWLY DISCOVERED USES (OFF-LABEL)
> Chronic hepatitis C, cocaine addiction, multiple sclerosis

ORIGINAL USES (ON-LABEL)
Influenza A, Parkinsonism, drug-induced extra pyramidal symptoms

BRAND NAME
Symmetrel

DRUG CLASS
Antiparkinson's, antiviral

DESCRIPTION
As an antiviral, amantadine blocks the uncoating of influenza A, preventing penetration of the virus. As an Antiparkinson's drug, it decreases the transmission of a chemical transmitter in the brain (dopamine).

POTENTIAL SIDE EFFECTS
Sudden decrease in blood pressure upon standing, insomnia, depression, anxiety, irritability, nausea, anorexia, constipation, diarrhea.

CAUTIONS
- Use with caution if you have liver disease, a history of eczematoid dermatitis, uncontrolled psychosis, or seizures.
- Reduced dosages are needed if you have decreased kidney function.
- Do not stop therapy suddenly if you have Parkinson's disease.
- Use with caution if you have congestive heart failure, are elderly (at more risk of side effects), or if you have peripheral edema or orthostatic hypotension.

- Avoid use if you have angle-closure glaucoma.
- Do not use this drug in the first trimester of pregnancy.

DRUG INTERACTIONS
Anticholinergic drugs, hydrochlorothiazide, triamterene, trimethoprim

FOOD INTERACTIONS
Alcohol

HERBAL INTERACTIONS
Quinine

PREGNANCY AND BREAST-FEEDING CAUTIONS
FDA Pregnancy Risk Category C. Excreted in breast milk; therapy not recommended during breast-feeding.

SPECIAL INFORMATION
Avoid getting up quickly from a sitting or lying down position when using this drug. If dizziness or lightheadedness occurs, notify your doctor. Blurred vision or reduced concentration may also occur.

AMIFOSTINE
(am-i-FOS-teen)

NEWLY DISCOVERED USES (OFF-LABEL)
Prevention of mucositis/stomatitis induced by cancer

ORIGINAL USES (ON-LABEL)
Cisplatin-induced kidney toxicity, radiation-induced dry mouth

BRAND NAME
Ethyol

DRUG CLASS
Cytoprotectant

DESCRIPTION
Amifostine helps to regulate use of the cancer chemotherapy drug, cisplatin. Specifically, the administration of this drug prior to the administration of cisplatin reduces kidney toxicities.

POTENTIAL SIDE EFFECTS
Flushing, low blood pressure, increased heart rate, shortness of breath, chills, dizziness, drowsiness, nausea / vomiting, sneezing, feeling of warmth/coldness, hiccups.

CAUTIONS
- Inform your doctor if you have an allergy to mannitol.
- Stop antihypertensives 24 hours before administration of this drug. Your blood pressure should be monitored during infusion of the drug.
- You should be adequately hydrated prior to taking this drug.
- If you are at risk for low calcium, you should be monitoring during therapy.

DRUG INTERACTIONS
Antihypertensives

FOOD INTERACTIONS
Unknown

HERBAL INTERACTIONS
Unknown

PREGNANCY AND BREAST-FEEDING CAUTIONS
FDA Pregnancy Risk Category C. Excretion in breast milk unknown. Breast-feeding is not advised with use of this drug.

AMIKACIN
(am-I-KAY-sin)

NEWLY DISCOVERED USES (OFF-LABEL)
Nocardiosis

ORIGINAL USES (ON-LABEL)
Treatment of serious bacterial infections resistant to gentamicin and tobramycin

BRAND NAME
Amikin

DRUG CLASS
Antibiotic (aminoglycoside)

DESCRIPTION
Amikacin inhibits the production of protein in bacteria, inhibiting their growth.

POTENTIAL SIDE EFFECTS
Reduced function of kidneys, deafness, nausea, diarrhea.

CAUTIONS

- Inform your doctor if you have had allergic reactions to other aminoglycosides such as gentamicin, tobramycin, neomycin, etc.
- This drug requires monitoring of kidney function during therapy. Kidney damage is usually reversible.
- Toxicity in the ears is proportional to dosage and duration of treatment. Tinnitus (ringing in the ears) or vertigo (dizziness) may become irreversible.

DRUG INTERACTIONS

Neuromuscular blocking drugs, other aminoglycosides, other kidney-toxic drugs (e.g. amphotericin, etc.) or ear-toxic drugs (e.g., furosemide, ethacrynic acid)

FOOD INTERACTIONS

Unknown

HERBAL INTERACTIONS

Unknown

PREGNANCY AND BREAST-FEEDING CAUTIONS

FDA Pregnancy Risk Category D. Excreted in breast milk. Consult with your doctor.

SPECIAL INFORMATION

This drug has a black box warning regarding ear, neuro-, and kidney toxicities.

AMILORIDE

(a-MIL-oh-ride)

NEWLY DISCOVERED USES (OFF-LABEL)

Ascites in cirrhosis, hyperaldosteronism, hypercalciuria, nephrogenic diabetes insipidus

ORIGINAL USES (ON-LABEL)

Congestive heart failure, high blood pressure

BRAND NAME

Midamor

DRUG CLASS

Diuretic (potassium-sparing)

DESCRIPTION
Amiloride interferes with sodium reabsorption in the kidneys and decreases potassium excretion from the body, while promoting fluid excretion.

POTENTIAL SIDE EFFECTS
Headache, fatigue, dizziness, increased potassium levels, dehydration, hyponatremia, breast swelling, nausea, diarrhea, vomiting, constipation, abdominal and gas pain, appetite changes, impotence, muscle cramps, weakness, cough, and shortness of breath.

CAUTIONS
- Do not use this drug if you have severe liver dysfunction.
- Your potassium levels should be monitored if you use this drug; it may cause increased levels. Do not take concurrent potassium supplementation or potassium-sparing drugs. Stop therapy if high levels of potassium occur.
- This drug should not be used if you have acute or chronic kidney insufficiency, or diabetic neuropathy.

DRUG INTERACTIONS
Triamterene, spironolactone, ACE inhibitors (e.g. captopril, ramipril, etc.), angiotension receptor antagonists (e.g., losartan, candesartan), digoxin, potassium preparations, cyclosporine, tacrolimus, indomethacin, amantadine, lithium, quinidine

FOOD INTERACTIONS
Take with food or meals to avoid stomach upset. Avoid eating large volumes of potassium-rich foods.

HERBAL INTERACTIONS
Unknown

PREGNANCY AND BREAST-FEEDING CAUTIONS
FDA Pregnancy Risk Category B. Excretion in breast milk unknown; therapy not recommended during breast-feeding.

SPECIAL INFORMATION
Notify your doctor if you experience muscle weakness, fatigue or muscle cramps.

This drug contains a black box warning regarding the potential of increased serum potassium levels.

AMINOCAPROIC ACID
(a-mee-noe-ka-PROE–ik AS-id)

NEWLY DISCOVERED USES (OFF-LABEL)
Hemophilia

ORIGINAL USES (ON-LABEL)
Excessive bleeding from fibrinolysis (breakdown of fibrin)

BRAND NAME
Amicar

DRUG CLASS
Hemostatic (anti-bleeding)

DESCRIPTION
This drug reduces the effects of bleeding.

POTENTIAL SIDE EFFECTS
Anorexia, nausea, gastric irritation, vomiting, low blood pressure, low heart rate, irregular heart rate, dizziness, headache, malaise, fatigue, rash, masculinization in females, adrenocortical insufficiency, decreased platelet function, various blood disorders, muscle weakness, weakness, ringing in ears, and nasal congestion.

CAUTIONS
- This drug may accumulate in your body if you have decreased kidney function.
- Kidney obstruction may occur related to clots in the kidney pelvis and ureters.
- Inform your doctor if you have cardiac, kidney, or liver disease.
- This drug may promote clotting.
- Neonate should not take this drug because benzyl alcohol is used as a preservative.

DRUG INTERACTIONS
Oral contraceptives, factor IX complex concentrated, anti-inhibitor complex

FOOD INTERACTIONS
Unknown

HERBAL INTERACTIONS
Unknown

PREGNANCY AND BREAST-FEEDING CAUTIONS
FDA Pregnancy Risk Category C. It is not known if this drug is excreted in breast milk. Refrain from breast-feeding while taking this drug.

SPECIAL INFORMATION
Inform your doctor if signs of bleeding occur. When standing up or sitting or lying down, change positions slowly to minimize dizziness.

AMIODARONE
(a-MEE-oh-da-rone)

NEWLY DISCOVERED USES (OFF-LABEL)
Atrial fibrillation, cardiac arrest, congestive heart failure

ORIGINAL USES (ON-LABEL)
Recurrent ventricular fibrillation (irregular heart rhythm) or unstable ventricular tachycardia (serious type of increased heart rate)

BRAND NAMES
Cordarone, Pacerone

DRUG CLASS
Antiarrhythmic

DESCRIPTION
Amiodarone blocks sodium and potassium channels at the cellular level in the heart, which regulates nerve activity in the heart. This effect helps regulate the rhythm of an abnormal heart rate.

POTENTIAL SIDE EFFECTS
Low blood pressure, congestive heart failure, low heart rate, heart conduction abnormalities, abnormal gait/difficulty walking, dizziness, fatigue, headache, malaise, impaired memory, involuntary movements, insomnia, peripheral neuropathy, sleep disturbances, tremor, photosensitivity, slate blue skin discoloration, low thyroid levels, libido decreased, nausea, vomiting, anorexia, constipation, elevations in tests for liver function, abdominal pain, blood clotting abnormalities, serious and potentially fatal liver toxicity, visual disturbances, corneal microdeposits, halo vision, lung toxicity, abnormal smell.

CAUTIONS

- Notify your doctor if you have an allergy to iodine or iodine type products.
- Use of this drug requires monitoring for lung toxicity and liver toxicity.
- Monitoring for low potassium or magnesium levels should be performed prior to initiation and throughout therapy.

DRUG INTERACTIONS

May increase effect of drugs that prolong the QT interval, affecting heart rate. For a comprehensive list of drugs that cause QT prolongation, see the following website: http://www.torsades.org/medical-pros/drug-lists/druglists.htm#). This drug strongly inhibits a specific set of liver enzymes that are responsible for the metabolism and clearance of other drugs. Thus, there are several potential drug interactions when amiodarone is administered with other drugs, often requiring dosage adjustments when they are administered in combination. As these are too numerous to list, you should always check with your doctor or pharmacist prior to starting a new medication while on this therapy.

HERBAL INTERACTIONS

St. John's wort

FOOD INTERACTIONS

Grapefruit juice increases absorption of oral amiodarone. Drinking grapefruit juice should be avoided during therapy.

PREGNANCY AND BREAST-FEEDING CAUTIONS

FDA Pregnancy Risk Category D. Amiodarone is excreted in breast milk and breast-feeding is not recommended during therapy.

SPECIAL INFORMATION

In January 2005, the FDA required that a Medication Guide be distributed directly to every patient to whom amiodarone tablets are dispensed. This brochure can be found at http://www.fda.gov/cder/Offices/ODS/labeling.htm and details specific information regarding serious safety issues with this drug. You should review this information prior to starting therapy.

AMITRIPTYLINE
(a-mee-TRIP-ti-leen)

NEWLY DISCOVERED USES (OFF-LABEL)
Chronic fatigue syndrome, chronic nausea and vomiting, chronic neuropathic pain, diabetic neuropathy, dyspepsia, fibromyalgia, interstitial cystitis, irritable bowel syndrome, migraine prevention, multiple sclerosis, panic disorder, post-herpetic neuralgia, posttraumatic stress disorder, pruritus, urticaria, vulvodynia

ORIGINAL USES (ON-LABEL)
Depression

BRAND NAME
Elavil

DRUG CLASS
Tricyclic antidepressant, anti-migraine

DESCRIPTION
Increases concentration of serotonin and/or norepinephrine in the central nervous system, which may alter mood and other symptoms.

POTENTIAL SIDE EFFECTS
Sudden drop in blood pressure upon standing from a sitting or lying down position, increased heart rate, changes in heart rhythm, restlessness, dizziness, insomnia, sedation, allergic rash, hives, photosensitivity reaction (skin reaction related to sun exposure), loss of hair, weight gain, dry mouth, constipation, urinary retention, various blood abnormalities, blurred vision, pupil widening, ocular pressure increase, ringing in the ears, numbness, tremor, sweating, withdrawal reactions.

CAUTIONS
- Do not use if you have been taking an MAO inhibitor such as phenelzine, tranylcypromine, or isocarboxazid within the past 14 days. When used with MAO-I's, fever, high blood pressure, increased heart rate, confusion, seizures, and deaths have been reported.
- Do not use this drug immediately after a heart attack.
- This drug can cause sedation, which may impair performance of tasks requiring alertness. Sedative effects may be additive with other drugs that cause similar effects.

- This drug may worsen psychosis or mania in patients with bipolar disease.
- Stop therapy with doctor permission and according to instructions (gradual taper) prior to elective surgery.
- Do not abruptly stop taking this medication; instead, taper gradually.
- Notify your doctor if you have low blood pressure, as this drug can cause low blood pressure episodes.
- Use with caution if you have urinary retention, history of cardiac disease, seizure disorders, diabetes, benign prostatic hyperplasia, narrow angle glaucoma, dry mouth, visual problems, constipation, or a history of bowel obstruction.
- The possibility of suicide attempt may persist until remission occurs.
- Use with caution if you have hyperthyroid disorder or if you are receiving thyroid supplementation.
- Use with caution if you have liver or kidney dysfunction, or if you are elderly.

DRUG INTERACTIONS

MAO inhibitors (e.g., phenelzine, tranylcypromine, isocarboxazid), ritonavir, bupropion, amphetamines, anticholinergics, sedatives, chlorpropamide, tolazamide, warfarin, fluoxetine, fluvoxamine, citalopram, escitalopram, paroxetine, sertraline, cimetidine, carbamazepine, haloperidol, smoking, methylphenidate, valproic acid, clonidine, venlafaxine, protease inhibitors, quinidine, diltiazem, verapamil, lithium, phenothiazines, drugs which prolong QT interval (see site: http://www.torsades.org/medical pros/drug-lists/drug-lists.htm#).

This drug is metabolized (inactivated) by specific set of liver enzymes. Several other drugs interfere with these liver enzymes, and thus may increase or decrease the clearance of amitriptyline from the body, potentially increasing the risk of side effects or decreasing effectiveness. When these drugs are given in combination with amitriptyline dosage adjustments may be needed. As these are too numerous to list, you should always check with your doctor or pharmacist prior to starting a new medication.

FOOD INTERACTIONS
Alcohol

HERBAL INTERACTIONS
Valerian, St. John's wort, kava kava, gotu kola

PREGNANCY AND BREAST-FEEDING CAUTIONS
FDA Pregnancy Risk Category C. This drug is excreted in the breast milk; breast-feeding is not recommended during therapy.

SPECIAL INFORMATION
May take four to six weeks for you to experience the full therapeutic effects. Avoid prolonged exposure to sunlight, and wear sunscreen.

In 2005, the FDA announced new labeling for antidepressants regarding the need to closely monitor for worsening of depression and for the potential of increased suicidal thinking or suicidal behavior during therapy. Although this recommendation applies to all patients (adults, children, adolescents) treated with antidepressants for any indication, this is of particular importance in patients being treated for depression.

Close observation may be especially important when antidepressant medications are started for the first time or when doses are changed. More information on this topic can be found at the following web site: http://www.fda.gov/cder/drug/antidepressants/default.htm

AMLODIPINE
(am-LOE-di-peen)

NEWLY DISCOVERED USES (OFF-LABEL)
Raynaud's syndrome

ORIGINAL USES (ON-LABEL)
Chest pain (angina), high blood pressure

BRAND NAME
Norvasc

DRUG CLASS
Antihypertensive (calcium channel blocker)

DESCRIPTION
Blocks calcium channels in the blood vessels and heart, preventing contraction of blood vessels, and allowing them to widen and relax.

POTENTIAL SIDE EFFECTS
Peripheral swelling due to fluid retention (edema), flushing, headache, dizziness, fatigue, nausea, gingival hyperplasia (swelling of the gum tissue).

CAUTIONS
- Dosage adjustments may be required if you have reduced kidney function.
- Use with caution if you have congestive heart failure, specific heart problems, edema, or increased brain pressure with brain tumors, of if you use beta-blockers or digoxin.
- Do not stop therapy suddenly.
- Elderly are at increased risk for lowered blood pressure and constipation.

DRUG INTERACTIONS
Itraconazole, ketoconazole, fluconazole, erythromycin, cyclosporine, sildenafil, tadalafil, and vardenafil, rifampin.

FOOD INTERACTIONS
Grapefruit juice

HERBAL INTERACTIONS
St. John's wort, dong quai, ephedra, yohimbe, ginseng, garlic

PREGNANCY AND BREAST-FEEDING CAUTIONS
FDA Pregnancy Risk Category C. It is not known if this drug is excreted in breast milk. Consult with your doctor prior to breast-feeding while taking this therapy.

AMOXICILLIN
(a-moks-i-SIL-in)

NEWLY DISCOVERED USES (OFF-LABEL)
Lyme disease, tonsillectomy

ORIGINAL USES (ON-LABEL)
Various bacterial infections

BRAND NAMES
Amoxil, Trimox

DRUG CLASS
Antibiotic (penicillin)

DESCRIPTION
Amoxicillin inhibits the production of the bacterial cell wall.

POTENTIAL SIDE EFFECTS
Hyperactivity, agitation, anxiety, insomnia, mild to severe, including some life-threatening rashes, nausea, vomiting, diarrhea, hemorrhagic colitis, various blood disorders, abnormal tests that monitor liver function, jaundice, crystals in the urine.

CAUTIONS
- Notify your doctor if you have an allergy to penicillins or cephalosporin antibiotics.
- Dose and/or frequency of administration should be adjusted if you have kidney impairment.
- Amoxil chewable tablets contain phenylalanine.
- Prolonged use of antibiotics may result in super-infection, resistance.

DRUG INTERACTIONS
Disulfiram, probenecid, warfarin, methotrexate, tetracyclines, chloramphenicol. If you are taking oral contraceptives, consult with pharmacist or doctor.

FOOD INTERACTIONS
Unknown

HERBAL INTERACTIONS
Khat

PREGNANCY AND BREAST-FEEDING CAUTIONS
FDA Pregnancy Risk Category B. Amoxicillin is excreted in breast milk. The American Academy of Pediatrics considers this drug compatible with breast-feeding.

SPECIAL INFORMATION
A high percentage of people with infectious mononucleosis have developed rashes during therapy with amoxicillin.

AMOXICILLIN-CLAVULANATE
(a-moks-i-SIL-in klav-yoo-LAN-ate)

NEWLY DISCOVERED USES (OFF-LABEL)
Diverticulitis, nocardiosis, peritonsillar abscess, tonsillectomy, tonsillitis

ORIGINAL USES (ON-LABEL)
Various bacterial infections

BRAND NAMES
Augmentin, Augmentin ES-600, Augmentin XR

DRUG CLASS
Antibiotic (penicillin)

DESCRIPTION
Amoxicillin inhibits the production of the bacterial cell wall. Clavulanic acid helps amoxicillin expand its spectrum of activity.

POTENTIAL SIDE EFFECTS
Diarrhea, diaper and skin rash, urticaria, abdominal discomfort, nausea, vomiting, vaginitis, moniliasis.

CAUTIONS
- Notify your doctor if you have an allergy to penicillins or cephalosporin antibiotics.
- Dose and/or frequency of administration should be adjusted if you have kidney impairment.
- Prolonged use of antibiotics may result in super-infection, resistance.
- Do not use if you have a history of cholestatic jaundice or hepatic dysfunction with amoxicillin-clavulanate.
- A high percentage of patients with infectious mononucleosis have developed a rash during therapy.
- The incidence of diarrhea is higher with amoxicillin-clavulanate than with amoxicillin alone.
- Due to differing content of clavulanic acid, *not all formulations are interchangeable.*
- Some products contain phenylalanine.

DRUG INTERACTIONS
Disulfiram, probenecid, allopurinol, warfarin, methotrexate, tetracyclines, chloramphenicol. If you are taking oral contraceptives, consult with your pharmacist or doctor.

FOOD INTERACTIONS
Unknown

HERBAL INTERACTIONS
Khat

PREGNANCY AND BREAST-FEEDING CAUTIONS
FDA Pregnancy Risk Category B. Amoxicillin is excreted into breast milk in low concentrations and is compatible. There are no human data pertaining to clavulanate and breast milk. Consult your doctor.

SPECIAL INFORMATION
Extended-release formulations should be taken with food. Two 250 mg tablets are not equivalent to a 500 mg tablet and two 500 mg tablets are not equivalent to a 1000 mg tablet in regards to amoxicillin. Some products contain phenylalanine.

AMPICILLIN
(am-pi-SIL-in)

NEWLY DISCOVERED USES (OFF-LABEL)
Cholera, food poisoning

ORIGINAL USES (ON-LABEL)
Various bacterial infections

BRAND NAME
Principen

DRUG CLASS
Antibiotic (penicillin)

DESCRIPTION
Amoxicillin inhibits the production of the cell wall of bacteria.

POTENTIAL SIDE EFFECTS
Hyperactivity, agitation, anxiety, insomnia, mild to severe, including some life-threatening rashes, nausea, vomiting, diarrhea, hemorrhagic colitis, various blood disorders, abnormal tests that monitor liver function, jaundice, crystals in the urine.

CAUTIONS
- Notify your doctor if you have an allergy to penicillins or cephalosporin antibiotics.
- Dose and/or frequency of administration should be adjusted if you have kidney impairment.
- Prolonged use of antibiotics may result in super-infection, resistance.

DRUG INTERACTIONS
Disulfiram, probenecid, warfarin, methotrexate, tetracyclines, chloramphenicol. If you are taking oral contraceptives, consult with pharmacist or doctor.

FOOD INTERACTIONS
Food decreases ampicillin absorption rate and may decrease ampicillin serum concentration.

HERBAL INTERACTIONS
Khat

PREGNANCY AND BREAST-FEEDING CAUTIONS
FDA Pregnancy Risk Category B. Amoxicillin is excreted in breast milk. The American Academy of Pediatrics considers this drug compatible with breast-feeding.

SPECIAL INFORMATION
Take on an empty stomach one hour before or two hours after meals.

AMPICILLIN/SULBACTAM
(am-pi SIL-in SUL-bak-tam)

NEWLY DISCOVERED USES (OFF-LABEL)
Acute otitis media, chronic otitis media, diverticulitis

ORIGINAL USES (ON-LABEL)
Various bacterial infections

BRAND NAME
Unasyn

DRUG CLASS
Antibiotic (penicillin and beta-lactamase inhibitor)

DESCRIPTION
Ampicillin inhibits the production of the bacterial cell wall. Sulbactam extends ampicillin's spectrum of activity related to bacteria.

POTENTIAL SIDE EFFECTS
Pain at injection site, thrombophlebitis (inflammation of the vein), rash, diarrhea, allergic reaction, nausea, vomiting, headache.

CAUTIONS
- Notify your doctor if you have an allergy to penicillins or cephalosporin antibiotics.
- Dose and/or frequency of administration should be adjusted if you have kidney impairment.
- Prolonged use of antibiotics may result in super-infection, resistance.
- A high percentage of patients with infectious mononucleosis have developed rash during therapy with ampicillin.

DRUG INTERACTIONS
Disulfiram, probenecid, warfarin, methotrexate, tetracyclines, chloramphenicol, allopurinol

FOOD INTERACTIONS
Unknown

HERBAL INTERACTIONS
Khat

PREGNANCY AND BREAST-FEEDING CAUTIONS
FDA Pregnancy Risk Category B. Ampicillin and sulbactam are excreted into breast milk in low concentrations. Consult your doctor.

ANAGRELIDE
(an-AG-gre-lide)

NEWLY DISCOVERED USES (OFF-LABEL)
Polycythemia vera

ORIGINAL USES (ON-LABEL)
Essential thrombocythemia (excessive platelets)

BRAND NAME
Agrylin

DRUG CLASS
Antiplatelet

DESCRIPTION
Reduces platelet production and inhibits the build-up of platelets.

POTENTIAL SIDE EFFECTS
Palpitations, chest pain, increased heart rate, diarrhea, abdominal pain, nausea, flatulence, vomiting, upset stomach, anorexia, head-

ache, edema, pain, dizziness, shortness of breath, rash, hives, numbness, black pain, malaise.

CAUTIONS
- Abrupt discontinuation may increase platelet counts, usually within four days.
- Inform your doctor if you have heart disease, or reduced liver or kidney function.
- Inform your doctor if you are pregnant or are planning to become pregnant.
- Requires monitoring of liver and kidney functioning, and blood parameters.
- Not for use if you have severe liver failure.

DRUG INTERACTIONS
Sucralfate

FOOD INTERACTIONS
Food slightly reduces absorption.

HERBAL INTERACTIONS
Gingko

PREGNANCY AND BREAST-FEEDING CAUTIONS
FDA Pregnancy Risk Category C. Excreted in breast milk. Consult doctor prior to breast-feeding if on this medication.

SPECIAL INFORMATION
Use effective contraception during therapy.

ANAKINRA
(an-a-KIN-ra)

NEWLY DISCOVERED USES (OFF-LABEL)
Juvenile rheumatoid arthritis

ORIGINAL USES (ON-LABEL)
Moderately- to severely-active rheumatoid arthritis in adult patients who have failed one or more disease-modifying anti-rheumatic drugs (DMARDs)

BRAND NAME
Kineret

DRUG CLASS

Antirheumatic, (interleukin-1 receptor antagonist, immuno-modulator)

DESCRIPTION

Anakinra binds to a certain receptor in the body that mediates a variety of immunological responses, including breakdown of cartilage and stimulation of bone absorption.

POTENTIAL SIDE EFFECTS

Headache, injection site reaction, nausea, diarrhea, infection, upper respiratory infection, abdominal pain, decreased white blood cells, sinusitis, flu-like symptoms.

CAUTIONS

- Not indicated for use if you have hypersensitivity to *E. coli*-derived proteins or anakinra.
- Not for use in active infections (including chronic or local infections) or in patients who are allergic to *E. Coli* proteins. Anakinra may increase your risk of developing infections. Stop therapy immediately if a serious infection develops. Asthmatics may be at increased risk of serious infections.
- Notify your doctor if you have significant blood abnormalities; this drug has been associated with uncommon, but significant decreases in blood parameters.
- Live vaccines should not be taken during therapy with this drug.
- If you are exposed to varicella virus, temporarily discontinue anakinra. Allergic-type reactions may occur.

DRUG INTERACTIONS

Tumor necrosis factor antagonists, (infliximab and thalidomide), etanercept

FOOD INTERACTIONS

Unknown

HERBAL INTERACTIONS

Unknown

PREGNANCY AND BREAST-FEEDING CAUTIONS

FDA Pregnancy Risk Category B. It is not known if this drug is excreted in breast milk. Consult your doctor.

SPECIAL INFORMATION

Seek medical attention if you experience signs and symptoms suggestive of blood disorders. Review and receive vaccines prior to starting therapy.

ANASTROZOLE
(an-AS-troe-zole)

NEWLY DISCOVERED USES (OFF-LABEL)
Infertility (male & female), McCune-Albright syndrome

ORIGINAL USES (ON-LABEL)
Advanced breast cancer in postmenopausal women with the disease progression following tamoxifen therapy; early ER-positive breast cancer in postmenopausal women; locally advanced or metastatic breast cancer (estrogen receptor-positive of hormone receptor unknown) in postmenopausal women.

BRAND NAME
Arimidex

DRUG CLASS
Antineoplastic (aromatase inactivator; aromatase inhibitor)

DESCRIPTION
The growths of some breast cancers are stimulated by estrogens. This drug suppresses the blood estrogen level by inhibiting aromatase, which controls the conversion of androstenedione to estrone, and testosterone to estradiol conversion is prevented.

POTENTIAL SIDE EFFECTS
Vasodilation (widening of blood vessels), pain, headache, depression, hot flashes, weakness, arthritis, muscle aches, sore throat, peripheral edema (swelling related to fluid retention), high blood pressure, weight gain, increased cough, bone pain, chest pain, pelvic pain, rash, hair loss, itching, high cholesterol levels, vomiting, constipation, abdominal pain, urinary tract infection, vulvovaginitis, vaginal bleeding, anemia, various blood disorders, increase in liver function tests, blood clots, osteoporosis, fracture, cataracts.

CAUTIONS
- Inform your doctor if you have increased cholesterol levels; total cholesterol and LDL-cholesterol increases have occurred.
- A reduction in bone mineral density may occur.
- Safety and efficacy in premenopausal women has not been established.

DRUG INTERACTIONS
Tamoxifen

FOOD INTERACTIONS
Unknown

HERBAL INTERACTIONS
Black cohosh, hops, natural licorice, red clover, thyme, dong quai

PREGNANCY AND BREAST-FEEDING CAUTIONS
FDA Pregnancy Risk Category D. Excretion in breast milk unknown. Consult your doctor.

ANTITHYMOCYTE GLOBULIN
(an-te-THY-moe-site GLOB-yu-lin)

Rabbit

NEWLY DISCOVERED USES (OFF-LABEL)
Aplastic anemia

ORIGINAL USES (ON-LABEL)
Acute rejection in kidney transplants (given with other immunosuppressant drugs)

BRAND NAME
Thymoglobulin (immune globulin)

DRUG CLASS
Immunosuppressant

DESCRIPTION
This drug suppresses the immune system. It is thought that antithymocyte globulin does this by eliminating antigen-reactive T-lymphocyte (known as killer cells) in the blood or by altering T-Cell function.

POTENTIAL SIDE EFFECTS
High blood pressure, increased heart rate, shortness of breath, nausea, yeast infections, urinary tract infection, various blood disorders, fever, swelling in limbs due to fluid retention (peripheral edema), chills, headache, rash, increased potassium levels, malaise, dizziness, abdominal pain, diarrhea, pain.

CAUTIONS
- Inform your doctor if you are allergic to rabbit proteins.
- Not for use during acute viral illness.

- Infusion may produce fever and chills. Premedication with corticosteroids, acetaminophen, and/or an antihistamine and/or slowing the infusion rate may reduce reaction incidence and intensity.
- Prolonged use may cause over-immunosuppression resulting in severe infections and may increase the incidence of other malignancies.

DRUG INTERACTIONS
Unknown

FOOD INTERACTIONS
Unknown

HERBAL INTERACTIONS
Unknown

PREGNANCY AND BREAST-FEEDING CAUTIONS
FDA Pregnancy Risk Category C. Excretion in breast milk is unknown. Consult your doctor.

SPECIAL INFORMATION
This drug has a black box warning stating that it should only be used by physicians experienced in immunosuppressive therapy for the management of kidney transplant patients.

APOMORPHINE
(a-poe-MOR-feen)

NEWLY DISCOVERED USES (OFF-LABEL)
Erectile dysfunction, hypoactive sexual desire disorder

ORIGINAL USES (ON-LABEL)
Parkinson's Disease

BRAND NAME
Apokyn

DRUG CLASS
Anti-Parkinson (dopamine receptor agonist, non ergot)

DESCRIPTION
The exact mechanism of this drug's action on Parkinson's disease is unknown. However, it is believed to be related to the stimula-

tion of post-synaptic dopamine D (2) receptors in the brain. Parkinson's disease is characterized by a reduction in dopamine levels.

POTENTIAL SIDE EFFECTS
Severe nausea and vomiting, headache, hallucinations, drowsiness, sedation, dizziness, decreased heart rate, low blood pressure, yawning, chest pain, confusion, edema, swelling of extremities, local injection site reaction, fainting.

CAUTIONS
- Not indicated for use in combination with serotonin 5-HT(3)-type receptor drugs, such as ondansetron, granisetron, dolasetron, palonosetron or alosetron.
- Use caution if you have cardiovascular disease or cerebrovascular disease.
- May affect your heart rate; use with caution if you are at risk for QT prolongation.
- May cause sudden drowsiness or falling asleep.
- This product contains metabisulfite. Notify your doctor if you have allergies to sulfites.
- Should be administered by subcutaneous route only, not for intravenous use.
- Use with caution in elderly, children, and asthmatics.
- Dosage adjustments and monitoring may be needed in reduced kidney and liver function.
- Use caution if you are predisposed to low blood pressure.

DRUG INTERACTIONS
Entacapone, tolcapone, alosetron, dolasetron, granisetron, ondansetron, palonosetron, antihypertensives, metoclopramide, antipsychotics, drugs prolonging the QT interval (see website: http://www.torsades.org/medical-pros/drug-lists/drug-lists.htm)

FOOD INTERACTIONS
Unknown

HERBAL INTERACTIONS
Unknown

PREGNANCY AND BREAST-FEEDING CAUTIONS
FDA Pregnancy Risk Category C. Excretion in breast milk unknown. This drug is not recommended during breast-feeding.

APROTININ
(a-proe-TYE-nin)

NEWLY DISCOVERED USES (OFF-LABEL)
Impaired hemostasis

ORIGINAL USES (ON-LABEL)
Reduction or prevention of blood loss in patients undergoing coronary artery bypass surgery

BRAND NAME
Trasylol

DRUG CLASS
Hemostatic (anti-bleeding)

DESCRIPTION
Aprotinin inhibits several aspects of the clotting process to prevent the breakdown of a protein called fibrin. This results in decreased bleeding.

POTENTIAL SIDE EFFECTS
Irregular heart rhythm, heart attack, heart failure, fever, mental confusion, phlebitis, increased potential for postoperative kidney dysfunction, shortness of breath, low blood pressure, pneumonia, abnormal liver function tests.

CAUTIONS
- Allergic reactions are more common with repeated use, especially when re-exposure is within six months.
- You should receive a test dose at least 10 minutes before loading dose.
- If you have a history of allergic reactions to drugs or other drugs, you may be more likely to develop a reaction to this drug.

DRUG INTERACTIONS
Succinylcholine, tubocurarine, thrombolytic drugs (alteplase and streptokinase), antihypertensives, ACE inhibitors

FOOD INTERACTIONS
Unknown

HERBAL INTERACTIONS
Unknown

PREGNANCY AND BREAST-FEEDING CAUTIONS
FDA Pregnancy Risk Category B. Excretion in breast milk unknown. Consult your doctor.

SPECIAL INFORMATION
This drug has a black box warning regarding the possibility of allergic type reactions and risk factors, such as re-exposure.

ARIPIPRAZOLE
(ay-ri-PIP-ray-zole)

NEWLY DISCOVERED USES (OFF-LABEL) ⎯⎯⎯⎯⎯
| Alzheimer's disease, restless legs syndrome

ORIGINAL USES (ON-LABEL)
Schizophrenia

BRAND NAMES
Abilify

DRUG CLASS
Antipsychotic

DESCRIPTION
Alters dopamine and serotonin levels in the brain, correcting imbalances that may contribute to psychiatric disorders.

CAUTIONS
- May cause decreases in blood pressure upon standing from a sitting or lying down position.
- Problems with esophageal motility and aspiration have been associated with antipsychotic use; use caution if you are at risk of pneumonia.
- May interfere with temperature regulation or mask toxicity of other drugs.
- Notify your doctor if you have diabetes or a history of drug abuse.
- May cause uncoordinated and uncontrolled muscle tremors and movements.

DRUG INTERACTIONS
Quinidine, amiodarone, cimetidine, delavirdine, fluoxetine, paroxetine, propafenone, ritonavir, ketoconazole, clarithromycin, ery-

thromycin, diltiazem, dirithromycin, disulfiram, fluvoxamine, indinavir, itraconazole, nefazodone, nevirapine, propoxyphene, quinupristin-dalfopristin, saquinavir, verapamil, zafirlukast, and zileuton, carbamazepine, phenobarbital, phenytoin, rifampin, and rifabutin.

This drug is metabolized (inactivated) by specific set of liver enzymes. Several other drugs interfere with these liver enzymes, and thus, may increase or decrease the clearance of aripiprazole from the body, effecting potential for side effects, and often requiring dosage adjustments when they are administered in combination. As these are too numerous to list, you should always check with your doctor or pharmacist prior to starting a new medication.

FOOD INTERACTIONS
Grapefruit juice

HERBAL INTERACTIONS
Kava kava, gotu kola, valerian, and St. John's wort

PREGNANCY AND BREAST-FEEDING CAUTIONS
FDA Pregnancy Risk Category C. As the excretion in breast milk is unknown, this drug is not recommended during breast-feeding.

SPECIAL INFORMATION
In 2005, the FDA published Health Advisories regarding the possible risk of death with atypical antipsychotics used to treat behavioral disorder in the elderly with dementia. A black box warning was added to the product labeling regarding this use.

ATENOLOL
(a-TEN-oh-lole)

NEWLY DISCOVERED USES (OFF-LABEL)

Alcohol withdrawal, chronic fatigue syndrome, congestive heart failure, essential tremor, migraine prevention, pheochromocytoma, prevention of recurrence and sudden death in ventricular tachycardia, supraventricular arrhythmia, supraventricular tachycardia, ventricular tachycardia

ORIGINAL USES (ON-LABEL)
High blood pressure, heart related chest pain (angina pectoris), after a heart attack

BRAND NAME
Tenormin

DRUG CLASS
Antianginal, antihypertensive, anti-migraine

DESCRIPTION
Atenolol stabilizes heart rate and reduces blood pressure.

POTENTIAL SIDE EFFECTS
Low blood pressure, decreased heart rate, chest pain, edema (swelling due to fluid retention), dizziness, fatigue, insomnia, lethargy, constipation, diarrhea, nausea, impotence, cold extremities.

CAUTIONS
- Not for use if you have certain lung or cardiac diseases.
- Do not stop therapy suddenly.
- Use caution if you are taking verapamil or diltiazem, as too-low heart rate may occur.
- Use cautiously if you are diabetic; this drug may mask signs of low blood sugar or thyroid problems.
- May cause fetal harm if used in pregnancy.
- Use cautiously if you have impaired kidney function or myasthenia gravis.

DRUG INTERACTIONS
Digoxin, verapamil, diltiazem, alpha blockers, alpha-adrenergic stimulants, reserpine, disopyramide, nondepolarizing muscle relaxants, theophylline, aluminum salts, barbiturates, calcium salts, cholestyramine, colestipol, penicillins, rifampin, salicylates, and sulfinpyrazone

FOOD INTERACTIONS
Atenolol levels may be decreased if taken with food.

HERBAL INTERACTIONS
Dong quai, ma huang, ephedra, yohimbe, ginseng, garlic

PREGNANCY AND BREAST-FEEDING CAUTIONS
FDA Pregnancy Risk Category D. Excreted in breast milk. Consult your doctor prior to breast-feeding during this therapy.

SPECIAL INFORMATION
This drug has a warning regarding the according of abrupt withdrawal in patients with heart disease.

ATOMOXETINE
(AT-oh-mox-e-teen)

NEWLY DISCOVERED USES (OFF-LABEL)
Nocturnal enuresis

ORIGINAL USES (ON-LABEL)
Attention deficit/hyperactivity disorder (ADHD)

BRAND NAME
Strattera

DRUG CLASS
Psychotherapeutic (selective norepinephrine reuptake inhibitor)

DESCRIPTION
The precise mechanism of this drug in the treatment of attention deficit/hyperactivity disorder (ADHD) is not fully known, but it is thought to be related to selective inhibition of norepinephrine.

POTENTIAL SIDE EFFECTS
Headache, upset stomach, constipation, insomnia, dry mouth, abdominal pain, vomiting, decreased appetite, nausea, cough, fatigue/lethargy, irritability, drowsiness, dizziness, painful menstruation, libido decreased, weight loss, diarrhea, erectile disturbance, ejaculatory disturbance, numbness, urinary retention/hesitation.

CAUTIONS

- Do not use with or within 14 days of using MAO inhibitor drugs, such as phenelzine, tranylcypromine, and isocarboxazid.
- Inform your doctor if you have narrow-angle glaucoma, reduced liver or kidney function (may need dosage adjustment), history of urinary retention, or bladder obstruction.
- May cause increased heart rate or blood pressure; use with caution if you have cardiac disease.
- When this drug is used by children, growth should be monitored during treatment.
- Safety and efficacy have not been evaluated in pediatric patients less than six years of age or with long-term use.

DRUG INTERACTIONS

MAO inhibitors, albuterol. This drug is metabolized by a specific set of liver enzymes. Several other drugs interfere with these liver enzymes, and thus, may increase or decrease the clearance of atomoxetine from the body, potentially increasing the risk of side effects or decreasing effectiveness. When these drugs are given in combination with atomoxetine, dosage adjustments may be needed. As these are too numerous to list, you should always check with your doctor or pharmacist prior to starting a new medication, herbal, or nonprescription product.

FOOD INTERACTIONS

Unknown

HERBAL INTERACTIONS

Unknown

PREGNANCY AND BREAST-FEEDING CAUTIONS

FDA Pregnancy Risk Category C. Excretion in breast milk unknown. Consult your doctor.

SPECIAL INFORMATION

You should use caution when driving or operating heavy machinery until effects of the drug are known. In February 2005, the FDA notified health care professionals about a new warning regarding the potential for severe liver injury in two patients who had been treated with atomoxetine for several months, both of whom recovered.

In September 2005, the labeling of this drug was revised to include a warning regarding the increased risk of suicide in children and adolescents receiving the drug. A medication guide is now required with each prescription.

ATORVASTATIN
(a-TORE-va-sta-tin)

NEWLY DISCOVERED USES (OFF-LABEL)
Alzheimer's disease, membranous nephropathy

ORIGINAL USES (ON-LABEL)
Cardiovascular disease in high-risk patients; hyperlipidemias by reducing total cholesterol, LDL-cholesterol, apolipoprotein B, and triglycerides; homozygous familial hypercholesterolemia and heterozygous familial hypercholesterolemia

BRAND NAME
Lipitor

DRUG CLASS
Anti-lipid (HMG-CoA reductase inhibitor)

DESCRIPTION
Lovastatin inhibits an enzyme that your body uses in the production of cholesterol.

POTENTIAL SIDE EFFECTS
Headache, chest pain, peripheral edema, insomnia, dizziness, rash, abdominal pain, constipation, diarrhea, upset stomach, urinary tract infection, increases in liver function tests, muscle aches, arthritis, back pain, sinusitis, sore throat, bronchitis, runny nose, infection, flu-like syndrome.

CAUTIONS
- Do not use this drug if you have active liver disease or if you have high levels of liver function tests.
- You should not consume large amounts of alcohol or have a history of liver disease if you want to use this drug.
- Your liver function should be monitored periodically during therapy.
- This drug can also cause severe muscles aches which are a symptom of a more serious disorder (rhabdomyolysis) in which the muscle fibers break down. If this disorder progresses,

decreases in kidney function may also occur. This risk is increased with concurrent use of drugs that increase atorvastatin levels.

DRUG INTERACTIONS

Azole antifungals, ciprofloxacin, clarithromycin, diclofenac, doxycycline, erythromycin, imatinib, isoniazid, nefazodone, nicardipine, propofol, protease inhibitors, quinidine, and verapamil. Cyclosporine, clofibrate, fenofibrate, gemfibrozil, levothyroxine, digoxin, ethinyl estradiol, cholestyramine, and niacin.

This drug is metabolized by a specific set of liver enzymes. Several other drugs interfere with these liver enzymes, and thus, may increase or decrease the clearance of atorvastatin from the body, potentially increasing the risk of side effects or decreasing effectiveness. When these drugs are given in combination with atorvastatin, dosage adjustments may be needed. As these are too numerous to list, you should always check with your doctor or pharmacist prior to starting a new medication, herbal, or nonprescription product.

FOOD INTERACTIONS

Grapefruit juice (greater than or equal to 1 quart/day) may increase toxicity.

HERBAL INTERACTIONS

St. John's wort

PREGNANCY AND BREAST-FEEDING CAUTIONS

FDA Pregnancy Risk Category X. Atorvastatin should not be used during breast-feeding.

SPECIAL INFORMATION

Before initiation of therapy with this drug, you should be placed on a standard cholesterol-lowering diet for six weeks and the diet should be continued during drug therapy. Report any signs of muscle pain, tenderness, or weakness to your doctor.

AURANOFIN
(Au-RANE-oh-fin)

NEWLY DISCOVERED USES (OFF-LABEL)
Juvenile rheumatoid arthritis, psoriatic arthritis

ORIGINAL USES (ON-LABEL)
Management of rheumatoid arthritis in patients that do not respond to or tolerate other drugs

BRAND NAME
Ridaura

DRUG CLASS
Antirheumatic (gold compound)

DESCRIPTION
Gold acts by several different methods in the treatment of arthritic diseases, it decreases serum rheumatoid factors and other substances in the blood which cause inflammation.

POTENTIAL SIDE EFFECTS
Itching, rash, mouth ulcers, conjunctivitis, protein in the urine, hives, hair loss, tongue swelling, blood in the urine, various blood disorders.

CAUTIONS
- Not for use in patients with kidney disease, history of blood abnormalities, congestive heart failure, serious skin reactions.
- Laboratory testing to monitor for blood abnormalities should be performed on a regular basis (monthly) during therapy.
- Use with caution in patients with kidney and liver impairment.

DRUG INTERACTIONS
Penicillamine, antimalarials, hydroxychloroquine, phenytoin, cytotoxic drugs, and immunosuppressants

FOOD INTERACTIONS
Unknown

HERBAL INTERACTIONS
Unknown

PREGNANCY AND BREAST-FEEDING CAUTIONS
FDA Pregnancy Risk Category C. Excreted in the breast milk. Do not use during breast-feeding.

SPECIAL INFORMATION
Notify your doctor if any of the following occur: itching, rash, sore mouth, metallic taste, easy bruising, nosebleed. Joint pain may be increased for 1 to 2 days after injection but will decrease with continued therapy. Maintain careful and regular oral hygiene during therapy.

AZATHIOPRINE
(ay-za-THYE-oh-preen)

NEWLY DISCOVERED USES (OFF-LABEL)

Atopic dermatitis, autoimmune hepatitis, bullous pemphigoid, Crohn's disease, dermatomyositis/polymyositis, liver fibrosis, multiple sclerosis, myasthenia gravis, oral lichen planus, pericarditis, primary biliary cirrhosis, psoriatic arthritis, therapy-resistant idiopathic thrombocytopenia purpura, therapy-resistant thrombotic thrombocytopenia purpura, sarcoidosis, ulcerative colitis, systemic lupus erythematosus (SLE), uveitis due to systemic disease

ORIGINAL USES (ON-LABEL)
Azathioprine is used in combination therapy to prevent the rejection of kidney transplant, to treat severe active rheumatoid arthritis unresponsive to other drugs, and to treat autoimmune diseases.

BRAND NAME
Imuran

DRUG CLASS
Antineoplastic/immunosuppressant

DESCRIPTION
This drug inhibits the production of cellular proteins and may also interfere with cellular metabolism by blocking cell division.

POTENTIAL SIDE EFFECTS
Fever, chills, hair loss, rash, nausea, vomiting, anorexia, diarrhea, leukopenia, thrombocytopenia, blood abnormalities such as anemia and pancytopenia, liver toxicity, muscle aches, shaking and tremors, shortness of breath, low blood pressure.

CAUTIONS

- Chronic suppression of the immune system increases the risk of developing secondary cancers.
- This drug may cause severe blood toxicities.
- Use with caution if you have liver disease or decreased kidney function.
- Some people have experienced severe nausea and vomiting accompanied by fever, diarrhea, muscle aches, increase in liver function tests. These symptoms develop within the first few weeks of therapy.

DRUG INTERACTIONS

Allopurinol, ACE inhibitors (such as captopril, lisinopril, etc.), warfarin, methotrexate, cyclosporine

FOOD INTERACTIONS

Unknown

HERBAL INTERACTIONS

Cat's claw and echinacea

PREGNANCY AND BREAST-FEEDING CAUTIONS

FDA Pregnancy Risk Category D. It is not known if this drug is excreted in breast milk. Breast-feeding during therapy with this drug is not recommended.

SPECIAL INFORMATION

If you experience stomach upset while taking this drug, divide doses or take with food. Notify your doctor if the following symptoms develop: fever, sore throat, mouth sores, signs of infection, pale stools, or dark urine. This drug has a black box warning regarding the increased risk of cancer associated with chronic suppression of the immune system. You should also be familiar with the adverse effects on blood factors.

AZITHROMYCIN
(az-ith-roe-MYE-sin)

NEWLY DISCOVERED USES (OFF-LABEL)

Chlamydia, diarrhea, drug-induced gingival enlargement, pelvic inflammatory disease, prevention of bacterial endocarditis

ORIGINAL USES (ON-LABEL)
Various bacterial infections

BRAND NAMES
Zithromax Tri-Pak, Zithromax Z-Pak

DRUG CLASS
Antibiotic (macrolide)

DESCRIPTION
This drug blocks the production of a certain type of protein in bacterial cells, limiting their growth.

POTENTIAL SIDE EFFECTS
Diarrhea, nausea, rash, abdominal pain, cramping, vomiting.

CAUTIONS
- Use caution if you have liver dysfunction (symptoms of liver problems may include jaundice, malaise, nausea, vomiting, abdominal colic, and fever). Discontinue use if liver dysfunction occurs.
- Use caution if you have developed a certain type of abnormal heart rhythm called QT prolongation prior to therapy.
- Safety and efficacy of this drug has not been established in children less than six months of age with acute bacterial infections of the ear, sinus or community-acquired pneumonia, or in children less than two years with tonsillitis.

DRUG INTERACTIONS
Pimozide, tacrolimus, phenytoin, ergot alkaloids, alfentanil, bromocriptine, carbamazepine, cyclosporine, digoxin, disopyramide, triazolam, nelfinavir, antacids containing aluminum or magnesium. Consult your pharmacist or physician before starting any new therapy.

FOOD INTERACTIONS
The suspension formulation, but not the tablet form, has increased absorption (46%) with food.

HERBAL INTERACTIONS
Unknown

PREGNANCY AND BREAST-FEEDING CAUTIONS
FDA Pregnancy Risk Category B. Azithromycin is excreted in the breast milk and may accumulate. Use with caution during breast-feeding.

SPECIAL INFORMATION

Take suspension formulation of this drug at least one hour before or two hours after meals. Tablets may be taken without regard to meals. Do not take aluminum or magnesium containing antacids at the same time with this drug. Do not cut, chew, or crush the tablets. Shake the suspension well before each use.

AZTREONAM
(AZ-tree-oh-nam)

NEWLY DISCOVERED USES (OFF-LABEL)
Treatment of traveler's diarrhea

ORIGINAL USES (ON-LABEL)
Urinary tract infections, lower respiratory tract infections, severe blood infections, skin and structure infections, intra-abdominal infections, endometritis and gynecological infections caused by susceptible bacteria

BRAND NAME
Azactam

DRUG CLASS
Antibiotic (monobactam)

DESCRIPTION
Aztreonam fights bacterial infections by inhibiting the growth of bacterial cell walls. Bacterial cells break down when the assembly of the wall is inhibited.

POTENTIAL SIDE EFFECTS
Rash, diarrhea, nausea, vomiting, and pain at injections site.

CAUTIONS
- Please notify doctor if you are allergic to other antibiotics, particularly penicillins or cephalosporins. Infrequently, there may be a cross-allergy between these drugs and aztreonam.
- May cause a severe inflammation of the lower colon (pseudomembranous colitis). Notify your doctor if severe diarrhea develops.

- Rare cases of serious skin reactions have occurred (epidermal necrolysis).
- Dosage adjustment is required if you have reduced kidney function.

DRUG INTERACTIONS
Cefoxitin, imipenem

FOOD INTERACTIONS
Unknown

HERBAL INTERACTIONS
Unknown

PREGNANCY AND BREAST-FEEDING CAUTIONS
FDA Pregnancy Risk Category B. Aztreonam is excreted in the breast milk. The American Academy of Pediatrics classifies this drug as compatible with breast-feeding.

BACLOFEN
(BAK-low-fen)

NEWLY DISCOVERED USES (OFF-LABEL)

Alcoholism (cravings & dependency), alcohol withdrawal, cluster headache treatment and prevention, cocaine addiction, Gilles de la Tourette syndrome, hiccups, migraine prevention, tension headache prevention

ORIGINAL USES (ON-LABEL)
Treatment of reversible spasticity associated with multiple sclerosis or spinal cord lesions and used intrathecally to treat intractable spasticity associated with spinal cord injury, multiple sclerosis, and other spinal disease (spinal ischemia or tumor, transverse myelitis, cervical spondylosis, degenerative myelopathy)

BRAND NAMES
Lioresal, Kemstro

DRUG CLASS
Skeletal muscle relaxant

DESCRIPTION
Relieves muscle spasticity by inhibiting the transmission of reflexes at the spinal cord level.

POTENTIAL SIDE EFFECTS

Drowsiness, vertigo, dizziness, psychiatric disturbances, and muscular weakness.

CAUTIONS

- Avoid abrupt discontinuation of the drug.
- Not for use in the elderly. The elderly are more likely to have central nervous system side effects at higher doses.
- Should be free of infection prior to receiving intrathecal injection with this drug.
- Dosage reduction may be necessary in patients with reduced kidney function.
- May aggravate symptoms of psychiatric disorders (e.g., schizophrenia, confusion, psychosis).

DRUG INTERACTIONS

Other drugs that cause depression of the central nervous system. Check with your pharmacist or doctor before starting new therapy.

FOOD INTERACTIONS

Avoid alcohol

HERBAL INTERACTIONS

Valerian, St. John's wort, kava kava, and gotu kola

PREGNANCY AND BREAST-FEEDING CAUTIONS

FDA Pregnancy Risk Category C. Baclofen is excreted into breast milk. The American Academy of Pediatrics classifies it as compatible with breast-feeding.

SPECIAL INFORMATION

This drug has a black box warning regarding the abrupt withdrawal of intrathecal baclofen. Sudden discontinuation may result in severe complications, including fever, rebound/exaggerated spasticity, muscle rigidity and severe muscle and kidney toxicity, which can lead to organ failure and possibly death.

BALSALAZIDE
(bal-SAL-a-zide)

NEWLY DISCOVERED USES (OFF-LABEL)
Treatment of Crohn's disease

ORIGINAL USES (ON-LABEL)
Mild to moderate active ulcerative colitis

BRAND NAME
Colazal

DRUG CLASS
Anti-inflammatory

DESCRIPTION
Balsalazide decreases gastric inflammation by blocking the production certain metabolites topically in the colon.

POTENTIAL SIDE EFFECTS
Headache, insomnia, fatigue, fever, abdominal pain, diarrhea, nausea, vomiting, muscle aches, rectal bleeding, flatulence, upset stomach, cough, anorexia, and respiratory infections.

CAUTIONS
- Notify your doctor if you have an abnormal narrowing or obstruction in the stomach called "pyloric stenosis," as this may cause balsalazide capsules to be retained in the stomach longer.
- Kidney toxicity has been observed with similar drugs. Notify your doctor if you have had kidney problems in the past.
- May aggravate symptoms of colitis.
- This drug is for use in adults only.

DRUG INTERACTIONS
Azathioprine, 6-mercaptopurine, antibiotics

FOOD INTERACTIONS
Unknown

HERBAL INTERACTIONS
Tamarind, tan-shen

PREGNANCY AND BREAST-FEEDING CAUTIONS
FDA Pregnancy Risk Category B. Only a limited amount of this drug is absorbed into the circulation and is rapidly excreted in the urine. It is not known if this drug is excreted in the breast milk. Use with caution if you are breast-feeding, as an allergic reaction (diarrhea) can occur in the nursing infant.

BENDROFLUMETHAZIDE
(Ben-dro-FLU-meth-a-zide)

NEWLY DISCOVERED USES (OFF-LABEL)
Nephrogenic diabetes insipidus

ORIGINAL USES (ON-LABEL)
High blood pressure, swelling due to fluid retention (edema)

BRAND NAME
Naturetin

DRUG CLASS
Blood pressure medication (thiazide diuretic)

DESCRIPTION
This drug increases the excretion of sodium and chloride in urine, thereby promoting fluid loss.

POTENTIAL SIDE EFFECTS
Potassium loss, nausea, vomiting, loss of appetite, upset stomach, diarrhea, electrolyte imbalances, gout, changes in blood sugar or cholesterol levels, sudden drop in blood pressure upon standing from sitting or lying down position (orthostatic hypotension), dizziness, photosensitivity (skin reaction related to sun exposure).

CAUTIONS
- Notify your doctor if you have allergies to sulfonamide drugs or if you have kidney disease, liver disease, diabetes, asthma, lupus, gout, or recently had surgery.
- Diabetics may require increased amounts of insulin or oral drugs commonly used to treat diabetes
- Your electrolyte levels should be monitored while using this drug; you may require potassium supplementation during therapy.
- This drug may cause dizziness and light-headedness when standing suddenly from a sitting or lying down position.

DRUG INTERACTIONS
ACE inhibitors (such as captopril, lisinopril, etc.), arsenic trioxide, calcitriol, calcium carbonate, cholestyramine, colestipol, digoxin, ketanserin, lithium, probenecid. Check with your phar-

macist or doctor before starting new medications, herbal products, or nonprescription drugs.

FOOD INTERACTIONS
Natural licorice

HERBAL INTERACTIONS
Ginkgo, gossypol, ma huang, ephedra

PREGNANCY AND BREAST-FEEDING CAUTIONS
Pregnancy Risk Category C/D according to manufacturer listings. Category D according to expert analysis. May suppress lactation. Consult your doctor.

SPECIAL INFORMATION
This medication can cause dizziness or drowsiness.

BENZTROPINE
(BENZ-troe-peen)

NEWLY DISCOVERED USES (OFF-LABEL)
Oculogyric crisis

ORIGINAL USES (ON-LABEL)
Drug-induced extrapyramidal effects (tremors, uncontrolled muscle movements), Parkinsonism, and for combination treatment of Parkinson's disease

BRAND NAME
Cogentin

DRUG CLASS
Anti-Parkinson's

DESCRIPTION
Benztropine inhibits the action of a chemical substance in the body that supplies nerve impulses in most tissues in the body. It also has antihistamine effects.

POTENTIAL SIDE EFFECTS
Increased heart rate, confusion, disorientation, memory impairment, rash, heat stroke, fever, dry mouth, nausea, vomiting, constipation, urinary retention, pain on urination, blurred vision, and dilation of the pupils.

CAUTIONS

- Do not use this drug if you have stomach or duodenal obstruction, peptic ulcers that cause stomach narrowing, bladder neck obstructions, myasthenia gravis.
- It should not be used in children under three years of age.
- Elderly patients (greater than 60 years of age) may be at greater risk of side effects.
- This drug can increase your risk of narrow-angle glaucoma and requires regular monitoring of the eyes.
- Use with caution if you have increased heart rate, low or high blood pressure, irregular heart rhythms, prostatic hyperplasia, or tendency toward urinary retention, liver or kidney disorders.
- This drug may cause confusion or hallucinations in patients with psychiatric disorders.

DRUG INTERACTIONS

Digoxin, levodopa, tacrine, donepezil, other anticholinergic or cholinergic drugs. Check with your pharmacist or doctor before starting any new therapy.

FOOD INTERACTIONS

Alcohol

HERBAL INTERACTIONS

Betel nut

PREGNANCY AND BREAST-FEEDING CAUTIONS

FDA Pregnancy Risk Category C. Not recommended during breast-feeding.

SPECIAL INFORMATION

As this drug may reduce the ability to sweat, you should avoid heat stroke by maintaining adequate hydration during periods of extremely hot weather or after extreme exercise. This risk is more pronounced in the elderly, alcoholics, and after prolonged outdoor exposure to the heat.

BETAMETHASONE
(bay-ta-METH-a-sone)

Injectable

NEWLY DISCOVERED USES (OFF-LABEL)

Premature labor (preterm)

ORIGINAL USES (ON-LABEL)
Rheumatic disorders (such as rheumatoid arthritis, osteoarthritis, joint inflammation), ocular conditions, gastrointestinal diseases, lung disorders, blood disorders, certain leukemias, endocrine disorders, and certain inflammatory conditions of the skin

BRAND NAME
Celestone

DRUG CLASS
Anti-inflammatory (corticosteroid)

DESCRIPTION
Betamethasone depresses the formation, release, and activity of elements involved in inflammation, such as prostaglandins, kinins, and histamine.

POTENTIAL SIDE EFFECTS
Tendon rupture, infection, skin atrophy, impaired wound healing, increased intraocular pressure, muscle weakness, sodium and fluid retention, potassium loss, high blood pressure, loss of muscle mass, peptic ulcer, increased sweating, menstrual irregularities.

CAUTIONS
- Do not use this drug if you are currently experiencing infections.
- This drug may cause immune suppression. Use with caution if you are immunocompromised, if you have infections or ocular herpes simplex. Avoid exposure to measles and chicken pox while on this drug. Consult your doctor prior to receiving vaccinations.
- Notify your doctor if you have hypothyroidism, cirrhosis, or ulcerative colitis.
- Prolonged use of steroids may promote the development of cataracts and glaucoma.

DRUG INTERACTIONS
Barbiturates, estrogens, ketoconazole, certain antibiotics, warfarin, digoxin, isoniazid

FOOD INTERACTIONS
Unknown

HERBAL INTERACTIONS
Unknown

PREGNANCY AND BREAST-FEEDING CAUTIONS
FDA Pregnancy Risk Category C. There are no human data available on the use of betamethasone in nursing mothers.

SPECIAL INFORMATION
The lowest possible dose should be used to control your condition while minimizing the risk of side effects. Psychiatric side effects have been reported (such as delusion, confusion, euphoria). Avoid receiving an injection of this drug in previously infected joints or an unstable joint.

BETAMETHASONE
(bay-ta-METH-a-sone)

Topical

NEWLY DISCOVERED USES (OFF-LABEL)
Canker sores, nasal polyps, oral lichen planus, otitis externa

ORIGINAL USES (ON-LABEL)
Inflammatory skin conditions including, but not limited to, seborrheic or atopic dermatitis, allergic states, or hypersensitivity reactions

BRAND NAMES
Bet-Val, Diprosone, Maxivate, Teladar

DRUG CLASS
Anti-inflammatory (topical corticosteroid)

DESCRIPTION
This drug depresses the formation, release, and activity of elements that contribute to inflammation, such as prostaglandins, kinins, and histamine.

POTENTIAL SIDE EFFECTS
Burning, itching, irritation, erythema, dryness, folliculitis, acne, numbness, crackening or tightening of the skin, secondary infection, skin atrophy. The risk of these side effects may occur more frequently if the area is covered with bandage or dressing.

CAUTIONS
- This drug should not be used alone to treat primary bacterial infections.

- There have been reports of adrenal suppression with chronic use of potent topical steroids such as betamethasone over large areas, particularly in children or with the addition of dressings that block airflow.
- Notify your doctor if you have decreased skin circulation.
- Discontinue if skin irritation or contact dermatitis occurs.
- Some areas of the body are more prone to atrophy changes, including the face, groin, and under the arms.
- Avoid contact with the eyes.

DRUG INTERACTIONS
Do not use with other topical products unless directed by your doctor.

FOOD INTERACTIONS
Unknown

HERBAL INTERACTIONS
Unknown

PREGNANCY AND BREAST-FEEDING CAUTIONS
FDA Pregnancy Risk Category C. There are no human data available on use of topical betamethasone in nursing mothers.

SPECIAL INFORMATION
Wash or soak the affected area prior to application. Apply topically in a light film, rub in gently. Do not cover with bandage or dressings unless directed by doctor. Notify your doctor if the condition gets worse.

BETAXOLOL
(be-TAKS-oh-lol)

NEWLY DISCOVERED USES (OFF-LABEL)
Chronic cardiac insufficiency

ORIGINAL USES (ON-LABEL)
Glaucoma, high blood pressure

BRAND NAMES
Betoptic S, Kerlone

DRUG CLASS
Antihypertensive (oral), anti-glaucoma (ocular) (selective beta-adrenergic blocker)

DESCRIPTION

Betaxolol blocks certain receptors in the heart, kidneys, and blood vessels, thereby stabilizing heart rate.

POTENTIAL SIDE EFFECTS

Ocular: Redness in the eye, unequal sizes of pupils, corneal inflammation and staining, decreased corneal sensitivity, eye pain, vision disturbances.

Oral: drowsiness, insomnia, decreased sexual ability, low heart rate, edema, congestive heart failure, reduced peripheral circulation, mental depression, diarrhea or constipation, nausea, vomiting, stomach discomfort, bronchospasm, cold extremities.

CAUTIONS

- Do not use if you have heart conditions such as congestive heart failure, cardiogenic shock, too low heart rate, or second- and third-degree heart block, sinus node dysfunction. Do not use if you are pregnant.
- Do not stop this medication suddenly; instead, taper use over a gradual period.
- May result in exaggerated responses such as increased heart rate, increased blood pressure, chest pain. Consult with your doctor about possible effects on the heart.
- May cause or mask the symptoms of low blood glucose levels in diabetics.
- Should be used cautiously in patients with lung disorders.
- Can cause fetal harm when administered in pregnancy.
- Dosage adjustment is required if you have severe kidney dysfunction or are in dialysis.

DRUG INTERACTIONS

This drug is metabolized (inactivated) by specific set of liver enzymes. Several other drugs interfere with these liver enzymes, and thus may increase or decrease the clearance of betaxolol from the body, increasing the risk of side effects, and often requiring dosage adjustments when they are administered in combination. As these are too numerous to list, you should always check with your doctor or pharmacist prior to starting a new medication.

Other interactions: digoxin, verapamil, diltiazem, reserpine, alpha-blockers (prazosin, terazosin), alpha-adrenergic stimulants (epinephrine, phenylephrine), ergot alkaloids, clonidine, disopyramide, nondepolarizing muscle relaxants, theophylline, aluminum salts, barbiturates, calcium salts, cholestyramine, colestipol, penicillins (ampicillin), rifampin, salicylates, and sulfinpyrazone, sulfonylureas (certain drugs used to treat diabetes).

HERBAL INTERACTIONS
Dong quai, ephedra, ma huang, yohimbe, or ginseng

FOOD INTERACTIONS
Unknown

PREGNANCY AND BREAST-FEEDING CAUTIONS
FDA Pregnancy Risk Category C. Betaxolol does enter breast milk. Consult your doctor prior to starting breast-feeding while on this therapy.

SPECIAL INFORMATION
Ocular: Temporary stinging is common with the use of ocular products. Notify your doctor if stinging does not stop. Do not touch the dropper to any surface. Do not use this product with contact lenses in your eyes.

BISOPROLOL
(bis-OH-proe-lol)

NEWLY DISCOVERED USES (OFF-LABEL)
Congestive heart failure, ventricular tachycardia, prevention of recurrence and sudden death

ORIGINAL USES (ON-LABEL)
High blood pressure

BRAND NAME
Zebeta

DRUG CLASS
Antihypertensive (beta selective blockers)

DESCRIPTION
Bisoprolol stabilizes heart rate and reduces blood pressure.

POTENTIAL SIDE EFFECTS
Drowsiness, insomnia, decreased sexual ability, low heart rate, edema (swelling due to fluid retention), congestive heart failure, reduced peripheral circulation, mental depression, diarrhea or constipation, nausea, vomiting, stomach discomfort.

CAUTIONS

- You should not use this drug if you have certain lung or cardiac diseases. Consult your doctor.
- Do not stop therapy suddenly.
- Use caution if you are taking verapamil or diltiazem, as too low heart rate may occur.
- Use cautiously if you are diabetic; this drug may mask signs of low blood sugar or thyroid problems.
- May cause fetal harm if used in pregnancy trimesters two and three.
- Use cautiously if you have impaired kidney function or myasthenia gravis.

DRUG INTERACTIONS

Digoxin, verapamil, diltiazem, reserpine, alpha-blockers (prazosin, terazosin), alpha-adrenergic stimulants (epinephrine, phenylephrine), ergot alkaloids, clonidine, disopyramide, nondepolarizing muscle relaxants, theophylline, aluminum salts, barbiturates, calcium salts, cholestyramine, colestipol, penicillins (ampicillin), rifampin, salicylates, and sulfinpyrazone, sulfonylureas (certain drugs used to treat diabetes).

This drug is metabolized (inactivated) by specific set of liver enzymes (cytochrome P450 enzymes 3A4). Several other drugs interfere with these liver enzymes, and thus, may increase or decrease the clearance of bisoprolol from the body, increasing the risk of side effects, and often requiring dosage adjustments when they are administered in combination. As these are too numerous to list, you should always check with your doctor or pharmacist prior to starting a new medication.

HERBAL INTERACTIONS

Dong quai, ephedra, yohimbe, ginseng

PREGNANCY AND BREAST-FEEDING CAUTIONS

FDA Pregnancy Risk Category C (manufacturer); D (2nd and 3rd trimesters-expert analysis). The excretion of bisoprolol in breast milk is unknown. Consult with your doctor before breast-feeding during therapy.

BIVALIRUDIN
(bye-VAL-I -roo-din)

NEWLY DISCOVERED USES (OFF-LABEL)
Heparin-induced thrombocytopenia

ORIGINAL USES (ON-LABEL)
Used in combination with aspirin in patients with unstable angina undergoing percutaneous transluminal coronary angioplasty (PTCA)

BRAND NAME
Angiomax

DRUG CLASS
Anticoagulant (thrombin inhibitor)

DESCRIPTION
Bivalirudin stops blood clots from forming by binding to thrombin, a component that is essential in clotting.

POTENTIAL SIDE EFFECTS
Lowered heart rate, changes in blood pressure, pain, headache, insomnia, nervousness, anxiety, nausea, vomiting, upset stomach, abdominal pain, pelvis pain, back pain, urinary retention, major hemorrhage (transfusion required), injection site pain.

CAUTIONS
- Do not use this drug if you are experiencing major bleeding.
- Notify your doctor if you are taking drugs other than aspirin which are known to affect blood clotting or bleeding times.
- Bleeding may occur at any site. Notify your doctor if you fall or have a sudden drop in blood pressure.
- Use with caution if you have any disease associated with increased risk of bleeding.

DRUG INTERACTIONS
Other drugs that affect bleeding or blood clot formation. Check with your doctor or pharmacist prior to starting any new prescription medication, herbal product, or nonprescription drug.

FOOD INTERACTIONS
Unknown

HERBAL INTERACTIONS
Unknown

PREGNANCY AND BREAST-FEEDING CAUTIONS
FDA Pregnancy Risk Category B. Excretion in breast milk is unknown. Consult your doctor.

BLEOMYCIN
(BLEE-o-mice-in)

NEWLY DISCOVERED USES (OFF-LABEL)
Keloids, oral leukoplakia (dysplasia)

ORIGINAL USES (ON-LABEL)
Various cancers

BRAND NAME
Blenoxane

DRUG CLASS
Antineoplastic

DESCRIPTION
Bleomycin prevents the growth or development of malignant cells by blocking the synthesis of DNA.

POTENTIAL SIDE EFFECTS
Raynaud's phenomenon, pain at the tumor site, skin redness, induration, mouth ulcers and inflammation, anorexia, weight loss, increased respiratory rate, lung disorders, acute fever reactions, allergy reactions characterized by decreased blood pressure, confusion, fever, chills, and wheezing, rash, skin thickening.

CAUTIONS
- Do not use this drug if you have severe pulmonary disease, or if you are pregnant.
- The risk of developing lung fibrosis is higher in the following groups: elderly patients; those receiving greater 400 units total of the drug; smokers; and patients with prior radiation therapy.
- Severe reactions (such as low blood pressure, mental confusion, fever, chills and wheezing) have been reported in less than 1% of lymphoma patients. Careful monitoring is needed during the first and second treatment if you have lymphoma.
- Check lungs prior to each treatment for signs of toxicity (such as shortness of breath, chest sounds during breathing). Chest x-rays should be performed to check for lung damage.

- Changes in kidney or liver function have occurred.
- Skin reactions are related to cumulative dose (after 150 to 200 units).

DRUG INTERACTIONS
Lomustine, cisplatin, digoxin, phenytoin

FOOD INTERACTIONS
Unknown

HERBAL INTERACTIONS
Unknown

PREGNANCY AND BREAST-FEEDING CAUTIONS
FDA Pregnancy Risk Category D. Excretion into breast milk is unknown. Do not breast-feed during therapy.

SPECIAL INFORMATION
This drug has a black box warning regarding the risk of severe lung toxicity, specifically, lung fibrosis. Although the risk seems highest in the elderly and with high doses, it has occurred at low doses and in all ages. Severe reactions are also possible.

BOTULINUM TOXIN TYPE A
(BOT-yoo-lin-num-TOKS-in type-aye)

NEWLY DISCOVERED USES (OFF-LABEL)

Cerebral palsy, essential tremor, migraine treatment and prevention, tension headache treatment and prevention, trigeminal neuralgia

ORIGINAL USES (ON-LABEL)
Strabismus (eye disorder of alignment) and blepharospasm (eyelid spasms) associated with dystonia (uncontrolled muscle movements), cervical dystonia to decrease the severity of abnormal head and neck pain, wrinkles of the face

BRAND NAMES
Botox, Botox cosmetic

DRUG CLASS
Neuromuscular blocker, ophthalmic

DESCRIPTION
Botulinum toxin A reduces muscle activity by blocking neuromuscular impulses on the nerve ends.

POTENTIAL SIDE EFFECTS
Ocular use: double vision, scleral perforation, eye dryness, drooping eyelid, vertical deviation of the eye, site reaction, eye irritation, tearing, local swelling, headache.

Other: Headache, difficulty swallowing, neck pain, upper respiratory infection, dizziness, speech disorder, fever, drowsiness, dry mouth, nausea, injection site reaction, back pain, hypertonia, weakness, facial pain, cough.

CAUTIONS
- This product contains a small amount of albumin from human sources.
- You should not use this drug if you are pregnant, if you have disease of neuromuscular transmission, or clotting problems, including therapeutic anticoagulation.
- Higher doses or more frequent administration may result in reduced efficacy.
- Use caution if you have inflammation, excessive weakness, or atrophy at the proposed injection site.
- Adequate contraception in women of childbearing age is needed.
- Do not use more frequently than every three months.

DRUG INTERACTIONS
Aminoglycosides and neuromuscular blocking drugs

FOOD INTERACTIONS
Unknown

HERBAL INTERACTIONS
Unknown

PREGNANCY AND BREAST-FEEDING CAUTIONS
FDA Pregnancy Risk Category C. Excretion in breast milk is unknown; the use of this therapy during breast-feeding is not recommended.

SPECIAL INFORMATION
Contact your doctor if you develop difficulties in swallowing, speech, or breathing.

BOTULINUM TOXIN TYPE B
(BOT-yoo-lin-num-TOKS-in type bee)

NEWLY DISCOVERED USES (OFF-LABEL)
Anal fissure

ORIGINAL USES (ON-LABEL)
Cervical dystonia, abnormal head and neck pain

BRAND NAME
Myobloc

DRUG CLASS
Neuromuscular blocker

DESCRIPTION
Botulinum toxin B reduces muscle activity by blocking neuro-muscular impulses on the nerve ends.

POTENTIAL SIDE EFFECTS
Dry mouth, difficulty swallowing, upset stomach, pain at injection site, dizziness, nausea, infection, flu syndrome, back pain, increased cough, runny nose.

CAUTIONS
- This product contains a small amount of albumin from human sources.
- Use cautiously if you have neuromuscular or neuropathic disorders.
- Use caution if you have inflammation, excessive weakness, or atrophy at the proposed injection site.
- Do not use more frequently than every three months.

DRUG INTERACTIONS
Aminoglycosides and neuromuscular blocking drugs

FOOD INTERACTIONS
Unknown

HERBAL INTERACTIONS
Unknown

PREGNANCY AND BREAST-FEEDING CAUTIONS
FDA Pregnancy Risk Category C. Excretion in breast milk is unknown; the use of this therapy during breast-feeding is not recommended.

BROMOCRIPTINE
(broe-moe-KRIP-teen)

NEWLY DISCOVERED USES (OFF-LABEL)

Mastalgia, male infertility, periodic limb movement disorder, premenstrual syndrome (PMS), therapy- psoriatic arthritis, Reiter's syndrome, rheumatoid arthritis, systemic lupus erythematosus (SLE)

ORIGINAL USES (ON-LABEL)

Amenorrhea (absence of menstruation) with or without galactorrhea (excessive or spontaneous milk flow), infertility or hypogonadism, prolactin-secreting cancers, increased prolactin levels, acromegaly, Parkinson's disease, pituitary tumors

BRAND NAME
Parlodel

DRUG CLASS
Anti-Parkinson's (dopamine agonist, ergot alkaloid)

DESCRIPTION
Bromocriptine inhibits the secretion of prolactin, a pituitary hormone that stimulates the secretion of milk. It also stimulates normal ovulation and menstruation cycles.

POTENTIAL SIDE EFFECTS
Headache, increased heart rate, dry mouth, irregular heart rate, constipation, diarrhea, drowsiness, psychosis, dizziness, fatigue, lightheadedness, nausea, anorexia, vomiting, abdominal cramps, low blood pressure upon standing from a sitting or lying down position, nasal congestion.

CAUTIONS
- Inform your doctor if you are allergic to ergot alkaloids, have uncontrolled high blood pressure, a history of or current heart disease, peripheral vascular disorders, psychosis, dementia, or are pregnant. Also inform your doctor if you have reduced kidney or liver function, or if you are taking medications to lower your blood pressure.
- Monitoring for cardiac effects during and immediately following pregnancy as a continuation of previous therapy.
- Pleural and peritoneal fibrosis have been reported with prolonged daily use.

- Cardiac valvular fibrosis has also been associated with ergot alkaloids.

DRUG INTERACTIONS

Antipsychotics, metoclopramide. This drug is metabolized by and affects a specific set of liver enzymes. Several other drugs are metabolized by these liver enzymes, and thus, may have increased or decreased clearance from the body, potentially increasing the risk of side effects or decreasing effectiveness. When these drugs are given in combination with bromocriptine dosage adjustments may be needed. You should always check with your doctor or pharmacist prior to starting a new medication, herbal, or nonprescription product.

FOOD INTERACTIONS

Alcohol (may increase gastric side effects or alcohol intolerance)

HERBAL INTERACTIONS

St. John's wort

PREGNANCY AND BREAST-FEEDING CAUTIONS

FDA Pregnancy Risk Category B. Do not breast-feed while taking this medication. Bromocriptine is excreted in breast milk.

SPECIAL INFORMATION

Use of this drug requires monitoring of blood pressure as well as liver, cardiac, and blood function. Dizziness or fainting may occur after the first dose. Avoid sudden changes from sleeping or sitting position. Use contraceptives other than oral contraceptives during therapy.

BUDESONIDE
(byoo-DES-oh-nide)

NEWLY DISCOVERED USES (OFF-LABEL)

Chronic otitis media, primary biliary cirrhosis (used with UDCA), sarcoidosis

ORIGINAL USES (ON-LABEL)

Asthma, Crohn's disease, rhinitis

BRAND NAMES
Entocort EC, Pulmicort Respules, Pulmicort Turbuhaler, Rhinocort Aqua

DRUG CLASS
Corticosteroid

DESCRIPTION
Budesonide prevents or controls inflammation at many sites in the body such as the gastrointestinal tract and lungs.

POTENTIAL SIDE EFFECTS
Headache, chest pain, emotional lability, nausea (oral capsule), abdominal pain, anorexia, diarrhea, respiratory infection, rhinitis, bronchitis, sudden loss of strength, edema (swelling related to fluid retention), high blood pressure, bruising, contact dermatitis, eczema, cervical low potassium levels, adrenal insufficiency, muscle aches, fracture, increased excessive tone of skeletal muscles, eye inflammation, eye infection, earache, ear infection, external ear infection, flu-like syndrome, herpes simplex.

CAUTIONS
- When taken in high doses for prolonged periods of time, this therapy may suppress your body's production and release of hormones from the adrenal gland.
- Orally-inhaled and intranasal corticosteroids may cause a reduced rate of growth in children. The lowest effective dose should be used. Growth rate in children taking prolonged therapy should be monitored.
- May suppress the immune system, increasing the risk of infection.
- Should be used with caution if you have high blood pressure, glaucoma, diabetes, hypertension, osteoporosis, peptic ulcer, cataracts, tuberculosis, or infections.
- While on therapy you should avoid contact with other persons who have chicken pox or shingles.
- Use caution if you have reduced liver function.

DRUG INTERACTIONS
Warfarin, cyclosporine, digoxin, isoniazid, diuretics, salicylates, aminogluthimide, barbiturates, cholestyramine, oral contraceptives, ephedrine, estrogens, phenytoin, ketoconazole, rifampin, macrolide antibiotics (e.g., erythromycin, clarithromycin, azithromycin, etc.). This drug is inactivated and cleared from the body by a specific set of liver enzymes called cytochrome P3A4.

Any drugs which prevent the action of these enzymes could cause higher levels of budesonide and require low doses of the drug during combination therapy. Consult your pharmacist or physician before starting any new therapy.

FOOD INTERACTIONS
Grapefruit juice, high fat meal (oral capsules)

HERBAL INTERACTIONS
St. John's wort

PREGNANCY AND BREAST-FEEDING CAUTIONS
FDA Pregnancy Risk Category C/B. Use with caution in breast-feeding; this drug enters breast milk.

SPECIAL INFORMATION
This drug has a black box warning regarding the proper transfer from oral corticosteroids to inhaled corticosteroids.

BUMETANIDE
(byoo-MET-a-nide)

NEWLY DISCOVERED USES (OFF-LABEL)
Nocturia

ORIGINAL USES (ON-LABEL)
Management of edema (swelling associated with fluid retention) associated with congestive heart failure, liver and kidney disease

BRAND NAME
Bumex

DRUG CLASS
Blood pressure medication (loop diuretic)

DESCRIPTION
Bumetanide helps your body excrete fluids by inhibiting reabsorption of sodium and chloride in the kidney.

POTENTIAL SIDE EFFECTS
Gout, electrolyte imbalances (low levels of sodium, potassium or chloride), reduced kidney function, dizziness, muscle cramps, ear problems (impaired hearing, discomfort), nausea, vomiting, fatigue, gastric irritation, headache, dehydration, dry mouth, itching, hives, sweating, chest pain.

CAUTIONS

- This drug can cause excessive loss of fluid and electrolytes; close medical supervision is required.
- Risk of serious ear problems are increased with severely reduced kidney function, high doses, and when used with other drugs that cause ear toxicities.
- Do not use this drug if you have a history of allergies to sulfonamides.
- Requires monitoring of electrolyte levels (such as potassium, sodium, magnesium, etc.).
- This drug may cause a skin reaction related to sun exposure.

DRUG INTERACTIONS

Digoxin, lithium, high dose aspirin and other salicylates, aminoglycosides (e.g., amikacin, gentamicin, tobramycin, etc.), warfarin, chloral hydrate, cisplatin, clofibrate, probenecid, nonsteroidal anti-inflammatory drugs (NSAIDs-indomethacin, etc.), other diuretics, cholestyramine, colestipol.

FOOD INTERACTIONS

Use of this drug may require potassium-rich foods or potassium supplements to maintain potassium balance.

HERBAL INTERACTIONS

Ephedra, yohimbe, ginseng, dong quai

PREGNANCY AND BREAST-FEEDING CAUTIONS

FDA Pregnancy Risk Category C (manufacturer), D (expert analysis). It is unknown if this drug is excreted in breast milk; use with caution.

SPECIAL INFORMATION

This drug has a black box warning regarding the need to perform frequent monitoring of electrolytes and kidney function during the first months of therapy and periodically thereafter.

BUPROPION
(byoo-PROE-pee-on)

NEWLY DISCOVERED USES (OFF-LABEL)

Attention deficit/hyperactivity disorder (ADHD), bipolar disorder, chronic neuropathic pain, diabetic neuropathy, female orgasmic disorder, hypoactive sexual desire disorder

ORIGINAL USES (ON-LABEL)
Treatment of depression (Wellbutrin) and used in combination therapy in smoking cessation (Zyban)

BRAND NAMES
Wellbutrin, Wellbutrin SR, Wellbutrin XL, Zyban

DRUG CLASS
Antidepressant, smoking deterrent (dopamine-reuptake inhibitor)

DESCRIPTION
Bupropion is used to manage depression and limit the cravings and other symptoms associated with nicotine withdrawal. The drug works by inhibiting the activity of certain chemicals in the brain.

POTENTIAL SIDE EFFECTS
Dizziness, headache, insomnia, nausea, dry mouth, sore throat, chest pain, agitation, anxiety, memory decreased, nervousness, itching, rash, sweating increased, anorexia, constipation, diarrhea, taste perversion, urinary frequency, joint aches, arthritis, muscle aches, tremor, double vision, ringing in ears, cough increased, abdominal pain, increased heart rate, sedation.

CAUTIONS
- Inform your doctor if you currently have or a history of seizures, anorexia, bulimia, liver or kidney dysfunction, high blood pressure, or heart disease.
- Do not use if you have used MAO inhibitors within 14 days or if you have suddenly stopped sedatives or chronic alcohol use.
- Elderly patients may need to be monitored while using this drug.
- Notify your doctor if you experience any changes in concentration or mental status.
- Wear protective clothing and sunscreen, as this drug has been associated with photosensitivity reactions (skin reactions related to sun exposure).

DRUG INTERACTIONS
Desipramine, paroxetine, sertraline, orphenadrine, thiotepa, cyclophosphamide, carbamazepine, nevirapine, phenobarbital, phenytoin, rifampin, amantadine, levodopa, tonavir, warfarin.

This drug is metabolized by a specific set of liver enzymes. Several other drugs interfere with these liver enzymes, and thus, may increase or decrease the clearance of bupropion from the body, potentially increasing the risk of side effects or decreasing effectiveness. When these drugs are given in combination with bupropion, dosage adjustments may be needed. As these are too numerous to list, you should always check with your doctor or pharmacist prior to starting a new medication, herbal, or nonprescription product.

FOOD INTERACTIONS
Alcohol

HERBAL INTERACTIONS
Valerian, St. John's wort, SAMe, gotu kola, kava kava

PREGNANCY AND BREAST-FEEDING CAUTIONS
FDA Pregnancy Risk Category B. This drug is excreted in breast milk. Breast-feeding is not recommended during therapy with this drug.

SPECIAL INFORMATION
Do not use Zyban and Wellbutrin concurrently, as they contain the same active ingredient.

Take immediate release formulations in equally divided doses (three or four times daily) to avoid risk of seizures. Do not chew or crush the XL or SR formulations. The bupropion XL formulation may be excreted in the stool. This is an empty shell which is not absorbed. The drug has been absorbed. This drug may cause significant sedation and drowsiness, which may impair your ability to perform tasks requiring judgment or motor or cognitive skills. If you experience a seizure while on this medication, stop immediately and report it to your doctor.

In January 2005, the FDA announced new labeling for antidepressants regarding the need to closely monitor for worsening of depression and for the potential of increased suicidal thinking or suicide behavior during therapy. Although this recommendation applies to all patients (adults, children, and adolescents) treated with antidepressants for any indication, this is of particular importance if you are being treated for depression.

BUSPIRONE
(byoo-SPYE-rone)

NEWLY DISCOVERED USES (OFF-LABEL)
Alcohol withdrawal, alcoholism (cravings & dependency), Alzheimer's disease, premenstrual disorder, social phobia

---

ORIGINAL USES (ON-LABEL)
Generalized anxiety disorder (GAD)

BRAND NAME
BuSpar

DRUG CLASS
Antianxiety

DESCRIPTION
Buspirone is used to help manage anxiety. It works by affecting the levels of certain neurotransmitters in the brain.

POTENTIAL SIDE EFFECTS
Dizziness, drowsiness, serotonin syndrome, confusion, rash, diarrhea, nausea, muscle weakness, numbness, tingling, incoordination, blurred vision, tunnel vision, increased sweating, allergic reactions, insomnia, dry mouth, fatigue.

CAUTIONS
- Safety and efficacy of this drug has not been established in children less than 18 years of age.
- This drug is not recommended if you have liver or kidney impairment.
- This drug does not prevent or treat withdrawal from benzodiazepines.
- Although this drug has a low potential for interfering with mental status and alertness, please use caution during initial therapy while operating machinery or performing tasks that require alertness.

DRUG INTERACTIONS
Cimetidine, fluoxetine, nefazodone, diazepam, alcohol, haloperidol, MAO inhibitors, trazodone.

This drug is metabolized by specific set of liver enzymes. Several other drugs interfere with these liver enzymes, and thus may increase or decrease the clearance of buspirone from the body, potentially increasing the risk of side effects or decreasing effectiveness. When these drugs are given in combination with buspirone, dosage adjustments may be needed. As these are too numerous to list, you should always check with your doctor or pharmacist prior to starting a new medication, herbal, or nonprescription product.

FOOD INTERACTIONS
Avoid drinking large amounts of grapefruit juice. Take consistently, always with or without food.

HERBAL INTERACTIONS
St. John's wort, valerian, gotu kola, and kava kava

PREGNANCY AND BREAST-FEEDING CAUTIONS
FDA Pregnancy Risk Category B. Excretion in breast milk is unknown. Breast-feeding is not recommended while using this drug.

SPECIAL INFORMATION
Avoid alcohol while using this drug.

CABERGOLINE
(ca-BER-goe-leen)

NEWLY DISCOVERED USES (OFF-LABEL)
Acromegaly

ORIGINAL USES (ON-LABEL)
Hyperprolactinemic (increased prolactin levels) disorders

BRAND NAME
Dostinex

DRUG CLASS
Ergot alkaloid and derivative

DESCRIPTION
Cabergoline inhibits the secretion of prolactin, a hormone secreted by the pituitary gland, by stimulating the release of dopamine.

POTENTIAL SIDE EFFECTS
Dizziness, fatigue, headache, constipation, nausea, somnolence, depression, low blood pressure upon standing from a sitting or lying position (orthostatic hypotension), vertigo, numbness, abdominal pain, upset stomach, vomiting.

CAUTIONS

- Orthostatic hypotension (a sudden decrease in blood pressure upon standing from a sitting or lying position) may occur if initial doses are greater than 1 mg.
- This drug is not indicated for the inhibition of the normal lactation after birth, since this has been associated with high blood pressure, seizures, and stroke.
- Do not take this drug if you are a post-partum woman who is breast-feeding or planning to breast-feed.
- Use with caution if you have reduced liver function.

DRUG INTERACTIONS

Antihypertensive medications (result in excessive lowering of blood pressure), metoclopramide, phenothiazines (antipsychotics).

FOOD INTERACTIONS

Unknown

HERBAL INTERACTIONS

Unknown

PREGNANCY AND BREAST-FEEDING CAUTIONS

FDA Pregnancy Risk Category B. It is not known if this drug is excreted in the breast milk, but its action would suppress normal physiologic lactation. Thus, it is not recommended during breast-feeding.

SPECIAL INFORMATION

Avoid sudden changes in posture and stand up slowly while using this drug.

CALCITONIN
(kal-si-TOE-nin)

NEWLY DISCOVERED USES (OFF-LABEL)

Bone cysts in children

ORIGINAL USES (ON-LABEL)

High calcium levels, postmenopausal osteoporosis, Paget's disease

BRAND NAME

Miacalcin

DRUG CLASS
Drug to reduce hypercalcemia (high calcium levels)

DESCRIPTION
This drug blocks the break down of bones and promotes the production of calcium, phosphate, sodium, magnesium and potassium.

POTENTIAL SIDE EFFECTS
Facial flushing, nausea, diarrhea, anorexia, swelling at injection site, frequent urination, back/joint pain, nasal bleeding/crusting following intranasal administration.

CAUTIONS
- Because allergic reactions may be a possibility, skin testing should be performed prior to starting therapy with calcitonin salmon. Inform your doctor if you are allergic to salmon protein or gelatin (used as a diluent).
- Excessive low levels of calcium may potentially cause cramping.
- A nasal exam should be performed prior to the initiation of therapy or after adverse events. If using the nasal spray, notify your doctor if significant nasal irritation occurs.

DRUG INTERACTIONS
Calcium, vitamin D

FOOD INTERACTIONS
Alcohol

HERBAL INTERACTIONS
Unknown

PREGNANCY AND BREAST-FEEDING CAUTIONS
FDA Pregnancy Risk Category C. Excretion in breast milk is unknown. In animals, this drug has suppressed the production of breast milk. Consult your doctor.

SPECIAL INFORMATION
If using the spray for the first time, activate the pump and press the pump six times until a faint spray is emitted.

CANDESARTAN
(kan-de-SAR-tan)

NEWLY DISCOVERED USES (OFF-LABEL) ⎯⎯⎯⎯⎯⎯
Diabetic nephropathy, migraine prevention, tension headache prevention

ORIGINAL USES (ON-LABEL)
Alone or in combination with other blood pressure drugs in treating essential hypertension

BRAND NAMES
Atacand

DRUG CLASS
Antihypertensive (angiotensin II receptor antagonist [ARB])

DESCRIPTION
Candesartan blocks the constriction of blood vessels and affects the body's secretion of aldosterone.

POTENTIAL SIDE EFFECTS
Flushing, increased heart rate, angina, dizziness, lightheadedness, drowsiness, headache, rash, increased levels of blood sugar, triglycerides, and uric acid, blood in the urine, back pain, weakness, upper respiratory tract infection, bronchitis, nose bleeds, increased sweating.

CAUTIONS
- Do not use if you have certain kidney problem, such as kidney artery stenosis.
- Do not use if you are pregnant in your second or third trimester.
- Lower doses are needed if you have liver impairment.

DRUG INTERACTIONS
Potassium supplements, potassium-sparing diuretics, lithium, trimethoprim

FOOD INTERACTIONS
Food reduces the time to reach maximum levels and increases the peak concentrations in the body.

HERBAL INTERACTIONS
Dong quai, ephedra, yohimbe, ginseng and garlic

PREGNANCY AND BREAST-FEEDING CAUTIONS
FDA Pregnancy Risk Category C in first trimester, category D in second and third trimesters. Do not use during second and third trimesters of pregnancy. This drug is excreted in breast milk. Breast-feeding while using this drug is not recommended.

SPECIAL INFORMATION
This drug has a black box warning regarding the fetal toxicities associated with the use of this drug class during the second and third trimesters of pregnancy. When pregnancy is detected, the drug should be discontinued as soon as possible.

CAPTOPRIL
(KAP-toe-pril)

NEWLY DISCOVERED USES (OFF-LABEL)
Cystinuria, dilated cardiomyopathy, idiopathic edema, hyperaldosteronism (diagnostic test), hypertensive crisis, pulmonary edema, Raynaud's Syndrome, rheumatoid arthritis, stroke risk reduction

ORIGINAL USES (ON-LABEL)
High blood pressure, congestive heart failure, after heart attacks, diabetic nephropathy

BRAND NAME
Capoten

DRUG CLASS
Blood pressure medication

DESCRIPTION
Captopril lowers blood pressure by inhibiting the production of chemicals that cause blood vessels to constrict. It also may cause the brain to release hormones that lower blood pressure.

POTENTIAL SIDE EFFECTS
Chest pain, too low blood pressure (especially after first dose), cough, fainting, headache, dizziness, fatigue, weakness, rash, abnormal taste, nausea, shortness of breath.

CAUTIONS
- Do not use if you have had tongue, lip, throat, or mouth swelling (symptoms of angioedema) after taking other drugs in

the same class or if you have these symptoms unrelated to drug therapy. Angioedema can occur at any time during treatment, but especially following the first dose. Report symptoms to your doctor.

- Do not use if you are pregnant in the second or third trimester.
- Do not use if you have certain kidney problems (kidney artery stenosis, decreased kidney function).
- Avoid rapid dosage increases, which may lead to kidney problems.

DRUG INTERACTIONS

Potassium supplements, co-trimoxazole (high dose), aluminum and magnesium containing antacids, iron, angiotension II receptor antagonists (candesartan, losartan, irbesartan, etc.) or potassium sparing diuretics (amiloride, spironolactone, triamterene), allopurinol, digoxin, lithium, and certain drugs used to treat diabetes.

Aspirin (high doses) or indomethacin may aggravate the beneficial effects of this drug.

FOOD INTERACTIONS

Captopril serum concentrations may be decreased if taken with food; take drug one hour before meals.

HERBAL INTERACTIONS

St. John's wort, capsaicin, dong quai, ephedra, yohimbe, ginseng, large amounts of natural licorice

PREGNANCY AND BREAST-FEEDING CAUTIONS

FDA Pregnancy Risk Category C for first trimester. FDA Pregnancy Risk Category D for second and third trimester. This drug is excreted in breast milk. The American Academy of Pediatrics considers this drug compatible with breast-feeding.

SPECIAL INFORMATION

Long-term use of captopril may result in a zinc deficiency, which can result in a decrease in taste perception. Report any vomiting, diarrhea, excessive perspiration, or dehydration to your physician. If any swelling of the face, lips, extremities, lips, tongue, throat or difficulty in breathing occurs or if a persistent dry cough develops it should be reported too. Separate ingestion of captopril with oral iron or antacids (containing magnesium and aluminum) by at least two hours. This drug has a black box warning regarding the fetal toxicities associated with the use of this drug class during the second and third trimesters of pregnancy.

CARBAMAZEPINE
(kar-ba-MAZ-e-peen)

NEWLY DISCOVERED USES (OFF-LABEL)
Alcohol withdrawal psychosis, Alzheimer's disease, benzodiazepine withdrawal, central neurogenic diabetes insipidus, chronic neuropathic pain, cocaine addiction, diabetes insipidus, diabetic neuropathy, hiccups, migraine prevention in children, multiple sclerosis, partial central diabetes insipidus, postpartum psychosis and lactation, post traumatic stress disorder (PTSD), schizoaffective disorder, vulvodynia

ORIGINAL USES (ON-LABEL)
Certain types of seizures (partial seizures, generalized tonic-clonic, mixed seizure patterns, or other partial or generalized seizures), trigeminal neuralgia

BRAND NAMES
Carbatrol, Epitol, Tegretol, Tegretol XR

DRUG CLASS
Anticonvulsant

DESCRIPTION
This drug is used to control seizures to treat certain pain syndromes.

POTENTIAL SIDE EFFECTS
Edema, congestive heart failure, fainting, slow heart rate, sedation, dizziness, fatigue, uncoordinated gait, rash, hives, severe skin reactions (e.g., toxic epidermal necrolysis, Stevens-Johnson syndrome), decreased sodium levels, fever, chills, nausea, vomiting, gastric distress, abdominal pain, urinary retention, kidney dysfunction, impotence, blood disorders (e.g., aplastic anemia, agranulocytosis, eosinophilia, leukopenia), changes in liver function, jaundice, liver failure, blurred vision, uncontrolled eye movements, lens opacities, eye irritation and inflammation, ringing in the ears.

CAUTIONS
- Not for use if you have marrow suppression or certain blood disorders. Potentially fatal blood cell abnormalities have been reported with the use of this drug.

- Do not use while taking MAO inhibitors; these drugs should be discontinued for a minimum of 14 days before carbamazepine is begun.
- Notify your doctor if you have a history of heart damage or liver disease.
- Severe skin reactions have been reported rarely, but may be serious. Report any sign of rash to your doctor immediately.
- Requires baseline assessment of blood, liver and kidney function, and eye exam.
- Elderly may have increased risk of SIADH-like (syndrome of inappropriate diuretic hormone).

DRUG INTERACTIONS
Protease inhibitors, cimetidine, clarithromycin, danazol, diltiazem, erythromycin, felbamate, fluoxetine, fluvoxamine, isoniazid, lamotrigine, metronidazole, propoxyphene, verapamil, fluconazole, itraconazole, ketoconazole, acetaminophen, lithium, benzodiazepines, citalopram, clozapine, corticosteroids, cyclosporine, doxycycline, ethosuximide, felbamate, felodipine, haloperidol, mebendazole, methadone, oral contraceptives, phenytoin, tacrolimus, theophylline, thyroid hormones, tricyclic antidepressants, valproic acid, warfarin, mefloquine.

This drug is metabolized by specific set of liver enzymes. Several other drugs interfere with these liver enzymes, and thus may increase or decrease the clearance of carbamazepine from the body, potentially increasing the risk of side effects or decreasing effectiveness. When these drugs are given in combination with carbamazepine, dosage adjustments may be needed. As these are too numerous to list, you should always check with your doctor or pharmacist prior to starting a new medication, herbal, or nonprescription product.

FOOD INTERACTIONS
Alcohol. Avoid concurrent use with grapefruit juice. Take with food.

HERBAL INTERACTIONS
Evening primrose, valerian, St. John's wort, kava kava, gotu kola, quinine

PREGNANCY AND BREAST-FEEDING CAUTIONS
FDA Pregnancy Risk Category D. This drug is excreted in breast milk. Consult your doctor prior to beginning breast-feeding.

SPECIAL INFORMATION

This drug has a black box warning regarding the potential for serious blood disorders. Requires baseline assessment of blood prior to the initiation of therapy and periodic monitoring thereafter.

CARBIDOPA-LEVODOPA
(kar-bi-DOE-pa lee-voe-DOE-pa)

NEWLY DISCOVERED USES (OFF-LABEL)
Periodic limb movement disorder, post-herpetic neuralgia

ORIGINAL USES (ON-LABEL)
Parkinson's disease

BRAND NAMES
Sinemet, Sinemet CR

DRUG CLASS
Dopamine agonist

DESCRIPTION
Levodopa is used to treat Parkinson's disease and some pain disorders. It works by circulating in the blood to the brain, where it is converted to dopamine. (A reduction in the concentration of dopamine is associated with Parkinson's disease.)

POTENTIAL SIDE EFFECTS
Anorexia, nausea, vomiting, abdominal pain, dry mouth, difficulty swallowing, taste disturbances, increased saliva production, difficulty walking, increased hand tremor, headache, dizziness, numbness, weakness, faintness, confusion, insomnia, nightmares, hallucinations, delusions, agitation, anxiety, malaise, fatigue, euphoria, decreased blood pressure upon standing from a sitting or lying down position (orthostatic hypotension), paranoid ideation, depression, urinary retention, on-off phenomenon (oscillation between improved clinical symptoms to abrupt loss of therapeutic effects).

CAUTIONS
- Inform your doctor if you have narrow angle glaucoma, if you have used MAO inhibitors within the prior 14 days, or if you have a history of melanoma or undiagnosed skin lesions.

- Use with caution if you have a history of cardiovascular disease, lung diseases, kidney, liver, or endocrine disease, or if you are at risk of low blood pressure.
- Abrupt discontinuation may cause worsening of Parkinson's disease.
- Elderly patients may be more sensitive to central nervous system effects of levodopa.
- Your doctor should observe you for depression with suicidal tendencies while you are taking this drug.
- This drug has been associated with a syndrome resembling neuroleptic malignant syndrome on withdrawal or significant dosage reduction after long-term use.
- Toxic reactions have occurred with dextromethorphan.
- Gastric bleeding has occurred in patients with a history of peptic ulcer.

DRUG INTERACTIONS

Iron, MAO inhibitors, antipsychotics (use antipsychotics with low dopamine blockade), benzodiazepines, L-methionine, phenytoin, pyridoxine, spiramycin, tacrine, antacids, metoclopramide, tricyclic antidepressants.

FOOD INTERACTIONS

High-protein diets may inhibit levodopa's efficacy; avoid high-protein foods. Protein in the diet should be distributed throughout the day to avoid fluctuations in levodopa absorption. May cause gastric upset; take with food. Avoid alcohol and high intakes of vitamin B6.

HERBAL INTERACTIONS

Kava kava

PREGNANCY AND BREAST-FEEDING CAUTIONS

FDA Pregnancy Risk Category C. Excretion in breast milk is unknown.

SPECIAL INFORMATION

The effects of this drug may be delayed (several weeks). Notify your doctor if uncontrollable movements of the face, eyelids, mouth, tongue, neck, arms, or legs occur.

CARBOPROST
(KAR-boe-prost)

NEWLY DISCOVERED USES (OFF-LABEL)
Cervical ripening, incomplete abortion, labor induction

ORIGINAL USES (ON-LABEL)
Abortion, postpartum hemorrhage

BRAND NAME
Hemabate

DRUG CLASS
Abortifacient (prostaglandin)

DESCRIPTION
This drug stimulates uterine contractions in a way similar to labor, resulting in expulsion of the products of conception. It is used to induce abortion between 13-20 weeks of pregnancy.

POTENTIAL SIDE EFFECTS
Diarrhea, vomiting, nausea, flushing, dizziness, headache, stomach cramps.

CAUTIONS
- Inform your doctor if you have asthma, blood pressure problems, cardiovascular, adrenal, kidney or liver disease, anemia, jaundice, diabetes, seizures, acute pelvic inflammatory disease, or uterine problems.

DRUG INTERACTIONS
Oxytocics (such as oxytocin, ergonovine maleate, methylergonovine maleate, etc.)

FOOD INTERACTIONS
Unknown

HERBAL INTERACTIONS
Unknown

PREGNANCY AND BREAST-FEEDING CAUTIONS
FDA Pregnancy Risk Category X. Excretion in breast milk is unknown; the opportunity for use is minimal. Consult your doctor.

CARVEDILOL
(KAR-ve-dil-ole)

NEWLY DISCOVERED USES (OFF-LABEL)

Ventricular tachycardia, prevention of recurrence and sudden death

ORIGINAL USES (ON-LABEL)

High blood pressure, mild to severe heart failure, left ventricular dysfunction following a myocardial infarction

BRAND NAME

Coreg

DRUG CLASS

Alpha-/beta-adrenergic blocker

DESCRIPTION

Carvedilol blocks a type of cell membrane, called beta-adrenergic receptors, in the heart to stabilize heart rate and reduce blood pressure.

POTENTIAL SIDE EFFECTS

Low blood pressure, dizziness, fatigue, changes in blood glucose, weight gain, diarrhea, weakness, low heart rate, headache, fever, increased liver function tests, gout, nausea, vomiting, impotence, back pain, joint pain, muscle aches, blurred vision, abnormal renal function, albuminuria, increased cough.

CAUTIONS

- Notify your doctor if you have cardiac failure, bronchial asthma, second- or third-degree AV block, sick sinus syndrome, severe low heart rate, severe liver impairment, or, in 2nd and 3rd trimester of pregnancy.
- Avoid driving or hazardous tasks during initiation of therapy.
- Avoid abrupt discontinuation. Dose should be tapered over 1-2 weeks.
- It may mask signs of thyroid problems.

DRUG INTERACTIONS

This drug is metabolized by specific set of liver enzymes (cytochrome P450 enzymes). Several other drugs interfere with these liver enzymes, and thus may increase or decrease the clearance of carvedilol from the body, potentially increasing the risk of side effects or decreasing effectiveness. When these drugs are given in combination with carvedilol, dosage adjustments may be needed. As these are too numerous to list, you should always check with your doctor or pharmacist prior to starting a new medication, herbal, or nonprescription product.

FOOD INTERACTIONS
Garlic

HERBAL INTERACTIONS
Dong quai, ephedra, yohimbe, and ginseng

PREGNANCY AND BREAST-FEEDING CAUTIONS
FDA Pregnancy Risk Category C (manufacturer); D (2nd and 3rd trimesters—expert analysis).

CEFOTAXIME
(sef-oh-TAKS-eem)

NEWLY DISCOVERED USES (OFF-LABEL)
Nocardiosis

ORIGINAL USES (ON-LABEL)
Susceptible infections in respiratory tract, skin and skin structure, bone and joint, urinary tract, gynecologic, and documented or suspected meningitis

BRAND NAME
Claforan

DRUG CLASS
Antibiotic (3rd generation cephalosporin)

DESCRIPTION
This drug inhibits the production of the cell walls of bacteria.

POTENTIAL SIDE EFFECTS
Rash, pruritus, diarrhea, nausea, vomiting, inflammation of the colon tissue, pain at injection site.

CAUTIONS
- Dosage may need to be reduced if you have severe kidney dysfunction.
- Prolonged use may result in superinfection.
- May cause colitis (inflammation of the colon tissue).

- Notify your doctor if you have had an allergic reaction to other cephalosporins or to a penicillin.

DRUG INTERACTIONS
Probenecid, furosemide, aminoglycosides (e.g., gentamicin, amikacin, tobramycin, etc.)

FOOD INTERACTIONS
Unknown

HERBAL INTERACTIONS
Unknown

PREGNANCY AND BREAST-FEEDING CAUTIONS
FDA Pregnancy Risk Category B. This drug is excreted in breast milk. The American Academy of Pediatrics classifies it as compatible with breast-feeding. Use with caution.

CEFOXITIN
(se-FOKS-i-tin)

NEWLY DISCOVERED USES (OFF-LABEL)
Diverticulitis

ORIGINAL USES (ON-LABEL)
Infections of the respiratory tract, skin and skin structure, bone and joint, urinary tract and gynecologic, intra-abdominal. Also used for septicemia and in the prevention of infections associated with surgery.

BRAND NAME
Mefoxin

DRUG CLASS
Antibiotic (2nd generation cephalosporin)

DESCRIPTION
This drug inhibits the production of bacterial cell walls.

POTENTIAL SIDE EFFECTS
Diarrhea, rash, nausea, itching

CAUTIONS
- Dosage may need to be reduced if you have severe kidney dysfunction.

- Prolonged use may result in superinfection.
- May cause colitis (inflammation of the colon tissue).
- Notify your doctor if you have had an allergic reaction to other cephalosporins or to a penicillin.

DRUG INTERACTIONS
Probenecid, furosemide, aminoglycosides (e.g., gentamicin, amikacin, tobramycin, etc.)

FOOD INTERACTIONS
Unknown

HERBAL INTERACTIONS
Unknown

PREGNANCY AND BREAST-FEEDING CAUTIONS
FDA Pregnancy Risk Category B. This drug is excreted in breast milk. The American Academy of Pediatrics classifies as compatible with breast-feeding. Use with caution.

CEFTRIAXONE
(sef-trye-AKS-one)

NEWLY DISCOVERED USES (OFF-LABEL)
Nocardiosis, prevention of meningococcal meningitis

ORIGINAL USES (ON-LABEL)
Infections of the lower respiratory tract, skin and skin structure, bone and joint, urinary tract and intra-abdominal area. Also used for septicemia and meningitis due to susceptible organisms, and Lyme disease (Stage II/III).

BRAND NAME
Rocephin

DRUG CLASS
Antibiotic (3rd generation cephalosporin)

DESCRIPTION
This drug inhibits the production of bacterial cell walls.

POTENTIAL SIDE EFFECTS
Rash, diarrhea, blood abnormalities, increases in liver function tests, warmth, tightness.

CAUTIONS
- Do not use in neonates with high bilirubin levels.
- Dosage may need to be reduced if you have severe kidney dysfunction.
- Prolonged use may result in superinfection.
- May cause colitis (inflammation of the colon tissue).
- Notify your doctor if you have had an allergic reaction to other cephalosporins or to a penicillin.

DRUG INTERACTIONS
Probenecid, aminoglycosides (such as gentamicin, amikacin, tobramycin)

FOOD INTERACTIONS
Unknown

HERBAL INTERACTIONS
Unknown

PREGNANCY AND BREAST-FEEDING CAUTIONS
FDA Pregnancy Risk Category B. This drug is excreted in breast milk. The American Academy of Pediatrics considers this drug compatible with breast-feeding. Use with caution.

CEPHALEXIN
(sef-a-LEKS-in)

NEWLY DISCOVERED USES (OFF-LABEL)
Diverticulitis

ORIGINAL USES (ON-LABEL)
Bacterial infections in the lower respiratory tract, skin and soft tissue, bone and joint and urinary tract. Also used to prevent bacterial endocarditis (in the heart).

BRAND NAMES
Biocef, Keflex

DRUG CLASS
Antibiotic (1st generation cephalosporin)

DESCRIPTION
This drug inhibits the production of bacterial cell walls.

POTENTIAL SIDE EFFECTS
Diarrhea, stomach upset, rash.

CAUTIONS
- Dosage may need to be reduced if you have severe kidney dysfunction.
- Prolonged use may result in superinfection.
- May cause colitis (inflammation of the colon tissue).
- Notify your doctor if you have had an allergic reaction to other cephalosporins or to a penicillin.

DRUG INTERACTIONS
Probenecid, furosemide, aminoglycosides (such as gentamicin, amikacin, tobramycin)

FOOD INTERACTIONS
Blood levels may be reduced if taken with food.

HERBAL INTERACTIONS
Unknown

PREGNANCY AND BREAST-FEEDING CAUTIONS
FDA Pregnancy Risk Category B. This drug is excreted in small amounts in breast milk.

SPECIAL INFORMATION
Discard refrigerated suspension formulations of this drug after two weeks.

CETIRIZINE
(se-TI-ra-zeen)

NEWLY DISCOVERED USES (OFF-LABEL)
Chemotherapy-induced anaphylaxis

ORIGINAL USES (ON-LABEL)
Perennial and seasonal allergic rhinitis and other allergic symptoms, including chronic hives

BRAND NAME
Zyrtec

DRUG CLASS
Antihistamine

DESCRIPTION
Cetirizine is primarily an allergy medication.

POTENTIAL SIDE EFFECTS
Headache, drowsiness, insomnia, fatigue, abdominal pain, dry mouth, diarrhea, nausea, nosebleeds, sore throat, bronchospasm.

CAUTIONS
- Inform your doctor if you have an allergy to hydroxyzine, glaucoma, peptic ulcer, or urinary retention.
- Use with caution if you have kidney or liver dysfunction, if you are elderly, or if you are a nursing mother.
- May cause drowsiness; use caution in tasks which require alertness.
- Safety and efficacy in pediatric patients less than 6 months have not been established.

DRUG INTERACTIONS
Central nervous system (CNS) depressants and anticholinergics

FOOD INTERACTIONS
Alcohol

HERBAL INTERACTIONS
Unknown

PREGNANCY AND BREAST-FEEDING CAUTIONS
FDA Pregnancy Risk Category B. Not recommended during breast-feeding.

CHLORAMBUCIL
(khlor-AM-byoo-sil)

NEWLY DISCOVERED USES (OFF-LABEL)
Membranous nephropathy, nephrotic syndrome, rheumatoid arthritis, systemic lupus erythematosus, uveitis

ORIGINAL USES (ON-LABEL)
Chronic lymphocytic leukemia and malignant lymphomas

BRAND NAME
Leukeran

DRUG CLASS
Antineoplastic

DESCRIPTION
This drug interacts with cellular DNA in the treatment of cancers and other diseases.

POTENTIAL SIDE EFFECTS
Tremors, muscular twitching, hives, nausea, vomiting, diarrhea, infertility, confusion, agitation, seizures, skin reactions, bone marrow suppression, liver toxicity, jaundice, lung fibrosis.

CAUTIONS
- Inform your doctor if you have had allergic reactions to other chemotherapy or alkylating drugs (such as cyclophosphamides, ifosfamide, mechlorethamine, etc.).
- Seizures have been associated with the use of this drug.
- Requires monitoring for bone marrow suppression and severe blood disorders.
- Should not be taken at full dose before four weeks after a full course of radiation or chemotherapy.

DRUG INTERACTIONS
Consult with your doctor prior to initiation of any new prescription medication, herbal drug, or nonprescription product.

FOOD INTERACTIONS
Unknown

HERBAL INTERACTIONS
Unknown

PREGNANCY AND BREAST-FEEDING CAUTIONS
FDA Pregnancy Risk Category D. Excretion in breast milk is unknown. Consult with doctor prior to initiation of breast-feeding.

SPECIAL INFORMATION
Review major toxicities with your doctor prior to initiation of therapy. Store the product in your refrigerator. This drug has a black box warning regarding the potential for bone marrow suppression. It is also mutagenic, teratogenic, and produces infertility. Inform your doctor immediately if any of the following occur: bleeding, fever, vomiting, skin rash, persistent cough, seizures, unusual lumps, yellow discoloration of skin or eyes.

CHLORHEXIDINE GLUCONATE
(klor-HEKS-I-deen GLOO-koe-nate)

NEWLY DISCOVERED USES (OFF-LABEL)

Drug-induced gingival enlargement

ORIGINAL USES (ON-LABEL)
Gingivitis, scaling and root planing procedures

BRAND NAMES
Peridex, PerioChip, PerioGard

DRUG CLASS
Antibacterial (oral rinse, chip)

DESCRIPTION
This drug binds to plaque-forming bacteria and interferes with their absorption into your teeth. It also binds to proteins in your saliva, reducing the spread of plaque.

POTENTIAL SIDE EFFECTS
Irritation of the mouth and tongue; change in taste; increase in tartar on teeth; staining of teeth, mouth, tooth fillings, and dentures or other mouth appliances.

CAUTIONS
- Keep out of your eyes, ears and mouth.
- May cause increase in supragingival calculus. This should be monitored with dental exams every six months.
- May cause staining of teeth, tongue, or oral tissues.
- Although changes in taste have occurred, this is usually not permanent.

DRUG INTERACTIONS
Consult with your doctor or dentist prior to starting any other oral rinse products.

FOOD INTERACTIONS
Unknown

HERBAL INTERACTIONS
Unknown

PREGNANCY AND BREAST-FEEDING CAUTIONS
FDA Pregnancy Risk Category B. Excretion in breast milk is unknown. Consult your doctor.

SPECIAL INFORMATION

Use as oral rinse for 30 seconds in the morning and evening after brushing teeth. Use one tablespoon. Do not ingest. Spit remaining material out after rinsing.

This information pertains to the use of the prescription product only and should not be inferred for the use of nonprescription formulations.

CHLOROQUINE
(klor-OH-kwin)

NEWLY DISCOVERED USES (OFF-LABEL)
Dermatomyositis/polymyositis, psoriatic arthritis, sarcoidosis

ORIGINAL USES (ON-LABEL)
Prevention and treatment of malaria, treatment of amebiasis

BRAND NAME
Aralen

DRUG CLASS
Antimalarial

DESCRIPTION
This drug interferes with the body's metabolism of parasites by inhibiting DNA and RNA enzymes.

POTENTIAL SIDE EFFECTS
Low blood pressure, changes in heart rhythm, headache, anorexia, nausea, vomiting, diarrhea, abdominal cramps, irreversible retinal damage, blurred vision, focusing difficulty, itching, skin changes.

CAUTIONS
- Not for use if you experience retinal or visual field changes.
- Inform your doctor if you have liver disease, G6PD (glucose-6-phosphate dehydrogenase) deficiency, alcoholism, or are taking other drugs which may damage the liver.
- May exacerbate psoriasis or porphyria.
- Requires monitoring for blood disorders if taken for prolonged periods.

- Irreversible retinopathy has occurred with long or high-dose therapy.
- Discontinue drug if any abnormality in the visual field or if muscular weakness develops during treatment. Knee and ankle reflexes may be periodically assessed.
- Use caution if you have pre-existing hearing damage; discontinue immediately if hearing defects are noted.

DRUG INTERACTIONS
Cimetidine, kaolin, magnesium trisilicate

FOOD INTERACTIONS
Alcohol

HERBAL INTERACTIONS
Hibiscus sabdariffa, lemon (citrus limetta), and tamarindus indica

PREGNANCY AND BREAST-FEEDING CAUTIONS
FDA Pregnancy Risk Category C. This drug is excreted in breast milk. Consult your doctor.

SPECIAL INFORMATION
May cause stomach upset; take with food. Immediately report visual or hearing changes or ringing in your ears to your doctor.

CHLORTHALIDONE
(klor-THAL-i-done)

NEWLY DISCOVERED USES (OFF-LABEL)
Nephrogenic diabetes insipidus, postmenopausal osteoporosis

ORIGINAL USES (ON-LABEL)
Mild to moderate high blood pressure, swelling due to fluid retention (edema)

BRAND NAME
Thalitone

DRUG CLASS
Blood pressure medication (thiazide diuretic)

DESCRIPTION
This drug increases the excretion of sodium and chloride in urine, thereby promoting fluid loss. It also promotes excretion of potas-

sium and bicarbonate, but decreases excretion of calcium and uric acid.

POTENTIAL SIDE EFFECTS
Potassium loss, nausea, vomiting, loss of appetite, upset stomach, diarrhea, electrolyte imbalances, gout, changes in blood sugar or cholesterol levels.

CAUTIONS
- Notify your doctor if you have allergies to sulfonamide drugs. Inform your doctor if you have kidney disease, liver disease, diabetes, asthma, lupus, gout, or recently had surgery.
- Diabetics may require increased amounts of insulin or oral drugs commonly used to treat diabetes.
- Requires monitoring of electrolytes, and may require potassium supplementation during therapy.
- May cause dizziness and light-headedness when standing suddenly from a sitting or lying down position.

DRUG INTERACTIONS
ACE inhibitors (such as captopril, lisinopril, etc.), arsenic trioxide, calcitriol, calcium carbonate, cholestyramine, colestipol, digoxin, ketanserin, lithium, probenecid. Check with your pharmacist or doctor before starting new medications, herbal products, or nonprescription drugs.

FOOD INTERACTIONS
Avoid excessive ingestion of natural licorice

HERBAL INTERACTIONS
Ginkgo, gossypol, ma huang, ephedra

PREGNANCY AND BREAST-FEEDING CAUTIONS
Pregnancy Risk Category C according to manufacturer. Category D according to expert analysis. May suppress lactation. The American Academy of Pediatrics considers this drug compatible with breast-feeding.

SPECIAL INFORMATION
This medication can cause dizziness or drowsiness.

CHLOROTHIAZIDE
(klor-oh-THYE-a-zide)

NEWLY DISCOVERED USES (OFF-LABEL)
Nephrogenic diabetes insipidus

ORIGINAL USES (ON-LABEL)
Mild to moderate high blood pressure, swelling due to fluid retention (edema)

BRAND NAME
Diuril

DRUG CLASS
Blood pressure medication (thiazide diuretic)

DESCRIPTION
This drug increases the excretion of sodium and chloride in urine, thereby promoting fluid loss. Also promotes excretion of potassium and bicarbonate, but decreases excretion of calcium and uric acid.

POTENTIAL SIDE EFFECTS
Potassium loss, nausea, vomiting, loss of appetite, upset stomach, diarrhea, electrolyte imbalances, gout, changes in blood sugar or cholesterol levels.

CAUTIONS
- Notify your doctor if you have allergies to sulfonamide drugs. Inform your doctor if you have kidney disease, liver disease, diabetes, asthma, lupus, gout, or recently had surgery.
- Diabetics may require increased amounts of insulin or oral drugs commonly used to treat diabetes.
- Requires monitoring of electrolytes, and may require potassium supplementation during therapy.
- May cause dizziness and light-headedness when standing suddenly from a sitting or lying down position.

DRUG INTERACTIONS
ACE inhibitors (captopril, lisinopril, etc.), arsenic trioxide, calcitriol, calcium carbonate, cholestyramine, colestipol, digoxin, ketanserin, lithium, probenecid. Check with your pharmacist or doctor before starting new medications, herbal products, or nonprescription drugs.

FOOD INTERACTIONS
Avoid excessive ingestion of natural licorice

HERBAL INTERACTIONS
Ginkgo, gossypol, ma huang, ephedra

PREGNANCY AND BREAST-FEEDING CAUTIONS
FDA Pregnancy Risk Category C according to manufacturer. Category D according to expert analysis. May suppress lactation. The American Academy of Pediatrics considers this drug compatible with breast-feeding.

SPECIAL INFORMATION
This medication can cause dizziness or drowsiness.

CHLORPROMAZINE
(klor-PROE-ma-zeen)

NEWLY DISCOVERED USES (OFF-LABEL)

Hyperemesis gravidarum (severe nausea and vomiting in pregnancy)

ORIGINAL USES (ON-LABEL)
Control of mania, treatment of schizophrenia, control of nausea and vomiting, relief of restlessness, intractable hiccups, and severe behavioral problems

BRAND NAME
Thorazine

DRUG CLASS
Antiemetic, antipsychotic (phenothiazine)

DESCRIPTION
This drug blocks dopamine receptors in the brain and depresses the release of certain hormones.

POTENTIAL SIDE EFFECTS
Low blood pressure upon standing from a sitting or lying down position, increased heart rate, dizziness, nonspecific QT changes, drowsiness, involuntary muscle spasm, akathisia, pseudoparkinsonism, photosensitivity (skin reaction related to sun exposure), dermatitis, skin pigmentation, lactation, breast engorgement, false-positive pregnancy test, loss of menstruation, dry mouth,

constipation, nausea, urinary retention, ejaculatory disorder, impotence, various blood disorders (e.g., agranulocytosis, eosinophilia, leukopenia, hemolytic anemia), jaundice, blurred vision, corneal and lens changes.

CAUTIONS
- May cause tardive dyskinesia, a syndrome characterized by involuntary, uncontrolled muscular movements. Also associated with neuroleptic malignant syndrome, including fever, muscle rigidity, irregular pulse rate, sweating, etc.
- Inform your doctor if you have heart, liver or kidney disease, or seizure disorder.
- This drug causes central nervous system depression and affects thermoregulation. Avoid extreme changes in heat.
- Significant decrease in blood pressure can occur.
- Contains sulfites that may cause allergic reactions.
- Increased confusion, memory loss, psychotic behavior, and agitation may occur.

DRUG INTERACTIONS
Additive central nervous system (CNS) depression when taken with other CNS depressants (narcotic analgesics, ethanol, barbiturates, cyclic antidepressants, antihistamines, or sedative-hypnotics). Anticholinergics, antihypertensives, lithium, trazodone, valproic acid, tricyclic antidepressants, chloroquine, propranolol, metoclopramide, bromocriptine,

Increased risk of irregular heart rhythm (QT prolongation) when administered with antiarrhythmics, cisapride, pimozide, sparfloxacin or other drugs which prolong QT intervals (http://www.torsades.org/medical-pros/drug-lists/drug-lists .htm#).

FOOD INTERACTIONS
Alcohol

HERBAL INTERACTIONS
St. John's wort, dong quai, kava kava, fotu kola, valerian

PREGNANCY AND BREAST-FEEDING CAUTIONS
FDA Pregnancy Risk Category C. This drug is excreted in breast milk. Consult your doctor.

SPECIAL INFORMATION
Do not stop taking this medication unless directed by your prescriber. Oral concentrate must be diluted in 2 to 4 ounces of

water, fruit juice, carbonated drinks, milk or pudding. Do not take antacid within one hour of taking medication. Avoid alcohol. Avoid excess sun exposure and use sun block. May cause drowsiness.

CHLORPROPAMIDE
(klor-PROE-pa-mide)

NEWLY DISCOVERED USES (OFF-LABEL)
Partial central diabetes insipidus

ORIGINAL USES (ON-LABEL)
Type 2 diabetes mellitus

BRAND NAME
Diabinese

DRUG CLASS
Antidiabetic, hypoglycemic (sulfonylurea)

DESCRIPTION
This drug stimulates insulin secretion.

POTENTIAL SIDE EFFECTS
Low blood sugar levels, nausea, vomiting, diarrhea, anorexia, itching, disulfiram-like reactions (flushing, nausea, vomiting, etc.), skin reactions, sweating, migraine.

CAUTIONS
Inform your doctor if you have reduced kidney or liver function.

DRUG INTERACTIONS
Acarbose, ammonium chloride, clofibrate, cotrimoxazole, diltiazem, NSAIDs, sulfadiazine, sulfamethoxazole, aspirin, beta- adrenergic blockers (e.g. propranolol, atenolol, etc.), chloramphenicol, chlorothiazide, fosphenytoin, phenytoin, hydrochlorothiazide, rifampin, rifapentine, sodium bicarbonate, chlorthalidone, fluoroquinolones, MAO inhibitors, androgens, anticoagulation, antifungals, fenfluramine, gemfibrozil, histamine-2 antagonists (e.g., cimetidine, ranitidine, etc.), magnesium salts, methyldopa, sulfonamides, tricyclic antidepressants, calcium channel blockers, barbiturates, anticoagulants. Many drugs affect blood glucose or interact with this drug, consult with your pharmacist or doctor

prior to starting a new medication, herbal, or non-prescription product.

FOOD INTERACTIONS
Disulfiram-like reactions occur when alcohol is consumed.

HERBAL INTERACTIONS
Bitter melon, eucalyptus, fenugreek, ginseng, glucomannan, guar gum, gymnema sylvestre, St. John's wort, glucosamine, licorice

PREGNANCY AND BREAST-FEEDING CAUTIONS
FDA Pregnancy Risk Category C. This drug is excreted in breast milk. Consult your doctor.

SPECIAL INFORMATION
You may take this medicine with food or milk to avoid stomach upset. Avoid using aspirin unless approved by your doctor. Avoid drinking alcohol while you are taking this medicine. Follow the diet provided by your doctor and take this medicine regularly to control your diabetes.

CILOSTAZOL
(sil-OH-sta-zol)

NEWLY DISCOVERED USES (OFF-LABEL)
Peripheral vascular disease and atherosclerosis in type 2 diabetes, prevention of recurrent stroke

ORIGINAL USES (ON-LABEL)
Intermittent claudication (pain and weakness in the legs while walking, usually related to problems with blood flow in the legs)

BRAND NAME
Pletal

DRUG CLASS
Antiplatelet (phosphodiesterase enzyme inhibitor)

DESCRIPTION
This drug promotes relaxation of the blood vessels. It works by inhibiting an important enzyme, phosphodiesterase III, that ultimately inhibits blood clotting and helps with healthy heart function.

POTENTIAL SIDE EFFECTS

Increased heart rate, sensation of rapid heart beat, dizziness, vertigo, abnormal stools, diarrhea, upset stomach, flatulence, nausea, cough, sore throat, abdominal pain, headache, infection, muscle aches, peripheral edema (swelling).

CAUTIONS

Not for use in heart failure. Use caution if you are receiving other drugs that affect platelet aggregation, if you have reduced liver function, or if you have severe underlying heart disease.

DRUG INTERACTIONS

Diltiazem, macrolide antibiotics (e.g., erythromycin, clarithromycin), omeprazole.

This drug is metabolized by specific set of liver enzymes. Several other drugs interfere with these liver enzymes, and thus may increase or decrease the clearance of cilostazol from the body, potentially increasing the risk of side effects or decreasing effectiveness. When these drugs are given in combination with cilostazol, dosage adjustments may be needed. As these are too numerous to list, you should always check with your doctor or pharmacist prior to starting a new medication, herbal, or nonprescription product.

FOOD INTERACTIONS

High fat meal increases absorption. Avoid grapefruit juice.

HERBAL INTERACTIONS

Unknown

PREGNANCY AND BREAST-FEEDING CAUTIONS

FDA Pregnancy Risk Category C. Excretion in breast milk is unknown. Not recommended during breast-feeding.

SPECIAL INFORMATION

This drug has a black box warning regarding that its use is contraindicated in all patients with heart failure, as it has been shown to decrease survival when compared to placebo.

CIMETIDINE
(sye-MET-i-deen)

NEWLY DISCOVERED USES (OFF-LABEL)
Chemotherapy induced anaphylaxis (prevention), chronic mucocutaneous candidiasis, dyspepsia, hyperparathyroid crisis, interstitial cystitis (therapy-resistant), non-genital warts, primary hyperparathyroidism, urticaria

ORIGINAL USES (ON-LABEL)
Short-term treatment of active duodenal ulcers and benign gastric ulcers, long-term prophylaxis of duodenal ulcer, gastric hypersecretory states, gastroesophageal reflux (GERD), prevention of upper gastric bleeding in critically ill patients

BRAND NAME
Tagamet

DRUG CLASS
Antihistamine (H2)

DESCRIPTION
This drug is used to treat ulcers and other gastric problems. It works by reducing gastric acid by inhibiting certain chemicals in gastric cells.

POTENTIAL SIDE EFFECTS
Headache, dizziness, agitation, drowsiness, diarrhea, nausea, and vomiting.

CAUTIONS
- Notify your doctor if you have allergies to cimetidine or other drugs in this class.
- Dosage adjustments may be required in kidney or liver impairment.
- Do not use for long-term treatment without doctor supervision.
- Mental confusion, delirium has occurred in the elderly or in individuals with impaired kidney function.
- Breast swelling (gynecomastia) has occurred rarely.

DRUG INTERACTIONS
Aminophylline, amphetamines, selected benzodiazepine (except lorazepam, oxazepam, temazepam), selected beta-blockers (except atenolol, betaxolol, bisoprolol, nadolol, penbutolol), calcium

channel blockers, citalopram, cyclosporine, dextromethorphan, diazepam, ergot derivatives, fluoxetine, fluvamine, lidocaine, methsuximide, mexiletine, mirtazapine, nateglinide, nefazodone, paroxetine, phenytoin, propranolol, risperidone, ritonavir, ropinirole, sertraline, sildenafil (and other PDE-5 inhibitors), tacrolimus, theophylline, thioridazine, warfarin, meperidine, metronidazole, moricizine, procainamide, propafenone, quinidine, quinolone antibiotics, tacrine, triamterene, ketoconazole, fluconazole, itraconazole (especially capsules), delvaridine, carmustine.

This drug inhibits a specific set of liver enzymes that are responsible for the metabolism (clearance or activation) of many other drugs, potentially increasing the risk of side effects or decreasing effectiveness. When these drugs are given in combination with cimetidine, dosage adjustments may be needed. As these are too numerous to list, you should always check with your doctor or pharmacist prior to starting a new medication, herbal drug, or nonprescription product.

FOOD INTERACTIONS
Unknown

HERBAL INTERACTIONS
St. John's wort

PREGNANCY AND BREAST-FEEDING CAUTIONS
FDA Pregnancy Risk Category B. Excreted in breast milk. Consult with your doctor.

SPECIAL INFORMATION
If taken with antacids, separate by taking one hour before or two hours after the antacid. Avoid excessive alcohol use with this drug.

This information pertains to the use of the prescription product only and should not be inferred for the use of nonprescription formulations.

CIPROFLOXACIN
(sip-roe-FLOKS-a-sin)

NEWLY DISCOVERED USES (OFF-LABEL)
Cholera, Crohn's disease, diverticulitis, gingivitis, granuloma inguinale, Legionnaire's disease, mycoplasma pneumonia, nonbacterial prostatitis, periodontitis, prevention of meningococcal meningitis

ORIGINAL USES (ON-LABEL)
Various bacterial infections in the lung, eye, sinuses, skin, and skin structure

BRAND NAMES
Ciloxan, Cipro, Cipro XR

DRUG CLASS
Antibiotic (quinolone)

DESCRIPTION
This drug is used to treat infections. It works by interfering with cellular enzymes, stopping the activity of DNA.

POTENTIAL SIDE EFFECTS
Dizziness, nausea, diarrhea, various blood disorders such as anemia, tremors, confusion, depression, nervousness, agitation, anxiety.

CAUTIONS
- Report to your doctor if you experience pain, inflammation or rupture of a tendon. Rest and refrain from exercise until you see a doctor. Tendon rupture can occur during or after therapy with this drug.
- Stop the medication at the first sign of a rash.
- Prolonged use may cause superinfection.
- May aggravate symptoms of myasthenia gravis.
- Inform your doctor if serious, persistent diarrhea develops.

DRUG INTERACTIONS
Iron, zinc, calcium, magnesium, aluminum, corticosteroids (increase risk of tendon rupture), antacids, electrolyte supplements, quinapril, sucralfate, certain antiarrhythmics, didanosine formulations (chewable/buffered tablets and pediatric powder for oral suspension), theophyllines, antacids, cyclosporine, cimetidine

FOOD INTERACTIONS
Dairy products or calcium-fortified juices. Serum caffeine levels may be increased.

HERBAL INTERACTIONS
Dong quai, St. John's wort

PREGNANCY AND BREAST-FEEDING CAUTIONS
FDA Pregnancy Risk Category C. May be excreted in breast milk. Do not use during breast-feeding.

SPECIAL INFORMATION
Extended release tablets cannot be crushed, split, or chewed. Take entire prescription even if feeling better. Maintain adequate hydration (2 to 3 L/day of fluids) to avoid concentrated urine and crystal formation. May cause increased sensitivity to sunlight; use sunblock, wear protective clothing and dark glasses. Report immediately any signs of rash, joint or back pain, difficulty breathing, easy bruising or bleeding, inflammation, or rupture of tendon.

CIPROFLOXACIN AND HYDROCORTISONE
(sip-roe-FLOKS-a-sin and hye-droe-KOR-ti-sone)

NEWLY DISCOVERED USES (OFF-LABEL)
Chronic otitis media

ORIGINAL USES (ON-LABEL)
Acute otitis externa

BRAND NAME
Cipro-HC

DRUG CLASS
Ear preparation (antibiotic/corticosteroid)

DESCRIPTION
Ciprofloxacin kills bacteria by interfering with the synthesis of bacterial DNA. Hydrocortisone helps resolve inflammation that accompanies bacterial infections.

POTENTIAL SIDE EFFECTS
Headache, itching, local irritation, dizziness.

CAUTIONS

- Notify your doctor if you have had allergies to ciprofloxacin or other quinolone antibiotics.
- Discontinue use if rash or signs of allergy develop.
- Do not use if tympanic membrane is perforated.
- Do not use if you have viral infections of the external canal including chicken pox, shingles, or herpes simplex infections.
- Not for use in the eyes or as an injection.
- Use of this product may result in overgrowth of nonsusceptible organisms. Notify your doctor if the infection does not appear to improve after one week of therapy.

DRUG INTERACTIONS
Unknown

FOOD INTERACTIONS
Unknown

HERBAL INTERACTIONS
Unknown

PREGNANCY AND BREAST-FEEDING CAUTIONS
FDA Pregnancy Risk Category C. Excretion in breast milk unknown. Consult your doctor.

SPECIAL INFORMATION
Shake well before using. Warm suspension by holding the bottle in your hands for one to two minutes to avoid dizziness after putting a cold solution in the ear canal. You should lie on your side with affected ear facing upward. Drops are put in affected ear. Maintain this position for 30 to 60 minutes to optimize absorption. Protect bottle from light. Do not contaminate dropper with contact from fingers, ear contents, or other sources.

CITALOPRAM
(sye-TAL-oh-pram)

NEWLY DISCOVERED USES (OFF-LABEL)

Alcoholism (cravings & dependency), Alzheimer's disease, bipolar disorder, diabetic neuropathy, fibromyalgia, panic disorder, pathological gambling, premenstrual dysphoric disorder (PMDD), premenstrual syndrome (PMS), post-traumatic stress syndrome (PTSD), obsessive-compulsive disorder, therapy-resistant PMDD, social phobia

ORIGINAL USES (ON-LABEL)
Depression

BRAND NAME
Celexa

DRUG CLASS
Antidepressant (selective serotonin reuptake inhibitor [SSRI])

DESCRIPTION
This drug is used in patients with depression. It works by inhibiting the reuptake of serotonin by neurons, thereby increasing levels of serotonin, an important chemical in mood disorders.

POTENTIAL SIDE EFFECTS
Somnolence, insomnia, nausea, dry mouth, diaphoresis, anxiety, anorexia, agitation, yawning, rash, pruritus, sexual dysfunction, diarrhea, stomach upset, vomiting, abdominal pain, tremor, weight gain, joint aches, muscle aches, cough, rhinitis, sinusitis, low sodium levels.

CAUTIONS
- Do not use concurrently with MAO inhibitors or within two weeks of discontinuing MAO-I.
- Inform your doctor if you have a history of mania or seizures, or if you have renal dysfunction.
- High-risk suicide-attempt patients should ask to be monitored during initiation of therapy.
- Has potential to impair cognitive/motor performance—should use caution operating hazardous machinery.
- Elderly patients with liver impairment should take lower dosages.
- Use with caution in renal insufficiency.

DRUG INTERACTIONS
MAO inhibitors or drugs with MAO inhibition (linezolid), amphetamines, buspirone, meperidine, nefazodone, serotonin agonists (sumatriptan), sibutramine, other SSRIs, sympathomimetics, ritonavir, tramadol, venlafaxine, loop diuretics, warfarin, aminoglutethimide, carbamazepine, phenytoin and rifampin, cyproheptadine.

This drug is metabolized by specific set of liver enzymes. Several other drugs interfere with these liver enzymes, and thus may increase or decrease the clearance of citalopram from the body, potentially increasing the risk of side effects or decreasing effectiveness. When these drugs are given in combination with citalopram, dosage adjustments may be needed. As these are too numerous to list, you should always check with your doctor or pharmacist prior to starting a new medication, herbal, or nonprescription product.

FOOD INTERACTIONS
Alcohol

HERBAL INTERACTIONS
Valerian, St. John's wort, SAMe, gotu kola, kava kava

PREGNANCY AND BREAST-FEEDING CAUTIONS
FDA Pregnancy Risk Category C. Excreted in breast milk. Breast-feeding is not advised while using this drug.

SPECIAL INFORMATION
In 2005, the FDA announced new labeling for antidepressants regarding the need to closely monitor for worsening of depression and for the potential of increased suicidal thinking or suicidal behavior during therapy. Although this recommendation applies to all patients (adults, children, adolescents) treated with antidepressants for any indication, this is of particular importance in patients being treated for depression. Discuss the latest information regarding this safety issue with your doctor prior to initiating therapy.

Close observation may be especially important when antidepressant medications are started for the first time or when doses are changed. More information on this topic can be found at the following web site: http://www.fda.gov/cder/drug/antidepressants/default.htm

Combination with other SSRIs, SSNRIs, tricyclic antidepressants, amphetamines, sympathomimetics, ritonavir, serotonin agonists (sumatriptan, etc.), and certain opiates carries an increased risk of serotonin syndrome. While taking this medication, check with your pharmacist or doctor before starting any new medication, herbal, or nonprescription product.

CLARITHOMYCIN
(kla-RITH-roe-mye-sin)

NEWLY DISCOVERED USES (OFF-LABEL)
Legionnaire's disease, Lyme disease, prevention of bacterial endocarditis

ORIGINAL USES (ON-LABEL)
Various infections

BRAND NAMES
Biaxin, Biaxin XL

DRUG CLASS
Antibiotic (macrolide)

DESCRIPTION
This drug stops the growth of bacteria by causing inhibition of protein production in the bacterial cell.

POTENTIAL SIDE EFFECTS
Headache, rash, abdominal pain, upset stomach, diarrhea, nausea, vomiting, abnormal taste, heartburn.

CAUTIONS
- Inform your doctor if you are allergic to macrolide antibiotics such as erythromycin, azithromycin.
- It should not be used in combination with ranitidine or bismuth citrate if you have a history of acute porphyria.
- Dosage adjustment is required with severe kidney impairment.
- Drugs in this class have been associated with various forms of abnormal heart rhythm, including QT prolongation, torsades de pointes.
- Use of antibiotics for prolonged periods may result in super infection.

- Safety and efficacy in children less than six months of age have not been established.

DRUG INTERACTIONS

Astemizole, cisapride, gatifloxacin, moxifloxacin, pimozide, sparfloxacin, thioridazine, type Ia and III antiarrhythmic drugs, mesoridazine, alfentanil, benzodiazepines, buspirone, calcium channel blockers, carbamazepine, cilostazol, clozapine, colchicine, cyclosporine, digoxin, disopyramide, ergot alkaloids, HMG-CoA reductase inhibitors, loratadine, methylprednisolone, rifabutin, tacrolimus, theophylline, valproate, vinblastine, vincristine, zopiclone, sildenafil, tadalafil, vardenafil, neuromuscular blocking drugs, warfarin, amprenavir, zafirlukast, clindamycin, lincomycin. zidovudine. This drug can potentially interact with many drugs. Consult with your pharmacist or doctor prior to starting prescription medications, herbals, or non-prescription drugs.

FOOD INTERACTIONS

Food delays absorption, but total absorption remains unchanged. May be taken with or without meals. May be taken with milk.

HERBAL INTERACTIONS

St. John's wort

PREGNANCY AND BREAST-FEEDING CAUTIONS

FDA Pregnancy Risk Category C. It is not known if this drug is excreted in breast milk. Consult with your doctor.

SPECIAL INFORMATION

Do not crush or chew XL tablets.

CLINDAMYCIN
(klin–da-MYE-sin)

Oral, Injectable

NEWLY DISCOVERED USES (OFF-LABEL)

Acute otitis media, diverticulitis, gingivitis, periodontitis, pharyngitis, pneumocystis jiroveci pneumonia, tonsillectomy, tonsillitis/peritonsillar abscess, toxoplasmosis in AIDS

ORIGINAL USES (ON-LABEL)

Various bacterial infections

BRAND NAMES
Cleocin, Clindamycin

DRUG CLASS
Antibiotic

DESCRIPTION
This drug inhibits the production of bacterial protein, thus stopping the growth of bacteria.

POTENTIAL SIDE EFFECTS
Decreased blood pressure, diarrhea, abdominal pain, hives, rash, pseudomembranous colitis, nausea, vomiting, sterile abscess at injection site, fungal overgrowth, allergic reaction, dryness, burning, itching, scaliness, headache, back pain, constipation, urinary tract infection.

CAUTIONS
- Inform your doctor if you have had pseudomembranous colitis or if you currently have intestinal disorders.
- Dosage adjustments are required in kidney or liver impairment.
- Can cause severe and possibly fatal colitis; report to your doctor if you have persistent diarrhea or severe abdominal cramps during therapy.
- Not for use in the treatment of meningitis.
- In prolonged therapy, may require monitoring of kidney and liver function.
- The prolonged use of antibiotics may result in superinfection.

DRUG INTERACTIONS
Erythromycin, kaolin-pectin, tubocurarine and pancuronium

FOOD INTERACTIONS
Unknown

HERBAL INTERACTIONS
St. John's wort

PREGNANCY AND BREAST-FEEDING CAUTIONS
FDA Pregnancy Risk Category B. Excreted in breast milk. The American Academy of Pediatrics considers this drug compatible with breast-feeding.

SPECIAL INFORMATION
This drug has a black box warning regarding the potential for developing pseudomembranous colitis, a severe and possibly fatal

inflammation of the lower intestines. Report any persistent diarrhea or abdominal pains to your doctor.

CLINDAMYCIN
(klin-da-MYE-sin)

Topical

NEWLY DISCOVERED USES (OFF-LABEL)

> Rosacea

ORIGINAL USES (ON-LABEL)
Acne

BRAND NAMES
Cleocin T, Clindagel, ClindaMax, Clindets

DRUG CLASS
Antibiotic

DESCRIPTION
This drug inhibits the production of bacterial protein, thus stopping the growth of bacteria.

POTENTIAL SIDE EFFECTS:
Skin reactions: burning, itching, dryness, redness, oiliness, peeling. Other: Colitis, blood diarrhea, abdominal pain.

CAUTIONS
- Inform your doctor if you have had pseudomembranous colitis or if you currently have intestinal disorders.
- Immediately report persistent diarrhea, bloody diarrhea, or abdominal pain to your doctor.

DRUG INTERACTIONS
Do not use other topical products unless instructed by your doctor.

FOOD INTERACTIONS
Unknown

HERBAL INTERACTIONS
Unknown

PREGNANCY AND BREAST-FEEDING CAUTIONS

FDA Pregnancy Risk Category B. Excreted in breast milk. The American Academy of Pediatrics considers this drug compatible with breast-feeding.

SPECIAL INFORMATION

This drug has a black box warning regarding the potential for developing pseudomembranous colitis, a severe and possibly fatal inflammation of the lower intestines. Report any persistent diarrhea or abdominal pains to your doctor.

For external use only. Avoid contact with eyes. Some products have alcohol base that may cause burning or stinging if applied near eyes. Use caution when applying near the mouth.

CLOBETASOL

(kloe-BAY-ta-sol)

NEWLY DISCOVERED USES (OFF-LABEL)

Bullous pemphigoid, canker sores, oral lichen planus, psoriasis

ORIGINAL USES (ON-LABEL)

Various skin conditions, including atopic dermatitis, dermatoses, eczema, inflammatory linear verrucous epidermal, psoriasis, psoriasis scalp

BRAND NAMES

Clobex, Cormax, Embeline, Olux, Temovate

DRUG CLASS

Anti-inflammatory (corticosteroid)

DESCRIPTION

Decrease formation, release, and activity of inflammation stimulators.

POTENTIAL SIDE EFFECTS

Acne-like skin changes, itching or mild skin rash, mild temporary stinging, irritation, local burning, redness, dryness, skin atrophy.

CAUTIONS

- Children are more susceptible to systemic absorption and toxicity.

- Should not be used in uncontrolled infection.
- Do not use clobetasol shampoo on face, groin, or under armpits. Avoid contact with the eyes and lips.
- Highly potent topical corticosteroids, such as this drug, have been shown to suppress the hypothalamic-pituitary-adrenal axis, reducing adrenal gland secretion.
- Do not use with a dressing that blocks airflow to the wound.

DRUG INTERACTIONS
Unknown

FOOD INTERACTIONS
Unknown

HERBAL INTERACTIONS
Unknown

PREGNANCY AND BREAST-FEEDING CAUTIONS
FDA Pregnancy Risk Category C. It is not known if the use of topical steroids would result in significant absorption to be excreted in breast milk in measurable quantities. Consult your doctor.

SPECIAL INFORMATION
This is for topical use only. Apply a small amount to the affected area. Allow the solution to dry before rubbing, washing, or putting on clothes. Do not put bandages, dressing, or cosmetics over the treated area unless directed by your doctor. Do not apply double doses, but if you miss a dose, apply it as soon as possible.

CLOMIPHENE
(kloe-mi-feen)

NEWLY DISCOVERED USES (OFF-LABEL)
Male infertility

ORIGINAL USES (ON-LABEL)
Treatment of ovulatory failure in patients desiring pregnancy

BRAND NAMES
Clomid, Serophene

DRUG CLASS
Ovulation stimulator

DESCRIPTION
This drug induces ovulation by stimulating the release of hormones.

POTENTIAL SIDE EFFECTS
Hot flashes, ovarian enlargement, blood clots, mental depression, headache, breast enlargement (males), breast discomfort (females), abnormal menstrual flow, ovarian cyst formation, distention, bloating, nausea, vomiting, liver toxicity, blurring of vision, double vision, visual floaters, visual after-images.

CAUTIONS
- Not for use if you have liver disease, abnormal uterine bleeding, enlargement or development of ovarian cyst, uncontrolled thyroid or adrenal dysfunction, pituitary tumor, or pregnancy.
- Multiple pregnancies, blurring or other visual symptoms, over stimulation of ovaries, and abdominal pain can occur with the use of this medication.

DRUG INTERACTIONS
Danazol, estradiol

FOOD INTERACTIONS
Unknown

HERBAL INTERACTIONS
Unknown

PREGNANCY AND BREAST-FEEDING CAUTIONS
FDA Pregnancy Risk Category X. Excretion in breast milk unknown. Not for use during breast-feeding.

SPECIAL INFORMATION
When used for female ovulation stimulation, the majority of patients who ovulate will do so after the first course of therapy. If ovulation does not occur after three courses of therapy, the need for this drug should be re-evaluated. Notify your doctor if bloating, stomach or pelvic pain, blurred vision, jaundice, hot flushes or vomiting occur.

CLOMIPRAMINE
(kloe-MI-pra-meen)

NEWLY DISCOVERED USES (OFF-LABEL)

Childhood anxiety, chronic fatigue syndrome, chronic neuropathic pain, diabetic neuropathy, narcolepsy, panic disorder, premenstrual dysphoric disorder (PMDD), premenstrual syndrome (PMS), premature ejaculation, post-traumatic stress syndrome disorder (PTSD)

ORIGINAL USES (ON-LABEL)
Obsessive-compulsive disorder (OCD)

BRAND NAME
Anafranil

DRUG CLASS
Antidepressant (tricyclic)

DESCRIPTION
This drug increases concentration of certain brain chemicals in the central nervous system; this alters mood and other symptoms.

POTENTIAL SIDE EFFECTS
Dizziness, drowsiness, headache, insomnia, nervousness, libido changes, dry mouth, constipation, increased appetite, nausea, weight gain, stomach upset, anorexia, abdominal pain, fatigue, tremor, sweating, low blood pressure, confusion, rash, diarrhea, difficult urination, blurred vision.

CAUTIONS
- Do not use if you have been taking an MAO inhibitor (such as phenelzine, tranylcypromine, isocarboxazid) within the past 14 days. When used with MAO-I's, fever, high blood pressure, increased heart rate, confusion, seizures, and deaths have been reported.
- Not for use immediately after a heart attack.
- Can cause sedation, which may impair performance of tasks requiring alertness. Sedative effects may be additive with other drugs that cause similar effects (central nervous system depressants).
- May worsen psychosis or mania in patients with bipolar disease.
- Stop therapy with doctor permission and according to instructions (gradual taper) prior to elective surgery.

- Do not abruptly stop medication, taper gradually.
- Notify your doctor if you have low blood pressure as this drug can cause low blood pressure episodes.
- Use with caution in patients with urinary retention, history of cardiac disease, seizure disorders, diabetes, benign prostatic enlargement, narrow angle glaucoma, dry mouth, visual problems, constipation, or a history of bowel obstruction.
- Possibility of suicide attempt may persist until remission occurs.
- Use with caution in patients with thyroid disease or those receiving thyroid supplementation.
- Use with caution if you have liver or kidney dysfunction of if you are elderly.

DRUG INTERACTIONS

This drug is metabolized by specific set of liver enzymes. Several other drugs interfere with these liver enzymes, and thus, may increase or decrease the clearance of clomipramine from the body, potentially increasing the risk of side effects or decreasing effectiveness. When these drugs are given in combination with clomipramine, dosage adjustments may be needed. As these are too numerous to list, you should always check with your doctor or pharmacist prior to starting a new medication, herbal, or nonprescription product.

MAO inhibitors (such as phenelzine, tranylcypromine, isocarboxazid), ritonavir, bupropion, amphetamines, anticholinergics, sedatives, chlorpropamide, tolazamide, warfarin, fluoxetine, fluvoxamine, citalopram, escitalopram, paroxetine, sertraline, cimetidine, carbamazepine, haloperidol, smoking, methylphenidate, valproic acid, clonidine, venlafaxine, protease inhibitors, quinidine, diltiazem, verapamil, lithium, phenothiazines, drugs which prolong QT interval (see website: http://www.torsades.org/medical-pros/drug-lists/drug-lists.htm#).

FOOD INTERACTIONS

Alcohol. Avoid grapefruit juice.

HERBAL INTERACTIONS

Valerian, St. John's wort, SAMe, kava kava

PREGNANCY AND BREAST-FEEDING CAUTIONS

FDA Pregnancy Risk Category C. Excreted in breast milk. Breast-feeding is not advised while using this drug.

SPECIAL INFORMATION
Avoid prolonged exposure to sunlight, wear sunscreen.

In 2005, the FDA announced new labeling for antidepressants regarding the need to closely monitor for worsening of depression and for the potential of increased suicidal thinking or suicidal behavior during therapy. Although this recommendation applies to all patients (adults, children, adolescents) treated with antidepressants for any indication, this is of particular importance in patients being treated for depression.

CLONAZEPAM
(kloe-NA-ze-pam)

NEWLY DISCOVERED USES (OFF-LABEL)

Burning mouth syndrome, essential tremor, Gilles de la Tourette syndrome, major depressive disorder, multiple sclerosis, periodic limb movement disorder, restless legs syndrome, social phobia, tinnitus, vertigo, West syndrome

ORIGINAL USES (ON-LABEL)
Certain seizure disorders, panic disorder

BRAND NAME
Klonopin

DRUG CLASS
Anticonvulsant, antianxiety (benzodiazepine)

DESCRIPTION
This drug helps control seizures by depressing nerve transmission in the motor cortex.

POTENTIAL SIDE EFFECTS
Drowsiness, sedation, lethargy, apathy, amnesia, memory impairment, confusion, crying, headache, slurred speech, constipation, dry mouth, changes in libido, urinary retention, vision changes, behavior problems, excitement, psychosis, increased salivation.

CAUTIONS
- Notify your doctor if you have an allergy to this drug or other benzodiazepines, if you have liver or kidney problems, mental depression, a history of drug dependence, narrow angle glau-

coma, lung disorders, increased salivation, a poor or problematic gag reflex, or are pregnant.
- Use with caution in the elderly or debilitated patients.
- If for chronic therapy, requires monitoring of blood and liver function.
- May cause anterograde amnesia and paradoxical reactions (such as excitability, stimulation).
- May cause significant drowsiness or sedation. Use caution when performing tasks that require alertness.
- Do not abruptly stop this medication, requires tapering of dose over gradual period.
- Prolonged use for anxiety may result in dependence.

DRUG INTERACTIONS
Valproate, other drugs which cause sedation or cause central nervous depression.

FOOD INTERACTIONS
May take with food or water if stomach upset occurs.

HERBAL INTERACTIONS
St. John's wort, valerian, kava kava, gotu kola

PREGNANCY AND BREAST-FEEDING CAUTIONS
FDA Pregnancy Risk Category D. Excreted in breast milk. Refrain from breast-feeding while taking this drug.

CLONIDINE
(KLON-i-deen)

NEWLY DISCOVERED USES (OFF-LABEL)
Attention deficit/hyperactivity disorder (ADHD), alcohol withdrawal, autism, chronic diarrhea, diabetic neuropathy, diagnostic test for pheochromocytoma, Gilles de la Tourette syndrome, irritable bowel syndrome (IBS), menopausal symptoms, polydipsia, post-herpetic neuralgia, Raynaud's syndrome, smoking cessation

ORIGINAL USES (ON-LABEL)
Management of mild to moderate high blood pressure

BRAND NAMES
Catapres, Catapres-TTS, Duraclon

DRUG CLASS

Antihypertensive (alpha-adrenergic agonist)

DESCRIPTION

This drug affects activity in the brain stem, reducing heart rate and blood pressure.

POTENTIAL SIDE EFFECTS

Drowsiness, dizziness, dry mouth, sudden drop in blood pressure upon standing from sitting or lying down position, headache, sedation, fatigue, lethargy, insomnia, nervousness, local skin reaction (patch), hyperpigmentation, edema, excoriation, impotence, weakness, sexual dysfunction, nausea, vomiting, constipation, dry throat.

CAUTIONS

- Do not discontinue this medication suddenly as rebound high blood pressure may occur and can be serious. Gradual withdrawal is needed if drug needs to be stopped.
- Notify your doctor if you have cardiac problems, recent heart attack or stroke, chronic kidney problems.
- Requires periodic eye examinations.
- Tolerance may develop to this drug.
- Discontinue within four hours of surgery then restart as soon as possible after.

DRUG INTERACTIONS

Antipsychotics, narcotic analgesics, nitroprusside, barbiturates, cyclosporine, tacrolimus, prazosin, tricyclic antidepressants, verapamil

FOOD INTERACTIONS

Alcohol

HERBAL INTERACTIONS

Dong quai if using clonidine for hypertension. Ephedra, yohimbe, ginseng, valerian, St. John's wort, kava kava, gotu kola.

PREGNANCY AND BREAST-FEEDING CAUTIONS

FDA Pregnancy Risk Category C. Excreted into breast milk. Breast-feeding is not recommended.

SPECIAL INFORMATION

Caution if driving or operation of machinery is needed. Apply patch to a hairless area of intact skin (upper arm, torso). Use a different site from previous application. If patch loosens, apply adhesive directly over the system to ensure good adherence. Do not stand suddenly from a sitting or lying down position. The epidural formulation has a black box warning stating that this drug is not recommended for pain management in obstetrical, post-partum, or peri-operative conditions.

CLOTRIMAZOLE
(kloe-TRIM-a-zole)

NEWLY DISCOVERED USES (OFF-LABEL)
Otitis externa

ORIGINAL USES (ON-LABEL)
Treatment of susceptible fungal infections of the skin and mouth

BRAND NAME
Clotrimazole

DRUG CLASS
Antifungal (oral troche, topical)

DESCRIPTION
This drug manages fungal infections by affecting the permeability of the fungal cell wall, limiting the cell's growth.

POTENTIAL SIDE EFFECTS
Skin redness, hives, nausea and vomiting (oral use), mild burning, irritation, stinging to skin or vaginal area, and vulvar/vaginal burning, abnormal liver function test (oral use).

CAUTIONS
- This drug should not be used to treat systemic fungal infections.
- Studies have not been done to establish the safety and effectiveness of clotrimazole lozenges (troches) in children less than three years of age.
- Avoid contact with eyes when using the topical formulation.

DRUG INTERACTIONS
Do not use with other topical or oral products unless directed by your doctor.

FOOD INTERACTIONS
Unknown

HERBAL INTERACTIONS
Unknown

PREGNANCY AND BREAST-FEEDING CAUTIONS
FDA Pregnancy Category B (topical); C (troches). Excretion in breast milk unknown. Consult your doctor.

SPECIAL INFORMATION
Troches should not be swallowed whole, but rather allowed to dissolve slowly in the mouth to achieve the maximal effect. Avoid contact with eyes. Avoid using wrappings or dressings that block airflow. Do not apply to infected areas. Not useful for treatment on scalp or nails.

This information applies to the prescription product only and is not applicable to nonprescription products.

CLOZAPINE
(KLOE-za-peen)

NEWLY DISCOVERED USES (OFF-LABEL)
Huntington's disease, Parkinson's disease, polydipsia

ORIGINAL USES (ON-LABEL)
Treatment of schizophrenia that has been unresponsive to other drugs, to reduce risk of recurrent suicidal behavior in schizophrenia

BRAND NAME
Clozaril

DRUG CLASS
Atypical antipsychotic

DESCRIPTION
This drug stabilizes levels of certain hormones by blocking specific receptors in the brain, including dopamine and serotonin.

POTENTIAL SIDE EFFECTS
Drowsiness, dizziness, constipation, weight gain, increased heart rate, urinary incontinence, chest pain, high blood pressure, increased heart rate, fainting, seizures, headache, nightmares, rash, anorexia, diarrhea, heartburn, dry mouth, various blood disorders (such as changes in white blood cells), elevations in tests

for liver function, tremor, rigidity, increased muscle activity, weakness, visual disturbances, sweating.

CAUTIONS

- Requires blood monitoring to screen for potentially serious and life-threatening blood disorders. Monitoring should occur prior to the initiation of therapy and on a routine basis throughout therapy. Based on the results of these tests, your doctor will decide to continue or stop the medication.
- Not for use if you have uncontrolled seizures or history of seizures or in combination with drugs that lower seizure threshold, certain blood disorders such as agranulocytosis, bone marrow suppression or history of blood disorders, or central nervous system depression.
- Do not discontinue suddenly; taper off over 1-2 weeks.
- Elderly patients may be at an increased risk for adverse reactions.
- Notify your doctor if you have urinary retention, benign prostatic hyperplasia, narrow-angle glaucoma, dry mouth, diabetes, visual problems, constipation, or history of bowel obstruction.
- May require dosage adjustment if you have decreased liver function.
- Rare cases of fatal blood clots, including in the lung and stroke have been associated with clozapine.

DRUG INTERACTIONS

Antihypertensives, benzodiazepines, risperidone, metoclopramide, epinephrine, citalopram, fluoxetine, fluvoxamine, sertraline, phenobarbital, ritonavir. This drug is metabolized (inactivated) by specific set of liver enzymes. Several other drugs interfere with these liver enzymes, and thus, may increase or decrease the clearance of clozapine from the body, potentially increasing the risk of side effects or decreasing effectiveness. When these drugs are given in combination with clozapine, dosage adjustments may be needed. As these are too numerous to list, you should always check with your doctor or pharmacist prior to starting a new medication.

FOOD INTERACTIONS

Alcohol. Limit caffeine intake.

HERBAL INTERACTIONS

Valerian, St. John's wort, gotu kola, kava kava

PREGNANCY AND BREAST-FEEDING CAUTIONS
FDA Pregnancy Risk Category B. This drug is excreted in breast milk. Breast-feeding is not recommended during therapy.

SPECIAL INFORMATION
This drug has a black box warning regarding the potential for serious, life-threatening blood disorders that have occurred during therapy. Blood monitoring must be performed prior to the initiation of therapy, during therapy, and for four weeks after the drug is stopped. This drug is only available through a restricted distribution program that ensures this monitoring. Other safety issues discussed in the black box are the potential for the development of serious cardiac effects (such as myocarditis, pericarditis, pericardial effusion, cardiomyopathy, and congestive heart failure).

CODEINE
(KOE-deen)

NEWLY DISCOVERED USES (OFF-LABEL)
Chronic diarrhea

ORIGINAL USES (ON-LABEL)
Treatment of mild to moderate pain; used as cough suppressant in lower doses

BRAND NAMES
No U.S. brand names available

DRUG CLASS
Analgesic (narcotic), cough suppressant

DESCRIPTION
Codeine is a narcotic derived from opium or morphine. It is used as a cough suppressant, analgesic, and hypnotic medication.

POTENTIAL SIDE EFFECTS
Drowsiness, constipation, low blood pressure, dizziness, light-headedness, false feeling of well being, malaise, rash, hives, dry mouth, anorexia, nausea, vomiting, liver toxicity, decreased urination, ureteral spasm, burning at injection site, weakness, blurred

vision, shortness of breath, physical and psychological dependence, histamine release.

CAUTIONS

- Use with caution if you have severe liver or kidney dysfunction.
- Use with caution if you have respiratory diseases including asthma, emphysema, and chronic obstructive pulmonary disease (COPD).
- Not for use to treat productive cough or for children younger than two years of age.

DRUG INTERACTIONS

This drug is metabolized (inactivated) by specific set of liver enzymes. Several other drugs interfere with these liver enzymes, and thus may increase or decrease the clearance of codeine from the body, and often requiring dosage adjustments when they are administered in combination. As these are too numerous to list, you should always check with your doctor or pharmacist prior to starting a new medication.

May severely increase toxicity of codeine when taken other drugs that cause central nervous system depression, tricyclic antidepressants, other narcotic analgesics, guanabenz, MAO inhibitors, and neuromuscular blockers.

FOOD INTERACTIONS

Alcohol

HERBAL INTERACTIONS

Valerian, St. John's wort, kava kava, gotu kola

PREGNANCY AND BREAST-FEEDING CAUTIONS

FDA Pregnancy Risk Category C/D (prolonged use or high doses at term). Excreted in breast milk. The American Academy of Pediatrics classifies this drug as compatible with breast-feeding. Check with your doctor before using in breast-feeding. Use caution.

SPECIAL INFORMAITON

May cause sedation and interfere with tasks that require alertness.

COLCHICINE
(KOL-chi-seen)

ORIGINAL USES (ON-LABEL)
Treatment and prevention of acute gouty arthritis attacks

BRAND NAMES
None

DRUG CLASS
Anti-gout, anti-inflammatory

DESCRIPTION
Colchicine reduces the production of lactic acid, which decreases the deposit of urate crystals in joints. Urate crystals are responsible for the inflammation and pain associated with gout.

POTENTIAL SIDE EFFECTS
Nausea, vomiting, diarrhea, abdominal pain, hair loss, nerve pain in the limbs, rash, muscle aches, blood disorders, anorexia.

CAUTIONS
- Do not use if you have hypersensitivity to colchicine or any component of the formulation.
- Not for use if you have serious kidney, gastrointestinal, liver, and/or cardiac disorders.
- Requires periodic blood tests during therapy to monitor for blood disorders and kidney function.
- For use with caution if you are debilitated or elderly, or if you have severe gastric, liver, or kidney disease.
- Severe local irritation can occur with injectable formulation.
- Decreases the absorption of vitamin B-12, may require supplementation with vitamins.

DRUG INTERACTIONS
Cyclosporine

FOOD INTERACTIONS
Unknown

HERBAL INTERACTIONS
Unknown

PREGNANCY AND BREAST-FEEDING CAUTIONS
FDA Pregnancy Risk Category C (oral), FDA Pregnancy Category D (Injectable form). Excreted in breast milk. The American Academy of Pediatrics considers this drug compatible with breast-feeding. Consult with your doctor.

SPECIAL INFORMATION
Contact your doctor if nausea, diarrhea or vomiting occurs. Stop taking this medication as soon as the gout pain is relieved or at the first sign of nausea, vomiting, stomach pain, or diarrhea.

COLESTIPOL
(koe-LES-ti-pole)

NEWLY DISCOVERED USES (OFF-LABEL)
> Primary biliary cirrhosis

ORIGINAL USES (ON-LABEL)
For combination use with other drugs in the management of primary hypercholesterolemia (increased total cholesterol levels)

BRAND NAME
Colestid

DRUG CLASS
Antilipemic (bile acid sequestrant)

DESCRIPTION
This drug is used to control cholesterol levels by affecting the activity of low-density lipoprotein (LDL) cholesterol.

POTENTIAL SIDE EFFECTS
Constipation, headache, dizziness, anxiety, vertigo, abdominal pain, stomach distention, belching, flatulence, nausea, vomiting, diarrhea.

CAUTIONS
- Do not take simultaneously with any other medications.
- Do not take this drug if you have high triglycerides, or gastric dysfunction (fecal impaction may occur and hemorrhoids may be worsened).
- Use caution if you have vitamin K deficiency (possible increased bleeding tendency).

- May interfere with normal absorption and digestion of fat and absorption of vitamins A, D, K, and E, and folic acid.

DRUG INTERACTIONS
This drug may reduce the absorption of numerous medications when administered simultaneously, including but not limited to: other drugs used to treat high cholesterol, diuretics, propranolol, corticosteroids, thyroid hormones, digoxin, valproic acid, nonsteroidal anti-inflammatory drugs, and troglitazone.

FOOD INTERACTIONS
May interfere with absorption of fat-soluble vitamins in diet.

HERBAL INTERACTIONS
Unknown

PREGNANCY AND BREAST-FEEDING CAUTIONS
FDA Pregnancy Risk Category C. Not recommended during breast-feeding.

SPECIAL INFORMATION
Give other medications one hour before or four hours after giving colestipol. Granules should be added to at least 90 mL of liquid and stirred until completely mixed.

CORTICOTROPIN
(cor-ti-COE-troe-pin)

NEWLY DISCOVERED USES (OFF-LABEL)
West syndrome

ORIGINAL USES (ON-LABEL)
Allergic states, collagen diseases, skin diseases, endocrine disorders, gastrointestinal diseases, blood disorders, nervous system disease, eye disease, rheumatic disease, lung disease

BRAND NAME
HP Acthar Gel

DRUG CLASS
Anterior pituitary hormone

DESCRIPTION
This drug stimulates the Boyd's adrenal cortex to secrete cortisol, corticosterone, aldosterone, and other hormones.

POTENTIAL SIDE EFFECTS

High blood pressure, congestive heart failure, change in heart rate, vertigo, headache, impaired wound healing, darkened spots of the skin, menstrual irregularities, abdominal distention, pancreatitis, muscle weakness, cataracts, glaucoma, sodium and fluid retention, potassium and calcium loss, swelling of feet or hands.

CAUTIONS

- Chronic therapy may result in irreversible adverse effects and increases the risk of allergic reactions.
- Therapy with this drug may mask the symptoms of infection and increase the susceptibility of infection via immuno-suppression.
- Psychiatric symptoms may develop or be aggravated.
- Diabetics may require increased doses of insulin or oral drugs to treat diabetes.

DRUG INTERACTIONS

Amphotericin B, hydrochlorothiazide, bupropion, fluoro-quinolones, itraconazole, rotavirus vaccine, testosterone, anthrax vaccine, aspirin, diuretics, barbiturates, phenytoin

FOOD INTERACTIONS

Avoid excessive real licorice ingestion.

HERBAL INTERACTIONS

Echinacea, saiboku-to, and ma huang

PREGNANCY AND BREAST-FEEDING CAUTIONS

FDA Pregnancy Risk Category C. Excretion in breast milk unknown. Consult doctor.

SPECIAL INFORMATION

Inform your doctor if any of the following develop: marked fluid retention, muscle weakness, abdominal pain, headache, or seizures.

CORTISONE

(KOR-ti-sone)

NEWLY DISCOVERED USES (OFF-LABEL)

Cluster headache treatment

ORIGINAL USES (ON-LABEL)
Management of adrenocortical insufficiency

BRAND NAME
Cortisone Acetate

DRUG CLASS
Anti-inflammatory (corticosteroid)

DESCRIPTION
This drug decreases inflammation by suppressing inflammatory mediators and affecting capillary permeability.

POTENTIAL SIDE EFFECTS
Insomnia, nervousness, increased appetite, indigestion, increased hair growth, diabetes mellitus, joint aches, cataracts, glaucoma, headache, impaired wound healing, thin fragile skin, loss of menstruation, sodium and fluid retention, loss of potassium or calcium, abdominal distention, nausea, vomiting.

CAUTIONS
- Chronic therapy may result in irreversible adverse effects and increases the risk of allergic reactions.
- Therapy with this drug may mask the symptoms of infection and increase the susceptibility of infection via immunosuppression.
- Psychiatric symptoms may develop or be aggravated.
- Diabetics may require increased doses of insulin or oral drugs to treat diabetes.

DRUG INTERACTIONS
Aminoglutethimide, barbiturates, cholestyramine, oral contraceptives, ephedrine, estrogens, phenytoin, ketoconazole, rifampin, oral anticoagulants, cyclosporine, isoniazid, diuretics, salicylates, somatrem, theophylline

FOOD INTERACTIONS
Caffeine intake should be limited while on this drug.

HERBAL INTERACTIONS
Unknown

PREGNANCY AND BREAST-FEEDING CAUTIONS
FDA Pregnancy Risk Category D. Excreted in breast milk. Consult your doctor.

SPECIAL INFORMATION
Prolonged therapy may result in suppression of adrenal gland function.

CROMOLYN
(KROE-moe-lin)

NEWLY DISCOVERED USES (OFF-LABEL)
Food allergy

ORIGINAL USES (ON-LABEL)
Inhalation: combination for the prevention of allergic disorders including asthma, prevention of exercise-induced bronchospasm. Nasal: prevention and treatment of seasonal allergies. Oral: systemic mastocytosis. Ocular: treatment of vernal keratoconjunctivitis, vernal conjunctivitis, and vernal keratitis.

BRAND NAMES
Crolom, Gastrocrom, Intal, NasalCrom (OTC), Opticrom

DRUG CLASS
Antiallergic (inhalation, nasal, ocular, oral)

DESCRIPTION
This drug prevents the release of histamine, a substance important in causing allergies or allergy-like symptoms, and leukotriene, a substance that causes vessel constriction in the lungs and difficulty breathing.

POTENTIAL SIDE EFFECTS
Inhaled: Unpleasant taste in mouth.

Nasal: increase in sneezing, burning, stinging, or irritation inside of nose, headache, hoarseness, cough, postnasal drip.

Ocular: Temporary burning and stinging.

Oral: Flushing, increased heart rate, anxiety, rash, hives, headache, insomnia, flatulence.

CAUTIONS
- This drug should not be used if you have acute asthma attacks.
- This drug should be used with caution if you have a history of irregular heart rhythm.
- Oral: Dosage adjustments may be needed in patients with decreased kidney or liver function.

DRUG INTERACTIONS
Unknown

FOOD INTERACTIONS
Oral: Should take at least 30 minutes before meals.

HERBAL INTERACTIONS
Unknown

PREGNANCY AND BREAST-FEEDING CAUTIONS
FDA Pregnancy Risk Category B. Excretion in breast milk unknown.

CYCLOBENZAPRINE
(sye-kloe-BEN-za-preen)

NEWLY DISCOVERED USES (OFF-LABEL)
Fibromyalgia

ORIGINAL USES (ON-LABEL)
Treatment of muscle spasm associated with acute painful musculoskeletal conditions

BRAND NAME
Flexeril

DRUG CLASS
Skeletal muscle relaxant

DESCRIPTION
Cyclobenzaprine relaxes muscles by which decreasing the activity of motor neurons.

POTENTIAL SIDE EFFECTS
Drowsiness, dizziness, dry mouth, increased heart rate, low blood pressure, fatigue, blurred vision, sweating, disorientation, insomnia.

CAUTIONS
- Notify your doctor if you have hyperthyroidism, congestive heart failure, irregular heart rhythm, urinary hesitancy, glaucoma, reduced liver function, or if recovering from a recent heart attack.
- Do not use at the same time or within 14 days of taking an MAO inhibitor. The combination may result in serious side effects (such as hypertensive crisis, seizures).
- May cause significant drowsiness, which may interfere with tasks requiring alertness.

DRUG INTERACTIONS

Tramadol, anticholinergics, MAO inhibitors, guanethidine. This drug is metabolized (inactivated) by a specific set of liver enzymes. Several other drugs interfere with these liver enzymes, and thus, may increase or decrease the clearance of cyclobenzaprine from the body, potentially increasing the risk of side effects or decreasing effectiveness. When these drugs are given in combination with cyclobenzaprine, dosage adjustments may be needed. As these are too numerous to list, you should always check with your doctor or pharmacist prior to starting a new medication.

FOOD INTERACTIONS

Alcohol

HERBAL INTERACTIONS

Valerian, kava, kava, gotu kola

PREGNANCY AND BREAST-FEEDING CAUTIONS

FDA Pregnancy Risk Category B. It is not known if this drug is excreted in breast milk. Consult your doctor.

SPECIAL INFORMATION

Avoid alcohol or other drugs that can cause sedation.

CYCLOPENTOLATE
(sye-cloe-PEN-toe-late)

Ophthalmic

NEWLY DISCOVERED USES (OFF-LABEL)
Uveitis

ORIGINAL USES (ON-LABEL)
Diagnostic procedures requiring mydriasis and cycloplegia

BRAND NAMES
AK-Pentolate (DSC); Cyclogyl; Cylate

DRUG CLASS
Anticholinergic, ophthalmic

DESCRIPTION
This drug causes pupil widening (mydriasis) and prevents pupil constriction (cycloplegia) during eye examinations.

POTENTIAL SIDE EFFECTS

Blurred vision, increased intraocular pressure, eye irritation, sedation, drowsiness, ataxia, fatigue, difficulty concentrating, irritability, and increased heart rate.

CAUTIONS

- Not for use if you have myasthenia gravis or narrow-angle glaucoma.
- Use with caution in patients with certain types of nerve pain (autonomic neuropathy).

DRUG INTERACTIONS

Belladonna alkaloids

FOOD INTERACTIONS

Unknown

HERBAL INTERACTIONS

Unknown

PREGNANCY AND BREAST-FEEDING CAUTIONS

FDA Pregnancy Category C. It is not known if this drug is excreted in the breast milk.

SPECIAL INFORMATION

Notify your doctor if you are using any medications for glaucoma.

CYCLOPHOSPHAMIDE
(sye-kloe-FOS-fa-mide)

NEWLY DISCOVERED USES (OFF-LABEL)

Autoimmune hemolytic anemia, bullous pemphigoid, chronic inflammatory demyelinating polyneuropathy, dermatomyositis/polymyositis, multiple sclerosis, myasthenia gravis, polyarteritis nodosa, therapy-resistant idiopathic thrombocytopenic purpura, therapy-resistant thrombotic thrombocytopenic purpura, rheumatoid arthritis, sarcoidosis, scleroderma, systemic lupus erythematosus (SLE), uveitis due to systemic disease

ORIGINAL USES (ON-LABEL)

Various cancers

BRAND NAMES
Cytoxan, Neosar

DRUG CLASS
Cancer chemotherapy (antineoplastic)

DESCRIPTION
This drug inhibits cell division, interfering with DNA production, and thus prevents cell growth and multiplication.

POTENTIAL SIDE EFFECTS
Hair loss, infertility, nausea, vomiting, loss of appetite, diarrhea, bladder bleeding and swelling, decreased platelets, anemia, cardiac toxicity, mouth ulcers, abdominal pain, loss of menstruation, various blood disorders, infection.

CAUTIONS
- Kidney and liver function may be assessed during therapy for adjusting doses.
- This therapy affects components in the blood (such as white blood cells), which can result in severe side effects. Blood testing should be performed on a regular basis during therapy.
- May affect heart function.
- This drug suppresses the immune system, which is essential in combating infections. Thus, this drug may interfere with normal wound healing and increase the risk of infection.
- Acute bleeding and swelling of the bladder may be common and can be severe in some patients. Drink ample fluids and urinate frequently to reduce the likelihood of developing these effects.

DRUG INTERACTIONS
Allopurinol, anesthetics, cimetidine, chloramphenicol, digoxin, doxorubicin, thiazide diuretics (such as hydrochlorothiazide). This drug is metabolized (inactivated) by specific set of liver enzymes. Several other drugs interfere with these liver enzymes, and thus, may increase or decrease the clearance of cyclophosphamide from the body, potentially increasing the risk of side effects or decreasing effectiveness. When these drugs are given in combination with cyclophosphamide, dosage adjustments may be needed. As these are too numerous to list, you should always check with your doctor or pharmacist prior to starting a new medication.

FOOD INTERACTIONS
Unknown

HERBAL INTERACTIONS
Black cohosh, dong quai (in estrogen-dependent tumors)

PREGNANCY AND BREAST-FEEDING CAUTIONS
FDA Pregnancy Risk Category D. Drug is excreted into the breast milk. Do not breast-feed while taking this drug.

SPECIAL INFORMATION
Take tablets on an empty stomach, unless stomach upset occurs, then take with food. Contraception is recommended during therapy for both men and women. Contact your doctor if any of the following occur: unusual bleeding, bruising, fever, chills, sore throat, cough, shortness of breath, seizures, mouth ulcers, yellow discoloration of the skin and eyes.

CYCLOSPORINE
(si-klo-SPOR- een)

NEWLY DISCOVERED USES (OFF-LABEL)
Allergen induced asthma, alopecia areata, aplastic anemia, autoimmune hemolytic anemia, autoimmune hepatitis, chronic inflammatory demyelinating polyneuropathy, dermatitis (atopic), dermatitis (chronic actinic), dermatomyositis/polymyositis, liver fibrosis, membranous nephropathy, myasthenia gravis, nephrotic syndrome, primary biliary cirrhosis, psoriatic arthritis, pterygium recurrence prevention, therapy-resistant idiopathic thrombocytopenic purpura, scleroderma, steroid dependent asthma, systemic lupus erythematosus (SLE), thrombotic thrombocytopenic purpura, ulcerative colitis, urticaria, uveitis

ORIGINAL USES (ON-LABEL)
For use in preventing transplanted organ rejection, psoriasis, and severe active rheumatoid arthritis

BRAND NAMES
Gengraf, Neoral, Sandimmune

DRUG CLASS
Immunosuppressant

DESCRIPTION
This is a potent immunosuppressant that prolongs the survival of transplant of various organs.

POTENTIAL SIDE EFFECTS

Dizziness, headache, numbness, swelling of the gums, nausea, kidney toxicity, bronchospasm, cough, shortness of breath, upper respiratory tract infection, joint aches, high blood pressure, flu-like syndrome, chest pain, flushing, depression, headache, tremor, abdominal pain, diarrhea, stomach upset, increased potassium levels, liver toxicity, seizures, decreased magnesium levels.

CAUTIONS

- May cause kidney toxicity, requires monitoring during therapy. Avoid other drugs that cause kidney toxicity.
- Conversion from one product to another is not recommended without the advice of your doctor or pharmacist.
- Requires close monitoring and periodic blood testing for liver and kidney function, blood factors, electrolytes, etc.

DRUG INTERACTIONS

NSAIDs, other drugs which can cause kidney toxicity (e.g., to-bramycin, gentamicin, melphalan, amphotericin B, ketoconazole, etc.), allopurinol, amiodarone, androgens, anticonvulsants, anti-fungals, beta-blockers, bosentan, bromocriptine, calcium channel blockers, colchicine, oral contraceptives, corticosteroids, fluoro-quinolones, foscarnet, macrolide antibiotics, metoclopramide, nafcillin, nefazodone, orlistat, probucol, sulfonamides, terbina-fine, ticlopidine, digoxin, etoposide, statins, methotrexate, potas-sium sparing diuretics, sirolimus.

This drug is metabolized by a specific set of liver enzymes. Several other drugs interfere with these liver enzymes, and thus may increase or decrease the clearance of cyclosporine from the body, potentially increasing the risk of side effects or decreasing effectiveness. When these drugs are given in combination with cyclosporine, dosage adjustments may be needed. As these are too numerous to list, you should always check with your doctor or pharmacist prior to starting a new medication, herbal, or nonprescription product.

FOOD INTERACTIONS

Take with food at the same time each day.

HERBAL INTERACTIONS

St. John's wort

PREGNANCY AND BREAST-FEEDING CAUTIONS
FDA Pregnancy Risk Category C. Excreted into breast milk. Consult your doctor.

SPECIAL INFORMATION
This drug has a black box warning regarding several complications associated with therapy, including but not limited to an increased risk of infection, kidney toxicity, and increased blood pressure. In addition, the black box describes the differences between different brand name products. Please review this with your doctor prior to the initiation of therapy.

CYCLOSPORINE
(si-klo-SPOR- een)

Ocular

NEWLY DISCOVERED USES (OFF-LABEL)
Uveitis

ORIGINAL USES (ON-LABEL)
To increase tear production in individuals who have suppressed tear production

BRAND NAME
Restasis

DRUG CLASS
Immune drug (ocular)

DESCRIPTION
Reduces eye inflammation, which is thought to modulate immunity.

POTENTIAL SIDE EFFECTS:
Eye burning, visual disturbances, swelling, discharge, eye pain, itching, stinging, foreign body sensation.

CAUTIONS
- Not for use if there is an active eye infection or if you have herpes keratitis.
- Do not use while wearing contact lenses. Remove them prior to instillation of drops and reinsert 15 minutes after administration.

DRUG INTERACTIONS
Do not use other eye products without consulting your doctor or pharmacist.

FOOD INTERACTIONS
Unknown

HERBAL INTERACTIONS
Unknown

PREGNANCY AND BREAST-FEEDING CAUTIONS
FDA Pregnancy Risk Category C. Excreted into breast milk. Consult your doctor.

SPECIAL INFORMATION
Do not allow the tip of the container to touch the eye or other surfaces as this may cause contamination and seed an infection.

CYPROHEPTADINE
(si-proe-HEP-ta-deen)

NEWLY DISCOVERED USES (OFF-LABEL)
Autism, post-traumatic stress syndrome (PTSD)

ORIGINAL USES (ON-LABEL)
Common seasonal and year-round allergies, use with other drugs to manage allergic type reactions

BRAND NAME
Periactin

DRUG CLASS
Antihistamine

DESCRIPTION
Cyproheptadine blocks the histamine and serotonin receptors in the gastrointestinal tract, blood vessels, and lungs.

POTENTIAL SIDE EFFECTS
Drowsiness, thickening of bronchial secretions, headache, tiredness, dizziness, increased appetite, nausea, diarrhea, dry mouth, muscle aches.

CAUTIONS
- Notify your doctor if you have narrow-angle glaucoma, prostate problems, bladder neck blockage, acute asthmatic at-

tacks, gastrointestinal tract blockage, or a stenosing peptic ulcer.

- Avoid use in combination with MAO inhibitors.
- Not for use in children less than two years old.
- Elderly patients are at increased risk for side effects.

DRUG INTERACTIONS
Other drugs that cause sedation (e.g., sedatives, anti-anxiety drugs, tranquilizers, narcotics, etc), MAO inhibitors (e.g., phenelzine, tranylcypromine, isocarboxazid)

FOOD INTERACTIONS
Alcohol

HERBAL INTERACTIONS
Unknown

FDA PREGNANCY CATEGORY/BREAST-FEEDING
FDA Pregnancy Category B. Excretion in breast milk is unknown. Because newborns have an increased sensitivity to antihistamines and the potential for side effects is increased, do not breast-feed during therapy with this drug.

SPECIAL INFORMATION
May cause drowsiness or dizziness, may interfere with tasks that require alertness.

DANAZOL
(DA-na-zole)

NEWLY DISCOVERED USES (OFF-LABEL) ——————
Autoimmune hemolytic anemia, dermatitis (chronic actinic), dysmenorrhea, gynecomastia, mastalgia, menorrhagia, menstrual migraine, premenstrual dysphoric disorder (PMDD), premenstrual syndrome (PMS), therapy-resistant idiopathic thrombocytopenic purpura

ORIGINAL USES (ON-LABEL)
Endometriosis, fibrocystic breast disease, and hereditary angioedema (recurrent allergic episodes which involve swelling of the skin, upper respiratory tract, and gastrointestinal tract)

BRAND NAME
Danocrine

DRUG CLASS
Hormone (androgen)

DESCRIPTION
This drug inhibits the release of hormones that are a part of the ovulation cycle. The decrease in the levels of these hormones results in a breakdown of endometrial tissue and also decreases the growth of abnormal breast tissue.

POTENTIAL SIDE EFFECTS
Acne, mild hair growth, hoarseness, weight gain, menstruation irregularities, flushing, sweating, liver dysfunction, vaginal dryness and irritation, emotional instability, reduction in breast size, changes in sperm count and motility.

CAUTIONS
- Not for use if you have undiagnosed abnormal genital bleeding, reduced liver, kidney, or heart function.
- Not for use in pregnancy or during breast-feeding. Pregnancy must be ruled out before starting this medication.
- Clot formation and life threatening of fatal stroke may occur with use of this medication.
- Use of this medication may result in serious liver events or serious high blood pressure.
- Before using for fibrocystic disease treatment, breast cancer should be ruled out.
- Use may increase the risk of certain cardiac disease, check with your doctor.
- Before using for fibrocystic disease, breast cancer must be excluded.
- Androgenic effects (masculinization) may not be reversible.

DRUG INTERACTIONS
Carbamazepine, cyclosporine, tacrolimus, warfarin, statin drugs such as lovastatin, pravastatin, anti-diabetic drugs. Danazol may lessen the action of hormonal contraceptives (birth control); it is recommended that you use other, non-hormonal contraception during therapy.

FOOD INTERACTIONS
Take this drug on an empty stomach. Avoid high-fat meals unless instructed by doctor.

HERBAL INTERACTIONS
Unknown

PREGNANCY AND BREAST-FEEDING CAUTIONS

FDA Pregnancy Risk Category X. Do not use in pregnancy or while breast-feeding.

SPECIAL INFORMATION

This drug has a black box warning regarding the risks of pregnancy, blood clots, long term therapy effects and high blood pressure related to increased pressure in the brain (benign intracranial hypertension). Pregnancy must be excluded as a possibility prior to initiation of therapy. During therapy a nonhormonal contraceptive method should be used. Report any signs and symptoms of intracranial hypertension to your doctor (such as headache, nausea, vomiting, vision changes.)

DAPSONE
(DAP-zone)

NEWLY DISCOVERED USES (OFF-LABEL)

Bullous pemphigoid, pneumocystis jiroveci pneumonia treatment and prevention

ORIGINAL USES (ON-LABEL)

Leprosy, dermatitis herpetiformis

BRAND NAMES

None

DRUG CLASS

Antibacterial (leprostatic)

DESCRIPTION

This drug weakens and kills the bacteria responsible for leprosy.

POTENTIAL SIDE EFFECTS

Headache, psychosis, insomnia, vertigo, numbness in limbs, nausea, vomiting, abdominal pain, anorexia, photosensitivity (skin reaction related to sun exposure), various blood disorders, blurred vision, ringing in the ears, fever, increased heart rate.

CAUTIONS

- Requires regular blood monitoring for side effects related to the blood.
- May cause severe liver problems.

- Wear protective clothing and sunscreen when spending time outdoors.

DRUG INTERACTIONS
Activated charcoal, didanosine, folic acid antagonists, para-aminobenzoic acid, probenecid, rifampin

FOOD INTERACTIONS
Unknown

HERBAL INTERACTIONS
Unknown

PREGNANCY AND BREAST-FEEDING CAUTIONS
FDA Pregnancy Risk Category C. Excreted in breast milk. Do not use during breast-feeding.

DESIPRAMINE
(des-IP-ra-meen)

NEWLY DISCOVERED USES (OFF-LABEL)
Attention deficit hyperactivity (ADHA), bulimia, chronic fatigue syndrome, chronic nausea and vomiting, chronic neuropathic pain, cocaine addiction, diabetic neuropathy, panic disorder, post-herpetic neuralgia, post-traumatic stress disorder (PTSD), stress incontinence, urge incontinence, vulvodynia

ORIGINAL USES (ON-LABEL)
Depression

BRAND NAME
Norpramin

DRUG CLASS
Antidepressant (tricyclic antidepressant)

DESCRIPTION
Desipramine is used to treat depression and other disorders. It works by increasing the levels of norepinephrine and serotonin in the body.

POTENTIAL SIDE EFFECTS
Dry mouth, sedation, dizziness, headache, nervousness, skin rash, tremors, hives, nausea, constipation, vision changes, sweating, lowered blood pressure, increased heart rate, decreased sodium

levels, suicidal ideation, changes in heart rhythm and conduction, blurred vision, weight gain, sexual dysfunction.

CAUTIONS

- Do not use if you have been taking an MAO inhibitor such as phenelzine, tranylcypromine, isocarboxazid within the past 14 days. When used with MAO-I's fever, high blood pressure, increased heart rate, confusion, seizures, and deaths have been reported.
- Not for use immediately after a heart attack.
- Can cause sedation that may impair performance of tasks requiring alertness. Sedative effects may be additive with other drugs that cause similar effects (CNS depressants).
- May worsen psychosis or mania in patients with bipolar disease.
- Do not abruptly stop medication; instead, taper gradually.
- Notify your doctor if you have low blood pressure as this drug can cause low blood pressure episodes.
- Use with caution if you have urinary retention, history of cardiac disease, seizure disorders, diabetes, benign prostatic hyperplasia, narrow angle glaucoma, dry mouth, visual problems, constipation, or a history of bowel obstruction.
- Possibility of suicidal behavior (see special information).
- Use with caution if you have hyperthyroidism or if you are receiving thyroid supplementation.
- Use with caution in patients with liver or kidney dysfunction and if you are elderly.

DRUG INTERACTIONS

MAO inhibitors (such as phenelzine, tranylcypromine, isocarboxazid), ritonavir, bupropion, amphetamines, anticholinergics, sedatives, chlorpropamide, tolazamide, warfarin, fluoxetine, fluvoxamine, citalopram, escitalopram, paroxetine, sertraline, cimetidine, carbamazepine, haloperidol, smoking, methylphenidate, valproic acid, clonidine, venlafaxine, protease inhibitors, quinidine, diltiazem, verapamil, lithium, phenothiazines may affect the levels of desipramine, drugs that prolong QT interval (see site: http://www.torsades.org/medical-pros/drug-lists/drug-lists.htm#)

This drug is metabolized (inactivated) by specific set of liver enzymes. Several other drugs interfere with these liver enzymes and thus may increase or decrease the clearance of desipramine from the body, potentially increasing the risk of side effects or decreasing effectiveness. When these drugs are given in combination with desipramine, dosage adjustments may be needed. As these are too numerous to list, you should always check with your doctor or pharmacist prior to starting a new medication.

FOOD INTERACTIONS
Alcohol, grapefruit juice

HERBAL INTERACTIONS
Valerian, St. John's wort, SAMe, kava kava

PREGNANCY AND BREAST-FEEDING CAUTIONS
FDA Pregnancy Risk Category C. Excreted in breast milk. Breast-feeding is not recommended during therapy with this drug.

SPECIAL INFORMATION
May take four to six weeks for the full therapeutic effects to be experienced. Avoid prolonged exposure to sunlight, wear sunscreen.

In 2005, the FDA announced new labeling for antidepressants regarding the need to closely monitor for worsening of depression and for the potential of increased suicidal thinking or suicidal behavior during therapy. Although this recommendation applies to all patients (adults, children, adolescents) treated with antidepressants for any indication, this is of particular importance in patients being treated for depression.

Close observation may be especially important when antidepressant medications are started for the first time or when doses are changed. More information on this topic can be found at the following web site: http://www.fda.gov/cder/drug/antidepressants/default.htm.

DESMOPRESSIN
(dez-mow-PREZ-in)

NEWLY DISCOVERED USES (OFF-LABEL)
Abnormal uterine bleeding, impaired hemostasis

ORIGINAL USES (ON-LABEL)
Nocturnal bedwetting (intranasal only), diabetes insipidus (intranasal, oral, injectable), hemophilia A (intranasal, injectable), von Willebrand's disease (intranasal, injectable)

BRAND NAMES
DDAVP, Minirin, Stimate

DRUG CLASS
Hormone

DESCRIPTION
This drug is a synthetic version of a human hormone (arginine vasopressin) that produces an anti-diuretic action and also decreases visceral smooth muscle activity.

POTENTIAL SIDE EFFECTS
Intranasal: abdominal pain, facial flushing, headache, nasal congestion, nausea, runny nose, nosebleed.

Injectable: abdominal pain, facial flushing, headache, nausea.

Oral: Increases in liver function tests.

CAUTIONS
- Not for use in the treatment of all types of hemophilia. Discuss with your doctor.
- Your doctor should provide a test dose of the intranasal product prior to starting therapy.
- May cause water intoxication. Ingest only enough fluid to satisfy thirst.
- May require urine monitoring if you are taking for diabetes insipidus.
- If using nasal product, notify your doctor prior to therapy if you have had nasal tissue scarring, blockage, surgery, congestion, cranial surgery.
- Tolerance may develop to the intranasal product when used for greater than 6 months.

DRUG INTERACTIONS
Carbamazepine, chlorpropamide

FOOD INTERACTIONS
Unknown

HERBAL INTERACTIONS
Unknown

PREGNANCY AND BREAST-FEEDING CAUTIONS
FDA Pregnancy Risk Category B. Excretion into the breast milk. Consult your doctor.

SPECIAL INFORMATION
Do not attempt to transfer contents of intranasal product from one bottle to the next. Review administration materials prior to therapy initiation. Notify your doctor if you develop a headache, shortness of breath, heartburn, nausea, abdominal cramps.

DESOGESTREL-ETHINYL ESTRADIOL
(des-oh-JES-trel ETH-in-il es-tra-DYE-ole)

NEWLY DISCOVERED USES (OFF-LABEL)
| Acne (women)

ORIGINAL USES (ON-LABEL)
Contraception

BRAND NAMES
Apri, Cyclessa, Desogen, Kariva, Mircette, Ortho-Cept

DRUG CLASS
Oral Contraceptives

DESCRIPTION
This drug inhibits ovulation by acting on the hypothalamus. Prevents secretion of two hormones important in the ovulation cycle: follicle stimulating hormone (FSH) and luteinizing hormone (LH).

POTENTIAL SIDE EFFECTS
Intermenstrual bleeding and irregularity, abdominal pain, diarrhea, nausea, vomiting, depression, dizziness, emotional lability, headache, migraine, nervousness, change in vision or ability to wear contact lenses, fluid retention, darkening of skin in areas, vaginal infections, hair loss. Increased risk of cardiac events, glucose intolerance, stroke, liver problems.

CAUTIONS
- Oral contraceptives do not protect against sexually transmitted diseases or HIV infection.
- Cardiovascular events increase if you are over 35 years of age and heavy smoker (at least 15 cigarettes daily), or have a history of cardiovascular disease or thromboembolic (blood clots) events. Thus, not for use in these patients.

- Not for use if you have decreased kidney, adrenal or liver function, diabetes with vascular involvement, history of or suspected breast cancer or estrogen dependent cancer, undiagnosed genital bleeding, liver tumor, severe high blood pressure, jaundice associated with pregnancy or prior birth control pill usage, headaches with neurological symptoms.
- Do not take if you are pregnant.
- Discuss cardiac and other risks with your doctor prior to starting therapy.

DRUG INTERACTIONS
Oral contraceptives, including this product, may interact with several drugs too numerous to list. Check with your pharmacist or doctor before starting any new medication, herbal product, or nonprescription drug.

FOOD INTERACTIONS
Grapefruit juice

HERBAL INTERACTIONS
St. John's wort, dong quai, black cohosh, saw palmetto, red clover, ginseng

PREGNANCY AND BREAST-FEEDING CAUTIONS
FDA Pregnancy Risk Category X. Do not use in pregnancy. Excreted in breast milk and not recommended during breast-feeding.

SPECIAL INFORMATION
Read the patient information brochure prior to therapy for important instructions regarding therapy and warnings (some black box).

DEXAMETHASONE
(deks-a-METH-a-sone)

Oral, Injectable

NEWLY DISCOVERED USES (OFF-LABEL)
Acute cisplatin-induced nausea and vomiting, bronchopulmonary dysplasia (in infants), canker sores, croup, cystic fibrosis, fetal distress, hirsutism, Ménière disease, oral lichen planus, premature labor (preterm), pharyngitis, prevention of post-op nausea and vomiting, therapy-resistant idiopathic thrombocytopenic purpura, sudden hearing loss, tonsillectomy, tonsillitis/peritonsillar abscess, varicella

ORIGINAL USES (ON-LABEL)
Management of allergic disorders, suppression test for diagnosis of Cushing's syndrome, cerebral edema, unresponsive shock

BRAND NAMES
Decadron, Dexameth, Dexone, Hexadrol

DRUG CLASS
Anti-inflammatory (corticosteroid)

DESCRIPTION
This drug decreases inflammation.

POTENTIAL SIDE EFFECTS
Insomnia, nervousness, increased appetite, indigestion, increased hair growth, diabetes mellitus, joint aches, cataracts, glaucoma, headache, impaired wound healing, thin fragile skin, loss of menstruation, sodium and fluid retention, loss of potassium or calcium, abdominal distention, nausea, vomiting.

CAUTIONS
- Chronic therapy may result in irreversible adverse effects and increases the risk of allergic reactions.
- Therapy with this drug may mask the symptoms of infection and increase the susceptibility of infection via immunosuppression.
- Psychiatric symptoms may develop or be aggravated.
- Diabetics may require increased doses of insulin or oral drugs to treat diabetes.
- Notify your doctor if you have hyperthyroidism, cirrhosis, nonspecific ulcerative colitis, hypertension, osteoporosis,

thromboembolic tendencies, congestive heart failure, convulsive disorders, myasthenia gravis, thrombophlebitis, peptic ulcer, or diabetes.

DRUG INTERACTIONS
Aminoglutethimide, barbiturates, cholestyramine, oral contraceptives, ephedrine, estrogens, phenytoin, ketoconazole, rifampin, oral anticoagulants, cyclosporine, isoniazid, diuretics, salicylates, somatrem, theophylline

FOOD INTERACTIONS
May cause stomach upset; take with food or snack.

HERBAL INTERACTIONS
Unknown

PREGNANCY AND BREAST-FEEDING CAUTIONS
FDA Pregnancy Risk Category C. Excreted in breast milk. Consult your doctor.

SPECIAL INFORMATION
Prolonged therapy may result in suppression of adrenal gland function.

Take single daily dose in morning prior to 9 a.m. Take multiple doses at evenly spaced intervals throughout the day.

DIAZEPAM
(dye-AZ-e-pam)

NEWLY DISCOVERED USES (OFF-LABEL)
Acute schizophrenia, labyrinthitis, Ménière's disease, multiple sclerosis, oculogyric crisis, tetanus

ORIGINAL USES (ON-LABEL)
Anxiety disorders, ethanol withdrawal symptoms, skeletal muscle relaxant, treatment of convulsive disorders, management of selected therapy-resistant epilepsy patients on stable regimens of antiepileptic drugs requiring intermittent use of diazepam to control episodes

BRAND NAMES
Diastat, Diazepam Intensol, Valium

DRUG CLASS
Antianxiety, anticonvulsant, sedative, muscle relaxant (benzo-diazepine)

DESCRIPTION
This drug acts on neurons at several sites within the body, including the spinal cord (muscle relaxation), brainstem (anticonvulsant), cerebellum, and cortical areas (emotional behavior).

POTENTIAL SIDE EFFECTS
Drowsiness, amnesia, slurred speech, rash, changes in libido, changes in salivation, constipation, nausea, incontinence, urinary retention, pain with injection, tremor, blurred vision, changes in vision, double vision, decrease in respiratory rate.

CAUTIONS
- Notify your doctor if you have narrow angle glaucoma, liver or kidney impairment, lung disease, depression, a history of drug dependence, or if you are over 65 years old or are pregnant.
- May increase the frequency of grand mal seizures.
- Associated with anterograde amnesia and paradoxical reactions.

DRUG INTERACTIONS
This drug is metabolized by a specific set of liver enzymes. Several other drugs interfere with these liver enzymes, and thus may increase or decrease the clearance of diazepam from the body, potentially increasing the risk of side effects or decreasing effectiveness. When these drugs are given in combination with diazepam, dosage adjustments may be needed. As these are too numerous to list, you should always check with your doctor or pharmacist prior to starting a new medication, herbal, or non-prescription product.

Diazepam potentiates the central nervous depressant effects of narcotic analgesics, barbiturates, phenothiazines, ethanol, antihistamines, MAO inhibitors, sedative-hypnotics, and cyclic antidepressants.

FOOD INTERACTIONS
Grapefruit juice. May be taken with food if stomach upset occurs.

HERBAL INTERACTIONS
St. John's wort, valerian, kava kava, gotu kola

PREGNANCY AND BREAST-FEEDING CAUTIONS
FDA Pregnancy Risk Category D. Excreted into the breast milk.
Refrain from breast-feeding while taking this drug.

SPECIAL INFORMATION
May cause drowsiness; avoid driving or other tasks that require
being alert. Avoid alcohol.

DIAZOXIDE
(dye-az-OKS-ide)

NEWLY DISCOVERED USES (OFF-LABEL)
Insulinomas

ORIGINAL USES (ON-LABEL)
Severe high blood pressure

BRAND NAME
Hyperstat IV

DRUG CLASS
Antihypertensive

DESCRIPTION
This drug relaxes blood vessels so as to induce changes in heart
rate and cardiac output that decrease blood pressure.

POTENTIAL SIDE EFFECTS
Sodium and water retention, nausea, headache, blurred vision,
decreased urination, swelling of feet or lower legs, weight gain
(rapid), electrolyte imbalances.

CAUTIONS
- Notify your doctor if you have an allergy to thiazide derivatives,
  or sulfonamides.
- Notify your doctor if you have fluid retention, gout, low blood
  pressure, impaired liver or kidney function, a recent stroke or
  heart attack.
- Requires frequent blood pressure monitoring.

DRUG INTERACTIONS
Hydralazine, sulfonylureas, thiazide diuretics such as hydrochlorothiazide, chlorothiazide.

FOOD INTERACTIONS
Unknown

HERBAL INTERACTIONS
Unknown

PREGNANCY AND BREAST-FEEDING CAUTIONS
FDA Pregnancy Risk Category C. Information not available. Consult your doctor.

DICLOFENAC SODIUM
(dye-KLOE-fen-ak)

Ocular

NEWLY DISCOVERED USES (OFF-LABEL)
Cystoid macular edema post-cataract surgery, uveitis

ORIGINAL USES (ON-LABEL)
Postoperative inflammation after cataract surgery, temporary relief of pain and photophobia after corneal refractive surgery

BRAND NAME
Voltaren Ophthalmic

DRUG CLASS
Anti-inflammatory [ocular nonsteroidal anti-inflammatory (NSAID)]

DESCRIPTION
This drug inhibits the production of prostaglandin, a chemical drug in the body responsible for inflammation and pain.

POTENTIAL SIDE EFFECTS
Temporary burning and stinging, inflammation of the cornea, increased ocular pressure, tearing, blurred vision, conjunctivitis, corneal deposits, corneal edema, eye discharge, eyelid swelling.

CAUTIONS
- Inform your doctor if you are allergic to aspirin or other NSAIDs.
- Patient should be monitored for a year after corneal refractive procedures for refractive stability.

- May increase bleeding time after ocular surgery. Use with caution if you are at increased risk of bleeding or you are taking medications that increase bleeding times.
- Use with topical steroids may delay healing.
- Corneal changes may occur with use such as thinning, ulcerations, and perforation. Discuss risk factors with your doctor.
- Use more than 24 hours prior to surgery or beyond 14 days post-surgery may increase risk of corneal adverse events.
- Do not use with contact lenses (except bandage hydrogel soft contact lens).

DRUG INTERACTIONS
Consult your doctor before using other ocular products. Drugs that affect bleeding times (such as warfarin, heparin, etc.).

FOOD INTERACTIONS
Unknown

HERBAL INTERACTIONS
Unknown

PREGNANCY AND BREAST-FEEDING CAUTIONS
FDA Pregnancy Risk Category C (Category D in third trimester). Consult with your doctor.

DICLOFENAC SODIUM
(dye-KLOE-fen-ak)

Oral

NEWLY DISCOVERED USES (OFF-LABEL)
Biliary colic, bursitis/tendonitis, dysmenorrhea, gout, juvenile rheumatoid arthritis, prevention of gallstone progression to acute cholecystitis

ORIGINAL USES (ON-LABEL)
Mild and chronic pain, actinic keratosis, ankylosing spondylitis, dysmenorrhea

BRAND NAMES
Voltaren, Voltaren-XR

DRUG CLASS
Pain reliever, anti-inflammatory [nonsteroidal anti-inflammatory (NSAID)]

DESCRIPTION
This drug inhibits the production of prostaglandin, a chemical drug in the body responsible for inflammation and pain.

POTENTIAL SIDE EFFECTS
Headache, dizziness, abdominal cramps, abdominal pain, constipation, diarrhea, increased liver enzymes.

CAUTIONS
- Not for use if you are allergic to aspirin or other NSAIDs.
- Not for use if you have active gastric/duodenal ulcer disease.
- Do not use during third trimester of pregnancy.
- Notify your doctor if you have congestive heart failure, asthma, dehydration, high blood pressure, decreased kidney or liver function, history of gastrointestinal (GI) disease, active gastric ulcer or bleeding, or are currently taking anticoagulants.
- Elderly are at higher risk of developing side effects.

DRUG INTERACTIONS
Digoxin, methotrexate, cyclosporine, lithium, insulin, sulfonylureas, potassium-sparing diuretics, warfarin, aspirin, thiazide diuretics, furosemide

FOOD INTERACTIONS
Alcohol (may increase stomach irritation)

HERBAL INTERACTIONS
Cat's claw, dong quai, evening primrose, feverfew, garlic, ginger, ginkgo, red clover, horse chestnut, green tea, ginseng

PREGNANCY AND BREAST-FEEDING CAUTIONS
FDA Pregnancy Risk Category B (Category D in third trimester). Excreted in breast milk. Consult with your doctor.

SPECIAL INFORMATION
Stop taking this drug (with doctor's approval) approximately 24 to 48 hours prior to surgical or dental procedures as it affects the body's ability to form blood clots and may increase bleeding time. In April 2005, the FDA announced the potential addition of a black box warning to the labeling of this class of drugs (NSAIDs), specifically regarding potential serious cardiac events and potentially life-threatening gastric adverse events.

DICYCLOMINE
(dye-SYE-kloe-meen)

NEWLY DISCOVERED USES (OFF-LABEL)
> Cancer treatment-induced mucositis/stomatitis

ORIGINAL USES (ON-LABEL)
Irritable bowel syndrome

BRAND NAMES
Bentyl, Bentylol, Di-Spaz

DRUG CLASS
Gastrointestinal antispasmodic

DESCRIPTION
This drug relieves smooth muscle spasms in the gastrointestinal tract.

POTENTIAL SIDE EFFECTS
Dry mouth, dizziness, blurred vision, nausea, light-headedness, drowsiness, weakness, nervousness.

CAUTIONS
- Inform your doctor if you have any of the following conditions: urinary blockage, gastric blockage, severe ulcerative colitis, reflux esophagitis, unstable cardiac disease, glaucoma, myasthenia gravis.
- Inform your doctor if you develop diarrhea, as this may be an early sign of intestinal obstruction.
- This drug may cause drowsiness or blurred vision, effects which can interfere with tasks that require alertness.

DRUG INTERACTIONS
Amantadine, certain antiarrhythmic drugs, nitrates and nitrites, cisapride, sympathomimetic drugs, tricyclic antidepressants, anti-glaucoma drugs, other drugs with anticholinergic activity, corticosteroids, extended release digoxin, metoclopramide, antacids. Check with your doctor or pharmacist prior to starting any new medication, herbal product, or nonprescription drug.

FOOD INTERACTIONS
Alcohol

HERBAL INTERACTIONS
Betel Nut

PREGNANCY AND BREAST-FEEDING CAUTIONS
FDA Pregnancy Risk Category B. Excreted in breast milk. Not recommended for use during breast-feeding.

SPECIAL INFORMATION
Dosage may need to be adjusted for individual needs. Do not take within two to three hours of taking antacids or medicine to stop diarrhea. This medicine may decrease sweating, causing you to get too hot. Be careful in hot weather, while you are exercising, or if using a sauna or whirlpool.

DILTIAZEM
(dil-TYE-a-zem)

NEWLY DISCOVERED USES (OFF-LABEL)
Anal fissure, dermatomyositis/polymyositis, esophageal motility disorders, migraine prevention, prevention of cyclosporine induced nephrotoxicity, premature labor (preterm), Raynaud's syndrome

ORIGINAL USES (ON-LABEL)
To treat essential hypertension (high blood pressure), chronic stable angina, or angina from coronary artery spasm

BRAND NAMES
Cardizem, Cartia XT, Dilacor XR, Diltia XT, Taztia XT, Tiazac

DRUG CLASS
Antianginal, antiarrhythmic, antihypertensive (calcium channel blocker)

DESCRIPTION
This drug blocks relaxes coronary vascular smooth muscle and increases oxygen delivery to the heart.

POTENTIAL SIDE EFFECTS
Edema, headache, low heart rate, dizziness, nervousness, vomiting, muscle aches, change in heart conduction, lightheadedness, constipation, nausea, shortness of breath, flushing.

CAUTIONS
- Do not use if you are allergic to this medication.
- Notify your doctor if you have had an allergic reaction to a drug in this class.

- Inform your doctor if you have low blood pressure, severe left ventricular dysfunction or other types of heart problems, liver or kidney dysfunction.
- Abrupt withdrawal may cause increased duration and frequency of chest pain.
- The elderly may be at greater risk of experiencing low blood pressure and constipation associated with this therapy.

DRUG INTERACTIONS
This drug is metabolized by a specific set of liver enzymes. Several other drugs interfere with these liver enzymes, and thus may increase or decrease the clearance of diltiazem from the body, potentially increasing the risk of side effects or decreasing effectiveness. When these drugs are given in combination with diltiazem, dosage adjustments may be needed. As these are too numerous to list, you should always check with your doctor or pharmacist prior to starting a new medication, herbal, or nonprescription product.

FOOD INTERACTIONS
Avoid alcohol, grapefruit. Take on an empty stomach.

HERBAL INTERACTIONS
St. John's wort, dong quai, ephedra, yohimbe, ginseng, garlic

PREGNANCY AND BREAST-FEEDING CAUTIONS
FDA Pregnancy Risk Category C. Excreted in breast milk. Consult your doctor.

SPECIAL INFORMATION
Do not crush or chew the extended release formulations.

DIVALPROEX
(DI-val-proe-ix)

NEWLY DISCOVERED USES (OFF-LABEL) ───────
Alcohol withdrawal, Alzheimer's disease, cocaine addiction, impulsive aggressive disorder, schizoaffective disorder

ORIGINAL USES (ON-LABEL)
Single drug or combination therapy for the treatment of seizures, to treat mania associated with bipolar disorder, and for migraine prophylaxis

BRAND NAMES
Depakote Delayed Release, Depakote ER, Depakote Sprinkle

DRUG CLASS
Anticonvulsant, antimanic, antimigraine

DESCRIPTION
This drug increases the body's response to a certain type of acid, decreasing the response to certain stimulus.

POTENTIAL SIDE EFFECTS
Somnolence, dizziness, tremor, uncoordinated gait, abnormal thinking, amnesia, nausea, stomach upset, diarrhea, abdominal pain, increased appetite, anorexia, changes in vision, weight gain, back pain, hair loss, chest pain, rash.

CAUTIONS
- Notify your doctor if you have liver impairment, are pregnant, are taking other anticonvulsants, or have HIV or cyto-megalovirus infections.
- Use may cause severe blood disorders (decrease in platelets and clotting), thus increasing risk of bleeding.
- Tremors may be a sign of toxicity.
- Life-threatening pancreatitis has been associated with use. Immediately report any signs of abdominal pain, nausea, vomiting, anorexia.
- Do not suddenly discontinue use of this drug, may increase seizure risk. Gradually decrease usage over time, if necessary.
- This medication may cause drowsiness. Use caution in activities requiring alertness or using other drugs or substances that decrease alertness.

DRUG INTERACTIONS
Clonazepam, diazepam, lamotrigine, nimodipine, phenobarbital, tricyclic antidepressants, phenytoin, carbamazepine, chlorpromazine, macrolides, felbamate, isoniazid, aspirin, clozapine, cholestyramine, acyclovir, mefloquine.

This drug is metabolized by a specific set of liver enzymes. Several other drugs interfere with these liver enzymes, and thus may increase or decrease the clearance of divalproex from the body, potentially increasing the risk of side effects or decreasing effectiveness. When these drugs are given in combination with divalproex dosage adjustments may be needed. As these are too numerous to list, you should always check with your doctor or pharmacist prior to starting a new medication, herbal, or non-prescription product.

FOOD INTERACTIONS
Avoid alcohol. If stomach upset occurs, take with food.

HERBAL INTERACTIONS
Evening primrose

PREGNANCY AND BREAST-FEEDING CAUTIONS
FDA Pregnancy Risk Category D. Excreted in breast milk. Consult your doctor.

SPECIAL INFORMATION
Do not chew capsules. Swallow whole. Sprinkle capsules may be opened and sprinkled on a small amount of soft food (applesauce, pudding) and swallowed immediately.

DOBUTAMINE
(doe-BYOO-ta-meen)

NEWLY DISCOVERED USES (OFF-LABEL)
Acute myocardial infarction, cardiac arrest, pulmonary edema

ORIGINAL USES (ON-LABEL)
Short-term management of cardiac decompensation

BRAND NAME
Dobutrex

DRUG CLASS
Vasopressor

DESCRIPTION
This drug increases the contractility of the heart and heart rate.

POTENTIAL SIDE EFFECTS
Increased heart rate, increased blood pressure, hypotension, fever, headache, numbness, nausea, slight decrease in serum potassium, local and inflammatory changes and pain from infiltration, skin necrosis (isolated cases), mild leg cramps, and shortness of breath.

CAUTIONS
• Notify your doctor if you have an allergy to sulfites (some formulations contain sodium metabisulfate).

- Notify your doctor if you have recently had a heart attack, have been diagnosed with idiopathic heart aorta or rhythm abnormalities.
- May cause changes in blood pressure and heart rhythm.

DRUG INTERACTIONS
Bretylium, guanethidine, anesthesia, tricyclic antidepressants

FOOD INTERACTIONS
Unknown

HERBAL INTERACTIONS
Unknown

PREGNANCY AND BREAST-FEEDING CAUTIONS
FDA Pregnancy Risk Category B. Excretion in breast milk is unknown.

SPECIAL INFORMATION
Requires close monitoring of heart function and blood pressure during therapy.

DONEPEZIL
(doh-NEP-e-zil)

NEWLY DISCOVERED USES (OFF-LABEL)
Brain trauma, Charles Bonnet syndrome

ORIGINAL USES (ON-LABEL)
Mild to moderate dementia of the Alzheimer's type

BRAND NAME
Aricept

DRUG CLASS
Alzheimer's (acetylcholinesterase inhibitor)

DESCRIPTION
This drug inhibits activity of the enzyme responsible for the breakdown of acetylcholine and thus increases the levels of acetylcholine. Acetylcholine deficiency may be the cause of Alzheimer's disease.

POTENTIAL SIDE EFFECTS
Headache, nausea, diarrhea, fainting, chest pain, changes in blood pressure or heart rhythm, fatigue, insomnia, dizziness, depres-

sion, abnormal dreams, bruising, anorexia, vomiting, weight loss, fecal incontinence, frequent urination, muscle cramps, arthritis, body pain

CAUTIONS
- May cause decrease in heart rate and/or heart block with or without a history of heart disease.
- Notify your doctor if you have heart disease, seizures, lung disease, asthma, ulcer disease, or bladder outlet obstruction.
- Notify your doctor that you are on this drug prior to any surgery.
- May cause diarrhea, nausea, and/or vomiting.

DRUG INTERACTIONS
This drug is metabolized by a specific set of liver enzymes. Several other drugs interfere with these liver enzymes, and thus may increase or decrease the clearance of donepezil from the body, potentially increasing the risk of side effects or decreasing effectiveness. When these drugs are given in combination with donepezil, dosage adjustments may be needed. As these are too numerous to list, you should always check with your doctor or pharmacist prior to starting a new medication, herbal, or nonprescription product.

FOOD INTERACTIONS
Unknown

HERBAL INTERACTIONS
St. John's wort

PREGNANCY AND BREAST-FEEDING CAUTIONS
FDA Pregnancy Risk Category C. Data regarding breast milk excretion are not available. Consult your doctor.

DOPAMINE
(DOE-pa-meen)

NEWLY DISCOVERED USES (OFF-LABEL)
Pulmonary edema

ORIGINAL USES (ON-LABEL)
Use in combination therapy for shock that persists after adequate fluid volume replacement

BRAND NAMES
None

DRUG CLASS
Vasopressor (adrenergic agonist)

DESCRIPTION
This drug reduces the heart's need for oxygen. It also increases blood flow to the kidneys and excretion of sodium.

POTENTIAL SIDE EFFECTS
Changes in heart rate, nausea, vomiting, chest pain, palpitations, shortness of breath, headache, lowered blood pressure.

CAUTIONS
- Notify your doctor if you have pheochromocytoma (disease of the adrenal glands), irregular heart rhythm, heart disease, recent heart attack, or allergies to sulfites.
- Requires close monitoring of urine output, blood pressure, and changes in skin temperature.

DRUG INTERACTIONS
MAO inhibitors, alpha and beta-adrenergic blockers, cocaine, general anesthetics, methyldopa, phenytoin, reserpine, tricyclic antidepressants.

FOOD INTERACTIONS
Unknown

HERBAL INTERACTIONS
Unknown

PREGNANCY AND BREAST-FEEDING CAUTIONS
FDA Pregnancy Risk Category C. Not known if excreted in breast milk. Consult your doctor.

DOXASOZIN
(doks-AY-zoe-sin)

NEWLY DISCOVERED USES (OFF-LABEL)
Nonbacterial prostatitis, preoperative preparation for pheochromocytoma

ORIGINAL USES (ON-LABEL)
High blood pressure or benign prostatic hyperplasia (enlarged prostate)

BRAND NAME
Cardura

DRUG CLASS
Antihypertensive (alpha-adrenergic blocker)

DESCRIPTION
This drug causes relaxation of veins and arterioles and a decrease in total vascular resistance and blood pressure.

POTENTIAL SIDE EFFECTS
Postural hypotension (sudden drop in blood pressure upon standing from sitting or lying down position), dizziness, headache, impotence, libido decreased, ejaculation disturbances, weakness, edema, fatigue, somnolence, nervousness, pain, vertigo, sexual dysfunction, abdominal pain, diarrhea, nausea, edema, fatigue, malaise.

CAUTIONS
- Do not use concurrently with phosphodiesterase-5 inhibitors (such as sildenafil, tadalafil, or vardenafil).
- Marked orthostatic hypotension (sudden drop in blood pressure when standing from sitting or lying down position), syncope, and loss of consciousness may occur with first dose (especially in patients taking beta blockers, diuretics, low sodium diets, or taking large first doses).
- Rarely, this drug class has been associated with priapism (painful erection).
- Avoid rapid increase in dose.
- Use with caution in patients with kidney or liver impairment.
- Does not affect levels of PSA (prostate specific antigen) a marker test used to diagnose prostate cancer.

DRUG INTERACTIONS
Beta-blockers, diuretics, ACE inhibitors, calcium channel blockers, sildenafil, tadalafil, vardenafil, NSAIDs

FOOD INTERACTIONS
Unknown

HERBAL INTERACTIONS
Saw palmetto, ephedrine, yohimbe, ginseng, garlic

PREGNANCY AND BREAST-FEEDING CAUTIONS
FDA Pregnancy Risk Category B. Excreted in breast milk. Consult your doctor prior to initiation of breast-feeding.

SPECIAL INFORMATION
Take dose at bedtime. Notify your doctor if dizziness or palpitations occur.

DOXEPIN
(DOKS-e-pin)

Oral

NEWLY DISCOVERED USES (OFF-LABEL)
Chronic fatigue syndrome, chronic nausea and vomiting, migraine prevention, urticaria

ORIGINAL USES (ON-LABEL)
Depression

BRAND NAMES
Prudoxin, Sinequan

DRUG CLASS
Antianxiety, tricyclic antidepressant

DESCRIPTION
Doxepin increases the levels of norepinephrine and serotonin in the body—two chemicals that affect mood—by preventing uptake of the chemicals by neurons in the brain.

POTENTIAL SIDE EFFECTS
Dry mouth, sedation, dizziness, headache, nervousness, skin rash, tremors, hives, nausea, constipation, vision changes, sweating, lowered blood pressure, increased heart rate, decreased sodium levels.

CAUTIONS
- Do not use if you have been taking an MAO inhibitor (such as phenelzine, tranylcypromine, isocarboxazid) within the past 14 days. When used with MAO-Is, fever, high blood pressure, increased heart rate, confusion, seizures, and deaths have been reported.
- Notify your doctor if you recently had a heart attack; not for use immediately after a heart attack.

- Can cause sedation, which may impair performance of tasks requiring alertness. Sedative effects may be additive with other drugs that cause similar effects.
- May worsen psychosis or mania in patients with bipolar disease.
- Stop therapy with doctor's permission and according to instructions (taper gradually) prior to elective surgery.
- Do not abruptly stop medication; instead, taper gradually.
- Notify your doctor if you have low blood pressure as this drug can cause low blood pressure episodes.
- Use with caution in patients with urinary retention, history of cardiac disease, seizure disorders, diabetes, benign prostatic hyperplasia, narrow-angle glaucoma, dry mouth, visual problems, constipation, or a history of bowel obstruction.
- Possibility of suicide attempt may persist until remission occurs.
- Use with caution in hyperthyroid patients or those receiving thyroid supplementation.
- Use with caution in patients with liver or kidney dysfunction and in elderly.

DRUG INTERACTIONS

MAO inhibitors (such as phenelzine, tranylcypromine, isocarboxazid), ritonavir, bupropion, amphetamines, anticholinergics, sedatives, chlorpropamide, tolazamide, warfarin, fluoxetine, fluvoxamine, citalopram, escitalopram, paroxetine, sertraline, cimetidine, carbamazepine, haloperidol, smoking, methylphenidate, valproic acid, clonidine, venlafaxine, protease inhibitors, quinidine, diltiazem, verapamil, lithium, phenothiazines may affect the levels of desipramine, drugs that prolong QT interval (see site: http://www.torsades.org/medical-pros/drug-lists/drug-lists.htm#).

This drug is metabolized (inactivated) by a specific set of liver enzymes. Several other drugs interfere with these liver enzymes and thus may increase or decrease the clearance of doxepin from the body, potentially increasing the risk of side effects or decreasing effectiveness. When these drugs are given in combination with doxepin, dosage adjustments may be needed. As these are too numerous to list, you should always check with your doctor or pharmacist prior to starting a new medication.

FOOD INTERACTIONS

Avoid alcohol, grapefruit juice.

HERBAL INTERACTIONS
Valerian, St. John's wort, SAMe, kava kava

PREGNANCY AND BREAST-FEEDING CAUTIONS
FDA Pregnancy Risk Category C. Excreted into breast milk. Refrain from breast-feeding while taking this medication.

SPECIAL INFORMATION
May take four to six weeks for the full therapeutic effects to be experienced. Avoid prolonged exposure to sunlight, wear sunscreen.

In 2005, the FDA announced new labeling for antidepressants regarding the need to closely monitor for worsening of depression and for the potential of increased suicidal thinking or suicidal behavior during therapy. Although this recommendation applies to all patients (adults, children, adolescents) treated with antidepressants for any indication, this is of particular importance in patients being treated for depression.

DOXORUBICIN
(dox-oh-ROOB-eh-sin)

NEWLY DISCOVERED USES (OFF-LABEL)
Pterygium recurrence prevention

ORIGINAL USES (ON-LABEL)
Treatment of various cancers

BRAND NAME
Adriamycin

DRUG CLASS
Antineoplastic

DESCRIPTION
This drug fights malignant cells by inhibiting DNA and RNA production, interrupting essential cell activity, causing toxicity and eventual cell death.

POTENTIAL SIDE EFFECTS
Nausea, vomiting, oral ulcers, blood disorders, fever, chills, hives, increased susceptibility to infections, cardiac toxicity may occur during therapy or after completion, nerve toxicity, seizures, hair loss, increased skin pigmentation.

CAUTIONS

- Notify your doctor if you have received previous anti-cancer therapy.
- This drug has significant effects on several components of the blood, particularly white blood cells that are essential in fighting infections. Thus, close monitoring of the blood is required during therapy.
- Immediately report any of the following to your doctor: bloody stools, severe infections.
- Irreversible cardiac toxicity has been related to therapy with this drug and is primarily cumulative dose related. Inform your doctor of any heart disease. Cardiac function will be monitored throughout and following therapy.
- Infusion reactions have occurred and most often occur with the first infusion.
- Liver toxicity has also been reported with this drug and requires monitoring.
- Treatment requires close monitoring and extensive laboratory testing.
- Urine may turn red for one to two days after the drug is administered.
- Do not receive any immunizations or vaccines without doctor/pharmacist approval.

DRUG INTERACTIONS

Cyclosporine, live vaccines, paclitaxel, phenobarbital, progesterone, streptozocin, verapamil, actinomycin, cyclophosphamide, mercaptopurine, digoxin, phenytoin, radiation

FOOD INTERACTIONS

Unknown

HERBAL INTERACTIONS

Unknown

PREGNANCY AND BREAST-FEEDING CAUTIONS

FDA Pregnancy Risk Category D. Excretion into breast milk is unknown. Breast-feeding is not recommended during therapy.

SPECIAL INFORMATION

This drug has a black box warning regarding the risk of severe tissue necrosis if the infusion infiltrates the tissue outside of the vein it is being administered in. In addition, the risks of cardiac, blood, and liver toxicity are described. Discuss all these risks with your doctor prior to the initiation of therapy.

DOXYCYCLINE
(doks-i-SYE-kleen)

NEWLY DISCOVERED USES (OFF-LABEL)
Chlamydia, gingivitis, Lyme arthritis, Lyme disease treatment and prevention, osteoarthritis, prevention of traveler's diarrhea, rheumatoid arthritis, rosacea

ORIGINAL USES (ON-LABEL)
Various bacterial infections

BRAND NAMES
Adoxa, Doryx, Doxy-100, Monodox, Periostat, Vibramycin, Vibra-Tabs

DRUG CLASS
Antibiotic (tetracycline)

DESCRIPTION
Doxycycline inhibits the formation of protein in susceptible bacteria. It may also cause changes in the membranes of the bacteria.

POTENTIAL SIDE EFFECTS
Skin reaction related to sun exposure (photosensitivity reaction), rash, hives, permanent discoloration of teeth (when administered during tooth development), anorexia, diarrhea, difficulty swallowing, various blood abnormalities, anemia, decreased kidney function, stomach upset.

CAUTIONS
- Not for use in children less than eight years of age, except in the treatment of anthrax.
- Not for use in patients with severe liver dysfunction.
- Sensitivity reactions are more likely to occur in patients with a history of asthma, allergies, hay fever, or hives.
- Not for use during pregnancy.
- Chronic use may result in super-infection, including oral or vaginal candidiasis.
- Avoid prolonged exposure to sunlight or tanning equipment.

DRUG INTERACTIONS
Digoxin, warfarin, antacids containing aluminum, calcium, or magnesium, iron, bismuth subsalicylate, barbiturates, zinc salts, phenytoin, sucralfate, didanosine, quinapril, mirtazapine, nateglinide, nefazodone, quinidine, sildenafil, tadalafil, varden-

afil, tacrolimus, venlafaxine, midazolam, triazolam, ergot alkaloids, lovastatin, simvastatin, mesoridazine, didanosine, quinapril, penthrane, oral anticoagulants and carbamazepine.

FOOD INTERACTIONS
Blood levels may be decreased if taken with food or milk. Administration with iron or calcium may decrease absorption. May decrease absorption of calcium, iron, magnesium, zinc, and amino acids. Avoid chronic alcohol ingestion.

HERBAL INTERACTIONS
Avoid St. John's wort; dong quai

PREGNANCY AND BREAST-FEEDING CAUTIONS
FDA Pregnancy Risk Category D. Do not use during second and third trimesters of pregnancy. Use of this drug during the last half of pregnancy may result in permanent teeth discoloration (grey-brown). Excreted in breast milk. Not recommended during breast-feeding.

SPECIAL INFORMATION
Avoid unnecessary exposure to sunlight; wear sunscreen. Drink adequate amounts of fluid when ingesting this drug to minimize irritation to the esophagus and stomach.

Although food may decrease the absorption of doxycycline, it may be necessary to take with food to prevent stomach upset. Doryx capsules may be opened and sprinkled on applesauce and swallowed immediately. Do not chew.

DRONABINOL
(droe-NAB-i-nol)

NEWLY DISCOVERED USES (OFF-LABEL)
Multiple sclerosis

ORIGINAL USES (ON-LABEL)
Chemotherapy-associated nausea and vomiting resistant to other antiemetics, to treat AIDS- and cancer-related appetite loss

BRAND NAME
Marinol

DRUG CLASS
Antiemetic

DESCRIPTION
While the exact action of this medication is not known, researchers believe it affects the centers of the brain that control vomiting.

POTENTIAL SIDE EFFECTS
Drowsiness, sedation, confusion, nausea, changes in vision, dizziness, increased appetite, dry mouth, depression, hallucinations, memory lapse, walking with an unsteady gait, increased heart rate, low blood pressure.

CAUTIONS
- Avoid use if you have a history of schizophrenia.
- Caution use if you have heart disease, liver disease, or seizure disorders.
- Decrease dosage in patients with poor liver function.
- This drug may have the potential for abuse.
- Patients should be monitored with first dose for psychotic reaction.
- This drug is the principal psychoactive substance in marijuana and may produce similar effects on the central nervous system. Notify your doctor if you have had an adverse event associated with this drug. Patients with no prior experience to this drug or *Cannabis* may require supervision initially.
- Older patients (more than 55 years) may be more susceptible to psychoactive effects.

DRUG INTERACTIONS
Alcohol, amphetamines, cocaine, anticholinergics, sedatives, antidepressants, antihistamines, disulfiram, fluoxetine, theophylline, barbiturates, and benzodiazepines

FOOD INTERACTIONS
Avoid alcohol. Do not take with fatty meals.

HERBAL INTERACTIONS
St. John's wort

PREGNANCY AND BREAST-FEEDING CAUTIONS
FDA Pregnancy Risk Category C. Excreted in breast milk. Breast-feeding not recommended during therapy.

SPECIAL INFORMATION
Tolerance may develop to the cardiac and subjective feelings after continued use. May cause dizziness and drowsiness; do not do tasks that require alertness or coordination. You should remain supervised after taking this medication.

DROPERIDOL
(droe-PER-I-dole)

NEWLY DISCOVERED USES (OFF-LABEL)
Acute schizophrenia, hyperemesis gravidarum, Ménière's disease

ORIGINAL USES (ON-LABEL)
To prevent or lessen nausea and vomiting associated with surgery or procedures

BRAND NAME
Inapsine

DRUG CLASS
Anti-nausea, antipsychotic

DESCRIPTION
Droperidol blocks a chemical substance in the brain (dopamine) which is associated with triggering nausea.

POTENTIAL SIDE EFFECTS
Prolongation of heart rhythm (QT prolongation), restlessness, anxiety, sedation, drowsiness. tremors, irregular and involuntary muscle movements, swelling of breasts, weight gain, constipation, low blood pressure (especially when standing quickly), increased heart rate, hallucinations, nausea, vomiting, painful urination.

CAUTIONS
- Do not use if you have known QT prolongation (prolonged uneven heart rate).
- May alter heart rhythm (QT prolongation and torsades de pointes), and in some cases may be fatal.
- Use extreme caution if you have low heart rate (less than 50 beats per minute), cardiac disease, concurrent MAO inhibitor therapy, or when used in combination with other drugs known to cause QT prolongation and electrolyte disturbances.

- Use with caution if you have bone marrow suppression, seizures, or severe liver disease.
- Use with caution if you have visual problems (especially glaucoma) decreased gastrointestinal motility, urinary retention, benign prostatic enlargement, or dry mouth.

DRUG INTERACTIONS
Other drugs that cause sedation (sedative/hypnotics) prolong QT (refer to website: http://www.torsades.org/medical-pros/drug-lists/printable-drug-list.cfm), cisapride, pimozide, diuretics, amphotericin B, cyclosporine, metoclopramide.

FOOD INTERACTIONS
Unknown

HERBAL INTERACTIONS
Unknown

PREGNANCY AND BREAST-FEEDING CAUTIONS
FDA Pregnancy Risk Category C. It is not known if this drug is excreted in breast milk. Do not breast-feed while taking this drug.

SPECIAL INFORMATION
In December 2001, the product information was revised to include a black box warning regarding the potential for QT Prolongation/Torsades de Pointes (heart rate abnormality) that may occur at or below recommended doses. Some cases have been fatal and have occurred in patients without known risk factors. Prior to starting therapy with this drug and for two to three hours after therapy is completed, patients should be monitored for underlying heart rate abnormalities.

DROSPIRENONE AND ETHINYL ESTRADIOL
(droh-SPYE-re-none ETH-in-il es-tra-DYE-ole)

NEWLY DISCOVERED USES (OFF-LABEL)
Premenstrual dysphoric disorder (PMDD), premenstrual syndrome (PMS)

ORIGINAL USES (ON-LABEL)
Contraception

BRAND NAME
Yasmin

DRUG CLASS
Oral Contraceptives

DESCRIPTION
This drug inhibits ovulation by preventing secretion of two hormones important in the ovulation cycle: follicle stimulating hormone (FSH) and luteinizing hormone (LH).

POTENTIAL SIDE EFFECTS
Intermenstrual bleeding and irregularity, abdominal pain, diarrhea, nausea, vomiting, depression, dizziness, emotional lability, headache, migraine, nervousness, change in vision or ability to wear contact lenses, fluid retention, darkening of skin in areas, vaginal infections, hair loss. Increased risk of cardiac events, glucose intolerance, stroke, liver problems.

CAUTIONS
- Oral contraceptives do not protect against sexually transmitted diseases or HIV infection.
- Cardiovascular events increase if you are over 35 years of age and a heavy smoker (at least 15 cigarettes daily), or have a history of cardiovascular disease or thromboembolic (blood clots) events.
- Not for use if you have decreased kidney, adrenal or liver function, diabetes with vascular involvement, history of or suspected breast cancer or estrogen dependent cancer, undiagnosed genital bleeding, liver tumor, severe high blood pressure, jaundice associated with pregnancy or prior birth control pill usage, or headaches with neurological symptoms.
- Do not take if you are pregnant.
- May increase potassium levels. Requires blood monitoring for potassium if taken with other drugs that can cause potassium accumulation, such as ACE inhibitors, potassium-sparing diuretics (spironolactone, heparin, NSAIDs). Check with your pharmacist or doctor before starting any new medication while taking this medication.
- Discuss cardiac and other risks with your doctor prior to starting therapy.

DRUG INTERACTIONS
Oral contraceptives, including this product, may interact with several drugs too numerous to list. Check with your pharmacist or doctor before starting any new medication, herbal product, or nonprescrip-

tion drug. Interacting drugs include but are not limited to the following: oral antibiotics, antifungals, warfarin, anticonvulsants, rifampin, bexarotene, bosentan, tizanidine, cyclosporine, anticoagulants, antidepressants, beta-blockers, caffeine, selegiline, modafinil, protease inhibitors.

In addition, because drospirenone can cause an increase in potassium levels, the risk for increased levels of potassium are greater when this drug is taken in combination with other potassium-sparing (does not excrete potassium) drugs, including but not limited to ACE inhibitors (such as captopril, enalapril, etc.), angiotensin II receptor blockers (such as losartan, candesartan), certain diuretics, and heparin.

FOOD INTERACTIONS
Caffeine

HERBAL INTERACTIONS
St. John's wort

PREGNANCY AND BREAST-FEEDING CAUTIONS
FDA Pregnancy Risk Category X. Do not use during pregnancy. Excreted in breast milk and not recommended during breast-feeding.

SPECIAL INFORMATION
Read the patient information brochure prior to therapy for important instructions regarding therapy and warnings.

DULOXETINE
(doo-LOX-e-teen)

NEWLY DISCOVERED USES (OFF-LABEL)
Fibromyalgia

ORIGINAL USES (ON-LABEL)
Diabetic peripheral neuropathic pain, major depressive disorder

BRAND NAME
Cymbalta

DRUG CLASS
Antidepressant (SSNRI—selective serotonin and norepinephrine reuptake inhibitor)

DESCRIPTION

This drug treats mood disorders and some pain disorders by preventing the reuptake of serotonin and norepinephrine in the neurons, resulting in increased levels of these chemicals in the brain and body.

POTENTIAL SIDE EFFECTS

Nausea, dry mouth, constipation, diarrhea, vomiting, decreased appetite, fatigue, dizziness, drowsiness, increased sweating, hot flushes, blurred vision, insomnia, sexual dysfunction, muscle cramps, muscle aches, headache, tremors, erectile dysfunction, cough, sore throat, increased blood pressure, activation of mania, numbness.

CAUTIONS

- Do not use if you have been taking an MAO inhibitor (such as phenelzine, tranylcypromine, isocarboxazid) within the past 14 days. When used with MAO-Is fever, high blood pressure, increased heart rate, confusion, seizures, and deaths have been reported.
- Combination with other selective serotonin reuptake inhibitors (SSRIs), selective serotonin norepinephrine reuptake inhibitors (SSNRIs), tricyclic antidepressants, amphetamines, sympathomimetics, ritonavir, serotonin agonists (sumatriptan, etc.), and certain opiates carries an increased risk of serotonin syndrome. While taking this medication, check with your pharmacist or doctor before starting any new medication, herbal, or nonprescription product.
- Notify your doctor if you have uncontrolled narrow-angle glaucoma, diabetes, high blood pressure, history of seizures, mania.
- You and your doctor should be attentive to worsening signs of depression with this drug.
- Do not stop this medication suddenly without medical supervision. Should be tapered over a gradual period.
- May cause liver toxicity.

DRUG INTERACTIONS

This drug is metabolized by a specific set of liver enzymes. Several other drugs interfere with these liver enzymes, and thus may increase or decrease the clearance of duloxetine from the body, potentially increasing the risk of side effects or decreasing effectiveness. When these drugs are given in combination with duloxetine, dosage adjustments may be needed. As these are too numerous to list, you should always check with your doctor or pharmacist prior to starting a new medication, herbal, or nonprescription product.

FOOD INTERACTIONS
Alcohol

HERBAL INTERACTIONS
Valerian, St. John's wort, kava kava, gotu kola, SAMe

PREGNANCY AND BREAST-FEEDING CAUTIONS
FDA Pregnancy Risk Category C. Breast-feeding is not recommended while taking duloxetine.

SPECIAL INFORMATION
In 2005, the FDA announced new labeling for antidepressants regarding the need to closely monitor for worsening of depression and for the potential of increased suicidal thinking or suicidal behavior during therapy. Although this recommendation applies to all patients (adults, children, adolescents) treated with antidepressants for any indication, this is of particular importance in patients being treated for depression.

Close observation may be especially important when antidepressant medications are started for the first time or when doses are changed. More information on this topic can be found at the following web site: http://www.fda.gov/cder/drug/antidepressants/default.htm

In October 2005, new safety data were added to the product labeling regarding the risk of liver toxicity, particularly in people with pre-existing liver disease.

ENALAPRIL
(e-NAL-a-pril)

NEWLY DISCOVERED USES (OFF-LABEL)
Diabetic nephropathy, dilated cardiomyopathy, membranous nephropathy, polydipsia, pulmonary edema

ORIGINAL USES (ON-LABEL)
Mild to severe blood pressure, congestive heart failure, post-heart attack

BRAND NAMES
Vasotec, Vasotec I.V.

DRUG CLASS
Blood pressure medication

DESCRIPTION
Enalapril lowers blood pressure by inhibiting the production of chemicals that cause blood vessels to constrict. It also may cause the brain to release hormones that lower blood pressure.

POTENTIAL SIDE EFFECTS
Chest pain, too low blood pressure (especially after first dose), cough, fainting, headache, dizziness, fatigue, weakness, rash, abnormal taste, nausea, shortness of breath.

CAUTIONS
- Do not use if you have had tongue, lip, throat, or mouth swelling (symptoms of angioedema) after taking other drugs in the same class, or if you have these symptoms unrelated to drug therapy. Angioedema can occur at any time during treatment, but especially following the first dose. Report symptoms to your doctor.
- Do not use with certain kidney problems (kidney artery stenosis, decreased kidney function).
- Do not use in pregnancy (second and third trimesters).
- Avoid rapid dosage increases, which may lead to kidney problems.

DRUG INTERACTIONS
Potassium supplements, cotrimoxazole (high dose), angiotension II receptor antagonists (candesartan, losartan, irbesartan, etc.) or potassium-sparing diuretics (amiloride, spironolactone, triamterene), digoxin, lithium, and certain drugs used to treat diabetes (sulfonylureas). Aspirin (high doses) may aggravate the beneficial effects of this drug.

FOOD INTERACTIONS
Unknown

HERBAL INTERACTIONS
St. John's wort, capsaicin, dong quai, ephedra, yohimbe, ginseng, large amounts of natural licorice

PREGNANCY AND BREAST-FEEDING CAUTIONS
FDA Pregnancy Risk Category C/D (not for use in second and third trimesters, may cause injury and death to fetus). Excreted in

breast milk. The American Academy of Pediatrics considers this drug compatible with breast-feeding.

SPECIAL INFORMATION
Report any vomiting, diarrhea, excessive perspiration, or dehydration to your physician. If any swelling of the face, lips, extremities, tongue, throat, or difficulty in breathing occurs or if persistent cough develops it should be reported, too.

This drug has a black box warning regarding potential injury to the fetus during second and third trimester.

EPLERENONE
(e-PLER-en-one)

NEWLY DISCOVERED USES (OFF-LABEL)
Prevention of proteinuria in type 2 diabetes

ORIGINAL USES (ON-LABEL)
High blood pressure; congestive heart failure, after heart attack

BRAND NAME
Inspra

DRUG CLASS
Blood pressure medication

DESCRIPTION
This drug lowers blood pressure by blocking a hormone in the body (aldosterone) that acts in the kidney, heart, and blood vessels.

POTENTIAL SIDE EFFECTS
Increase in triglyceride levels, dizziness, fatigue, changes in kidney function, low potassium levels, low sodium levels, diarrhea, cough, flu-like syndrome.

CAUTIONS
- Safety has not been established in children or patients with liver problems.
- Do not use if you have high potassium levels or renal problems.
- Do not use with potassium supplements or potassium-sparing diuretics, as this increases the risk of high potassium levels.

DRUG INTERACTIONS

High potassium levels may occur if this drug is used in combination with ACE inhibitors (captopril, enalapril, etc.), angiotension II receptor antagonists (losartan, candesartan, etc.), potassium supplements, potassium-sparing diuretics, ketoconazole, itraconazole, erythromycin, fluconazole, saquinavir, and verapamil increase eplerenone levels.

Aminoglutethimide, some anti-inflammatory (nonsteroidals), carbamazepine, nafcillin, nevirapine, phenobarbital, phenytoin, and rifamycins may decrease the effects of eplerenone.

FOOD INTERACTIONS

Grapefruit juice

HERBAL INTERACTIONS

St. John's wort

PREGNANCY AND BREAST-FEEDING CAUTIONS

FDA Pregnancy Risk Factor B. Excretion in breast milk is unknown. Therapy during breast-feeding not recommended.

EPOETIN ALPHA
(e-POE-e-tin AL-fa)

NEWLY DISCOVERED USES (OFF-LABEL)

Aplastic anemia, therapy-resistant anemia, uremic pruritus

ORIGINAL USES (ON-LABEL)

Anemia related to the following: zidovudine therapy, chronic kidney failure including dialysis and nondialysis, and cancer chemotherapy. To reduce the need for blood transfusions in surgery patients

BRAND NAMES

Epogen, Procrit

DRUG CLASS

Colony-stimulating factor, recombinant human erythropoietin

DESCRIPTION

Epoetin alpha stimulates the production of red blood cells.

POTENTIAL SIDE EFFECTS

High blood pressure, headache, fever, nausea, muscle aches, swelling due to fluid retention, chest pain, fatigue, seizures, vomiting, diarrhea, loss of energy and strength, diarrhea, fever.

CAUTIONS

- Not for use if you have uncontrolled high blood pressure.
- This product contains human albumin and is not for use if allergic to albumin (human) or mammalian cell-derived products.
- Use with caution if you have a history of seizures or high blood pressure. Blood pressure should be controlled before therapy starts and monitored closely throughout treatment.
- Dialysis patients may require preventive therapy for blood clots.
- Requires blood monitoring regularly during therapy.

DRUG INTERACTIONS

Unknown

FOOD INTERACTIONS

Unknown

PREGNANCY AND BREAST-FEEDING CAUTIONS

FDA Pregnancy Risk Category C. Excretion in breast milk is unknown. Refrain from breast-feeding during therapy with this drug.

SPECIAL INFORMATION

Not useful for the treatment of anemia due to sudden causes (acute onset).

ERYTHROMYCIN
(er-ith-roe-MYE-sin)

NEWLY DISCOVERED USES (OFF-LABEL)

Acne, chancroid, cholera, diarrhea due to *Campylobacter*, gingivitis, granuloma inguinale, impetigo, Lyme disease, lymphogranuloma venereum, periodontitis

ORIGINAL USES (ON-LABEL)

Various bacterial infections

BRAND NAMES

Akne-Mycin, E.E.S., Eryc, Ery-Tab, Erythrocin

DRUG CLASS

Antibiotic (macrolide) oral, topical, intravenous, eye

DESCRIPTION

Erythromycin interferes with the production of protein in the bacteria cell.

POTENTIAL SIDE EFFECTS

Systemic: Irregular heart rate (ventricular arrhythmias, QT prolongation), headache, fever, seizures, rash, abdominal pain, cramping, nausea, oral yeast infection, vomiting, jaundice, inflammation at the injection site, weakness, cough. Topical: skin reactions including redness, peeling itching, dryness.

CAUTIONS

- Do not use if you have pre-existing liver disease and use with caution if you have reduced liver function.
- Do not use concomitantly with ergot derivatives, pimozide, astemizole, or cisapride.
- May aggravate weakness symptoms if you have myasthenia gravis.

DRUG INTERACTIONS

Cisapride, gatifloxacin, moxifloxacin, pimozide, sparfloxacin, thioridazine, alfentanil, benzodiazepines (such as diazepam, flurazepam, etc.), warfarin, buspirone, carbamazepine, cyclosporine, digoxin, ergotamine and ergotamine-like drugs, disopyramide, felodipine, fluoroquinolones (such as ciprofloxacin, norfloxacin, etc.), statins (such as lovastatin, fluvastatin, etc.), methylprednisolone, rifampin, theophylline. For a complete list of drugs that cause QT prolongation visit website (http://www.torsades.org/ medical-pros/drug-lists/printable-drug-list.cfm).

FOOD INTERACTIONS

Avoid alcohol. The absorption of some erythromycin formulations are affected by food. Erythromycin stearate should be taken at least two hours before or after a meal. Erythromycin estolate, erythromycin ethylsuccinate and erythromycin base may be taken without regard to meals.

HERBAL INTERACTIONS

St. John's wort

PREGNANCY AND BREAST-FEEDING CAUTIONS

FDA Pregnancy Risk Category B. Excreted in breast milk. This drug is considered compatible with breast-feeding by the American Academy of Pediatrics.

ESCITALOPRAM
(es-sye-TAL-oh-pram)

NEWLY DISCOVERED USES (OFF-LABEL)
Premenstrual dysphoric disorder (PMDD)

ORIGINAL USES (ON-LABEL)
Depression, generalized anxiety disorder

BRAND NAME
Lexapro

DRUG CLASS
Antidepressant (selective serotonin reuptake inhibitor [SSRI])

DESCRIPTION
This drug inhibits serotonin reuptake by neurons, promoting increases in levels of serotonin, an important neurotransmitter in mood disorders.

POTENTIAL SIDE EFFECTS
Somnolence, insomnia, nausea, dry mouth, sweating, anxiety, anorexia, agitation, yawning, rash, itching, sexual dysfunction, diarrhea, stomach upset, vomiting, abdominal pain, tremor, weight gain, joint aches, muscle aches, cough, rhinitis, sinusitis, low sodium levels.

CAUTIONS
- Do not use concurrently with MAO inhibitors or within two weeks of discontinuing MAO-I.
- Inform your doctor if you have a history of mania or seizures, or if you have kidney dysfunction.
- Use caution if you are a high-risk suicide attempt patient during initiation of therapy.
- Has potential to impair cognitive/motor performance; you should use caution operating hazardous machinery.
- Elderly patients with liver impairment should receive lower dosages.
- Use with caution in kidney insufficiency.

DRUG INTERACTIONS
MAO inhibitors or drugs with MAO inhibition (linezolid), amphetamines, buspirone, meperidine, nefazodone, serotonin agonists (sumatriptan), sibutramine, other SSRIs, sympathomimetics, ritonavir, tramadol, venlafaxine, loop diuretics, warfarin, amino-

glutethimide, carbamazepine, phenytoin and rifampin, cyproheptadine.

This drug is metabolized by a specific set of liver enzymes. Several other drugs interfere with these liver enzymes, and thus may increase or decrease the clearance of escitalopram from the body, potentially increasing the risk of side effects or decreasing effectiveness. When these drugs are given in combination with escitalopram, dosage adjustments may be needed. As these are too numerous to list, you should always check with your doctor or pharmacist prior to starting a new medication, herbal, or nonprescription product.

FOOD INTERACTIONS
Alcohol

HERBAL INTERACTIONS
Valerian, St. John's wort, SAMe, gotu kola, kava kava

PREGNANCY AND BREAST-FEEDING CAUTIONS
FDA Pregnancy Risk Category C. Excreted in breast milk. Do not use while breast-feeding.

SPECIAL INFORMATION
In 2005, the FDA announced new labeling for antidepressants regarding the need to closely monitor for worsening of depression and for the potential of increased suicidal thinking or suicidal behavior during therapy. Although this recommendation applies to all patients (adults, children, adolescents) treated with antidepressants for any indication, this is of particular importance in patients being treated for depression. Discuss the latest information regarding this safety issue with your doctor prior to initiating therapy.

Close observation may be especially important when antidepressant medications are started for the first time or when doses are changed. More information on this topic can be found at the following web site: http://www.fda.gov/cder/drug/antidepressants/default.htm.

Combination with other SSRIs, SSNRIs, tricyclic antidepressants, amphetamines, sympathomimetics, ritonavir, serotonin agonists (sumatriptan, etc.), and certain opiates carries an increased risk of serotonin syndrome. While taking this medication, check with your pharmacist or doctor before starting any new medication, herbal, or nonprescription product.

ESMOLOL
(ES-moe-lol)

NEWLY DISCOVERED USES (OFF-LABEL)
Acute myocardial infarction, aortic aneurysm, pheochromocytoma, unstable angina

ORIGINAL USES (ON-LABEL)
Increased or abnormal heart rate, high blood pressure

BRAND NAME
Brevibloc

DRUG CLASS
Blood pressure medication (selective beta-1 blocker)

DESCRIPTION
Esmolol blocks beta-1 receptors found in the heart and blood vessels.

POTENTIAL SIDE EFFECTS
Low blood pressure, sweating, shortness of breath, dizziness, somnolence, confusion, headache, nausea.

CAUTIONS
- Do not use if you have too low heart rate or blood pressure, bronchial asthma, certain types of heart failure, or pregnancy (second and third trimester).
- Use with caution in patients with certain types of lung (bronchospastic) disease.
- Use with caution in diabetics because it can mask symptoms of too low blood glucose levels.
- Use caution if you have kidney function problems, thyroid disease, peripheral vascular disease, myasthenia gravis.

DRUG INTERACTIONS
Esmolol may increase the effects or the potential for toxicity when given with verapamil, digoxin, or theophylline. Morphine may increase esmolol blood levels. Effects may be decreased when used with aluminum hydroxide, barbiturates, cholestyramine, colestipol, certain pain drugs (nonsteroidal anti-inflammatory drugs), penicillins (ampicillin), rifampin. Beta-blockers may decrease the effect of some drugs used to treat diabetes (chlorpropamide, tolazamide, glipizide, glimepiride)

FOOD INTERACTIONS
Unknown

HERBAL INTERACTIONS
Unknown

PREGNANCY AND BREAST-FEEDING CAUTIONS
FDA Pregnancy Risk Category C, D (second and third trimester).
Can cause serious decreases in fetal heart rate when administered
in the third trimester of pregnancy or at delivery. Excretion in
breast milk is unknown.

ETHACRYNIC ACID
(eth-a-KRIN-ik-AS-id)

NEWLY DISCOVERED USES (OFF-LABEL)
Hypertension, nephrogenic diabetes insipidus

ORIGINAL USES (ON-LABEL)
Management of swelling with water retention (edema) associated
with congestive heart failure, liver or kidney disease

BRAND NAME
Edecrin

DRUG CLASS
Blood pressure medication (loop diuretic)

DESCRIPTION
This drug decreases absorption of sodium and chloride in the kidneys, causing an increased clearance of water and electrolytes
from the body.

POTENTIAL SIDE EFFECTS
Lowered blood pressure upon standing (orthostatic hypotension),
dehydration, numbness, dizziness, lightheadedness, various skin
rashes, skin reactions related to sun exposure (photosensitivity), increased levels of glucose or uric acid, decreased levels of potassium
or chloride, nausea, vomiting, anorexia, gastric irritation, urinary
bladder spasm, weakness, hearing impairment, ringing in the ears,
decrease in kidney function.

CAUTIONS
- Watch for warning signs of dehydration: dryness of mouth,
  thirst, anorexia, weakness, muscle cramps or pain, increased
  heart rate, irregular heart rhythm, vomiting.

- Use may result in imbalance in electrolytes (potassium, sodium, magnesium).

DRUG INTERACTIONS
Lithium, propranolol, cisplatin, clofibrate, probenecid

FOOD INTERACTIONS
Unknown

HERBAL INTERACTIONS
Ginseng

PREGNANCY AND BREAST-FEEDING CAUTIONS
FDA Pregnancy Category B (Category D if used for high blood pressure that develops during pregnancy). Excretion in breast milk is unknown. Not recommended for use during breast-feeding.

SPECIAL INFORMATION
Rise slowly from sitting or lying position to avoid dizziness. Avoid long periods of exercise. This drug will increase urination; take early in day to prevent frequent need to urinate during the bedtime hours.

ETHAMBUTOL
(e-THAM-byoo-tole)

NEWLY DISCOVERED USES (OFF-LABEL)
Mycobacterium avium complex in AIDS

ORIGINAL USES (ON-LABEL)
Tuberculosis and other similar bacterial (mycobacteria) diseases in combination with other antituberculosis drugs

BRAND NAME
Myambutol

DRUG CLASS
Antitubercular

DESCRIPTION
This drug suppresses multiplication of the bacteria that causes tuberculosis by interfering with its production.

POTENTIAL SIDE EFFECTS
Headache, confusion, disorientation, malaise, fever, dizziness, rash, itching, acute gout, possible hallucinations, joint pain,

abdominal pain, anorexia, nausea, vomiting, various blood reactions, increase in liver function tests, peripheral nerve inflammation, optic nerve inflammation.

CAUTIONS

- Do not use if you have optic nerve inflammation.
- Stop immediately if any of the following occur: changes in vision, color blindness, or visual defects (effects normally reversible, but reversal may require up to a year). Requires regular assessment of vision during therapy.
- During long-term therapy, requires regular testing of kidney and liver function and for abnormalities of the blood.
- Not recommended in children less than 13 years old.
- Dosages should be reduced if kidney function is decreased.

DRUG INTERACTIONS

Absorption is decreased when taken with aluminum salts. Avoid taking aluminum-containing antacids for at least four hours following ethambutol.

FOOD INTERACTIONS

Unknown

HERBAL INTERACTIONS

Unknown

PREGNANCY AND BREAST-FEEDING CAUTIONS

FDA Pregnancy Risk Category C. Excreted in breast milk. The American Academy of Pediatrics considers this drug compatible with breast-feeding.

SPECIAL INFORMATION

This drug may be used along with other medications.

ETIDRONATE
(e-ti-DROE-nate)

NEWLY DISCOVERED USES (OFF-LABEL)

Bone loss reduction in spinal cord injury, prevention of osteoporosis due to glucocorticoids

ORIGINAL USES (ON-LABEL)

Paget's disease, heterotopic ossification to spinal cord injury or after total hip replacement, increased calcium levels associated with cancer

BRAND NAME
Didronel

DRUG CLASS
Bisphosphonate

DESCRIPTION
This drugs acts upon bone tissue, inhibiting the breakdown of
bone tissue.

POTENTIAL SIDE EFFECTS
Constipation, nausea, mouth ulcers, liver problems, low magnesium levels, low phosphate levels, shortness of breath, changes in
taste sensation, fever, fluid overload.

CAUTIONS
- Can cause local irritation of the esophagus. Contact your doc-
  tor if you develop difficulty swallowing, pain on swallowing,
  chest pain, or new or worsening heartburn.
- Take with full glass of water to avoid esophageal or stomach ir-
  ritation.
- If stomach irritation occurs, the dose may be given as two doses.
- Not for use if you have esophageal problems or problems with
  esophageal emptying.
- Requires monitoring of blood levels of minerals (such as cal-
  cium, phosphate, etc.).
- Maintain adequate nutrition, especially vitamin D and calcium.

DRUG INTERACTIONS
Calcium supplements, antacids, warfarin.

FOOD INTERACTIONS
To ensure best absorption of this drug, food, especially those high
in calcium (such as milk and milk products) should be avoided
within two hours of taking the drug. Vitamins or antacids which
are high in metals (such as magnesium, aluminum, calcium, or
iron) should be avoided within two hours of taking this drug.

HERBAL INTERACTIONS
Unknown

PREGNANCY AND BREAST-FEEDING CAUTIONS
FDA Pregnancy Risk Category C. It is not known whether this
drug is excreted in breast milk. Avoid during breast-feeding.

ETODOLAC
(ee-toe-DOE-lak)

NEWLY DISCOVERED USES (OFF-LABEL)
Gout

ORIGINAL USES (ON-LABEL)
Osteoarthritis, rheumatoid arthritis, juvenile rheumatoid arthritis

BRAND NAMES
Lodine, Lodine XL

DRUG CLASS
Pain reliever, anti-inflammatory [nonsteroidal anti-inflammatory (NSAID)]

DESCRIPTION
This drug inhibits the production of prostaglandin, a chemical drug in the body responsible for inflammation and pain.

POTENTIAL SIDE EFFECTS
Abdominal cramps, nausea, stomach upset, diarrhea, flatulence, weakness, stomach irritation, blurred vision, ringing in the ears, constipation.

CAUTIONS
- Not for use if you are allergic to aspirin or other NSAIDs.
- Not for use if you have active gastric/duodenal ulcer disease.
- Do not use during third trimester of pregnancy.
- Ask physician about use if you have the following medical problems: high blood pressure, dehydration, decreased kidney or liver function, history of gastric disease.
- Elderly are at higher risk of developing side effects.

DRUG INTERACTIONS
Aspirin, lithium, methotrexate, digoxin, cyclosporine (nephrotoxicity), diuretics, some anti-hypertensives, and warfarin (bleeding)

FOOD INTERACTIONS
Alcohol

HERBAL INTERACTIONS
Cat's claw, dong quai, evening primrose, feverfew, garlic, ginger, ginkgo, red clover, horse chestnut, green tea, ginseng

PREGNANCY AND BREAST-FEEDING CAUTIONS

FDA Pregnancy Risk Category C. FDA Pregnancy Category D in third trimester. Not known if excreted in breast milk. Do not breast-feed during therapy with this drug.

Stop taking this drug approximately 24 to 48 hours prior to surgical or dental procedures as it affects the body's ability to form blood clots and may increase bleeding time. In April 2005, the FDA announced the potential addition of a black box warning to the labeling of this class of drugs (NSAIDs), specifically regarding potential serious cardiac events and potentially life-threatening gastric adverse events.

FAMCICLOVIR
(fam-SYE-kloe-veer)

NEWLY DISCOVERED USES (OFF-LABEL)
Hepatitis B, polyarteritis nodosa

ORIGINAL USES (ON-LABEL)
Acute herpes zoster (shingles) and recurrent episodes of genital herpes, treatment of recurrent herpes simplex in immunocompetent patients

BRAND NAME
Famvir

DRUG CLASS
Antiviral

DESCRIPTION
Famciclovir is changed in the body to its active compound, penciclovir triphosphate, which interferes with an enzyme responsible for the production of herpes simplex virus-2.

POTENTIAL SIDE EFFECTS
Fatigue, dizziness, headache, diarrhea, vomiting, constipation, abdominal pain, nausea, painful menstruation, flatulence, migraine, itching, rash, sinus inflammation, sore throat

CAUTIONS
- Dosage needs to be adjusted if you have kidney problems and in some patients with liver disease.

- Safety and efficacy have not been established in children less than 18 years of age.

DRUG INTERACTIONS
Cimetidine, digoxin, probenecid, theophylline

FOOD INTERACTIONS
Unknown

HERBAL INTERACTIONS
Unknown

PREGNANCY AND BREAST-FEEDING CAUTIONS
FDA Pregnancy Risk Category B. Excretion in breast milk is not known, but it is suspected to pass into the breast milk. Do not take during breast-feeding.

SPECIAL INFORMATION
Therapy is most effective when therapy is started within 72 hours after the appearance of the first lesion (herpes infections).

This information pertains to the prescription products only.

FAMOTIDINE
(fa-MOE-ti-deen)

NEWLY DISCOVERED USES (OFF-LABEL)
Chemotherapy induced (prevention) anaphylaxis, prevention of recurrence of upper gastrointestinal (GI) bleeding

ORIGINAL USES (ON-LABEL)
Treatment of duodenal ulcer, benign gastric ulcer, gastro-esophageal reflux disease (GERD), pathological hypersecretory conditions

BRAND NAME
Pepcid

DRUG CLASS
Antihistamine, gastric ulcer (H2 blocker; histamine H2 antagonist)

DESCRIPTION
This drug inhibits gastric acid secretion.

POTENTIAL SIDE EFFECTS
Headache, dizziness, dry mouth.

CAUTIONS
- May require reduced doses if you have impaired kidney function.
- Injectable form (multidose vials) contains benzyl alcohol.

DRUG INTERACTIONS
Ketoconazole, itraconazole

FOOD INTERACTIONS
Alcohol. May be taken without regard to meals.

HERBAL INTERACTIONS
Unknown

PREGNANCY AND BREAST-FEEDING CAUTIONS
FDA Pregnancy Risk Category B. Excreted in breast milk. Breast-feeding not recommended due to limited human data.

FELODIPINE
(fe-LOE-di-peen)

NEWLY DISCOVERED USES (OFF-LABEL)
Congestive heart failure, prevention of cyclosporine induced nephrotoxicity, Raynaud's syndrome

---

ORIGINAL USES (ON-LABEL)
High blood pressure

BRAND NAME
Plendil

DRUG CLASS
Antihypertensive (calcium channel blocker)

DESCRIPTION
This drug produces a relaxation of coronary vascular smooth muscle, increasing oxygen delivery to the heart.

POTENTIAL SIDE EFFECTS

Headache, peripheral edema, increased heart rate, constipation, flushing.

CAUTIONS

- Notify your doctor if you have had an allergic reaction to a drug in this class.
- Inform your doctor if you have low blood pressure, severe left ventricular dysfunction or other types of heart problems, liver or kidney dysfunction.
- Abrupt withdrawal may cause increased duration and frequency of chest pain.
- The elderly may be at greater risk of experiencing low blood pressure and constipation associated with this therapy.

DRUG INTERACTIONS

This drug is metabolized by a specific set of liver enzymes. Several other drugs interfere with these liver enzymes, and thus may increase or decrease the clearance of felodipine from the body, potentially increasing the risk of side effects or decreasing effectiveness. When these drugs are given in combination with felodipine, dosage adjustments may be needed. As these are too numerous to list, you should always check with your doctor or pharmacist prior to starting a new medication, herbal, or nonprescription product.

FOOD INTERACTIONS

Alcohol. High fat-carbohydrate meals, grapefruit juice.

HERBAL INTERACTIONS

St. John's wort, dong quai, ephedra, yohimbe, ginseng, garlic

PREGNANCY AND BREAST-FEEDING CAUTIONS

FDA Pregnancy Risk Category C. Excreted in breast milk. Consult your doctor.

SPECIAL INFORMATION

Do not crush or chew.

FENOFIBRATE
(fen-oh-FYE-brate)

NEWLY DISCOVERED USES (OFF-LABEL)
Gout

ORIGINAL USES (ON-LABEL)
In combination with dietary therapy for the treatment of adults
with very high serum triglyceride levels (types IV and V hyperlipidemia) who are at risk of pancreatitis and who do not respond
adequately to dietary measures alone. In combination with dietary
therapy to reduce low-density lipoprotein cholesterol (LDL-C),
total cholesterol (total-C), triglycerides, and apolipoprotein B (apo
B) in adult patients with primary hypercholesterolemia or mixed
dyslipidemia (Fredrickson types IIa and IIb).

BRAND NAMES
Antara, Lofibra, TriCor

DRUG CLASS
Antilipemic (fibric acid)

DESCRIPTION
Fenofibrate breaks down lipoproteins and clears triglycerides
from the blood.

POTENTIAL SIDE EFFECTS
Pancreatitis, gallstones, muscle aches, diarrhea, nausea, constipation, abnormal elevations in liver function tests, liver toxicity, respiratory disorder, abdominal pain, back pain, headache, muscle
incoordination, changes in blood factors.

CAUTIONS
- Do not use if you have liver or severe kidney dysfunction in-
  cluding primary biliary cirrhosis and unexplained persistent
  liver function abnormalities.
- Inform your doctor if you have pre-existing gallbladder disease.
  This drug may increase the risk of gallstones.
- Report any muscle tenderness or weakness, especially if accom-
  panied by fever and malaise, to your doctor.
- May cause liver toxicity, manifested by increases in liver func-
  tion tests.
- Dosages are reduced in kidney dysfunction and the elderly.

- Therapy should be withdrawn if an adequate response is not obtained after two months of therapy at the maximal daily dose.
- Requires monitoring of lipids, liver function, and blood factors prior to initiation and periodically during therapy.

DRUG INTERACTIONS
Sulfonylureas, warfarin, HMG-CoA reductase inhibitors such as lovastatin, atorvastatin, ezetimibe, cyclosporine, bile acid sequestrants

FOOD INTERACTIONS
Capsules should be taken with food. Tablets may be taken with or without food.

HERBAL INTERACTIONS
Unknown

PREGNANCY AND BREAST-FEEDING CAUTIONS
FDA Pregnancy Risk Category C. Excreted in breast milk. Breast-feeding not recommended due to potential toxicity.

SPECIAL INFORMATION
Take fenofibrate at least one hour before or four to six hours after the administration of bile acid sequestrants.

FILGRASTIM
(fil-GRA-stim)

NEWLY DISCOVERED USES (OFF-LABEL)
Agranulocytosis, HIV

ORIGINAL USES (ON-LABEL)
Stimulation of white blood cell production in people with reduced counts due to malignancies, those receiving therapy which are known to reduce certain types of white blood cells; severe chronic neutropenia (reduced neutrophils); those receiving bone marrow transplantation (BMT); or undergoing peripheral blood progenitor cell (PBPC) collection

BRAND NAME
Neupogen

DRUG CLASS
Blood formation (colony-stimulating factor)

DESCRIPTION

This drug stimulates the production, maturation, and activation of neutrophils (a type of white blood cell) to combat low white blood cell counts and to reduce the risk of complications associated with those conditions, such as infection.

POTENTIAL SIDE EFFECTS

Nausea, vomiting, skeletal pain, hair loss, diarrhea, fever, mouth ulcers, fatigue, anorexia, shortness of breath, headache, cough, skin rash, chest pain, weakness, sore throat, constipation.

CAUTIONS

- Requires close monitoring of blood factors before, during, and after therapy.
- Has rarely produced cardiac events. Patients with pre-existing cardiac conditions should be monitored closely.
- May produce severe bone pain which requires pain therapy. Notify your doctor if this begins to develop.
- May affect thyroid function.
- Not for use in the period 12 to 24 hours before to 24 hours after administration of cytotoxic chemotherapy.
- May potentially act as a growth factor for any tumor type, particularly myeloid malignancies.
- Allergic-type reactions have happened with first given doses and later doses, occurring most frequently with intravenous administration and within 30 minutes of the infusion. May require the administration of antihistamines, steroids, bronchodilators, and/or epinephrine.

DRUG INTERACTIONS

Lithium. Consult your doctor or pharmacist before starting any new medication, herbal preparation or nonprescription product.

FOOD INTERACTIONS

Unknown

HERBAL INTERACTIONS

Unknown

PREGNANCY AND BREAST-FEEDING CAUTIONS

FDA Pregnancy Risk Category C. Excretion in breast milk unknown. Consult your doctor prior to initiation of breast-feeding during therapy with this drug.

SPECIAL INFORMATION

Read provided patient information brochure.

FINASTERIDE
(fi-NAS-teer-ide)

NEWLY DISCOVERED USES (OFF-LABEL)
Acne in women, hirsutism

ORIGINAL USES (ON-LABEL)
Treatment of male pattern hair loss. Treatment of symptomatic benign prostatic hyperplasia (BPH).

BRAND NAMES
Propecia, Proscar

DRUG CLASS
Antiandrogen

DESCRIPTION
Inhibits 5-alpha reductase, an enzyme responsible for the conversion of testosterone to dihydrotestosterone. This effect markedly suppresses serum dihydrotestosterone levels.

POTENTIAL SIDE EFFECTS
Erectile dysfunction, impotence, decreased sex drive, decreased ejaculatory volume, breast tenderness or enlargement, skin rash, lip swelling, testicular pain.

CAUTIONS
- Not for use if you are pregnant, and children should not use this drug.
- Notify your doctor if you have liver dysfunction.
- Patients with a large residual urinary volume or severely diminished urinary flow for obstructive uropathy may not be candidates.
- A minimum of six months of treatment may be necessary to determine whether an individual will have a response to finasteride.
- Patients with benign prostate hyperplasia (BPH) should be monitored for prostate cancer before starting therapy with this drug and periodically during therapy.

DRUG INTERACTIONS
Check with your doctor or pharmacist prior to starting any new medication, herbal product, or nonprescription drug.

FOOD INTERACTIONS
Unknown

HERBAL INTERACTIONS
St. John's wort, saw palmetto

PREGNANCY AND BREAST-FEEDING CAUTIONS
FDA Pregnancy Risk Category X. Pregnant women or women who may become pregnant should avoid contact with crushed or broken tablets. Not recommended during breast-feeding.

FLUCONAZOLE
(floo-KOE-na-zole)

NEWLY DISCOVERED USES (OFF-LABEL)
| Endophthalmitis |

ORIGINAL USES (ON-LABEL)
Treatment of various fungal and yeast infections

BRAND NAME
Diflucan

DRUG CLASS
Antifungal

DESCRIPTION
This drug interferes with the production of fungal cell membrane and inhibits cell membrane formation.

POTENTIAL SIDE EFFECTS
Headache, rash, nausea, vomiting, abdominal pain, diarrhea, upset stomach, taste perversion, serious skin reactions, liver toxicity.

CAUTIONS
- Do not take this drug at the same time as cisapride.
- Notify your doctor if you have impaired liver or kidney function or if you have developed liver problems while taking other antifungals.
- This drug has caused (rarely) serious problems with liver function or skin reactions and may require monitoring during multiple dose therapy. Notify your doctor immediately if you develop abdominal pain, jaundice (yellowing of skin), dark urine, or rash.

DRUG INTERACTIONS
Rifampin, cisapride, amiodarone, selected benzodiazepines, calcium channel blockers, citalopram, cyclosporine, diazepam, ergot

derivatives, fluoxetine, glimepiride, glipizide, statin drugs (such as lovastatin, atorvastatin, etc.), methsuximide, mirtazapine, nateglinide, nefazodone, phenytoin, pioglitazone, propranolol, rosiglitazone, sertraline, sildenafil, tadalafil, tacrolimus, venlafaxine, warfarin.

This drug has strong inhibitory action on a specific set of liver enzymes (cytochrome P450 enzymes 3A4). Several other drugs are metabolized (cleared from the body or activated) by these liver enzymes, and thus, their levels may be increased or decreased when administered with fluconazole. In some cases, these drugs should not be given during fluconazole therapy (such as cisapride), in other cases, when these drugs are given in combination, dosage adjustments may be needed. As these are too numerous to list, you should always check with your doctor or pharmacist prior to starting a new medication, herbal, or nonprescription product.

FOOD INTERACTIONS
May be taken with or without regard to food.

HERBAL INTERACTIONS
Unknown

PREGNANCY AND BREAST-FEEDING CAUTIONS
FDA Pregnancy Risk Category C. Excreted in breast milk. Consult your doctor.

SPECIAL INFORMATION
This drug is often used as single dose therapy to treat some vaginal yeast infections.

FLUDROCORTISONE
(floo-droe-KOR-ti-sone)

NEWLY DISCOVERED USES (OFF-LABEL)
Chronic fatigue syndrome, orthostatic hypotension

ORIGINAL USES (ON-LABEL)
Used as a partial replacement therapy for primary and secondary adrenocortical insufficiency in Addison's disease and for the treatment of salt-losing adrenogenital syndrome

BRAND NAME
Florinef

DRUG CLASS
Mineralocorticoid

DESCRIPTION
Fludrocortisone promotes increased absorption of sodium and loss of potassium from the kidneys.

POTENTIAL SIDE EFFECTS
High blood pressure, edema (swelling due to fluid retention), headache, dizziness, acne, rash, bruising, menstrual irregularities, suppression of growth, high glucose levels, adrenal gland suppression, peptic ulcer, muscle weakness, cataracts, sweating, congestive heart failure, seizures.

CAUTIONS
- Not advised for off-labeled indications because of ability to cause marked sodium retention. Discuss with your doctor prior to initiation of therapy.
- Therapy with this drug may mask the symptoms of infection and increase the susceptibility of infection via immuno-suppression.
- Chronic use may be associated with the development of cataracts.
- Taper the dose gradually when therapy is discontinued.
- Check with your doctor prior to receiving vaccinations or immunizations.
- Watch for sodium retention and potassium loss.

DRUG INTERACTIONS
Anabolic steroids, barbiturates, phenytoin, estrogens, amphotericin B, potassium sparing diuretics, warfarin, anti-diabetic drugs, insulin, digoxin, aspirin.

FOOD INTERACTIONS
Unknown

HERBAL INTERACTIONS
Unknown

PREGNANCY AND BREAST-FEEDING CAUTIONS
FDA Pregnancy Risk Category C. Excretion in breast milk is unknown.

SPECIAL INFORMATION
Notify your doctor if dizziness, severe or continuing headaches, swelling of feet or lower legs, or unusual weight gain develops. If on chronic therapy, you may require monitoring of blood pressure and signs of edema.

FLUOCINONIDE
(floo-oh-SIN-oh-nide)

NEWLY DISCOVERED USES (OFF-LABEL)
Canker sores

ORIGINAL USES (ON-LABEL)
Various skin conditions, including atopic dermatitis, dermatoses, eczema, inflammatory skin diseases, psoriasis

BRAND NAMES
Fluonex, Lidex, Lidex-E

DRUG CLASS
Anti-inflammatory (corticosteroid)

DESCRIPTION
This drug decreases the formation, release, and activity of inflammation stimulators.

POTENTIAL SIDE EFFECTS
Acne-like skin changes, itching or mild skin rash, mild temporary stinging, irritation, local burning, redness, dryness, skin atrophy.

CAUTIONS
- Children are more susceptible to systemic absorption and toxicity.
- Should not be used in uncontrolled infection.
- Do not use gel on face, groin, or under armpits. Avoid contact with the eyes and lips.
- Highly potent topical corticosteroids, such as this drug, have been shown to suppress the hypothalamic-pituitary-adrenal axis, reducing adrenal gland secretion.
- Do not use with a dressing that blocks airflow.

DRUG INTERACTIONS
Unknown

FOOD INTERACTIONS
Unknown

HERBAL INTERACTIONS
Unknown

PREGNANCY AND BREAST-FEEDING CAUTIONS
FDA Pregnancy Risk Category C. It is not known if the use of topical steroids would result in significant absorption to be excreted in breast milk in measurable quantities. Consult your doctor.

SPECIAL INFORMATION
This is for topical use only. Apply a small amount to the affected area. Allow the solution to dry before rubbing, washing, or putting on clothes. Do not put bandages, dressing, or cosmetics over the treated area unless directed by your doctor. Do not apply double doses, but if you miss a dose, apply it as soon as possible.

FLUOXETINE
(floo-OKS-e-teen)

NEWLY DISCOVERED USES (OFF-LABEL)
Attention deficit/hyperactivity disorder (ADHD), alcoholism (cravings & dependence), Alzheimer's disease, anorexia nervosa, bipolar disorder, childhood anxiety, chronic fatigue syndrome, fibromyalgia, impulsive aggressive disorder, migraine prevention, stroke (motor control), multiple sclerosis, narcolepsy, nocturnal enuresis, premature ejaculation, posttraumatic stress disorder (PTSD), Raynaud's syndrome, schizoaffective disorder, social phobia, tension headache prevention, vasovagal syncope

ORIGINAL USES (ON-LABEL)
Major depressive disorder, obsessive compulsive disorder, bulimia nervosa, panic disorder, premenstrual dysphoric disorder

BRAND NAMES
Prozac, Prozac Weekly, Sarafem

DRUG CLASS
Antidepressant (selective serotonin reuptake inhibitor)

DESCRIPTION
This drug inhibits the reuptake of serotonin at the neuron and thus increases levels of serotonin in the body and in the brain.

POTENTIAL SIDE EFFECTS

Abnormal thinking, anxiety, dizziness, headache, decreased libido, manic reaction, nervousness, somnolence, excessive sweating, abdominal pain, anorexia, constipation, diarrhea, dry mouth, upset stomach, nausea, vomiting, urinary frequency, rhinitis, abnormal vision, fever, flu-syndrome, pain, weight loss, low sodium levels, changes in blood glucose, abnormal dreams, rash, sexual dysfunction, sinusitis.

CAUTIONS

- Use may be associated with the development of suicidal thinking and behavior (see special information section).
- Do not use if you have been taking an MAO inhibitor (such as phenelzine, tranylcypromine, isocarboxazid) within the past 14 days. When used with MAO-Is fever, high blood pressure, increased heart rate, confusion, seizures, and deaths have been reported.
- Gradually decrease in dosage upon discontinuation of therapy.
- Notify your doctor if you have a history of mania, seizures, and alcoholism.
- Use caution if you have liver dysfunction, or kidney insufficiency, or if you are elderly.
- Concurrent use of aspirin or other non-steroidal anti-inflammatory drugs (NSAIDs) may increase the risk of bleeding.

DRUG INTERACTIONS

MAO inhibitors (such as phenelzine, isocarboxazid, or linezolid), selegiline, warfarin, cimetidine, linezolid, cyproheptadine, metoclopramide, sibutramine, tramadol, phenytoin, L-tryptophan, tricyclic antidepressants (such as nortriptyline, amitriptyline, imipramine, etc.), benzodiazepines (such as diazepam, flurazepam, etc.), beta-blockers, buspirone, carbamazepine, clozapine, cyclosporine, haloperidol, lithium, olanzapine, phenothiazines, propafenone, ritonavir, trazodone.

This drug is metabolized by and affects a specific set of liver enzymes. Several other drugs interfere with these liver enzymes, and thus may increase or decrease the clearance of fluoxetine from the body, potentially increasing the risk of side effects or decreasing effectiveness. When these drugs are given in combination with fluoxetine, dosage adjustments may be needed in either or both drugs. As these are too numerous to list, you should always check with your doctor or pharmacist prior to starting a new medication, herbal, or nonprescription product.

FOOD INTERACTIONS
May be given with or without food. Avoid alcohol.

HERBAL INTERACTIONS
Valerian, St. John's wort, SAMe, kava kava

PREGNANCY AND BREAST-FEEDING CAUTIONS
FDA Pregnancy Risk Category C. Excreted in breast milk. Not recommended during breast-feeding.

SPECIAL INFORMATION
In 2005, the FDA announced new labeling for antidepressants regarding the need to closely monitor for worsening of depression and for the potential of increased suicidal thinking or suicidal behavior during therapy. Although this recommendation applies to all patients (adults, children, adolescents) treated with antidepressants for any indication, this is of particular importance in patients being treated for depression. Discuss the latest information regarding this safety issue with your doctor prior to initiating therapy.

Close observation may be especially important when antidepressant medications are started for the first time or when doses are changed. More information on this topic can be found at the following web site: http://www.fda.gov/cder/drug/antidepressants/default.htm.

FLURBIPROFEN
(flure-BI-proe-fen)

Oral

NEWLY DISCOVERED USES (OFF-LABEL)
Ankylosing spondylitis, dysmenorrhea, periodontitis

ORIGINAL USES (ON-LABEL)
Osteoarthritis, rheumatoid arthritis

BRAND NAME
Ansaid

DRUG CLASS
Non-steroidal anti-inflammatory (NSAID)

DESCRIPTION

This drug inhibits the production of prostaglandin, a chemical drug in the body responsible for inflammation and pain.

POTENTIAL SIDE EFFECTS

Abdominal cramps, nausea, stomach upset, diarrhea, flatulence, weakness, stomach irritation, blurred vision, ringing in the ears, constipation.

CAUTIONS

- Not for use if you are allergic to aspirin or other NSAIDs.
- Not for use if you have active gastric/duodenal ulcer disease.
- Do not use during third trimester of pregnancy.
- Ask your physician about use if you have any of the following medical problems: high blood pressure, dehydration, decreased kidney or liver function, history of gastric disease.
- Elderly are at higher risk of developing side effects.

DRUG INTERACTIONS

Aspirin, lithium, methotrexate, digoxin, cyclosporine diuretics, some anti-hypertensives, warfarin, amiodarone, fluoxetine, glimepiride, glipizide, nateglinide, phenytoin, pioglitazone, rosiglitazone, sertraline, warfarin.

FOOD INTERACTIONS

Alcohol

HERBAL INTERACTIONS

Cat's claw, dong quai, evening primrose, feverfew, garlic, ginger, ginkgo, red clover, horse chestnut, green tea, ginseng

PREGNANCY AND BREAST-FEEDING CAUTIONS

FDA Pregnancy Risk Category C (D in the third trimester). Excreted in breast milk, nursing not recommended.

SPECIAL INFORMATION

Stop taking this drug (with doctor's approval) approximately 24 to 48 hours prior to surgical or dental procedures as it affects the body's ability to form blood clots and may increase bleeding time. In April 2005, the FDA announced the potential addition of a black box warning to the labeling of this class of drugs (NSAIDs), specifically regarding potential serious cardiac events and potentially life-threatening gastric adverse events.

FLUTAMIDE
(FLOO-ta-mide)

NEWLY DISCOVERED USES (OFF-LABEL)

Acne in women, congenital adrenal hyperplasia, hirsutism, McCune-Albright syndrome

ORIGINAL USES (ON-LABEL)
Treatment of metastatic prostatic carcinoma in combination therapy with LHRH agonist analogues

BRAND NAME
Eulexin

DRUG CLASS
Antineoplastic (anti-androgen)

DESCRIPTION
This drug inhibits androgen uptake in target tissues such as the prostate, which is androgen sensitive.

POTENTIAL SIDE EFFECTS
Hot flashes, loss of libido, impotence, diarrhea, nausea, vomiting, breast swelling (gynecomastia), liver toxicity, reduced sperm motility resulting in impaired fertility, green or amber discoloration of urine, photosensitivity reactions (skin reaction related to sun exposure).

CAUTIONS
- Not for use if you have severe liver dysfunction or pregnancy. Ask your doctor to perform liver function tests prior to and periodically during therapy. Approximately half of the reported liver toxicity cases occurred within the first three months of therapy. Discontinue therapy if jaundice develops.
- Not for use in women.
- Inform your doctor if you have glucose-6 phosphate dehydrogenase deficiency, hemoglobin M disease, or smoke.
- Wear sunscreen or protective clothing when in sunlight. Avoid prolonged exposure to sun.

DRUG INTERACTIONS
Warfarin

FOOD INTERACTIONS
None

HERBAL INTERACTIONS
St. John's wort, chaparral, comfrey, eucalyptus, germander, jin bu huan, kava, pennyroyal, skullcap

PREGNANCY AND BREAST-FEEDING CAUTIONS
FDA Pregnancy Risk Category D. Excretion in breast milk unknown. Breast-feeding is not recommended.

SPECIAL INFORMATION
Contents of capsule may be opened and mixed with applesauce, pudding, or other soft foods; mixing with a beverage is not recommended, however. This drug has a black box warning regarding the potential for liver toxicity and failure. Report any symptoms of liver toxicity to your doctor, including jaundice, nausea, abdominal pain, fatigue, anorexia, etc.

FLUTICASONE
(floo-TIK-a-sone)

Inhalant

NEWLY DISCOVERED USES (OFF-LABEL)

Cystic fibrosis

ORIGINAL USES (ON-LABEL)
Inhalation: Maintenance treatment of asthma as preventive therapy. It is also indicated for patients requiring oral corticosteroid therapy for asthma to assist in total discontinuation or reduction of total oral dose.

BRAND NAMES
Flovent, Flovent HFA, Flovent Rotadisk

DRUG CLASS
Corticosteroid (inhalant or nasal spray)

DESCRIPTION
This drug has medium potency as an anti-inflammatory drug, and has some limited ability to suppress adrenal secretions when applied topically. Inhaled fluticasone's effectiveness is due to its direct local effect.

POTENTIAL SIDE EFFECTS
Oral inhalation: Headache, fever, nausea/vomiting, viral gastric infection, diarrhea, abdominal discomfort/pain, muscle injury,

musculoskeletal pain, back problems, upper respiratory tract infection, throat irritation, nasal congestion, sore throat, viral infection.

Nasal inhalation: Headache, sore throat, nausea/vomiting, epistaxis, asthma symptoms, cough, aches and pains, flu-like symptoms.

CAUTIONS
- Inhaled fluticasone should not be used for primary treatment of acute asthma attacks.
- May cause hypercorticism or suppression of hypothalamic-pituitary-adrenal (HPA) axis, particularly in younger children or in patients receiving high doses for prolonged periods. HPA axis suppression may lead to adrenal crisis.
- Particular care is required if you are being transferred from oral or injection corticosteroids to inhaled products due to possible adrenal insufficiency or withdrawal from steroids, including an increase in allergic symptoms.
- Concurrent use of ritonavir (and potentially other strong inhibitors of specific liver enzymes) may increase fluticasone levels and effects on HPA suppression.
- Controlled clinical studies have shown orally-inhaled and intranasal corticosteroids may cause a reduction in growth velocity in children.
- May suppress the immune system, so you may be more susceptible to infection. Use with caution, if you use this drug at all, if you have systemic infections, active or quiescent tuberculosis infection or ocular herpes simplex. Avoid exposure to chickenpox and measles.
- Flovent Rotadisk contains lactose; very rare allergic reactions have been reported in patients with severe milk protein allergy.

DRUG INTERACTIONS
This drug is metabolized by a specific set of liver enzymes. Several other drugs interfere with these liver enzymes, and thus may increase or decrease the clearance of fluticasone from the body, potentially increasing the risk of side effects or decreasing effectiveness. When these drugs are given in combination with fluticasone, dosage adjustments may be needed. As these are too numerous to list, you should always check with your doctor or pharmacist prior to starting a new medication, herbal, or nonprescription products

FOOD INTERACTIONS
Unknown

HERBAL INTERACTIONS
St. John's wort

PREGNANCY AND BREAST-FEEDING CAUTIONS
FDA Pregnancy Risk Category C. Excretion in breast milk unknown. Consult your doctor.

SPECIAL INFORMATION
Fluticasone is not indicated for the relief of acute bronchospasm. The inhaled products have a black box warning which describes the need for special care in patients who are transferred from systemic (oral or injectable) steroids to inhaled products that are less absorbed. A sudden decrease in dose due to lesser absorption may result in fatal suppression of the hypothalamus-pituitary-adrenal function and cause an adrenal crisis. This particularly applies to patients that are maintained on at least 20 mg daily (or its equivalent).

FLUVOXAMINE
(floo-VOKS-a-meen)

NEWLY DISCOVERED USES (OFF-LABEL)
Alcoholism (cravings & dependence), childhood anxiety, generalized anxiety disorder, migraine prevention, nocturnal enuresis, panic disorder, premenstrual dysphoric disorder (PMDD), premenstrual syndrome (PMS), social phobia

ORIGINAL USES (ON-LABEL)
Obsessive-compulsive disorder

BRAND NAME
Luvox

DRUG CLASS
Serotonin reuptake inhibitor

DESCRIPTION
This drug inhibits the reuptake of serotonin at the neuron and thus increases the levels of serotonin in the body and in the brain.

POTENTIAL SIDE EFFECTS
Palpitations, anxiety, dizziness, headache, insomnia, nervousness, somnolence, tremor, excessive sweating, anorexia, constipation, dry mouth, upset stomach, swallowing difficulty, flatulence, nausea, vomiting, abnormal ejaculation, urinary problems, changes in vision, changes in taste, flu-syndrome, low sodium levels.

CAUTIONS
- Use may be associated with the development of suicidal thinking and behavior (see special information section).
- Do not use if you have been taking an MAO inhibitor (such as phenelzine, tranylcypromine, isocarboxazid) within the past 14 days. When used with MAO-Is fever, high blood pressure, increased heart rate, confusion, seizures, and deaths have been reported.
- Gradually decrease in dosage upon discontinuation of therapy.
- Notify your doctor if you have a history of mania, seizures, alcoholism.
- Use caution with liver dysfunction, or kidney insufficiency, or in elderly patients.
- Concurrent use of aspirin or other non-steroidal anti-inflammatory drugs (NSAIDs) may increase the risk of bleeding.

DRUG INTERACTIONS
MAO inhibitors (such as phenelzine, isocarboxazid, or linezolid), warfarin, cimetidine, metoclopramide, sibutramine, tramadol, phenytoin, smoking, L-tryptophan, tricyclic antidepressants, benzodiazepines (such as diazepam, flurazepam, temazepam, etc.), beta-blockers (such as propranolol, etc.), buspirone, carbamazepine, cisapride, clozapine, diltiazem, haloperidol, lithium, methadone, NSAIDs, olanzapine, phenothiazines, pimozide, ropivacaine, glimepiride, tolbutamide, sumatriptan, tacrine, theophylline.

This drug is metabolized by and affects a specific set of liver enzymes. Several other drugs interfere with these liver enzymes, and thus may increase or decrease the clearance of fluvoxamine from the body, potentially increasing the risk of side effects or decreasing effectiveness. When these drugs are given in combination with fluvoxamine, dosage adjustments may be needed in either or both drugs. As these are too numerous to list, you should always check with your doctor or pharmacist prior to starting a new medication, herbal, or nonprescription product.

FOOD INTERACTIONS
May be given with or without food. Avoid alcohol.

HERBAL INTERACTIONS
Valerian, St. John's wort, SAMe, kava kava

PREGNANCY AND BREAST-FEEDING CAUTIONS
FDA Pregnancy Risk Category C. Excreted in breast milk. Not recommended during breast-feeding.

SPECIAL INFORMATION
In 2005, the FDA announced new labeling for antidepressants regarding the need to closely monitor for worsening of depression and for the potential of increased suicidal thinking or suicidal behavior during therapy. Although this recommendation applies to all patients (adults, children, adolescents) treated with antidepressants for any indication, this is of particular importance in patients being treated for depression. Discuss the latest information regarding this safety issue with your doctor prior to initiating therapy.

Close observation may be especially important when antidepressant medications are started for the first time or when doses are changed. More information on this topic can be found at the following web site: http://www.fda.gov/cder/drug/antidepressants/default.htm

FONDAPARINUX
(fon-da-PARE-i-nuks)

NEWLY DISCOVERED USES (OFF-LABEL)
Heparin-induced thrombocytopenia

ORIGINAL USES (ON-LABEL)
Prevents deep vein thrombosis (DVT-clotting) in patients undergoing surgery for hip replacement, knee replacement, or hip fracture surgery (including extended prevention following hip fracture surgery), treatment of acute pulmonary embolism (PE), treatment of acute DVT without PE

BRAND NAME
Arixtra

DRUG CLASS
Anticoagulant (factor Xa inhibitor)

DESCRIPTION
This drug inhibits factor Xa, which interrupts blood clotting and inhibits thrombin formation and clot development.

POTENTIAL SIDE EFFECTS
Bleeding, insomnia, dizziness, confusion, headache, rash, nausea, constipation, vomiting, diarrhea, upset stomach, urinary tract infection, anemia, bruising, fever, swelling due to fluid retention, potassium loss, low blood pressure.

CAUTIONS
- Notify your doctor if you have kidney dysfunction, gastrointestinal disease, weigh less than 110 pounds, active major bleeding or bleeding disorders, high blood pressure, bacterial endocarditis, or certain blood disorders. Inform your doctor if you are taking other drugs which affect bleeding.
- Patients with recent or anticipated epidural or spinal anesthesia are at risk of spinal or epidural bleeding and subsequent paralysis.

DRUG INTERACTIONS
Anticoagulants, antiplatelet drugs, drotrecogin alfa, NSAIDs, salicylates, and thrombolytic drugs (drugs which break blood clots) may enhance the anticoagulant effect and/or increase the risk of bleeding.

FOOD INTERACTIONS
Unknown

HERBAL INTERACTIONS
Alfalfa, anise, bilberry, bladderwrack, bromelain, cat's claw, celery, coleus, cordyceps, dong quai, evening primrose oil, fenugreek, feverfew, garlic, ginger, ginkgo biloba, ginseng (American/Panax/Siberian), grape seed, green tea, guggul, horse chestnut seed, horseradish, licorice, prickly ash, red clover, reishi, sweet clover, turmeric, white willow

PREGNANCY AND BREAST-FEEDING CAUTIONS
FDA Pregnancy Risk Category B. Excretion in breast milk unknown. Consult your doctor.

SPECIAL INFORMATION
This drug has a black box warning regarding the risk of spinal bleeding and paralysis when this drug is used when spinal/epidural anesthesia is administered.

FOSCARNET
(fos-KAR-net)

NEWLY DISCOVERED USES (OFF-LABEL)

Acyclovir-resistant varicella zoster in HIV, outer retinal necrosis

ORIGINAL USES (ON-LABEL)

Treatment of herpes virus infections suspected to be caused by acyclovir-resistant or ganciclovir-resistant strains (CMV); this occurs almost exclusively in immunocompromised persons who have received prolonged treatment for a herpes virus infection. Treatment of CMV retinitis in persons with AIDS.

BRAND NAME

Foscavir

DRUG CLASS

Antiviral

DESCRIPTION

This drug inhibits viral reproduction by interfering with the production of DNA in the virus.

POTENTIAL SIDE EFFECTS

Fever, headache, seizure, electrolyte disorders (such as calcium, magnesium, phosphate, or potassium), nausea, diarrhea, vomiting, anemia, kidney dysfunction.

CAUTIONS

- Requires reduced dosage in kidney failure.
- Kidney impairment occurs to some degree in the majority of patients and can occur at any time. It is usually reversible within one week following dose adjustment or discontinuation of therapy.
- Your kidney function should be closely monitored.
- Imbalance of serum electrolytes or minerals may occur.
- Patients with a low calcium levels or decreased kidney function may experience perioral tingling, numbness, or seizures. Seizures have been experienced by up to 10% of AIDS patients.

DRUG INTERACTIONS

Ciprofloxacin (or other fluoroquinolones) increases seizure potential. Cyclosporine, other drugs known to affect kidneys adversely (such as amphotericin B, intravenous pentamidine, aminoglycosides, etc.), pentamidine, protease inhibitors (such as ritonavir, saquinavir).

FOOD INTERACTIONS
Unknown

HERBAL INTERACTIONS
Unknown

PREGNANCY AND BREAST-FEEDING CAUTIONS
FDA Pregnancy Risk Category C. Excretion in breast milk unknown. Breast-feeding not recommended during therapy.

SPECIAL INFORMATION
Saline infusions before and after foscarnet infusion help to minimize the risk of kidney damage. This drug has a black box warning regarding kidney impairment as a potential side effect. This requires frequent monitoring and dosage adjustments if needed. In addition, the black box warning details the possibility of seizures associated with electrolyte imbalances.

FUROSEMIDE
(fyoor-OH-se-mide)

NEWLY DISCOVERED USES (OFF-LABEL)
Acute asthma, allergen-induced asthma, ascites in cirrhosis, aspirin-sensitive asthma, bronchopulmonary dysplasia (in infants), chronic asthma, membranous nephropathy, nocturia, prevention of exercise-induced bronchospasm, steroid-dependent asthma.

ORIGINAL USES (ON-LABEL)
Management of edema (swelling from water retention) associated with congestive heart failure and liver or kidney disease, treatment of high blood pressure

BRAND NAME
Lasix

DRUG CLASS
Blood pressure medication (loop diuretic)

DESCRIPTION

This drug decreases reabsorption of sodium and chloride in the kidneys, causing an increased clearance of water and electrolytes (sodium chloride, magnesium, and calcium) from the body.

POTENTIAL SIDE EFFECTS

Lowered blood pressure upon standing (orthostatic hypotension), dehydration, numbness, dizziness, lightheadedness, various skin rashes, skin reactions related to sun exposure (photosensitivity), increased levels of glucose or uric acid, decreased levels of potassium or chloride, nausea, vomiting, anorexia, gastric irritation, urinary bladder spasm, weakness, hearing impairment, ringing in the ears, decrease in kidney function.

CAUTIONS

- Do not use if you are allergic to certain types of sulfa drugs.
- The risk of kidney or ear side effects are increased if used with other drugs that have similar side effects.
- Watch for warning signs of dehydration: dryness of mouth, thirst, anorexia, weakness, muscle cramps or pain, increased heart rate, irregular heart rhythm, vomiting.
- Use may result in imbalance in electrolytes (potassium, sodium, magnesium).

DRUG INTERACTIONS

Lithium, propranolol, cisplatin, clofibrate, probenecid

HERBAL INTERACTIONS

Dong quai, yohimbe, ginseng, garlic. Limit intake of natural licorice.

PREGNANCY AND BREAST-FEEDING CAUTIONS

FDA Pregnancy Risk Category C. Excreted in breast milk. No reports of adverse effects. Use with caution.

SPECIAL INFORMATION

May be taken with food or milk. Rise slowly from sitting or lying position to avoid dizziness. Avoid long periods of exercise. This drug will increase urination; take early in day to prevent frequent need to urinate during the bedtime hours.

GABAPENTIN
(GA-ba-pen-tin)

NEWLY DISCOVERED USES (OFF-LABEL)
Alcohol withdrawal, attention deficit hyperactivity disorder (ADHD), chronic neuropathic pain, cocaine addiction, diabetic peripheral neuropathy, generalized anxiety disorder (GAD), fibromyalgia, menopause, migraine prevention, panic disorder, post-traumatic stress disorder (PTSD), social phobia, trigeminal neuralgia

ORIGINAL USES (ON-LABEL)
Post-herpetic neuralgia, epilepsy

BRAND NAME
Neurontin

DRUG CLASS
Anticonvulsant

DESCRIPTION
This drug is used to control seizures, possibly by slowing transmission of excitatory chemicals in the brain.

POTENTIAL SIDE EFFECTS
Drowsiness, dizziness, muscle incoordination, fatigue, fever, emotional lability, nausea, upset stomach, dry mouth, double vision, blurred vision.

CAUTIONS
- Avoid abrupt discontinuation of therapy.
- Use with caution if you have renal impairment, or if you are elderly.
- Use with caution when operating heavy machinery or driving.
- Monitor for possible mood disturbances or psychological changes when using this drug in children.

DRUG INTERACTIONS
Cimetidine may increase the levels of gabapentin. Gabapentin may increase the levels of norethindrone if given concurrently. Caution use with other drugs that may cause sedation (such as sedatives, alcohol).

FOOD INTERACTIONS
Alcohol

HERBAL INTERACTIONS
Evening primrose, valerian, St. John's wort, kava kava, and gotu kola

PREGNANCY AND BREAST-FEEDING CAUTIONS
FDA Pregnancy Risk Category C. Excretion in breast milk unknown. Nursing is not recommended.

GALANTAMINE
(guh-LANT-tah-meen)

NEWLY DISCOVERED USES (OFF-LABEL)
Brain trauma

ORIGINAL USES (ON-LABEL)
Mild to moderate dementia of the Alzheimer's type

BRAND NAME
Reminyl

DRUG CLASS
Alzheimer's (acetylcholinesterase inhibitor)

DESCRIPTION
This drug blocks the activity of the enzyme responsible for breakdown of acetylcholine, thereby increasing the levels of acetylcholine. Acetylcholine deficiency may be the cause of Alzheimer's disease.

POTENTIAL SIDE EFFECTS
Dizziness, headache, depression, insomnia, somnolence, tremor, nausea, vomiting, diarrhea, anorexia, abdominal pain, upset stomach, urinary tract infection, bloody urine, weight loss, fatigue, anemia, fainting, heart rate decrease.

CAUTIONS
- Notify your doctor if you have kidney or liver impairment, bladder outlet obstruction, asthma, lung disease, gastric ulcers, or if you are taking NSAIDs.
- May exaggerate the effects of certain anesthetics. Notify your doctor that you are taking this drug prior to any surgery or procedure.
- Notify your doctor if you have heart disease, particularly that which includes heart conduction problems or heart rhythm.

DRUG INTERACTIONS

Succinylcholine, bethanecol, cimetidine, ketoconazole, paroxetine, erythromycin.

This drug is metabolized by a specific set of liver enzymes. Several other drugs interfere with these liver enzymes, and thus may increase or decrease the clearance of galantamine from the body, potentially increasing the risk of side effects or decreasing effectiveness. When these drugs are given in combination with galantamine, dosage adjustments may be needed. As these are too numerous to list, you should always check with your doctor or pharmacist prior to starting a new medication, herbal, or nonprescription product.

FOOD INTERACTIONS

Take with morning and evening meal to reduce stomach upset.

HERBAL INTERACTIONS

St. John's wort

PREGNANCY AND BREAST-FEEDING CAUTIONS

FDA Pregnancy Risk Category B. Data regarding breast milk excretion are not available. Consult your doctor.

SPECIAL INFORMATION

If taking solution, read patient information sheet for proper administration.

In 2005, new safety data were added to the product labeling regarding death, which occurred in patients with cognitive impairment.

GATIFLOXACIN
(gat-ih-FLOX-uh-sin)

Oral, Injectable

NEWLY DISCOVERED USES (OFF-LABEL)
Acute otitis media (therapy-resistant)

ORIGINAL USES (ON-LABEL)

Various bacterial infections in the lung, eye, sinuses, skin, and skin structure

BRAND NAME
Tequin

DRUG CLASS
Antibiotic (quinolone)

DESCRIPTION
This drug is used to fight bacteria. It works by halting DNA replication, repair, recombination, and transposition in bacterial cells.

POTENTIAL SIDE EFFECTS
Headache, dizziness, nausea, diarrhea, vaginitis, abnormal dream, tremor, change in heart rate (see QT prolongation in caution), tendon rupture.

CAUTIONS
- Notify your doctor if you have any problems now or recently with irregular heart rates, low potassium levels, seizures, or heart attack.
- Gatifloxacin has affected heart rate rhythm (QT prolongation) in some patients and should be avoided if you have this problem, have low potassium levels, or are taking certain antiarrhythmics. Check with your doctor prior to starting any new drug while on this medication.
- Report to your doctor if you experience pain, inflammation or rupture of a tendon. Rest and refrain from exercise until you see a doctor. Tendon rupture can occur during or after therapy with this drug.
- Report any episodes of changes in heart rate or fainting spells.
- Stop the medication at the first sign of a rash.
- Prolonged use may cause superinfection.
- May aggravate symptoms of myasthenia gravis.
- Inform your doctor if serious, persistent diarrhea develops.

DRUG INTERACTIONS
Iron, zinc, calcium, magnesium, aluminum, corticosteroids (increase risk of tendon rupture), antacids, electrolyte supplements, quinapril, sucralfate, certain antiarrhythmics, didanosine formulations (chewable/buffered tablets and pediatric powder for oral suspension), theophylline, cimetidine, anticoagulants (such as warfarin, etc.).

If administered with other drugs that can cause QT prolongation (potentially serious changes in heart rhythm) may increase risk of this occurring. For a comprehensive list of drugs known and suspected to cause these effects, refer to the following website: (http://www.torsades.org/medical-pros/drug-lists/drug-lists .htm#). While taking this medication, consult with your pharmacist or doctor for interactions prior to starting any new medication, new herbal product, or nonprescription drug.

FOOD INTERACTIONS
May be taken with or without food. Do not take with dairy products or calcium-fortified juices.

HERBAL INTERACTIONS
Unknown

PREGNANCY AND BREAST-FEEDING CAUTIONS
FDA Pregnancy Risk Category C. May be excreted in breast milk. Do not use during breast-feeding.

SPECIAL INFORMATION
Take four hours before or eight hours after didanosine, multiple vitamins, antacids, or other products containing magnesium, aluminum, iron or zinc. May cause dizziness or lightheadedness; use caution with tasks that require alertness.

GEMIFLOXACIN
(je-mi-FLOKS-a-sin)

NEWLY DISCOVERED USES (OFF-LABEL)
Legionnaire's disease

ORIGINAL USES (ON-LABEL)
Various bacterial infections in the lungs

BRAND NAME
Factive

DRUG CLASS
Antibiotic (quinolone)

DESCRIPTION
This drug is used to fight bacteria. It works by halting DNA replication, repair, recombination, and transposition in bacterial cells.

POTENTIAL SIDE EFFECTS
Rash, diarrhea, nausea, liver function test increases.

CAUTIONS

- Notify your doctor if you have any problems now or recently with irregular heart rates, low potassium levels, seizures, or heart attack.
- This drug has affected heart rate rhythm (QT prolongation) in some patients and should be avoided if you have this problem, have low potassium levels, or are taking certain antiarrhythmics. Check with your doctor prior to starting any new drug while on this medication.
- Report to your doctor if you experience pain, inflammation or rupture of a tendon. Rest and refrain from exercise until you see a doctor. Tendon rupture can occur during or after therapy with this drug.
- Report any episodes of changes in heart rate or fainting spells.
- Stop the medication at the first sign of a rash.
- Prolonged use may cause superinfection.
- Inform your doctor of allergies to antibiotics, specifically other drugs in this class.
- May aggravate symptoms of myasthenia gravis.
- Inform your doctor if serious, persistent diarrhea develops.

DRUG INTERACTIONS

Iron, zinc, calcium, magnesium, aluminum, corticosteroids (increase risk of tendon rupture), antacids, electrolyte supplements, quinapril, sucralfate, certain antiarrhythmics, theophylline, cimetidine, anticoagulants (such as warfarin, etc.).

If administered with other drugs that can cause QT prolongation (potentially serious changes in heart rhythm) may increase risk of this occurring. For a comprehensive list of drugs known and suspected to cause these effects, refer to the following website: (http://www.torsades.org/medical-pros/drug-lists/drug-lists.htm#). While taking this medication, consult with your pharmacist or doctor for interactions prior to starting any new medication, new herbal product, or nonprescription drug.

FOOD INTERACTIONS

May be taken with or without food. Do not take with dairy products or calcium-fortified juices.

HERBAL INTERACTIONS

Unknown

PREGNANCY AND BREAST-FEEDING CAUTIONS

FDA Pregnancy Risk Category C. May be excreted in breast milk. Do not use during breast-feeding.

SPECIAL INFORMATION

Take four hours before or eight hours after multiple vitamins, antacids, or other products containing magnesium, aluminum, iron or zinc. May cause dizziness or lightheadedness, caution with tasks that require alertness.

GENTAMICIN
(jen-ta-MYE-sin)

NEWLY DISCOVERED USES (OFF-LABEL)

Diverticulitis, Ménière's disease, otitis externa

ORIGINAL USES (ON-LABEL)

Injectable: Treatment of various bacterial infections, including bone infections, abdominal and urinary tract infections, respiratory tract infections, skin and soft tissue infection, endocarditis, septicemia. Topically: Treatment of skin and ocular infections.

BRAND NAMES

Garamycin, Genoptic, Gentacidin, Gentak

DRUG CLASS

Antibiotic (aminoglycoside—ophthalmic, topical, injectable)

DESCRIPTION

This drug interferes with bacterial protein production by destroying the bacterial cell membrane.

POTENTIAL SIDE EFFECTS

Neurotoxicity (vertigo, ataxia), gait instability, ototoxicity (auditory and vestibular), nephrotoxicity, decreased creatinine clearance, edema, skin itching, reddening of skin, and rash.

CAUTIONS

- Inform your doctor if you are allergic to other drugs in this class (such as tobramycin, amikacin, kanamycin, etc.) or allergic to sulfites (which may be contained in some products).
- Injectable: Requires monitoring of kidney and hearing function and blood levels. May cause neurotoxicity. Elderly patients may be at higher risk of toxicities.

- Injectable: Is not intended for long-term use due to toxicity.
- Prolonged use may result in superinfection or resistance.
- Avoid use in patients who have kidney insufficiency, vestibular or cochlear (ear) impairment, myasthenia gravis, low calcium levels, and conditions that depress neuromuscular transmission.

DRUG INTERACTIONS

Injectable: penicillins, cephalosporins, amphotericin B, loop diuretics (e.g. furosemide, bumetanide), neuromuscular blocking drugs.

Topical, eye formulations: Do not use with other topical or eye formulations without consulting your doctor.

FOOD INTERACTIONS

Unknown

HERBAL INTERACTIONS

Unknown

PREGNANCY AND BREAST-FEEDING CAUTIONS

FDA Pregnancy Risk Category C. Excreted in breast milk. Consult your doctor.

SPECIAL INFORMATION

Black box warning: Injectable drugs in this drug class have been associated with significant kidney or ear toxicity. Although kidney damage may be reversible, ear toxicity may not be reversible. Monitoring of levels and kidney function are required.

Topical: For external use only. Wash hands after application.

Eye Formulations (Cream, drops): Do not touch container to objects. May cause temporary stinging or blurring of vision after application. Consult doctor about contact lenses wear. Tilt head back to apply drops, place medication in eye and close eyes. Apply light finger pressure on tear gland for one minute after application.

GLYCOPYRROLATE
(glye-koe-PYE-roe-late)

NEWLY DISCOVERED USES (OFF-LABEL)
Drooling in cerebral palsy, Ménière's disease

ORIGINAL USES (ON-LABEL)
Used before surgery to inhibit salivation and excessive secretions of the respiratory tract and to reduce the volume and acidity of gastric secretions, used in combination for the treatment of peptic ulcer

BRAND NAMES
Robinul, Robinul Forte

DRUG CLASS
Antispasmodic, gastrointestinal (anticholinergic)

DESCRIPTION
This drug blocks the action of acetylcholine, a neurotransmitter, at receptor sites in smooth muscle, secretor glands, and the central nervous system.

POTENTIAL SIDE EFFECTS
Dry skin, constipation, dry throat, dry mouth. Irritation at injection site, dry nose, and decreased sweating, increased sensitivity to light, decreased flow of breast milk, difficulty swallowing, irregular heart rhythm, low heart rate, headache, flushing, nervousness, urinary retention, blurred vision, pupils widening, nasal stuffiness, glaucoma.

CAUTIONS
- Inform your doctor if you have ulcerative colitis, narrow-angle glaucoma, acute hemorrhage, increased heart rate, urinary obstruction, paralytic ileus, obstructive disease of the gastric tract, myasthenia gravis.
- Use with caution in elderly, patients with autonomic neuropathy, liver or kidney disease, ulcerative colitis, hyperthyroidism, cardiac disease, prostatic hypertrophy, hiatal hernia.

DRUG INTERACTIONS
Amantadine, other anticholinergic drugs, digoxin, atenolol, phenothiazines, tricyclic antidepressants, levodopa.

FOOD INTERACTIONS
Take 30 to 60 minutes prior to a meal.

HERBAL INTERACTIONS
Unknown

PREGNANCY AND BREAST-FEEDING CAUTIONS
FDA Pregnancy Risk Category B. Excretion in breast milk is unknown. Consult your doctor.

SPECIAL INFORMATION
Maintain good oral hygiene habits, because decreases in saliva may increase the chance of cavities. Because this drug may cause drowsiness or blurred vision, observe caution while performing tasks that need mental alertness. Notify your doctor if the following occurs: skin rash, flushing, eye pain, or difficulty urinating or sensitivity to light.

GOSERELIN
(GOE-se-rel-in)

NEWLY DISCOVERED USES (OFF-LABEL)
Chronic pelvic pain, dysmenorrhea, pelvic congestion, premenstrual dysphoric disorder (PMDD), therapy-resistant PMDD, premenstrual syndrome (PMS)

ORIGINAL USES (ON-LABEL)
Breast cancer, endometrial thinning, endometriosis, prostate cancer

BRAND NAME
Zoladex

DRUG CLASS
Cancer chemotherapy

DESCRIPTION
Goserelin suppresses the release of hormones from the pituitary gland, which decreases their effect on various tissues such as the ovaries and breasts.

POTENTIAL SIDE EFFECTS
Headache, emotional lability, depression, pain, insomnia, hot flashes, sexual dysfunction, vaginitis, decreased libido (women), breast enlargement or pain, lower urinary symptoms (men), vaginitis, difficult or painful sexual intercourse (women), sweat-

ing, fatigue (men), dizziness, rash, anorexia, nausea, sore throat (women).

CAUTIONS
- Temporary worsening of signs and symptoms may occur within the first few weeks of treatment, usually an increase in cancer-related pain.
- Urinary tract obstruction and spinal cord compression have been reported.
- Irreversible decreases in bone density may occur.

DRUG INTERACTIONS
Unknown

FOOD INTERACTIONS
Unknown

HERBAL INTERACTIONS
Unknown

PREGNANCY AND BREAST-FEEDING CAUTIONS
FDA Pregnancy Risk Category X. Non-hormonal contraception should be used during therapy. Should not be used while breast-feeding.

SPECIAL INFORMATION
In women, menstruation should stop during goserelin therapy. You should notify your doctor if regular menstruation continues.

GUANFACINE
(GWAHN-fa-seen)

NEWLY DISCOVERED USES (OFF-LABEL)
Attention deficit/hyperactivity (ADHD), Gilles de la Tourette syndrome

ORIGINAL USES (ON-LABEL)
High blood pressure

BRAND NAME
Tenex

DRUG CLASS
Antihypertensive (alpha-adrenergic agonist)

DESCRIPTION
This drug reduces blood pressure.

POTENTIAL SIDE EFFECTS
Dry mouth, drowsiness, muscle incoordination, dizziness, headache, impotence, constipation, fatigue, low heart rate, increased urinary frequency or urination at night, changes in taste.

CAUTIONS
- Requires dosage reduction in impaired kidney function.
- Notify your doctor if you have had recent heart attack, chronic kidney or liver dysfunction, severe cardiac disease.
- Because this drug can cause significant sedation, be cautious performing tasks that require alertness.
- Do not suddenly stop this medication.
- Not recommended for the treatment of acute high blood pressure in pregnancy.

DRUG INTERACTIONS
Amitriptyline, bupropion, desipramine, imipramine, nortriptyline, phenobarbital

FOOD INTERACTIONS
Avoid excessive ingestion of natural licorice, yohimbine.

HERBAL INTERACTIONS
Ma huang, ephedra

PREGNANCY AND BREAST-FEEDING CAUTIONS
FDA Pregnancy Risk Category B. The excretion of this drug in breast milk is unknown. Consult your doctor.

SPECIAL INFORMATION
Tolerance for alcohol may be decreased. Take at bedtime.

HALOPERIDOL
(ha-loe-PER-I-dole)

NEWLY DISCOVERED USES (OFF-LABEL)
Alzheimer's disease, autism, hiccups, prevention of post-op nausea and vomiting

ORIGINAL USES (ON-LABEL)
Psychotic disorders, Tourette's syndrome, severe behavioral problems in children, hyperactivity

BRAND NAMES
Haldol, Haldol Decanoate

DRUG CLASS
Antipsychotic (butyrophenone)

DESCRIPTION
Researchers believe that antipsychotics work by blocking dopamine receptors in the brain, reducing levels of dopamine, which stabilizes mental activity.

POTENTIAL SIDE EFFECTS
Motor restlessness, uncontrolled voluntary movements, excessive involuntary movements, increased heart rate, low blood pressure, sedation, headache, confusion, lethargy, rash, menstrual irregularities, anorexia, constipation, diarrhea, dry mouth, blurred vision, may cause changes in heart rhythm (prolongation of QT interval in cardiac monitoring), various blood disorders.

CAUTIONS
- Not for use if you have Parkinson's disease, severe central nervous system depression, bone marrow suppression, severe heart or liver disease. Use caution if you have cardiovascular disease, predisposition to seizures, subcortical brain damage, kidney or lung disease (especially if you are at risk for pneumonia).
- Use caution if you have breast cancer or other prolactin-dependent tumors, decreased GI motility, urinary retention, benign prostatic hypertrophy, dry mouth, or visual problems.
- May cause tardive dyskinesia, a syndrome characterized by involuntary, irregular muscle movements. The risk of developing these effects and the potential for irreversibility are increased as the dose and length of treatment increase.
- May cause extrapyramidal symptoms (such as uncontrolled tremors, motor restlessness, etc.).
- May increase prolactin levels, interfere with thermoregulation, predisposing patients, particularly the elderly, to heat stroke.

DRUG INTERACTIONS
This drug effects and is metabolized by specific set of liver enzymes. Several other drugs also interfere with or are metabolized by these liver enzymes, and thus may increase or decrease the clearance of haloperidol from the body, potentially increasing the risk of side effects or decreasing effectiveness. Haloperidol may also affect the risk of side effects with other medications. Some-

times, these combinations are not recommended. When these drugs are given in combination with haloperidol, dosage adjustments may be needed. As these are too numerous to list, you should always check with your doctor or pharmacist prior to starting a new medication, herbal, or nonprescription product.

In addition, the administration of this drug with other drugs that affect the QT interval, should be avoided. See the following website for a list of drugs associated with this effect: http://www.torsades.org/medical-pros/drug-lists/drug-lists.htm#

FOOD INTERACTIONS
Unknown

HERBAL INTERACTIONS
Valerian, St. John's wort, kava kava, gotu kola, betel nut, ginkgo biloba

PREGNANCY AND BREAST-FEEDING CAUTIONS
FDA Pregnancy Risk Category C. Excreted in breast milk; not recommended during breast-feeding.

SPECIAL INFORMATION
Sound-alike/look-alike issues: Haloperidol may be confused with Halostein. Haldol may be confused with Halcion, Halenol, Halog, Halotensin, Stadol. Haloperidol safety and efficacy has not been established in children less than three years of age.

May alter cardiac conduction—life threatening arrhythmias have occurred at therapeutic doses of antipsychotic.

HYDRALAZINE
(hye-DRAL-a-zeen)

NEWLY DISCOVERED USES (OFF-LABEL)
Aortic valve regurgitation, congestive heart failure, pulmonary hypertension

ORIGINAL USES (ON-LABEL)
Management of moderate to severe high blood pressure, congestive heart failure, high blood pressure secondary to pregnancy or during delivery, primary pulmonary hypertension

BRAND NAMES
None

DRUG CLASS
Blood pressure medication (vasodilator)

DESCRIPTION
This drug causes widening of blood vessels, which decreases blood pressure.

POTENTIAL SIDE EFFECTS
Increased heart rate, angina pectoris, paradoxical high blood pressure, peripheral swelling in limbs, increased intracranial pressure, anxiety, disorientation, depression, rash, anorexia, nausea, vomiting, diarrhea, difficulty in urination, impotence, rheumatoid arthritis, muscle cramps, weakness, tremor, conjunctivitis, nasal congestion, dyspnea, drug-induced lupus-like syndrome, sweating.

CAUTIONS
- Avoid this drug if you have mitral valve rheumatic heart disease.
- Use with caution if you have severe kidney disease, coronary arterial disease, pulmonary hypertension.
- May cause drug-induced lupus-like syndrome, especially kidney dysfunction, at greater than 200mg/day.

DRUG INTERACTIONS
Propranolol, metoprolol

FOOD INTERACTIONS
Food enhances the absorption of hydralazine. Avoid alcohol.

HERBAL INTERACTIONS
Dong quai, ephedra, yohimbe, ginseng, garlic

PREGNANCY AND BREAST-FEEDING CAUTIONS
FDA Pregnancy Risk Category C. Excreted in breast milk. No reports of adverse effects.

HYDROCHLORTHIAZIDE
(hye-droe-klor-oh-THYE-a-zide)

NEWLY DISCOVERED USES (OFF-LABEL)
Nephrogenic diabetes insipidus

ORIGINAL USES (ON-LABEL)
High blood pressure, swelling due to fluid retention (edema)

BRAND NAMES
Esidrix, Ezide, HydroDIURIL, Microzide

DRUG CLASS
Blood pressure medication (thiazide diuretic)

DESCRIPTION
This drug increases the excretion of sodium and chloride in urine, thereby promoting fluid loss. Also promotes excretion of potassium and bicarbonate, but decreases excretion of calcium and uric acid.

POTENTIAL SIDE EFFECTS
Potassium loss, nausea, vomiting, loss of appetite, upset stomach, diarrhea, electrolyte imbalances, gout, changes in blood sugar or cholesterol levels, sudden drop in blood pressure upon standing from sitting or lying down position (orthostatic hypotension), dizziness, photosensitivity (skin reaction related to sun exposure).

CAUTIONS
- Notify your doctor if you have allergies to sulfonamide drugs, because this drug is not for use in these patients. Inform your doctor if you have kidney disease, liver disease, diabetes, asthma, lupus, gout, or recently had surgery.
- Diabetics may require increased amounts of insulin or oral drugs commonly used to treat diabetes.
- Requires monitoring of electrolytes, and may require potassium supplementation during therapy.
- May cause dizziness and light-headedness when standing suddenly from a sitting or lying down position.

DRUG INTERACTIONS
ACE inhibitors (such as captopril, lisinopril, etc.), arsenic trioxide, calcitriol, calcium carbonate, cholestyramine, colestipol, digoxin, ketanserin, lithium, probenecid. Check with your phar-

macist or doctor before starting new medications, herbal products, or nonprescription drugs.

FOOD INTERACTIONS
Avoid excessive ingestion of natural licorice.

HERBAL INTERACTIONS
Ginkgo, gossypol, ma huang, ephedra

PREGNANCY AND BREAST-FEEDING CAUTIONS
Category C according to manufacturer. Category D according to expert analysis. May suppress lactation. The American Academy of Pediatrics considers this drug compatible with breast-feeding. Consult your doctor.

SPECIAL INFORMATION
This medication can cause dizziness or drowsiness.

HYDROCORTISONE
(Hi-dro-KOR-ti-sone)

Injectable

NEWLY DISCOVERED USES (OFF-LABEL)
Chronic fatigue syndrome, congenital adrenal hyperplasia

ORIGINAL USES (ON-LABEL)
Treatment of various allergic and various inflammatory disorders, including those of the skin, endocrine system, gastrointestinal, lung, rheumatic, blood, management of adrenocortical insufficiency.

BRAND NAME
Cortef

DRUG CLASS
Anti-inflammatory (corticosteroid)

DESCRIPTION
This drug decreases inflammation by suppressing inflammation and also can suppress the immune system.

POTENTIAL SIDE EFFECTS
Insomnia, nervousness, increased appetite, indigestion, increased hair growth, diabetes mellitus, joint aches, cataracts, glaucoma,

headache, impaired wound healing, thin fragile skin, loss of menstruation, sodium and fluid retention, loss of potassium or calcium, abdominal distention, nausea, vomiting.

CAUTIONS
- Chronic therapy may result in irreversible adverse effects and increases the risk of allergic reactions.
- Therapy with this drug may mask the symptoms of infection and increase the susceptibility of infection via immunosuppression.
- Psychiatric symptoms may develop or be aggravated.
- Diabetics may require increased doses of insulin or oral drugs to treat diabetes.
- Notify your doctor if you have bacterial or viral infections, hyperthyroidism, cirrhosis, nonspecific ulcerative colitis, hypertension, osteoporosis, thromboembolic tendencies, congestive heart failure, convulsive disorders, myasthenia gravis, thrombophlebitis, peptic ulcer, diabetes.
- Acute adrenal insufficiency may occur with abrupt withdrawal after long-term therapy or with stress.
- Use the smallest possible dose, and for the shortest possible period of time.

DRUG INTERACTIONS
Aminoglutethimide, barbiturates, cholestyramine, oral contraceptives, ephedrine, estrogens, phenytoin, ketoconazole, rifampin, oral anticoagulants, cyclosporine, isoniazid, diuretics, salicylates, somatrem, theophylline.

FOOD INTERACTIONS
Unknown

HERBAL INTERACTIONS
Unknown

PREGNANCY AND BREAST-FEEDING CAUTIONS
FDA Pregnancy Risk Category D. Excreted in breast milk. Consult your doctor.

SPECIAL INFORMATION
Prolonged therapy may result in suppression of adrenal gland function.

HYDROFLUMETHAZIDE
(hi-dro-FLU-meth-a-zide)

NEWLY DISCOVERED USES (OFF-LABEL)
Nephrogenic diabetes insipidus

ORIGINAL USES (ON-LABEL)
High blood pressure, swelling due to fluid retention (edema)

BRAND NAME
Diucardin

DRUG CLASS
Blood pressure medication (thiazide diuretic)

DESCRIPTION
This drug increases the excretion of sodium and chloride in urine, thereby promoting fluid loss. Also promotes excretion of potassium and bicarbonate, but decreases excretion of calcium and uric acid.

POTENTIAL SIDE EFFECTS
Potassium loss, nausea, vomiting, loss of appetite, upset stomach, diarrhea, electrolyte imbalances, gout, changes in blood sugar or cholesterol levels, sudden drop in blood pressure upon standing from sitting or lying down position (orthostatic hypotension), dizziness, photosensitivity (skin reaction related to sun exposure).

CAUTIONS
- Notify your doctor if you have allergies to sulfonamide drugs. Also inform your doctor if you have kidney disease, liver disease, diabetes, asthma, lupus, gout, or recently had surgery.
- Diabetics may require increased amounts of insulin or oral drugs commonly used to treat diabetes.
- Requires monitoring of electrolytes, and may require potassium supplementation during therapy.
- May cause dizziness and light-headedness when standing suddenly from a sitting or lying down position.

DRUG INTERACTIONS
ACE inhibitors (such as captopril, lisinopril, etc.), arsenic trioxide, calcitriol, calcium carbonate, cholestyramine, colestipol, digoxin, ketanserin, lithium, probenecid. Check with your pharmacist or doctor before starting new medications, herbal products, or nonprescription drugs.

FOOD INTERACTIONS
Avoid excessive ingestion of natural licorice.

HERBAL INTERACTIONS
Ginkgo, gossypol, ma huang, ephedra

PREGNANCY AND BREAST-FEEDING CAUTIONS
Pregnancy Risk Category C/D according to manufacturer listings. Pregnancy Risk Category D according to expert analysis. May suppress lactation. Consult your doctor.

SPECIAL INFORMATION
This medication can cause dizziness or drowsiness.

HYDROXYCHLOROQUINE
(hye-droks-ee-KLOR-oh-kwin)

NEWLY DISCOVERED USES (OFF-LABEL)
Lyme arthritis, psoriatic arthritis

ORIGINAL USES (ON-LABEL)
Suppression and treatment of acute attacks of malaria, treatment of systemic lupus erythematosus (SLE) and rheumatoid arthritis

BRAND NAME
Plaquenil

DRUG CLASS
Antimalarial, antirheumatic

DESCRIPTION
This drug interferes with the metabolism of parasites by binding to and inhibiting DNA and RNA enzymes.

POTENTIAL SIDE EFFECTS
Irritability, nervousness, nightmares, bleaching of hair, nausea, vomiting, diarrhea, abdominal cramps, various blood disorders, skin reactions, skeletal muscle weakness, visual disturbances (changes in focusing, accommodation, blurred vision, corneal edema or deposits, retinal edema).

CAUTIONS
- Not for use if you have retinal or visual field changes.
- Inform your doctor if you have liver disease, G6PD (glucose-6-

phosphate dehydrogenase) deficiency, alcoholism, or are taking other drugs which may damage the liver.
- May aggravate psoriasis or porphyria.
- Requires monitoring for blood disorders if taken for prolonged periods.
- Irreversible retinal damage has occurred with long or high-dose therapy. Progress of damage may continue even after the drug is stopped.
- Discontinue drug if any abnormality in vision occurs or if muscular weakness develops during treatment. Knee and ankle reflexes may be periodically assessed.

DRUG INTERACTIONS
Digoxin

FOOD INTERACTIONS
May be taken with food or milk. Avoid alcohol, may cause gastric irritation.

HERBAL INTERACTIONS
Unknown

PREGNANCY AND BREAST-FEEDING CAUTIONS
FDA Pregnancy Risk Category C. Excreted in breast milk. Consult your doctor.

SPECIAL INFORMATION
Eye exams and blood monitoring should be conducted before therapy is started and periodically during therapy.

HYDROXYUREA
(hye-droks-ee-yoor-EE-a)

NEWLY DISCOVERED USES (OFF-LABEL)
Polycythemia vera, thalassemia, thrombocythemia

ORIGINAL USES (ON-LABEL)
Certain cancers (such as melanoma, squamous cell carcinoma, ovarian cancer, etc.), sickle cell anemia (to reduce the frequency of painful crises and decrease the need for blood transfusions)

BRAND NAMES
Droxia, Hydrea, Mylocel

DRUG CLASS
Antineoplastic, antimetabolite

DESCRIPTION
This drug, used to treat cancers, may work by interfering with the production of DNA in the cancerous cells.

POTENTIAL SIDE EFFECTS
Headache, dizziness, confusion, rashes, mouth ulcers, anorexia, kidney toxicity, fever, chills, malaise, abnormalities in liver function tests, acute lung reactions, fever, chills, sore throat, diarrhea, bruising, various blood disorders, post-irradiation reactions, weight gain, bleeding.

CAUTIONS
- Not for use if you have severe anemia or bone marrow suppression in certain blood disorders (decreased white blood cells, etc.), if you are pregnant or have severe kidney impairment or mouth ulcers.
- The elderly may require reduced dosages as they are more susceptible to side effects.
- Requires monitoring for blood disorders, liver and kidney function prior to and periodically during therapy.

DRUG INTERACTIONS
Zidovudine, zalcitabine, didanosine, fluorouracil, cytarabine, stavudine, live vaccine

FOOD INTERACTIONS
Unknown

HERBAL INTERACTIONS
Unknown

PREGNANCY AND BREAST-FEEDING CAUTIONS
FDA Pregnancy Risk Category D. Excreted in breast milk. Not for use during breast-feeding.

SPECIAL INFORMATION
Capsules could be emptied into water, but they will not dissolve completely.

There is a black box warning for this drug when regarding serious and sometimes life-threatening adverse effects (such as blood disorders, secondary leukemias). Discuss the risks of therapy with doctor prior to initiation of therapy.

IBUPROFEN
(eye-byoo-PROE-fen)

NEWLY DISCOVERED USES (OFF-LABEL)
Kidney stones, lumbar puncture induced headache, membranous nephropathy, periodontitis, renal colic, ureteral stones

ORIGINAL USES (ON-LABEL)
Inflammatory diseases, rheumatoid arthritis, mild to moderate pain or fever or dysmenorrhea

BRAND NAMES
Motrin, Ultraprin

DRUG CLASS
Pain reliever, anti-inflammatory (nonsteroidal anti-inflammatory [NSAID])

DESCRIPTION
Ibuprofen inhibits the production of prostaglandin, a chemical drug in the body responsible for inflammation and pain.

POTENTIAL SIDE EFFECTS
Abdominal cramps, nausea, stomach upset, diarrhea, flatulence, weakness, stomach irritation, blurred vision, ringing in the ears, constipation.

CAUTIONS
- Not for use if you are allergic to aspirin or other NSAIDs.
- Not for use if you have active gastric/duodenal ulcer disease.
- Do not use during third trimester of pregnancy.
- Ask physician about use if you have the following medical problems: high blood pressure, dehydration, decreased kidney or liver function, history of gastric disease.
- Elderly are at higher risk of developing side effects.
- Do not exceed 3200mg/day.

DRUG INTERACTIONS
Aspirin, lithium, methotrexate, digoxin, cyclosporine (nephrotoxicity), diuretics, some anti-hypertensives, and warfarin (bleeding)

FOOD INTERACTIONS
Peak serum concentration decreases with food.

HERBAL INTERACTIONS

Cat's claw, dong quai, evening primrose, feverfew, garlic, ginger, ginkgo, red clover, horse chestnut, green tea, ginseng

PREGNANCY AND BREAST-FEEDING CAUTIONS

FDA Pregnancy Risk Category B (D if in 3rd trimester). Excreted in breast milk. Consult your doctor.

SPECIAL INFORMATION

Stop taking this drug (with doctor's approval) approximately 24 to 48 hours prior to surgical or dental procedures, as it affects the body's ability to form blood clots and may increase bleeding time. In April 2005, the FDA announced the potential addition of a black box warning to the labeling of this class of drugs (NSAIDs), specifically regarding potential serious cardiac events and potentially life-threatening gastric adverse events.

This information refers only to the use of the prescription product.

IMIPENEM-CILASTATIN
(i-mi-PEN-em sye-la-STAT-in)

NEWLY DISCOVERED USES (OFF-LABEL)
Diverticulitis, nocardiosis

ORIGINAL USES (ON-LABEL)
Various bacterial infections of the respiratory tract, urinary tract, intra-abdominal, gynecological, bone and joint, skin structure

BRAND NAME
Primaxin

DRUG CLASS
Antibiotic, (carbapenem)

DESCRIPTION
Impinem kills bacteria by inhibiting the synthesis of bacterial cells. Cilastatin reduces the accumulation of imipenem in the kidney, thus reducing toxicity.

POTENTIAL SIDE EFFECTS
Nausea, diarrhea, vomiting, local reaction, confusion, tremors, seizures, dizziness.

CAUTIONS
- Dosage requires adjustment in impaired kidney function and the elderly.
- Prolonged use may result in superinfection.
- Has been associated with central nervous system (CNS) adverse effects including confusional states and seizures with increased risk of these events in kidney dysfunction. Inform your doctor if you have a history of seizures or allergy to penicillins.
- Not recommended in pediatric CNS infections.
- Contains benzyl alcohol.

DRUG INTERACTIONS
Cyclosporine, ganciclovir, probenecid

FOOD INTERACTIONS
Unknown

HERBAL INTERACTIONS
Unknown

PREGNANCY AND BREAST-FEEDING CAUTIONS
FDA Pregnancy Risk Category C. Excretion in breast milk. Consult your doctor.

SPECIAL INFORMATION
Periodic testing of kidney, liver and blood function tests should be performed. Monitor for signs of allergy during first dose.

IMIPRAMINE
(im-IP-ra-meen)

NEWLY DISCOVERED USES (OFF-LABEL)
Attention deficit hyperactivity disorder (ADHD), bulimia, chronic fatigue syndrome, chronic nausea and vomiting, diabetic neuropathy, irritable bowel syndrome (IBS), migraine prevention, mixed incontinence, multiple sclerosis, nocturia, panic disorder, post-traumatic stress disorder (PTSD), retrograde ejaculation, stress incontinence, urge incontinence

---

ORIGINAL USES (ON-LABEL)
Depression, childhood bedwetting (enuresis)

BRAND NAMES
Tofranil, Tofranil-PM

DRUG CLASS
Tricyclic antidepressant

DESCRIPTION
This drug is used to treat depression and other disorders. It works by increasing the levels of norepinephrine and serotonin in the body by inhibiting uptake of these chemicals by neurons.

POTENTIAL SIDE EFFECTS
Dry mouth, sedation, dizziness, headache, nervousness, skin rash, tremors, hives, nausea, constipation, vision changes, sweating, lowered blood pressure, increased heart rate, decreased sodium levels, suicidal ideation, changes in heart rhythm and conduction, blurred vision, weight gain, sexual dysfunction.

CAUTIONS
- Do not use if you have been taking an MAO inhibitor (such as phenelzine, tranylcypromine, isocarboxazid) within the past 14 days. When used with MAO-Is fever, high blood pressure, increased heart rate, confusion, seizures, and deaths have been reported.
- Not for use immediately after a heart attack.
- Can cause sedation which may impair performance of tasks requiring alertness. Sedative effects may be additive with other drugs that cause similar effects (central nervous system depressants).
- May worsen psychosis or mania in patients with bipolar disease.
- Stop therapy with doctor permission and according to instructions (gradual taper) prior to elective surgery.
- Do not abruptly stop medication; taper gradually.
- Notify your doctor if you have low blood pressure as this drug can cause low blood pressure episodes.
- Use with caution if you have urinary retention, history of cardiac disease, seizure disorders, diabetes, benign prostatic hyperplasia, narrow-angle glaucoma, dry mouth, visual problems, constipation, or a history of bowel obstruction.
- Possibility of suicide attempt may persist until remission occurs.
- Use with caution in hyperthyroid patients or those receiving thyroid supplementation.
- Use with caution if you have liver or kidney dysfunction or are elderly.

DRUG INTERACTIONS

MAO inhibitors (such as phenelzine, tranylcypromine, isocarboxazid), ritonavir, bupropion, amphetamines, anticholinergics, sedatives, chlorpropamide, tolazamide, warfarin, fluoxetine, fluvoxamine, citalopram, escitalopram, paroxetine, sertraline, cimetidine, carbamazepine, haloperidol, smoking, methylphenidate, valproic acid, clonidine, venlafaxine, protease inhibitors, quinidine, diltiazem, verapamil, lithium, phenothiazines may affect the levels of imipramine, drugs which prolong QT interval (see website: http://www.torsades.org/medicalpros/drug-lists/drug-lists.htm#).

This drug is inactivated by a specific set of liver enzymes. Several other drugs interfere with these liver enzymes, and thus, may increase or decrease the clearance of imipramine from the body, potentially increasing the risk of side effects or decreasing effectiveness. When these drugs are given in combination with imipramine, dosage adjustments may be needed. As these are too numerous to list, you should always check with your doctor or pharmacist prior to starting a new medication.

FOOD INTERACTIONS

Alcohol, grapefruit juice

HERBAL INTERACTIONS

Valerian, St. John's wort, SAMe, kava kava

PREGNANCY AND BREAST-FEEDING CAUTIONS

FDA Pregnancy Risk Category D. Excreted in breast milk. Breast-feeding is not recommended during therapy with this drug.

SPECIAL INFORMATION

May take four to six weeks for the full therapeutic effects to be experienced. Avoid prolonged exposure to sunlight, wear sunscreen.

In 2005, the FDA announced new labeling for antidepressants regarding the need to closely monitor for worsening of depression and for the potential of increased suicidal thinking or suicidal behavior during therapy. Although this recommendation applies to all patients (adults, children, adolescents) treated with antidepressants for any indication, this is of particular importance in patients being treated for depression.

IMIQUIMOD
(i-mi-KWI-mod)

NEWLY DISCOVERED USES (OFF-LABEL)
Hemangioma, non-genital warts

ORIGINAL USES (ON-LABEL)
External genital and perianal warts/condyloma acuminata

BRAND NAME
Aldara

DRUG CLASS
Skin and mucous membrane; topical skin product

DESCRIPTION
Imiquimod works by acting on the body's cytokines, regulatory proteins released by cells of the immune system.

POTENTIAL SIDE EFFECTS
Skin redness, itching, erosion, burning, flaking, swelling, scabbing, fungal infection, upper respiratory infection, pain, headache, increased cholesterol levels, diarrhea, upset stomach, eczema, induration, ulceration, vesicles, sinusitis, sore throat.

CAUTIONS
- Not recommended for treatment of urethral, intravaginal, cervical, rectal, or intra-anal human papilloma viral disease.
- Not intended for ophthalmic use.
- Not recommended until genital/perianal tissue is healed from any previous drug or surgical treatment.
- May aggravate inflammatory conditions of the skin.
- May increase sunburn susceptibility.
- Safety and efficacy in immunosuppressed patients have not been established.

DRUG INTERACTIONS
Consult with your doctor before using other topical treatments.

FOOD INTERACTIONS
Unknown

HERBAL INTERACTION
Unknown

PREGNANCY AND BREAST-FEEDING CAUTIONS
FDA Pregnancy Risk Category C. Excretion in breast milk is unknown. Consult your doctor.

SPECIAL INFORMATION

This drug may weaken condoms and vaginal diaphragms. Concurrent use is not recommended. Avoid contact with eyes, for external use only. Do not cover with dressing, bandages, or wrapping. Avoid sexual contact while cream is on the skin. Wash the area six to ten hours after the application of the cream. This drug does not provide cure, new warts may develop during therapy. Uncircumcised males who are treating warts under the foreskin should retract the foreskin and clean area daily.

IMMUNE GLOBULIN IGG
(EH-mune GLOB-ewe-lyn)

NEWLY DISCOVERED USES (OFF-LABEL)
Guillain-Barre syndrome, multiple sclerosis, outer retinal necrosis

ORIGINAL USES (ON-LABEL)
Prevention or modification of hepatitis A, measles, varicella (chicken pox), rubella, immunoglobulin deficiency

BRAND NAME
BayGam

DRUG CLASS
Immune globulin

DESCRIPTION
Provides passive immunity by inactivating various bacteria, viruses, and fungi. "Passive immunity" is immunity acquired by the transfer of antibodies from another individual, as through injection or placental transfer to a fetus.

POTENTIAL SIDE EFFECTS
Flushing, angioedema (tongue, lip, and/or throat swelling), chills, lethargy, fever, hives, skin redness, nausea, vomiting, pain, tenderness and muscle stiffness at injection site, muscle aches, allergic reactions.

CAUTIONS
- Inform your doctor if you have an allergy to the preservative thimerosal or any component of the formulation or if you have a deficiency of immunoglobulin A.

- Periodic monitoring of kidney function is recommended.
- Intramuscular injections in patients are not recommended for patients with certain blood disorders (such as thrombocytopenia or clotting disorders).
- This product is made from human sources (such as plasma and plasma sources) and carries the risk of infection, though minimized through procedures during production.
- Skin testing should not be performed because irritation can occur, leading to false positives.
- Immune globulin should not be used to control outbreaks of measles.
- Not for intravenous administration.

DRUG INTERACTIONS
Do not take this drug within three months of live virus vaccines.

FOOD INTERACTIONS
Unknown

HERBAL INTERACTIONS
Unknown

PREGNANCY AND BREAST-FEEDING CAUTIONS
FDA Pregnancy Risk Category C. Excretion in breast milk is not known. Not recommended in breast-feeding.

SPECIAL INFORMATION
Report to your doctor if any of the following occur: sudden weight gain, decrease urine output, fluid retention, edema, and/or shortness of breath. Discuss benefits and risks of therapy.

IMMUNE GLOBULIN IVIG
(EH-mune GLOB-ewe-lyn)

NEWLY DISCOVERED USES (OFF-LABEL)
Bullous pemphigoid, complicated mononucleosis/Epstein-Barr, dermatomyositis/polymyositis, tonsillitis and peritonsillar abscess (therapy-resistant)

ORIGINAL USES (ON-LABEL)
Immunoglobulin deficiency, certain blood disorders (idiopathic thrombocytopenic purpura), certain leukemias, bone marrow transplantation, HIV infection in children, Kawasaki disease

BRAND NAMES
Octagam, Gamimune N, Gamunex, Polygam S/D, Venoglobulin S

DRUG CLASS
Immune globulin

DESCRIPTION
This drug provides passive immunity by inactivating various bacteria, viruses, and fungi. "Passive immunity" is immunity acquired by the transfer of antibodies from another individual, as through injection or placental transfer to a fetus.

POTENTIAL SIDE EFFECTS
Flushing, angioedema (tongue, lip, and/or throat swelling), chills, lethargy, fever, hives, skin redness, nausea, vomiting, pain, tenderness and muscle stiffness at injection site, muscle aches, allergic reactions.

CAUTIONS
- Periodic monitoring of kidney function is recommended as this drug may cause kidney toxicity.
- Rare cases of aseptic meningitis have been reported after therapy with this drug.
- This product is made from human sources (such as plasma and plasma sources) and carry the risk of infection, though minimized through procedures during production.
- Skin testing should not be performed because irritation can occur, leading to false positives.

DRUG INTERACTIONS
Do not administer within three months of live virus vaccines.

FOOD INTERACTIONS
Unknown

HERBAL INTERACTIONS
Unknown

PREGNANCY AND BREAST-FEEDING CAUTIONS
FDA Pregnancy Risk Category C. Excretion in breast milk is not known. Not recommended during breast-feeding.

SPECIAL INFORMATION
Report to your doctor if any of the following occur: sudden weight gain, decrease urine output, fluid retention, edema, and/or shortness of breath. Discuss benefits and risks of therapy.

INDAPAMIDE
(in-DAP-ah-mide)

NEWLY DISCOVERED USES (OFF-LABEL)

Central diabetes insipidus, hypercalciuria, nephrogenic diabetes insipidus

ORIGINAL USES (ON-LABEL)

High blood pressure, swelling (edema) due to fluid retention in congestive heart failure

BRAND NAME

Lozol

DRUG CLASS

Blood pressure medication (thiazide diuretic)

DESCRIPTION

This drug increases the excretion of sodium and chloride in urine, thereby promoting fluid loss. Also promotes excretion of potassium and bicarbonate, but decreases excretion of calcium and uric acid.

POTENTIAL SIDE EFFECTS

Potassium loss, nausea, vomiting, loss of appetite, upset stomach, diarrhea, electrolyte imbalances, gout, changes in blood sugar or cholesterol levels, sudden drop in blood pressure upon standing from sitting or lying down position (orthostatic hypotension), dizziness, photosensitivity (skin reaction related to sun exposure).

CAUTIONS

- Notify your doctor if you have allergies to sulfonamide drugs. Inform your doctor if you have kidney disease, liver disease, diabetes, asthma, lupus, gout, or recently had surgery.
- Diabetics may require increased amounts of insulin or oral drugs commonly used to treat diabetes.
- Requires monitoring of electrolytes, and may require potassium supplementation during therapy.
- May cause dizziness and light-headedness when standing suddenly from a sitting or lying down position.

DRUG INTERACTIONS

ACE inhibitors (such as captopril, lisinopril, etc.), arsenic trioxide, calcitriol, calcium carbonate, cholestyramine, colestipol, digoxin, ketanserin, lithium, probenecid. Check with your phar-

macist or doctor before starting new medications, herbal products, or nonprescription drugs.

FOOD INTERACTIONS
Avoid excessive ingestion of natural licorice

HERBAL INTERACTIONS
Ginkgo, gossypol, ma huang, ephedra

PREGNANCY AND BREAST-FEEDING CAUTIONS
Pregnancy Risk Category B according to manufacturer. Pregnancy Risk Category D according to expert analysis. Excretion in breast milk unknown. Consult your doctor.

INDOMETHACIN
(in-doe-METH-a-sin)

NEWLY DISCOVERED USES (OFF-LABEL)

Acute cholecystitis, cluster headache treatment, intraventricular hemorrhage, nephrogenic diabetes insipidus, pericarditis, preterm labor, sunburn

ORIGINAL USES (ON-LABEL)
Management of inflammatory diseases and rheumatoid disorders, moderate pain, acute gouty arthritis, acute bursitis/tendonitis, osteoarthritis, ankylosing spondylitis, intravenous form used as alternative to surgery for closure of patent ductus arteriosus in neonates

BRAND NAMES
Indocin, Indocin I.V., Indocin SR

DRUG CLASS
Analgesic, nonsteroidal anti-inflammatory (NSAID), anti-gout

DESCRIPTION
This drug inhibits prostaglandin production, a substance responsible for the development of inflammation and pain.

POTENTIAL SIDE EFFECTS
Headache, dizziness, fatigue, vertigo, depression, nausea, esophageal pain, abdominal pain, heartburn, inhibition of blood clotting, ringing in the ears.

CAUTIONS

- Do not use if patient has the following: allergy to indomethacin or NSAIDs, asthma, hives, gastric bleeding, ulcer disease, impaired kidney function, thrombocytopenia, pregnant in third trimester.
- Use caution if you have congestive heart failure, high blood pressure, dehydration, decreased kidney function, history of gastric disease, receiving anticoagulants or corticosteroids.
- When given with other drugs that can cause ulcers, may increase risk of ulcers (examples: other NSAIDs, steroids, etc.).
- May interfere with the effectiveness of drugs used for managing blood pressure.

DRUG INTERACTIONS

Cyclosporine, digoxin, lithium, methotrexate, ACE inhibitors (captopril, lisinopril, ramipril), probenecid, potassium-sparing diuretics (aldactone, spironolactone)

FOOD INTERACTIONS

Take with food to minimize stomach upset.

HERBAL INTERACTIONS

Cat's claw, dong quai, evening primrose, feverfew, garlic, ginger, ginkgo, red clover, horse chestnut, green tea, ginseng

PREGNANCY AND BREAST-FEEDING CAUTIONS

FDA Pregnancy Risk Category B (FDA Pregnancy Category Risk D if in third trimester). Excreted in breast milk; use with caution.

SPECIAL INFORMATION

In April 2005, the FDA issued a boxed warning regarding the potential for serious adverse cardiac events and serious, gastric adverse events associated with the use of this class of drugs. The FDA also issued a drug safety alert and had requested manufacturers to revise product labeling and provide medication guides regarding cardiovascular and gastrointestinal risks.

INFLIXIMAB
(in-FLIKS-e-mab)

NEWLY DISCOVERED USES (OFF-LABEL)

Juvenile rheumatoid arthritis, Kawasaki disease, psoriasis, sarcoidosis

ORIGINAL USES (ON-LABEL)
Ankylosing spondylitis, moderate to severe or fistulizing Crohn's disease, rheumatoid arthritis

BRAND NAME
Remicade

DRUG CLASS
Disease modifying antirheumatic (monoclonal antibody)

DESCRIPTION
This drug affects the inflamed area of the intestine and joints of patients with rheumatoid arthritis.

POTENTIAL SIDE EFFECTS
Headache, fatigue, insomnia, depression, rash, nausea, diarrhea, abdominal pain, urinary tract infection, infusion reactions, joint pain, back pain, upper respiratory infection, cough, sinusitis, sore throat, development of antinuclear antibodies, infection, development of antibodies to double-stranded DNA, high blood pressure, pain, fatigue, fever, itching, stomach upset, bronchitis, shortness of breath, yeast infection.

CAUTIONS
- Hypersensitivity to murine proteins or any component of the formulation.
- Reduced doses required in moderate or severe congestive heart failure.
- Serious infections have been reported. Caution should be exercised when considering the use of infliximab if you have a chronic infection or history of recurrent infection.
- If serious infection or sepsis develops, infliximab should be discontinued.
- Patients should be evaluated for latent tuberculosis infection with a tuberculin skin test prior to the initiation of therapy.
- Severe liver reactions have been reported during treatment.
- Notify your doctor if you have a history of blood abnormalities.
- Autoimmune antibodies and a lupus-like syndrome have been reported.

DRUG INTERACTIONS
Anakinra

FOOD INTERACTIONS
Unknown

HERBAL INTERACTIONS
Unknown

PREGNANCY AND BREAST-FEEDING CAUTIONS
FDA Pregnancy Risk Category C. Excretion into breast milk unknown. Consult your doctor.

SPECIAL INFORMATION
This drug has a black box warning for the potential development of tuberculosis, invasive fungal infections, and other infections during the therapy with this drug. You should be evaluated for latent tuberculosis infection with a tuberculin skin test. If latent tuberculosis infection is present, it should be treated prior to when therapy was initiated.

INTERFERON ALFA-2A
(in-ter-FEER-on AL-fa too-aye)

NEWLY DISCOVERED USES (OFF-LABEL)
Hemangioma in children, liver cirrhosis, liver fibrosis

ORIGINAL USES (ON-LABEL)
Certain types of leukemia, AIDS-related Kaposi's sarcoma, chronic hepatitis C

BRAND NAME
Roferon-A

DRUG CLASS
Immune response modulator (interferon)

DESCRIPTION
This drug works by acting against the reproduction of tumor cells and modulating the immune response in the body.

POTENTIAL SIDE EFFECTS
The incidence of reactions may vary depending upon the condition that the drug is being used to treat. The following side effects have been reported with use: headache, depression, irritability, insomnia, dizziness, numbness, increased triglyceride levels, confusion, anxiety, difficulty concentrating, changes in taste and/or smell, injection site reaction, hair loss, rash, dry skin, itching, bruising, nausea, vomiting, diarrhea, anorexia, abdominal pain,

flatulence, liver pain, bleeding of the gums, eye irritation, menstrual irregularities, flu-like syndrome, fatigue, muscle aches, fever, chills, sweating, leg cramps, malaise, rash, throat irritation, sleep disturbances, weight loss, chest pain, runny nose, involuntary movements, cough, changes in heart rhythm.

CAUTIONS

- Not for use if you have autoimmune hepatitis, visceral AIDS-related Kaposi's, or liver decomposition.
- Notify your doctor if you are depressed or have a history of depression, seizure disorders, brain tumor or cancer involving the brain, heart disease, psoriasis, sarcoidosis, kidney or liver impairment, diabetes, thyroid disease, heart problems, autoimmune disease, had an organ transplant, taking drugs which affect the immune system.
- May cause severe psychiatric adverse events, including severe depression or suicidal ideation.
- Treatment should be discontinued in patients with worsening or persistently severe signs/symptoms of autoimmune problems, infections, heart problems, or neuropsychiatric disorders.
- You should receive an eye exam before initiating therapy. If you have underlying eye problems these should be monitored closely during therapy.
- Requires close monitoring and blood testing for effectiveness and toxicity.
- Due to differences in dosage, patients should not change brands of interferons.
- Contains benzyl alcohol. Notify your doctor if you have had reactions to this drug. Benzyl alcohol has been associated with serious toxicity when used in infants.

DRUG INTERACTIONS

Theophylline, ACE inhibitors, clozapine, warfarin, zidovudine, prednisone, erythropoietin, melphalan, interleukin-2. There are numerous drugs that may have the potential to interact with interferons. Consult your doctor or pharmacist prior to starting any new medication, herbal product, or nonprescription drug.

FOOD INTERACTIONS

Unknown

HERBAL INTERACTIONS

Unknown

PREGNANCY AND BREAST-FEEDING CAUTIONS

FDA Pregnancy Risk Category C. Excreted in breast milk. Not for use while breast-feeding.

SPECIAL INFORMATION

This drug has a black box warning that emphasizes the potential for significant reactions that may occur, including psychiatric, autoimmune, cardiac and infectious disorders. Interferons may cause or aggravate fatal or life threatening disorders of this nature. Completely read patient information brochure.

INTERFERON ALFA-2B
(in-ter-FEER-on AL-fa-too-bee)

NEWLY DISCOVERED USES (OFF-LABEL)

Keloids, Liver cirrhosis, liver fibrosis, myelofibrosis, Peyronie's disease, polyarteritis nodosa, polycythemia vera, thrombocythemia

ORIGINAL USES (ON-LABEL)

Chronic hepatitis B, Condyloma acuminate, hairy cell leukemia, AIDS-related Kaposi's sarcoma, chronic hepatitis C, malignant melanoma, follicular non-Hodgkin's lymphoma

BRAND NAME

Intron A

DRUG CLASS

Immune response modulator (interferon)

DESCRIPTION

This drug works by acting against the reproduction of tumor cells and modulating the immune response in the body.

POTENTIAL SIDE EFFECTS

Flu-like symptoms, chest pain, fever, depression, fatigue, headache, rash, hair loss, decreased calcium levels, increased blood glucose, loss of menstruation, liver toxicity, loss of smell, anorexia, nausea, vomiting, diarrhea, various blood disorders, injection site reaction, increased triglyceride levels, weakness, muscle and joint aches, rigors, cough, high blood pressure, sore throat, shortness of breath, anxiety, skin reactions, decreased libido, loose stools, nasal congestion, confusion, depression, dizziness, rash, chills, fatigue, fever, flu-like syndrome, abdominal pain, anorexia, changes in taste sensation, shortness of breath.

CAUTIONS

- Not for use if you have autoimmune hepatitis, visceral AIDS-related Kaposi's, and liver decomposition.
- Notify your doctor if you are depressed or have a history of depression, seizure disorders, brain tumor or cancer involving the brain, heart disease, psoriasis, sarcoidosis, kidney or liver impairment, diabetes, thyroid disease, heart problems, autoimmune disease, lung disorders, had an organ transplant, taking drugs which affect the immune system.
- May cause severe psychiatric adverse events, including severe depression or suicidal ideation.
- You should receive an eye exam before initiating therapy. If you have underlying eye problems these should be monitored closely during therapy.
- Treatment should be discontinued if you have worsening or persistently severe signs/symptoms of autoimmune problems, infections, heart problems, or neuropsychiatric disorders.
- Contains benzyl alcohol. Notify your doctor if you have had reactions to this drug. Benzyl alcohol has been associated with serious toxicity when used in infants.
- Requires close monitoring and blood testing for effectiveness and toxicity.
- Due to differences in dosage, patients should not change brands of interferons.

DRUG INTERACTIONS

Theophylline, zidovudine. There are numerous drugs that may have the potential to interact with interferons. Consult your doctor or pharmacist prior to starting any new medication, herbal product, or nonprescription drug.

FOOD INTERACTIONS

Unknown

HERBAL INTERACTIONS

Unknown

PREGNANCY AND BREAST-FEEDING CAUTIONS

FDA Pregnancy Risk Category C. Excreted in breast milk. Do not use this drug while breast-feeding.

SPECIAL INFORMATION

This drug has a black box warning that emphasizes the potential for significant reactions that may occur, including psychiatric, autoimmune, cardiac and infectious disorders. Interferons may cause or aggravate fatal or life threatening disorders of this nature. Completely read patient information brochure.

IPRATROPIUM
(i-pra-TROE-pee-um)

NEWLY DISCOVERED USES (OFF-LABEL)

Acute asthma, bronchopulmonary dysplasia, chronic asthma, cystic fibrosis, exercise-induced bronchospasm, pulmonary edema

ORIGINAL USES (ON-LABEL)

Used in bronchospasm associated with chronic obstructive lung disease, bronchitis, and emphysema. Symptomatic relief of nasal symptoms associated with the common cold and allergies.

BRAND NAMES

Atrovent, Atrovent HFA

DRUG CLASS

Anticholinergic (bronchodilator)

DESCRIPTION

This drug blocks the action of a certain neurotransmitter at sites in the body's bronchial smooth muscle, causing relaxation of the lung airways.

POTENTIAL SIDE EFFECTS

Bronchitis, upper respiratory tract infection, dizziness, nausea, dry mouth, urinary tract infection, nasal congestion, shortness of breath, bronchospasm, sore throat, inflammation of the nasal passages, nose bleed, nasal dryness.

CAUTIONS

- Notify your doctor if you are allergic to soy lecithin or related food products such as soybean and peanut (for use of inhalation aerosol).
- Not indicated for the initial treatment of acute episodes of bronchospasm.

- Notify your doctor if you have myasthenia gravis, narrow-angle glaucoma, benign prostatic hyperplasia (BPH), or bladder neck obstruction.
- Immediately report any of the following symptoms to your doctor: hives, swollen tongue, rash, throat swelling.

DRUG INTERACTIONS
Increased toxicity with anticholinergics or drugs with anticholinergic properties. Consult with doctor or pharmacist regarding these drugs.

FOOD INTERACTIONS
Unknown

HERBAL INTERACTIONS
Unknown

PREGNANCY AND BREAST-FEEDING CAUTIONS
FDA Pregnancy Risk Category B. Excretion in breast milk is unknown. Consult with your doctor.

SPECIAL INFORMATION
Do not spray aerosol into eyes. If this occurs it may result in blurred vision, worsening or narrow-angle glaucoma, or eye pain. Shake well before each use and rinse mouth after each use to decrease the risk of dry mouth. To prime the nasal spray pump, press down seven times. If used regularly, no further priming is necessary. If not used for at least 24 hours, the pump will require two primes. If not used for at least seven days, the pump will again require seven primes.

ISONIAZID
(eye-soe-NYE-a-zid)

NEWLY DISCOVERED USES (OFF-LABEL)
Multiple sclerosis

ORIGINAL USES (ON-LABEL)
Treatment of susceptible and latent tuberculosis infections.

BRAND NAME
Nydrazid

DRUG CLASS
Antitubercular

DESCRIPTION

This drug acts against bacteria. It may work by the inhibition of mycolic acid production, resulting in disruption of the bacterial cell wall.

POTENTIAL SIDE EFFECTS

Loss of appetite, nausea, vomiting, stomach pain, increases in liver function tests, weakness, peripheral nerve pain, dizziness, slurred speech, lethargy, progressive liver damage, hyperreflexia.

CAUTIONS

- Notify your doctor if you have acute liver disease or previous history of liver damage during isoniazid therapy.
- Use caution if you have kidney impairment and chronic liver disease.
- Severe and sometimes fatal liver toxicity may occur or develop even after many months of treatment.
- Immediately report any of the following symptoms to your doctor, such as fatigue, weakness, malaise, anorexia, nausea, or vomiting.
- Some patients may require concurrent pyridoxine therapy.
- Periodic eye exams are recommended.
- Dosage adjustment is necessary if you have liver impairment.

DRUG INTERACTIONS

Rifampin, acetaminophen, carbamazepine, chlorzoxazone, disulfiram, enflurane, phenytoin, ketoconazole, theophylline. This drug has the potential to interact with several drugs that are activated or cleared by the liver. As these are too numerous to list, you should always check with your doctor or pharmacist prior to starting a new medication, herbal, or nonprescription product.

FOOD INTERACTIONS

Avoid alcohol. May decrease folic acid absorption. Avoid foods containing tyramine (such as certain fish, tuna, etc.).

HERBAL INTERACTIONS

Unknown

PREGNANCY AND BREAST-FEEDING CAUTIONS

FDA Pregnancy Risk Category C. Excreted into the breast milk and is probably compatible.

SPECIAL INFORMATION

Should be taken one hour before or two hours after meals on an empty stomach.

This drug has a black box warning regarding the potential for severe and sometimes fatal hepatitis that may occur during and many months after treatment. Risk is related to age and increases with daily alcohol consumption. Monitoring of changes in liver function may be required at regular intervals. Report any signs of liver problems to your doctor immediately (such as dark urine, abdominal pain, yellowing discoloration of the skin and eyes, etc.).

ISOPROTERENOL
(eye-soe-proe-TER-e-nole)

NEWLY DISCOVERED USES (OFF-LABEL)
Pulmonary embolism

ORIGINAL USES (ON-LABEL)
Certain types of irregular heart rhythms (ventricular arrhythmia, bradyarrhythmias), used to control heart rate until pacemaker insertion

BRAND NAME
Isuprel

DRUG CLASS
Adrenergic agonist, bronchodilator, sympathomimetic

DESCRIPTION
This drug triggers relaxation of bronchial, gastrointestinal, and uterus smooth muscle. It also increases heart rate and contractibility and allows for relaxation of certain blood vessels.

POTENTIAL SIDE EFFECTS
Decreased heart rate, high blood pressure, low blood pressure, chest palpitation, headache, nervousness, restlessness, serum glucose increased, serum potassium decreased, nausea, vomiting, shortness of breath.

CAUTIONS
- Do not use if you are allergic to sulfites.
- Avoid if you have any of the following: angina, pre-existing cardiac heart beat irregularities, increased heart rate, or heart rhythm disorders caused by cardiac glycoside intoxication.

- Use caution if you are elderly, diabetic, or have kidney or cardiovascular disease, seizure disorders, or excessive levels of thyroid.

DRUG INTERACTIONS
Use with other drugs that increase blood pressure will increase risk of high blood pressures and cause headaches. Use with general anesthetics may cause irregular heartbeat.

FOOD INTERACTIONS
Unknown

HERBAL INTERACTIONS
Ephedra, yohimbe

PREGNANCY AND BREAST-FEEDING CAUTIONS
FDA Pregnancy Risk Category C. No human data available. Animal data indicate moderate risk. Drug excretion in breast milk unknown.

SPECIAL INFORMATION
Excessive or prolonged use may result in decreased effectiveness.

ISOSORBIDE DINITRATE
(eye-soe-SOR-bide dye-NYE-trate)

NEWLY DISCOVERED USES (OFF-LABEL)
Congestive heart failure

ORIGINAL USES (ON-LABEL)
Treatment and prevention of angina pectoris

BRAND NAMES
Dilatrate-SR, Isochron, Isordil, Sorbitrate

DRUG CLASS
Antianginal (nitrate)

DESCRIPTION
This drug reduces cardiac oxygen demand by decreasing cardiac pressure in the left ventricle (heart chamber) and decreasing resistance in the blood vessels. Relaxes coronary arteries and improves blood flow to regions that are poorly oxygenated.

POTENTIAL SIDE EFFECTS

Low blood pressure, cardiovascular collapse, increased heart rate, shock, flushing, peripheral swelling, headache, lightheadedness, dizziness, restlessness, nausea, vomiting, bowel incontinence, dry mouth, urinary incontinence, weakness, blurred vision, cold sweat.

CAUTION

- Notify your doctor if you have an allergy to any nitrates, or are concurrently using sildenafil, tadalafil, or vardenafil.
- Inform your doctor if you have angle-closure glaucoma, liver or kidney problems, cardiac problems, or recent head trauma or cerebral hemorrhage, severe anemia.
- May cause lowered blood pressure upon standing from a sitting or lying down position.
- Tolerance to effects of the drug may develop.

DRUG INTERACTIONS

Do not administer sildenafil, tadalafil, or vardenafil within 24 hours of a nitrate preparation. Calcium channel blockers (such as verapamil, nifedipine, diltiazem, etc.), dihydroergotamine.

FOOD INTERACTIONS

Unknown

HERBAL INTERACTIONS

Unknown

PREGNANCY AND BREAST-FEEDING CAUTIONS

FDA Pregnancy Risk Category C. Excretion in breast milk is unknown. Consult your doctor.

SPECIAL INFORMATION

Abrupt withdrawal may result in angina. Tolerance may develop and your doctor may need to adjust dose or change drug. Do not crush or chew sublingual tablets. Do not crush chewable tablets before taking. Dissolve sublingual tablets under the tongue, do not swallow.

ISOSORBIDE MONONITRATE
(eye-soe-SOR-bide mon-oh-NYE-trate)

NEWLY DISCOVERED USES (OFF-LABEL)
Congestive heart failure

ORIGINAL USES (ON-LABEL)
For treatment and prevention of angina pectoris

BRAND NAMES
Imdur, ISMO, Monoket

DRUG CLASS
Antianginal (nitrate)

DESCRIPTION
This drug reduces cardiac oxygen demand by decreasing cardiac pressure in the left ventricle (heart chamber) and decreasing resistance in the blood vessels. Relaxes coronary arteries and improves blood flow to regions that are poorly oxygenated.

POTENTIAL SIDE EFFECTS
Low blood pressure, cardiovascular collapse, increased heart rate, shock, flushing, peripheral swelling, headache, lightheadedness, dizziness, restlessness, nausea, vomiting, bowel incontinence, dry mouth, urinary incontinence, weakness, blurred vision, cold sweat.

CAUTIONS
- Notify your doctor if you have an allergy to any nitrates, or are concurrently using sildenafil, tadalafil, or vardenafil.
- Inform your doctor if you have angle-closure glaucoma, liver or kidney problems, cardiac problems, or recent head trauma or cerebral hemorrhage, severe anemia.
- May cause lowered blood pressure upon standing from a sitting or lying down position.
- Tolerance to effects of the drug may develop.

DRUG INTERACTIONS
Do not administer sildenafil, tadalafil, or vardenafil within 24 hours of a nitrate preparation. Calcium channel blockers (such as verapamil, nifedipine, diltiazem, etc.), dihydroergotamine.

FOOD INTERACTIONS
Unknown

HERBAL INTERACTIONS
Unknown

PREGNANCY AND BREAST-FEEDING CAUTIONS
FDA Pregnancy Risk Category C. Excretion in breast milk is unknown. Consult your doctor.

SPECIAL INFORMATION
Abrupt withdrawal may result in angina. Tolerance may develop and your doctor may need to adjust dose or change drug. Do not crush or chew extended release tablets. Not for sublingual use.

ISOTRETINOIN
(eye-soe-TRET-i-noyn)

NEWLY DISCOVERED USES (OFF-LABEL)
Leukoplakia, oral lichen planus, prevention of recurrence of oral cancer

ORIGINAL USES (ON-LABEL)
Severe acne unresponsive to conventional therapy

BRAND NAMES
Accutane, Claravis

DRUG CLASS
Acne product (vitamin A derivative)

DESCRIPTION
This drug reduces the size of fatty glands and reduces fat production. It also regulates cell proliferation and differentiation.

POTENTIAL SIDE EFFECTS
Increased heart rate, headache, visual disturbances, malaise, nervousness, dry lips, dry skin, hair abnormalities, skin peeling, increased susceptibility to sunburn, itching, nausea, fatigue, suicidal ideation.

CAUTIONS
- Notify your doctor if you are pregnant, are allergic to parabens, vitamin A, or other retinoids, have diabetes mellitus, increased triglyceride levels, or pancreatitis.
- Not for use during pregnancy. Requires two negative pregnancy tests; effective contraceptive used at least one month prior to

starting therapy, during therapy, and for at least one month after discontinuing therapy, and prescriptions can only be written for one month supply at a time.

- Not to be used if you are a woman in childbearing age unless complying with effective contraceptive methods, and patients must commit to using two forms of birth control.
- Patients must be enrolled in the manufacturer sponsored and FDA approved monitoring programs.
- Depression, psychosis, aggressive or violent behavior, and rarely suicidal thoughts and actions have been reported during use.

DRUG INTERACTIONS
Corticosteroids, phenytoin, tetracycline, carbamazepine

FOOD INTERACTIONS
Take with food.

HERBAL INTERACTIONS
Dong quai, St. John's wort, and additional vitamin A supplements

PREGNANCY AND BREAST-FEEDING CAUTIONS
FDA Pregnancy Risk Category X. Excretion in breast milk is unknown. Use during breast-feeding is not recommended.

SPECIAL INFORMATION
This drug has a black box warning describing the known teratogenic effects when taken during pregnancy. In addition, it describes the restricted dispensing program that requires signed patient consent and counseling along with negative pregnancy tests prior to the initiation of therapy. Additional information is also provided regarding the risk of suicidal ideation. Read the complete patient brochure and discuss these risks with your doctor.

In 2005, the FDA notified health professionals and patients regarding the approval of a strengthened isotretinoin management program called iPledge, designed to minimize pregnancy exposures.

ISOXSUPRINE
(eye-SOKS-syoo-preen)

NEWLY DISCOVERED USES (OFF-LABEL)
Dysmenorrhea, premature labor

ORIGINAL USES (ON-LABEL)
Peripheral vascular diseases, such as arteriosclerosis obliterans and Raynaud's disease

BRAND NAME
Vasodilan

DRUG CLASS
Vasodilator

DESCRIPTION
This drug relaxes blood vessels primarily in the skeletal muscle to improve blood flow to these areas.

POTENTIAL SIDE EFFECTS
Low blood pressure, increased heart rate, chest pain, nausea, vomiting, abdominal pain, dizziness, weakness, severe rash.

CAUTIONS
- Not for use if you have arterial bleeding or heart disease, if you are immediately postpartum, premature labor with infection, or with premature detachment of placenta.
- Notify your doctor if you have/had bleeding disorders, chest pain, glaucoma, or stroke.
- Discontinue use if rash appears.

DRUG INTERACTIONS
Unknown

FOOD INTERACTIONS
Unknown

HERBAL INTERACTIONS
Unknown

PREGNANCY AND BREAST-FEEDING CAUTIONS
FDA Pregnancy Risk Category C. Excreted in breast milk. Consult your doctor.

ISRADIPINE
(iz-RA-di-peen)

NEWLY DISCOVERED USES (OFF-LABEL)
Prevention of cyclosporine-induced nephrotoxicity

ORIGINAL USES (ON-LABEL)
High blood pressure

BRAND NAMES
Dynacirc, Dynacirc CR

DRUG CLASS
Cardiac (calcium channel blocker)

DESCRIPTION
This drug inhibits calcium ions from entering the "slow channels" vascular smooth muscle and heart tissue. This produces a relaxation of coronary vessels, which reduces blood pressure.

POTENTIAL SIDE EFFECTS
Headache, swelling, sensation of changes in heart rate, flushing, increased heart rate, dizziness, fatigue, rash, nausea, abdominal discomfort, diarrhea, urinary frequency, shortness of breath.

CAUTIONS
- Notify your doctor if you have had an allergic reaction to a drug in this class.
- Inform your doctor if you have low blood pressure, severe left ventricular dysfunction or other types of heart problems, liver or kidney dysfunction.
- Abrupt withdrawal may cause increased duration and frequency of chest pain.
- The elderly may be at greater risk of experiencing low blood pressure and constipation associated with this therapy.

DRUG INTERACTIONS
Amiodarone, itraconazole, barbiturates, beta-blockers, calcium salts, cimetidine, ranitidine, rifampin, lovastatin.

This drug is metabolized by and affects a specific set of liver enzymes. Several other drugs interfere with these liver enzymes, and thus may increase or decrease the clearance of isradipine from the body, potentially increasing the risk of side effects or decreasing effectiveness. When these drugs are given in combination with isradipine, dosage adjustments may be needed. As these are too numerous to list, you should always check with your doctor or pharmacist prior to starting a new medication, herbal, or non-prescription product.

FOOD INTERACTIONS
Avoid grapefruit juice.

HERBAL INTERACTIONS
St. John's wort, dong quai, ephedra, yohimbe, ginseng, and garlic

PREGNANCY AND BREAST-FEEDING CAUTIONS
FDA Pregnancy Risk Category C. Excreted in breast milk. Consult your doctor.

SPECIAL INFORMATION
Report any dizziness, shortness of breath, palpitation, or edema.

ITRACONAZOLE
(i-tra-KOE-na-zole)

NEWLY DISCOVERED USES (OFF-LABEL)

Blepharitis, endophthalmitis, mucocutaneous candidiasis in AIDS

ORIGINAL USES (ON-LABEL)
Treatment of various fungal and yeast infections

BRAND NAME
Sporanox

DRUG CLASS
Antifungal

DESCRIPTION
This drug interferes with the production of fungal cell membrane and inhibits cell membrane formation.

POTENTIAL SIDE EFFECTS
Headache, nausea, diarrhea, vomiting, abdominal pain, rash, taste perversion, liver toxicity.

CAUTIONS
- Notify your doctor if you have heart failure or other cardiac conditions, as this risk for serious side effects is increased.

- Serious liver toxicity has rarely occurred; not recommended for patients with active liver disease or elevated liver enzymes tests.
- Capsules and oral solution should not be used interchangeably. There are differences in absorption characteristics between the two formulations.
- Dosage requires adjustment in impaired kidney or liver function. Requires monitoring of liver function and potassium levels during long-term therapy.
- Notify your doctor if numbness or tingling occurs.

DRUG INTERACTIONS

This drug has strong inhibitory action on a specific set of liver enzymes (cytochrome P450 enzymes 3A4). Several other drugs are metabolized (cleared from the body or activated) by these liver enzymes, and thus their levels may be increased or decreased when administered with itraconazole. In some cases, these drugs should not be given during itraconazole therapy (such as cisapride); in other cases, when these drugs are given in combination, dosage adjustments may be needed. As these are too numerous to list, you should always check with your doctor or pharmacist prior to starting a new medication, herbal, or nonprescription product.

This drug requires a certain level of stomach acidity to be absorbed. Thus, when stomach acidity is decreased by the administration of other drugs (such as antacids, drugs used to treat stomach ulcers by reducing gastric acidity, such as ranitidine, famotidine, cimetidine, omeprazole, pantoprazole, etc.), this decreases the absorption of itraconazole. Take antacids one hour before or two hours after itraconazole.

FOOD INTERACTIONS

Avoid grapefruit juice, orange juice. Take oral capsules with food, and take the solution without food.

HERBAL INTERACTIONS

St. John's wort

PREGNANCY AND BREAST-FEEDING CAUTIONS

FDA Pregnancy Risk Category C. Excreted in breast milk. Breast-feeding is not recommended during therapy.

SPECIAL CONSIDERATIONS

This drug has a black box warning that describes the risks of serious heart effects when administered with certain interacting drugs. In addition, the black box warning cites problems in patients with heart failure. Because of these serious potential effects, it is important to establish just cause for use of this drug. If being used for nail fungal infections, it is recommended that laboratory testing of nails be performed prior to initiation therapy with this drug. Women of childbearing age should use effective contraception during therapy and for at least one menstrual cycle after stopping therapy. Consult with your doctor.

IVERMECTIN
(eye-ver-MEK-tin)

NEWLY DISCOVERED USES (OFF-LABEL)

Pediculosis capitis, scabies

ORIGINAL USES (ON-LABEL)
Treatment of intestinal strongyloidiasis (hookworm) and the immature form of onchocerciasis

BRAND NAME
Stromectol

DRUG CLASS
Anthelmintic (for parasitic worms)

DESCRIPTION
This drug is used to kill parasitic worms.

POTENTIAL SIDE EFFECTS
Low blood pressure, dizziness, headache, drowsiness, itching, rash, abdominal pain, diarrhea, changes in liver function, muscle aches, blurred vision, tremor, hives.

CAUTIONS
- Skin and/or systemic reactions called Mazzotti reactions can occur in patients with onchocerciasis; symptoms include joint aches, edema (swelling), ocular damage, swollen lymph glands, and fever.
- Serious and fatal encephalopathy has been reported rarely during ivermectin treatment for loiasis.

DRUG INTERACTIONS
Consult your doctor.

FOOD INTERACTIONS
Orange juice

HERBAL INTERACTIONS
Unknown

PREGNANCY AND BREAST-FEEDING CAUTIONS
FDA Pregnancy Risk Category C. Excreted into breast milk. Breast-feeding not recommended during therapy.

SPECIAL INFORMATION
Periodical eye exams should be performed. Take with water. Repeated stool examinations may be needed to document clearance of infection (strongyloidiasis). Other infections may require retreatment.

KETOCONAZOLE
(kee-toe-KOE-na-zole)

NEWLY DISCOVERED USES (OFF-LABEL)
Cushing's syndrome, hirsutism, hypercalciuria

ORIGINAL USES (ON-LABEL)
Treatment of various systemic and skin fungal infections

BRAND NAME
Nizoral

DRUG CLASS
Antifungal

DESCRIPTION
Ketoconazole interferes with the building of triglycerides and phospholipids in fungi, so the cell membrane is not made.

POTENTIAL SIDE EFFECTS
Itching, nausea, abdominal pain, severe irritation, hair loss, abnormal hair texture, scalp pustules, and mild skin dryness.

CAUTIONS
- Do not use if you have fungal meningitis infections or with ergotamine type drugs, astemizole, lovastatin, midazolam, simvastatin, triazolam, and cisapride.
- Use with caution if you have impaired liver function; this drug may cause liver toxicity.

- High doses of ketoconazole may suppress adrenal gland function or the production of testosterone.

DRUG INTERACTIONS

Ketoconazole blocks a specific set of liver enzymes (cytochrome P450 enzymes) that are useful for the metabolism or promote the clearance of other drugs from the body. Ketoconazole interferes with these liver enzymes, and thus, may increase or decrease the clearance of these drugs from the body, often requiring dosage adjustments when they are administered in combination.

Amiodarone, amphetamines, benzodiazepines, beta-blockers, buspirone, busulfan, calcium channel blockers, cyclosporine, sirolimus, tacrolimus, digoxin, docetaxel, HMG-CoA reductase inhibitors (lovastatin, pravastatin, etc.), methylprednisolone, phenytoin, quinolones, trimetrexate, warfarin, sidenafil, tadalafil, vardenafil, and zolpidem. (This list is not comprehensive and you should check with your pharmacist for a complete listing). Carbamazepine, didanosine, isoniazid, phenobarbital, phenytoin, rifabutin, and rifampin, protease inhibitors.

Ketoconazole needs gastric acidity in the stomach to be absorbed. The use of antacids, histamine-2 blockers (such as cimetidine, ranitidine, famotidine) and proton pump inhibitors (such as omeprazole, pantoprazole, etc.) may reduce the extent of absorption by lessening the gastric acid production in the stomach. Give these products at least two hours after ketoconazole is taken.

FOOD INTERACTIONS

Avoid alcohol, may cause disulfiram-like reaction (flushing, sweating, increased heart rate, nausea, vomiting). Avoid alcohol ingestion for at least 48 hours after the last dose of ketoconazole.

HERBAL INTERACTIONS

St. John's wort

PREGNANCY AND BREAST-FEEDING CAUTIONS

FDA Pregnancy Risk Category C. Excreted in breast milk. It is not recommended for use in women who are breast-feeding.

SPECIAL INFORMATION

This drug has a black box warning regarding the possible adverse event of liver toxicity. Monitoring of liver function should be performed during therapy. Take with food to minimize stomach upset.

This information pertains to the use of the prescription product only and should not be inferred for the use of nonprescription formulations.

KETOPROFEN
(kee-toe-PROE-fen)

NEWLY DISCOVERED USES (OFF-LABEL)
Ankylosing spondylitis, gout, membranous nephropathy, periodontitis

ORIGINAL USES (ON-LABEL)
Acute and long-term treatment for rheumatoid arthritis and osteoarthritis, primary dysmenorrhea, mild to moderate pain, and fever reduction

BRAND NAME
Oruvail

DRUG CLASS
Nonsteroidal anti-inflammatory (NSAID)

DESCRIPTION
This drug is a pain reliever and anti-inflammatory drug.

POTENTIAL SIDE EFFECTS
Upset stomach, headache, dizziness, rash, itching, diarrhea, nausea, constipation, abdominal pain, flatulence.

CAUTIONS
- Not for use if you are allergic to aspirin or other NSAIDs.
- Not for use if you have active gastric/duodenal ulcer disease.
- Do not use during third trimester of pregnancy.
- Ask physician about use if you have the following medical problems: high blood pressure, dehydration, decreased kidney or liver function, history of gastric disease.
- Elderly are at higher risk of developing side effects.
- Do not exceed 300 mg/day.
- Discuss with your doctor about temporarily stopping this medication prior to dental procedures and surgery.

DRUG INTERACTIONS
Aspirin, lithium, methotrexate, digoxin, cyclosporine (nephrotoxicity), diuretics, some anti-hypertensives, and warfarin (bleeding).

FOOD INTERACTIONS
Unknown

HERBAL INTERACTIONS
Unknown

PREGNANCY AND BREAST-FEEDING CAUTIONS
FDA Pregnancy Risk Category B (D if in third trimester). Excreted in breast milk. Consult your doctor.

SPECIAL INFORMATION
In April 2005, the FDA announced the potential addition of a black box warning to the labeling of this class of drugs (NSAIDs), specifically regarding potential serious cardiac events and potentially life-threatening gastric adverse events. There is a Medication Guide for patients regarding the potential for cardiac and gastric adverse events associated with the use of this class of drugs.

KETOROLAC
(KEE-toe-role-ak)

Ophthalmic

NEWLY DISCOVERED USES (OFF-LABEL)
Uveitis

ORIGINAL USES (ON-LABEL)
Temporary relief of ocular itching due to seasonal allergies, post-surgical inflammation after cataract surgery, reduction of ocular pain and photophobia (light sensitivity) after incisional refractive surgery, reduction of ocular pain, burning, and stinging after corneal refractive surgery

BRAND NAMES
Acular, Acular LS

DRUG CLASS
Ocular (nonsteroidal anti-inflammatory [NSAID])

DESCRIPTION
This drug decreases the production of prostaglandin, a stimulator of pain and inflammation.

POTENTIAL SIDE EFFECTS

Burning, stinging, ocular irritation and pain, corneal edema (swelling), allergic reactions, keratitis (inflammation of the cornea).

CAUTIONS

- Inform your doctor if you are allergic to other NSAIDs or aspirin.
- Not for use if you have nasal polyps, or experienced angioedema, or bronchospastic reactions to other NSAIDS. Not for use in active or a history of peptic ulcer disease, gastric bleeding, advanced kidney disease, and cerebrovascular bleeding.
- May increase bleeding time associated with ocular surgery, and may slow healing time.
- Adverse corneal effects, such as corneal thinning and erosion, may occur. Use for greater than 24 hours before surgery or more than two weeks after surgery increases this risk.
- Do not administer while wearing contact lenses.

DRUG INTERACTIONS

Do not use with other ocular products without consulting your doctor.

FOOD INTERACTIONS

Alcohol

HERBAL INTERACTIONS

Unknown

PREGNANCY AND BREAST-FEEDING CAUTIONS

FDA Pregnancy Risk Category C. Consult with doctor prior to breast-feeding.

KETOROLAC
(KEE-toe-role-ak)

Oral

NEWLY DISCOVERED USES (OFF-LABEL) ——————

Gout, kidney stones, preterm labor, renal colic, ureteral stones

ORIGINAL USES (ON-LABEL)

Short-term (not greater than five days) use for moderate-severe pain

BRAND NAME
Toradol

DRUG CLASS
Nonsteroidal anti-inflammatory (NSAID)

DESCRIPTION
This drug inhibits the activity of an enzyme responsible for the production of prostaglandins, thus decreasing the production of prostaglandin, a chemical in the body responsible for inflammation and pain.

POTENTIAL SIDE EFFECTS
Headache, stomach pain and upset, nausea, edema, dizziness, drowsiness, diarrhea. Peptic ulcers, gastrointestinal bleeding.

CAUTIONS
- Notify your doctor if you are allergic to aspirin or other NSAIDs.
- Do not use during third trimester of pregnancy.
- This drug has been associated with causing significant gastrointestinal complications, including peptic ulcers, bleeding or perforation.
- Contraindicated for use with other NSAIDs or aspirin.
- Reduced doses required in elderly (greater than 65 years) or patients less than 110 pounds.
- Ask physician about use if you have the following medical problems: high blood pressure, dehydration, decreased kidney or liver function, history of or active gastric disease.
- Not for labor and delivery or preventive pain prior to surgery.
- Total therapy is not to exceed five days.

DRUG INTERACTIONS
Cyclosporine, digoxin, lithium, methotrexate, ACE inhibitors (captopril, lisinopril, ramipril), probenecid, potassium-sparing diuretics (aldactone, spironolactone), aspirin, other NSAIDs, some anti-hypertensives, warfarin.

FOOD INTERACTIONS
Alcohol

HERBAL INTERACTIONS
Cat's claw, dong quai, evening primrose, feverfew, garlic, ginger, red clover, horse chestnut, green tea, and ginseng

PREGNANCY AND BREAST-FEEDING CAUTIONS
FDA Pregnancy Risk Category B (D if in third trimester). Excreted in breast milk. Consult your doctor.

SPECIAL INFORMATION

In April 2005, the FDA announced the potential addition of a black box warning to the labeling of this class of drugs (NSAIDs), specifically regarding potential serious cardiac events and potentially life-threatening gastric adverse events. You should discuss these new safety changes in labeling with your doctor.

This drug has a black box warning, which limits the use for therapy to 5 days with maximum daily doses (40 mg orally, 120 mg intravenously) to minimize risk of adverse events. Other risks discussed in the black box warning section regard the risk for bleeding, contraindication for use in patients with kidney impairment, not for use as pre-operative pain relief, and the contraindication for use as an intrathecal and epidural.

LABETALOL
(la-BET-a-lole)

NEWLY DISCOVERED USES (OFF-LABEL)

Pheochromocytoma (add-on treatment)

ORIGINAL USES (ON-LABEL)

Treatment of mild to severe high blood pressure. The intravenous form is used to treat severe high blood pressure crisis.

BRAND NAMES

Normodyne, Trandate

DRUG CLASS

Blood pressure medication (alpha-blocker, beta-blocker)

DESCRIPTION

Labetalol acts on specific receptors in the cardiac system to reduce blood pressure.

POTENTIAL SIDE EFFECTS

Dizziness, nausea, low blood pressure, numbness, scalp tingling, upset stomach, ejaculatory failure, impotence, increase in liver function tests, nasal congestion.

CAUTIONS

- Avoid use when heart rate is too low, in heart block, cardiogenic shock, asthma, cardiac failure, or pregnancy.

- Paradoxical increase in blood pressure may occur.
- Patient should remain lying down during and for three hours after intravenous administration.
- Use with caution in impaired liver function.
- May mask signs and symptoms of low blood glucose levels.
- Avoid abrupt discontinuation.
- Concurrent use with verapamil, diltiazem, or digoxin could cause too slow heart rate or heart block.

DRUG INTERACTIONS
Aluminum and aluminum salts, barbiturates, inhaled anesthetics, cholestyramine, colestipol, NSAIDs, penicillins, other drugs used for blood pressure or those that effect the specific liver enzyme group (P2D6) responsible for metabolizing labetalol

FOOD INTERACTIONS
Food increases serum levels of labetalol.

HERBAL INTERACTIONS
Dong quai, ephedra, yohimbe, ginseng, large quantities of natural licorice, garlic

PREGNANCY AND BREAST-FEEDING CAUTIONS
FDA Pregnancy Risk Category C. FDA Pregnancy Risk Category D in second and third trimester of pregnancy. Excreted in breast milk. Contact doctor for approval of use during breast-feeding.

LAMIVUDINE
(la-MI-vyoo-deen)

NEWLY DISCOVERED USES (OFF-LABEL)
Liver cirrhosis, liver fibrosis

ORIGINAL USES (ON-LABEL)
HIV infection in combination with other antiretroviral drugs, chronic hepatitis B

BRAND NAMES
Epivir; Epivir-HBV

DRUG CLASS
Antiviral (antiretroviral; nucleoside reverse transcriptase inhibitor [NRTI])

DESCRIPTION
Inhibits RNA- and DNA-dependent activities in cell production.

POTENTIAL SIDE EFFECTS
Headache, nerve pain, insomnia, dizziness, depressive disorders, nausea, diarrhea, vomiting, anorexia, abdominal pain, abdominal cramps, upset stomach, musculoskeletal pain, muscle aches, joint aches, nasal signs and symptoms, cough, malaise, fever, chills, rash.

CAUTIONS
- You should take a reduced dosage if you have kidney impairment.
- Do not use as monotherapy in treatment of HIV.
- Treatment of hepatitis B in the presence of unrecognized/untreated HIV may lead to rapid HIV resistance.
- Lactic acidosis (excessive lactic acid in the blood) and severe liver problems have been reported with this drug. Pregnancy, obesity, and/or prolonged therapy may increase the risk of lactic acidosis and liver damage.
- Requires monitoring of liver function during and for several months after therapy in patients with both HIV and HBV.

DRUG INTERACTIONS
Zidovudine, sulfamethoxazole/trimethoprim, ribavirin, adefovir, didanosine, stavudine, zalcitabine, zalcitabine

FOOD INTERACTIONS
May take with or without food.

HERBAL INTERACTIONS
Unknown

PREGNANCY AND BREAST-FEEDING CAUTIONS
FDA Pregnancy Risk Category C. Excreted in breast milk. Do not breast-feed during therapy.

SPECIAL INFORMATION
This drug has a black box warning regarding complications associated with therapy, particularly the risk of developing lactic acidosis and liver problems. In addition, it is noted that Epivir HBV and Epivir do not contain the same amount of lamivudine and should be used for their respective indications.

LAMOTRIGINE
(la-MOE-tri-jeen)

NEWLY DISCOVERED USES (OFF-LABEL)
Borderline personality disorder, chronic neuropathic pain, diabetic neuropathy, multiple sclerosis, post-traumatic stress disorder (PTSD), trigeminal neuralgia, West syndrome

ORIGINAL USES (ON-LABEL)
Use in combination therapy for the treatment of generalized seizure (Lennox-Gastaut syndrome) in children older than 2 years, used as sole therapy for partial seizures, and maintenance treatment for bipolar disorder

BRAND NAME
Lamictal

DRUG CLASS
Anticonvulsant

DESCRIPTION
The exact mechanism by which lamotrigine acts as an anticonvulsant drug is not known. It may prevent electrochemical impulses in the brain.

POTENTIAL SIDE EFFECTS
Headache, anorexia, muscle incoordination, dizziness, increased cough, double vision, somnolence, nausea, painful menstruation, blurred vision, runny nose, depression, anxiety, irritability, confusion, allergic-type rash, abdominal pain, diarrhea, upset stomach, constipation, vaginitis, tremor, muscle aches, involuntary rapid movement of the eyeball, neck pain, eczema, insomnia, flu syndrome, and fever.

CAUTIONS
- Serious skin rashes requiring hospitalization have occurred. Use with caution, especially in children.
- Caution in patients with impaired kidney, liver, or cardiac function.
- Do not stop this drug suddenly; the dose should be tapered over a period of two weeks unless safety issues are involved.
- May affect melanin levels in the eye with long-term use.

DRUG INTERACTIONS
Acetaminophen, carbamazepine, oral contraceptives, oxcarbazepine, primidone, phenytoin, valproic acid, phenobarbital

FOOD INTERACTIONS
Avoid alcohol

HERBAL INTERACTIONS
Evening primrose, ginkgo

PREGNANCY AND BREAST-FEEDING CAUTIONS
FDA Pregnancy Risk Category C. Excreted in breast milk; not recommended during breast-feeding.

SPECIAL INFORMATION
This drug has a black box warning regarding the potential for serious rashes in children and adults.

LANSOPRAZOLE
(lan-SOE-pra-zole)

NEWLY DISCOVERED USES (OFF-LABEL)
Laryngitis, stress-related mucosal disease

ORIGINAL USES (ON-LABEL)
Short-term treatment of active duodenal ulcers; maintenance treatment of healed duodenal ulcers; part of *H. pylori* treatment regimen; treatment of gastric ulcer, gastroesophageal reflux disease (GERD), erosive esophagitis, and hypersecretory (increased gastric acid secretion) conditions (such as Zollinger-Ellison syndrome)

BRAND NAMES
Prevacid, Prevacid IV, Prevacid SoluTabs

DRUG CLASS
Gastrointestinal (proton pump inhibitor)

DESCRIPTION
Lansoprazole decreases gastric acid secretion by inhibiting an intracellular "acid" (proton) pump, which is the final step in gastric acid production.

POTENTIAL SIDE EFFECTS
Diarrhea, abdominal pain.

CAUTIONS
• Dosage reductions may be required in severe liver dysfunction.

DRUG INTERACTIONS
Carbamazepine, phenytoin, rifampin, atazanavir, indinavir, itraconazole, ketoconazole, warfarin, ampicillin, clarithromycin, digoxin.

FOOD INTERACTIONS
Avoid cranberry juice.

HERBAL INTERACTIONS
Ginkgo biloba

PREGNANCY AND BREAST-FEEDING CAUTIONS
FDA Pregnancy Risk Factor Category B. Excretion in breast milk unknown. Breast-feeding is not recommended.

SPECIAL INFORMATION
Lansoprazole works best if taken before eating, especially before breakfast.

Lansoprazole capsules and granules should not be crushed or chewed.

Prevacid SoluTabs contain phenylalanine.

LEFLUNOMIDE
(le-FLOO-noh-mide)

NEWLY DISCOVERED USES (OFF-LABEL)
Psoriasis, psoriatic arthritis

ORIGINAL USES (ON-LABEL)
Active rheumatoid arthritis

BRAND NAME
Arava

DRUG CLASS
Antirheumatic

DESCRIPTION
This drug inhibits the production of pyrimidine, which promotes anti-inflammatory effects.

POTENTIAL SIDE EFFECTS
Diarrhea, nausea, respiratory tract infection, high blood pressure, rash, urinary tract infection, headache, dizziness, chest pain, hair

loss, itching, dry skin, upset stomach, abnormal liver enzymes tests, abdominal pain, mouth ulcers, vomiting, low potassium levels, weight loss, muscle aches, leg cramps, joint disorders, increased cough, bronchitis.

CAUTIONS

- Do not use this drug in pregnancy. Pregnancy must be excluded prior to initiation of therapy. Reliable use of contraception in women of childbearing age should be ensured during therapy. Pregnancy must be avoided during and prior to completion of the drug elimination procedure after leflunomide treatment.

- Leflunomide has been associated with liver toxicity. Monitoring of blood factors and liver function is recommended during therapy. The use of this drug in impaired liver function is not recommended.

- Not recommended for use in patients with severe immune deficiency, bone marrow dysplasia, or with an uncontrolled infection.

DRUG INTERACTIONS

Methotrexate, rifampin, cholestyramine, charcoal, NSAIDs (nonsteroidal anti-inflammatory drugs), tolbutamide, other drugs known to cause liver toxicity.

FOOD INTERACTIONS

Unknown

HERBAL INTERACTIONS

Unknown

PREGNANCY AND BREAST-FEEDING CAUTIONS

FDA Pregnancy Risk Category X. Not known if this drug is excreted in breast milk. Breast-feeding is not recommended.

SPECIAL INFORMATION

This drug has a black box warning regarding the contraindication of pregnancy (see cautions).

LEPIRUDIN
(leh-puh-ROO-din)

NEWLY DISCOVERED USES (OFF-LABEL)
Add-on therapy for unstable angina in patients with heparin-induced conditions, add-on therapy in myocardial infraction in patients with heparin-induced conditions
---

ORIGINAL USES (ON-LABEL)
For anticoagulation in patients with heparin-induced thrombocytopenia (HIT)

BRAND NAME
Refludan

DRUG CLASS
Anticoagulant

DESCRIPTION
Lepirudin directly inhibits thrombin, a substance needed to form blood clots.

POTENTIAL SIDE EFFECTS
Anemia, bleeding, heart failure, fever, eczema, rash, gastric bleeding, rectal bleeding, increase in laboratory tests used to monitor liver function, blood in urine, bloody nose, bronchospasm, difficulty breathing, shortness of breath, and cough are possible in non-HIT populations.

CAUTIONS
- This product is made from hirudins; avoid if you are sensitive to hirudins.
- Use extreme caution with the following conditions: recent large puncture or biopsy, abnormal blood vessels or organs, recent cardiac procedures, severe uncontrolled high blood pressure, bacterial endocarditis, advanced kidney impairment, recent major surgery, recent major bleeding.
- Requires strict monitoring of blood testing in prolonged therapy.

DRUG INTERACTIONS
Other drugs that affect the formation of blood clots increase risk of bleeding complications.

FOOD INTERACTIONS
Unknown

HERBAL INTERACTIONS

Cat's claw, dong quai, evening primrose, feverfew, garlic, ginger, gingko, red clover, horse chestnut, green tea, ginseng

PREGNANCY AND BREAST-FEEDING CAUTIONS

FDA Pregnancy Risk Category B. Excretion in breast milk unknown. Breast-feeding is probably compatible.

SPECIAL INFORMATION

Administered only by intravenous formulation.

LETROZOLE

(LET-roe-zole)

NEWLY DISCOVERED USES (OFF-LABEL)

Delayed puberty in boys, infertility, male infertility

ORIGINAL USES (ON-LABEL)

Breast cancer in post-menopausal women

BRAND NAME

Femara

DRUG CLASS

Antineoplastic (aromatase inhibitor)

DESCRIPTION

This drug decreases estrogen levels in the body. As some breast cancers are estrogen stimulated or maintained by estrogens, the growth of the cancer may be inhibited by the action of this drug.

POTENTIAL SIDE EFFECTS

Lower limb edema (swelling due to fluid retention), high blood pressure, headache, insomnia, nausea, constipation, diarrhea, vomiting, decreased appetite, abdominal pain, bone pain, back pain, muscle aches, limb pain, shortness of breath, cough, hot flashes, fatigue, chest pain, decreased weight, breast pain, weakness, hair loss, post-mastectomy lymphedema (swelling of the lymph glands).

CAUTIONS

- May impair fertility.
- May cause abnormal elevations in liver function tests.

DRUG INTERACTIONS
Tamoxifen

FOOD INTERACTIONS
Unknown

HERBAL INTERACTIONS
Unknown

PREGNANCY AND BREAST-FEEDING CAUTIONS
FDA Pregnancy Risk Category D. Excretion in breast milk is unknown. Breast-feeding is not recommended.

SPECIAL INFORMATION
Due to side effects, use caution when doing tasks that require alertness. Report chest pain, pressure, palpitations, and/or extremity swelling; numbness, weakness or loss of strength in any part of your body; difficulty speaking; vaginal bleeding or unusual signs of bleeding; breathing difficulties; severe nausea; and skin rash to your doctor.

LEUPROLIDE
(loo-PROE-lide)

NEWLY DISCOVERED USES (OFF-LABEL)
Abnormal uterine bleeding, chronic pelvic pain, dysmenorrhea, hirsutism, menorrhagia, menstrual migraine, ovulation induction for in-vitro fertilization (IVF), pelvic congestion, premenstrual dysphoric disorder (PMDD), therapy-resistant PMDD

ORIGINAL USES (ON-LABEL)
Palliative treatment of advanced prostate cancer, initial treatment for endometriosis, preoperative treatment of anemia caused by uterine fibroids, and central precocious puberty

BRAND NAMES
Eligard, Lupron, Lupron Depot, Lupron Depot-Ped, Viadur

DRUG CLASS
Chemotherapy, gonadotropin releasing hormone analog

DESCRIPTION
This drug decreases levels of testosterone and estrogen. (It may cause increased testosterone and estrogen levels at the beginning of treatment.)

POTENTIAL SIDE EFFECTS
Angina, atrial fibrillation, deep vein thrombosis, abnormal thinking, agitation, amnesia, confusion, hair loss, bruising, bone density
decreased, breast enlargement, breast tenderness, dehydration,
anorexia, appetite increased, diarrhea, difficulty swallowing, inflammation of the glans penis, impotence, urinary frequency during the night, penile shrinkage, increased time to form blood clots,
abnormal liver function tests, abscess, leg cramps, congestive heart
failure, myalgia, numbness, weakness, decreased kidney function.

CAUTIONS
- Do not use during vaginal bleeding, pregnancy, breast-feeding.
- Long-term use of greater than six months may decrease bone
  density.

DRUG INTERACTIONS
Unknown

FOOD INTERACTIONS
Unknown

HERBAL INTERACTIONS
Unknown

PREGNANCY AND BREAST-FEEDING CAUTIONS
FDA Pregnancy Risk Category X. Do not use during pregnancy.
Do not use while breast-feeding.

SPECIAL INFORMATION
Patient information brochures are available with each injection
kit. When used to treat prostate cancer, may cause increased bone
pain and difficulty urinating during the first few weeks of treatment. May also cause hot flashes, irritation and itching at the injection site.

LEVAMISOLE
(lee-VAM-i-sole)

NEWLY DISCOVERED USES (OFF-LABEL)
Nephrotic syndrome

ORIGINAL USES (ON-LABEL)
Combination therapy with fluorouracil for Dukes stage C colon
cancer

BRAND NAME
Ergamisol

DRUG CLASS
Antineoplastic (immune modulator)

DESCRIPTION
This drug is used to treat cancer. Its mechanism of action is unknown.

POTENTIAL SIDE EFFECTS
Nausea, diarrhea, metallic taste, headache, numbness, mouth ulcers, edema, fatigue, fever, dizziness, severe blood disorders (see cautions), hair loss, skin reactions, muscle aches, joint aches, drowsiness, infection.

CAUTIONS
- Severe and life-threatening blood disorders (agranulocytosis) can occur with flu-like symptoms or asymptomatically with the use of this drug. Frequent blood monitoring is required.
- Liver function testing and electrolyte monitoring is recommended periodically during therapy.

DRUG INTERACTIONS
Phenytoin, warfarin, fluorouracil

FOOD INTERACTIONS
Avoid alcohol.

HERBAL INTERACTIONS
Unknown

PREGNANCY AND BREAST-FEEDING CAUTIONS
FDA Pregnancy Risk Category C. Excretion into breast milk is unknown, and breast-feeding is not recommended.

SPECIAL INFORMATION
Immediately report flu-like symptoms or malaise to your doctor.

LEVETIRACETAM
(lee-va-tye-RA-se-tam)

NEWLY DISCOVERED USES (OFF-LABEL)
Bipolar disorder, tension headache prevention

ORIGINAL USES (ON-LABEL)
Used in combination with other drugs in the treatment of partial onset seizures in adults with epilepsy

BRAND NAME
Keppra

DRUG CLASS
Anticonvulsant

DESCRIPTION
This drug is used mainly to control seizures. Its mechanism of action is unknown.

POTENTIAL SIDE EFFECTS
Drowsiness, headache, weakness, infection, chest pain, amnesia, muscle incoordination, depression, dizziness, bruising, rash, anorexia, abdominal pain, constipation, diarrhea, decreased red blood cells, decreased white blood cells, numbness, muscle aches, back pain, tremors, double vision, ear infections, sore throat, runny nose, cough, and sinus infection.

CAUTIONS
- Side effects may be severe. Contact doctor if the following occur: extreme drowsiness, fatigue, problems with muscle coordination (trouble walking and moving), psychosis (sudden aggression, anger, anxiety, depression, irritability), hallucinations, and depression.
- Do not stop the drug suddenly. Taper the dose gradually to prevent an increase in seizures.
- Use with caution if you have reduced kidney function.

DRUG INTERACTIONS
Unknown

FOOD INTERACTIONS
Food does not affect the amount of this drug absorbed but does decrease the maximum levels of the drug reached.

HERBAL INTERACTIONS
Evening primrose, ginkgo

PREGNANCY AND BREAST-FEEDING CAUTIONS
FDA Pregnancy Risk Category C. Excreted into breast milk; not recommended for use by women who are breast-feeding.

SPECIAL INFORMATION

Swallow tablets whole. Do not chew or crush tablets. If using solution, a medicine dropper or cup should be used to measure. Do not use a teaspoon.

LEVOFLOXACIN
(lee-voe-FLOKS-a-sin)

NEWLY DISCOVERED USES (OFF-LABEL)

Nonbacterial prostatitis

ORIGINAL USES (ON-LABEL)

Treatment of infections caused by susceptible organisms, postexposure prevention for anthrax. The ophthalmic formulation is indicated for the treatment of bacterial conjunctivitis.

BRAND NAMES

Levaquin, Quixin

DRUG CLASS

Antibiotic (quinolone)

DESCRIPTION

This drug fights infections by interfering with cellular enzymes, halting DNA replication, repair, recombination, and transposition.

POTENTIAL SIDE EFFECTS

Dizziness, headache, nausea, diarrhea, constipation

CAUTIONS

- Report to your doctor if you experience pain, inflammation or rupture of a tendon. Rest and refrain from exercise until you see a doctor. Tendon rupture can occur during or after therapy with this drug.
- Stop the medication at the first sign of a rash.
- May cause changes in blood glucose levels, monitor blood glucose in diabetics.
- Prolonged use may cause superinfection.
- May aggravate symptoms of myasthenia gravis.
- Inform your doctor if serious, persistent diarrhea develops.

DRUG INTERACTIONS
Iron, zinc, calcium, magnesium, aluminum, corticosteroids (increase risk of tendon rupture), antacids, electrolyte supplements, quinapril, sucralfate, certain antiarrhythmics, didanosine formulations (chewable/buffered tablets and pediatric powder for oral suspension), theophyllines, antacids, cyclosporine, cimetidine

FOOD INTERACTION
Dairy products or calcium-fortified juices. Serum caffeine levels may be increased. May be taken without regard to meals.

HERBAL INTERACTIONS
Unknown

PREGNANCY AND BREAST-FEEDING CAUTIONS
FDA Pregnancy Risk Category C. May be excreted in breast milk. Do not use during breast-feeding.

SPECIAL INFORMATION
May cause increased sensitivity to sunlight; use sunblock, wear protective clothing and dark glasses. Report immediately any signs of rash, joint or back pain, difficulty breathing, easy bruising or bleeding, inflammation, or rupture of tendon.

Ocular formulation: Do not touch tip of container to other surfaces. Do not wear contact lenses during treatment. May cause temporary burning and stinging, blurred vision.

LEVONORGESTREL-ETHINYL ESTRADIOL
(LEE-voe-nor-jes-trel ETH-in-il es-tra-DYE-ole)

NEWLY DISCOVERED USES (OFF-LABEL)
Abnormal uterine bleeding, acne, amenorrhea, dysmenorrhea, endometriosis, hirsutism, menopausal symptoms, menorrhagia, polycystic ovary syndrome

ORIGINAL USES (ON-LABEL)
Prevention of pregnancy

BRAND NAMES
Levlen, Levora, Nordette, Portia, Seasonale

DRUG CLASS
Contraceptive (estrogen and progestin combination)

DESCRIPTION
This drug inhibits ovulation. It prevents secretion of hormones important in the ovulation cycle: follicle stimulating hormone (FSH) and luteinizing hormone (LH). In addition, the cervical mucus of the vagina changes, becoming an environment hostile for sperm.

POTENTIAL SIDE EFFECTS
Intermenstrual bleeding and irregularity, abdominal pain, diarrhea, nausea, vomiting, depression, dizziness, emotional lability, headache, migraine, nervousness, change in vision or ability to wear contact lenses, fluid retention, darkening of skin in areas, vaginal infections, hair loss. Increased risk of cardiac events, glucose intolerance, stroke, liver problems.

CAUTIONS
- Oral contraceptives do not protect against sexually transmitted diseases or HIV infection.
- Cardiovascular events increase if you are over 35 years of age and heavy smoker (at least 15 cigarettes daily), or have a history of cardiovascular disease or thromboembolic (blood clots) events.
- Not for use if you have decreased kidney, adrenal or liver function, diabetes with vascular involvement, history of or suspected breast cancer or estrogen dependent cancer, undiagnosed genital bleeding, liver tumor, severe high blood pressure, jaundice associated with pregnancy or prior birth control pill usage, headaches with neurological symptoms.
- Do not take if you are pregnant.
- Discuss cardiac and other risks with your doctor prior to starting therapy.

DRUG INTERACTIONS
Oral contraceptives, including this product, may interact with several drugs too numerous to list. Check with your pharmacist or doctor before starting any new medication, herbal product, or nonprescription drug.

FOOD INTERACTIONS
Grapefruit juice

HERBAL INTERACTIONS
St. John's wort, dong quai, black cohosh, saw palmetto, red clover, ginseng

PREGNANCY AND BREAST-FEEDING CAUTIONS
FDA Pregnancy Risk Category X. Do not use in pregnancy. Excreted in breast milk and not recommended during breast-feeding.

SPECIAL INFORMATION
Read the patient information brochure prior to therapy for important instructions regarding therapy.

LEVONORGESTREL-RELEASING INTRAUTERINE SYSTEM
(LEE-voe-nor-jes-trel)

NEWLY DISCOVERED USES (OFF-LABEL)
  Menorrhagia

ORIGINAL USES (ON-LABEL)
Prevention of pregnancy

BRAND NAME
Mirena

DRUG CLASS
Contraceptive

DESCRIPTION
This is an intrauterine device which releases the drug locally, resulting in changes in the local cervical mucus of the vagina, developing an environment hostile for sperm.

POTENTIAL SIDE EFFECTS
Abdominal pain, nausea, vomiting, acne, skin disorder, headache, depression, nervousness, lowered heart rate, high blood pressure, fainting.

CAUTIONS
- Not recommended for use if you have a history of ectopic pregnancy or condition that would increase the risk of ectopic pregnancy.
- Does not protect against HIV infection or other sexually transmitted diseases.
- Discuss with your doctor the risks associated with the possibility of intrauterine pregnancy, including septic abortion, con-

tinuation of pregnancy, long-term effects and congenital anomalies.

- Infections and sepsis (severe infection of the blood) have been rarely reported after insertion of this system. Report any severe abdominal or pelvic pain immediately to your doctor.
- Not for use if you have pelvic inflammatory disease (PID) or are at increased risk of developing PID.
- May alter your bleeding pattern for the first three to six months with stabilization afterward.
- This system may become partially embedded in or perforate the local tissue making it less effective or more difficult to remove.
- Not for use in women who have a history of or currently have breast cancer.
- Discuss all risks of adverse events and mortality with your doctor prior to insertion.
- You may be at increased risk of bacterial endocarditis (infection of the heart) if you have congenital heart disease or valvular heart disease.
- Any local vaginal or cervical infection should be treated and cleared prior to insertion.
- Requires periodic monitoring during use and should be replaced every five years.
- Report to your doctor any development of pain, odorous discharge, bleeding, fever, lesions, or sores.
- Requires glucose monitoring in diabetics.

DRUG INTERACTIONS

Contraceptives, including this product, may interact with several drugs too numerous to list. Check with your pharmacist or doctor before starting any new medication, herbal product, or nonprescription drug.

FOOD INTERACTIONS

Unknown

HERBAL INTERACTIONS

Unknown

PREGNANCY AND BREAST-FEEDING CAUTIONS

FDA Pregnancy Risk Category X. Do not use in pregnancy. Excreted in breast milk and not recommended during breast-feeding.

SPECIAL INFORMATION

Read the patient information brochure prior to therapy for important instructions regarding therapy.

This refers only to use of the prescription formulation of the drug.

LIDOCAINE
(LYE-doe-kane)

Topical

NEWLY DISCOVERED USES (OFF-LABEL)

Anal fissure, cancer treatment-induced mucositis/stomatitis, chronic neuropathic pain, diabetic neuropathy, migraine treatment (intranasally—this requires special formulation compounding by your pharmacist)

ORIGINAL USES (ON-LABEL)

To reduce local pain relief of various skin disorders, including minor burns, abrasions, sunburn, pain on mucous membranes

BRAND NAMES

Anestacon, Xylocaine

DRUG CLASS

Local anesthetic

DESCRIPTION

This drug inhibits the sensory nerve impulses to deaden sensation on the skin.

POTENTIAL SIDE EFFECTS

Burning, stinging, tenderness, hives.

CAUTIONS

- Use the lowest effective dose to avoid increased systemic absorption and high blood levels, which may increase the risk of non-local side effects.
- Not for use in patients with high blood levels of methohemoglobin.
- Patients with severe liver impairment are at increased risk of developing toxic blood levels because they clear the drug more slowly from the body. This is less likely with topical application, but use the minimal effective dose not for prolonged periods.

Use lower amounts in debilitated or the elderly, or small children.

- Topical anesthetics may affect swallowing and increase the risk of choking. Avoid eating for one hour after using these products in the mouth.
- Inform your doctor of any allergies to other anesthetics prior to use. Some products also contain tartrazine or sulfite, which has been associated with allergic type symptoms.
- For external application only. Do not use in the eyes.

DRUG INTERACTIONS
Do not use other topical drugs without the advice of your doctor or pharmacist.

FOOD INTERACTIONS
Unknown

HERBAL INTERACTIONS
Unknown

PREGNANCY AND BREAST-FEEDING CAUTIONS
FDA Pregnancy Risk Category B. Excreted in breast milk. Consult your doctor.

SPECIAL INFORMATION
Use on the tongue or inner cheek tissue (buccal) may cause local numbness. Take care not to bite this area. Avoid chewing gum or eating for one hour after use.

LISINOPRIL
(lyse-IN-oh-pril)

NEWLY DISCOVERED USES (OFF-LABEL)
Diabetic nephropathy, diabetic retinopathy, membranous nephropathy, migraine prevention

ORIGINAL USES (ON-LABEL)
For the treatment of high blood pressure, congestive heart failure, after heart attacks

BRAND NAMES
Prinivil, Zestril

DRUG CLASS
Blood pressure medication

DESCRIPTION
Lisinopril lowers blood pressure by inhibiting the production of chemicals that cause blood vessels to constrict. It also may cause the brain to release hormones that lower blood pressure.

POTENTAL SIDE EFFECTS
Chest pain, too low blood pressure (especially after first dose), cough, fainting, headache, dizziness, fatigue, weakness, rash, abnormal taste, nausea, shortness of breath.

CAUTIONS
- Do not use if you have had tongue, lip, throat, or mouth swelling (symptoms of angioedema) after taking other drugs in the same class or if you have these symptoms unrelated to drug therapy. Angioedema can occur at any time during treatment, but especially following the first dose. Report symptoms to your doctor.
- Do not use in pregnant patients who are in the second or third trimester.
- Do not use with certain kidney problems (kidney artery stenosis, decreased kidney function).
- Avoid rapid dosage increases that may lead to kidney problems.

DRUG INTERACTIONS
Potassium supplements, cotrimoxazole (high dose), angiotension II receptor antagonists (candesartan, losartan, irbesartan, etc.) or potassium sparing diuretics (amiloride, spironolactone, triamterene), digoxin, lithium, and certain drugs used to treat diabetes (sulfonylureas). Aspirin (high doses) or indomethacin may aggravate the beneficial effects of this drug.

FOOD INTERACTIONS
Unknown

HERBAL INTERACTIONS
St. John's wort, capsaicin, dong quai, ephedra, yohimbe, ginseng, ma huang, large amounts of natural licorice

PREGNANCY AND BREAST-FEEDING CAUTIONS
FDA Pregnancy Risk Category C for first trimester. FDA Pregnancy Risk Category D for second and third trimester. Excreted in breast milk. No reports of use during breast-feeding.

SPECIAL INFORMATION

Report any vomiting, diarrhea, excessive perspiration, or dehydration to your physician. If any swelling of the face, lips, extremities, lips, tongue, throat or difficulty in breathing occurs or if a persistent dry cough develops it should be reported too.

LITHIUM
(LITH-ee-um)

NEWLY DISCOVERED USES (OFF-LABEL)

Cluster headache prevention, neutropenia, schizoaffective disorder

ORIGINAL USES (ON-LABEL)

To manage bipolar disorders, for the treatment and prevention of mania in patients with bipolar disorder.

BRAND NAMES

Eskalith, Eskalith CR, Lithobid

DRUG CLASS

Psychiatric

DESCRIPTION

Lithium affects the levels of the chemicals serotonin and norepinephrine in the body.

POTENTIAL SIDE EFFECTS

Dizziness, sedation, anorexia, nausea, drowsiness, sedation, diarrhea, dry mouth, weight gain, tremor, blurred vision.

CAUTIONS

- Do not use in patients with severe heart or kidney disease, or in severe dehydration. Use with caution in patients with mild to moderate heart or kidney disease.
- Do not use if you are pregnant.
- Lithium toxicity is related to drug levels in the body and can occur at normal doses.
- Some elderly patients may be more sensitive to the effects of lithium.
- Long-term use can decrease kidney function.

DRUG INTERACTIONS

Carbamazepine, diltiazem, fluoxetine, fluvoxamine, haloperidol, MAO inhibitors, phenytoin, tricyclic antidepressants (amitriptyline, nortriptyline, imipramine, desipramine, etc.), verapamil, acetazolamide, theophylline diuretics, losartan, tetracycline, celecoxib, some nonsteroidal anti-inflammatory drugs, ACE inhibitors (captopril, lisinopril, enalapril, etc.), sibutramine, chlorpromazine.

FOOD INTERACTIONS

Caffeine

HERBAL INTERACTIONS

Herbal diuretics; plantain

PREGNANCY AND BREAST-FEEDING CAUTIONS

FDA Pregnancy Risk Category D. Lithium is excreted in breast milk. Avoid using lithium in pregnancy or while breast-feeding.

SPECIAL INFORMATION

May upset stomach; take immediately after meals or with food or milk.

If signs or symptoms of toxicity occur, contact your doctor. These include diarrhea, vomiting, unsteady walking, tremor, drowsiness, muscle weakness.

Drink plenty of fluid (eight to 12 glasses of water daily) to avoid dehydration.

LORAZEPAM
(lore-AZ-ee-pam)

NEWLY DISCOVERED USES (OFF-LABEL)

Acute cisplatin-induced nausea and vomiting, acute schizophrenia, alcohol withdrawal, labyrinthitis, oculogyric crisis, panic attack, tension headache treatment

ORIGINAL USES (ON-LABEL)

Management of anxiety disorders or short-term relief of the symptoms of anxiety or anxiety associated with depressive symptoms, intravenous lorazepam is used for certain types of seizures, preanesthesia for desired amnesia and in combination therapy to prevent vomiting

BRAND NAMES
Ativan, Lorazepam Intensol

DRUG CLASS
Antianxiety, anticonvulsant, sedative (benzodiazepine)

DESCRIPTION
Lorazepam is used to manage excitable states in patients. It works by binding to specific benzodiazepine receptors.

POTENTIAL SIDE EFFECTS
Sedation, respiratory depression, low blood pressure, confusion, dizziness, skin reaction, rash, weight gain/loss, nausea, changes in appetite, weakness, nasal congestion, hyperventilation, amnesia, sedation, light headedness, sleepiness, dry mouth, blurred vision, double vision.

CAUTIONS
- Notify your doctor if you have had an allergic reaction to other benzodiazepines.
- Not for use if you have acute narrow-angle glaucoma, sleep apnea, or severe respiratory depression.
- Careful monitoring or reduced doses are needed in elderly or debilitated patients and those with liver or kidney impairment.
- Inform your doctor if you have a respiratory disease or impaired gag reflux.
- Prolonged use can result in dependence. Inform your doctor if you have a history of drug dependence.
- Caution in operating machinery or driving due to sedative properties of lorazepam.
- Use caution in patients using other central nervous system depressants or psychoactive drugs.
- This drug may cause amnesia.
- Paradoxical reactions, including hyperactive or aggressive behavior have been reported with this drug class.
- Use caution if you have depression, particularly if you have suicidal risk.
- Do not stop therapy abruptly. Acute withdrawal symptoms on discontinuation or reduction in dose can occur.
- Lorazepam should only be used as a hypnotic drug only after evaluation of potential causes of sleep disturbance.

DRUG INTERACTIONS
Other central nervous system (CNS) depressants, scopolamine, loxapine, levodopa, oral contraceptives, theophylline, probenecid, rifampin, digoxin, phenytoin, neuromuscular blocking drugs.

FOOD INTERACTIONS
Alcohol

HERBAL INTERACTIONS
Valerian, St. John's wort, kava kava, gotu kola

PREGNANCY AND BREAST-FEEDING CAUTIONS
FDA Pregnancy Risk Category D. Excreted in the breast milk and is not for use while breast-feeding.

SPECIAL INFORMATION
May result in drowsiness. Avoid driving or other tasks that require alertness. May be taken with food if stomach upset occurs. Do not stop therapy abruptly or change dose without notifying your doctor.

LOSARTAN
(loe-SAR-tan)

NEWLY DISCOVERED USES (OFF-LABEL)
Raynaud's syndrome

ORIGINAL USES (ON-LABEL)
High blood pressure, diabetic nephropathy in patients with type 2 diabetes mellitus and a history of high blood pressure, reduction of stroke risk in patients with high blood pressure and cardiac impairment (left ventricular hypertrophy)

BRAND NAME
Cozaar

DRUG CLASS
Blood pressure medication (angiotensin II receptor antagonist [ARB])

DESCRIPTION
Losartan works by blocking the substance that causes fluid retention and blood vessels to constrict.

POTENTIAL SIDE EFFECTS
Low blood pressure, sudden drop in blood pressure upon standing, fatigue, dizziness, fever, low blood sugar levels, diarrhea, urinary tract infection, anemia, weakness, back pain, cough, cellulitis, gastritis, weight gain, abdominal pain, nausea, knee pain, bronchitis, upper respiratory infection, flu-like syndrome.

CAUTIONS

- Do not use with certain kidney problems (kidney artery stenosis).
- Do not use in pregnant patients who are in the second or third trimester.
- Lower doses needed in patients with liver impairment.

DRUG INTERACTIONS

Potassium supplements, cimetidine, phenobarbital, and potassium-sparing diuretics, lithium, indomethacin, drugs that inhibit metabolism of specific liver enzymes (cytochrome P3A4- ketoconazole, etc.). Drugs that affect liver enzymes may interact with this drug.

FOOD INTERACTIONS

Unknown

HERBAL INTERACTIONS

St. John's wort, dong quai, ephedra, yohimbe, garlic, ginseng

PREGNANCY AND BREAST-FEEDING CAUTIONS

FDA Pregnancy Risk Category C for first trimester. FDA Pregnancy Risk Category D for second and third trimester. Excretion in breast milk unknown. No reports of the use of this drug during breast-feeding.

LOVASTATIN
(LOE-va-sta-tin)

NEWLY DISCOVERED USES (OFF-LABEL)
Peripheral artery disease

ORIGINAL USES (ON-LABEL)

In combination with dietary changes to reduce increased total and LDL-cholesterol levels, primary prevention of coronary artery disease (patients without symptomatic disease with average to moderately elevated total and LDL-cholesterol and below average HDL-cholesterol), coronary heart disease. In combination with dietary measure to treat adolescent patients (10–17 years of age, females greater than one year past the date of menstruation), high cholesterol levels related to certain types of hereditary disease.

BRAND NAMES
Altocor[DSC], Altoprev, Mevacor

DRUG CLASS
Anti-lipid (HMG-CoA reductase inhibitor)

DESCRIPTION
Lovastatin inhibits a substance (HMG-CoA reductase) that is an important factor in the production of cholesterol.

POTENTIAL SIDE EFFECTS
Headache, dizziness, rash, abdominal pain, constipation, diarrhea, upset stomach, flatulence, nausea, muscle aches.

CAUTIONS
- Not for use if you have active liver disease, are pregnant or breast-feeding.
- May cause increases in laboratory tests used to monitor liver function. These tests should be performed before and every 4–6 weeks during the first 12–15 months of therapy and periodically thereafter.
- Can also cause severe muscles aches that are a symptom of a more serious disorder (rhabdomyolysis) in which the muscle fibers break down. If this disorder progresses, decreases in kidney function may also occur. Risk is increased with the combination use of clarithromycin, danazol, diltiazem, fluvoxamine, indinavir, nefazodone, nelfinavir, ritonavir, verapamil, troleandomycin, cyclosporine, fibric acid derivatives, erythromycin, niacin, azole antifungals, or large quantities of grapefruit juice.

DRUG INTERACTIONS
Azole antifungals, ciprofloxacin, clarithromycin, diclofenac, doxycycline, erythromycin, imatinib, isoniazid, nefazodone, nicardipine, propofol, protease inhibitors, quinidine, and verapamil. Stop lovastatin therapy during concurrent clarithromycin, erythromycin, itraconazole, or ketoconazole therapy. Cyclosporine, clofibrate, fenofibrate, gemfibrozil, niacin, warfarin, levothyroxine may be increased by lovastatin. Digoxin, norethindrone, and ethinyl estradiol levels, cholestyramine.

FOOD INTERACTIONS
Avoid intake of large quantities of grapefruit juice (greater than or equal to 1 quart/day); may increase toxicity.

HERBAL INTERACTIONS
St. John's wort

PREGNANCY AND BREAST-FEEDING CAUTIONS
FDA Pregnancy Risk Category X. Lovastatin should not be used during breast-feeding.

SPECIAL INFORMATION
Before initiation of therapy, patients should be placed on a standard cholesterol-lowering diet for six weeks and the diet should be continued during drug therapy. Take as directed, with food at evening meal. Report any signs of muscle pain, tenderness, or weakness to doctor. Extended release tablets (Altoprev) should be swallowed whole; do not chew, crush, or cut.

MAGNESIUM SULFATE
(mag-NEE-zhum SUL-fate)

Injection

NEWLY DISCOVERED USES (OFF-LABEL)

Cardiac arrest, premature labor (preterm), tachycardia in children, Torsades de Pointes, ventricular tachycardia

ORIGINAL USES (ON-LABEL)
Treatment and prevention of low magnesium levels, seizure prevention in severe pre-eclampsia or eclampsia, pediatric acute nephritis (inflammation of the kidney)

BRAND NAME
Magnesium Sulfate

DRUG CLASS
Electrolyte supplement (injection)

DESCRIPTION
When taken orally, magnesium promotes bowel evacuation by expanding the colon. When given by injection, magnesium decreases the level of a certain neurotransmitter in the body's motor nerve terminals and acts on the muscular tissue of the heart to strengthen the heart's performance.

POTENTIAL SIDE EFFECTS
Changes in blood pressure and heart rate with rapid administration. Flushing, sweating, depressed reflexes, flaccid paralysis, low temperatures, cardiac and central nervous system (CNS) depression.

CAUTIONS
- Inform your doctor if you have heart disease or damage, kidney or liver problems, myasthenia gravis, other neuromuscular disease, or Addison's disease.
- Requires monitoring of serum magnesium level, respiratory rate, deep tendon reflex, and kidney function.

DRUG INTERACTIONS
Neuromuscular blockers (such as tubocurarine, vecuronium, succinylcholine)

FOOD INTERACTIONS
Unknown

HERBAL INTERACTIONS
Unknown

PREGNANCY AND BREAST-FEEDING CAUTIONS
FDA Pregnancy Risk Category B. Consult your doctor regarding breast-feeding.

SPECIAL INFORMATION
This information does not apply to oral formulations.

MECAMYLAMINE
(meh-CAM-el-ah-mean)

NEWLY DISCOVERED USES (OFF-LABEL)
Smoking cessation

ORIGINAL USES (ON-LABEL)
Used in the treatment of moderately severe to severe high blood pressure and in uncomplicated malignant high blood pressure

BRAND NAME
Inversine

DRUG CLASS
Antihypertensive

DESCRIPTION
This drug inhibits the chemical acetylcholine in nerves in the body, causing a decrease in blood pressure.

POTENTIAL SIDE EFFECTS
Postural hypotension (sudden drop in blood pressure related to standing up from a sitting or lying down position), drowsiness, seizures, confusion, sexual ability decreased, dry mouth, loss of appetite, nausea, discomfort upon urination, uncontrolled movements of hands, arms, legs or face, blurred vision, enlarged pupils, shortness of breath.

CAUTION
- Not for use if you have coronary insufficiency, pyloric stenosis, glaucoma, uremia, recent heart attack.
- Inform your doctor if you are currently taking sulfonamides or antibiotics that cause neuromuscular blockade.
- Notify your doctor if you have impaired kidney function, prostatic hyperplasia, or bladder obstruction.
- Do not stop abruptly.
- This drug rarely produces several central nervous system effects (such as tremor, involuntary movements). The risk of these effects is increased by large doses or the use of therapy in kidney dysfunction or cerebral insufficiency.

DRUG INTERACTIONS
Sulfonamides and antibiotics that cause neuromuscular blockade, anesthesia, other antihypertensives

FOOD INTERACTIONS
Unknown

HERBAL INTERACTIONS
Unknown

PREGNANCY AND BREAST-FEEDING CAUTIONS
FDA Pregnancy Risk Category C. Not recommended during breast-feeding.

SPECIAL INFORMATION
This information only applies to prescription products.

MECLIZINE
(MEH-cle-zeen)

NEWLY DISCOVERED USES (OFF-LABEL)
Ménière's disease

ORIGINAL USES (ON-LABEL)
Prevention and treatment of symptoms of motion sickness; management of vertigo with diseases affecting the vestibular system

BRAND NAME
Antivert

DRUG CLASS
Antiemetic, antihistamine

DESCRIPTION
Meclizine decreases the nausea, vomiting and dizziness of motion sickness. It works by limiting the excitability of the middle ear and blocking conduction in the middle ear pathways.

POTENTIAL SIDE EFFECTS
Slight to moderate drowsiness, thickening of the bronchial secretions, headache, fatigue, nervousness, appetite increase, weight gain, nausea, joint aches, sore throat.

CAUTIONS
- Notify your doctor if you have angle-closure glaucoma, prostatic hyperplasia, pyloric or duodenal obstruction, or bladder neck obstruction.
- Use caution in hot weather and during exercise.
- Elderly may be at risk for anticholinergic side effects such as glaucoma, prostatic hyperplasia, constipation, and gastric obstructive disease.
- Discontinue use after one to two weeks if vertigo does not respond.

DRUG INTERACTIONS
Increased risk of toxicity with concurrent use of central nervous depressants (alcohol, narcotics), neuroleptics, and anticholinergics. Consult your doctor or pharmacist prior to starting a new medication, herbal product, or nonprescription drug.

FOOD INTERACTIONS
Alcohol

HERBAL INTERACTIONS
Unknown

PREGNANCY AND BREAST-FEEDING CAUTIONS
FDA Pregnancy Risk Category B. Excretion into breast milk is unknown. Breast-feeding is not recommended while using meclizine.

MECLOFENAMATE
(meh-clo-phen-A-mate)

NEWLY DISCOVERED USES (OFF-LABEL)
Psoriatic arthritis

ORIGINAL USES (ON-LABEL)
Treatment of inflammatory disorders, rheumatoid and osteo-arthritis, mild to moderate pain, painful menstruation

BRAND NAME
Meclomen

DRUG CLASS
Pain reliever (nonsteroidal anti-inflammatory [NSAID])

DESCRIPTION
This drug inhibits the production of prostaglandin by decreasing the activity of the enzyme responsible for its production. Prostaglandins are known mediators of pain and inflammation.

POTENTIAL SIDE EFFECTS
Dizziness, skin rash, abdominal cramps, heartburn, indigestion, headache, nervousness, itching, fluid retention, vomiting, ringing in the ears (tinnitus).

CAUTIONS
- Notify your doctor if you have an allergy to other NSAIDs or aspirin.
- Inform your doctor if you have gastric bleeding, congestive heart failure, high blood pressure, dehydration, decreased kidney or liver function, history of gastric disease or those receiving anticoagulants.
- Elderly are at high risk of adverse effects from NSAIDs.
- Use the lowest effective dose for the shortest duration possible.
- Central nervous system adverse effects such as confusion, agitation, and hallucinations are generally seen in overdose or high dose situations and may occur at lower doses in elderly patients.
- Withhold for at least four to six hours prior to surgical or dental procedures.
- May cause changes in kidney function.

DRUG INTERACTIONS
Anticoagulants (warfarin, heparins), other antiplatelet drugs (ticlopidine, clopidogrel, aspirin, abciximab, dipyridamole,

eptifibatide, tirofiban), cyclosporine, lithium, corticosteroids, methotrexate, antihypertensive drugs (such as ACE inhibitors, angiotensin antagonists, diuretics and hydralazine), cholestyramine, colestipol

FOOD INTERACTIONS
Alcohol

HERBAL INTERACTIONS
Unknown

PREGNANCY AND BREAST-FEEDING CAUTIONS
FDA Pregnancy Risk Category B, Pregnancy Risk Category D in third trimester. Excreted in breast milk. Consult your doctor.

MEDROXYPROGESTERONE ACETATE
(me-DROKS-ee-proe-JES-te-rone
AS-eh-tate)

Oral

NEWLY DISCOVERED USES (OFF-LABEL)
Chronic pelvic pain, endometriosis, hirsutism, McCune-Albright syndrome, menopausal symptoms, pelvic congestion, polycystic ovary, precocious puberty

ORIGINAL USES (ON-LABEL)
Endometrial cancer, kidney cancer, secondary amenorrhea or abnormal uterine bleeding due to hormonal imbalance, reduction of endometrial hyperplasia in non-hysterectomized postmenopausal women receiving conjugated estrogens

BRAND NAME
Provera

DRUG CLASS
Progestin

DESCRIPTION
This drug prevents ovulation by blocking the secretion of pituitary hormones. It also causes endometrial thinning.

POTENTIAL SIDE EFFECTS
Dizziness, headache, nervousness, decreased libido, menstrual irregularities (bleeding, amenorrhea, or both), abdominal pain/discomfort, weight changes, weakness, leg cramps, joint aches.

CAUTIONS
- Notify your doctor if you have heart problems or disease. When this drug is used in combination with estrogens, it may increase risk of cardiac problems, stroke, or blood clots.
- Notify your doctor immediately if you develop sudden partial or complete vision loss, sudden onset of vision changes, or migraine. Will require an eye exam immediately.
- Notify your doctor if you have any diseases that may be aggravated by fluid retention (including asthma, epilepsy, migraine, diabetes, or renal dysfunction).
- Notify your doctor if you have depression or a history of depression.
- This drug should be discontinued at least 4–6 weeks prior to surgeries associated with an increased risk of blood clots or during periods of prolonged immobilization.
- Notify your doctor if you develop abdominal pain, jaundice, dark urine.

DRUG INTERACTIONS
Consult your doctor or pharmacist prior to starting any new prescription medication, herbal product, or nonprescription drug while on this therapy.

FOOD INTERACTIONS
Absorption increased if the oral tablet is taken with food.

HERBAL INTERACTIONS
Unknown

PREGNANCY RISK
FDA Pregnancy Risk Category X. Excreted in breast milk. Consult your doctor.

SPECIAL INFORMATION
This drug has a black box warning regarding the teratogenic effects when used in pregnancy.

MEDROXYPROGESTERONE CONTRACEPTIVE INJECTION
(me-DROKS-ee-proe-JES-te-rone)

NEWLY DISCOVERED USES (OFF-LABEL)
Endometriosis, menorrhagia, premenstrual syndrome (PMS)

ORIGINAL USES (ON-LABEL)
Long-term contraceptive in women (injectable administered every three months)

BRAND NAME
Depo-Provera

DRUG CLASS
Contraceptive (progestin)

DESCRIPTION
This drug prevents ovulation by blocking the secretion of pituitary hormones. It also causes endometrial thinning.

POTENTIAL SIDE EFFECTS
Dizziness, headache, nervousness, decreased libido, menstrual irregularities (bleeding, amenorrhea, or both), abdominal pain/discomfort, weight changes, weakness, leg cramps, joint aches.

CAUTIONS
- Prolonged use may result in a loss of bone mineral density (BMD), which may not be completely reversible once the drug is stopped. Long-term use (more than two years) should be limited to situations where other birth control methods are inadequate.
- Notify your doctor if you have heart problems or disease. When this drug is used in combination with estrogens, it may increase your risk of cardiac problems, stroke, or blood clots.
- Notify your doctor immediately if you develop sudden partial or complete vision loss, sudden onset of vision changes, or migraine. Will require an eye exam immediately.
- Notify your doctor if you have any diseases that may be aggravated by fluid retention (including asthma, epilepsy, migraine, diabetes, or renal dysfunction).
- Notify your doctor if you have depression or a history of depression.

- This drug should be discontinued at least 4–6 weeks prior to surgeries associated with an increased risk of blood clots or during periods of prolonged immobilization.
- Notify your doctor if you develop abdominal pain, jaundice, dark urine.
- You will experience disruption of menstrual bleeding patterns initially, which will regulate as therapy continues. Report heavy or continuous bleeding to your doctor.

DRUG INTERACTIONS

Because of the potential for significant drug interactions and loss of contraceptive effectiveness, consult your doctor or pharmacist prior to starting any new prescription medication, herbal product, or nonprescription drug while on this therapy.

FOOD INTERACTIONS

Unknown

HERBAL INTERACTIONS

Unknown

PREGNANCY RISK

FDA Pregnancy Risk Category X. Excreted in breast milk. Consult your doctor.

SPECIAL INFORMATION

It is not known if the use of this drug during adolescence or early adulthood, when bone building is critical, will reduce peak bone mass and increase the risk of fractures in later life. This drug should be used as a long-term birth control method (more than two years) only if other birth control methods are inadequate. This drug has a black box warning regarding the teratogenic effects when used in pregnancy.

MEFENAMIC ACID
(me-fe-NAM-ik AS-id)

NEWLY DISCOVERED USES (OFF-LABEL)

Menstrual migraine, premenstrual dysphoric disorder (PMDD), premenstrual syndrome (PMS)

ORIGINAL USES (ON-LABEL)
Short-term relief of mild to moderate pain including primary painful menstruation and lower back pain

BRAND NAME
Ponstel

DRUG CLASS
Pain reliever, anti-inflammatory (nonsteroidal anti-inflammatory [NSAID])

DESCRIPTION
This drug inhibits the production of prostaglandin, a chemical in the body responsible for inflammation and pain.

POTENTIAL SIDE EFFECTS
Headache, nervousness, dizziness, itching, rash, fluid retention, abdominal cramps, nausea, vomiting, bleeding, ringing in the ears (tinnitus), increased liver function tests.

CAUTIONS
- Not for use if you are allergic to aspirin or other NSAIDs.
- Not for use if you have active gastric/duodenal ulcer disease.
- Do not use during third trimester of pregnancy.
- Ask physician about use if you have any of the following medical problems: high blood pressure, dehydration, decreased kidney or liver function, history of gastric disease.

DRUG INTERACTIONS
Aspirin, lithium, steroids, methotrexate, digoxin, cyclosporine (kidney toxicity), diuretics, some antihypertensives, and warfarin (bleeding). CYP2C8/9 inhibitors may increase the effect of mefenamic acid.

FOOD INTERACTIONS
Alcohol

HERBAL INTERACTIONS
Cat's claw, dong quai, evening primrose, feverfew, garlic, ginger, ginkgo, red clover, horse chestnut, green tea, ginseng

PREGNANCY AND BREAST-FEEDING CAUTIONS
FDA Pregnancy Risk Category C. FDA Pregnancy Risk Category D in third trimester. Not known if excreted in breast milk. Do not breast-feed during therapy with this drug.

SPECIAL INFORMATION

Stop taking this drug (with your doctor's approval) approximately 24 to 48 hours prior to surgical or dental procedures as it affects the body's ability to form blood clots and may increase bleeding time. In April 2005, the FDA announced the potential addition of a black box warning to the labeling of this class of drugs (NSAIDs), specifically regarding potential serious cardiac events and potentially life-threatening gastric adverse events.

MEGESTROL ACETATE
(mee-GES-trawl)

NEWLY DISCOVERED USES (OFF-LABEL)
| Menopausal symptoms

ORIGINAL USES (ON-LABEL)

Palliative treatment of certain cancers (such as breast and endometrial), appetite enhancer

BRAND NAME

Megace

DRUG CLASS

Antineoplastic, hormone

DESCRIPTION

This drug is used to treat cancer. It interferes with the normal estrogen cycle, affects a hormone called luteinizing hormone, and may also have direct effect on the endometrium in endometrial cancers.

POTENTIAL SIDE EFFECTS

Weight gain, blood clots, nausea, breakthrough menstrual bleeding, headache, back pain, abdominal pain, breast tenderness.

CAUTIONS

- Notify your doctor if you have diabetes, a current problem with or a history of blood clots, or if you are pregnant. Do not become pregnant while taking this medication.
- Elderly women may develop vaginal bleeding or discharge.

DRUG INTERACTIONS

Dofetilide

FOOD INTERACTIONS

Unknown

HERBAL INTERACTIONS
Black cohosh, dong-quai

PREGNANCY AND BREAST-FEEDING CAUTIONS
FDA Pregnancy Risk Category X. Excreted in the breast milk. Do not use while breast-feeding.

SPECIAL INFORMATION
Contraceptive measures are recommended during therapy.

MELOXICAM
(mel-OKS-I-kam)

NEWLY DISCOVERED USES (OFF-LABEL)
Ankylosing spondylitis, gout, periodontitis

ORIGINAL USES (ON-LABEL)
Relief of signs and symptoms of osteoarthritis and rheumatoid arthritis

BRAND NAME
Mobic

DRUG CLASS
Pain reliever (non-steroidal anti-inflammatory)

DESCRIPTION
Meloxicam blocks prostaglandin, a chemical in the body responsible for inflammation and pain.

POTENTIAL SIDE EFFECTS
Edema, headache, dizziness, rash, diarrhea, stomach upset, nausea, flatulence, abdominal pain, upper respiratory infection, flu-like symptoms.

CAUTIONS
- Not for use if allergic to aspirin or other NSAIDs.
- Not for use in active gastric/duodenal ulcer disease.
- Do not use during third trimester of pregnancy.
- Ask physician about use if you have any of the following medical problems: high blood pressure, dehydration, decreased kidney or liver function, history of gastric disease.
- Elderly are at higher risk of developing side effects.

DRUG INTERACTIONS
Aspirin, corticosteroids, lithium, methotrexate, digoxin, cyclosporine (increased risk of kidney toxicity), diuretics, some antihypertensives, and warfarin (bleeding), heparins, ticlopidine, Clopidogrel, dipyridamole, Eptifibatide, tirofiban, cholestyramine.

FOOD INTERACTIONS
Avoid ethanol, may enhance stomach irritation.

HERBAL INTERACTIONS
Unknown

PREGNANCY AND BREAST-FEEDING CAUTIONS
FDA Pregnancy Risk Category C. In third trimester FDA Pregnancy Risk Category D. Excretion in breast milk is unknown. Do not use during breast-feeding.

SPECIAL INFORMATION
In April 2005, the FDA announced the potential addition of a black box warning to the labeling of this class of drugs (NSAIDs), specifically regarding potential serious cardiac events and potentially life-threatening gastric adverse events.

MEMANTINE
(me-MAN-teen)

NEWLY DISCOVERED USES (OFF-LABEL)
Diabetic neuropathy

ORIGINAL USES (ON-LABEL)
Alzheimer's disease

BRAND NAME
Namenda

DRUG CLASS
N-Methyl-D-aspartate receptor antagonist

DESCRIPTION
This drug has been shown to have beneficial effects on symptoms of Alzheimer's disease.

POTENTIAL SIDE EFFECTS

Dizziness, confusion, headache, hallucination, somnolence, constipation, vomiting, coughing, shortness of breath, high blood pressure, back pain, pain, fatigue.

CAUTIONS

- Dose reduction may be needed if you have impaired kidney function.
- The acidity of urine affects the blood levels of this drug. Less acidic (alkaline or basic) urine results in a lower excretion rate of the drug from the body and thus, higher levels of the drug. Urine acidity may be affected by diet, drugs (such as sodium bicarbonate).

DRUG INTERACTIONS

Hydrochlorothiazide, triamterene, cimetidine, ranitidine, quinidine, nicotine, carbonic anhydrase inhibitors (such as acetazolamide), sodium bicarbonate.

FOOD INTERACTIONS

May be taken with or without food.

HERBAL INTERACTIONS

Unknown

PREGNANCY AND BREAST-FEEDING CAUTIONS

FDA Pregnancy Risk Category B. Excretion in breast milk unknown. Consult your doctor.

SPECIAL INFORMATION

Requires gradual dosage titration.

MERCAPTOPURINE
(mer-kap-toe-PYOOR-een)

NEWLY DISCOVERED USES (OFF-LABEL)

Autoimmune hepatitis, Crohn's disease, psoriatic arthritis

ORIGINAL USES (ON-LABEL)

Maintenance and induction therapy of acute lymphoblastic leukemia (ALL)

BRAND NAME

Purinethol

DRUG CLASS
Antineoplastic

DESCRIPTION
This drug blocks DNA and RNA synthesis by incorporating itself into DNA and RNA and hindering the synthesis process.

POTENTIAL SIDE EFFECTS
Various blood disorders, liver toxicity, fever, hyperpigmentation, rash, increased uric acid, nausea, vomiting, diarrhea, mouth inflammation and ulcers, anorexia, stomach pain, kidney toxicity.

CAUTIONS
- Use with caution if you have bone marrow suppression or toxicity.
- Use caution with other liver-toxic drugs.
- Patients with genetic deficiency of thiopurine methyltransferase (TPMT) or concurrent therapy with drugs that may inhibit TPMT (olsalazine) or xanthine oxidase (allopurinol) may be sensitive to blood toxic effects.
- May be associated with increased risk of pancreatitis when used in patients who have inflammatory bowel disease.

DRUG INTERACTIONS
Allopurinol, trimethoprim-sulfamethoxazole, aminosalicylates (olsalazine, mesalamine, sulfasalazine), warfarin, hepatotoxic drugs as well as any other drugs that could potentially alter the metabolic function of the liver, could produce higher mercaptopurine levels and greater toxicities.

FOOD INTERACTIONS
Unknown

HERBAL INTERACTIONS
Unknown

PREGNANCY AND BREAST-FEEDING CAUTIONS
FDA Pregnancy Risk Category D. Excreted in breast milk. Do not use during breast-feeding.

SPECIAL INFORMATION
Contraceptive measures are recommended for both men and women during therapy. Inform your doctor immediately if any of the following occur: sore throat, chills, nausea, vomiting, unusual bleeding or bruising, yellow discoloration of the skin or eyes, abdominal or flank pain, swelling of the legs or feet. Maintain adequate fluid intake.

MEROPENEM
(MIRO-pen-em)

NEWLY DISCOVERED USES (OFF-LABEL)
Nocardiasis

ORIGINAL USES (ON-LABEL)
Various bacterial infections of the respiratory tract, urinary tract, intra-abdominal, gynecological, bone and joint, skin structure

BRAND NAME
Merrem IV

DRUG CLASS
Antibiotic (carbapenem)

DESCRIPTION
This drug kills bacteria by inhibiting the production of bacteria cell walls.

POTENTIAL SIDE EFFECTS
Headache, rash, diarrhea, nausea/vomiting, oral yeast infection, inflammation at the injection site, changes in liver function, blood disorders.

CAUTIONS
- Dosage requires adjustment in patients who have impaired kidney function and the elderly.
- Prolonged use may result in superinfection.
- Has been associated with central nervous system adverse effects including confusional states and seizures with increased risk of these events in kidney dysfunction. Inform your doctor if you have a history of seizures or allergy to penicillins or other antibiotics.
- Notify your doctor if persistent diarrhea occurs during or soon after completing therapy.
- May require specific lab testing during prolonged therapy.

DRUG INTERACTIONS
Probenecid, valproic acid

FOOD INTERACTIONS
Unknown

HERBAL INTERACTIONS
Unknown

PREGNANCY AND BREAST-FEEDING CAUTIONS
FDA Pregnancy Risk Category B. Excretion into breast milk is unknown. Consult your doctor.

METFORMIN
(met-FOR-min)

NEWLY DISCOVERED USES (OFF-LABEL)
Polycystic ovary syndrome, prevention of type 2 diabetes

ORIGINAL USES (ON-LABEL)
Non-insulin dependent diabetes mellitus

BRAND NAMES
Glucophage, Glucophage XR, Riomet

DRUG CLASS
Antidiabetic

DESCRIPTION
This drug decreases glucose production in the liver, decreasing intestinal absorption of glucose and improving insulin sensitivity.

POTENTIAL SIDE EFFECTS
Diarrhea, nausea, vomiting, flatulence, abdominal discomfort, headache, low blood glucose.

CAUTIONS
- Lactic acidosis (increased levels of lactic acid in the blood) may be characterized by initial symptoms of malaise, muscle aches, breathing difficulty, increased sedation, abdominal distress. Report any of these symptoms to your doctor immediately.
- If you are a diabetic, follow the diet and exercise plan as prescribed by your doctor.
- Notify your doctor if you have impaired kidney or liver function. May require monitoring of kidney function.
- This drug needs to be temporarily stopped if you are having surgery or a procedure that requires the administration of a contrast dye. Discuss the best possible way to do this with your doctor.
- May decrease vitamin B12 levels.
- Elderly may require reduced dosing.

DRUG INTERACTIONS

Glyburide, alcohol, amiloride, digoxin, morphine, procainamide, quinidine, quinine, ranitidine, triamterene, trimethoprim, vancomycin, furosemide, cimetidine, contrast dyes, nifedipine

FOOD INTERACTIONS

Take on an empty stomach.

HERBAL INTERACTIONS

Guar gum, fenugreek, glucomannan, psyllium, bitter melon, St. John's wort, ginseng, eucalyptus, gymnema sylvestre, and excessive ingestion of natural licorice

PREGNANCY AND BREAST-FEEDING CAUTIONS

FDA Pregnancy Risk Category B. Excretion in breast milk unknown. Consult your doctor.

SPECIAL INFORMATION

Discuss the aspects of diet and exercise and regular testing of blood glucose. Avoid excessive alcohol intake. The extended release tablets should be swallowed whole and not crushed or chewed. This drug has a black box warning regarding the risk of developing lactic acidosis.

METHAZOLAMIDE
(meth-a-ZOE-la-mide)

NEWLY DISCOVERED USES (OFF-LABEL)

Ménière's disease

ORIGINAL USES (ON-LABEL)

Glaucoma

BRAND NAME

Neptazane

DRUG CLASS

Anti-glaucoma (carbonic anhydrase inhibitor)

DESCRIPTION

This drug slows abnormal and excessive discharge from central nervous system neurons. This action results in a decreased pressure in the eyeball.

POTENTIAL SIDE EFFECTS

Malaise, fever, mental depression, drowsiness, dizziness, nervousness, headache, confusion, fatigue, trembling, itching, rash, electrolyte disturbances, nausea, vomiting, diarrhea, constipation, weight loss, dry mouth, urinary frequency, crystals in urine, blood disorders.

CAUTIONS

- Notify your doctor if you have an allergy to sulfonamides (antibacterials or diuretics) prior to therapy with this drug, as this drug should not be taken in patients with sulfonamide allergies.
- Not for use if you have liver disease or insufficiency (may result in coma), with decreased sodium and or potassium levels, adrenocortical insufficiency, severe kidney disease or dysfunction, or severe lung obstruction.
- Not for long-term use in non-congestive angle-closure glaucoma.
- Requires blood monitoring during therapy to screen for blood disorders.
- Malaise, tiredness, and muscle aches are indicative of excessive doses and acidosis in elderly patients.

DRUG INTERACTIONS

Diuretics, steroids, digoxin, salicylates, primidone, lithium, amphetamines, quinidine, procainamide, methenamine, phenobarbital.

FOOD INTERACTIONS

Unknown

HERBAL INTERACTIONS

Unknown

PREGNANCY AND BREAST-FEEDING CAUTIONS

FDA Pregnancy Risk Category C. Excretion in breast milk unknown. Breast-feeding is not recommended while using this drug.

SPECIAL INFORMATION

If stomach upset occurs, take with food.

METHIMAZOLE
(meth-IM-a-zole)

NEWLY DISCOVERED USES (OFF-LABEL)
Thyroid crisis

ORIGINAL USES (ON-LABEL)
Hyperthyroidism

BRAND NAME
Tapazole

DRUG CLASS
Antithyroid

DESCRIPTION
This drug inhibits the synthesis of thyroid hormones.

POTENTIAL SIDE EFFECTS
Headache, vertigo, drowsiness, depression, hives, itching, nausea, vomiting, stomach distress, taste changes, joint aches, hair loss, bruising.

CAUTIONS
- Some serious but rare blood disorders may occur with the use of this drug. Report any symptoms to your doctor that may suggest these are developing including, hay fever, unusual bleeding, vomiting, jaundice, sore throat, skin rash, fever, general malaise.
- Requires periodic monitoring of thyroid function and bleeding times.

DRUG INTERACTIONS
Warfarin

FOOD INTERACTIONS
Unknown

HERBAL INTERACTIONS
Unknown

PREGNANCY AND BREAST-FEEDING CAUTIONS
FDA Pregnancy Risk Category D. Excreted in breast milk. Consult your doctor.

METHOTREXATE
(meth-oh-TREKS-ate)

NEWLY DISCOVERED USES (OFF-LABEL)
Abortion, ankylosing spondylitis, dermatomyositis/polymyositis, ectopic pregnancy, Felty's syndrome, food poisoning, Lyme arthritis, multiple sclerosis, polyarteritis nodosa, primary biliary cirrhosis, psoriatic arthritis, sarcoidosis, scleroderma, steroid dependent asthma, systemic lupus erythematosus, temporal arteritis, urticaria, uveitis

ORIGINAL USES (ON-LABEL)
Treatment of various cancers, psoriasis, rheumatoid arthritis

BRAND NAMES
Rheumatrex, Trexall

DRUG CLASS
Antineoplastic, antimetabolite, folate antagonist, immunosuppressant

DESCRIPTION
This drug inhibits cellular DNA synthesis, repair and replication by inhibiting an important enzyme. This stops cells from rapidly reproducing in cancer patients. The mechanism of action in rheumatoid arthritis patients is not known, but it does exhibit effects on immune activity.

POTENTIAL SIDE EFFECTS
Ulcers in the mouth, blood disorders (decreased white blood cells), nausea, abdominal discomfort, malaise, fatigue, chills, fever, dizziness, decreased resistance to infection, anorexia, drowsiness, headache, blurred vision, changes in vision, liver toxicity, rash, serious skin reactions, increased susceptibility to infections.

CAUTIONS
- Notify your doctor if you have severe kidney or liver impairment, pre-existing profound bone marrow suppression with psoriasis or rheumatoid arthritis, alcoholic liver disease, AIDS, or pre-existing blood disorders.
- Not for use if you are pregnant.
- Bone and soft tissue necrosis may occur following radiation treatment.

- Painful plaque erosions may occur when used as psoriasis treatment.
- Use with caution if you have peptic ulcer disease, ulcerative colitis, or pre-existing bone marrow suppression.
- May cause inflammation of the lungs; report any symptoms of shortness of breath or breathing difficulties to your doctor.
- The elderly may be at increased risk of side effects and toxicity.
- Report any of the following symptoms to your doctor immediately: vomiting, diarrhea, mouth ulcers, rash.
- Requires periodic testing of liver function before and during therapy.

DRUG INTERACTIONS
Salicylates, sulfonamides, probenecid, high dose penicillins, cytarabine, mercaptopurine, tetracycline, chloramphenicol, broad spectrum antibiotics, folic acid, trimethoprim/sulfamethoxazole, cyclosporine, and NSAIDs (such as ibuprofen, indomethacin, naprosyn, etc.), methotrexate and live virus vaccines can result in vaccinia infections, other drugs which are potentially toxic to the liver (azathioprine, retinoids, sulfasalazine). Do not take corticosteroids within 12 hours of taking methotrexate.

FOOD INTERACTIONS
Avoid alcohol, caffeine

HERBAL INTERACTIONS
Echinacea

PREGNANCY RISK
FDA Pregnancy Risk Category X. Excreted in breast milk. Do not use methotrexate while pregnant or breast-feeding.

SPECIAL INFORMATION
This drug has a black box warning that describes and discusses serious toxic reactions associated with therapy. Please review these potential side effects with your doctor prior to the initiation of therapy.

METHYLERGONOVINE
(meth-il-er-goe-NOE-veen)

NEWLY DISCOVERED USES (OFF-LABEL)
Incomplete abortion

ORIGINAL USES (ON-LABEL)
Prevention/treatment of postpartum and post-abortion bleeding caused by uterine loss of muscle tone

BRAND NAME
Methergine

DRUG CLASS
Uterine active

DESCRIPTION
This drug causes sustained uterine smooth muscle contractions, shortening the third stage of labor.

POTENTIAL SIDE EFFECTS
High blood pressure, headache, nausea, vomiting, transient pain, shortness of breath, dizziness, ringing in the ears, increased sweating.

CAUTIONS
- Should not be routinely administered via the intravenous route.
- Should be used cautiously if you have sepsis, certain types of vascular disease, or with kidney or liver impairment.

DRUG INTERACTIONS
Antipsychotics, metoclopramide, beta blockers, ergot derivatives, MAOIs, SSRIs, TCAs, nefazodone, sumatriptan, trazodone, buspirone, sumatriptan, peripheral vasoconstrictors.

This drug is metabolized by specific set of liver enzymes. Several other drugs interfere with these liver enzymes, and thus may increase or decrease the clearance of this drug from the body, potentially increasing the risk of side effects or decreasing effectiveness. When these drugs are given in combination with methylergonovine, dosage adjustments may be needed. As these are too numerous to list, you should always check with your doctor or pharmacist prior to starting a new medication, herbal, or nonprescription product.

FOOD INTERACTIONS
Unknown

HERBAL INTERACTIONS
Unknown

PREGNANCY AND BREAST-FEEDING CAUTIONS
FDA Pregnancy Risk Category C. This drug is not to be used during pregnancy because of its propensity to cause sustained, tetanic

uterine contractions, resulting in loss of oxygen to the fetus. It is only intended for use after delivery. Excreted into the breast milk. Consult your doctor.

METHYLPHENIDATE
(meth-il-FEN-i-date)

NEWLY DISCOVERED USES (OFF-LABEL)
Autism, bipolar disorder, brain tumor, familial male precocious puberty (sexual hyperactivity), multiple sclerosis

ORIGINAL USES (ON-LABEL)
Treatment of attention-deficit/hyperactivity disorder (ADHD), narcolepsy

BRAND NAMES
Concerta, Metadate CD, Metadate ER, Methylin, Methylin ER, Ritalin, Ritalin LA, Ritalin-SR

DRUG CLASS
Central nervous system stimulant, nonamphetamine

DESCRIPTION
This drug stimulates the central nervous system by blocking the reuptake of dopamine and stimulating the cerebral cortex and surrounding structures in a way similar to amphetamines.

POTENTIAL SIDE EFFECTS
Depression, dizziness, vomiting, cough increased, headache, insomnia, drowsiness, hair loss, rash, growth retardation, anorexia, nausea, blurred vision, change in heart rhythm, high blood pressure.

CAUTIONS
- Not for use if you have marked anxiety, tension, agitation, glaucoma, Tourette's syndrome, or tics.
- Do not use during or within 14 days following MAO inhibitor therapy.
- This drug has a high potential for abuse/psychic dependence. Do not stop this medication abruptly.
- Notify your doctor if you have bipolar disorder, diabetes mellitus, heart disease, seizure disorders, insomnia, porphyria, severe depression, or mild high blood pressure.

- May worsen symptoms of behavior and thought disorder in psychotic patients.
- Therapy has been associated with growth suppression.
- The brand, Concerta, of this drug does not change shape in the esophagus, stomach or intestinal tract and thus should not be given to anyone with pre-existing gastrointestinal narrowing.

DRUG INTERACTIONS
MAO inhibitors, venlafaxine, phenytoin, phenobarbital, tricyclic antidepressants, warfarin, clonidine or sibutramine.

FOOD INTERACTIONS
Alcohol

HERBAL INTERACTIONS
Ephedra, yohimbe

PREGNANCY AND BREAST-FEEDING CAUTIONS
FDA Pregnancy Risk Category C. Excretion in breast milk is unknown. Do not breast-feed during therapy.

SPECIAL INFORMATION
Each brand has specific instructions regarding dosing and timing. Consult with your pharmacist regarding this information. This drug has a black box warning regarding the risk of dependence when used in patients with a history of drug dependence or alcoholism.

METHYLPREDNISOLONE
(meth-il-pred-NIS-oh-lone)

NEWLY DISCOVERED USES (OFF-LABEL)
Acute spinal cord injury, chronic obstructive lung disease, drug-induced anaphylaxis, juvenile rheumatoid arthritis, membranous nephropathy, optic neuritis, respiratory distress syndrome, sudden hearing loss, urticaria, uveitis

ORIGINAL USES (ON-LABEL)
Various disorders of endocrine nature, collagen disease, skin disease, allergic states, gastrointestinal disorders, lung diseases, blood disorders, nervous system, certain leukemias and lymphomas, and blood disorders. Also used to prevent/treat graft-versus-host disease after allogeneic bone marrow transplantation

BRAND NAMES
Depo-Medrol, Medrol, Solu-Medrol

DRUG CLASS
Corticosteroid

DESCRIPTION
This drug decreases inflammation by suppressing white blood cell migration and reversing capillary permeability.

POTENTIAL SIDE EFFECTS
Edema, high blood pressure, insomnia, headache, acne, skin atrophy, diabetes mellitus, adrenal suppression, increased lipid levels, pituitary-adrenal axis suppression, low potassium, sodium and water retention, peptic ulcer, nausea, vomiting, increased white blood cell (transient), joint aches, fractures, glaucoma, infections, allergic reactions.

CAUTIONS
- Steroid use may mask some signs of infection and may make you more susceptible to infections. Avoid contact with individuals who have chicken pox or measles.
- Contact your doctor before receiving any vaccinations.
- Inform your doctor if you have had or might have tuberculosis.
- Prolonged use of steroids may promote the development of cataracts, glaucoma, or ocular infections.
- May cause high blood pressure and fluid and sodium retention.
- Use with caution if you have hyperthyroidism, cirrhosis, liver impairment, nonspecific ulcerative colitis, high blood pressure, osteoporosis, blood clot risk, congestive heart failure, convulsive disorders, myasthenia gravis, peptic ulcer, diabetes, glaucoma, cataracts, or tuberculosis, and increased age.

DRUG INTERACTIONS
Phenytoin, phenobarbital, rifampin, diuretics, insulin, vaccinations, calcium

FOOD INTERACTIONS
Alcohol may increase irritation of gastric mucosa; limit caffeine intake.

HERBAL INTERACTIONS
St. John's wort, cat's claw, echinacea

PREGNANCY AND BREAST-FEEDING CAUTIONS
FDA Pregnancy Risk Category C. Excretion in breast milk unknown. Consult your doctor.

METOCLOPRAMIDE
(met-oh-kloe-PRA-mide)

NEWLY DISCOVERED USES (OFF-LABEL)

Hyperemesis gravidarum, migraine, nephrogenic diabetes insipidus

ORIGINAL USES (ON-LABEL)
Diabetic gastric stasis, gastroesophageal reflux disease (GERD)

BRAND NAME
Reglan

DRUG CLASS
Antiemetic, prokinetic

DESCRIPTION
This drug blocks dopamine receptors in the central nervous system to prevent nausea and vomiting.

POTENTIAL SIDE EFFECTS
Restlessness, drowsiness, extrapyramidal symptoms (neurological side effects), diarrhea, weakness, rash, breast tenderness, nausea

CAUTIONS
- Use in patients who have Parkinson's disease or history of mental illness has been associated with extrapyramidal symptoms and depression. Extrapyramidal symptoms are characterized by involuntary movements of the limbs, facial grimacing, rhythmic protrusion of the tongue, etc.
- Extrapyramidal reactions typically occur within the first 24–48 hours of use and risk is higher in children and adults more than 30 years of age and at higher doses.
- Neuroleptic malignant syndrome (such as severe high blood pressure, tremors, etc.) has been reported (rare) with metoclopramide use.
- May cause transient elevations in serum aldosterone. Use with caution if you are at risk of fluid overload.
- Use caution if you have seizure history.
- Withdrawal symptoms may result (rare) upon abrupt discontinuation.
- Dose must be adjusted if you have kidney impairment.

DRUG INTERACTIONS
Anticholinergics, antipsychotics, opiates, cimetidine, cyclosporine, levodopa, MAO inhibitors.

FOOD INTERACTIONS
Alcohol

HERBAL INTERACTIONS
Unknown

PREGNANCY AND BREAST-FEEDING CAUTIONS
FDA Pregnancy Risk Category B. Excreted into breast milk. The American Academy of Pediatrics classifies metoclopramide as a drug for which the effect on a nursing infant is unknown but may be of concern.

SPECIAL INFORMATION
Immediately notify your doctor if involuntary movements of the eyes, face, or limbs occur. May produce drowsiness; use caution when performing tasks that require alertness. Take medication 30 minutes before meals.

METOLAZONE
(me-TOLE-a-zone)

NEWLY DISCOVERED USES (OFF-LABEL)
Nephrogenic diabetes insipidus, premenstrual dysphoric disorder (PMDD)

ORIGINAL USES (ON-LABEL)
Mild to moderate high blood pressure, edema in congestive heart failure, and nephrotic syndrome, or impaired kidney function

BRAND NAMES
Mykrox, Zaroxolyn

DRUG CLASS
Antihypertensive (diuretic)

DESCRIPTION
This drug inhibits the absorption of sodium in the kidney. This causes increased excretion of sodium, water, potassium, and hydrogen ions.

POTENTIAL SIDE EFFECTS

Dizziness, sensation of rapid heart beat, sudden drop in blood pressure upon standing from a sitting or lying down position, chest pain, headache, fatigue, lethargy, malaise, low potassium, impotence, reduced libido, nausea, vomiting, increased urinary frequency at night, muscle cramps, spasm, eye itching, ringing in the ears, cough, sinus congestion.

CAUTIONS

- Inform your doctor if you are allergic to thiazide diuretics or sulfonamide drugs.
- Not for use if you have anuria (absence of urination) or if you are pregnant.
- Use with caution in patients with kidney or liver disease, gout, lupus, erythematosus, or diabetes mellitus.
- Some products may contain tartrazine.
- Mykrox is not bioequivalent to Zaroxolyn and should not be interchanged for one another.
- Electrolyte disturbances and orthostatic hypotension (dizziness upon standing) can occur.

DRUG INTERACTIONS

Loop diuretics, ACE inhibitors (such as captopril, enalapril, etc.), cyclosporine, thiazide diuretics, lithium, neuromuscular blocking drugs, cholestyramine, colestipol, NSAIDs.

FOOD INTERACTIONS

Unknown

HERBAL INTERACTIONS

Dong quai, St. John's wort, ephedra, yohimbe, garlic, ginseng, natural licorice

PREGNANCY AND BREAST-FEEDING CAUTIONS

Pregnancy Risk Category B (manufacturer) or D (expert analysis). Excreted in breast milk. Consult your doctor.

METOPROLOL
(me-toe-PROE-lole)

NEWLY DISCOVERED USES (OFF-LABEL)

Dilated cardiomyopathy, essential tremor, migraine prevention, migraine prevention in children, pheochromocytoma, prevention of recurrence and sudden death in ventricular tachycardia, ventricular tachycardia

---

ORIGINAL USES (ON-LABEL)
High blood pressure, angina pectoris, heart attack, stable congestive heart failure

BRAND NAMES
Lopressor, Toprol-XL

DRUG CLASS
Antihypertensive (beta-blocker)

DESCRIPTION
This drug decreases heart rate, cardiac contractility, blood pressure, and the heart's oxygen demand.

POTENTIAL SIDE EFFECTS
Decreased heart rate, drowsiness, insomnia, sexual dysfunction, edema, congestive heart failure, reduced peripheral circulation, mental depression, diarrhea, constipation, nausea, bronchospasm.

CAUTIONS
- Inform your doctor if you have heart conditions (such as congestive heart failure, cardiogenic shock, too low heart rate, or second- and third-degree heart block, sinus node dysfunction), are pregnant, or have lung/breathing problems.
- Do not stop this medication suddenly; taper over a gradual period.
- May cause or mask the symptoms of low blood glucose levels in diabetics.
- May mask signs of thyroid problems.
- Not indicated for high blood pressure emergencies.
- Immediately report to your doctor any signs of swelling of the extremities, sudden weight gain, changes in breathing, night cough.

DRUG INTERACTIONS
Barbiturates, cholestyramine, colestipol, rifampin, calcium channel blockers, cimetidine, oral contraceptives, diphenhydramine,

flecainide, hydralazine, hydroxychloroquine, MAO inhibitors, NSAIDs, propafenone, selective serotonin reuptake inhibitors (such as fluoxetine, paroxetine, etc.), quinidine, ciprofloxacin, thyroid hormones, clonidine, epinephrine, ergot alkaloids, lidocaine, prazosin, oral sulfonylureas (drugs used to treat diabetes)

FOOD INTERACTIONS
Take at the same time each day.

HERBAL INTERACTIONS
Dong quai, ephedra, yohimbe, ginseng, garlic

PREGNANCY AND BREAST-FEEDING CAUTIONS
FDA Pregnancy Risk Category C (manufacturer), D second and third trimesters (expert analysis). Excreted in breast milk. Consult your doctor.

SPECIAL INFORMATION
This drug has a black box warning regarding the avoidance of abrupt withdrawal in those with heart disease.

METRONIDAZOLE
(me-troe-NI-da-zole)

NEWLY DISCOVERED USES (OFF-LABEL)
Crohn's disease, diverticulitis, gingivitis, hepatic encephalopathy, periodontitis, tetanus

ORIGINAL USES (ON-LABEL)
Treatment of susceptible anaerobic bacterial and protozoal infections, topical treatment of inflammatory lesions and rosacea, bacterial vaginosis and vaginitis due to susceptible organisms (vaginal preparations)

BRAND NAMES
Flagyl, Flagyl ER, MetroCream, MetroGel, MetroLotion, MetroGel Vaginal

DRUG CLASS
Antibiotic, antiprotozoal, amebicide

DESCRIPTION
Metronidazole interacts with DNA to disrupt their structure and break DNA strands, ultimately causing cell death.

POTENTIAL SIDE EFFECTS

Uncoordinated gait, confusion, dizziness, hives, disulfiram-like reaction (flushing, nausea, vomiting), nausea, vomiting, constipation, diarrhea, metallic taste, darkened urine, blood disorders (low white blood cell count), weakness, flu-like syndrome.

Vaginal preparation: stomach cramps, abdominal cramps, vaginitis, vaginal itching or swelling.

Topical preparation: skin redness, itching, rash, dryness, worsening of rosacea.

CAUTIONS

- Notify your doctor if you have kidney or liver impairment, a history of seizures, blood disorders, or congestive heart failure.
- Therapy should be discontinued if seizures or numbness develops. Dose may need adjustment in elderly.
- May need to monitor blood for potential blood disorders (oral and intravenous formulations).
- Carcinogenic potential has been demonstrated in animal studies with chronic oral administration in rats and mice.
- Intravaginal preparations: Avoid contact with eyes. Gel may contain ingredients that cause burning or stinging.
- Topical preparation: Avoid contact with eyes. For external use only.

DRUG INTERACTIONS

Cimetidine, benzodiazepines, calcium channel blockers, cyclosporine, mirtazapine, nateglinide, nefazodone, sildenafil, tacrolimus, venlafaxine, lithium, phenytoin, phenobarbital, warfarin.

FOOD INTERACTIONS

- Concurrent use of alcohol and metronidazole should be avoided as it can cause a disulfiram reaction (such as nausea, vomiting, flushing).
- Flagyl ER should be taken on an empty stomach, at least one hour before or two hours after meals.

HERBAL INTERACTIONS

Unknown

PREGNANCY AND BREAST-FEEDING CAUTIONS

FDA Pregnancy Risk Category B. May be contraindicated in first trimester. Excreted into breast milk. Unnecessary exposure to metronidazole in breast-feeding infants should be avoided. Consult your doctor if you are breast-feeding.

SPECIAL INFORMATION

This drug has a black box warning regarding a carcinogenic effect noted in animals. Avoid unnecessary use (oral and injection). Vaginal formulation: Do not engage in sexual intercourse during therapy.

Topical formulation: Cleanse affected areas prior to application. Wait until medication dries before applying cosmetics to your face.

MEXILETINE
(MEKS-i-le-teen)

NEWLY DISCOVERED USES (OFF-LABEL)
Chronic neuropathic pain, diabetic neuropathy, myotonic dystrophy

ORIGINAL USES (ON-LABEL)
Life-threatening ventricular arrhythmias

BRAND NAME
Mexitil

DRUG CLASS
Antiarrhythmic

DESCRIPTION
This drug stabilizes heart rhythm by inhibiting sodium flow into cardiac tissue.

POTENTIAL SIDE EFFECTS
Chest pain, palpitations, dizziness, lightheadedness, tremor, nervousness, coordination difficulties, changes in sleep patterns, headache, blurred vision, fatigue, weakness, nausea, vomiting, diarrhea, constipation, dry mouth, changes in appetite, abnormal liver function tests.

CAUTIONS
- May worsen heart rate rhythm. Requires initiation of therapy in a hospital setting.
- A large study suggested that patients who had recent heart attacks and were treated with this drug experienced an increased risk of mortality.

- Requires close monitoring and possible dose reduction in patients with decreased liver function. May cause liver toxicity evidenced by increases in liver function tests.
- Rarely has caused changes in blood parameters and seizures.
- The blood level of this drug is affected by the acidity of the urine. Avoid drugs that alter urinary pH.

DRUG INTERACTIONS
Atropine, narcotics, cimetidine, fluvoxamine, phenytoin, metoclopramide, propafenone, rifampin, urinary acidifiers or alkalinizers, theophylline

FOOD INTERACTIONS
Caffeine. Take with food or an antacid.

HERBAL INTERACTIONS
Unknown

PREGNANCY AND BREAST-FEEDING CAUTIONS
FDA Pregnancy Risk Category C. Excreted in breast milk. Do not breast-feed during therapy.

SPECIAL INFORMATION
Report severe or persistent abdominal pain, nausea, vomiting, yellowing of eyes or skin, pale stools, dark urine, or persistent fever, sore throat, bleeding or bruising. Avoid changes in diet that could affect urinary acidity/alkalinity. This drug has a black box warning regarding mortality risks associated with other types of antiarrhythmics. It should be reserved for use in patients with life-threatening ventricular arrhythmias.

MIDAZOLAM
(MID-aye-zoe-lam)

NEWLY DISCOVERED USES (OFF-LABEL)
Alcohol withdrawal, seizures in children

ORIGINAL USES (ON-LABEL)
Preoperative sedation, conscious sedation prior to diagnostic/radiographic procedures, intensive care unit sedation (continuous), IV anesthesia (induction and maintenance)

BRAND NAME
Versed

DRUG CLASS
Benzodiazepine

DESCRIPTION
This drug induces sedation.

POTENTIAL SIDE EFFECTS
Drowsiness, dizziness, confusion, low blood pressure, pain/local injection site reactions, physical and psychological dependence with prolonged use, amnesia.

CAUTIONS
- May cause respiratory depression, respiratory arrest and requires appropriate resuscitative equipment and personnel for monitoring during drug administration.
- Some formulations (injection) contain benzyl alcohol—requiring slower rate of administration.
- As this drug is a central nervous system depressant, notify your doctor if you are taking other central nervous system (CNS) depressants, sedatives, or psychoactive drugs.
- Risk of dependence and acute withdrawal symptoms upon discontinuation.

DRUG INTERACTIONS
CNS depressants: Alcohol, barbiturates, narcotic analgesics, other sedatives, Aminoglutethimide, carbamazepine, nafcillin, nevirapine, phenobarbital, phenytoin, and rifamycins (rifampin, rifabutin, etc.), azole antifungals (fluconazole, ketoconazole), ciprofloxacin, clarithromycin, diclofenac, doxycycline, erythromycin, imatinib, isoniazid, nefazodone, nicardipine, propofol, protease inhibitors, quinidine, and verapamil, saquinavir, theophylline.

This drug is metabolized by a specific set of liver enzymes. Several other drugs interfere with these liver enzymes, and thus may increase or decrease the clearance of midazolam from the body, potentially increasing the risk of side effects or decreasing effectiveness. When these drugs are given in combination with midazolam, dosage adjustments may be needed. As these are too numerous to list, you should always check with your doctor or pharmacist prior to starting a new medication, herbal, or nonprescription product.

FOOD INTERACTIONS
Alcohol, grapefruit juice

HERBAL INTERACTIONS
St. John's wort, valerian, gotu kola, echinacea, kava kava

PREGNANCY RISK
FDA Pregnancy Risk Category D. Excreted into breast milk. Consult your doctor.

SPECIAL INFORMATION
This drug has a black box warning that describes the potential for respiratory depression/arrest. This drug should only be used in settings that can provide continuous monitoring for respiratory and cardiac function.

MIDODRINE
(MI-doe-dreen)

NEWLY DISCOVERED USES (OFF-LABEL)

Chronic fatigue syndrome, partial retrograde ejaculation, post-spinal injury ejaculation

ORIGINAL USES (ON-LABEL)
To treat symptomatic orthostatic hypotension

BRAND NAME
ProAmatine

DRUG CLASS
Blood pressure medication (alpha-adrenergic agonist)

DESCRIPTION
This drug increases the tone of blood vessels, resulting in a rise of blood pressure in patients who have orthostatic hypotension (low blood pressure upon standing from a sitting or lying down position).

POTENTIAL SIDE EFFECTS
Numbness and tingling, goosebumps, itching, rash, painful urination, high blood pressure, chills, headache, confusion, dry mouth, anxiety, rash.

CAUTIONS
- Not recommended if you have high blood pressure associated with lying down. Requires blood pressure monitoring.

- Inform your doctor if you have diabetes, visual problems, urinary retention, or liver or kidney dysfunction.
- Requires monitoring of liver and kidney function prior to and periodically during therapy.
- Notify your doctor if you sense a decrease in your pulse.

DRUG INTERACTIONS
Fludrocortisone, beta-blockers, digoxin, psychotherapeutics, other drugs which affect alpha receptors. Consult your doctor and pharmacist prior to initiation of therapy with other drugs, herbal products, or nonprescription medications.

FOOD INTERACTIONS
Unknown

HERBAL INTERACTIONS
Unknown

PREGNANCY AND BREAST-FEEDING CAUTIONS
FDA Pregnancy Risk Category C. Excretion in breast milk is unknown. Consult your doctor.

SPECIAL INFORMATION
Should take this drug during the day while you will be upright. Do not take after the evening meal or less than four hours before bedtime. This drug has a black box warning regarding the risk of significant high blood pressure and thus should be used only in those with considerable impairment.

MIFEPRISTONE
(mi-FE-pris-tone)

NEWLY DISCOVERED USES (OFF-LABEL)
Abortion, Cushing's syndrome, endometriosis, labor induction, late abortion, uterine fibroids

ORIGINAL USES (ON-LABEL)
Medical termination of intrauterine pregnancy through day 49 of pregnancy

BRAND NAME
Mifeprex

DRUG CLASS
Abortifacient, antiprogestin

DESCRIPTION

This drug, when used in termination of pregnancy, causes contraction of myometrium, the muscular wall of the uterus.

POTENTIAL SIDE EFFECTS

Vaginal bleeding, uterine cramping, headache, dizziness, abdominal pain, nausea, vomiting, diarrhea, fatigue, fever, insomnia, anxiety, uterine hemorrhage, vaginitis, pelvic pain, decreased hemoglobin, anemia, back pain, rigors, leg pain, weakness, sinusitis, viral infection.

CAUTIONS

- Not for use if you have chronic adrenal failure, porphyrias, ectopic pregnancy, undiagnosed adnexal mass, certain blood or bleeding disorder or currently taking anticoagulant or long-term corticosteroid therapy.
- Do not use when more than 49 days into the pregnancy, or if intrauterine device is in place.
- You should be provided with information regarding access to emergency medical services when taking this drug.
- An agreement form regarding the risks of this drug must be reviewed and signed before initiation of therapy.
- Bleeding occurs and should be expected, but may require treatment.
- Safety and effectiveness have not been determined in women with high blood pressure, heart, lung, or kidney disease, diabetes mellitus, or heavy smokers.

DRUG INTERACTIONS

Other progestins. This drug is metabolized by a specific set of liver enzymes. Several other drugs interfere with these liver enzymes, and thus may increase or decrease the clearance of mifepristone from the body, potentially increasing the risk of side effects or decreasing effectiveness. When these drugs are given in combination with mifepristone, dosage adjustments may be needed. As these are too numerous to list, you should always check with your doctor or pharmacist prior to starting a new medication, herbal, or nonprescription product.

FOOD INTERACTIONS

Avoid grapefruit juice

HERBAL INTERACTIONS

St. John's wort

PREGNANCY AND BREAST-FEEDING CAUTIONS
FDA Pregnancy Risk Category X. Excretion in breast milk unknown. Do not use during breast-feeding.

SPECIAL INFORMATION
Review patient information and agreement form with your doctor prior to initiation of therapy. This drug has a black box warning regarding the risk of incomplete abortion and the potential need for surgical intervention. In 2005, the product labeling was revised to include warning regarding the potential for serious bacterial infections.

MILRINONE
(MIL-ri-none)

NEWLY DISCOVERED USES (OFF-LABEL)
Cardiac arrest, pulmonary edema, therapy-resistant cardiogenic shock

ORIGINAL USES (ON-LABEL)
Short-term intravenous therapy of congestive heart failure

BRAND NAME
Primacor

DRUG CLASS
Cardiac (phosphodiesterase enzyme inhibitor)

DESCRIPTION
This drug increases the output of the heart in patients with decreased heart function. It also relaxes the blood vessels to make the heart pump more easily and efficiently.

POTENTIAL SIDE EFFECTS
Irregular heart rhythm, low blood pressure, increased heart rate, chest pain, headache, pain at infusion site, numbness or tingling of extremities, or difficulty breathing.

CAUTIONS
- On rare occasions, this drug has caused life-threatening changes in heart rhythm, most often occurring in the presence of pre-existing arrhythmias, metabolic abnormalities, abnormal digoxin levels, and catheter insertion.

- Not recommended for use in patients who have recently had heart attacks.
- Requires close monitoring of blood pressure, electrolytes, and heart rate.
- Only for intravenous administration.

DRUG INTERACTIONS
Unknown

FOOD INTERACTIONS
Unknown

HERBAL INTERACTIONS
Unknown

PREGNANCY AND BREAST-FEEDING CAUTIONS
FDA Pregnancy Risk Category C. Excretion in breast milk unknown. Consult your doctor.

MINOCYCLINE
(min-OH-sik-leen)

NEWLY DISCOVERED USES (OFF-LABEL)
Legionnaire's disease, Lyme disease, mycoplasma pneumonia, nocardiosis, rheumatoid arthritis, rosacea

ORIGINAL USES (ON-LABEL)
Treatment of various bacterial infections, acne

BRAND NAMES
Dynacin, Minocin

DRUG CLASS
Antibiotic (tetracycline derivative)

DESCRIPTION
This drug inhibits the production of bacterial proteins by hindering essential cell function.

POTENTIAL SIDE EFFECTS
Dizziness, upset stomach, photosensitivity reaction (see cautions), itching, discoloration of teeth and enamel (young children), nausea, diarrhea, abdominal cramps, liver toxicity.

CAUTIONS

- Inform your doctor if you have a history of allergies to other antibiotics in this class or if you have liver or kidney problems.
- If used during tooth development may cause permanent discoloration of the tooth enamel.
- It should not be used in young children (under 8 years of age).
- Not for use during pregnancy.
- May retard skeletal development and bone growth with greatest risk for children less than four years and those receiving high doses.
- Dosages may be reduced in kidney impairment.
- May cause photosensitivity reactions (skin reaction related to sun exposure). Wear sunscreen and protective clothing during sun exposure.
- Chronic use may result in superinfection.
- Notify your doctor if persistent diarrhea develops.
- Do not use outdated tetracycline products.

DRUG INTERACTIONS
Warfarin, certain antibiotics (check with doctor or pharmacist), methoxyflurane, oral contraceptives, isotretinoin.

FOOD INTERACTIONS
Unknown

HERBAL INTERACTIONS
Unknown

PREGNANCY AND BREAST-FEEDING CAUTIONS
FDA Pregnancy Risk Category D. Excreted in breast milk. Do not use during breast-feeding.

MIRTAZAPINE
(mir-TAZ-a-peen)

NEWLY DISCOVERED USES (OFF-LABEL)

Charles Bonnet syndrome, fibromyalgia, insomnia, migraine prevention, obsessive-compulsive disorder (OCD), panic disorder, premenstrual dysphoric disorder (PMDD), post-traumatic stress disorder (PTSD)

ORIGINAL USES (ON-LABEL)
The treatment of depression

BRAND NAMES
Remeron, Remeron SolTab

DRUG CLASS
Antidepressant (alpha-2 antagonist)

DESCRIPTION
This drug increases the release of norepinephrine and serotonin, two chemicals that affect mood levels.

POTENTIAL SIDE EFFECTS
Dry mouth, constipation, increased appetite, weight gain, flu-syndrome, muscle aches, abnormal dreams, agitation, anxiety, somnolence, abnormal thinking, increases in blood pressure.

CAUTIONS
- Do not use within 14 days of MAO inhibitors.
- Notify your doctor if you have a seizure disorder.
- May cause sedation, and impair tasks requiring alertness.
- May worsen psychosis in some patients with bipolar disease.
- The possibility of suicide is always present in patients with severe depression.
- Notify your doctor if you have kidney or liver impairment.
- SolTab formulation contains phenylalanine.

DRUG INTERACTIONS
Alcohol, diazepam. This drug is metabolized by a specific set of liver enzymes. Several other drugs interfere with these liver enzymes, and thus may increase or decrease the clearance of mirtazapine from the body, potentially increasing the risk of side effects or decreasing effectiveness. When these drugs are given in combination with mirtazapine, dosage adjustments may be needed. As these are too numerous to list, you should always check with your doctor or pharmacist prior to starting a new medication, herbal, or nonprescription product.

FOOD INTERACTIONS
Alcohol

HERBAL INTERACTIONS
St. John's wort, valerian, SAMe, kava kava.

PREGNANCY RISK
FDA Pregnancy Risk Category C. Excretion in breast milk unknown. Do not breast-feed during therapy.

SPECIAL INFORMATION
This drug has a warning that both adult and children with major depression may experience worsening of their depression and/or the emergence of suicidal thinking and behavior (suicidality), whether or not they are taking antidepressant medications. The warning recommends patients being treated with antidepressants be observed closely for clinical worsening and suicidality, especially at the beginning of a course of drug therapy, or at the time of dose changes.

MISOPROSTOL
(mye-soe-PROST-ole)

NEWLY DISCOVERED USES (OFF-LABEL)
Abortion, cervical ripening, chronic constipation, labor induction, late abortion

ORIGINAL USES (ON-LABEL)
Prevention of NSAID-induced gastric ulcers. Medical termination of pregnancy at less than 49 days. (Used in conjunction with mifepristone. Labeled use in mifepristone package insert.)

BRAND NAME
Cytotec

DRUG CLASS
Prostaglandin

DESCRIPTION
This drug replaces the protective prostaglandins that are destroyed during prostaglandin-inhibiting therapies (NSAIDs). It has also been shown to induce uterine contractions.

POTENTIAL SIDE EFFECTS
Diarrhea, abdominal pain, nausea, flatulence, headache, stomach upset, vomiting, constipation.

CAUTIONS
- Does not reduce the risk of duodenal ulcers during NSAID therapy.
- Ulcer therapy: Not to be used in pregnant women or women of childbearing potential unless woman is capable of complying with effective contraceptive measures. Requires negative preg-

nancy test two weeks prior to the initiation of therapy, oral and written warnings of the risks of this drug must be provided prior to initiation of therapy. Initiate therapy only on the second or third day of the next normal menstrual period.

- Diarrhea is dose related and usually occurs early in the course of therapy, typically resolving with continued therapy, but sometimes requires stopping the drug.

DRUG INTERACTIONS
Antacids

FOOD INTERACTIONS
Incidence of diarrhea may be lessened by taking right after meals.

HERBAL INTERACTIONS
Unknown

PREGNANCY AND BREAST-FEEDING CAUTIONS
FDA Pregnancy Risk Category X. Misoprostol induces abortion after oral or vaginal administration early in pregnancy through its potent uterine stimulant effects. However, when used later during second and third trimesters, it has been shown efficacious for labor induction and cervical ripening. This drug should not be used during breast-feeding because of the potential for severe diarrhea in the nursing infant.

SPECIAL INFORMATION
Ulcer therapy: Requires written and oral patient counseling. Begin therapy only on second or third day of the next normal menstrual period. This drug has a black box warning regarding its abortifacient properties. Uterine rupture has been reported when this drug has been used to induce labor or abortion beyond the eighth week of pregnancy.

MITOMYCIN
(mye-toe-MYE-sin)

NEWLY DISCOVERED USES (OFF-LABEL)
Pterygium recurrence prevention

ORIGINAL USES (ON-LABEL)
Treatment of cancers of the stomach or pancreas, bladder cancer, breast cancer, or colorectal cancer

BRAND NAME
Mutamycin

DRUG CLASS
Antineoplastic

DESCRIPTION
This drug is used primarily to treat cancers by blocking DNA and RNA synthesis.

POTENTIAL SIDE EFFECTS
Severe blood disorders (such as reduction of red blood cells, platelets, white blood cells, etc.), lung and kidney toxicity, fever, anorexia, nausea, vomiting, bone marrow suppression.

CAUTIONS
- Notify your doctor if you have recently received radiation therapy or have liver problems.
- Hemolytic-uremic syndrome, a serious complication and potentially fatal, occurs in some patients receiving long-term therapy.
- May cause ulceration, necrosis, cellulites, and tissue sloughing if infiltrated during administration.
- May cause kidney toxicity.

DRUG INTERACTIONS
Vinca alkaloids or doxorubicin may enhance heart toxicity when co-administered with mitomycin.

FOOD INTERACTIONS
Unknown

HERBAL INTERACTIONS
Black cohosh, dong quai in estrogen-dependent tumors

PREGNANCY AND BREAST-FEEDING CAUTIONS
FDA Pregnancy Risk Category D. Excreted in breast milk and is not compatible with breast-feeding.

SPECIAL INFORMATION
This drug has a black box warning regarding bone marrow suppression, which may be severe and predispose to infection. This drug requires regular monitoring of blood for complications and toxicities.

MITOTANE
(MYE-toe-tane)

NEWLY DISCOVERED USES (OFF-LABEL)
Cushing's syndrome

ORIGINAL USES (ON-LABEL)
Treatment of inoperable adrenal cortical cancers.

BRAND NAME
Lysodren

DRUG CLASS
Antineoplastic, antiadrenal

DESCRIPTION
This drug is primarily used to treat certain cancers. It decreases the production of cortisol in the adrenal cortex (glands), thus suppressing the adrenal cortex.

POTENTIAL SIDE EFFECTS
Increased blood pressure, sudden decrease in blood pressure upon standing from a prolonged sitting or lying down position, lethargy, vision changes, generalized aching, central nervous system depression, dizziness, skin rash, anorexia, nausea, vomiting, diarrhea, weakness.

CAUTIONS
- Monitoring for neurotoxicity is required for prolonged therapy.
- The administration of steroids may be required as the adrenal glands are suppressed during therapy.
- Notify your doctor if any of the following symptoms occur: nausea, vomiting, loss of appetite, diarrhea, mental depression, skin rash or darkening of the skin.
- Contraceptive measures are recommended during therapy.

DRUG INTERACTIONS
Barbiturates, warfarin, spironolactone, phenytoin, corticosteroids.

FOOD INTERACTIONS
Alcohol

HERBAL INTERACTIONS
Unknown

PREGNANCY AND BREAST-FEEDING CAUTIONS
FDA Pregnancy Risk Category C. Excreted in breast milk. Do not breast-feed during therapy.

SPECIAL INFORMATION
May cause drowsiness; use caution when driving or performing tasks that require alertness. This drug has a black box warning regarding the need to temporarily discontinue therapy after shock or severe trauma.

MODAFINIL
(moe-DAF-i-nil)

NEWLY DISCOVERED USES (OFF-LABEL)
Attention deficit/hyperactivity disorder (ADHD), brain trauma, chronic fatigue syndrome, cocaine addiction, fibromyalgia, multiple sclerosis, Parkinson's disease, seasonal affective disorder

ORIGINAL USES (ON-LABEL)
Increases wakefulness in patients with excessive daytime sleepiness associated with narcolepsy

BRAND NAME
Provigil

DRUG CLASS
Central nervous system stimulant (nonamphetamine)

DESCRIPTION
This drug promotes wakefulness.

POTENTIAL SIDE EFFECTS
Nervousness, dizziness, depression, anxiety, diarrhea, nausea, anorexia, vomiting, sore throat, runny nose, lung disorder, headache, insomnia, numbness, dry mouth, changes in blood pressure.

CAUTIONS
- Inform your doctor if you have a history of psychosis or cardiac problems. May require periodic monitoring of blood pressure.
- Requires dosage reduction in liver impairment and in the elderly.

- Stimulants may affect ability to perform certain tasks, affecting judgment, thinking, or motor skills. Should assess effects before driving or operating machinery.
- Oral contraceptives may lose efficacy.
- Stimulants may unmask tics in patients with coexisting Tourette's syndrome.

DRUG INTERACTIONS

Diazepam, mephenytoin, phenytoin, propanolol, warfarin, oral contraceptives, cyclosporine, theophylline, phenobarbital, carbamazepine, rifampin. This drug is metabolized by a specific set of liver enzymes (cytochrome P450 enzymes 3A4) and affects other enzymes (cytochrome P450 1A2, 2B6 and 3A4). Several other drugs are metabolized or also interfere with these liver enzymes, and thus may increase or decrease the clearance of modafinil from the body, potentially increasing the risk of side effects or decreasing effectiveness. Modafinil also has the ability to effect the clearance of other drugs from the body. When these drugs are given in combination with modafinil, dosage adjustments may be needed. As these are too numerous to list, you should always check with your doctor or pharmacist prior to starting a new medication, herbal, or nonprescription product.

FOOD INTERACTIONS

Food may delay absorption by approximately one hour. Avoid alcohol.

HERBAL INTERACTIONS

Unknown

PREGNANCY AND BREAST-FEEDING CAUTIONS

FDA Pregnancy Risk Category C. Excretion in breast milk unknown. Consult your doctor.

SPECIAL INFORMATION

To be taken during the day to avoid insomnia. Because of the increased potential for drug interactions, consult your pharmacist or doctor prior to starting any new medication, herbal, or nonprescription product.

MONTELUKAST
(mon-te-LOO-kast)

NEWLY DISCOVERED USES (OFF-LABEL)
Nasal polyps, urticaria

ORIGINAL USES (ON-LABEL)
Prevention and chronic treatment of asthma in adults and children (at least one year of age) and the relief of symptoms of seasonal allergies in adults and children (at least two years of age)

BRAND NAME
Singulair

DRUG CLASS
Asthma (leukotriene receptor antagonist)

DESCRIPTION
This drug acts on leukotrienes, a substance which is responsible for causing constriction and difficulty breathing in the lungs.

POTENTIAL SIDE EFFECTS
Headache, dizziness, fatigue, fever, rash, dental pain, gastroenteritis, abdominal pain, weakness, nasal congestion, upper respiratory infection, flu-like symptoms, upset stomach.

CAUTIONS
- This medication has not been approved by the FDA for the reversal of bronchospasm in acute asthma attacks.

DRUG INTERACTIONS
This drug is metabolized (inactivated) by a specific set of liver enzymes. Several other drugs interfere with these liver enzymes, and thus may increase or decrease the clearance of montelukast from the body, and often requiring dosage adjustments when they are administered in combination. As these are too numerous to list, you should always check with your doctor or pharmacist prior to starting a new medication.

FOOD INTERACTIONS
Unknown

HERBAL INTERACTIONS
St. John's wort

FDA PREGNANCY CATEGORY/BREAST-FEEDING
FDA Pregnancy Category C. It is not known if this drug is excreted in breast milk. Use with caution in breast-feeding.

SPECIAL INFORMATION
Chewable tablets contain phenylalanine. This medication is not useful for an acute asthma attack. Take medication according to your doctor's instructions, even if you are not symptomatic.

MORPHINE
(MOR-feen)

NEWLY DISCOVERED USES (OFF-LABEL)
Pulmonary edema

ORIGINAL USES (ON-LABEL)
Relief of moderate to severe acute and chronic pain difficulty breathing associated with lung edema and certain types of heart failure, used to produce anesthesia in heart surgery

BRAND NAMES
DepoDur, Duramorph, Kadian, MS Contin, Oramorph SR

DRUG CLASS
Opiate agonists

DESCRIPTION
Morphine is an opium extract used as an analgesic, a light anesthetic, or a sedative.

POTENTIAL SIDE EFFECTS
Sedation, respiratory depression, dependence (physical and physiological), low blood pressure, sweating, constipation.

CAUTIONS
- The dosing and schedule of administration should be individualized to the type of pain you are experiencing, route of administration, degree of tolerance for opioids, age, weight, and medical condition.
- Tolerance or drug dependence may result from extended use.
- Elderly may be particularly susceptible to the central nervous system depressant effects and constipating effects of narcotics.

DRUG INTERACTIONS

Other central nervous system depressants (phenothiazines, anxiolytics, sedatives, hypnotics, or alcohol), dextroamphetamine, diuretics, MAO inhibitors (avoid using within 14 days of MAOIs), meperidine.

FOOD INTERACTIONS

Alcohol

HERBAL INTERACTIONS

Valerian, St. John's wort, kava kava, gotu kola

PREGNANCY AND BREAST-FEEDING CAUTIONS

FDA Pregnancy Risk Category C. Excreted in breast milk. Consult your doctor.

SPECIAL INFORMATION

Do not substitute one brand product for another without doctor notification.

MOXIFLOXACIN
(moxs-i-FLOKS-a-sin)

Oral, Injectable

NEWLY DISCOVERED USES (OFF-LABEL)

Legionnaire's disease

ORIGINAL USES (ON-LABEL)

Various bacterial infections in the lung, eye, sinuses, skin, and skin structure

BRAND NAMES

Avelox, Vigamox

DRUG CLASS

Antibiotic (quinolone)

DESCRIPTION

This drug is used to fight bacterial infections. It works by interfering with cellular enzymes, halting DNA replication, repair, recombination, and transposition.

POTENTIAL SIDE EFFECTS

Dizziness, nausea, diarrhea, various blood disorders (anemia, changes in white blood cells, etc.), tremors, confusion, depression, nervousness, agitation, anxiety, changes in heart rhythm (QT prolongation, see caution section).

CAUTIONS

- Notify your doctor if you have any problems now or recently with irregular heart rates, low potassium levels, seizures, or heart attack.
- Moxifloxacin has affected heart rate rhythm (QT prolongation) in some patients and should be avoided in patients who have this problem, have low potassium levels, or who are taking certain antiarrhythmics. Check with your doctor prior to starting any new drug while on this medication.
- Report to your doctor if you experience pain, inflammation or rupture of a tendon. Rest and refrain from exercise until you see a doctor. Tendon rupture can occur during or after therapy with this drug.
- Report any episodes of changes in heart rate or fainting spells.
- Stop the medication at the first sign of a rash.
- Prolonged use may cause superinfection.
- May aggravate symptoms of myasthenia gravis.
- Inform your doctor if serious, persistent diarrhea develops.

DRUG INTERACTIONS

Iron, zinc, calcium, magnesium, aluminum, corticosteroids (increase risk of tendon rupture), antacids, electrolyte supplements, quinapril, sucralfate, certain antiarrhythmics, didanosine formulations (chewable/buffered tablets and pediatric powder for oral suspension), theophylline, cimetidine, anticoagulants (such as warfarin, etc.). If administered with other drugs that can cause QT prolongation (potentially serious changes in heart rhythm) may increase risk of this occurring. For a comprehensive list of drugs known and suspected to cause these effects, refer to the following website: (http://www.torsades.org/medical-pros/drug-lists/drug-lists.htm#). While taking this medication, consult with your pharmacist or doctor for interactions prior to starting any new medication, new herbal product, or nonprescription drug.

FOOD INTERACTIONS

May be taken with or without food. Do not take with dairy products or calcium fortified juices.

HERBAL INTERACTIONS

Unknown

PREGNANCY AND BREAST-FEEDING CAUTIONS
FDA Pregnancy Risk Category C. May be excreted in breast milk.
Do not use during breast-feeding.

SPECIAL INFORMATION
Take four hours before or eight hours after didanosine, multiple
vitamins, antacids, or other products containing magnesium, aluminum, iron, or zinc. May cause dizziness or lightheadedness,
caution with tasks that require alertness.

MYCOPHENOLATE MOFETIL
(mye-koe-FEN-oh-late MAH-feh-till)

NEWLY DISCOVERED USES (OFF-LABEL)
Autoimmune hepatitis, bullous pemphigoid, chronic inflammatory demyelinating polyneuropathy, dermatitis (atopic),
dermatomyositis/polymyositis, myasthenia gravis, oral lichen
planus, therapy-resistant idiopathic thrombocytopenia purpura, scleroderma, systemic lupus erythematosus, uveitis

ORIGINAL USES (ON-LABEL)
Use in combination therapy with immunosuppressive drugs in
the prevention of organ rejection for kidney, heart, or liver transplants

BRAND NAMES
CellCept, Myfortic

DRUG CLASS
Immunosuppressant

DESCRIPTION
This drug stops transplant rejection by suppressing the immune
system and preventing inflammation triggered by the immune
system.

POTENTIAL SIDE EFFECTS
Diarrhea, leukopenia (decreased white blood cells), sepsis, vomiting, higher frequency of certain types of infections (such as op-
portunistic infections), pain, abdominal pain, fever, anemia,
urinary tract infection, blood disorders, changes in blood pressure, back pain, increased heart rate, nausea, changes in lipid levels, changes in glucose levels, dizziness, anxiety.

CAUTIONS

- Patients receiving immunosuppressants may be at increased risk of developing certain types of cancer (such as lymphoma) and increased susceptibility to infection.
- Notify your doctor if you have active peptic ulcers, Lesch-Nyhan, or Kelley-Seegmiller syndrome.
- Requires a negative serum or urine pregnancy test (sensitivity of at least 50 IU/mL) within one week prior to initiating therapy. Requires effective contraception during therapy and six weeks after completion. Causes teratogenic effects in animals.
- Severe blood disorders have occurred and requires periodic monitoring during therapy.
- Report any evidence of infection to your doctor, as well as unexpected bruising, bleeding or other signs suggesting bone marrow depression.
- Toxicity may be increased in those with kidney impairment.
- Do not crush or chew tablets.
- May cause gastrointestinal perforation (rarely) or bleeding.
- Oral suspension contains aspartame.

DRUG INTERACTIONS

Acyclovir, ganciclovir, probenecid, azathioprine (increases risk of bone marrow suppression), antacids, cholestyramine, live vaccines, oral contraceptives, trimethoprim/sulfamethoxazole

FOOD INTERACTIONS

Oral forms should be taken on an empty stomach.

HERBAL INTERACTIONS

Cat's claw and echinacea

PREGNANCY AND BREAST-FEEDING CAUTIONS

FDA Pregnancy Risk Category C. Excretion in breast milk is unknown. Not recommended for use while breast-feeding.

SPECIAL INFORMATION

CellCept and Myfortic should not be used interchangeably due to differences in drug absorption. This drug has a black box warning describing the increased risk of lymphoma and increased susceptibility to infection may be related to immunosuppression.

NABUMETONE
(na-BYOO-me-tone)

NEWLY DISCOVERED USES (OFF-LABEL)
Juvenile rheumatoid arthritis

ORIGINAL USES (ON-LABEL)
Management of osteoarthritis and rheumatoid arthritis

BRAND NAME
Relafen

DRUG CLASS
Analgesic (nonsteroidal anti-inflammatory [NSAID])

DESCRIPTION
This drug inhibits the production of prostaglandin by decreasing the activity of the enzyme responsible for its production. Prostaglandins are known mediators of pain and inflammation.

POTENTIAL SIDE EFFECTS
Dizziness, skin rash, abdominal cramps, heartburn, indigestion, headache, nervousness, itching, fluid retention, vomiting.

CAUTIONS
- Notify your doctor if you have an allergy to other NSAIDs or aspirin.
- Inform your doctor if you have gastric bleeding, congestive heart failure, high blood pressure, dehydration, decreased kidney or liver function, history of gastric disease or those receiving anticoagulants.
- Elderly are at high risk of adverse effects from NSAIDs.
- May be associated with photosensitivity reactions (skin reaction related to sun exposure).
- Use the lowest effective dose for the shortest duration possible.
- May cause changes in kidney or liver function, fluid retention.

DRUG INTERACTIONS
Anticoagulants (warfarin, heparins), other antiplatelet drugs (ticlopidine, clopidogrel, aspirin, abciximab, dipyridamole, eptifibatide, tirofiban), cyclosporine, lithium, corticosteroids, methotrexate, antihypertensive drugs (such as ACE inhibitors, angiotensin antagonists, diuretics and hydralazine), cholestyramine, colestipol

FOOD INTERACTIONS
May be taken without regard to meals.

HERBAL INTERACTIONS
Cat's claw, dong quai, evening primrose, feverfew, garlic, ginger, ginkgo, red clover, horse chestnut, green tea, ginseng

PREGNANCY AND BREAST-FEEDING CAUTIONS
FDA Pregnancy Risk Category C, D (third trimester). Excreted in breast milk. Refrain from breast-feeding while taking this drug.

SPECIAL INFORMATION
In 2005, the FDA requested that manufacturers of all prescription NSAIDs revise their product labeling to include a black box warning regarding the potential for serious adverse cardiac events and potentially life-threatening gastric adverse events associated with the use. In addition, this class of drugs is not to be used in patients who have recently undergone coronary artery bypass surgery. A medication guide regarding this new information should be dispensed at each prescription.

NADOLOL
(nay-DOE-lole)

NEWLY DISCOVERED USES (OFF-LABEL)
Migraine prevention, prevention of bleeding in cirrhosis, portal hypertension

ORIGINAL USES (ON-LABEL)
To treat hypertension and angina pectoris

BRAND NAME
Cogard

DRUG CLASS
Antianginal, antihypertensive (beta-blocker)

DESCRIPTION
This drug decreases heart rate, cardiac contractility, blood pressure, and heart oxygen demand.

POTENTIAL SIDE EFFECTS
Decreased heart rate, dizziness, reduced peripheral circulation, chest pain, mental depression, lightheadedness, rash, hair loss,

changes in blood glucose and lipids, increased potassium levels, nausea, vomiting, constipation, anorexia, impotence, weakness, wheezing, bronchospasm, pulmonary edema, decreased tear production, decreased visual acuity.

CAUTIONS

- Inform your doctor if you have heart conditions (such as congestive heart failure, cardiogenic shock, too low heart rate, or second- and third-degree heart block, sinus node dysfunction), are pregnant, have kidney dysfunction, or have lung/breathing problems.
- Do not stop this medication suddenly, taper over a gradual period.
- May cause or mask the symptoms of low blood glucose levels in diabetics.
- May mask signs of thyroid problems.
- Not indicated for high blood pressure emergencies.
- Immediately report to your doctor any signs of swelling of the extremities, sudden weight gain, changes in breathing, night cough.
- May require dosage adjustment in kidney impairment.

DRUG INTERACTIONS

Barbiturates, cholestyramine, colestipol, rifampin, calcium channel blockers, diphenhydramine, flecainide, hydroxychloroquine, MAO-inhibitors, NSAIDs, quinidine, thyroid hormones, warfarin, clonidine, epinephrine, ergot alkaloids, prazosin, oral sulfonylureas (drugs used to treat diabetes), theophylline

FOOD INTERACTIONS

May be taken without regard to meals.

HERBAL INTERACTIONS

Dong quai, ephedra, garlic, yohimbine, ginseng, and licorice

PREGNANCY AND BREAST-FEEDING CAUTIONS

FDA Pregnancy Risk Category C (manufacturer) D second and third trimesters (expert analysis). Excreted in breast milk. Consult your doctor.

SPECIAL INFORMATION

This drug has a black box warning regarding the avoidance of abrupt withdrawal in those with heart disease.

NAFARELIN
(NAF-a-re-lin)

NEWLY DISCOVERED USES (OFF-LABEL)
Dysmenorrhea, ovulation induction for in-vitro fertilization, premenstrual dysphoric disorder (PMDD), therapy-resistant PMDD, premenstrual syndrome (PMS)

ORIGINAL USES (ON-LABEL)
Treatment of endometriosis and of central precocious puberty in children of both sexes

BRAND NAME
Synarel

DRUG CLASS
Gonadotropin-releasing hormone

DESCRIPTION
This drug stimulates the release of two types of hormones from the pituitary.

POTENTIAL SIDE EFFECTS
Hot flashes, decrease in libido, vaginal dryness, headaches, emotional lability, insomnia, acne, muscle aches, reduced breast size, edema, weight gain, nasal irritation.

CAUTIONS
- When used to treat central precocious puberty, it is important that diagnosis is firmly established prior to the initiation of therapy.
- Requires regular monitoring.
- Notify your doctor if regular menstruation persists.
- A small bone loss in bone density may occur. If you are at risk for decreased bone mineral content, please notify your doctor. These would include chronic alcohol use, chronic tobacco use, strong family history of osteoporosis, chronic use of drugs that may affect bone density (such as certain anticonvulsants, corticosteroids). Discuss these risks with your doctor prior to therapy.
- Retreatment for endometriosis is not recommended.
- Ovarian cysts have occurred during treatment for endometriosis.
- May significantly increase serum lipid levels.

DRUG INTERACTIONS
Consult your doctor. Do not use nasal decongestant for at least two hours after using nafarelin spray.

FOOD INTERACTIONS
Unknown

HERBAL INTERACTIONS
Unknown

PREGNANCY AND BREAST-FEEDING CAUTIONS
FDA Pregnancy Risk Category X. Excreted in breast milk. Do not use during breast-feeding.

SPECIAL INFORMATION
Use of non-hormonal contraceptive is suggested. Full compliance is important. Avoid sneezing during or immediately after dosing, as this may impair absorption.

NALMEFENE
(NAL-me-feen)

NEWLY DISCOVERED USES (OFF-LABEL)
Pruritus

ORIGINAL USES (ON-LABEL)
To cause complete or partial reversal of opioid drug effects, to manage a known or suspected opioid overdose

BRAND NAME
Revex

DRUG CLASS
Antidote (opiate antagonist)

DESCRIPTION
Prevents or reverses respiratory depression, sedation, and low blood pressure induced by opiates by antagonizing the opioid receptor sites.

POTENTIAL SIDE EFFECTS
Nausea, vomiting, increased heart rate, changes in blood pressure, post-operative pain, fever, dizziness, headache, chills.

CAUTIONS

- May precipitate acute withdrawal in patients who are addicted to opioids.
- If the opioid being treated is long acting, respiratory depression may recur once the effects of this drug wear off. Patients should be monitored until it is certain that respiratory depression will not recur.
- The reversal of opioids has been associated with significant adverse events, including serious lung and heart problems (such as pulmonary edema, cardiac instability, low blood pressure).

DRUG INTERACTIONS
Flumazenil

FOOD INTERACTIONS
Unknown

HERBAL INTERACTIONS
Unknown

PREGNANCY AND BREAST-FEEDING CAUTIONS
FDA Pregnancy Risk Category B. Excreted in breast milk. Consult your doctor.

NALOXONE
(nal-OKS-one)

NEWLY DISCOVERED USES (OFF-LABEL)
Primary biliary cirrhosis

ORIGINAL USES (ON-LABEL)
To completely or partially reverse opioid depression, to diagnose a suspected opioid tolerance or acute opioid overdose

BRAND NAME
Narcan

DRUG CLASS
Antidote (opiate antagonist)

DESCRIPTION
This drug reverses the effects of narcotics.

POTENTIAL SIDE EFFECTS
Changes in blood pressure, shortness of breath, increased heart rate, irritability, anxiety, tremor, seizures, changes in heart rate, nausea, vomiting, diarrhea.

CAUTIONS
- Inform your doctor if you have heart disease.
- May precipitate withdrawal symptoms in patients addicted to opiates (such as pain, hypertension, sweating, agitation, irritability).
- Requires close monitoring during administration and for a period after administration.
- Not effective in reversing respiratory depression for nonopioid drugs.

DRUG INTERACTIONS
Narcotic analgesics

FOOD INTERACTIONS
Unknown

HERBAL INTERACTIONS
Unknown

PREGNANCY AND BREAST-FEEDING CAUTIONS
FDA Pregnancy Risk Category C. It is not known if this drug is excreted in breast milk. Not recommended for use during breast-feeding.

NALTREXONE
(nal-TREKS-one)

NEWLY DISCOVERED USES (OFF-LABEL)
Binge eating disorder, pathological gambling, primary biliary cirrhosis, pruritus, smoking cessation

ORIGINAL USES (ON-LABEL)
To reverse the effects of opiates, to treat alcohol dependence

BRAND NAMES
Naltrexone, ReVia

DRUG CLASS
Antidote (opioid antagonist)

DESCRIPTION
This drug prevents or reverses respiratory depression, sedation, and low blood pressure induced by opiates.

POTENTIAL SIDE EFFECTS
Nausea, headache, dizziness, nervousness, fatigue, insomnia, vomiting, anxiety, drowsiness, depression, suicidal ideation, irritability, increased energy, rash, abdominal cramps, anorexia, diarrhea, constipation, delayed ejaculation, muscle/joint pain, nasal congestion, vision changes, chills, increased thirst.

CAUTIONS
- Not for use in patients with a narcotic dependence, current use of opioid analgesics, acute opioid withdrawal, failure to pass naloxone challenge, acute or chronic liver failure.
- Use may result in liver toxicity. Discuss these risks with your doctor.
- Must be opioid free for 7–10 days prior to administration as determined by urine analysis.
- Risk of suicide may continue to be increased even with this therapy.

DRUG INTERACTIONS
Thioridazine, opioid-containing products

FOOD INTERACTIONS
Unknown

HERBAL INTERACTIONS
Unknown

PREGNANCY AND BREAST-FEEDING CAUTIONS
FDA Pregnancy Risk Category C. Excretion in breast milk unknown. Not recommended for use while breast-feeding.

SPECIAL INFORMATION
This drug has a black box warning describing the risk of liver injury with high doses. You should wear an identification bracelet indicating that you are using this drug.

This information refers only to use of the prescription product.

NAPROXEN
(na-PROKS-en)

NEWLY DISCOVERED USES (OFF-LABEL)
Membranous nephropathy, menorrhagia, periodontitis, premenstrual dysphoric disorder (PMDD), premenstrual syndrome (PMS)

ORIGINAL USES (ON-LABEL)
Management of inflammatory disease and rheumatoid disorders, acute gout, mild to moderate pain, dysmenorrhea, fever, migraine headache.

BRAND NAMES
Anaprox (DS), EC-Naprosyn, Naprelan, Naprosyn

DRUG CLASS
Pain reliever, anti-inflammatory (nonsteroidal anti-inflammatory [NSAID])

DESCRIPTION
This drug inhibits prostaglandin synthesis by decreasing the activity of the enzyme responsible for the production of prostaglandins. Prostaglandins are a known mediator in the body of pain and inflammation.

POTENTIAL SIDE EFFECTS
Abdominal cramps, nausea, stomach upset, diarrhea, flatulence, weakness, stomach irritation, blurred vision, ringing in the ears, constipation.

CAUTIONS
- Not for use if you are allergic to aspirin or other NSAIDs.
- Not for use if you have active gastric/duodenal ulcer disease.
- Do not use during third trimester of pregnancy.
- Ask physician about use if you have any of the following medical problems: high blood pressure, dehydration, decreased kidney or liver function, history of gastric disease.
- Elderly are at higher risk of developing side effects.

DRUG INTERACTIONS
Aspirin, lithium, methotrexate, digoxin, cyclosporine (nephrotoxicity), diuretics, some anti-hypertensives, and warfarin (bleeding). Other NSAIDs.

FOOD INTERACTIONS
Take with food to minimize upset stomach.

HERBAL INTERACTIONS
Cat's claw, dong quai, evening primrose, feverfew, garlic, ginger, ginkgo, red clover, horse chestnut, green tea, ginseng.

PREGNANCY AND BREAST-FEEDING CAUTIONS
FDA Pregnancy Risk Category B (D if in third trimester). Excreted in breast milk. Consult your doctor.

SPECIAL INFORMATION
Stop taking this drug (with doctor's approval) approximately 48 to 72 hours prior to surgical or dental procedures as it affects the body's ability to form blood clots and may increase bleeding time.

In April 2005, the FDA announced the potential addition of a black box warning to the labeling of this class of drugs (NSAIDs), specifically regarding potential serious cardiac events and potentially life-threatening gastric adverse events.

NEDOCROMIL
(ne-doe-KROE-mil)

Inhaled

NEWLY DISCOVERED USES (OFF-LABEL)
Prevention of exercise-induced bronchospasm

ORIGINAL USES (ON-LABEL)
To treat mild or moderate bronchial asthma as a maintenance therapy

BRAND NAME
Tilade

DRUG CLASS
Allergy medication (inhalation)

DESCRIPTION
This drug inhibits the activity of a variety of inflammatory cell types associated with asthma. It also inhibits the release of histamine, leukotrienes, and slow-reacting substances of allergic reactions.

POTENTIAL SIDE EFFECTS

Nausea, vomiting, abdominal pain, upset stomach, diarrhea, cough, bronchospasm, sore throat, sinusitis, upper respiratory infection, shortness of breath, increased sputum, unpleasant taste, headache, chest pain, fever.

CAUTIONS

- If reduction of oral or inhaled steroid therapy occurs, you should be monitored by your doctor.
- Do not use as a bronchodilator for reversal of acute bronchospasm.
- If bronchospasm occurs immediately after inhalation, stop therapy and use alternative treatment.

DRUG INTERACTIONS

Unknown

FOOD INTERACTIONS

Unknown

HERBAL INTERACTIONS

Unknown

PREGNANCY AND BREAST-FEEDING CAUTIONS

FDA Pregnancy Risk Category B. Excretion in breast milk is unknown. Consult your doctor.

SPECIAL INFORMATION

Prime each inhaler with three pumps prior to the first use. Must re-prime if the canister remains unused for more than seven days. Full therapeutic effect may not be realized for at least one week after starting therapy.

NEFAZODONE
(nef–AY-zoe-done)

NEWLY DISCOVERED USES (OFF-LABEL)
Social phobia

ORIGINAL USES (ON-LABEL)
Depression

BRAND NAME
Serzone

DRUG CLASS
Antidepressant (serotonin reuptake inhibitor/antagonist)

DESCRIPTION
This drug increases the levels of important chemicals in the brain.

POTENTIAL SIDE EFFECTS
Headache, drowsiness, insomnia, agitation, dizziness, xerostomia, nausea, constipation, weakness, bradycardia, hypotension, peripheral edema, postural hypotension, chills, fever, incoordination, lightheadedness, pruritus, rash, breast pain, impotence, gastroenteritis, vomiting, dyspepsia, diarrhea, urinary frequency, urinary retention, hematocrit decreased, arthralgia, hypertonia, parenthesis, blurred vision, abnormal vision, eye pain, visual field defect, tinnitus, bronchitis, cough, dyspnea, pharyngitis, flu syndrome, infection.

CAUTIONS
- Not for use if you have liver injury, active liver disease, or if you have elevated liver function tests.
- May cause serious, life-threatening liver toxicity. Immediately report any signs or symptoms of liver injury to your doctor, including jaundice, dark urine, and abdominal pain.
- Do not begin therapy if an MAO inhibitor has been taken within the previous 14 days.
- Notify your doctor if you recently had a heart attack, have a history of seizures, have liver or kidney disease, have heart disease, low blood pressure, are taking carbamazepine, cisapride, pimozide, triazolam, or alprazolam.
- May cause an increase in sedation.
- May increase the risk of suicidal behavior, requiring monitoring.

DRUG INTERACTIONS
This drug is metabolized by a specific set of liver enzymes. Several other drugs interfere with these liver enzymes, and thus may increase or decrease the clearance of nefazodone from the body, potentially increasing the risk of side effects or decreasing effectiveness. When these drugs are given in combination with nefazodone, dosage adjustments may be needed. As these are too numerous to list, you should always check with your doctor or pharmacist prior to starting a new medication, herbal, or non-prescription product.

FOOD INTERACTIONS
Take on an empty stomach, food decreases absorption. Avoid alcohol.

HERBAL INTERACTIONS
Valerian, St. John's wort, SAMe, kava kava

PREGNANCY AND BREAST-FEEDING CAUTIONS
FDA Pregnancy Risk Category C. Excreted in breast milk. Consult your doctor.

SPECIAL INFORMATION
This drug has a black box warning describing the potential risk of serious, life-threatening liver failure associated with drug therapy. In addition, in 2005, the FDA announced new labeling for antidepressants regarding the need to closely monitor for worsening of depression and for the potential of increased suicidal thinking or suicidal behavior during therapy. Although this recommendation applies to all patients (adults, children, adolescents) treated with antidepressants for any indication, this is of particular importance in patients being treated for depression. Discuss the latest information regarding this safety issue with your doctor prior to initiating therapy.

Close observation may be especially important when antidepressant medications are started for the first time or when doses are changed. More information on this topic can be found at the following web site: http://www.fda.gov/cder/drug/antidepressants/default.htm

NICARDIPINE
(nye-KAR-de-peen)

NEWLY DISCOVERED USES (OFF-LABEL)
Essential tremor, premature labor, Raynaud's syndrome

ORIGINAL USES (ON-LABEL)
Chronic stable angina, essential hypertension (high blood pressure)

BRAND NAME
Cardene, Cardene IV, Cardene SR

DRUG CLASS
Antianginal, antihypertensive (calcium channel blocker)

DESCRIPTION
This drug relaxes coronary vascular smooth muscle and increases oxygen delivery to the heart.

POTENTIAL SIDE EFFECTS
Flushing, palpitations, change in heart rate, peripheral edema, nausea and weakness, constipation, dizziness, lightheadedness, headache.

CAUTIONS
- Notify your doctor if you have had an allergic reaction to a drug in this class.
- Inform your doctor if you have low blood pressure, severe left ventricular dysfunction or other types of heart problems, liver or kidney dysfunction.
- Abrupt withdrawal may cause increased duration and frequency of chest pain.
- The elderly may be at greater risk of experiencing low blood pressure and constipation associated with this therapy.

DRUG INTERACTIONS
This drug is metabolized by a specific set of liver enzymes (cytochrome P450 enzymes 3A4). Several other drugs interfere with these liver enzymes, and thus may increase or decrease the clearance of nicardipine from the body, potentially increasing the risk of side effects or decreasing effectiveness. When these drugs are given in combination with nicardipine, dosage adjustments may be needed. As these are too numerous to list, you should always check with your doctor or pharmacist prior to starting a new medication, herbal, or nonprescription product.

FOOD INTERACTIONS
Avoid alcohol and grapefruit juice. Do not take with high fat breakfast.

HERBAL INTERACTIONS
St. John's wort, ephedra, dong quai, yohimbine, ginseng, garlic

PREGNANCY AND BREAST-FEEDING CAUTIONS
FDA Pregnancy Risk Category C. Excreted in breast milk. Consult your doctor.

SPECIAL INFORMATION
The sustained release form should be taken with food (not a fatty meal). Do not crush. Limit caffeine intake. Notify your doctor if symptoms of angina do not improve.

NIFEDIPINE
(nye-FED-i-peen)

NEWLY DISCOVERED USES (OFF-LABEL)
Dysmenorrhea, kidney stones, myotonic dystrophy, premature labor, prevention of cyclosporine-induced nephrotoxicity, ureteral stones

ORIGINAL USES (ON-LABEL)
To treat angina and hypertension (sustained release only), hypertension

BRAND NAMES
Adalat CC, Apo-Nifed (PA), Novo-Nifedin, Nu-Nifed, Procardia

DRUG CLASS
Antianginal, antihypertensive (calcium channel blocker)

DESCRIPTION
This drug relaxes coronary vascular smooth muscle and increases oxygen delivery to the heart.

POTENTIAL SIDE EFFECTS
Flushing, peripheral edema, dizziness/lightheadedness/giddiness, headache, nausea/heartburn, weakness, increased cough, gout, lower heart rate, fatigue, lethargy, constipation, weakness.

CAUTIONS
- Routine use of this drug in emergency high blood pressure is not recommended.
- Do not take this drug sublingually (under the tongue).
- Notify your doctor if you have had an allergic reaction to a drug in this class.
- Inform your doctor if you have low blood pressure, severe left ventricular dysfunction or other types of heart problems, liver or kidney dysfunction.
- Abrupt withdrawal may cause increased duration and frequency of chest pain.

- The elderly may be at greater risk of experiencing low blood pressure and constipation associated with this therapy.

DRUG INTERACTIONS

This drug is metabolized by a specific set of liver enzymes. Several other drugs interfere with these liver enzymes, and thus may increase or decrease the clearance of nifedipine from the body, potentially increasing the risk of side effects or decreasing effectiveness. When these drugs are given in combination with nifedipine, dosage adjustments may be needed. As these are too numerous to list, you should always check with your doctor or pharmacist prior to starting a new medication, herbal, or nonprescription product.

FOOD INTERACTIONS

Alcohol, grapefruit juice. Do not take Adalat CC with high-fat meals; take on an empty stomach.

HERBAL INTERACTIONS

St. John's wort, ephedra, yohimbine, garlic

PREGNANCY AND BREAST-FEEDING CAUTIONS

FDA Pregnancy Risk Category C. Excreted in breast milk. Consult your doctor.

SPECIAL INFORMATION

Sustained release products should not be crushed or chewed. The shell of sustained release tablets may appear intact in stool. This is no cause for concern.

NIMODIPINE
(nye-MOE-di-peen)

NEWLY DISCOVERED USES (OFF-LABEL)
Essential tremor

ORIGINAL USES (ON-LABEL)

Reduction of cerebral infarction (stroke) and improvement of outcome after subarachnoid bleeding

BRAND NAME

Nimotop

DRUG CLASS
Cardiac (calcium channel blocker)

DESCRIPTION
This drug relaxes coronary vascular smooth muscle and increases oxygen delivery to the heart.

POTENTIAL SIDE EFFECTS
Decrease in blood pressure, changes in heart rate, sweating, dizziness, flushing, headache, nausea, feelings of warmth.

CAUTIONS
- If low blood pressure occurs, medication may need to be discontinued.
- Not for use in pregnancy, during breast-feeding, or if you have severe liver impairment.

DRUG INTERACTIONS
This drug is metabolized by a specific set of liver enzymes. Several other drugs interfere with these liver enzymes, and thus may increase or decrease the clearance of nimodipine from the body, potentially increasing the risk of side effects or decreasing effectiveness. When these drugs are given in combination with nimodipine, dosage adjustments may be needed. As these are too numerous to list, you should always check with your doctor or pharmacist prior to starting a new medication, herbal, or nonprescription product.

FOOD INTERACTIONS
Avoid grapefruit juice.

HERBAL INTERACTIONS
St. John's wort, ephedra, yohimbine, ginseng, garlic

PREGNANCY AND BREAST-FEEDING CAUTIONS
FDA Pregnancy Risk Category C. Excreted in breast milk. Do not breast-feed during therapy with this drug.

NITROGLYCERIN
(nye-troe-GLI-ser-in)

Transdermal, Topical

NEWLY DISCOVERED USES (OFF-LABEL)
Anal fissure, Raynaud's syndrome

ORIGINAL USES (ON-LABEL)
Angina pectoris

BRAND NAMES
Minitran, Nitrek, Nitro-Dur, Nitro-Bid, Transderm-Nitro

DRUG CLASS
Antianginal

DESCRIPTION
This drug reduces cardiac oxygen demand by decreasing cardiac pressure in the left ventricle (heart chamber) and decreasing resistance in the vessels. It relaxes coronary arteries and improves blood flow to regions that are poorly oxygenated.

POTENTIAL SIDE EFFECTS
Low blood pressure, cardiovascular collapse, increased heart rate, shock, flushing, peripheral swelling, headache, lightheadedness, dizziness, restlessness, nausea, vomiting, bowel incontinence, dry mouth, urinary incontinence, weakness, blurred vision, cold sweat.

CAUTIONS
- Notify your doctor if you have an allergy to any nitrates, or are concurrently using sildenafil, tadalafil, or vardenafil.
- Inform your doctor if you have angle-closure glaucoma, liver or kidney problems, cardiac problems, or recent head trauma or cerebral hemorrhage, severe anemia.
- May cause lowered blood pressure upon standing from a sitting or lying down position.
- Tolerance to effects of the drug may develop.
- Not for immediate relief of anginal attacks.
- Use caution when discarding patches as there is enough residual nitroglycerin in the product to be a potential hazard for children and pets.

DRUG INTERACTIONS
Do not administer sildenafil, tadalafil, or vardenafil within 24 hours of a nitrate preparation. Calcium channel blockers (such as verapamil, nifedipine, diltiazem, etc.), dihydroergotamine.

FOOD INTERACTIONS
Unknown

HERBAL INTERACTIONS
Unknown

PREGNANCY AND BREAST-FEEDING CAUTIONS
FDA Pregnancy Risk Category C. Excretion in breast milk is unknown. Consult your doctor.

SPECIAL INFORMATION
Do not change from one brand to another without consulting your doctor or pharmacist.

Topical: Do not use fingers to apply ointment, use applicator or dose measuring paper. Do not rub or massage area. One inch of ointment contains approximately 15 mg of nitroglycerin.

NITROGLYCERIN
(nye-troe-GLI-ser-in)

IV

NEWLY DISCOVERED USES (OFF-LABEL)

Acute myocardial infarction, cocaine-induced acute coronary syndrome, congestive heart failure, hypertensive crisis, left ventricular dysfunction, pulmonary edema, severe hypertension

---

ORIGINAL USES (ON-LABEL)
Angina pectoris (acute treatment), congestive heart failure (especially when associated with acute heart attacks), pulmonary hypertension, high blood pressure emergencies occurring during surgery (especially during cardiovascular surgery)

BRAND NAME
Nitro-Bid IV

DRUG CLASS
Antianginal, antihypertensive

DESCRIPTION
This drug reduces cardiac oxygen demand by decreasing cardiac pressure in the left ventricle (heart chamber) and decreasing resistance in the vessels. It relaxes coronary arteries and improves blood flow to regions that are poorly oxygenated.

POTENTIAL SIDE EFFECTS
Low blood pressure, cardiovascular collapse, increased heart rate, shock, flushing, peripheral swelling, headache, lightheadedness, dizziness, restlessness, nausea, vomiting, bowel incontinence, dry mouth, urinary incontinence, methemoglobinemia, weakness, blurred vision, cold sweat.

CAUTIONS
- Notify your doctor if you have an allergy to any nitrates, or are concurrently using sildenafil, tadalafil, or vardenafil.
- Inform your doctor if you have angle-closure glaucoma, liver or kidney problems, cardiac problems, or recent head trauma or cerebral hemorrhage, severe anemia.
- May cause lowered blood pressure upon standing from a sitting or lying down position.
- Tolerance to effects of the drug may develop.

DRUG INTERACTIONS
Do not administer sildenafil, tadalafil, or vardenafil within 24 hours of a nitrate preparation. Aspirin, calcium channel blockers (such as verapamil, nifedipine, diltiazem), dihydroergotamine.

FOOD INTERACTIONS
Unknown

HERBAL INTERACTIONS
Unknown

PREGNANCY AND BREAST-FEEDING CAUTIONS
FDA Pregnancy Risk Category C. Excretion in breast milk is unknown. Consult your doctor.

NITROGLYCERIN
(nye-troe-GLI-ser-in)

Oral, SL

NEWLY DISCOVERED USES (OFF-LABEL)
Acute myocardial infarction, anal fissure, cocaine-induced acute coronary syndrome, hypertensive crisis, pulmonary edema, Raynaud's syndrome, severe hypertension

ORIGINAL USES (ON-LABEL)
Angina pectoris (acute treatment), congestive heart failure (associated with acute heart attacks), pulmonary hypertension, high blood pressure emergencies occurring during surgery (especially during cardiovascular surgery)

BRAND NAMES
Nitro-Time, Nitrogard, NitroQuick, Nitrostat, Nitro-Tab

DESCRIPTION
This drug reduces cardiac oxygen demand by decreasing cardiac pressure in the left ventricle (heart chamber) and decreasing resistance in the vessels. It relaxes coronary arteries and improves blood flow to regions that are poorly oxygenated.

POTENTIAL SIDE EFFECTS
Low blood pressure, cardiovascular collapse, increased heart rate, shock, flushing, peripheral swelling, headache, lightheadedness, dizziness, restlessness, nausea, vomiting, bowel incontinence, dry mouth, urinary incontinence, weakness, blurred vision, cold sweat.

CAUTIONS
- Notify your doctor if you have an allergy to any nitrates, or are concurrently using sildenafil, tadalafil, or vardenafil.
- Inform your doctor if you have angle-closure glaucoma, liver or kidney problems, cardiac problems, or recent head trauma or cerebral hemorrhage, severe anemia.
- Do not use extended release preparations in patients with GI hypermotility or malabsorptive syndrome.
- May cause lowered blood pressure upon standing from a sitting or lying down position.
- Tolerance to effects of the drug may develop.

DRUG INTERACTIONS

Do not administer sildenafil, tadalafil, or vardenafil within 24 hours of a nitrate preparation. Aspirin, calcium channel blockers (such as verapamil, nifedipine, diltiazem), dihydroergotamine.

FOOD INTERACTIONS

- Low blood pressure may occur when nitrates are taken one hour or more after alcohol ingestion.
- Take oral preparations on an empty stomach with a glass of water.

HERBAL INTERACTIONS

Unknown

PREGNANCY AND BREAST-FEEDING CAUTIONS

FDA Pregnancy Risk Category C. Excretion in breast milk is unknown. Consult your doctor.

SPECIAL INFORMATION

Do not change from one brand to another without consulting your doctor or pharmacist.

May cause headache and dizziness, notify your doctor if this persists. Aspirin or acetaminophen may be useful in providing relief. Keep tablets in original container. Sublingual tablets: Dissolve tablet under your tongue, do not swallow. Take at first sign of chest pain. Do not wait for the pain to become severe. If pain is unrelieved after five minutes, take another one. Repeat this again. Contact your doctor if pain persists.

NITROPRUSSIDE
(nye-tro-PRUS-ide)

NEWLY DISCOVERED USES (OFF-LABEL)

Aortic aneurysm, cardiogenic shock, congestive heart failure, mitral valve regurgitation, pulmonary edema

ORIGINAL USES (ON-LABEL)

Hypertensive crisis, to reduce bleeding during surgery, acute congestive heart failure

BRAND NAME

Nitropress

DRUG CLASS
Antihypertensive

DESCRIPTION
This drug relaxes smooth muscle of the blood vessels, inducing a decrease in blood pressure. It acts primarily more on veins than arteries.

POTENTIAL SIDE EFFECTS
Changes in heart rate, rapid decrease in blood pressure, abdominal pain, sweating, dizziness, muscle weakness, nausea, restlessness, irritation at infusion site.

CAUTIONS
- Requires careful monitoring to ensure that excessive lowering of blood pressure does not occur.
- Infusion of this drug may generate cyanide toxicity or accumulation of methemoglobin in the blood. Requires monitoring during therapy.

DRUG INTERACTIONS
Drugs which affect blood pressure.

FOOD INTERACTIONS
Unknown

HERBAL INTERACTIONS
Unknown

PREGNANCY AND BREAST-FEEDING CAUTIONS
FDA Pregnancy Risk Category C. Excretion in breast milk not known. Not recommended during breast-feeding.

SPECIAL INFORMATION
This drug has a black box warning regarding specific instructions for dilution and administration. In addition, warnings include the potential for rapid decreases in blood pressure, requiring close monitoring during infusions to prevent serious adverse events. This drug has also been shown to cause increased levels of cyanide in the blood.

NOREPINEPHRINE
(nor-ep-i-NEF-rin)

NEWLY DISCOVERED USES (OFF-LABEL)
Pulmonary edema

ORIGINAL USES (ON-LABEL)
To restore blood pressure in acute hypotensive (low-blood pressure) episodes

BRAND NAME
Levophed

DRUG CLASS
Vasopressor (used to treat shock)

DESCRIPTION
This drug is a powerful stimulant of alpha- and beta-receptors in the cardiac system, causing increases in blood pressure by causing the blood vessels to constrict.

POTENTIAL SIDE EFFECTS
Decreased heart rate, anxiety, headache, necrosis at the injection site.

CAUTIONS
- Alert your doctor if you have allergies to bisulfites.
- Not for use if you have low blood pressure due to decreased blood volume.
- Not for use if you have mesenteric or peripheral vascular blood clots.
- Requires blood pressure monitoring.
- Avoid infusion into leg veins.

DRUG INTERACTIONS
Tricyclic antidepressants, MAO inhibitors, antihistamines, beta-blockers, guanethidine, ergot alkaloids, reserpine, methyldopa, alpha-blockers, and atropine

FOOD INTERACTIONS
Unknown

HERBAL INTERACTIONS
Unknown

PREGNANCY AND BREAST-FEEDING CAUTIONS
FDA Pregnancy Risk Category C. Excretion in breast milk is unknown. Do not breast-feed during therapy.

NORETHINDRONE ACETATE-ETHINYL ESTRADIOL
(NOR-eth-in-drone As-eh-tate ETH-in-il es-tra DYE-ole)

NEWLY DISCOVERED USES (OFF-LABEL)

Abnormal uterine bleeding, dysmenorrhea, endometriosis, hirsutism, menopausal symptoms, menorrhagia, perimenopausal symptoms, polycystic ovary

ORIGINAL USES (ON-LABEL)
Prevention of pregnancy, treatment of acne

BRAND NAMES
Estrostep, Junel, Loestrin, Microgestin

DRUG CLASS
Contraceptive (estrogen and progestin combination)

DESCRIPTION
This drug inhibits ovulation. It prevents the secretion of two hormones important in the ovulation cycle: follicle stimulating hormone (FSH) and luteinizing hormone (LH). In addition, the cervical mucus of the vagina changes, becoming hostile for sperm.

POTENTIAL SIDE EFFECTS
Intermenstrual bleeding and irregularity, abdominal pain, diarrhea, nausea, vomiting, depression, dizziness, emotional lability, headache, migraine, nervousness, change in vision or ability to wear contact lenses, fluid retention, darkening of skin in areas, vaginal infections, hair loss. Increased risk of cardiac events, glucose intolerance, stroke, liver problems

CAUTIONS
- Oral contraceptives do not protect against sexually transmitted diseases or HIV infection.
- Cardiovascular events increase if you are over 35 years of age and a heavy smoker (at least 15 cigarettes daily), or have a history of cardiovascular disease or thromboembolic (blood clots) events. Thus, not for use in these patients.
- Not for use in patients with decreased kidney, adrenal or liver function, diabetes with vascular involvement, history of or suspected breast cancer or estrogen dependent cancer, undiagnosed genital bleeding, liver tumor, severe high blood pressure,

jaundice associated with pregnancy or prior birth control pill usage, headaches with neurological symptoms.

- Do not take if you are pregnant.
- Discuss cardiac and other risks with your doctor prior to starting therapy.

DRUG INTERACTIONS
Oral contraceptives, including this product, may interact with several drugs too numerous to list. Check with your pharmacist or doctor before starting any new medication, herbal product, or nonprescription drug.

FOOD INTERACTIONS
Grapefruit juice

HERBAL INTERACTIONS
St. John's wort, dong quai, black cohosh, saw palmetto, red clover, ginseng

PREGNANCY AND BREAST-FEEDING CAUTIONS
FDA Pregnancy Risk Category X. Do not use in pregnancy. Excreted in breast milk and not recommended during breast-feeding.

SPECIAL INFORMATION
Read the patient information brochure prior to therapy for important instructions regarding therapy.

NORETHINDRONE ACETATE
(NOR-eth-in-drone As-eh-tate)

NEWLY DISCOVERED USES (OFF-LABEL)
Dysmenorrhea, menorrhagia, premenstrual syndrome (PMS)

ORIGINAL USES (ON-LABEL)
Loss of menstruation (amenorrhea), endometriosis, abnormal uterine bleeding

BRAND NAME
Aygestin

DRUG CLASS
Progestin

DESCRIPTION

This hormone is necessary to increase the receptivity of the endometrioses for implantation. Once an embryo is implanted, progesterones act to maintain pregnancy. They also inhibit uterine contractions.

POTENTIAL SIDE EFFECTS

Changes in weight, nausea, vomiting, depression, dizziness, emotional lability, headache, fluid retention, changes in vision, migraine

CAUTIONS

- Report any of loss of vision or vision changes to your doctor immediately.
- Do not take if you are pregnant.
- Discuss cardiac and other risks with your doctor prior to starting therapy.
- Fluid retention may occur.

DRUG INTERACTIONS

Rifampin. Check with your pharmacist or doctor before starting any new medication, herbal product, or nonprescription drug.

FOOD INTERACTIONS

If stomach upset occurs, take with food.

HERBAL INTERACTIONS

Unknown

PREGNANCY AND BREAST-FEEDING CAUTIONS

FDA Pregnancy Risk Category X. Do not use in pregnancy. Excreted in breast milk and not recommended during breast-feeding.

SPECIAL INFORMATION

Read the patient information brochure prior to therapy for important instructions regarding therapy and black box warnings regarding adverse events associated with use during first four months of pregnancy.

NORFLOXACIN
(nor-FLOKS-a-sin)

NEWLY DISCOVERED USES (OFF-LABEL)
Traveler's diarrhea

ORIGINAL USES (ON-LABEL)
Uncomplicated urinary tract infections, prostatitis, and cystitis caused by susceptible bacteria; sexually transmitted disease caused by *N. gonorrhoeae*

BRAND NAME
Noroxin

DRUG CLASS
Antibiotic (quinolone)

DESCRIPTION
This drug interferes with cellular enzymes, halting DNA replication, repair, recombination, and transposition.

POTENTIAL SIDE EFFECTS
Dizziness, nausea, diarrhea, headache.

CAUTIONS
- Report to your doctor if you experience pain, inflammation or rupture of a tendon. Rest and refrain from exercise until you see a doctor. Tendon rupture can occur during or after therapy with this drug.
- Stop the medication at the first sign of a rash.
- Prolonged use may cause superinfection.
- May aggravate symptoms of myasthenia gravis.
- Inform your doctor if serious, persistent diarrhea develops.
- May require dosage adjustment if you have kidney impairment.
- Crystalluria (crystals in urine have developed). Drink ample fluids to ensure hydration and adequate urinary output. Do not exceed recommended dose.

DRUG INTERACTIONS
Inhibits CYP1A2 (strong), 3A4 (moderate). Iron, zinc, calcium, magnesium, aluminum, corticosteroids (increase risk of tendon rupture), antacids, electrolyte supplements, quinapril, sucralfate, certain antiarrhythmics, didanosine formulations (chewable/buffered tablets and pediatric powder for oral suspension), theophyllines, antacids, cyclosporine, cimetidine.

FOOD INTERACTIONS
Take at least one hour prior to or at least two hours after meals or ingestion of milk. Dairy products or calcium-fortified juices. Caffeine levels may be increased.

HERBAL INTERACTIONS
St. John's wort, dong quai, zinc

PREGNANCY AND BREAST-FEEDING CAUTIONS
FDA Pregnancy Risk Category C. May be excreted in breast milk. Do not use during breast-feeding.

SPECIAL INFORMATION
Take antacids or sucralfate three to four hours after giving norfloxacin. Take entire prescription even if feeling better. Maintain adequate hydration (2 to 3 L/day of fluids) to avoid concentrated urine and crystal formation. May cause increased sensitivity to sunlight; use sun block, wear protective clothing and dark glasses. Report immediately any signs of rash, joint or back pain, difficulty breathing, easy bruising or bleeding, inflammation, or rupture of tendon.

NORGESTIMATE-ETHINYL ESTRADIOL
(nor-JES-ti-mate ETH-in-il es-tra-DYE-ole)

NEWLY DISCOVERED USES (OFF-LABEL)
Abnormal uterine bleeding, amenorrhea, dysmenorrhea, endometriosis, hirsutism, menopausal symptoms, menorrhagia, perimenopausal symptoms, polycystic ovary

ORIGINAL USES (ON-LABEL)
Prevention of pregnancy, acne in females greater than 15 years of age

BRAND NAMES
MonoNessa, Ortho-Cyclen, Ortho Tri-Cyclen, Ortho Tri-Cyclen Lo, Sprintec

DRUG CLASS
Contraceptive (estrogen and progestin combination)

DESCRIPTION

This drug inhibits ovulation. It prevents the secretion of two hormones important in the ovulation cycle: follicle stimulating hormone (FSH) and luteinizing hormone (LH). In addition, the cervical mucus of the vagina changes, becoming hostile for sperm.

POTENTIAL SIDE EFFECTS

Intermenstrual bleeding and irregularity, abdominal pain, diarrhea, nausea, vomiting, depression, dizziness, emotional lability, headache, migraine, nervousness, change in vision or ability to wear contact lenses, fluid retention, darkening of skin in areas, vaginal infections, hair loss. Increased risk of cardiac events, glucose intolerance, stroke, liver problems.

CAUTIONS

- Oral contraceptives do not protect against sexually transmitted diseases or HIV infection.
- Cardiovascular events increase if you are over 35 years of age and a heavy smoker (at least 15 cigarettes daily), or have a history of cardiovascular disease or thromboembolic (blood clots) events.
- Not for use in patients with decreased kidney, adrenal or liver function, diabetes with vascular involvement, history of or suspected breast cancer or estrogen dependent cancer, undiagnosed genital bleeding, liver tumor, severe high blood pressure, jaundice associated with pregnancy or prior birth control pill usage, headaches with neurological symptoms.
- Do not take if you are pregnant.
- Discuss cardiac and other risks with your doctor prior to starting therapy.

DRUG INTERACTIONS

Oral contraceptives, including this product, may interact with several drugs too numerous to list. Check with your pharmacist or doctor before starting any new medication, herbal product, or nonprescription drug.

FOOD INTERACTIONS

Grapefruit juice

HERBAL INTERACTIONS

St. John's wort, dong quai, black cohosh, saw palmetto, red clover, ginseng

PREGNANCY AND BREAST-FEEDING CAUTIONS
FDA Pregnancy Risk Category X. Do not use in pregnancy. Excreted in breast milk and not recommended during breast-feeding.

SPECIAL INFORMATION
Read the patient information brochure prior to therapy for important instructions regarding therapy.

NORGESTREL-ETHINYL ESTRADIOL
(nor-JES-trel ETH-in-il es-tra-DYE-ole)

NEWLY DISCOVERED USES (OFF-LABEL)
Abnormal uterine bleeding, amenorrhea, dysmenorrhea, endometriosis, hirsutism, menorrhàgia, polycystic ovary

ORIGINAL USES (ON-LABEL)
Prevention of pregnancy

BRAND NAMES
Cryselle, Lo/Ovral, Low-Ogestrel, Ogestrel, Ovral

DRUG CLASS
Contraceptive (estrogen and progestin combination)

DESCRIPTION
This drug inhibits ovulation. It prevents the secretion of two hormones important in the ovulation cycle: follicle stimulating hormone (FSH) and luteinizing hormone (LH). In addition, the cervical mucus of the vagina changes, becoming hostile for sperm.

POTENTIAL SIDE EFFECTS
Intermenstrual bleeding and irregularity, abdominal pain, diarrhea, nausea, vomiting, depression, dizziness, emotional lability, headache, migraine, nervousness, change in vision or ability to wear contact lenses, fluid retention, darkening of skin in areas, vaginal infections, hair loss. Increased risk of cardiac events, glucose intolerance, stroke, liver problems.

CAUTIONS
• Oral contraceptives do not protect against sexually transmitted diseases or HIV infection.

- Cardiovascular events increase if you are over 35 years of age and a heavy smoker (at least 15 cigarettes daily), or have a history of cardiovascular disease or thromboembolic (blood clots) events. Thus, not for use in these patients.
- Not for use if you have decreased kidney, adrenal or liver function, diabetes with vascular involvement, history of or suspected breast cancer or estrogen dependent cancer, undiagnosed genital bleeding, liver tumor, severe high blood pressure, jaundice associated with pregnancy or prior birth control pill usage, headaches with neurological symptoms.
- Do not take if you are pregnant.
- Discuss cardiac and other risks with your doctor prior to starting therapy.

DRUG INTERACTIONS
Oral contraceptives, including this product, may interact with several drugs too numerous to list. Check with your pharmacist or doctor before starting any new medication, herbal product, or nonprescription drug.

FOOD INTERACTIONS
Grapefruit juice

HERBAL INTERACTIONS
St. John's wort, dong quai, black cohosh, saw palmetto, red clover, ginseng

PREGNANCY AND BREAST-FEEDING CAUTIONS
FDA Pregnancy Risk Category X. Do not use in pregnancy. Excreted in breast milk and not recommended during breast-feeding.

SPECIAL INFORMATION
Read the patient information brochure prior to therapy for important instructions regarding therapy.

NORTRIPTYLINE
(nor-TRIP-ti-leen)

NEWLY DISCOVERED USES (OFF-LABEL)
Chronic fatigue syndrome, chronic nausea and vomiting, chronic neuropathic pain, diabetic neuropathy, migraine prevention, multiple sclerosis, panic disorder, post-herpetic neuralgia, premenstrual dysphoric disorder (PMDD), premenstrual syndrome (PMS), post-traumatic stress syndrome (PTSD), smoking cessation, stress incontinence, urge incontinence, vulvodynia

ORIGINAL USES (ON-LABEL)
Depression

BRAND NAMES
Aventyl, Pamelor

DRUG CLASS
Antidepressant (tricyclic)

DESCRIPTION
Nortriptyline increases the levels of norepinephrine and serotonin in the body by inhibiting uptake of these chemicals by neurons.

POTENTIAL SIDE EFFECTS
Dry mouth, sedation, dizziness, headache, nervousness, skin rash, tremors, hives, nausea, constipation, vision changes, sweating, lowered blood pressure, increased heart rate, decreased sodium levels suicidal ideation, changes in heart rhythm and conduction, blurred vision, weight gain.

CAUTIONS
- Do not use if you have been taking an MAO inhibitor (such as phenelzine, tranylcypromine, isocarboxazid) within the past 14 days. When used with MAO-Is fever, high blood pressure, increased heart rate, confusion, seizures, and deaths have been reported.
- Not for use immediately after a heart attack.
- Can cause sedation that may impair performance of tasks requiring alertness. Sedative effects may be additive with other drugs that cause similar effects (central nervous system depressants).

- May worsen psychosis or mania in patients with bipolar disease.
- Stop therapy with doctor permission and according to instructions (gradual taper) prior to elective surgery.
- Do not abruptly stop medication; taper gradually.
- Notify your doctor if you have low blood pressure as this drug can cause low blood pressure episodes.
- Use with caution in patients with urinary retention, history of cardiac disease, seizure disorders, diabetes, benign prostatic hyperplasia, narrow-angle glaucoma, dry mouth, visual problems, constipation, or a history of bowel obstruction.
- Possibility of suicide attempt may persist until remission occurs.
- Use with caution in hyperthyroid patients or those receiving thyroid supplementation.
- Use with caution in patients with liver or kidney dysfunction and in elderly.

DRUG INTERACTIONS
MAO inhibitors (such as phenelzine, tranylcypromine, isocarboxazid), ritonavir, bupropion, amphetamines, anticholinergics, sedatives, chlorpropamide, tolazamide, warfarin, fluoxetine, fluvoxamine, citalopram, escitalopram, paroxetine, sertraline, cimetidine, carbamazepine, haloperidol, smoking, methylphenidate, valproic acid, clonidine, venlafaxine, protease inhibitors, quinidine, diltiazem, verapamil, lithium, phenothiazines may affect the levels of desipramine, drugs which prolong QT interval (see site: http://www.torsades.org/medical- pros/drug-lists/drug-lists.htm#).

This drug is metabolized (inactivated) by specific set of liver enzymes. Several other drugs interfere with these liver enzymes, and thus may increase or decrease the clearance of nortriptyline from the body, potentially increasing the risk of side effects or decreasing effectiveness. When these drugs are given in combination with nortriptyline, dosage adjustments may be needed. As these are too numerous to list, you should always check with your doctor or pharmacist prior to starting a new medication.

FOOD INTERACTIONS
Alcohol, grapefruit juice

HERBAL INTERACTIONS
Valerian, St. John's wort, SAMe, kava kava

PREGNANCY AND BREAST-FEEDING CAUTIONS
FDA Pregnancy Risk Category D. Excreted in breast milk. Breast-feeding is not recommended during therapy with this drug.

SPECIAL INFORMATION
May take four to six weeks for the full therapeutic effects to be experienced. Avoid prolonged exposure to sunlight, wear sunscreen.

OCTREOTIDE
(ok-TREE-oh-tide)

NEWLY DISCOVERED USES (OFF-LABEL)
Acute upper gastrointestinal bleeding, chronic diarrhea, irritable bowel syndrome (IBS)

ORIGINAL USES (ON-LABEL)
To control symptoms in metastatic carcinoid and vasoactive intestinal peptide-secreting tumors, for pancreatic tumors, gastrinoma, secretory diarrhea, and acromegaly

BRAND NAMES
Sandostatin, Sandostatin LAR

DRUG CLASS
Antidiarrheal, antisecretory (somatostatin analog)

DESCRIPTION
This drug mimics a natural drug in the body, somatostatin. It also decreases growth hormone in acromegaly (abnormal enlargement of limbs caused by excessive secretion of growth hormone after maturity).

POTENTIAL SIDE EFFECTS
Decreased heart rate, irregular heart rhythms, chest pain, shortness of breath, changes in blood pressure or blood glucose, diarrhea, abdominal pain, flatulence, constipation, nausea, flushing, edema, fatigue, headache, dizziness, jaundice, hepatitis, liver toxicity, rash, hives, gallbladder abnormalities (such as stones, sludge, decreased contractility).

CAUTIONS
- Has been associated with several, potentially severe gallbladder complications. Notify your doctor if you have a history of or currently have gallbladder problems.

- Reduced dosage may be needed if you are elderly, have decreased kidney function or currently on dialysis.
- May require monitoring to determine therapeutic response, or changes in blood .glucose, thyroid, cardiac and liver function
- Dietary fat absorption may be altered during therapy and may require assessment.
- If you are taking insulin or sulfonylurea, dosages may need to be reduced.

DRUG INTERACTIONS
Insulin or sulfonylurea antidiabetic drugs, bromocriptine, cyclosporine, codeine

FOOD INTERACTIONS
This drug alters the absorption of fat in the diet and vitamin B 12 levels, and periodically requires monitoring of this effect. Schedule injections between meals to decrease gastrointestinal effects.

HERBAL INTERACTIONS
Unknown

PREGNANCY AND BREAST-FEEDING CAUTIONS
FDA Pregnancy Risk Category B. Excreted in breast milk. Do not breast-feed during therapy,

OLANZAPINE
(oh-LAN-za-peen)

NEWLY DISCOVERED USES (OFF-LABEL)
Alzheimer's disease, autism, borderline personality disorder, Huntington's disease

ORIGINAL USES (ON-LABEL)
Treatment of schizophrenia and acute mania episodes associated with bipolar disorder

BRAND NAMES
Zyprexa, Zyprexa Zydis

DRUG CLASS
Atypical antipsychotic

DESCRIPTION
This drug affects multiple neurotransmitters in the brain, including serotonin, dopamine, and histamine.

POTENTIAL SIDE EFFECTS
Headache, somnolence, insomnia, agitation, nervousness, dizziness, upset stomach, constipation, weight gain, increased blood glucose, weakness, sudden drop in blood pressure upon standing, increased heart rate, peripheral edema, uncontrolled muscle movements, parkinsonian events, amnesia, euphoria, rash, bruising, dry mouth, joint ache, neck rigidity, twitching, increased triglycerides/cholesterol levels, increased glucose levels, liver toxicity.

CAUTIONS
- May worsen narrow-angle glaucoma, or myasthenia gravis.
- Zyprexa Zydis tablets contain phenylalanine.
- Has demonstrated increased mortality in elderly patients when used for off-label treatment of dementia in elderly patients.
- Notify your doctor if you plan to become pregnant, if you have heart disease; cerebrovascular disease or conditions that predispose to low blood pressure, history of seizures, thyroid disease, liver disease, increased cholesterol or triglycerides levels, diabetes.
- Neuroleptic malignant syndrome (NMS), a potentially fatal complex, has been reported with antipsychotic drugs. Report any of the following symptoms to your doctor immediately: fever, muscle rigidity, altered mental status, irregular heart rate, increased heart rate.
- Has been reported to cause significant increases in blood glucose levels, causing diabetes that requires treatment.
- May disrupt regulation of body temperature. Avoid dehydration, particularly during strenuous exercise or extreme heat.
- Patients with bipolar depression/schizophrenia may be at increased risk of suicidial thinking.

DRUG INTERACTIONS
This drug is metabolized by a specific set of liver enzymes. Several other drugs interfere with these liver enzymes, and thus may increase or decrease the clearance of olanzapine from the body, potentially increasing the risk of side effects or decreasing effectiveness. When these drugs are given in combination with olanzapine, dosage adjustments may be needed. As these are too numerous to list, you should always check with your doctor or pharmacist prior to starting a new medication, herbal, or non-prescription product.

FOOD INTERACTIONS
Avoid alcohol; it may increase sedation.

HERBAL INTERACTIONS
Dong quai, St. John's wort, kava kava, gotu kola, valerian

PREGNANCY AND BREAST-FEEDING CAUTIONS
FDA Pregnancy Risk Category C. Excreted in breast milk. Do not breast-feed during therapy.

SPECIAL INFORMATION
This drug has a black box warning describing the risk of increased mortality when the drug has been used for off-label treatment of dementia in the elderly.

OLANZAPINE-FLUOXETINE
(oh-LAN-za-peen flu-ox-eh-TEEN)

NEWLY DISCOVERED USES (OFF-LABEL)
Borderline personality disorder

ORIGINAL USES (ON-LABEL)
Treatment of depressive episodes associated with bipolar disorder

BRAND NAME
Symbyax

DRUG CLASS
Atypical antipsychotic-antidepressant (selective serotonin reuptake inhibitor)

DESCRIPTION
This drug affects multiple neurotransmitters in the brain, including serotonin, dopamine, and histamine. It inhibits the reuptake of serotonin at the neuron and thus increases the levels of serotonin in the body and in the brain.

POTENTIAL SIDE EFFECTS
Headache, somnolence, insomnia, agitation, nervousness, dizziness, upset stomach, constipation, weight gain, increased blood glucose, weakness, sudden drop in blood pressure upon standing, increased heart rate, peripheral edema, uncontrolled muscle movements, parkinsonian events, amnesia, euphoria, rash, bruis-

ing, dry mouth, joint ache, neck rigidity, twitching, increased triglycerides/cholesterol levels, increased glucose levels, liver toxicity.

Abnormal thinking, anxiety, dizziness, decreased libido, abnormal vision, fever, flu-syndrome, pain, low sodium levels, changes in blood glucose, abnormal dreams, rash, sexual dysfunction, sinusitis.

CAUTIONS

- Use may be associated with the development of suicidal thinking and behavior (see special information section).
- Do not use if you have been taking an MAO inhibitor (such as phenelzine, tranylcypromine, isocarboxazid) within the past 14 days. When used with MAO-Is fever, high blood pressure, increased heart rate, confusion, seizures, and deaths have been reported.
- Gradually decrease in dosage upon discontinuation of therapy.
- May worsen narrow-angle glaucoma, or myasthenia gravis.
- Has demonstrated increased mortality in elderly patients when used for off-label treatment of dementia in elderly patients.
- Notify your doctor if you plan to become pregnant, if you have heart disease, or if you have cerebrovascular disease or conditions that predispose to low blood pressure, a history of mania, seizures, alcoholism, thyroid disease, or if you have liver or kidney disease, increased cholesterol or triglycerides levels, or diabetes.
- Neuroleptic malignant syndrome (NMS), a potentially fatal complex, has been reported with antipsychotic drugs. Report any of the following symptoms to your doctor immediately: fever, muscle rigidity, altered mental status, irregular heart rate, increased heart rate.
- Has been reported to cause significant increases in blood glucose levels, causing diabetes that requires treatment.
- May disrupt regulation of body temperature. Avoid dehydration, particularly during strenuous exercise or extreme heat.
- Patients with bipolar depression/schizophrenia may be at increased risk of suicidal thinking.
- Concurrent use of aspirin or other non-steroidal anti-inflammatory drugs (NSAIDs) may increase the risk of bleeding.

DRUG INTERACTIONS

This drug is metabolized by and affects a specific set of liver enzymes. Several other drugs interfere with these liver enzymes, and thus may increase or decrease the clearance of olanzapine/fluoxetine from the body, potentially increasing the risk of side effects or decreasing effectiveness. When these drugs are given in combination with olanzapine/fluoxetine, dosage adjustments may be needed. As these are too numerous to list, you should always check with your doctor or pharmacist prior to starting a new medication, herbal, or nonprescription product.

FOOD INTERACTIONS
Avoid alcohol; it may increase sedation.

HERBAL INTERACTIONS
Dong quai, St. John's wort, kava kava, gotu kola, valerian

PREGNANCY AND BREAST-FEEDING CAUTIONS
FDA Pregnancy Risk Category C. Excreted in breast milk. Do not breast-feed during therapy.

SPECIAL INFORMATION
This drug has a black box warning describing the risk of increased mortality when the drug has been used for off-label treatment of dementia in the elderly.

In 2005, the FDA announced new labeling for antidepressants regarding the need to closely monitor for worsening of depression and for the potential of increased suicidal thinking or suicidal behavior during therapy. Although this recommendation applies to all patients (adults, children, adolescents) treated with antidepressants for any indication, this is of particular importance in patients being treated for depression. Discuss the latest information regarding this safety issue with your doctor prior to initiating therapy.

Close observation may be especially important when antidepressant medications are started for the first time or when doses are changed.

This information pertains to the use of the prescription product only and should not be inferred for the use of nonprescription formulations.

OMEPRAZOLE
(oh-ME-pray-zol)

NEWLY DISCOVERED USES (OFF-LABEL)
Acute upper gastrointestinal (GI) bleeding, cystic fibrosis, hiccups, laryngitis, prevention of upper gastrointestinal bleeding recurrence

ORIGINAL USES (ON-LABEL)
Treatment of active duodenal ulcer disease, active benign gastric ulcer, gastroesophageal reflux disease (GERD), erosive esophagitis, hypersecretory conditions. Also used in combination with other drugs for the eradication of *H. pylori* in the stomach to reduce the risk of duodenal ulcer recurrence.

BRAND NAMES
Prilosec, Zegerid

DRUG CLASS
Proton pump inhibitor

DESCRIPTION
This drug inhibits the last step of gastric acid production by suppressing gastric acid secretion via the inhibition of a specific enzyme system in the stomach. This enzyme system is referred to as the acid (proton) pump in the stomach mucosa and this class of drugs is called the "proton pump inhibitors."

POTENTIAL SIDE EFFECTS
Headache, dizziness, diarrhea, abdominal pain, nausea, vomiting, constipation, rash, cough.

CAUTIONS
- Inform your doctor if you have allergies to any drugs in this class.
- Long-term treatment has resulted in atrophic gastritis.
- Absorption may be increased in the elderly.
- Zegerid use is contraindicated in patients with metabolic alkalosis and low calcium levels.
- Relief of symptoms with use of this drug does not exclude gastric cancer.

DRUG INTERACTIONS
Benzodiazepines, carbamazepine, phenytoin, warfarin, amiodarone, citalopram, diazepam, fluoxetine, glimepiride, glipizide,

methsuximide, nateglinide, phenytoin, pioglitazone, propranolol, rosiglitazone, sertraline, aminoglutethimide, rifampin, atazanavir, indinavir, itraconazole, ketoconazole, clarithromycin, sucralfate.

This drug affects other drugs metabolized by a specific set of liver enzymes, and thus may increase or decrease the clearance of these drugs from the body, potentially increasing the risk of side effects or decreasing effectiveness. When these drugs are given in combination with omeprazole, dosage adjustments may be needed. As these are too numerous to list, you should always check with your doctor or pharmacist prior to starting a new medication, herbal, or nonprescription product.

FOOD INTERACTIONS
Take before eating. Avoid alcohol.

HERBAL INTERACTIONS
St. John's wort, ginkgo biloba

PREGNANCY AND BREAST-FEEDING CAUTIONS
FDA Pregnancy Risk Category C. Excreted in breast milk. Therapy not recommended during breast-feeding.

SPECIAL INFORMATION
Swallow capsules whole, do not chew, open, or split.

ONDANSETRON
(on-DAN-se-tron)

NEWLY DISCOVERED USES (OFF-LABEL)

Alcoholism (cravings & dependence), tardive dyskinesia (drug induced), multiple sclerosis, pruritus, schizophrenia, uremic pruritus

ORIGINAL USES (ON-LABEL)
To prevent nausea and vomiting associated with certain cancer chemotherapy and total body radiation therapy, prevention and treatment of post-operative nausea and vomiting

BRAND NAMES
Zofran, Zofran ODT

DRUG CLASS
Antiemetic (serotonin antagonist)

DESCRIPTION
This drug blocks serotonin centrally in the brain.

POTENTIAL SIDE EFFECTS
Changes in blood pressure, anxiety, agitation, dizziness, drowsiness, sedation, headache, malaise, fatigue, chills, shivering, abdominal pain, constipation, diarrhea, dry mouth, cold sensation, numbness, itching, urinary retention, weakness, increase in liver function tests.

CAUTIONS
- Orally-disintegrating tablets contain phenylalanine.
- This drug does not increase gastric motility.
- May require reduced dosages in elderly patients.

DRUG INTERACTIONS
This drug is metabolized by a specific set of liver enzymes (cytochrome P450 enzymes). Several other drugs interfere with these liver enzymes, and thus may increase or decrease the clearance of ondansetron from the body, potentially increasing the risk of side effects or decreasing effectiveness. When these drugs are given in combination with ondansetron, dosage adjustments may be needed. As these are too numerous to list, you should always check with your doctor or pharmacist prior to starting a new medication, herbal, or nonprescription product.

FOOD INTERACTIONS
Take without regard to meals.

HERBAL INTERACTIONS
St. John's wort

PREGNANCY AND BREAST-FEEDING CAUTIONS
FDA Pregnancy Risk Category B. Excretion in breast milk is unknown. Not recommended to breast-feed while taking ondansetron.

ORLISTAT
(OR-li-stat)

NEWLY DISCOVERED USES (OFF-LABEL)
Prevention in type 2 diabetes

ORIGINAL USES (ON-LABEL)
Management of obesity

BRAND NAME
Xenical

DRUG CLASS
Lipase inhibitor

DESCRIPTION
This drug inhibits the absorption of dietary fats by inhibiting the activity of the enzyme responsible for breaking down fats into absorbable units. This drug acts in the stomach and small intestine.

POTENTIAL SIDE EFFECTS
Oily spotting, flatus with discharge, fecal urgency, fatty/oily stool, oily evacuation, increased defecation, fecal incontinence, abdominal pain, gum disorder, diarrhea, nausea, rectal pain, tooth disorder, vomiting, rash, back pain, muscle aches, menstrual irregularity, influenza, ear infection, sleep disorder, urinary tract infection.

CAUTIONS
- While taking this medication, you must comply with dietary guidelines as instructed by your doctor. Side effects may increase if a high fat diet is ingested.
- Requires supplementation with fat soluble vitamins (A, D, E, and K) to ensure adequate nutrition.
- Notify your doctor if you have a history of urinary or kidney stones.
- If you are diabetic, this therapy may require a dosage adjustment in your diabetic medications.

DRUG INTERACTIONS
Warfarin, cyclosporine, fat-soluble vitamins, pravastatin

FOOD INTERACTIONS
Do not take with high fat diet.

HERBAL INTERACTIONS
Cholecalciferol, vitamin E, beta carotene, linoleic acid

PREGNANCY AND BREAST-FEEDING CAUTIONS
FDA Pregnancy Risk Category B. Excretion in breast milk unknown. Breast-feeding is not recommended during therapy.

SPECIAL INFORMATION
You should be on a nutritionally balanced, reduced calorie diet that contains approximately 30% of calories from fat. Daily intake of fat, carbohydrate, and protein should be distributed over the three main meals. Read patient brochure completely prior to starting therapy.

OXCARBAZEPINE
(ox-car-BAZ-e-peen)

NEWLY DISCOVERED USES (OFF-LABEL)
Chronic neuropathic pain, diabetic neuropathy, trigeminal neuralgia

ORIGINAL USES (ON-LABEL)
To treat partial seizures in adults and children (4–16 years of age) with epilepsy

BRAND NAME
Trileptal

DRUG CLASS
Anticonvulsant

DESCRIPTION
This drug blocks sensitive sodium channels, inhibiting the repeated firing and release of neurotransmitters. Thus, it stabilizes seizure activity.

POTENTIAL SIDE EFFECTS
Headache, dizziness, somnolence, anxiety, uncoordinated gait, vertigo, insomnia, tremor, amnesia, emotional lability, nervousness, agitation, abnormal thinking, nausea, vomiting, abdominal pain, diarrhea, upset stomach, constipation, upper respiratory infection, double vision, uncontrolled eye movements, changes in taste sensation, fatigue.

CAUTIONS
- Low blood levels of sodium may occur; thus, it requires periodic monitoring during therapy.
- Do not abruptly stop this medication as it may increase the frequency of seizures.
- Notify your doctor if you have had previous allergies with carbamazepine, if you have reduced kidney function, or previous problems with low sodium.
- May have significant effects on cognitive function, including slowing, difficultly with concentration, and speech or language problems, fatigue, and coordination problems.

DRUG INTERACTIONS
Phenytoin, phenobarbital, carbamazepine, phenytoin, valproic acid, verapamil, felodipine, oral contraceptives, calcium channel

blockers, benzodiazepines, cyclosporine, pimozide, protease inhibitors, quinidine, sirolimus, and tacrolimus.

This drug affects a specific set of liver enzymes (cytochrome P450 enzymes 2C19, 3A4/5). Several other drugs are metabolized and cleared from the body by these liver enzymes, and thus may be increased or decreased in the body, potentially increasing the risk of side effects or decreasing effectiveness. When these drugs are given in combination with oxcarbamazepine, dosage adjustments may be needed. As these are too numerous to list, you should always check with your doctor or pharmacist prior to starting a new medication, herbal, or nonprescription product.

FOOD INTERACTIONS
Avoid alcohol, may increase central nervous system depression.

HERBAL INTERACTIONS
St. John's wort, primrose, valerian, kava kava, gotu kola

PREGNANCY AND BREAST-FEEDING CAUTIONS
FDA Pregnancy Risk Category C. Excreted in breast milk. Do not breast-feed during therapy with this drug.

SPECIAL INFORMATION
Oral contraceptive may be less effective while you are taking this medication. Therefore, you will need to use a back-up form of birth control. In 2005, new information was added to the warnings and precautions of the product labeling regarding the risk of serious skin reactions in both children and adults. Discuss these potential risks with your doctor.

PAMIDRONATE
(pa-mi-DROE-nate)

NEWLY DISCOVERED USES (OFF-LABEL)
Ankylosing spondylitis, bone loss reduction in spinal cord injury, hyperparathyroid crisis, McCune-Albright syndrome, postmenopausal osteoporosis, prevention of glucocorticoid-induced osteoporosis, primary and secondary hyperparathyroidism

ORIGINAL USES (ON-LABEL)
Hypercalcemia (increased calcium levels) associated with malignancy, bone lesions that are associated with breast cancer or multiple myeloma, Paget's disease

BRAND NAME
Aredia

DRUG CLASS
Biphosphonate

DESCRIPTION
This drug reduces bone breakdown by increasing bone mineral density.

POTENTIAL SIDE EFFECTS
Increase in blood pressure, abdominal pain, acid reflux, constipation, dry mouth, nausea, vomiting, diarrhea, low calcium levels, low potassium levels, changes in kidney function, joint aches, bone pain, muscle aches, coughing, shortness of breath, sinusitis, fatigue, fever, pain, anxiety, headache, insomnia, fainting, increased heart rate, changes in heart rate and regularity.

CAUTIONS
- May cause impairment of kidney function. Require monitoring during therapy. Notify your doctor if you have kidney problems prior to therapy.
- Low calcium levels have occurred and may require supplemental calcium administration.
- May require blood monitoring.
- Osteonecrosis (breakdown of the bone) of the jaw has occurred in cancer patients when taking pamidronate with chemotherapy and corticosteroids.

DRUG INTERACTIONS
Consult your doctor or pharmacist prior to starting a new medication, herbal, or nonprescription product.

FOOD INTERACTIONS
Unknown

HERBAL INTERACTIONS
Unknown

PREGNANCY AND BREAST-FEEDING CAUTIONS
FDA Pregnancy Risk Category D. Excretion in breast milk not known. Do not breast-feed during therapy.

SPECIAL INFORMATION

In 2005, the manufacturer notified health professionals and patients regarding the possibility of osteonecrosis (bone breakdown) in the jaw, mainly in cancer patients who received intravenous bisphosphonates. You should receive a dental examination prior to the initiation of therapy and avoid invasive dental procedure during therapy.

PANTOPRAZOLE
(pant-OH-pray-zoll)

NEWLY DISCOVERED USES (OFF-LABEL)
Laryngitis, stress-related mucosal disease, prevention of recurrence of upper gastrointestinal (GI) bleeding

ORIGINAL USES (ON-LABEL)
Short-term treatment of active duodenal ulcers; maintenance treatment of healed duodenal ulcers, part of *H. pylori* treatment regimen, treatment of gastric ulcer, gastroesophageal reflux disease (GERD), erosive esophagitis

BRAND NAMES
Protonix, Protonix IV

DRUG CLASS
Gastrointestinal (proton pump inhibitor)

DESCRIPTION
This drug decreases gastric acid secretion by blocking the final step in gastric acid production.

POTENTIAL SIDE EFFECTS
Diarrhea, abdominal pain, abnormal dreams

CAUTIONS
- Dosage reductions may be required if you have severe liver dysfunction.
- Inform your doctor if you have allergies to any drugs in this class.
- Long-term treatment has resulted in atrophic gastritis.
- Absorption may be increased in the elderly.
- Relief of symptoms with use of this drug does not exclude gastric cancer.

DRUG INTERACTIONS

This drug affects other drugs metabolized by a specific set of liver enzymes, and thus may increase or decrease the clearance of these drugs from the body, potentially increasing the risk of side effects or decreasing effectiveness. When these drugs are given in combination with pantoprazole, dosage adjustments may be needed. As these are too numerous to list, you should always check with your doctor or pharmacist prior to starting a new medication, herbal, or nonprescription product.

FOOD INTERACTIONS

Avoid alcohol.

HERBAL INTERACTIONS

St. John's wort, ginkgo biloba

PREGNANCY AND BREAST-FEEDING CAUTIONS

FDA Pregnancy Risk Category B. Excreted in breast milk. Therapy not recommended during breast-feeding.

SPECIAL INFORMATION

Antacids may be taken during therapy with this drug.

PAPAVERINE
(pa-PAV-er-een)

NEWLY DISCOVERED USES (OFF-LABEL)

Erectile dysfunction

ORIGINAL USES (ON-LABEL)

To treat various conditions associated with spasm of smooth muscle, including vascular spasm associated with acute heart attacks, angina pectoris, peripheral and lung blood clots, and peripheral or cerebral vascular disease

BRAND NAME

Para-Time S.R.

DRUG CLASS

Vasodilator

DESCRIPTION

This drug acts directly on all smooth muscle. During spasms, it causes a relaxation effect. This relaxation occurs in the vascular blood system, bronchial (lung) muscle, and in the gastric, biliary, and urinary tracts.

POTENTIAL SIDE EFFECTS
Nausea, abdominal discomfort, anorexia, constipation, skin rash, vertigo, headache, flushing of skin, diarrhea.

CAUTIONS
- Notify your doctor if you have glaucoma, certain types of heart problems (such as atrioventricular heart block).
- Local injections in the penis for impotence have resulted in priapism (such as prolonged painful erection).
- Discontinue this medication if any liver allergic reactions or changes in liver function occur (such as jaundice).

DRUG INTERACTIONS
Levodopa

FOOD INTERACTIONS
Unknown

HERBAL INTERACTIONS
Unknown

PREGNANCY AND BREAST-FEEDING CAUTIONS
FDA Pregnancy Risk Category C. Excretion in breast milk not known. Consult your doctor.

PAROXETINE
(pa-ROKS-e-teen)

NEWLY DISCOVERED USES (OFF-LABEL)
Attention deficit/hyperactivity disorder (ADHD), alcoholism (cravings and dependence), Alzheimer's disease, chronic fatigue syndrome, diabetic neuropathy, fibromyalgia, menopausal symptoms, nocturnal enuresis, premature ejaculation, pruritus, stuttering, vasovagal syncope

ORIGINAL USES (ON-LABEL)
Depression, panic disorders with or without agoraphobia, obsessive-compulsive disorder, social anxiety disorder, generalized anxiety disorder, post-traumatic stress disorder (PTSD), premenstrual mood disorders.

BRAND NAMES
Paxil, Paxil CR

DRUG CLASS
Antidepressant (selective serotonin reuptake inhibitor)

DESCRIPTION
This drug inhibits the reuptake of serotonin at the neuron, increasing the levels of serotonin in the body and in the brain.

POTENTIAL SIDE EFFECTS
Increased sweating, headache, somnolence, dizziness, insomnia, nausea, dry mouth, constipation, diarrhea, ejaculatory disturbances, muscle weakness, sudden drop in blood pressure upon standing from a sitting or lying position, nervousness, anxiety, yawning, abnormal dreams, rash, decreased libido, flatulence, vomiting, upset stomach, urinary frequency, impotence, tremor, muscle aches and pain, low sodium levels.

CAUTIONS
- Use may be associated with the development of suicidal thinking and behavior (see special information section).
- Do not use if you have been taking an MAO inhibitor (phenelzine, tranylcypromine, isocarboxazid) within the past 14 days. When used with MAO-Is fever, high blood pressure, increased heart rate, confusion, seizures, and deaths have been reported.
- Gradually decrease in dosage upon discontinuation of paroxetine therapy.
- Notify your doctor if you have a history of mania, seizures, or alcoholism.
- Use caution if you have liver dysfunction, or kidney insufficiency, or in elderly patients.
- Concurrent use of aspirin or other non-steroidal anti-inflammatory drugs (NSAIDs) may increase the risk of bleeding.

DRUG INTERACTIONS
MAO inhibitors (such as phenelzine, isocarboxazid, or linezolid), selegiline, phenothiazines (thioridazine or mesoridazine; wait at least five weeks after discontinuation of paroxetine before starting phenothiazines), amphetamines, buspirone, meperidine, nefazodone, sumatriptan, sibutramine, sympathomimetics, ritonavir, tramadol, venlafaxine, alprazolam, diazepam, carbamazepine, carvedilol, clozapine, cyclosporine, dextromethorphan, digoxin, haloperidol, lovastatin, simvastatin, phenytoin, propafenone, theo-

phylline, trazodone, tricyclic antidepressants, valproic acid, lithium, bumetanide, furosemide, torsemide, warfarin, sumatriptan, naratriptan, rizatriptan, and zolmitriptan, cyproheptadine.

This drug is metabolized by a specific set of liver enzymes. Several other drugs interfere with these liver enzymes, and thus may increase or decrease the clearance of paroxetine from the body, potentially increasing the risk of side effects or decreasing effectiveness. When these drugs are given in combination with paroxetine, dosage adjustments may be needed. As these are too numerous to list, you should always check with your doctor or pharmacist prior to starting a new medication, herbal, or nonprescription product.

FOOD INTERACTIONS
Alcohol

HERBAL INTERACTIONS
Valerian, St. John's wort, SAMe, kava kava

PREGNANCY AND BREAST-FEEDING CAUTIONS
FDA Pregnancy Category C. Excreted in breast milk. Not recommended during breast-feeding.

SPECIAL INFORMATION
In 2005, the FDA announced new labeling for antidepressants regarding the need to closely monitor for worsening of depression and for the potential of increased suicidal thinking or suicidal behavior during therapy. Although this recommendation applies to all patients (adults, children, adolescents) treated with antidepressants for any indication, this is of particular importance in patients being treated for depression. Discuss the latest information regarding this safety issue with your doctor prior to initiating therapy.

Close observation may be especially important when antidepressant medications are started for the first time or when doses are changed. More information on this topic can be found at the following web site: http://www.fda.gov/cder/drug/antidepressants/default.htm

Combination with other SSRIs, SSNRIs, tricyclic antidepressants, amphetamines, sympathomimetics, ritonavir, serotonin agonists (sumatriptan), and certain opiates carries an increased risk of serotonin syndrome. While taking this medication, check with your pharmacist or doctor before starting any new medication, herbal, or nonprescription product.

In 2005, product labeling was revised regarding new information about the use of this drug during first trimester of pregnancy, suggesting increased risk of congenital malformations. Discuss these risks with your doctor.

PEGINTERFERON ALFA-2A
(peg-in-ter-FEER-on AL-fa-too-aye)

NEWLY DISCOVERED USES (OFF-LABEL)
Therapy-resistant hepatitis C

ORIGINAL USES (ON-LABEL)
To treat chronic hepatitis C as monotherapy or in combination with ribavirin in adult patients with liver disease who have not been previously treated with interferon alpha

BRAND NAME
Pegasys

DRUG CLASS
Antiviral

DESCRIPTION
This drug is effective by acting against the reproduction of viral cells and by modulating the immune response in the body.

POTENTIAL SIDE EFFECTS
Injection site inflammation, dry mouth, increased sweating, flushing, fatigue, headache, tremors, fever, weight decrease, abdominal pain, chest pain, malaise, dizziness, nausea, anorexia, diarrhea, vomiting, abdominal pain, upset stomach, constipation, blood disorders, insomnia, depression, anxiety, impaired concentration, agitation, nervousness, menstrual disorders, sore throat, hair loss, itching, rash, dry skin, increased triglycerides levels.

CAUTIONS
- May cause severe psychiatric adverse events, including severe depression or suicidal thinking. Inform your doctor if you have had prior psychiatric disorders or are currently being treated for a psychiatric disorder.

- Notify your doctor if you are depressed or have a history of depression, seizure disorders, brain tumor or cancer involving the brain, heart disease, psoriasis, sarcoidosis, kidney or liver impairment, diabetes, thyroid disease, heart problems, autoimmune disease, had an organ transplant, taking drugs which affect the immune system.
- You should receive an eye exam before initiating therapy. If you have underlying eye problems these should be monitored closely during therapy.
- Requires close monitoring and blood testing for effectiveness and toxicity.
- Due to differences in dosage, patients should not change brands of interferons.

DRUG INTERACTIONS
ACE inhibitors, clozapine, erythropoietin, methadone, fluorouracil, theophylline, zidovudine, warfarin, melphan, prednisone

FOOD INTERACTIONS
Avoid alcohol use in hepatitis C.

HERBAL INTERACTIONS
Unknown

PREGNANCY AND BREAST-FEEDING CAUTIONS
FDA Pregnancy Risk Category C. Excretion into breast milk not known. Breast-feeding not recommended during therapy.

SPECIAL INFORMATION
This drug has a black box warning that emphasizes the potential for significant reactions that may occur, including psychiatric, autoimmune, cardiac and infectious disorders. Interferons may cause or aggravate fatal or life-threatening disorders of this nature. Completely read patient information brochure.

PEGINTERFERON ALFA-2B
(peg-in-ter-FEER-on AL-fa-too-bee)

NEWLY DISCOVERED USES (OFF-LABEL)
Liver cirrhosis (with ribavirin), liver fibrosis (with ribavirin), therapy-resistant hepatitis C, thrombocythemia

ORIGINAL USES (ON-LABEL)
To treat chronic hepatitis C as monotherapy or in combination with ribavirin in adult patients with liver disease who have not been previously treated with interferon alpha

BRAND NAME
PEG-intron

DRUG CLASS
Antiviral

DESCRIPTION
This drug is effective by acting against the reproduction of viral cells and by modulating the immune response in the body.

POTENTIAL SIDE EFFECTS
Injection site inflammation, dry mouth, increased sweating, flushing, fatigue, headache, tremors, fever, weight decrease, abdominal pain, chest pain, malaise, dizziness, nausea, anorexia, diarrhea, vomiting, abdominal pain, upset stomach, constipation, blood disorders, insomnia, depression, anxiety, impaired concentration, agitation, nervousness, menstrual disorders, sore throat, hair loss, itching, rash, dry skin, increased triglycerides levels.

CAUTIONS
- May cause severe psychiatric adverse events, including severe depression or suicidal ideation. Inform your doctor if you have had prior psychiatric disorders or are currently being treated for a psychiatric disorder.
- Notify your doctor if you are depressed or have a history of depression, seizure disorders, brain tumor or cancer involving the brain, heart disease, psoriasis, sarcoidosis, kidney or liver impairment, diabetes, thyroid disease, heart problems, autoimmune disease, had an organ transplant, taking drugs which affect the immune system.
- You should receive an eye exam before initiating therapy. If you have underlying eye problems these should be monitored closely during therapy.
- Requires close monitoring and blood testing for effectiveness and toxicity.
- Due to differences in dosage, patients should not change brands of interferons.

DRUG INTERACTIONS
ACE inhibitors, clozapine, erythropoietin, fluorouracil, theophylline, zidovudine, warfarins, melphan, prednisone

FOOD INTERACTIONS
Avoid alcohol use in hepatitis C.

HERBAL INTERACTIONS
Unknown

PREGNANCY AND BREAST-FEEDING CAUTIONS
FDA Pregnancy Risk Category C. Excretion into breast milk not known. Breast-feeding not recommended during therapy.

SPECIAL INFORMATION
This drug has a black box warning that emphasizes the potential for significant reactions that may occur, including psychiatric, autoimmune, cardiac and infectious disorders. Interferons may cause or aggravate fatal or life-threatening disorders of this nature. Completely read patient information brochure.

PENICILLAMINE
(pen-ah-SILL-AMINE)

NEWLY DISCOVERED USES (OFF-LABEL)
  Scleroderma

ORIGINAL USES (ON-LABEL)
Wilson's disease, chronic lead poisoning, stone formation in the urine (cystinuria), and in patients with severe, active rheumatoid arthritis who have failed conventional therapy

BRAND NAMES
Cuprimine, Depen

DRUG CLASS
Chelating-antidote

DESCRIPTION
This drug works by removing copper and lead from the body by binding to the metals and forming a complex that is then excreted. It appears to suppress disease activity.

POTENTIAL SIDE EFFECTS
Generalized itching, rash, hives, anorexia, upset stomach, nausea, vomiting, diarrhea, changes in taste perception, blood disorders (see cautions), blood in urine, protein in urine, ringing in ears, vision changes, fever, joint aches, oral ulcerations.

CAUTIONS

- Not for use during pregnancy (except for treatment of Wilson's disease and certain cases of cystinuria).
- Notify your doctor if you have a history of kidney impairment, penicillin allergies, or penicillamine related-blood disorders (such as aplastic anemia or agranulocytosis).
- Not for chronic lead poisoning if lead substances are still evident in gastrointestinal tract.
- Associated with significant blood disorders requiring periodic monitoring during therapy. Not for use with gold therapy, antimalarial or other drugs known to cause serious blood disorders (such as phenylbutazone).
- Notify your doctor if you develop bloody urine, shortness of breath upon exertion, unexplained cough, wheezing, blurred vision, changes in vision, fever, rash.
- When used for urinary stones, an annual x-ray for kidney stones is recommended.
- Requires periodic liver function monitoring if taken longer than six months.
- May require supplemental pyridoxine or iron therapy during therapy.

DRUG INTERACTIONS

Other drugs known to cause serious blood disorders (such as cytotoxic drugs, phenylbutazone), digoxin, gold therapy, iron salts

FOOD INTERACTIONS

Mineral supplements

HERBAL INTERACTIONS

Unknown

PREGNANCY AND BREAST-FEEDING CAUTIONS

FDA Pregnancy Risk Category C. Excretion in breast milk. Do not breast-feed while taking this drug.

SPECIAL INFORMATION

Separate iron supplements by at least two hours with administration of penicillamine.

PENICILLIN
(Pen-eh-sill-in)

NEWLY DISCOVERED USES (OFF-LABEL) ────────
| Lyme disease |

ORIGINAL USES (ON-LABEL)
Treatment of various bacterial infections

BRAND NAMES
Bicillin, Penicillin VK, Pfizerpen, Veetids

DESCRIPTION
This drug fights bacteria by inhibiting the production of the bacterial cell wall.

POTENTIAL SIDE EFFECTS
Mild to severe, including some life-threatening rashes, nausea, vomiting, diarrhea, hemorrhagic colitis, various blood disorders, jaundice, crystals in the urine.

CAUTIONS
- Notify your doctor if you have an allergy to penicillins or cephalosporin antibiotics.
- Dose and/or frequency of administration should be adjusted if you have kidney impairment.
- Prolonged use of antibiotics may result in superinfection, resistance.

DRUG INTERACTIONS
Disulfiram, probenecid, warfarin, methotrexate, tetracyclines, chloramphenicol, aminoglycosides, heparin, diuretics. If you are taking oral contraceptives, consult with pharmacist or doctor.

FOOD INTERACTIONS
Penicillin V tabs: Take without regard to meals.

HERBAL INTERACTIONS
Khat

PREGNANCY AND BREAST-FEEDING CAUTIONS
FDA Pregnancy Risk Category B. Excreted in breast milk. Consult your doctor.

SPECIAL INFORMATION
Report any sign of a rash to your doctor.

PENTOSAN POLYSULFATE
(PEN-toe-san pol-i-SUL-fate)

NEWLY DISCOVERED USES (OFF-LABEL)
Hypercalciuria

ORIGINAL USES (ON-LABEL)
Relief of bladder pain or discomfort due to interstitial cystitis

BRAND NAME
Elmiron

DRUG CLASS
Analgesic, urinary

DESCRIPTION
This drug adheres to the bladder surface to alleviate symptoms of
interstitial cystitis, a chronic inflammatory condition resulting in
reduced bladder capacity.

POTENTIAL SIDE EFFECTS
Headache, stomach discomfort, diarrhea, nausea, hair loss, rash,
malaise, pelvic pain, changes in liver function, vomiting, mouth
ulcers, colitis, inflammation of the esophagus, gastritis, anemia,
weight changes, edema, muscle or joint aches, dizziness, numbness, insomnia, sweating, urinary urgency.

CAUTIONS
Has a weak potential effect to cause bleeding, and thus you should
notify your doctor if you are taking other drugs that increase the
risk of bleeding (such as warfarin, heparin, etc.) or if you have
conditions that would increase your risk of bleeding (such as
stomach ulcers, aneurysms, diverticulitis, etc.).

DRUG INTERACTIONS
Heparin, warfarin, high-dose NSAIDs or aspirin, streptokinase

FOOD INTERACTIONS
Take with water at least one hour before meals or two hours after
meals.

HERBAL INTERACTIONS
Unknown

PREGNANCY AND BREAST-FEEDING CAUTIONS
FDA Pregnancy Risk Category B. Excretion in breast milk unknown. Consult your doctor.

SPECIAL INFORMATION

No studies have been done beyond six months, so the risks/benefits are not known in long-term use.

PENTOXIFYLLINE
(pen-TOKS-i-fi-leen)

NEWLY DISCOVERED USES (OFF-LABEL)

Alcoholic hepatitis, recurrent canker sores, sarcoidosis

ORIGINAL USES (ON-LABEL)

Used for the treatment of intermittent claudication in people with chronic occlusive arterial disease of the limbs

BRAND NAMES

Pentoxil, Trental

DRUG CLASS

Blood viscosity reducer

DESCRIPTION

This drug reduces blood viscosity and improves blood flow to the affected areas and improves oxygen delivery to tissues.

POTENTIAL SIDE EFFECTS

Flushing, abdominal discomfort, upset stomach, belching, bloating, nausea, vomiting, dizziness, headache.

CAUTIONS

- Notify your doctor if you have recently experienced bleeding in the eye or brain or if you have intolerance to caffeine, theophylline, or theobromine.
- If you are taking warfarin, you may require more frequent monitoring.
- Requires periodic monitoring of blood, particularly if you have risk factors that may be complicated by bleeding, such as peptic ulcers, recent surgeries, etc.
- May require periodic monitoring of blood pressure.

DRUG INTERACTIONS

Histamine-2 antagonists (such as cimetidine, ranitidine, etc.), warfarin (see cautions), theophylline, antihypertensive medications (may result in blood pressure decreases)

FOOD INTERACTIONS
Take with meals.

HERBAL INTERACTIONS
Unknown

PREGNANCY AND BREAST-FEEDING CAUTIONS
FDA Pregnancy Risk Category C. Excreted in breast milk. Not recommended while breast-feeding.

SPECIAL INFORMATION
Must be swallowed whole; do not chew or crush.

PERGOLIDE
(PER-go-lide)

NEWLY DISCOVERED USES (OFF-LABEL)
Acromegaly, hyperprolactinemia, periodic limb movement disorder, restless legs syndrome

ORIGINAL USES (ON-LABEL)
Used in combination treatment with levodopa/carbidopa in the management of Parkinson's disease

BRAND NAME
Permax

DRUG CLASS
Anti-Parkinson's (dopamine)

DESCRIPTION
This drug stimulates dopamine receptors in the nigrostriatal system (a bundle of nerve fibers). The release of dopamine is important action in controlling Parkinson's disease movements and symptoms.

POTENTIAL SIDE EFFECTS
Dizziness, hallucinations, involuntary muscle movements, somnolence, confusion, nausea, constipation, rhinitis, low blood pressure, peripheral swelling, chest pain, palpitations, fainting, low blood pressure, insomnia, pain, anxiety, psychosis, extrapyramidal symptoms, incoordination, rash, diarrhea, stomach upset, abdominal pain, anorexia, dry mouth, vomiting, abnormal vision, double vision, shortness of breath, flu syndrome.

CAUTIONS

- Low blood pressure may be sudden, particularly when standing from a sitting or lying down position, and is most likely during initial treatment. May be avoided by a gradual increase in dosage. Avoid stopping this drug suddenly as a syndrome similar to malignant hypertension may occur, characterized by elevated temperature, muscle rigidity, altered consciousness.
- Inform your doctor if you have history of arrhythmias (irregular heart beats), hallucinations, or mental illness.
- The elderly and patients with decreased kidney function are at increased risk of developing side effects, most notably confusion, somnolence, and peripheral swelling.

DRUG INTERACTIONS

MAO inhibitors, dopamine agonists (such as neuroleptics, phenothiazines), metoclopramide, sibutramine.

This drug is metabolized by a specific set of liver enzymes. Several other drugs interfere with these liver enzymes, and thus may increase or decrease the clearance of pergolide from the body, potentially increasing the risk of side effects or decreasing effectiveness. When these drugs are given in combination with pergolide, dosage adjustments may be needed. As these are too numerous to list, you should always check with your doctor or pharmacist prior to starting a new medication, herbal, or nonprescription product.

FOOD INTERACTIONS

Alcohol

HERBAL INTERACTIONS

Unknown

PREGNANCY AND BREAST-FEEDING CAUTIONS

FDA Pregnancy Risk Category B. Excretion in breast milk unknown; breast-feeding is not recommended.

SPECIAL INFORMATION

In 2003, cardiac changes were identified in a small number of individuals on pergolide therapy. Warnings section has been updated in the package insert. In addition, this drug has been reported to cause somnolence.

PHENELZINE
(FEN-el-zeen)

NEWLY DISCOVERED USES (OFF-LABEL)
Bulimia, migraine prevention, panic disorder

ORIGINAL USES (ON-LABEL)
Treatment of atypical, nonendogenous, or neurotic depression

BRAND NAME
Nardil

DRUG CLASS
Antidepressant (monoamine oxidase inhibitor)

DESCRIPTION
This drug inhibits the activity of a certain enzyme, thereby increasing the concentration of norepinephrine, dopamine, and serotonin, important neurotransmitters in mood and behavior.

POTENTIAL SIDE EFFECTS
Sudden drop in blood pressure upon standing from sitting or lying down position, swelling from fluid retention, dizziness, headache, drowsiness, sleep disturbances, rash, itching, decreased sexual ability, increased sodium levels, dry mouth, constipation, weight gain, urinary retention, decreased white blood cells, liver toxicity, weakness, tremor, blurred vision, glaucoma, sweating.

CAUTIONS
- Should not be used in uncontrolled high blood pressure, pheochromocytoma (tumor on adrenal glands resulting in excessive adrenal secretions of adrenaline), liver disease, congestive heart failure.
- Should not be used concurrently with sympathomimetics (and related compounds), central nervous system depressants, alcohol, other antidepressants, meperidine, bupropion, buspirone, guanethidine, serotonergic drugs (including SSRIs), general anesthesia, and spinal anesthesia.
- Should not be used within five weeks of fluoxetine discontinuation, or two weeks of other antidepressant discontinuation.
- Coadministration with foods that contain high amounts of tryptamine, tryptophan, dopamine, chocolate, or caffeine may lead to serious increased blood pressure.

- Notify your doctor if you are hyperactive, hyperexcitable, or have glaucoma, bipolar disorder, mania, seizure disorders, or low blood pressure.
- May worsen psychotic symptoms in some patients.
- Do not use with the nonprescription cold product dextromethorphan.
- Prior to any surgery or procedures, notify your dentist or doctor that you are taking this medication. May require temporary discontinuation.

DRUG INTERACTIONS

Serious drug interactions may occur with tricyclic antidepressants, venlafaxine, trazodone, dexfenfluramine, sibutramine, lithium, meperidine, fenfluramine, dextromethorphan, SSRIs (such as fluoxetine, paroxetine, citalopram, etc.), barbiturates, amphetamines, other stimulants (methylphenidate), levodopa, metaraminol, hypoglycemic drugs, bupropion, tramadol, reserpine, decongestants (pseudoephedrine) (also see cautions). Check with your doctor or pharmacist prior to starting any new medication, nonprescription drug, or herbal product.

FOOD INTERACTIONS

Severe increases in blood pressure may occur if MAO inhibitors, such as phenelzine, are taken with foods containing tyramine. Avoid foods containing tryptophan, dopamine, chocolate, and caffeine. Alcoholic beverages containing tyramine can also cause a severe hypertensive response when taken with phenelzine. Alcohol should be avoided.

HERBAL INTERACTIONS

New Zealand prickly spinach, ginseng

PREGNANCY AND BREAST-FEEDING CAUTIONS

FDA Pregnancy Risk Category C. Excretion in breast milk unknown. Not recommended during breast-feeding.

SPECIAL INFORMATION

This drug has a black box warning regarding the increased risk of suicidal thinking and behavior in children, adolescents, and adults with major depressive disorder. Discuss these risks with your doctor.

PHENOXYBENZAMINE
(fen-oks-see-BEN-za-meen)

NEWLY DISCOVERED USES (OFF-LABEL)
Benign prostatic hypertrophy

ORIGINAL USES (ON-LABEL)
Pheochromocytoma (increased excretion of adrenal gland secretions) including high blood pressure, sweating, increased heart rate

BRAND NAME
Dibenzyline

DRUG CLASS
Antihypertensive (alpha-adrenergic blocking)

DESCRIPTION
Phenoxybenzamine produces long-lasting blockade of alpha-adrenergic receptors in exocrine glands and smooth muscle. It also relaxes the urethra and increases the opening of the bladder.

POTENTIAL SIDE EFFECTS
Decreased blood pressure upon standing from sitting or lying down position, increased heart rate, syncope, shock, fatigue, headache, confusion, vomiting, nausea, diarrhea, dry mouth, inhibition of ejaculation, weakness, nasal congestion.

CAUTIONS
- Not recommended for patients where a fall in blood pressure would be undesirable.
- Not for concurrent use with phosphodiesterase-5 inhibitors including sildenafil, tadalafil, or vardenafil because of additive lowered blood pressure effects.
- Elderly are at increased risk of adverse effects.
- Notify your doctor if you have kidney impairment, cerebral or coronary arteriosclerosis, or respiratory tract infection.

DRUG INTERACTIONS
Sildenafil, vardenafil, tadalafil, alpha-adrenergic agonists

FOOD INTERACTIONS
Alcohol

HERBAL INTERACTIONS
Unknown

PREGNANCY AND BREAST-FEEDING CAUTIONS

FDA Pregnancy Risk Category C. Excretion in breast milk unknown. Consult your doctor.

SPECIAL INFORMATION

Gastrointestinal irritation can be reduced by giving in divided doses.

PHENTOLAMINE
(fen-TOLE-a-meen)

NEWLY DISCOVERED USES (OFF-LABEL)

Dyspareunia, erectile dysfunction, hypoactive sexual desire disorder

ORIGINAL USES (ON-LABEL)

For diagnosis of pheochromocytoma and treatment of severe high blood pressure caused by increased levels of sympathomimetic amines, treatment of necrosis due to extravasations

BRAND NAMES

Regitine, Rogitine

DRUG CLASS

Antihypertensive, diagnostic, antidote

DESCRIPTION

This drug reduces blood pressure and relaxes blood vessels. It works by blocking alpha-adrenergic receptors to prevent binding of epinephrine and norepinephrine.

POTENTIAL SIDE EFFECTS

Decreased blood pressure or sudden drop in blood pressure upon standing from sitting or lying down position, increased heart rate, irregular heart rate, flushing, weakness, dizziness, nausea and vomiting, nasal stuffiness.

CAUTIONS

- Inform your doctor if you have peptic ulcer, gastritis, increased heart rate or a history of irregular heart beats, kidney impairment, coronary or cerebral arteriosclerosis.

- Heart attacks or cerebrovascular spasm and stroke have occurred; they are usually associated with prolonged lowered blood pressure.
- Notify your doctor if you are taking phosphodiesterase-5 (PDE-5) inhibitors (sildenafil, tadalafil, vardenafil).

DRUG INTERACTIONS
Sildenafil, tadalafil, vardenafil, ephedrine and epinephrine

FOOD INTERACTIONS
Unknown

HERBAL INTERACTIONS
Unknown

PREGNANCY AND BREAST-FEEDING CAUTIONS
FDA Pregnancy Risk Category C. Excretion in breast milk unknown. Consult your doctor.

PHENYLEPHRINE
(fen-ill-EPH-rhine)

Injection

NEWLY DISCOVERED USES (OFF-LABEL)
Priapism

ORIGINAL USES (ON-LABEL)
Treatment of vascular failure in shock, shock-like states due to various causes, or drug-induced hypotension (low blood pressure)

BRAND NAME
Neo-Synephrine

DRUG CLASS
Vasopressor

DESCRIPTION
This drug is a powerful stimulant of alpha-receptors in the cardiac system, causing increases in blood pressure by causing the blood vessels to constrict.

POTENTIAL SIDE EFFECTS
Headache, reflex low blood pressure, excitability, restlessness.

CAUTIONS
- Not for use if you have severe high blood pressure.
- Notify your doctor if you have thyroid disease, low heart rate, cardiac disease, including heart block, heart attack, severe arteriosclerosis.
- Some products contain sulfites; notify your doctor if you have a sulfite allergy.

DRUG INTERACTIONS
Bretylium, guanethidine, MAO Inhibitors (such as phenelzine, tranylcypromine). Consult with your doctor or pharmacist before starting any new therapy with prescription medications, non-prescription medications, or herbal products.

FOOD INTERACTIONS
Unknown

HERBAL INTERACTIONS
Unknown

PREGNANCY AND BREAST-FEEDING CAUTIONS
FDA Pregnancy Risk Category C. Excretion into breast milk is unknown. Breast-feeding not recommended during therapy.

This information refers to use of prescription product only.

PHENYTOIN
(FEN-i-toyn)

NEWLY DISCOVERED USES (OFF-LABEL)

Acute spinal cord injury, chronic neuropathic pain, multiple sclerosis, neuropathy, prevention of recurrence and sudden death in ventricular tachycardia, ventricular tachycardia

---

ORIGINAL USES (ON-LABEL)
Complex partial seizures, to prevent seizures following head trauma/neurosurgery

BRAND NAME
Dilantin

DRUG CLASS
Anticonvulsant, antiarrhythmic

DESCRIPTION

This drug decreases seizure activity by increasing or decreasing flow of sodium ions across cell membranes in the motor cortex. Also affects conduction of the heart.

POTENTIAL SIDE EFFECTS

Uncontrolled eye movements, slurred speech, confusion, dizziness, fatigue, vision changes, rash, increase in glucose levels, diabetes, nausea, vomiting, diarrhea, swelling of the gums, liver injury, blood disorders, taste changes.

CAUTIONS

- Notify your doctor if you have low blood pressure, porphyria, liver dysfunction, too low heart rate or other cardiac conditions.
- This drug requires periodic blood testing to determine effectiveness and toxicity. At excessive blood levels, toxic effects may occur, including sedation, confusion, and gross coordination.
- Do not abruptly discontinue this medication as it may precipitate seizures.
- Notify your doctor immediately if you develop a rash.

DRUG INTERACTIONS

Felbamate, gabapentin, topiramate, allopurinol, amiodarone, diltiazem, nifedipine, cimetidine, disulfiram, methylphenidate, metronidazole, omeprazole, SSRIs, ticlopidine, tricyclic antidepressants, trazodone, trimethoprim, ciprofloxacin, barbiturates, sedatives, antidepressants, narcotic analgesics, and benzodiazepines, delavirdine, fluconazole, gemfibrozil, ketoconazole, nicardipine, NSAIDs, pioglitazone, sulfonamides, fluvoxamine, isoniazid, omeprazole, acetazolamide, lithium, valproic acid, warfarin, estrogens, oral contraceptives. Phenytoin may increase the metabolism of barbiturates, carbamazepine, ethosuximide, felbamate, lamotrigine, tiagabine, topiramate, and zonisamide.

There are numerous drug interactions with this drug; consult your doctor or pharmacist prior to starting therapy with any prescription or nonprescription drug, or herbal product.

FOOD INTERACTIONS

Avoid alcohol. Take with food to avoid stomach upset. Phenytoin may decrease calcium, folic acid, and vitamin D levels.

HERBAL INTERACTIONS

Evening primrose, valerian, St. John's wort, kava kava, gotu kola

PREGNANCY AND BREAST-FEEDING CAUTIONS
FDA Pregnancy Risk Category D. Excreted in breast milk. Do not breast-feed during therapy.

SPECIAL INFORMATION
Do not change brands or dosage form without consulting your doctor or pharmacist.

Maintain good oral hygiene. An alternative method of contraception should be considered.

PIMECROLIMUS
(pie-meh-CROW-lie-mus)

NEWLY DISCOVERED USES (OFF-LABEL)
Alopecia areata

ORIGINAL USES (ON-LABEL)
Mild to moderate atopic dermatitis

BRAND NAME
Elidel

DRUG CLASS
Topical immunomodulator

DESCRIPTION
This drug modifies inflammatory responses in the skin.

POTENTIAL SIDE EFFECTS
Local skin burning, skin infection, upper abdominal pain, sore throat, diarrhea.

CAUTIONS
- Use the minimum amount of product to control symptoms.
- The safety of long term use is not known, do not use continuously. Discontinue use after signs and symptoms have resolved.
- If no improvement occurs after six weeks of treatment or the condition worsens, notify your doctor.
- Should not be used in someone with a weakened immune system.
- Should not be used in children less than two years of age.
- Do not apply to skin with active infection.

• Minimize or avoid exposure to natural or artificial sunlight.

DRUG INTERACTIONS
Check with your doctor or pharmacist prior to starting a new medication, herbal, or nonprescription product.

FOOD INTERACTIONS
Unknown

HERBAL INTERACTIONS
Unknown

PREGNANCY AND BREAST-FEEDING CAUTIONS
FDA Pregnancy Risk Category C. Excretion in breast milk is not known. Breast-feeding is not recommended.

SPECIAL INFORMATION
In 2005, the FDA issued a public health advisory regarding a potential cancer risk associated with the use of this product when applied to the skin, and thus this product is only intended for short-term use as a second line drug in people who have not responded to other drugs. Most cancer data has originated in animal studies. Discuss these risks with your doctor.

PIMOZIDE
(PI-moe-zide)

NEWLY DISCOVERED USES (OFF-LABEL)
Autism

ORIGINAL USES (ON-LABEL)
Suppression of severe motor and phonic tics in people with Tourette's syndrome who have failed to respond satisfactorily to standard treatment

BRAND NAME
Orap

DRUG CLASS
Antipsychotic

DESCRIPTION
Pimozide appears to block dopamine receptors in the central nervous system.

POTENTIAL SIDE EFFECTS

Dry mouth, constipation, muscle tightness, drowsiness, sedation, akathisia, rigidity, speech disorder, involuntary muscle movements, depression, visual disturbances, impotence, headache, increased salivation, abnormal dreams, rash, changes in heart rate.

CAUTIONS

- Not for use in the treatment of simple tics or tics other than those associated with Tourette's syndrome. Not for use with drugs that may cause motor and phonic tics.
- Notify your doctor if you have congenital long QT syndrome, a history of cardiac arrhythmias (irregular heart rhythm), or are taking other QT prolonging drugs. A test to determine if you have changes in heart rhythm (electrocardiogram) will be performed before you start the drug and periodically during therapy.
- You may be tested for low potassium or low magnesium levels prior to initiation of the drug.
- Not for use with macrolide antibiotics (such as clarithromycin, erythromycin, azithromycin, dirithromycin, and troleandomycin), azole antifungals (such as itraconazole and ketoconazole), protease inhibitors (such as ritonavir, saquinavir, indinavir and nelfinavir), nefazodone, sertraline.
- May impair mental and/or physical abilities such as driving a car or operating machinery.
- Inform your doctor if you have liver or kidney impairment.
- May lower the seizure threshold.

DRUG INTERACTIONS

Pimozide prolongs the QT interval on electrocardiograms. An additive effect on the QT interval would be anticipated if pimozide is taken with other drugs that prolong the QT interval including phenothiazines, tricyclic antidepressants and antiarrhythmics. The list of drugs that affect the QT interval are listed at the following url: http://www.torsades.org/medical-pros/ drug-lists/drug lists.htm#

This drug is metabolized by a specific set of liver enzymes (cytochrome P450 enzymes 1A2, 3A4). Several other drugs interfere with these liver enzymes, and thus may increase or decrease the clearance of pimozide from the body, potentially increasing the risk of side effects or decreasing effectiveness. When these drugs are given in combination with pimozide, dosage adjustments may be needed. As these are too numerous to list, you should always check with your doctor or pharmacist prior to starting a new medication, herbal, or nonprescription product.

FOOD INTERACTIONS
Grapefruit juice

HERBAL INTERACTIONS
Unknown

PREGNANCY AND BREAST-FEEDING CAUTIONS
FDA Pregnancy Risk Category C. It is not known whether or not pimozide is excreted in breast milk. Consult your doctor regarding breast-feeding.

PINDOLOL
(PIN-doe-lole)

NEWLY DISCOVERED USES (OFF-LABEL)
Obsessive-compulsive disorder, panic disorder

ORIGINAL USES (ON-LABEL)
Hypertension

BRAND NAME
Visken

DRUG CLASS
Antihypertensive (beta-blocker)

DESCRIPTION
This drug decreases heart rate, cardiac contractility, blood pressure, and heart oxygen demand.

POTENTIAL SIDE EFFECTS
Chest pain, edema, nightmares/vivid dreams, dizziness, insomnia, fatigue, nervousness, anxiety, rash, itching, nausea, abdominal discomfort, weakness, numbness, joint aches, shortness of breath.

CAUTIONS
- Inform your doctor if you have heart conditions (such as congestive heart failure, cardiogenic shock, too low heart rate, or second- and third-degree heart block, sinus node dysfunction), are pregnant, or have lung/breathing problems.

- Do not stop this medication suddenly; taper over a gradual period, particularly under doctor's instructions prior to elective
  surgery.
- May cause or mask the symptoms of low blood glucose levels in
  diabetics.
- May mask signs of thyroid problems.
- Not indicated for high blood pressure emergencies.
- Immediately report to your doctor any signs of swelling of the
  extremities, sudden weight gain, changes in breathing, night
  cough.

DRUG INTERACTIONS

This drug is metabolized by a specific set of liver enzymes (cytochrome P450 enzymes). Several other drugs interfere with these
liver enzymes, and thus may increase or decrease the clearance of
pindolol from the body, potentially increasing the risk of side effects or decreasing effectiveness. When these drugs are given in
combination with pindolol, dosage adjustments may be needed.
As these are too numerous to list, you should always check with
your doctor or pharmacist prior to starting a new medication,
herbal, or nonprescription product.

FOOD INTERACTIONS
Unknown

HERBAL INTERACTIONS
Dong quai, ephedra, yohimbe, and ginseng

PREGNANCY AND BREAST-FEEDING CAUTIONS
FDA Pregnancy Risk Category B. Excreted in breast milk. Consult
your doctor.

SPECIAL INFORMATION
May be taken with or without meals.

PIOGLITAZONE
(pye-oh-GLI-ta-zone)

NEWLY DISCOVERED USES (OFF-LABEL)
Prevention of cardiovascular disease in type 2 diabetes,
prevention in type 2 diabetes

ORIGINAL USES (ON-LABEL)

Type 2 Diabetes – monotherapy and combination therapy, combination therapy with sulfonylureas, metformin, or insulin are indicated when monotherapy with diet and exercise are inadequate for control

BRAND NAME

Actos

DRUG CLASS

Antidiabetic (thiazolidinedione hypoglycemic)

DESCRIPTION

Lowers blood sugar by improving response to insulin.

POTENTIAL SIDE EFFECTS

Headache, tooth disorder, aggravated diabetes, sore throat, sinusitis, upper respiratory infection, edema, muscle aches, increases in HDL cholesterol, decreases in triglycerides, too low glucose levels, weight gain, anemia.

CAUTIONS

- Active liver disease or elevated liver function tests.
- Inform your doctor if you have a history of jaundice or liver disease, if you currently have anemia or edema, or certain types of cardiac disease (class III or class IV congestive heart failure).
- May result in resumption of ovulation if you are premenopausal but not ovulating.
- Requires periodic monitoring of liver function and blood glucose parameters.
- May cause too low blood glucose levels.
- There is a possibility of fluid retention leading to or exacerbating congestive heart failure with combined therapy of pioglitazone and insulin.

DRUG INTERACTIONS

Delavirdine, fluconazole, gemfibrozil, ketoconazole, nicardipine, NSAIDs, sulfonamides, itraconazole, carbamazepine, phenobarbital, phenytoin, rifampin, rifapentine, secobarbital, oral contraceptives, bile acid sequestrants.

This drug is metabolized by and induces a specific set of liver enzymes (cytochrome P450 enzymes). Several other drugs interfere with these liver enzymes, and thus may increase or decrease the clearance of pioglitazone from the body, potentially increasing the risk of side effects or decreasing effectiveness. When these drugs are given in combination with pioglitazone, dosage adjustments may be needed. As these are too numerous to list, you should always check with your doctor or pharmacist prior to starting a new medication, herbal, or nonprescription product.

FOOD INTERACTIONS
May take without regard to meals.

HERBAL INTERACTIONS
St. John's wort, chromium, garlic, gymnema

PREGNANCY AND BREAST-FEEDING CAUTIONS
FDA Pregnancy Risk Category C. Excretion in the breast milk is unknown. Therapy not recommended for those who are breast-feeding.

SPECIAL INFORMATION
If you miss a dose, do not double the dose the next day. When used in combination with insulin or other oral antidiabetic drugs, the risk of developing too low blood glucose is possible. Discuss risks and signs and symptoms with your doctor. Immediately report to your doctor any development of sudden weight gain, swelling, shortness of breath, nausea, vomiting, abdominal pain, fatigue, dark urine, or jaundice.

PIPERACILLIN AND TAZOBACTAM SODIUM
(pi-PER-a-sil-in and ta-zoe-BAK-tam SOW-dee-um)

NEWLY DISCOVERED USES (OFF-LABEL)
Diverticulitis

ORIGINAL USES (ON-LABEL)
Treatment of various bacterial infections, including those located in the lower respiratory tract (community-acquired pneumonia, nosocomial pneumonia), urinary tract, skin and skin structure, gynecological, bone and joints, intra-abdominal (appendicitis with rupture/abscess, peritonitis) and of the blood.

BRAND NAME
Zosyn

DRUG CLASS
Antibiotic (penicillin and beta-lactamase inhibitor)

DESCRIPTION
Piperacillin inhibits bacterial cell wall synthesis by binding to penicillin-binding proteins. Tazobactam inhibits beta-lactamases, enzymes that would normally metabolize penicillins, and thus extends their antibacterial activity.

POTENTIAL SIDE EFFECTS
Pain at injection site, thrombophlebitis (inflammation of the vein), rash, diarrhea, allergic reaction, nausea, vomiting, headache.

CAUTIONS
- Notify your doctor if you have an allergy to penicillins or cephalosporin antibiotics.
- Dose and/or frequency of administration should be adjusted in kidney impairment.
- Prolonged use of antibiotics may result in superinfection, resistance.

DRUG INTERACTIONS
Disulfiram, probenecid, warfarin, methotrexate, tetracyclines, chloramphenicol, allopurinol

FOOD INTERACTIONS
Unknown

HERBAL INTERACTIONS
Unknown

PREGNANCY AND BREAST-FEEDING CAUTIONS
FDA Pregnancy Risk Category B. Excreted in breast milk. Consult your doctor.

PRAMIPEXOLE
(pram-eh-PEX-oll)

NEWLY DISCOVERED USES (OFF-LABEL)
Restless legs syndrome

ORIGINAL USES (ON-LABEL)
Parkinson's disease

BRAND NAMES
Mirapex

DRUG CLASS
Antiparkinson

DESCRIPTION
This drug stimulates dopamine receptors in the brain to increase dopamine levels. A deficiency in dopamine levels is thought to be linked to Parkinson's disease.

POTENTIAL SIDE EFFECTS
Weakness, general edema, nausea, constipation, dizziness, drowsiness (see cautions), confusion, amnesia, vision changes, hallucinations, sudden drop in blood pressure when standing from a sitting or lying down position.

CAUTIONS
- May cause liver toxicity, requiring periodic monitoring of liver function.
- May cause sudden sleep attacks during activities of daily living. Discuss these effects with your doctor prior to initiation of therapy. You should not drive or participate in potentially dangerous activities until you have experience with this drug or contacted your doctor.
- Notify your doctor if you have kidney impairment as it will require dosage reduction.

DRUG INTERACTIONS
Carbidopa/levodopa, selegiline, amantadine, cimetidine, probenecid, cimetidine, ranitidine, diltiazem, triamterene, verapamil, quinidine, quinine, phenothiazines, metoclopramide

FOOD INTERACTIONS
Unknown

HERBAL INTERACTIONS
Unknown

PREGNANCY AND BREAST-FEEDING CAUTIONS
FDA Pregnancy Risk Category C. Excretion into breast milk is unknown. Breast-feeding not recommended during therapy.

SPECIAL INFORMATION
Avoid alcohol during therapy.

PRAVASTATIN
(PRA-va-stat-in)

NEWLY DISCOVERED USES (OFF-LABEL)
Peripheral artery disease

ORIGINAL USES (ON-LABEL)
Primary and secondary prevention of coronary events, hyperlipidemia (high levels of lipids)

BRAND NAME
Pravachol

DRUG CLASS
Anti-lipid (HMG-CoA reductase inhibitor)

DESCRIPTION
This drug inhibits an enzyme that is an important factor in the production of cholesterol.

POTENTIAL SIDE EFFECTS
Dizziness, headache, stomach cramps or discomfort, diarrhea, flatulence, nausea, vomiting, muscle aches, localized pain, common cold, cough, chest pain, fatigue, flu syndrome.

CAUTIONS
- Not for use in active liver disease or in patients with high levels of liver function tests.
- You should not consume large amounts of alcohol or have a history of liver disease.
- Liver function should be monitored before initiation and periodically during therapy.
- May require reduced doses in impaired kidney function.
- Can also cause severe muscle aches which are a symptom of a more serious disorder (rhabdomyolysis) in which the muscle fibers break down. If this disorder progresses, decreases in kidney function may also occur. This risk is increased with concurrent use of drugs that increase pravastatin levels.

DRUG INTERACTIONS
Azole antifungals, ciprofloxacin, colestipol, cholestyramine, fibric acid drugs (such as gemfibrozil), niacin, protease inhibitors (such as ritonavir, saquinavir, etc.). Check with your doctor or pharmacist prior to starting any new medication, herbal product, or nonprescription drug.

FOOD INTERACTIONS
Grapefruit juice. Avoid excessive intake of alcohol.

HERBAL INTERACTIONS
St. John's wort

PREGNANCY AND BREAST-FEEDING CAUTIONS
FDA Pregnancy Risk Category X. Pravastatin should not be used during breast-feeding.

SPECIAL INFORMATION
Before initiation of therapy, patients should be placed on a standard cholesterol-lowering diet for six weeks and the diet should be continued during drug therapy. Report any signs of muscle pain, tenderness, or weakness to your doctor.

PRAZIQUANTEL
(pray-zi-KWON-tel)

NEWLY DISCOVERED USES (OFF-LABEL)
Cestodiasis

ORIGINAL USES (ON-LABEL)
Infections (schistosomiasis) due to all species of *Schistosoma*

BRAND NAME
Biltricide

DRUG CLASS
Anthelmintic

DESCRIPTION
This drug causes strong contractions and paralysis of worm musculature, resulting in detachment of suckers from the blood vessel walls.

POTENTIAL SIDE EFFECTS
Malaise, headache, dizziness, abdominal discomfort, hives (rarely), rise in temperature. Side effects are more frequent and serious in patients with heavy worm burden.

CAUTIONS
- Not for use if you have ocular infection.
- Notify your doctor if you have liver impairment.

- May cause dizziness or drowsiness. Do not drive a car or operate machinery on the day of treatment and the following day.
- If brain involvement/infection is present, requires hospitalization.

DRUG INTERACTIONS
Histamine-2 antagonists: cimetidine, ranitidine, famotidine, nizatidine. Inform your doctor of other medications that you are taking prior to initiating therapy.

FOOD INTERACTIONS
Avoid taking with grapefruit products.

HERBAL INTERACTIONS
Unknown

PREGNANCY AND BREAST-FEEDING CAUTIONS
FDA Pregnancy Risk Category B. Excreted in breast milk. Do not nurse on the day of treatment and for 72 hours afterward.

SPECIAL INFORMATION
Take with liquid during meals. Do not chew tablets.

PRAZOSIN
(PRA-zoe-sin)

NEWLY DISCOVERED USES (OFF-LABEL)
Benign prostate hyperplasia (BPH), congestive heart failure, preoperative preparation for pheochromocytoma, post-traumatic stress disorder (PTSD), Raynaud's syndrome

ORIGINAL USES (ON-LABEL)
Treatment of hypertension

BRAND NAME
Minipress

DRUG CLASS
Antihypertensive (alpha-adrenergic blockers)

DESCRIPTION
This drug relaxes veins and arterioles and decreases total vascular resistance and blood pressure.

POTENTIAL SIDE EFFECTS
Dizziness, sensation of unusual heart beats, headache, drowsiness, rash, decreased energy, nausea, urinary frequency, fainting, depression, dry mouth, diarrhea, constipation, nasal congestion, nose bleeds, blurred vision, red eye, vertigo, edema, lack of energy, weakness.

CAUTIONS
- Do not use concurrently with phosphodiesterase-5 inhibitors (such as sildenafil, tadalafil, or vardenafil).
- Marked orthostatic hypotension (sudden drop in blood pressure when standing from sitting or lying down position), syncope, and loss of consciousness may occur with first dose (especially in patients taking beta-blockers, diuretics, low sodium diets or taking larger first doses greater than 1 mg).
- Rarely, this drug class has been associated with priapism (painful erection).
- Avoid rapid increase in dose.
- Use with caution in patients with kidney impairment.

DRUG INTERACTIONS
Beta-blockers, diuretics, calcium channel blockers, ACE inhibitors, and other antihypertensive medications, tricyclic antidepressants, low-potency antipsychotics, NSAIDs, cimetidine, indomethacin, verapamil, clonidine

FOOD INTERACTIONS
Alcohol

HERBAL INTERACTIONS
Dong quai, ephedra, yohimbe, ginseng, saw palmetto, garlic

PREGNANCY AND BREAST-FEEDING CAUTIONS
FDA Pregnancy Risk Category C. Excretion in breast milk unknown. Consult your doctor.

SPECIAL INFORMATION
Take dose at bedtime. Notify doctor if dizziness or palpitations occur.

PREDNISOLONE
(pred-NISS-oh-lone)

Oral, Injectable

NEWLY DISCOVERED USES (OFF-LABEL)
Alcoholic hepatitis, cystic fibrosis, liver fibrosis, muscular dystrophy, nasal polyps, primary biliary cirrhosis, urticaria (therapy-resistant)

ORIGINAL USES (ON-LABEL)
Treatment of various allergic and various inflammatory disorders, including those of the skin, endocrine system, gastrointestinal, lung, rheumatic, blood

BRAND NAMES
Predalone, Prelone

DRUG CLASS
Anti-inflammatory, corticosteroid

DESCRIPTION
This drug decreases inflammation and suppresses the immune system by reducing activity and volume of the lymphatic system.

POTENTIAL SIDE EFFECTS
Insomnia, nervousness, increased appetite, indigestion, increased hair growth, diabetes mellitus, joint aches, cataracts, glaucoma, headache, impaired wound healing, thin fragile skin, loss of menstruation, sodium and fluid retention, loss of potassium or calcium, abdominal distention, nausea, vomiting.

CAUTIONS
- Chronic therapy may result in irreversible adverse effects.
- Therapy with this drug may mask the symptoms of infection and increase the susceptibility of infection via immunosuppression.
- Psychiatric symptoms may develop or be aggravated.
- Diabetics may require increased doses of insulin or oral drugs to treat diabetes.
- Notify your doctor if you have bacterial or viral infections, hyperthyroidism, cirrhosis, nonspecific ulcerative colitis, hypertension, osteoporosis, thromboembolic tendencies, congestive heart failure, convulsive disorders, myasthenia gravis, thrombophlebitis, peptic ulcer, diabetes.
- Acute adrenal insufficiency may occur with abrupt withdrawal after long-term therapy or with stress.

- Use the smallest possible dose, and for the shortest possible period of time.

DRUG INTERACTIONS
Aminoglutethimide, barbiturates, cholestyramine, oral contraceptives, ephedrine, estrogens, phenytoin, ketoconazole, rifampin, oral anticoagulants, cyclosporine, isoniazid, diuretics, salicylates, somatrem, theophylline

FOOD INTERACTIONS
Caffeine intake should be limited. May cause stomach upset; take with food or snack.

HERBAL INTERACTIONS
Unknown

PREGNANCY AND BREAST-FEEDING CAUTIONS
FDA Pregnancy Risk Category C. Excreted in breast milk. Consult your doctor.

SPECIAL INFORMATION
Prolonged therapy may result in suppression of adrenal gland function. Take single daily dose in morning prior to 9 a.m. Take multiple doses at evenly spaced intervals throughout the day. Increase dietary intake of pyridoxine, vitamin C, vitamin D, folate, calcium, and phosphorus. Monitor blood pressure, blood glucose and electrolytes.

PREDNISONE
(pred-NIS-zone)

Oral, Injectable

NEWLY DISCOVERED USES (OFF-LABEL)
Alopecia areata, autoimmune hepatitis, bullous pemphigoid, canker sores (recurrent), complicated mononucleosis/Epstein-Barr, cystic fibrosis in children, drug-induced anaphylaxis, hemosiderosis, kidney stones, muscular dystrophy, myasthenia gravis, nasal polyps, pneumocystis jiroveci pneumonia, polyarteritis nodosa, polymyalgia rheumatica, sudden hearing loss, thrombotic thrombocytopenic purpura, ureteral stones, urticaria, West syndrome

ORIGINAL USES (ON-LABEL)
Treatment of various allergic and various inflammatory disorders, including those of the skin, endocrine system, gastrointestinal, lung, rheumatic, blood.

BRAND NAMES
Deltasone, Liqui-PRED, Meticorten, Orasone, Sterapred

DRUG CLASS
Anti-inflammatory, corticosteroid

DESCRIPTION
This drug decreases inflammation and suppresses the immune system by reducing activity and volume of the lymphatic system.

POTENTIAL SIDE EFFECTS
Insomnia, nervousness, increased appetite, indigestion, increased hair growth, diabetes mellitus, joint aches, cataracts, glaucoma, headache, impaired wound healing, thin fragile skin, loss of menstruation, sodium and fluid retention, loss of potassium or calcium, abdominal distention, nausea, vomiting.

CAUTIONS
- Chronic therapy may result in irreversible adverse effects.
- Therapy with this drug may mask the symptoms of infection and increase the susceptibility of infection via immunosuppression.
- Psychiatric symptoms may develop or be aggravated.
- Diabetics may require increased doses of insulin or oral drugs to treat diabetes.
- Notify your doctor if you have bacterial or viral infections, hyperthyroidism, cirrhosis, nonspecific ulcerative colitis, hypertension, osteoporosis, thromboembolic tendencies, congestive heart failure, convulsive disorders, myasthenia gravis, thrombophlebitis, peptic ulcer, diabetes.
- Acute adrenal insufficiency may occur with abrupt withdrawal after long-term therapy or with stress.
- Use the smallest possible dose, and for the shortest possible period of time.

DRUG INTERACTIONS
Aminoglutethimide, barbiturates, cholestyramine, oral contraceptives, ephedrine, estrogens, phenytoin, ketoconazole, rifampin, oral anticoagulants, cyclosporine, isoniazid, diuretics, salicylates, somatrem, theophylline

FOOD INTERACTIONS
Caffeine intake should be limited. May cause stomach upset; take with food or snack.

HERBAL INTERACTIONS
Unknown

PREGNANCY AND BREAST-FEEDING CAUTIONS
FDA Pregnancy Risk Category C. Excreted in breast milk. Consult your doctor.

SPECIAL INFORMATION
Prolonged therapy may result in suppression of adrenal gland function. Take single daily dose in morning prior to 9 a.m. Take multiple doses at evenly spaced intervals throughout the day. Increase dietary intake of pyridoxine, vitamin C, vitamin D, folate, calcium, and phosphorus. Monitor blood pressure, blood glucose and electrolytes.

PREGABALIN
(pre-GAB-a-lin)

NEWLY DISCOVERED USES (OFF-LABEL)
Epilepsy seizures, fibromyalgia, generalized anxiety disorder, social phobia

ORIGINAL USES (ON-LABEL)
To manage pain associated with diabetic peripheral neuropathy, post-herpetic neuralgia, and used in combination with other drugs for the treatment of partial onset seizure disorder in adults

BRAND NAME
Lyrica

DRUG CLASS
Analgesic, anticonvulsant

DESCRIPTION
This drug inhibits the release of excitatory neurotransmitters.

POTENTIAL SIDE EFFECTS
Peripheral edema, chest pain, dizziness, abnormal gait, neuropathy, dry mouth, constipation, flatulence, vomiting, tremor, twitching, blurred vision, diplopia, visual abnormalities, weight gain.

CAUTIONS

- Use caution in tasks that require alertness, as this drug may cause drowsiness.
- Notify your doctor if you develop visual changes, muscle pain or weakness.
- Inform your doctor if you have congestive heart failure, high blood pressure, kidney dysfunction.
- Avoid abrupt cessation; gradually decrease dosage according to your doctor's instructions.

DRUG INTERACTIONS
Central nervous system depressants, barbiturates, narcotic analgesics, and other sedative drugs.

FOOD INTERACTIONS
Unknown

HERBAL INTERACTIONS
Valerian, St. John's wort, kava kava, gotu kola

PREGNANCY AND BREAST-FEEDING CAUTIONS
FDA Pregnancy Risk Category C. Excretion in breast milk unknown. Do not breast-feed while taking this drug.

SPECIAL INFORMATION
May be taken with or without food.

PRIMIDONE
(PRI-mi-done)

NEWLY DISCOVERED USES (OFF-LABEL)
Essential tremor, febrile seizure prevention

ORIGINAL USES (ON-LABEL)
To manage seizures (grand mal, psychomotor, and focal)

BRAND NAME
Mysoline

DRUG CLASS
Anticonvulsant (barbiturate)

DESCRIPTION
This drug raises the body's electroshock or chemoshock seizure threshold and thus alters seizure patterns.

POTENTIAL SIDE EFFECTS
Anorexia, nausea, changes in vision, vertigo, uncoordinated gait, drowsiness, fatigue, rash, blood disorders (anemia, etc.).

CAUTIONS
- Do not stop this medication suddenly as it may precipitate seizures.
- May take several weeks to assess full therapeutic effects.
- Requires periodic blood monitoring.
- Causes drowsiness, thus use caution while driving or operating machinery.
- Notify your doctor if you have kidney, liver, or lung problems.

DRUG INTERACTIONS
Carbamazepine, phenytoin, ethosuximide, valproic acid, beta-blockers (such as propranolol, etc.), corticosteroids, doxycycline, estrogens, oral contraceptives, felodipine, methadone, metronidazole, nifedipine, quinidine, theophylline griseofulvin.

This drug is metabolized by and affects a specific set of liver enzymes (cytochrome P450 enzymes). Several other drugs interfere with these liver enzymes, and thus may increase or decrease the clearance of primidone from the body or vice versa, potentially increasing the risk of side effects or decreasing effectiveness. When these drugs are given in combination with primidone, dosage adjustments may be needed. As these are too numerous to list, you should always check with your doctor or pharmacist prior to starting a new medication, herbal, or nonprescription product.

FOOD INTERACTIONS
Unknown

HERBAL INTERACTIONS
Valerian, St. John's wort, kava kava, gotu kola

PREGNANCY AND BREAST-FEEDING CAUTIONS
FDA Pregnancy Risk Category D. Excreted into breast milk. Do not breast-feed during therapy.

SPECIAL INFORMATION
Notify your doctor if skin rash or fever occurs.

PROCHLORPERAZINE
(proe-klor-PER-a-zeen)

NEWLY DISCOVERED USES (OFF-LABEL)
Hyperemesis gravidarum

ORIGINAL USES (ON-LABEL)
To manage severe nausea and vomiting, schizophrenia, and short-term treatment of generalized non-psychotic anxiety

BRAND NAMES
Compazine, Compro

DRUG CLASS
Antiemetic

DESCRIPTION
This drug blocks transmission of several chemical neurotransmitters, and affects metabolism, body temperature, wakefulness, vasomotor tone and vomiting.

POTENTIAL SIDE EFFECTS
Changes in blood pressure and heart rate, lowered blood pressure upon standing from a sitting or lying down position, uncontrolled muscle movements, dizziness, rash, changes in heart rate or regularity.

CAUTIONS
- Not for use in children less than 2 years or less than 20 pounds. Use in children less than 5 years only after other anti-emetics (anti-vomiting) have failed.
- May cause drowsiness; use caution if driving or performing tasks requiring high levels of mental alertness.
- Notify your doctor if you have allergies to tartrazine dye or have a seizure disorder. This drug may decrease seizure threshold.
- Elderly are at an increased risk of developing irreversible tardive dyskinesia (uncontrolled muscle movements, tics) or orthostatic hypotension (lowered blood pressure upon standing from sitting or lying down position).
- Has been known to cause confusion, memory loss, psychotic behavior, and agitation.
- Has rarely caused a potentially fatal syndrome called neuroleptic malignant syndrome, characterized by fever, muscle rigidity,

altered mental status, irregular blood pressure, increased heart rate, sweating, irregular heart rate.

DRUG INTERACTIONS
Chloroquine, propranolol, sulfadoxine-pyrimethamine, tricyclic antidepressants, barbiturates, carbamazepine, benztropine, lithium, other central nervous system depressants such as alcohol, narcotics, metoclopramide, bromocriptine, guanethidine, guanadrel, levodopa, epinephrine

FOOD INTERACTIONS
Caffeine. Take with food or water.

HERBAL INTERACTIONS
Dong quai, St. John's wort, kava kava, gotu kola, valerian

PREGNANCY AND BREAST-FEEDING CAUTIONS
FDA Pregnancy Risk Category C. Excreted into breast milk. Breast-feeding not recommended while taking this drug.

SPECIAL INFORMATION
May need to supplement riboflavin in diet. Rectal suppositories may contain coconut and palm oil. Prochlorperazine is not recommended for use as an antipsychotic due to its decreased efficacy.

PROMETHAZINE
(proe-METH-a-zeen)

NEWLY DISCOVERED USES (OFF-LABEL)
Hyperemesis gravidarum

ORIGINAL USES (ON-LABEL)
To treat allergic conditions, vomiting, motion sickness, postoperative pain (in combination with other drugs), and anaphylaxis (in combination with other drugs), also used as a sedative and an anesthetic (in combination with other drugs)

BRAND NAMES
Phenadoz, Phenergan, Promethegan

DRUG CLASS
Antiemetic (anti-nausea, vomiting), antihistamine, sedative

DESCRIPTION
Promethazine blocks dopamine, alpha and histamine receptors to reduce nausea and vomiting, and produce sedation.

POTENTIAL SIDE EFFECTS
Drowsiness, sedation, blurred vision, confusion, dizziness, disorientation, extrapyrimadal symptoms, ringing in the ears, incoordination, fatigue, euphoria, nervousness, double vision, insomnia, tremors, changes in blood pressure or heart rate, dry mouth.

CAUTIONS
- Not for use in coma, treatment of lower respiratory tract symptoms (including asthma) in children less than 2 years of age.
- Avoid other drugs that cause respiratory depression.
- When used in children older than 2 years, the lowest possible dose should be used.
- Has rarely caused a potentially fatal syndrome called neuroleptic malignant syndrome, characterized by fever, muscle rigidity, altered mental status, irregular blood pressure, increased heart rate, sweating, irregular heart rate.
- Notify your doctor if you have sulfonamide allergies, Reye's syndrome, heart disease, impaired liver function, asthma, sleep apnea, a history of seizures, or concurrently taking narcotics or local anesthetics. Promethazine can lower the seizure threshold.
- Elderly are at an increased risk of side effects, particularly tremors, uncontrolled muscle movements.

DRUG INTERACTIONS
This drug is metabolized by a specific set of liver enzymes (cytochrome P450 enzymes). Several other drugs interfere with these liver enzymes, and thus may increase or decrease the clearance of promethazine from the body, potentially increasing the risk of side effects or decreasing effectiveness. When these drugs are given in combination with promethazine, dosage adjustments may be needed. As these are too numerous to list, you should always check with your doctor or pharmacist prior to starting a new medication, herbal, or nonprescription product.

FOOD INTERACTIONS
Unknown

HERBAL INTERACTIONS
St. John's wort, kava kava, gotu kola

PREGNANCY AND BREAST-FEEDING CAUTIONS

FDA Pregnancy Risk Category C. Excretion in breast milk is unknown. Breast-feeding while taking this drug is not recommended.

SPECIAL INFORMATION

This drug has a black box warning describing that it should not be used in children less than 2 years of age because of the potential for fatal respiratory depression. In addition, when used in children older than two years of age, the lowest effective dose should be used. (See cautions.)

PROPANTHELINE
(proe-PAN-the-leen)

NEWLY DISCOVERED USES (OFF-LABEL)
Ménière's disease

ORIGINAL USES (ON-LABEL)
Used in combination with other drugs to treat peptic ulcer

BRAND NAME
Pro-Banthine

DRUG CLASS
Gastrointestinal antispasmodic (anticholinergic)

DESCRIPTION
This drug decreases gastric motion via action on the smooth muscle in the gastrointestinal tract. It also has an antisecretory effect. In addition, it affects other areas of the body including the biliary tract, urinary tract, pupil, and heart rate.

POTENTIAL SIDE EFFECTS
Dry mouth, altered taste perception, nausea, upset stomach, heartburn, constipation, bloated feeling, urinary hesitancy and retention, blurred vision, headache, flushing, drowsiness, changes in heart rate.

CAUTIONS
- May cause decreased sweating and thereby increase the risk of impaired thermoregulation and heat stroke.
- Report any signs of diarrhea or changes in mental behavior to your doctor.

- The elderly may experience paradoxical reactions (such as excitement, agitation, etc.).
- Notify your doctor if you have heart disease, liver or kidney impairment, glaucoma, lung disease, or asthma.

DRUG INTERACTIONS
Amantadine, atenolol, digoxin, phenothiazines, tricyclic antidepressants

FOOD INTERACTIONS
Take 30 minutes prior to meals.

HERBAL INTERACTIONS
Unknown

PREGNANCY AND BREAST-FEEDING CAUTIONS
FDA Pregnancy Risk Category C. Excreted in breast milk. Do not use during breast-feeding.

PROPRANOLOL
(proe-PRAN- oh-lole)

NEWLY DISCOVERED USES (OFF-LABEL)

Aortic aneurysm, dilated cardiomyopathy, hyperthyroidism, portal hypertension, prevention of bleeding in cirrhosis, post-traumatic stress disorder (PTSD), thyroid crisis

ORIGINAL USES (ON-LABEL)
Cardiac arrhythmias (irregular heart rate), myocardial infarction (heart attacks), hypertrophic subaortic stenosis, pheochromocytoma, high blood pressure, prevention of migraines, angina pectoris, essential tremor

BRAND NAMES
Inderal, Inderal LA, InnoPran XL, Propranolol Intensol

DRUG CLASS
Antianginal, anti-arrhythmic, antihypertensive, antimigraine (beta-blocker)

DESCRIPTION
This drug decreases heart rate, cardiac contractility, blood pressure, and heart oxygen demand.

POTENTIAL SIDE EFFECTS
Decreased heart rate, dizziness, reduced peripheral circulation, chest pain, mental depression, lightheadedness, amnesia, emotional lability, rash, hair loss, various skin disorders (such as exfoliative dermatitis, psoriasiform eruptions), changes in blood glucose and lipids, increased potassium levels, nausea, vomiting, constipation, anorexia, impotence, various blood disorders (such as agranulocytosis, thrombocytopenia, thrombocytopenic purpura), weakness, wheezing, pharyngitis, bronchospasm, pulmonary edema, decreased tear production, decreased visual acuity.

CAUTIONS
- Inform your doctor if you have heart conditions (such as congestive heart failure, cardiogenic shock, too low heart rate, or second- and third-degree heart block, sinus node dysfunction), are pregnant, or have lung/breathing problems.
- Do not stop this medication suddenly, taper over a gradual period.
- May cause or mask the symptoms of low blood glucose levels in diabetics.
- May mask signs of thyroid problems.
- Not indicated for high blood pressure emergencies.
- Immediately report to your doctor any signs of swelling of the extremities, sudden weight gain, changes in breathing, night cough.

DRUG INTERACTIONS
Barbiturates, cholestyramine, colestipol, rifampin, calcium channel blockers, cimetidine, oral contraceptives, diphenhydramine, flecainide, haloperidol, hydralazine, hydroxychloroquine, furosemide, bumetanide, NSAIDs, phenothiazines, propafenone, quinidine, ciprofloxacin, thyroid hormones, warfarin, clonidine, epinephrine, ergot alkaloids, gabapentin, lidocaine, prazosin, oral sulfonylureas (drugs used to treat diabetes), theophylline.

FOOD INTERACTIONS
Take at the same time every day.

HERBAL INTERACTIONS
Dong quai, ephedra, yohimbe, ginseng, natural licorice, saw palmetto, garlic

PREGNANCY AND BREAST-FEEDING CAUTIONS
FDA Pregnancy Risk Category C (manufacturer); D 2nd and 3rd trimesters (expert analysis). Excreted in breast milk. Consult doctor.

SPECIAL INFORMATION
This drug has a black box warning regarding the avoidance of abrupt withdrawal in patients with heart disease.

QUETIAPINE
(kwe-TYE-a-peen)

NEWLY DISCOVERED USES (OFF-LABEL)
Alzheimer's disease, Huntington's disease

ORIGINAL USES (ON-LABEL)
Treatment of schizophrenia

BRAND NAME
Seroquel

DRUG CLASS
Atypical antipsychotic

DESCRIPTION
This drug affects chemical neurotransmitters in the brain, including serotonin, dopamine, and histamine.

POTENTIAL SIDE EFFECTS
Headache, sudden drop in blood pressure upon standing from a sitting or lying down position, somnolence, weight gain, increased heart rate, dizziness, rash, abdominal pain, constipation, dry mouth, upset stomach, back pain, weakness, sore throat, cough, shortness of breath, increases in triglycerides or cholesterol, increased prolactin levels, increases in liver function tests, priapism (prolonged painful erection).

CAUTIONS
- Reduced doses may be needed if you have liver impairment.
- Has demonstrated increased mortality in elderly patients when used for off-label treatment of dementia in elderly patients.
- Not for use in central nervous system depression, bone marrow suppression, blood dyscrasias, severe liver disease, coma.

- Notify your doctor if you plan to become pregnant, if you have heart disease, cerebrovascular disease or conditions that predispose to low blood pressure, history of seizures, thyroid disease, liver disease, increased cholesterol or triglycerides levels, diabetes.
- Neuroleptic malignant syndrome (NMS), a potentially fatal complex, has been reported with antipsychotic drugs. Report any of the following symptoms to your doctor immediately: fever, muscle rigidity, altered mental status, irregular heart rate, increased heart rate.
- Has been reported to cause significant increases in blood glucose levels, causing diabetes that requires treatment.
- Report any vision changes to your doctor, particularly blurred vision. May require regular eye exams to monitor for the development of cataracts.
- Patients with schizophrenia may be at increased risk of suicidal thinking.
- May disrupt regulation of body temperature. Avoid dehydration, particularly during strenuous exercise or extreme heat.

DRUG INTERACTIONS
This drug is metabolized by a specific set of liver enzymes (cytochrome P450 enzymes 3A4). Several other drugs interfere with these liver enzymes, and thus may increase or decrease the clearance of quetiapine from the body, potentially increasing the risk of side effects or decreasing effectiveness. When these drugs are given in combination with quetiapine, dosage adjustments may be needed. As these are too numerous to list, you should always check with your doctor or pharmacist prior to starting a new medication, herbal, or nonprescription product.

FOOD INTERACTIONS
Serum levels may be increased when taken with food. Avoid alcohol.

HERBAL INTERACTIONS
St. John's wort, valerian, kava kava, gotu kola

PREGNANCY AND BREAST-FEEDING CAUTIONS
FDA Pregnancy Risk Category C. Excretion in breast milk is not known. Do not breast-feed during therapy.

SPECIAL INFORMATION
This drug has a black box warning describing the risk of increased mortality when the drug has been used for off-label treatment of dementia in the elderly.

RAMIPRIL
(ra-MI-pril)

NEWLY DISCOVERED USES (OFF-LABEL)
Diabetic nephropathy

ORIGINAL USES (ON-LABEL)
To reduce risk of cardiac events, high blood pressure, congestive heart failure, after heart attacks

BRAND NAME
Altace

DRUG CLASS
Blood pressure

DESCRIPTION
Ramipril lowers blood pressure by inhibiting the production of chemicals that cause blood vessels to constrict.

POTENTIAL SIDE EFFECTS
Chest pain, too low blood pressure (especially after first dose), cough, fainting, headache, dizziness, fatigue, weakness, rash, abnormal taste, nausea, shortness of breath.

CAUTIONS
- Do not use if you have had tongue, lip, throat, or mouth swelling (symptoms of angioedema) after taking other drugs in the same class or if you have these symptoms unrelated to drug therapy. Angioedema can occur at any time during treatment, but especially following the first dose. Report symptoms to your doctor.
- Do not use in pregnant patients who are in the second or third trimester.
- Do not use with certain kidney problems (kidney artery stenosis, decreased kidney function).
- Avoid rapid dosage increases, which may lead to kidney problems.

DRUG INTERACTIONS
Potassium supplements, cotrimoxazole (high dose), angiotension II receptor antagonists (candesartan, losartan, irbesartan, etc.) or potassium sparing diuretics (amiloride, spironolactone, triamterene), digoxin, lithium, and certain drugs used to treat dia-

betes (sulfonylureas). Aspirin (high doses) or indomethacin may aggravate the beneficial effects of this drug.

FOOD INTERACTIONS
Unknown

HERBAL INTERACTIONS
St. John's wort, capsaicin, dong quai, ephedra, yohimbe, ginseng, large amounts of natural licorice

PREGNANCY AND BREAST-FEEDING CAUTIONS
FDA Pregnancy Risk Category C for first trimester. FDA Pregnancy Category D for second and third trimester. Excreted in breast milk. Do not use this drug during breast-feeding.

SPECIAL INFORMATION
Report vomiting, diarrhea, excessive perspiration, or dehydration; also sore throat, fever, swelling of face, lips, tongue, or if difficulty in breathing occurs or if persistent cough develops; may cause lightheadedness during first few days of therapy; if a cough develops which is bothersome, consult physician. Capsule is usually swallowed whole but may be sprinkled on applesauce or mixed in water or juice.

RANITIDINE
(rah-NIT-a-deen)

NEWLY DISCOVERED USES (OFF-LABEL)
Chemotherapy-induced anaphylaxis, prevention of recurrence of upper gastrointestinal (GI) bleeding, urticaria

ORIGINAL USES (ON-LABEL)
Short-term treatment of active duodenal ulcers and benign gastric ulcers, long-term prophylaxis of duodenal ulcer, erosive esophagitis, gastric hypersecretory states, gastroesophageal reflux (GERD), prevention of upper gastric bleeding in critically ill patients

BRAND NAME
Zantac, Zantac EFFERdose

DRUG CLASS
Antihistamine (H2)

DESCRIPTION
This drug reduces gastric acid secretion, gastric volume and hydrogen ion (acidity) concentration by competitively inhibiting histamine at histamine-2 receptors in gastric cells.

POTENTIAL SIDE EFFECTS
Headache, agitation, drowsiness, diarrhea, nausea, and vomiting, blood disorders.

CAUTIONS
- Notify your doctor if you have allergies to other drugs in this class.
- Dosage adjustments may be required in kidney or liver impairment. May cause changes in liver function tests, requiring testing.
- Do not use for long term treatment without doctor supervision.
- Mental confusion and delirium have occurred in the elderly or in individuals with impaired kidney function.

DRUG INTERACTIONS
Antacids, metoclopramide, diazepam, sulfonylureas, theophylline, warfarin.

This drug inhibits a specific set of liver enzymes that are responsible for the metabolism (clearance or activation) of many other drugs, potentially increasing the risk of side effects or decreasing effectiveness. When these drugs are given in combination with cimetidine, dosage adjustments may be needed. As these are too numerous to list, you should always check with your doctor or pharmacist prior to starting a new medication, herbal product, or nonprescription drug.

FOOD INTERACTIONS
May be taken without regard to food.

HERBAL INTERACTIONS
St. John's wort

PREGNANCY AND BREAST-FEEDING CAUTIONS
FDA Pregnancy Risk Category B. Excreted in breast milk. Consult with your doctor.

SPECIAL INFORMATION
If taken with antacids separate by taking one hour before or two hours after the antacid. Avoid excessive alcohol use with this drug.

This information refers to the use of the prescription product only.

RETEPLASE
(Re-te-plase)

NEWLY DISCOVERED USES (OFF-LABEL)
Toxic shock syndrome

ORIGINAL USES (ON-LABEL)
For the management of acute myocardial infarction (heart attack) to reduce mortality

BRAND NAME
Retavase

DRUG CLASS
Fibrinolytic

DESCRIPTION
This drug generates plasmin, which breaks down fibrin (fibrinolysis) in a thrombus (clot).

POTENTIAL SIDE EFFECTS
Injection site reaction, bleeding, changes in heart rhythm and rate.

CAUTIONS
- Not for use if you have an increased risk for bleeding (such as recent surgery, stroke, aneurysm, brain tumor, active internal bleeding, severe uncontrolled high blood pressure). Discuss these risks with your doctor.
- Requires blood testing for bleeding tendencies before administration.

DRUG INTERACTIONS
Warfarin, heparins, aspirin, aminocaproic acid, nitroglycerin, dipyridamole, abciximab, vitamin K antagonist, drugs that affect clotting and bleeding.

FOOD INTERACTIONS
Unknown

HERBAL INTERACTIONS
Cat's claw, dong quai, evening primrose, feverfew, red clover, horse chestnut, garlic, green tea, ginseng, and gingko

PREGNANCY AND BREAST-FEEDING CAUTIONS
FDA Pregnancy Risk Category C. Excretion into breast milk is unknown; do not breast-feed while using this drug.

SPECIAL INFORMATION
Watch for signs of bleeding and bruising; report to your doctor.

RIBAVIRIN
(rye-ba-VYE-rin)

NEWLY DISCOVERED USES (OFF-LABEL)

Influenza A and B treatment, liver cirrhosis, liver fibrosis, therapy-resistant hepatitis C, viral hemorrhagic fever

ORIGINAL USES (ON-LABEL)
Inhalation: treatment of severe lower respiratory tract infections due to respiratory syncytial virus (RSV), in infants and children.

Oral: Used in combination with interferon alfa-2b or peginterferon alfa-2b for treatment of chronic hepatitis C in patients with liver disease who have received previous treatment with or relapsed after interferon therapy.

BRAND NAMES
Rebetol, Ribasphere, Virazole

DRUG CLASS
Antiviral

DESCRIPTION
This drug blocks the reproduction of RNA and DNA in viruses. It also exhibits inhibitory activity against influenza.

POTENTIAL SIDE EFFECTS
Inhalation: Fatigue, headache, insomnia, nausea, anorexia, anemia.

Oral (in combination therapy with interferon alpha-2b): Agitation, anxiety, emotional lability, impaired concentration, depression, dizziness, insomnia, nervousness, hair loss, itching, rash, dry skin, increased sweating, abdominal pain, anorexia, constipation, diarrhea, upset stomach, nausea, vomiting, anemia, joint aches, muscle pain and aches, fever, cough, sore throat, change in taste sensation, headache, dry mouth, injection site reaction.

CAUTIONS

- This drug can cause malformations in fetuses and is not for use if you are pregnant or trying to conceive with a male patient who is on therapy. If of childbearing age, you must use at least two forms of effective contraception during therapy and for six months after therapy is completed. Requires negative pregnancy test to start therapy. Pregnancy testing should be performed monthly during therapy and for six months after therapy is completed.
- This drug should not be used in patients with pancreatitis.

ORAL:

- Notify your doctor if you have sarcoidosis, lung disease, heart disease, or history of psychiatric disorders.
- Primary toxicity is hemolytic anemia, occurring in 10% of those who receive this drug, usually occurring within one to two weeks of initiation of therapy. Requires blood testing before therapy begins and periodically during therapy.
- Heart attacks have been reported in patients with drug-induced anemia. Notify your doctor if you have heart disease prior to the initiation of therapy. Cardiac status should be monitored during therapy.
- This drug should not be used in patients with decreased kidney function.
- Not for use as monotherapy in the treatment of hepatitis C.
- Not for use in patients with autoimmune hepatitis, anemia, or severe heart disease.
- Safety and efficacy not established in organ transplant patients, certain types of liver disease, concurrent hepatitis B or HIV, or patients less than three years old.
- Requires periodic testing during therapy for blood disorders, liver function, thyroid function, and pregnancy.

INHALATION:

- Not for use in patients requiring ventilation. Not for use in adults.
- Should be used cautiously in people with underlying chronic obstructive pulmonary disease (COPD), asthma, congenital heart disease.
- Requires monitoring of respiratory function during therapy.

DRUG INTERACTIONS

Oral: antacids containing magnesium, aluminum, and simethicone, zidovudine, stavudine.

FOOD INTERACTIONS

High-fat meals may ease absorption and blood levels (oral formulations). May take capsules with or without food, but should be consistent. Should take capsules with food if taking with peginterferon alfa-2b. Tablets should be taken with food.

HERBAL INTERACTIONS

Unknown

PREGNANCY AND BREAST-FEEDING CAUTIONS

FDA Pregnancy Risk Category X. Excretion in breast milk is unknown. Do not breast-feed during therapy.

SPECIAL INFORMATION

All formulations of this drug have a black box warning that describes various risks associated with therapy (see cautions). Read the Medication Safety Guide prior to therapy and discuss such risks with your doctor.

RIBAVIRIN/INTERFERON

(rye-ba-VYE-rin in-ter-FEER-on)

NEWLY DISCOVERED USES (OFF-LABEL)

Therapy-resistant hepatitis C

ORIGINAL USES (ON-LABEL)

Treatment of chronic hepatitis C

BRAND NAMES

Copegus, Rebetron

DRUG CLASS

Antiviral

DESCRIPTION

This drug inhibits the reproduction of RNA and DNA in viruses.

POTENTIAL SIDE EFFECTS

Agitation, anxiety, emotional lability, impaired concentration, depression, dizziness, insomnia, nervousness, hair loss, itching, rash, dry skin, increased sweating, abdominal pain, anorexia, constipation, diarrhea, upset stomach, nausea, vomiting, anemia, joint aches, muscle pain and aches, fever, cough, sore throat, change in taste sensation, headache, dry mouth, injection site reaction, increased triglycerides, changes in blood glucose.

CAUTIONS

- This drug can cause malformations in fetuses and is not for use if you are pregnant or trying to conceive with a male patient who is on therapy. If of childbearing age, you must use at least two forms of effective contraception during therapy and for six months after therapy is completed. Requires negative pregnancy test to start therapy. Pregnancy testing should be performed monthly during therapy and for six months after therapy is completed.
- This drug should not be used in patients with pancreatitis.
- Notify your doctor if you have sarcoidosis, lung disease, heart disease, a history of psychiatric disorders, if you are depressed or have a history of depression, seizure disorders, brain tumor or cancer involving the brain, heart disease, psoriasis, kidney or liver impairment, diabetes, thyroid disease, heart problems, autoimmune disease, had an organ transplant, taking drugs which affect the immune system.
- Primary toxicity is hemolytic anemia, occurring in 10% of those who receive this drug, usually occurring within one to two weeks of initiation of therapy. Requires blood testing before therapy begins and periodically during therapy.
- Heart attacks have been reported in patients with drug-induced anemia. Notify your doctor if you have heart disease prior to the initiation of therapy. Cardiac status should be monitored during therapy.
- This drug should not be used in people with decreased kidney function.
- Not for use in patients with autoimmune hepatitis, anemia, or severe heart disease, visceral AIDS-related Kaposi's, and liver decomposition.
- Safety and efficacy not established in organ transplant patients, certain types of liver disease, concurrent hepatitis B or HIV, or patients less than 3 years old.
- Requires periodic testing during therapy for blood disorders, liver function, thyroid function, and pregnancy.
- May cause severe psychiatric adverse events, including severe depression or suicidal ideation.

- Treatment should be discontinued in patients with worsening or persistently severe signs/symptoms of autoimmune problems, infections, heart problems, or neuropsychiatric disorders.
- Should receive an eye exam before initiating therapy. If you have underlying eye problems these should be monitored closely during therapy.

DRUG INTERACTIONS

Antacids containing magnesium, aluminum, and simethicone, zidovudine, stavudine. Theophylline, ACE inhibitors, clozapine, warfarin, zidovudine, prednisone, erythropoietin, melphalan, interleukin-2. There are numerous drugs that may have the potential to interact with interferons. Consult your doctor or pharmacist prior to starting any new medication, herbal product, or nonprescription drug.

FOOD INTERACTIONS

May take capsules with or without food, but should be consistent. Should take capsules with food if taking with peginterferon alfa-2b.

HERBAL INTERACTIONS

Unknown

PREGNANCY AND BREAST-FEEDING CAUTIONS

FDA Pregnancy Risk Category X. Excretion in breast milk is unknown. Do not breast-feed during therapy.

SPECIAL INFORMATION

This drug has a black box warning that describes various risks associated with ribavirin therapy (see cautions of ribavirin) and interferons, including psychiatric, autoimmune, cardiac and infectious disorders. Interferons may cause or aggravate fatal or life-threatening disorders of this nature. Completely read patient information brochure.

Read the Medication Safety Guide prior to therapy and discuss such risks with your doctor.

RIFAMPIN
(ri-FAM-pin)

NEWLY DISCOVERED USES (OFF-LABEL)

Diverticulitis, pharyngitis, tonsillitis/peritonsillar abscess

ORIGINAL USES (ON-LABEL)
Treatment of various bacterial infections, specifically tuberculosis, and carriers of *Neisseria meningitides*

BRAND NAME
Rifadin

DRUG CLASS
Anti-infective

DESCRIPTION
Inhibits DNA and RNA activity in the bacterial cells, preventing reproduction and replication.

POTENTIAL SIDE EFFECTS
Flu-like syndrome, various blood disorders, skin reactions, liver reaction, shortness of breath, headache, flushing, itching, hives, muscular weakness, changes in vision.

CAUTIONS
- Requires careful monitoring of liver function as this drug has been associated with significant damage to the liver. Report any symptoms of liver problems to your doctor, including dark urine, abdominal pain, nausea, loss of appetite.
- The possibility of resistance or tolerance to this medication may develop.
- Requires laboratory monitoring prior to initiation of therapy and during therapy.
- Will cause red-orange discoloration of body fluids, including urine, sputum, sweat, and tears. May permanently stain soft contact lenses.
- This drug has been associated with various blood disorders (such as anemia, decrease in red blood cells).
- Avoid missing doses.
- Interacts with oral contraceptives or other types of hormonal contraceptives. Discuss contraceptive alternatives with doctor.

DRUG INTERACTIONS
This drug affects the metabolism of other drugs by a specific set of liver enzymes, and thus may increase the clearance of other drugs from the body, decreasing effectiveness. When these drugs are given in combination with rifampin, dosage adjustments may be needed or other alternative drug therapy is required. As these are too numerous to list, you should always check with your doctor or pharmacist prior to starting a new medication, herbal, or nonprescription product.

FOOD INTERACTIONS
Food increases absorption. Take on an empty stomach, either one hour prior to or two hours after a meal, with a full glass of water.

HERBAL INTERACTIONS
Unknown

PREGNANCY AND BREAST-FEEDING CAUTIONS
FDA Pregnancy Risk Category C. Excreted in breast milk. Not recommended during breast-feeding.

RIFAXIMIN
(rif-AX-i-min)

NEWLY DISCOVERED USES (OFF-LABEL)
> Diverticulitis

ORIGINAL USES (ON-LABEL)
To treat travelers' diarrhea caused by noninvasive strains of *E. coli*

BRAND NAME
Xifaxan

DRUG CLASS
Antibiotic

DESCRIPTION
This drug inhibits the production of bacterial proteins.

POTENTIAL SIDE EFFECTS
Flatulence, headache, abdominal pain, urge to defecate, nausea, constipation, fever, vomiting.

CAUTIONS
- Do not use for diarrhea associated with fever and blood in stool.
- Effectiveness has not been determined in the treatment of diarrhea due to bacteria other than *E. coli.*
- Consider alternative therapy if symptoms persist after 24–48 hours of treatment.
- Not useful for other types of infections.

DRUG INTERACTIONS
Consult with doctor or pharmacist prior to initiation of therapy with any herbal, medication or nonprescription drug.

FOOD INTERACTIONS
May be taken without regard to meals.

HERBAL INTERACTIONS
Unknown

PREGNANCY AND BREAST-FEEDING CAUTIONS
FDA Pregnancy Risk Category C. Excreted in breast milk. Breast-feeding while on this drug is not recommended.

RILUZOLE
(RIL-yoo-zole)

NEWLY DISCOVERED USES (OFF-LABEL) ───────────
  Huntington's disease

ORIGINAL USES (ON-LABEL)
Treatment of amyotrophic lateral sclerosis (ALS)

BRAND NAME
Rilutek

DRUG CLASS
Glutamate inhibitor

DESCRIPTION
This drug relaxes muscles and has sedative effects.

POTENTIAL SIDE EFFECTS
Headache, abdominal pain, nausea, vomiting, upset stomach, anorexia, diarrhea, depression, dizziness, dry mouth, itching, decreased lung function, high blood pressure, weight loss, peripheral edema, joint aches.

CAUTIONS
- Inform your doctor if you have or have had liver disease. This therapy requires regular monitoring of liver function due to possible liver toxicity.
- Report any illness that results in fever to your doctor.
- Inform your doctor if you have kidney impairment.
- The elderly, women and Japanese patients may require dosage adjustments.
- May make you dizzy or cause somnolence. Be careful when operating machinery or driving.

DRUG INTERACTIONS
This drug is metabolized by a specific set of liver enzymes (cytochrome P450 enzymes 1A2). Several other drugs interfere with these liver enzymes, and thus may increase or decrease the clearance of riluzole from the body, potentially increasing the risk of side effects or decreasing effectiveness. When these drugs are given in combination with riluzole, dosage adjustments may be needed. As these are too numerous to list, you should always check with your doctor or pharmacist prior to starting a new medication, herbal, or nonprescription product.

FOOD INTERACTIONS
Avoid high-fat meals and charbroiled foods. Riluzole should be taken at least one hour before or two hours after a meal.

HERBAL INTERACTIONS
Unknown

PREGNANCY AND BREAST-FEEDING CAUTIONS
FDA Pregnancy Risk Category C. Excretion in breast milk is unknown. Consult your doctor.

SPECIAL INFORMATION
Avoid alcohol. Monitoring of serum aminotransferases should be performed before and during treatment.

RISEDRONATE
(ris-ED-roe-nate)

NEWLY DISCOVERED USES (OFF-LABEL)
Hypercalciuria

ORIGINAL USES (ON-LABEL)
To treat or prevent osteoporosis in postmenopausal women as well as in glucocorticoid-induced osteoporosis. To treat Paget's disease of the bone

BRAND NAME
Actonel

DRUG CLASS
Bisphosphonate

DESCRIPTION
Inhibits bone resorption, leading to an indirect increase in bone mineral density.

POTENTIAL SIDE EFFECTS
Joint aches, back pain, pain, abdominal pain, high blood pressure, bruising, muscle aches, bone pain, leg cramps, depression, insomnia, vertigo, sore throat, shortness of breath, cataracts, urinary tract infection, headache, rash, diarrhea, flu-like symptoms, nausea, dizziness, chest pain, constipation, sinusitis, peripheral edema.

CAUTIONS
- You cannot take this drug if you have low blood calcium levels, severe kidney impairment, if you have esophageal abnormalities which delay esophageal emptying, or are unable to stand or sit upright for at least 30 minutes.
- To reduce the potential of esophageal irritation or ulceration and to ensure that the drug reaches the stomach, you must take with a full glass of water and remain upright for at least 30 minutes after taking.
- Requires periodic monitoring of bone and laboratory tests.
- This therapy may cause upper gastrointestinal disorders such as difficulty swallowing, esophageal ulcer, or gastric ulcer. Notify your doctor if you develop difficulty swallowing, pain upon swallowing, chest pain, or persistent or worsening heartburn.
- Requires adequate calcium and vitamin D intake or such supplements.

DRUG INTERACTIONS
Calcium supplements and antacids interfere with absorption of risedronate (take at a separate time of day).

FOOD INTERACTIONS
Food may reduce absorption. Should be taken before the first food or drink of the day other than water.

HERBAL INTERACTIONS
Unknown

PREGNANCY AND BREAST-FEEDING CAUTIONS
FDA Pregnancy Risk Category C. Excretion in breast milk unknown. Refrain from breast-feeding while taking this drug.

RISPERIDONE
(RIS-peer-i-dohn)

NEWLY DISCOVERED USES (OFF-LABEL)
. Alzheimer's disease, autism, Gilles de la Tourette syndrome, obsessive-compulsive disorder (OCD)

ORIGINAL USES (ON-LABEL)
To manage psychotic disorders such as chronic schizophrenia and bipolar disorder, also used to treat AIDS-related psychosis

BRAND NAMES
Risperdal, Risperdal M-TAB

DRUG CLASS
Antipsychotic

DESCRIPTION
Risperidone works by decreasing abnormal excitement in the brain. It affects brain receptors for serotonin and dopamine, two neurohormones.

POTENTIAL SIDE EFFECTS
Sleepiness; sleeplessness; agitation; anxiety; uncontrolled movements; headache; and nasal stuffiness.

CAUTIONS
- People taking this drug for longer than six to eight weeks must be reevaluated at least every two months.
- May increase blood sugar levels (hyperglycemia). Tell your doctor immediately if you have any of the following high blood sugar symptoms: extreme thirst, frequent urination, extreme hunger, blurred vision, or weakness.
- If you are having surgery, including dental surgery, tell the doctor or dentist that you are taking this drug.
- May make you drowsy and affect your judgment. Be careful when driving a car or operating machinery.
- Alcohol can add to the drowsiness caused by this drug.
- May make your skin sensitive to sunlight. Avoid unnecessary or prolonged exposure to sunlight.
- May interfere with the body's temperature-regulating mechanism. Avoid extreme heat or cold.

- This drug increases the risk of developing diabetes for people who have schizophrenia.

DRUG INTERACTIONS
Levodopa, dopamine agonists, carbamazepine, clozapine, blood-pressure-lowering drugs, central nervous system depressants

FOOD INTERACTIONS
Unknown

HERBAL INTERACTIONS
St. John's wort, ma huang, yohimbe, ginkgo, ginseng, evening primrose oil

PREGNANCY AND BREAST-FEEDING CAUTIONS
FDA Pregnancy Risk Category C. Refrain from breast-feeding while taking this drug.

SPECIAL INFORMATION
Tell your doctor if you use or have ever used street drugs or large amounts of alcohol and if you have or have ever had Alzheimer's disease, difficulty swallowing, phenylketonuria, breast cancer, angina (chest pain), irregular heartbeat, problems with blood pressure, heart failure, a heart attack, a stroke, seizures, kidney or liver disease, or if you or anyone in your family has or has ever had diabetes.

RITUXIMAB
(ri-TUK-si-mab)

NEWLY DISCOVERED USES (OFF-LABEL)
Autoimmune hemolytic anemia, chronic inflammatory demyelinating polyneuropathy, chronic neuropathic pain, therapy-resistant idiopathic thrombocytopenic purpura, therapy-resistant thrombotic thrombocytopenic purpura

ORIGINAL USES (ON-LABEL)
B-cell non-Hodgkin's lymphoma

BRAND NAME
Rituxan

DRUG CLASS
Monoclonal antibody

DESCRIPTION
This drug is a genetically engineered human monoclonal antibody that acts on the surface of normal and malignant lymphocytes and causes them to decompose.

POTENTIAL SIDE EFFECTS
Fever, chills, infection, headache, abdominal pain, pain, back pain, throat irritation, blood pressure changes, nausea, diarrhea, vomiting, blood disorders, changes in blood glucose, edema, muscle aches, joint pain, dizziness, anxiety, increased cough, bronchospasm, rash, night sweats, itching, hives, infusion reactions, tumor lysis syndrome (see cautions), skin reactions, changes in heart rhythm, kidney toxicity.

CAUTIONS
- Notify your doctor if you have allergies to mouse proteins.
- Severe infusion related reactions have been reported (77% following first dose).
- Notify your doctor if you have a history or currently have hepatitis B, hepatitis, heart or lung disease, with high numbers of circulating malignant cells.
- Requires periodic monitoring of blood to determine toxicities.
- Tumor lysis syndrome leading to acute kidney failure requiring dialysis may occur 12–24 hours following the first dose.
- Severe skin reactions have been reported, (usually 1–13 weeks following treatment).

DRUG INTERACTIONS
Rituximab, cisplatin. Do not receive vaccinations or immunizations without checking with your doctor or pharmacist first.

FOOD INTERACTIONS
Unknown

HERBAL INTERACTIONS
Unknown

PREGNANCY AND BREAST-FEEDING CAUTIONS
FDA Pregnancy Risk Category C. Excretion in breast milk unknown. Refrain from breast-feeding while taking this drug.

SPECIAL INFORMATION
Black box warning for fatal infusion reactions, tumor lysis syndrome, and severe skin reactions.

RIVASTIGMINE
(ri-va-STIG-meen)

NEWLY DISCOVERED USES (OFF-LABEL)
Brain trauma

ORIGINAL USES (ON-LABEL)
To treat mild to moderate dementia from Alzheimer's disease

BRAND NAME
Exelon

DRUG CLASS
Cholinergic

DESCRIPTION
Inhibits cholinesterase, the enzyme which is responsible for the breakdown of acetylcholine, thereby increasing acetylcholine in the central nervous system.

POTENTIAL SIDE EFFECTS
Nausea, dizziness, vomiting, anorexia, upset stomach, weight loss, fatigue, asthenia, diarrhea, abdominal pain, constipation, insomnia, confusion, anxiety, hallucination, aggressive reaction.

CAUTIONS
- Notify your doctor if you have liver or kidney impairment, peptic ulcers, have heart problems, seizure disorders, urinary obstruction, asthma, underlying lung disease, or are taking NSAIDs.
- Significant gastric effects (such as nausea, vomiting, anorexia, peptic ulcers, bleeding, and weight loss) occur more frequently in women and during the titration phase.

DRUG INTERACTIONS
This drug is metabolized by a specific set of liver enzymes (cytochrome P450 enzymes). Several other drugs interfere with these liver enzymes, and thus may increase or decrease the clearance of rivastigmine from the body, potentially increasing the risk of side effects or decreasing effectiveness. When these drugs are given in combination with rivastigmine, dosage adjustments may be needed. As these are too numerous to list, you should always check with your doctor or pharmacist prior to starting a new medication, herbal, or nonprescription product.

FOOD INTERACTIONS
Take with meals in divided dose in the morning and the evening.

HERBAL INTERACTIONS
Unknown

PREGNANCY AND BREAST-FEEDING CAUTIONS
FDA Pregnancy Risk Category B. Excretion in breast milk unknown. Consult your doctor.

SPECIAL INFORMATION
If treatment is disrupted for more than several days, reinstate at the lowest daily dose.

RIZATRIPTAN
(rye-za-TRIP-tan)

NEWLY DISCOVERED USES (OFF-LABEL)
Migraine treatment in children

ORIGINAL USES (ON-LABEL)
Acute treatment of migraine with or without aura

BRAND NAMES
Maxalt, Maxalt-MLT

DRUG CLASS
Anti-migraine

DESCRIPTION
This drug stimulates serotonin receptors in the cranial arteries, which causes constriction of blood vessels and a relief of migraine symptoms.

POTENTIAL SIDE EFFECTS
Blood pressure increases, chest pain, sensation of unusual heart beats, dizziness, drowsiness, fatigue, skin flushing, mild increases in growth hormone, hot flashes, nausea, abdominal pain, dry mouth, shortness of breath.

CAUTIONS
- Only for patients with clear diagnosis of migraine. Not for preventive treatment of migraine headaches.

- Notify your doctor of cardiac problems, particularly chest pain, irregular heart rhythm, uncontrolled blood pressure. Also notify your doctor if you have basilar or hemiplegic migraine.
- First dose may be given in healthcare setting.
- May make you drowsy and affect your judgment. Be careful when driving a car or operating machinery.
- You should be monitored for blood pressure changes.
- Alcohol may have added central nervous toxicity.
- Oral disintegrating tablets contain phenylalanine.
- Cerebral bleeding, stroke or other brain vascular events have been reported with this drug class.
- Do not use during or within two weeks of MAO inhibitors; or within 24 hours of treatment with another 5-HT1 agonist, or ergot-containing or ergot-like medication.
- Use with caution in patients that are elderly, with liver or kidney impairment.
- Do not use in patients with signs and symptoms of reduced arterial flow (ischemic bowel, Raynaud's disease) which could be exacerbated by vasospasm.
- Reconsider diagnosis of migraine if you have no response to initial dose.

DRUG INTERACTIONS
5-HT1 agonists, ergot containing drugs (dihydroergotamine, methysergide), propranolol, selective serotonin reuptake inhibitors (fluoxetine, fluvoxamine, paroxetine, sertraline), MAO inhibitors, nonselective MAO inhibitors, sibutramine

FOOD INTERACTIONS
Food delays absorption but does not affect overall extent of absorption.

HERBAL INTERACTIONS
Unknown

PREGNANCY AND BREAST-FEEDING CAUTIONS
FDA Pregnancy Risk Category C. Excretion in breast milk is unknown. Consult your doctor.

SPECIAL INFORMATION
The initial dose should be given in a setting where the response may be monitored (medical setting). Redosing should be separated by at least two hours. No more than 30 mg used in any 24-hour period. Patients taking propranolol should take a reduced dose.

For orally disintegrating tablets: Do not remove blister from outer pouch until just prior to dosing. Place tablet on tongue, where it will dissolve and be swallowed with saliva.

ROSIGLITAZONE
(roh-si-GLI-ta-zone)

NEWLY DISCOVERED USES (OFF-LABEL)
Prevention of cardiovascular disease in type 2 diabetes, prevention in type 2 diabetes

ORIGINAL USES (ON-LABEL)
Type 2 Diabetes—monotherapy and combination therapy, combination therapy with sulfonylureas, metformin, or insulin are indicated when monotherapy with diet and exercise are inadequate for control.

BRAND NAME
Avandia

DRUG CLASS
Antidiabetic (thiazolidinedione hypoglycemic)

DESCRIPTION
This drug lowers blood sugar by improving response to insulin.

POTENTIAL SIDE EFFECTS
Fatigue, headache, diarrhea, sinusitis, upper respiratory infection, anemia, back pain, edema, muscle aches, increases in HDL cholesterol, increases in triglycerides, increases in LDL cholesterol, too low glucose levels, weight gain.

CAUTIONS
- Active liver disease or elevated liver function tests.
- Inform your doctor if you have a history of jaundice or liver disease, if you currently have anemia or edema, or certain types of cardiac disease (class III or class IV congestive heart failure).
- May result in resumption of ovulation if you are premenopausal but not ovulating.
- Requires periodic monitoring of liver function and blood glucose parameters.
- May cause too low blood glucose levels.

- There is a possibility of fluid retention leading to or exacerbating congestive heart failure with combined therapy of pioglitazone and insulin.

DRUG INTERACTIONS

Delavirdine, fluconazole, gemfibrozil, ketoconazole, nicardipine, NSAIDs, sulfonamides, itraconazole, carbamazepine, phenobarbital, phenytoin, rifampin, rifapentine, secobarbital, oral contraceptives, bile acid sequestrants.

This drug is metabolized by a specific set of liver enzymes (cytochrome P450 enzymes). Several other drugs interfere with these liver enzymes, and thus may increase or decrease the clearance of rosiglitazone from the body, potentially increasing the risk of side effects or decreasing effectiveness. When these drugs are given in combination with rosiglitazone, dosage adjustments may be needed. As these are too numerous to list, you should always check with your doctor or pharmacist prior to starting a new medication, herbal, or nonprescription product.

FOOD INTERACTIONS

May take without regard to meals.

HERBAL INTERACTIONS

St. John's wort, chromium, garlic, gymnema

PREGNANCY AND BREAST-FEEDING CAUTIONS

FDA Pregnancy Risk Category C. Excretion in the breast milk is unknown. Therapy not recommended for those who are breast-feeding.

SPECIAL INFORMATION

If you miss a dose, do not double the dose the next day. When used in combination with insulin or other oral antidiabetic drugs, the risk of developing too low blood glucose is possible. Discuss risks and signs and symptoms with your doctor. Immediately report to your doctor any development of sudden weight gain, swelling, shortness of breath, nausea, vomiting, abdominal pain, fatigue, dark urine, or jaundice.

SARGRAMOSTIM
(sar-GRAM-oh-stim)

NEWLY DISCOVERED USES (OFF-LABEL)
Aplastic anemia, agranulocytosis, HIV

ORIGINAL USES (ON-LABEL)
Recovery of blood factors after bone marrow transplantation, peripheral stem cell transplantation

BRAND NAME
Leukine

DRUG CLASS
Colony-stimulating factor (blood factor)

DESCRIPTION
This drug stimulates the production of several important factors in the blood for promoting immune response against the growth of cancer cells or recovery of cells after chemotherapy.

POTENTIAL SIDE EFFECTS
Increased or decreased blood pressure, bleeding, increased heart rate, headache, numbness, insomnia, anxiety, rash, hair loss, itching, nausea, diarrhea, vomiting, abdominal pain, mouth ulcers, stomach upset, anorexia, difficulty swallowing, constipation, increased bilirubin, changes in blood, bone pain, muscle aches, sore throat, shortness of breath, fever, infection, weight loss.

CAUTIONS
- This product is produced from yeast-derived products and thus should not be used by persons allergic to yeasts.
- Notify your doctor if you have cardiac problems, fluid retention, lung disorders, liver or kidney impairment. Notify your doctor if you are receiving chemotherapy or radiation.
- Contains benzyl alcohol.
- May cause rapid increase in platelets.

DRUG INTERACTIONS
Lithium, corticosteroids

FOOD INTERACTIONS
Unknown

HERBAL INTERACTIONS
Unknown

PREGNANCY AND BREAST-FEEDING CAUTIONS
FDA Pregnancy Risk Category C. Excretion in breast milk is unknown. Consult your doctor.

SPECIAL INFORMATION
Requires extensive laboratory monitoring.

SCOPOLAMINE
(skoe-POL-a-meen)

NEWLY DISCOVERED USES (OFF-LABEL)

Prevention of post-op nausea and vomiting (add-on)

ORIGINAL USES (ON-LABEL)
Injection: preoperative medication to produce amnesia, sedation, and decrease salivary and respiratory secretions.

Ophthalmic: produce cycloplegia (paralysis of the ciliary muscle of the eye) and dilates pupils; treatment of iridocyclitis.

Oral: symptomatic treatment of postencephalitic parkinsonism and paralysis agitans; inhibits excessive motility of genitourinary or gastrointestinal tract.

Transdermal: prevention of nausea/vomiting associated with anesthesia or opiate pain meds; prevention of motion sickness.

BRAND NAMES
Scopace, Transderm Scōp, Buscopan, Transderm-V

DRUG CLASS
Anticholinergic

DESCRIPTION
This drug blocks the action of acetylcholine, an important chemical neurotransmitter, in smooth muscle, secretory glands and the central nervous system. The drug's action increases cardiac output, dries secretions and antagonizes histamine and serotonin.

POTENTIAL SIDE EFFECTS
Drowsiness, sudden drop in blood pressure upon standing from a sitting or lying down position, confusion, constipation, dry throat, pain on urination, blurred vision, fatigue, increased intraocular pressure.

CAUTIONS

- Notify your doctor if you have narrow-angle glaucoma, acute hemorrhage, paralytic ileus, gastrointestinal or urinary obstruction, thyroid disorders, heart or heart rate problems, tachycardia, myasthenia gravis.
- Adverse central nervous effects occur more often in patients with liver or kidney impairment.

DRUG INTERACTIONS

Other anticholinergic drugs (such as tricyclic antidepressants, belladonna alkaloids, antihistamines, etc.), central nervous system depressants, acetaminophen, levodopa, ketoconazole, digoxin, riboflavin, and potassium chloride in wax matrix preparations.

FOOD INTERACTIONS
Unknown

HERBAL INTERACTIONS
Unknown

PREGNANCY AND BREAST-FEEDING CAUTIONS
FDA Pregnancy Risk Category C. Excreted in breast milk. Consult your doctor.

SPECIAL INFORMATION
Scopolamine hydrobromide should not be interchanged with scopolamine butylbromide formulations. Dosages are not equivalent. Apply patch behind the ear.

SELEGILINE
(se-LE-ji-leen)

NEWLY DISCOVERED USES (OFF-LABEL)
Major depressive disorder, periodic limb movement disorder, smoking cessation

ORIGINAL USES (ON-LABEL)
Used in combination with other drugs to manage Parkinsonian patients in which levodopa/carbidopa therapy is deteriorating.

BRAND NAME
Eldepryl

DRUG CLASS
Anti-Parkinson's (MAO type B inhibitor)

DESCRIPTION
This drug increases dopamine levels. Dopamine deficiency is one of the causes of Parkinson's disease.

POTENTIAL SIDE EFFECTS
Nausea, dizziness, lightheadedness, confusion, hallucinations, dry mouth, vivid dreams, involuntary muscle movements, headache.

CAUTIONS
- Inform your doctor if you are currently taking meperidine.
- Increased risk of nonselective MAO inhibition occurs with doses greater than 10 mg.
- Addition to levodopa may result in an exacerbation of levodopa adverse effects; a decrease in levodopa dose may be necessary.

DRUG INTERACTIONS
This drug is metabolized by a specific set of liver enzymes (cytochrome P450 enzymes). Several other drugs interfere with these liver enzymes, and thus may increase or decrease the clearance of selegiline from the body, potentially increasing the risk of side effects or decreasing effectiveness. When these drugs are given in combination with selegiline, dosage adjustments may be needed. As these are too numerous to list, you should always check with your doctor or pharmacist prior to starting a new medication, herbal, or nonprescription product.

FOOD INTERACTIONS
If using higher doses (greater than 10 mg) avoid beverages containing tyramine (wine, beer). Selegiline may cause sudden severe high blood pressure when taken with foods with high tyramine. Small amounts of caffeine may produce irregular heartbeat or high blood pressure and can interact with this medication for up to two weeks after stopping its use.

HERBAL INTERACTIONS
Valerian, St. John's wort, SAMe, kava kava

PREGNANCY AND BREAST-FEEDING CAUTIONS
FDA Pregnancy Risk Category C. Excretion in breast milk unknown. Consult your doctor.

SPECIAL INFORMATION
Notify your doctor if severe headache, and other atypical or unusual symptoms develop.

SERTRALINE
(SER-tra-leen)

NEWLY DISCOVERED USES (OFF-LABEL)
Attention deficit hyperactivity (ADHD), alcoholism (cravings and dependence), Alzheimer's disease, bulimia, childhood anxiety, chronic fatigue syndrome, migraine prevention, nocturnal enuresis, premature ejaculation, seasonal affective disorder

ORIGINAL USES (ON-LABEL)
Treatment of major depression, obsessive compulsive disorder, panic disorder, post-traumatic stress disorder, premenstrual dysphoric disorder, social anxiety disorder

BRAND NAME
Zoloft

DRUG CLASS
Antidepressant (selective serotonin reuptake inhibitor)

DESCRIPTION
This drug inhibits the reuptake of serotonin at the neuron and thus increases the levels of serotonin in the body and in the brain. Serotonin is a chemical that affects mood levels.

POTENTIAL SIDE EFFECTS
Insomnia, solomnence, dizziness, headache, fatigue, dry mouth, diarrhea, nausea, ejaculatory disturbances, palpitations, agitation, anxiety, nervousness, rash, decreased libido, constipation, anorexia, upset stomach, flatulence, urinary disorders, tremors, numbness, visual difficulty, abnormal vision, increased sweating, ringing in the ears, changes in weight, low sodium levels, decrease in uric acid levels.

CAUTIONS
- Notify your doctor if you have a latex allergy as the dropper of the concentrated solution formulation contains dry natural rubber.
- Use may be associated with the development of suicidal ideation and behavior (see special information section).
- Do not use if you have been taking an MAO inhibitor (e.g., phenelzine, tranylcypromine, isocarboxazid) within the past 14 days. Wait 5 weeks after stopping sertraline before starting a

nonselective MAO inhibitor and 2 weeks before starting sertraline after stopping a MAO inhibitor. When used with MAO-Is fever, high blood pressure, increased heart rate, confusion, seizures, and deaths have been reported.

- Gradually decrease dosage upon discontinuation of therapy.
- Notify your doctor if you have a history of mania, seizures, alcoholism.
- Use caution with liver dysfunction, or kidney insufficiency, or in elderly patients.
- Concurrent use of aspirin or other non-steroidal anti-inflammatory drugs (NSAIDs) may increase the risk of bleeding.

DRUG INTERACTIONS
MAO inhibitors (such as phenelzine, isocarboxazid, or linezolid), selegiline, warfarin, cimetidine, linezolid, metoclopramide, sibutramine, tramadol, phenytoin, l-tryptophan, tricyclic antidepressants (such as amitriptyline, nortriptyline, imipramine, etc.), benzodiazepines (such as diazepam, flurazepam, temazepam, etc.), carbamazepine, clozapine, lithium, NSAIDs, pimozide, tolbutamide, glimepiride, sumatriptan, zolpidem.

This drug is metabolized by and affects a specific set of liver enzymes (cytochrome P450 enzymes). Several other drugs interfere with these liver enzymes, and thus may increase or decrease the clearance of sertraline from the body, potentially increasing the risk of side effects or decreasing effectiveness. When these drugs are given in combination with sertraline, dosage adjustments may be needed in either or both drugs. As these are too numerous to list, you should always check with your doctor or pharmacist prior to starting a new medication, herbal, or nonprescription product.

FOOD INTERACTIONS
May be given with or without food. Avoid alcohol.

HERBAL INTERACTIONS
Valerian, St. John's wort, SAMe, kava kava

PREGNANCY AND BREAST-FEEDING CAUTIONS
FDA Pregnancy Risk Category C. Excreted in breast milk. Not recommended during breast-feeding.

SPECIAL INFORMATION
In 2005, the FDA announced new labeling for antidepressants regarding the need to closely monitor for worsening of depression and for the potential of increased suicidal thinking or suicidal be-

havior during therapy. Although this recommendation applies to all patients (adults, children, adolescents) treated with antidepressants for any indication, this is of particular importance in patients being treated for depression. Discuss the latest information regarding this safety issue with your doctor prior to initiating therapy.

Close observation may be especially important when antidepressant medications are started for the first time or when doses are changed. More information on this topic can be found at the following web site: http://www.fda.gov/cder/drug/antidepressants/default.htm

SIBUTRAMINE
(si-BYOO-tra-meen)

NEWLY DISCOVERED USES (OFF-LABEL)
Binge eating disorder

ORIGINAL USES (ON-LABEL)
Management of obesity

BRAND NAME
Meridia

DRUG CLASS
Anorexiant

DESCRIPTION
This drug blocks the uptake of several neurotransmitters in the neurons, including norepinephrine and serotonin.

POTENTIAL SIDE EFFECTS
Headache, back pain, flu syndrome, abdominal pain, increased heart rate, migraine, anorexia, constipation, increased appetite, nausea, stomach upset, joint aches, dry mouth, insomnia, nervousness, anxiety, depression, runny nose, sore throat, sinusitis, increased cough, rash, painful menstruation.

CAUTIONS
- Use is not recommended during or within two weeks of MAO inhibitors. Should not be used concurrently with other centrally acting appetite suppressants or drugs which increase serotonin levels (such as some antidepressants, etc.).

- Inform your doctor if you have current or a history of drug abuse or dependence, anorexia nervosa, bulimia nervosa, uncontrolled or poorly controlled high blood pressure, congestive heart failure, irregular heart beats, and stroke.
- Inform your doctor if you have impaired kidney or liver function, bleeding tendencies or taking drugs which affect bleeding, seizure disorders, or narrow-angle glaucoma.
- Initial and regular monitoring of blood pressure and pulse are needed to detect substantial increases in blood pressure.
- Serious, potentially fatal toxicities may occur when thyroid hormones (at dosages above usual daily hormonal requirements) are used in combination with sympathomimetic amines to induce weight loss.

DRUG INTERACTIONS

Serotonergic drugs, drugs that raise blood pressure, tricyclic antidepressants, ketoconazole. This drug is metabolized by a specific set of liver enzymes (cytochrome P450 enzymes 3A4). Several other drugs interfere with these liver enzymes, and thus may increase or decrease the clearance of sibutramine from the body, potentially increasing the risk of side effects or decreasing effectiveness. When these drugs are given in combination with sibutramine, dosage adjustments may be needed. As these are too numerous to list, you should always check with your doctor or pharmacist prior to starting a new medication, herbal, or nonprescription product.

FOOD INTERACTIONS

May be given without regard to meals.

HERBAL INTERACTIONS

St. Johns wort, tryptophan

PREGNANCY AND BREAST-FEEDING CAUTIONS

FDA Pregnancy Risk Category C. Excretion in breast milk unknown. Notify your doctor if you are breast-feeding.

SPECIAL INFORMATION

Notify your doctor if you develop a rash, hives, or other allergic reactions.

Recommended only for obese patients in the presence of other risk factors such as high blood pressure, diabetes, and/or lipid disorders.

SILDENAFIL
(sil-DEN-a-fil)

NEWLY DISCOVERED USES (OFF-LABEL)

Anal fissure, dyspareunia, esophageal motility disorders, female orgasmic disorder secondary to SSRI use, pulmonary hypertension

ORIGINAL USES (ON-LABEL)
Erectile dysfunction

BRAND NAME
Viagra

DRUG CLASS
Impotence drugs (5-phosphodiesterase inhibitors)

DESCRIPTION
This drug causes smooth muscle relaxation and flow of blood to the corpus cavernosum (erectile tissue of the penis).

POTENTIAL SIDE EFFECTS
Headache, stomach upset, diarrhea, nasal congestion, abnormal vision, flushing, dizziness, rash, urinary tract infection.

CAUTIONS
- Seek medical attention if prolonged erection (greater than four hours) occurs.
- There is a potential risk of a cardiac event associated with sexual activity in some patients. This drug is not for use in such patients. Discuss these risks with your doctor prior to initiation of therapy.
- May require lower doses in reduced kidney or liver function.
- Inform your doctor if you have an anatomical deformation of the penis or conditions that may put you at an increased risk for priapism (prolonged, painful erections greater than six hours), including but not limited to sickle cell anemia, multiple myeloma, and leukemia.
- Do not use nitrates in any form. See the following website for a list of such drugs (http://www.fda.gov/medwatch/safety/1998/viagra.htm). Check with your pharmacist or doctor before starting a new medication, herbal product or nonprescription drug while taking this drug.

- Use with other erectile dysfunction treatments is not recommended.

DRUG INTERACTIONS
Nitrates (see cautions), alpha-blockers (such as doxazosin, terazosin, etc.), heparin, phenytoin, carbamazepine, phenobarbital, rifampin, antihypertensives, amlodipine, beta-blockers (such as propranolol, etc.), cimetidine, diuretics, ketoconazole, itraconazole, erythromycin, protease inhibitors, tacrolimus.

This drug is metabolized by a specific set of liver enzymes (cytochrome P450 enzymes 3A4). Several other drugs interfere with these liver enzymes, and thus may increase or decrease the clearance of sildenafil from the body, potentially increasing the risk of side effects or decreasing effectiveness. When these drugs are given in combination with sildenafil, dosage adjustments may be needed. As these are too numerous to list, you should always check with your doctor or pharmacist prior to starting a new medication, herbal, or nonprescription product.

FOOD INTERACTIONS
Grapefruit juice, high fat meal. Avoid substantial alcohol intake.

HERBAL INTERACTIONS
St. John's wort

PREGNANCY AND BREAST-FEEDING CAUTIONS
FDA Pregnancy Risk Category B. Not for use in women, and not recommended during breast-feeding.

SPECIAL INFORMATION
This medication is to be taken by mouth one hour prior to sexual activity. May be used anytime from four hours to 30 minutes before. Do not take sildenafil within four hours of taking an alpha-blocker (may result in significant low blood pressure). This drug does not protect against sexually transmitted diseases. Do not take more than once daily.

In 2005, the FDA reported a safety alert that described changes in the product labeling for all drugs in this class. Specifically, the changes were based on a small number of post-marketing reports of sudden vision loss, attributed to NAION (non arteritis ischemic optic neuropathy), a condition where blood flow is blocked to the optic nerve. FDA advises patients to stop taking these medicines, and call a doctor or healthcare provider right away if they experience sudden or decreased vision loss in one or both eyes.

SIMVASTATIN
(SIM-va-stat-in)

NEWLY DISCOVERED USES (OFF-LABEL)
Membranous nephropathy, multiple sclerosis, peripheral artery disease, postmenopausal osteoporosis

ORIGINAL USES (ON-LABEL)
Cardiovascular disease, coronary heart disease prophylaxis, familial combined hyperlipidemia, familial dysbetalipoproteinemia, heterozygous familial hypercholesterolemia, homozygous familial hypercholesterolemia, hyperlipidemia, mixed dyslipidemia, primary hypercholesterolemia, stroke prophylaxis

BRAND NAME
Zocor

DRUG CLASS
Anti-lipid drug (HMG-CoA reductase inhibitor)

DESCRIPTION
This drug inhibits an enzyme (HMG-CoA reductase) that is an important factor in the production of cholesterol.

POTENTIAL SIDE EFFECTS
Headache, diarrhea, upset stomach, flatulence, rash, muscle aches.

CAUTIONS
- Not for use in active liver disease or in patients with high levels of liver function tests.
- You should not consume large amounts of alcohol or have a history of liver disease.
- Liver function should be monitored before initiation and periodically during therapy.
- May require reduced doses in impaired kidney function.
- Can also cause severe muscle aches which are a symptom of a more serious disorder (rhabdomyolysis) in which the muscle fibers break down. If this disorder progresses, decreases in kid-

ney function may also occur. This risk is increased with concurrent use of drugs that increase simvastatin levels.

DRUG INTERACTIONS
Azole antifungals, ciprofloxacin, clarithromycin, diclofenac, doxycycline, erythromycin, imatinib, isoniazid, nefazodone, nicardipine, propofol, protease inhibitors, quinidine, verapamil, cyclosporine, clofibrate, fenofibrate, gemfibrozil, levothyroxine, digoxin, ethinyl estradiol, cholestyramine, and niacin.

This drug is metabolized by a specific set of liver enzymes (cytochrome P450 enzymes, 3A4). Several other drugs interfere with these liver enzymes, and thus may increase or decrease the clearance of simvastatin from the body, potentially increasing the risk of side effects or decreasing effectiveness. When these drugs are given in combination with simvastatin, dosage adjustments may be needed. As these are too numerous to list, you should always check with your doctor or pharmacist prior to starting a new medication, herbal, or nonprescription product.

FOOD INTERACTIONS
Grapefruit juice. Avoid excessive intake of alcohol.

HERBAL INTERACTIONS
St. John's wort

PREGNANCY AND BREAST-FEEDING CAUTIONS
FDA Pregnancy Risk Category X. Simvastatin should not be used during breast-feeding.

SPECIAL INFORMATION
Before initiation of therapy, patients should be placed on a standard cholesterol-lowering diet for six weeks and the diet should be continued during drug therapy. Report any signs of muscle pain, tenderness, or weakness to your doctor.

SIROLIMUS
(sear-OH-le-mus)

NEWLY DISCOVERED USES (OFF-LABEL)
Psoriasis

ORIGINAL USES (ON-LABEL)
To prevent rejection of organ transplant

BRAND NAME
Rapamune

DRUG CLASS
Immunosuppressant

DESCRIPTION
This drug suppresses the immune system and inhibits antibody production to prevent organ rejection after transplant.

POTENTIAL SIDE EFFECTS
Headache, insomnia, tremor, acne, rash, constipation, abdominal pain, diarrhea, stomach upset, nausea, vomiting, anemia, edema, increased cholesterol levels, changes in potassium levels, weight gain, shortness of breath, back or chest pain, fever, pain, muscle or joint aches, increased blood pressure.

CAUTIONS
- Certain lung diseases and infections have developed in patients receiving immunosuppressants including sirolimus.
- Increased risk of infection.
- May cause increased lipid or cholesterol levels, requiring treatment of these effects.
- May impair kidney function or fertility.
- Requires monitoring of sirolimus concentrations in the blood and various other laboratory tests during therapy to gauge effectiveness or development of organ rejection.

DRUG INTERACTIONS
This drug is metabolized by a specific set of liver enzymes (cytochrome P450 enzymes 3A4). Several other drugs interfere with these liver enzymes, and thus may increase or decrease the clearance of sirolimus from the body, potentially increasing the risk of side effects or decreasing effectiveness. When these drugs are given in combination with sirolimus, dosage adjustments may be needed. As these are too numerous to list, you should always check with your doctor or pharmacist prior to starting a new medication, herbal, or nonprescription product.

FOOD INTERACTIONS
High-fat meal, grapefruit juice

HERBAL INTERACTIONS
St. John's wort

PREGNANCY AND BREAST-FEEDING CAUTIONS
FDA Pregnancy Risk Category C. Excreted in breast milk. Breast-feeding is not recommended.

SPECIAL INFORMATION
This drug has a black box warning regarding the increased risk of infection as a result of suppressing the immune system. In addition, the warnings also address a potential increase in mortality in some liver transplant patients who also received tacrolimus. Severe adverse events have also occurred in certain lung transplant patients. The use of this drug is not recommended in liver or lung transplant patients.

SODIUM BICARBONATE
(SOW-dee-um bye-KAR-bun-ate)

Intravenous

NEWLY DISCOVERED USES (OFF-LABEL)
Cardiac arrest, nephrotoxicity due to coronary procedures and CT scan

ORIGINAL USES (ON-LABEL)
Management of metabolic acidosis, makes urine less acidic (alkalinization), treatment of increased potassium, management of overdose of certain drugs (such as tricyclic antidepressants and aspirin)

BRAND NAMES
Sodium Bicarbonate (IV)

DRUG CLASS
Electrolyte supplement, parenteral; sodium salt

DESCRIPTION
Once administered in the body, sodium bicarbonate breaks down to provide bicarbonate ion, which neutralizes hydrogen ion concentration and raises blood and urinary pH (makes it less acidic).

POTENTIAL SIDE EFFECTS
Increased sodium levels, decreased calcium or potassium levels, aggravation of congestive heart failure (due to sodium administration), fluid overload, edema, local site infusion problems.

CAUTIONS

- Not for use in individuals with increased sodium levels, decreased calcium levels, and unknown abdominal pain.
- Avoid too rapid administration, particularly in infants and children less than two years of age.
- Avoid extravasation (leakage outside of vein into the tissues surrounding the intravenous site), tissue necrosis.
- May cause sodium retention especially if kidney function is impaired.
- Notify your doctor if you have congestive heart failure, edema, liver or kidney failure.

DRUG INTERACTIONS

Lithium, chlorpropamide, salicylates, methotrexate, tetracyclines, flecainide, quinidine, mecamylamine

FOOD INTERACTIONS

Unknown

HERBAL INTERACTIONS

Unknown

PREGNANCY AND BREAST-FEEDING CAUTIONS

FDA Pregnancy Risk Category C. Consult your doctor. Excretion in breast milk not known.

SPIRONOLACTONE
(speer-on-oh-LAK-tone)

NEWLY DISCOVERED USES (OFF-LABEL)

Acne, congestive heart failure, familial male precocious puberty, hair loss in women, hirsutism, premenstrual dysphoric syndrome (PMDD), premenstrual syndrome (PMS), polycystic ovary syndrome

---

ORIGINAL USES (ON-LABEL)

Management of high blood pressure or edema associated with excessive aldosterone. Primary increased aldosterone levels, cirrhosis of the liver accompanied by edema or ascites, low potassium levels

BRAND NAME

Aldactone

DRUG CLASS
Antihypertensive; (diuretic, potassium-sparing)

DESCRIPTION
This drug increases sodium chloride and water excretion while conserving potassium.

POTENTIAL SIDE EFFECTS
Edema, drowsiness, lethargy, rash, hives, increased hair growth, breast swelling (men), breast pain (men), increased potassium levels, decreased sodium levels, anorexia, nausea, cramping, diarrhea, liver toxicity.

CAUTIONS
- Notify your doctor if you have increased potassium levels, are pregnant, have kidney or liver impairment, taking other potassium-sparing diuretics (such as triamterene, amiloride).
- Avoid potassium supplements, potassium containing salt substitutes, a diet rich in potassium, or other drugs that can cause increased potassium levels.
- Breast swelling is often related to dose and duration of therapy.

DRUG INTERACTIONS
Other potassium-sparing diuretics, potassium supplements, ACE inhibitors, angiotension receptor antagonists (ACE inhibitors), cotrimoxazole (high dose), salicylates, cholestyramine, digoxin, mitotane

FOOD INTERACTIONS
Food increases absorption.

HERBAL INTERACTIONS
Avoid excessive ingestion of natural licorice.

PREGNANCY AND BREAST-FEEDING CAUTIONS
FDA Pregnancy Risk Category C/D. Enters breast milk. Consult your doctor.

SPECIAL INFORMATION
This drug has a black box warning regarding the development of tumors when administered for chronic periods in rats. Avoid unnecessary use of the product.

STREPTOKINASE
(strep-toe-KYE-nase)

NEWLY DISCOVERED USES (OFF-LABEL)
Pleural effusion

ORIGINAL USES (ON-LABEL)
Treatment of recent severe or massive deep vein thrombosis (blood clots), pulmonary emboli (blood clots), myocardial infarction, and occluded arteriovenous cannulas

BRAND NAME
Streptase

DRUG CLASS
Thrombolytic

DESCRIPTION
This drug breaks up fibrin in blood clots, thereby dissolving the clot.

POTENTIAL SIDE EFFECTS
Bleeding (minor and major), allergic type reactions, severe drop in blood pressure.

CAUTIONS
- Not for use if you have an increased risk for bleeding (such as recent surgery, stroke, aneurysm, brain tumor, active internal bleeding, severe uncontrolled high blood pressure, etc.). Discuss these risks with your doctor.
- Requires blood testing for bleeding tendencies before administration (such as international normalized ratio, prothrombin time, etc.).
- Your doctor should watch all bleeding sites and sites of injection.
- May cause allergic reaction.
- Rare cases of pancreatitis have occurred with the use of this drug.
- Resistance to the effects of this drug have been known to occur in situations where prior administration has occurred within a year or in patients with streptococcal infections.

DRUG INTERACTIONS
Warfarin, heparins, aspirin, dipyridamole, abciximab, vitamin K antagonist, drugs that affect clotting and bleeding

FOOD INTERACTIONS
Unknown

HERBAL INTERACTIONS
Garlic, green tea, cat's claw, dong quai, evening primrose, feverfew, red clover, horse chestnut, ginseng, ginkgo

PREGNANCY AND BREAST-FEEDING CAUTIONS
FDA Pregnancy Risk Category C. Excretion in breast milk unknown. Not recommended during breast-feeding.

STREPTOMYCIN
(strep-toe-MY-sin)

NEWLY DISCOVERED USES (OFF-LABEL)
Ménière's disease

ORIGINAL USES (ON-LABEL)
Treatment of tuberculosis and various bacterial infections

BRAND NAME
Streptomycin Sulfate

DRUG CLASS
Antibiotic (aminoglycoside)

DESCRIPTION
This drug inhibits the production of protein in susceptible bacteria.

POTENTIAL SIDE EFFECTS
Nerve toxicity (dose-related), nausea, vomiting , vertigo, numbness of the face, fever, hives, blood disorders.

CAUTION
- Inform your doctor if you have had allergic reactions to other aminoglycosides (such as gentamicin, tobramycin, neomycin, etc.).
- Requires monitoring of kidney function during therapy. Kidney damage is usually reversible.
- Toxicity of the ears is proportional to dosage and duration of treatment. Tinnitus (ringing in the ears) or vertigo (dizziness) may become irreversible.

DRUG INTERACTIONS
Neuromuscular blocking drugs, other aminoglycosides, other kidney-toxic drugs (such as amphotericin, etc.) or ear-toxic drugs (such as furosemide, ethacrynic acid)

FOOD INTERACTIONS
Unknown

HERBAL INTERACTIONS
Unknown

PREGNANCY AND BREAST-FEEDING CAUTIONS
FDA Pregnancy Risk Category D. Excreted in breast milk. Consult with your doctor.

SPECIAL INFORMATION
This drug has a black box warning regarding ear, neuro- and kidney toxicities.

SUCRALFATE
(soo-KRAL-fate)

NEWLY DISCOVERED USES (OFF-LABEL)
Esophagitis, gastric ulcer, NSAID-induced ulcer, prevention of cancer treatment-induced mucositis/stomatitis, prevention of gastric ulcer, stress related mucosal disease, vaginal ulceration

ORIGINAL USES (ON-LABEL)
Short-term management of duodenal ulcers, maintenance of duodenal ulcers

BRAND NAME
Carafate

DRUG CLASS
Gastrointestinal

DESCRIPTION
This drug affects proteins to form a paste-like, adhesive substance which acts as a coating that protects the stomach lining against pepsin, peptic acid and bile salts.

POTENTIAL SIDE EFFECTS
Constipation, nausea, indigestion, dizziness, headache, rash.

CAUTIONS
- Notify your doctor if you have impaired kidney function or are on dialysis.
- May alter the absorption of some drugs.

DRUG INTERACTIONS
Digoxin, phenytoin, warfarin, ketoconazole, quinidine, tetracycline, theophylline, cimetidine, fluoroquinolone antibiotics (such as ciprofloxacin, levofloxacin, etc.), l-thyroxine, ranitidine. Administer drugs two hours before giving sucralfate.

FOOD INTERACTIONS
Decreased absorption of vitamin A, vitamin D, vitamin E and vitamin K.

HERBAL INTERACTIONS
Unknown

PREGNANCY AND BREAST-FEEDING CAUTIONS
FDA Pregnancy Risk Category B. Excreted in breast milk. Consult your doctor.

SULFASALAZINE
(sul-fa-SAL-a-zeen)

NEWLY DISCOVERED USES (OFF-LABEL)
Ankylosing spondylitis, psoriatic arthritis

ORIGINAL USES (ON-LABEL)
Management of ulcerative colitis, rheumatoid arthritis

BRAND NAMES
Azulfidine, Azulfidine EN-tabs

DRUG CLASS
Anti-inflammatory (5-aminosalicylic acid derivative)

DESCRIPTION
This drug decreases inflammation in the colon. It does this by inhibiting the production of prostaglandins, a known mediator of inflammation and pain.

POTENTIAL SIDE EFFECTS
Anorexia, headache, nausea, vomiting, gastric distress, skin rash, itching, hives, fever, various anemias.

CAUTIONS

- Notify your doctor if you have intestinal or urinary obstruction, impaired kidney or liver function, blood disorders, asthma, G6PD deficiency, porphyria, or allergies to sulfonamides.
- Contact your doctor immediately if you develop sore throat, fever, pallor, rash, or jaundice, as these may be indications of serious blood disorders.
- Periodic blood testing and urine analysis are required during therapy.
- Reversible oligospermia (reduced number of sperm in semen) and male infertility have been associated with the use of this drug. Typically, these effects reverse when the drug is discontinued.
- Requires adequate fluid intake to avoid the formation of crystals/stones in the urine.
- May produce an orange-yellow discoloration of skin/urine.

DRUG INTERACTIONS

Phenytoin, oral antidiabetic drugs, warfarin

FOOD INTERACTIONS

May impair folate absorption. Take after meals.

HERBAL INTERACTIONS

Dong quai, St. John's wort (due to increased photosensitivity)

PREGNANCY AND BREAST-FEEDING CAUTIONS

FDA Pregnancy Risk Category B. Excreted in breast milk. Consult your doctor.

SPECIAL INFORMATION

May permanently discolor soft contact lenses.

SULFASOXAZOLE
(sul-fi-SOKS-a-zole)

NEWLY DISCOVERED USES (OFF-LABEL)
Prevention of recurrent otitis media

ORIGINAL USES (ON-LABEL)
Treatment of urinary tract infections, otitis media, chlamydia

BRAND NAME
Gantrisin

DRUG CLASS
Antibiotic (sulfonamide derivative)

DESCRIPTION
This drug interferes with bacterial growth by inhibiting the production of bacterial folic acid, which is necessary for cell wall construction.

POTENTIAL SIDE EFFECTS
Photosensitivity (skin reaction related to sun exposure), abdominal pain, anorexia, thyroid function disturbances, bloody urine, crystals in the urine, fever, headache, dizziness, diarrhea, constipation, anemia, blood disorders, dyslipidemia, insomnia, tremor, rash.

CAUTIONS
- Notify your doctor if you have allergies to sulfonamide-type drugs.
- Not for use in infants less than two months of age, pregnant women at term, or women nursing infants less than two months of age.
- This drug may cause severe skin reactions, that although rare, may cause death. Discontinue this drug at the first sign of rash and notify your doctor immediately.
- Rash, sore throat, fever, joint pain, pallor, jaundice may be an early sign of serious reactions.
- Report any cough; shortness of breath may be indicative of a hypersensitivity reaction to the respiratory tract.
- Not for use in the treatment of group A beta-hemolytic streptococcal infections.
- Report chronic, persistent diarrhea that develops during or shortly after the completion of therapy.
- Notify your doctor if you have impaired kidney or liver function.
- May require periodic blood testing.

DRUG INTERACTIONS
Warfarin, thiopental, methotrexate, sulfonylureas

FOOD INTERACTIONS
Interferes with folate absorption.

HERBAL INTERACTIONS
Dong quai, St. John's wort (due to increased photosensitivity)

PREGNANCY AND BREAST-FEEDING CAUTIONS
FDA Pregnancy Risk Category C. Excreted in breast milk. Not recommended during breast-feeding.

SULINDAC
(sul-IN-dak)

NEWLY DISCOVERED USES (OFF-LABEL)
Amnioreduction, premature labor

ORIGINAL USES (ON-LABEL)
Management of inflammatory disease, rheumatoid disorders, acute gouty arthritis, bursitis

BRAND NAME
Clinoril

DRUG CLASS
Pain reliever, anti-inflammatory drug (nonsteroidal anti-inflammatory drug [NSAID])

DESCRIPTION
Inhibits the production of prostaglandin, a chemical drug in the body responsible for inflammation and pain.

POTENTIAL SIDE EFFECTS
Abdominal cramps, nausea, stomach upset, diarrhea, flatulence, weakness, stomach irritation, blurred vision, ringing in the ears, constipation.

CAUTIONS
- Not for use if allergic to aspirin or other NSAIDs.
- Not for use in active gastric/duodenal ulcer disease.
- Do not use during third trimester of pregnancy.
- Ask physician about use if you have the following medical problems: high blood pressure, dehydration, decreased kidney or liver function, history of gastric disease.
- Elderly are at higher risk of developing side effects.

DRUG INTERACTIONS
Aspirin, lithium, methotrexate, digoxin, cyclosporine (kidney toxicity), diuretics, some anti-hypertensives, and warfarin (bleeding)

FOOD INTERACTIONS
Avoid alcohol (increased gastric mucosal irritation)

HERBAL INTERACTIONS
Cat's claw, horse chestnut, dong quai, evening primrose, feverfew, garlic, ginger, ginseng, green tea, red clover (due to additive antiplatelet actions)

PREGNANCY AND BREAST-FEEDING CAUTIONS
FDA Pregnancy Risk Category B. FDA Pregnancy Risk Category D in third trimester. Not known if excreted in breast milk. Do not breast-feed during therapy with this drug.

SPECIAL INFORMATION
Stop taking this drug (with doctor's approval) approximately 24 to 48 hours prior to surgical or dental procedures as it affects the body's ability to form blood clots and may increase bleeding time. In April 2005, the FDA announced the potential addition of a black box warning to the labeling of this class of drugs (NSAIDs), specifically regarding potential serious cardiac events and potentially life-threatening gastric adverse events.

SUMATRIPTAN
(soo-ma-TRIP-tan)

NEWLY DISCOVERED USES (OFF-LABEL)
Lumbar puncture induced headache, migraine treatment in children

ORIGINAL USES (ON-LABEL)
Acute treatment of migraine with or without aura, acute treatment of cluster headaches (injectable)

BRAND NAME
Imitrex

DRUG CLASS
Antimigraine (serotonin 5-HT$_4$ receptor agonist)

DESCRIPTION
Stimulates serotonin receptors in the cranial arteries which causes constriction of blood vessels and a relief of migraine symptoms.

POTENTIAL SIDE EFFECTS

Injection: Blood pressure increases, chest pain, sensation of unusual heart beats, dizziness, drowsiness, fatigue, skin flushing, mild increases in growth hormone, hot flashes, nausea, abdominal pain, dry mouth, shortness of breath.

Nasal Spray: bad taste, nausea, vomiting, dizziness, nasal discomfort.

Tablets: chest pain/tightness/heaviness/pressure, neck, throat and jaw pain/tightness/pressure, numbness.

CAUTIONS

- Only for patients with clear diagnosis of migraine. Not for preventive treatment of migraine headaches.
- Notify your doctor of cardiac problems, particularly chest pain, irregular heart rhythm, uncontrolled blood pressure. Also notify your doctor if you have basilar or hemiplegic migraine.
- First dose may be given in healthcare setting.
- May make you drowsy and affect your judgment. Be careful when driving a car or operating machinery.
- Patients should be monitored for blood pressure changes.
- Alcohol may have added central nervous system toxicity.
- Cerebral bleeding, stroke or other brain vascular events have been reported with this drug class.
- Cardiac events and stroke have been reported with 5-HT1 agonist use.
- Do not use during or within 2 weeks of MAO inhibitors, or within 24 hours of treatment with another 5-HT1 agonist, or ergot-containing or ergot-like medication.
- Use with caution in patients that are elderly, with liver or kidney impairment.
- Do not use in patients with signs and symptoms of reduced arterial flow (ischemic bowel, Raynaud's disease) which could be exacerbated by vasospasm.
- Reconsider diagnosis of migraine if no response to initial dose.

DRUG INTERACTIONS

5-HT1 agonists, ergot-containing drugs (dihydroergotamine, methysergide), propranolol, selective serotonin reuptake inhibitors (fluoxetine, fluvoxamine, paroxetine, sertraline), MAO inhibitors, nonselective MAO inhibitors, sibutramine

FOOD INTERACTIONS

Take without regard to meals.

HERBAL INTERACTIONS
Unknown

PREGNANCY AND BREAST-FEEDING CAUTIONS
FDA Pregnancy Risk Category C. Excreted in breast milk. Consult your doctor.

SPECIAL INFORMATION
Injectable product requires education. May use second dose of nasal spray within two hours after first dose. However, do not use second nasal spray without consulting doctor. Do not use more than 40 mg of nasal spray in any 24-hour period. Redosing should be separated by at least two hours. No more than 200 (oral) mg used in any 24-hour period. Patients taking propranolol should take a reduced dose.

TACROLIMUS
(ta-KROE-li-mus)

NEWLY DISCOVERED USES (OFF-LABEL)
> Alopecia areata, blepharitis, dermatomyositis/polymyositis, keratoconjunctivitis sicca in graft vs. host disease, oral lichen planus, uveitis, varicella, vitiligo

ORIGINAL USES (ON-LABEL)
Oral/injection: Prevention of rejection of liver or kidney transplantation

Topical: Moderate to severe atopic dermatitis

BRAND NAMES
Prograf, Protopic

DRUG CLASS
Immunosuppressant

DESCRIPTION
This drug inhibits the activation and promotion of T-lymphocytes, which can destroy target cells, and thus suppresses cellular immunity.

POTENTIAL SIDE EFFECTS
Oral, injection: Headache, tremor, insomnia, numbness, diarrhea, nausea, constipation, liver function tests, anorexia, vomiting, high

blood pressure, kidney function, changes in potassium levels, increases in glucose, low magnesium levels, blood disorders (such as anemia, etc.), abdominal pain, pain, fever, ascites, peripheral edema, shortness of breath, itching, rash.

Topical: Headache, fever, skin burning, itching, redness, increased cough, flu-like symptoms, allergic reaction.

CAUTIONS
- Notify your doctor if you have an allergy to castor oil.
- Has caused post-transplant diabetes and may require monitoring. Also has been associated with nerve or kidney toxicity, particularly with high doses.
- Requires dose adjustment in kidney or liver impairment.
- Requires periodic monitoring during therapy with laboratory testing.
- May increase risk of infection.

DRUG INTERACTIONS
Including but not limited to: potassium-sparing diuretics (such as spironolactone, etc.), drugs which may cause kidney toxicity (such as amikacin, gentamicin, tobramycin, etc.), metoclopramide, antacids, calcium channel blockers (such as diltiazem, nicardipine, nifedipine, etc.), antifungal drugs (such as fluconazole, itraconazole, etc.), macrolides (such as clarithromycin, erythromycin, etc.).

This drug is metabolized by a specific set of liver enzymes. Several other drugs interfere with these liver enzymes, and thus may increase or decrease the clearance of tacrolimus from the body, potentially increasing the risk of side effects or decreasing effectiveness. When these drugs are given in combination with tacrolimus, dosage adjustments may be needed. As these are too numerous to list, you should always check with your doctor or pharmacist prior to starting a new medication, herbal, or nonprescription product.

FOOD INTERACTIONS
Avoid high fat meals and grapefruit juice.

HERBAL INTERACTIONS
St. John's wort

PREGNANCY AND BREAST-FEEDING CAUTIONS
FDA Pregnancy Risk Category C. Excreted in breast milk. Do not use during breast-feeding.

SPECIAL INFORMATION
This drug has a black box warning regarding the risk of developing lymphoma when used as an immunosuppressant.

TADALAFIL
(tah-DA-la-fil)

NEWLY DISCOVERED USES (OFF-LABEL)
| Pulmonary hypertension

ORIGINAL USES (ON-LABEL)
Erectile dysfunction

BRAND NAME
Cialis

DRUG CLASS
Impotence drugs (5-phosphodiesterase inhibitors)

DESCRIPTION
This drug causes smooth muscle relaxation and flow of blood to the corpus cavernosum (erectile tissue of the penis).

POTENTIAL SIDE EFFECTS
Headache, stomach upset, diarrhea, nasal congestion, abnormal vision, flushing, dizziness, rash, urinary tract infection.

CAUTIONS
- Seek medical attention if prolonged erection (greater than four hours) occurs.
- There is a potential risk of a cardiac event associated with sexual activity in some patients. This drug is not for use in such patients. Discuss these risks with your doctor prior to initiation of therapy.
- May require lower doses in reduced kidney or liver function.
- Inform your doctor if you have an anatomical deformation of the penis or conditions that may put you at an increased risk for priapism (prolonged, painful erections greater than six hours), including but not limited to sickle cell anemia, multiple myeloma, and leukemia.
- Do not use nitrates in any form. See the following website for a list of such drugs (http://www.fda.gov/medwatch/safety/1998/viagra.htm). Check with your pharmacist or doctor before

starting a new medication, herbal product or nonprescription drug while taking this drug.

- Use with other erectile dysfunction treatments is not recommended.

DRUG INTERACTIONS

Nitrates (see cautions), alpha-blockers (such as doxazosin, terazosin, etc.), antacids, bendroflumethiazide, enalapril, metoprolol, heparin, phenytoin, carbamazepine, phenobarbital, rifampin, antihypertensives, amlodipine, beta-blockers (such as propranolol, etc.), simetidine, diuretics, ketoconazole, itraconazole, erythromycin, protease inhibitors.

This drug is metabolized by specific set of liver enzymes (cytochrome P450 enzymes 3A4). Several other drugs interfere with these liver enzymes, and thus may increase or decrease the clearance of tadalafil from the body, potentially increasing the risk of side effects or decreasing effectiveness. When these drugs are given in combination with tadalafil, dosage adjustments may be needed. As these are too numerous to list, you should always check with your doctor or pharmacist prior to starting a new medication, herbal, or nonprescription product.

FOOD INTERACTIONS

Grapefruit juice. Avoid substantial alcohol intake. May be taken with or without food.

HERBAL INTERACTIONS

St. John's wort

PREGNANCY AND BREAST-FEEDING CAUTIONS

FDA Pregnancy Risk Category B. Not for use in women; not recommended during breast-feeding.

SPECIAL INFORMATION

This medication is to be taken by mouth one hour prior to sexual activity. Do not take with an alpha-blocker (may result in significant low blood pressure). This drug does not protect against sexually transmitted diseases. Do not take more than once daily.

In 2005, the FDA reported a safety alert that described changes in the product labeling for all drugs in this class. Specifically, the changes were based on a small number of post-marketing reports of sudden vision loss, attributed to NAION (non arteritis ischemic optic neuropathy), a condition where blood flow is blocked to the optic nerve. FDA advises patients to stop taking these medicines, and call a doctor or healthcare provider right away if they experience sudden or decreased vision loss in one or both eyes.

TAMOXIFEN
(ta-MOKS-I-fen)

NEWLY DISCOVERED USES (OFF-LABEL)
Gynecomastia, infertility, female infertility, mastalgia, McCune-Albright syndrome

ORIGINAL USES (ON-LABEL)
Treatment of advanced or metastatic breast cancer, reduce the incidence of breast cancer in women at high risk, reduce risk of invasive breast cancer in women with ductal carcinoma, metastatic female and male breast cancer, treatment of melanoma, desmoid tumors

BRAND NAME
Nolvadex

DRUG CLASS
Antineoplastic

DESCRIPTION
This drug binds to estrogen receptors on tumors, decreasing production of DNA and inhibiting estrogen effects.

POTENTIAL SIDE EFFECTS
Increased bone and tumor pain, hot flashes, loss of menstruation, altered menstruation, nausea, cough, edema, fatigue, muscle pain, ovarian cysts, fluid retention, vaginal discharge, weight loss, skin changes, liver toxicity.

CAUTIONS
- Notify your doctor if you are pregnant or plan to get pregnant, have a history of blood clots, or are currently taking warfarin.
- May cause increased calcium levels, uterine or endometrial cancer, blood clots.
- Report any abnormal vaginal bleeding to your doctor, even after you have stopped the drug.
- Decreased visual acuity, retinopathy, corneal changes, and cataracts have been reported.
- Requires blood monitoring during therapy.

DRUG INTERACTIONS
Allopurinol, cyclosporine, warfarin, diltiazem, letrozole, rifampin, aminoglutethimide, bromocriptine, medroxyprogesterone.

This drug is metabolized by a specific set of liver enzymes (cytochrome P450 enzymes). Several other drugs interfere with these liver enzymes, and thus may increase or decrease the clearance of tamoxifen from the body, potentially increasing the risk of side effects or decreasing effectiveness. When these drugs are given in combination with tamoxifen, dosage adjustments may be needed. As these are too numerous to list, you should always check with your doctor or pharmacist prior to starting a new medication, herbal, or nonprescription product.

FOOD INTERACTIONS
Unknown

HERBAL INTERACTIONS
Black cohosh, dong quai in estrogen-dependent tumors

PREGNANCY AND BREAST-FEEDING CAUTIONS
FDA Pregnancy Risk Category D. Excreted in breast milk. Do not breast-feed during therapy.

SPECIAL INFORMATION
This drug has a black box warning that warns of the possible development of uterine malignancies, stroke and pulmonary embolism when used to reduce risk of breast cancer. Pregnancy should be avoided for two months after treatment has been discontinued. For sexually active women of childbearing age, initiate treatment during menstruation.

TAMSULOSIN
(tam-SOO-loe-sin)

NEWLY DISCOVERED USES (OFF-LABEL)
Ureteral stones

ORIGINAL USES (ON-LABEL)
Treatment of signs and symptoms of benign prostatic hyperplasia (enlargement)

BRAND NAME
Flomax

DRUG CLASS
Prostate (alpha-adrenergic blocking)

DESCRIPTION
This drug increases smooth muscle tone in the prostate and the bladder neck, leading to improvement of urine flow and decreased symptoms associated with prostate enlargement.

POTENTIAL SIDE EFFECTS
Headache, dizziness, drowsiness, insomnia, decreased libido, runny nose, sore throat, increased cough, sinusitis, diarrhea, nausea, abnormal ejaculation, infection, back pain, chest pain, orthostatic hypotension (sudden drop in blood pressure).

CAUTIONS
- Not intended for use as a blood pressure medication.
- Marked orthostatic hypotension (sudden drop in blood pressure when standing from sitting or lying down position), syncope, and loss of consciousness may occur with first dose (especially in patients taking beta blockers, diuretics, low sodium diets or taking large first doses).
- Rarely, this drug class has been associated with priapism (painful erection).
- Avoid rapid increase in dose.
- Use with caution in patients with kidney or liver impairment.
- Does not affect levels of PSA (prostate specific antigen), a marker test used to diagnose prostate cancer.

DRUG INTERACTIONS
Cimetidine, digoxin, theophylline

FOOD INTERACTIONS
Take one half hour before the same meal each day.

HERBAL INTERACTIONS
Saw palmetto

PREGNANCY AND BREAST-FEEDING CAUTIONS
FDA Pregnancy Risk Category B. Not indicated for use in women. No data in breast milk.

TEGASEROD
(teg-a-SER-od)

NEWLY DISCOVERED USES (OFF-LABEL)
Gastroesophageal reflux disease (GERD)

ORIGINAL USES (ON-LABEL)
Short term treatment of irritable bowel in women whose primary bowel symptom is constipation

BRAND NAME
Zelnorm

DRUG CLASS
Gastrointestinal (serotonin 5-HT$_4$ receptor agonist)

DESCRIPTION
This drug promotes the release of neurotransmitters in the intestine to promote peristalsis (motility) and intestinal secretion.

POTENTIAL SIDE EFFECTS
Headache, dizziness, migraine, abdominal pain, diarrhea, nausea, flatulence, back pain, joint aches.

CAUTIONS
- Inform your doctor if you have diarrhea, liver impairment, a history of bowel obstruction, gallbladder disease, suspected sphincter of Oddi dysfunction, or abdominal adhesions.
- Treatment should not be started in patients with diarrhea or in those who experience diarrhea frequently.
- Notify your doctor immediately if you develop severe diarrhea, or diarrhea with severe cramping, abdominal pain, or dizziness.

DRUG INTERACTIONS
Digoxin

FOOD INTERACTIONS
Take 30 minutes before a meal.

HERBAL INTERACTIONS
Unknown

PREGNANCY AND BREAST-FEEDING CAUTIONS
FDA Pregnancy Risk Category B. Excretion in breast milk unknown, breast-feeding is not recommended during therapy.

The FDA and Novartis notified healthcare professionals of an important drug warning for serious consequences of diarrhea and a precaution for rare reports of ischemic colitis in post-marketing use of Zelnorm. http://www.fda.gov/medwatch/SAFETY/2004/safety04.htm

TELMISARTAN
(tell-miss-SAR-tan)

NEWLY DISCOVERED USES (OFF-LABEL)
Diabetic nephropathy

ORIGINAL USES (ON-LABEL)
For the treatment of high blood pressure

BRAND NAME
Micardis

DRUG CLASS
Blood pressure medication (angiotensin II receptor antagonist [ARB])

DESCRIPTION
This drug blocks the constriction of blood vessels and affects aldosterone secretion.

POTENTIAL SIDE EFFECTS
Dizziness, diarrhea, sore throat, rash, upper respiratory infection.

CAUTIONS
- Notify your doctor if you have biliary obstructive disorders or liver impairment.
- Not for use in pregnant patients who are in the second or third trimester.
- Avoid use in dehydrated patients.

DRUG INTERACTIONS
Digoxin, triamterene, potassium supplements

FOOD INTERACTIONS
Unknown

HERBAL INTERACTIONS
Ma huang, yohimbine, limit intake of natural licorice

PREGNANCY AND BREAST-FEEDING CAUTIONS

FDA Pregnancy Risk Category C in first trimester, Category D in second and third trimesters. Do not use during second and third trimesters of pregnancy. Excreted in breast milk. Breast-feeding is not recommended.

SPECIAL INFORMATION

This drug has a black box warning regarding the fetal toxicities associated with the use of this drug class during the second and third trimesters of pregnancy. If pregnancy is detected, the drug should be discontinued as soon as possible.

TERAZOSIN
(ter-AY–zoe-sin)

NEWLY DISCOVERED USES (OFF-LABEL)

Nonbacterial prostatitis

ORIGINAL USES (ON-LABEL)

Management of mild to moderate hypertension, benign prostate enlargement

BRAND NAME

Hytrin

DRUG CLASS

Antihypertensive, prostate (alpha-adrenergic blocking)

DESCRIPTION

This drug blocks alpha-1 adrenergic receptors, causing a reduction in blood pressure. It also reduces the smooth muscle tone in the prostate and bladder neck, and thus decreases urethral resistance, relieves obstruction, and improves urine flow.

POTENTIAL SIDE EFFECTS

Palpitations, increased heart rate, dizziness, nervousness, numbness, drowsiness, nausea, joint ache, shortness of breath, nasal congestion, sinusitis, headache, swelling in the limbs, postural hypotension (sudden drop in blood pressure upon standing from a sitting or lying down position), vision changes, weight gain, decrease in cholesterol levels.

CAUTIONS

- Inform your doctor if you have kidney dysfunction, allergies to other drugs in this class (such as prazosin, doxazosin, etc.), or if you are taking phosphodiesterase-5 inhibitors (such as sildenafil, tadalafil, or vardenafil).
- Orthostatic hypotension (a sudden drop in blood pressure upon standing from a sitting or lying down position), fainting, and loss of consciousness may occur with first dose.
- Avoid rapid increase in dose.
- Screen for prostate cancer prior to therapy for prostate enlargement.
- In treatment up to two years, does not affect blood concentrations of prostate specific antigen (PSA), a marker used to diagnose prostate cancer.

DRUG INTERACTIONS

Other antihypertensives, verapamil, NSAIDs, calcium channel blockers.

FOOD INTERACTIONS

Avoid alcohol, especially those who flush after drinking alcohol

HERBAL INTERACTIONS

Dong quai, ephedra, yohimbe, ginseng, saw palmetto, garlic

PREGNANCY AND BREAST-FEEDING CAUTIONS

FDA Pregnancy Risk Category C. Excretion in breast milk unknown. Consult your doctor.

SPECIAL INFORMATION

Should rise slowly after prolonged sitting or lying down. Report to your doctor any weight gain or painful, persistent erection.

TERBUTALINE
(ter-BYOO-ta-leen)

NEWLY DISCOVERED USES (OFF-LABEL)

Dysmenorrhea, external cephalic version, fetal distress, preterm labor, priapism

ORIGINAL USES (ON-LABEL)

Treatment of asthma and bronchospasm

BRAND NAME
Brethine

DRUG CLASS
Bronchodilator, (beta-agonist)

DESCRIPTION
This drug relaxes bronchial smooth muscle by selective action on beta 2-receptors with less effect on heart rate.

POTENTIAL SIDE EFFECTS
Nervousness, increased heart rate, high blood pressure, restlessness, dizziness, lightheadedness, serum glucose increased, serum potassium decreased, trembling, muscle cramps, weakness.

CAUTIONS
- Before therapy, notify your doctor if you have heart disease, particularly irregular heart rhythm, seizure disorders, diabetes, glaucoma, thyroid disease, or low potassium levels.
- May cause elevation in blood pressure, heart rate, and result in central nervous system stimulation.

DRUG INTERACTIONS
Beta-blockers, MAO inhibitors and tricyclic antidepressants.

FOOD INTERACTIONS
Unknown

HERBAL INTERACTIONS
Ephedra, yohimbe

PREGNANCY AND BREAST-FEEDING CAUTIONS
FDA Pregnancy Risk Category B. Excreted in breast milk. Consult your doctor.

TESTOLACTONE
(tes-toe-LAK-tone)

NEWLY DISCOVERED USES (OFF-LABEL)
Congenital adrenal hyperplasia, McCune-Albright syndrome, precocious puberty

ORIGINAL USES (ON-LABEL)
Treatment of advanced or disseminated breast cancer

BRAND NAME
Teslac

DRUG CLASS
Antineoplastic (androgen)

DESCRIPTION
This drug blocks the production of estradiol and estrone by interfering with steroid activity.

POTENTIAL SIDE EFFECTS
Numbness, tongue swelling or redness, anorexia, nausea, vomiting, limb aches, hair loss, changes in blood pressure, numbness in fingers or toes.

CAUTIONS
- Not for use in the treatment of breast cancer in men.
- Notify your doctor if you miss a dose.
- Contraceptive measures are recommended during therapy if premenopausal.
- Prolonged use may be associated with liver toxicity and may require monitoring.
- Notify your doctor if you have kidney, liver, or heart problems.
- Notify your doctor if numbness of fingers, toes, or face occurs.

DRUG INTERACTIONS
Warfarin, heparins

FOOD INTERACTIONS
Unknown

HERBAL INTERACTIONS
Saw palmetto

PREGNANCY AND BREAST-FEEDING CAUTIONS
FDA Pregnancy Risk Category C. Excreted in breast milk. Do not use during breast-feeding.

SPECIAL INFORMATION
Plasma calcium levels may be monitored while taking this drug. Desired response may take as long as three months.

TESTOSTERONE
(tes-TOS-ter-one)

NEWLY DISCOVERED USES (OFF-LABEL)
Female hypoactive sexual desire disorder

ORIGINAL USES (ON-LABEL)
Treatment of delayed male puberty, male hypogonadism, inoperable female breast cancer

BRAND NAMES
Androderm, AndroGel, Delatestryl, Depo-Testosterone, Striant, Testim, Testoderm, Testoderm with Adhesive, Testopel

DRUG CLASS
Androgen

DESCRIPTION
This drug promotes the growth and development of the male sex organ and maintains secondary sex characteristics in males who have biological problems related to sexual development.

POTENTIAL SIDE EFFECTS
Flushing, swelling related to fluid retention, aggressive behavior, mental depression, sleeplessness, hair growth, loss of menstruation, breast soreness, breast swelling, prostate enlargement, liver toxicity, changes in lipid levels.

Topical: application site irritation.

CAUTIONS
- Notify your doctor if you have heart, liver, or kidney disease, prostate enlargement with obstruction, undiagnosed genital bleeding; males: breast or prostate cancer.
- Androderm (testosterone patch) should not be used in women.
- Not for use in pregnancy.
- May require monitoring for prostate cancer (in adults) or bone growth (in children). May cause liver toxicity, worsen sleep apnea.

DRUG INTERACTIONS
Oral anticoagulants, corticosteroids, insulin.

This drug is metabolized by a specific set of liver enzymes (cytochrome P450 enzymes). Several other drugs interfere with these liver enzymes, and thus may increase or decrease the clearance of testosterone from the body, potentially increasing the risk of side effects or decreasing effectiveness. When these drugs are given in combination with testosterone, dosage adjustments may be needed. As these are too numerous to list, you should always check with your doctor or pharmacist prior to starting a new medication, herbal, or nonprescription product.

FOOD INTERACTIONS
Unknown

HERBAL INTERACTIONS
St. John's wort

PREGNANCY AND BREAST-FEEDING CAUTIONS
FDA Pregnancy Risk Category X. Excreted in breast milk. Do not use during breast-feeding.

SPECIAL INFORMATION
Requires periodic testing for liver function, prostate cancer, lipid levels, and blood disorders.

TETRACYCLINE
(tet-ra-SYE-kleen)

NEWLY DISCOVERED USES (OFF-LABEL)
Bullous pemphigoid, Legionnaire's disease, rosacea

ORIGINAL USES (ON-LABEL)
Treatment of various bacterial infections. Used in combination with other drugs to treat *H. pylori* related gastric ulcers

BRAND NAMES
Sumycin, Wesmycin

DRUG CLASS
Antibiotic

DESCRIPTION
This drug inhibits the production of bacterial proteins by binding to parts of the proteins that are essential to cell function.

POTENTIAL SIDE EFFECTS
Dizziness, upset stomach, photosensitivity reaction (see cautions), itching, discoloration of teeth and enamel (young children), nausea, diarrhea, abdominal cramps, liver toxicity.

CAUTIONS

- Inform your doctor if you have a history of allergies to other antibiotics in this class or if you have liver or kidney problems.
- If used during tooth development may cause permanent discoloration of the tooth enamel. Thus, should not be used in young children (under eight years of age).
- Not for use during pregnancy.
- May retard skeletal development and bone growth with greatest risk for children less than four years and those receiving high doses.
- Dosages may be reduced in kidney impairment.
- May cause photosensitivity reactions (skin reaction related to sun exposure). Wear sunscreen and protective clothing during sun exposure.
- Chronic use may result in superinfection.
- Notify your doctor if persistent diarrhea develops.
- Do not use outdated tetracycline products.

DRUG INTERACTIONS

Benzodiazepines, calcium channel blockers, cisapride, cyclosporine, ergot alkaloids, selected HMG-CoA reductase inhibitors, mirtazapine, nateglinide, nefazodone, pimozide, quinidine, sildenafil, tacrolimus, venlafaxine, calcium, magnesium, or aluminum containing antacids, iron, zinc, sodium bicarbonate sucralfate, didanosine, quinapril, aminoglutethimide, carbamazepine, nafcillin, nevirapine, phenobarbital, phenytoin, rifamycins, cholestyramine, colestipol, oral contraceptives, digoxin, insulin, isotretinoin

FOOD INTERACTIONS

Avoid concurrent administration with dairy products or metal containing products (such as calcium, iron, zinc, aluminum, magnesium). Take at least two hours before or after tetracycline.

HERBAL INTERACTIONS

Zinc

PREGNANCY AND BREAST-FEEDING CAUTIONS

FDA Pregnancy Risk Category D. Excreted in breast milk. Do not use during breast-feeding.

SPECIAL INFORMATION

Take on an empty stomach, at least one hour prior to or two hours after meals.

THALIDOMIDE
(tha-LI-doe-mide)

NEWLY DISCOVERED USES (OFF-LABEL)

Ankylosing spondylitis, Crohn's disease, gastrointestinal bleeding, myelofibrosis, pruritus, sarcoidosis, scleroderma, systemic lupus erythematosus, ulcerative colitis

ORIGINAL USES (ON-LABEL)
Treatment and maintenance of the skin manifestations of erythema nodosum leprosum

BRAND NAME
Thalomid

DRUG CLASS
Immune modulator

DESCRIPTION
This drug triggers immunosuppression, possibly by suppressing production of the antibody called tumor necrosis factor alpha (TNF-alpha).

POTENTIAL SIDE EFFECTS
Dizziness, insomnia, nervousness, nerve pain, numbness, somnolence, tremor, orthostatic hypotension (a sudden drop in blood pressure upon standing from a sitting or lying down position), vertigo, acne, nail disorder, itching, rash, sweating, anorexia, constipation, diarrhea, dry mouth, flatulence, liver function, nausea, oral yeast infection, tooth pain, blood in urine, impotence, anemia and other blood disorders, swelling in limbs, changes in cholesterol levels and liver function tests, sore throat, inflammation of the sinuses, abdominal pain, back pain, chills, fever, headache, malaise, neck pain, neck rigidity, pain.

CAUTIONS
- This drug is a known teratogen (induces severe abnormalities in fetuses exposed during pregnancy) and is not for use during pregnancy or in women of childbearing age unless alternative therapies have been deemed inappropriate. A negative pregnancy test is required 24 hours prior to the initiation of therapy. Pregnancy tests will be performed weekly during the first month of use and monthly thereafter in women with regular menstruation and every two weeks in women with irregular

menstruation. Oral and written warnings must be provided and signed prior to initiation of therapy. Discuss these materials and risks with your doctor and appropriate contraceptive measures required during therapy. Similar risks and requirements are in place for male patients.

- May cause significant decreases in white blood cell count and requires monitoring to determine this complication.
- This drug can only be prescribed by a doctor registered in a special program designed to ensure the safe use of this drug.
- Serious skin reactions have been reported with this drug (such as Stevens Johnson Syndrome). Stop the medication and notify your doctor if a rash develops.
- Notify your doctor if you have decreased kidney or liver function, neurological disorders, heart disease, HIV infection, a history of seizures, or constipation.
- Use caution in patients with a history of seizures, concurrent therapy with drugs that alter seizure threshold, or conditions that predispose to seizures.
- May cause a photosensitivity reaction related to sun exposure. Wear sunscreen and protective clothing.

DRUG INTERACTIONS
Sedatives, anakinra, barbiturates, chlorpromazine, reserpine

FOOD INTERACTIONS
Alcohol

HERBAL INTERACTIONS
Cat's claw

PREGNANCY AND BREAST-FEEDING CAUTIONS
FDA Pregnancy Risk Category X. Excretion in breast milk unknown. Do not breast-feed while taking this drug.

SPECIAL INFORMATION
This drug has a black box warning which describes the teratogenic potential of the drug when administered during pregnancy. In addition, thalidomide is approved only under a special distribution program, the "System for Thalidomide Education and Prescribing Safety" (STEPS) and prescribing and dispensing of thalidomide is restricted to prescribers and pharmacists registered with the program. No more than a four-week supply is dispensed at one time and prescriptions must be filled within seven days.

THEOPHYLLINE
(theo-FILL-in)

NEWLY DISCOVERED USES (OFF-LABEL)
Bronchopulmonary dysplasia (in infants), Cheyne-Stokes respiration, cystic fibrosis in children, neonatal apnea

ORIGINAL USES (ON-LABEL)
Treatment and prevention of bronchial asthma and reversible bronchospasm associated with chronic bronchitis and emphysema

BRAND NAMES
Bronkodyl, Quibron-T, Theo-24, Theochron, Theolair

DRUG CLASS
Bronchodilator (xanthine derivative)

DESCRIPTION
This drug relaxes smooth muscle of the bronchi and lung blood vessels, induces fluid excretion, and lowers the sphincter pressure in the esophagus.

POTENTIAL SIDE EFFECTS
Increased heart rate, nausea, headache, insomnia, irritability, restlessness.

CAUTIONS
- Requires blood monitoring to determine effectiveness and toxicity. Too high serum levels of this drug are associated with toxic side effects, ranging from less serious effects such as nausea and vomiting, to more serious effects such as changes in heart rhythm or seizures.
- Prior to therapy, notify your doctor if you have irregular heart rhythms, heart disease, liver dysfunction, high blood pressure, congestive heart failure, alcoholism, peptic ulcers, esophageal problems.
- Notify your doctor if any of the following symptoms develop: nausea, vomiting, insomnia, jitteriness, headache, rash, severe gastric pain, restlessness, irregular heart beat.

DRUG INTERACTIONS
This drug has several drug interactions, some of which are listed below. This list is not comprehensive; it is advised that you check

with your pharmacist or physician prior to starting any new prescription medication, herbal product, or nonprescription drug.

Aminogluthethimide, nonselective beta-blockers (such as propranolol, etc.), barbiturates, charcoal, phenytoin, ketoconazole, rifampin, smoking, sulfinpyrazone, carbamazepine, isoniazid, loop diuretics, allopurinol, beta-blockers, calcium channel blockers, cimetidine, oral contraceptive, corticosteroids, disulfiram, ephedrine, influenza virus vaccine, interferon, macrolide antibiotics, mexiletine, quinolone antibiotics, thyroid hormones.

FOOD INTERACTIONS
Low carbohydrate, high protein diet. Charcoal broiled beef. Take on an empty stomach.

HERBAL INTERACTIONS
Unknown

PREGNANCY AND BREAST-FEEDING CAUTIONS
FDA Pregnancy Risk Category C. Excretion into breast milk. Consult your doctor.

SPECIAL INFORMATION
Do not crush or chew extended-release dosage forms. Take at the same time without food each day. Do not change from one brand to another without consulting your doctor or pharmacist.

THIOTEPA
(thye-oh-TEP-a)

NEWLY DISCOVERED USES (OFF-LABEL)
Prevention of recurrence of pterygium

ORIGINAL USES (ON-LABEL)
To treat several types of cancers and lymphomas

BRAND NAME
Thioplex

DRUG CLASS
Antineoplastic (alkylating)

DESCRIPTION
Reacts with DNA to inhibit the production of DNA, RNA, and protein.

POTENTIAL SIDE EFFECTS
Dizziness, headache, blurred vision, skin reactions, pain at injection site, hair loss, nausea, vomiting, abdominal pain, anorexia, pain upon urination, urinary retention, fatigue, weakness, fever, suppression of various blood parameters (myelosuppression).

CAUTIONS
- This drug is highly toxic to certain factors of the blood (such as white blood cells, red blood cells, etc.) and requires weekly monitoring of blood to determine toxicity.
- Notify your doctor if you are pregnant or plan to become pregnant. This drug is not for use during pregnancy.
- Reduced dosages are needed in liver or kidney dysfunction, or in bone marrow damage.

DRUG INTERACTIONS
Succinylcholine, neuromuscular blockers, or other drugs known to affect bone marrow function. This represents a numerous list, so consult your doctor or pharmacist prior to initiation of therapy with other prescription medications, herbal products, or non-prescription products.

FOOD INTERACTIONS
Alcohol

HERBAL INTERACTIONS
Black cohosh, dong quai when treating estrogen-dependent tumors

PREGNANCY AND BREAST-FEEDING CAUTIONS
FDA Pregnancy Risk Category D. Excreted in breast milk. Do not breast-feed during therapy.

SPECIAL INFORMATION
Contraceptive measures are recommended during therapy. Inform your doctor if signs of bleeding or infection develop.

TIAGABINE
(tie-GA-been)

NEWLY DISCOVERED USES (OFF-LABEL)
Chronic neuropathic pain, fibromyalgia, generalized anxiety disorder (GAD), impulsive aggressive disorder, migraine prevention, multiple sclerosis, neuropathy, panic disorder, post-traumatic stress disorder (PTSD)

ORIGINAL USES (ON-LABEL)
Use in combination treatment in partial seizures

BRAND NAME
Gabitril

DRUG CLASS
Anticonvulsant

DESCRIPTION
Decreases seizure frequency by enhancing certain neurotransmitter activity (gabanergic).

POTENTIAL SIDE EFFECTS
Dizziness, drowsiness, nausea, weakness, nervousness, difficulty with concentration, insomnia, abnormal gait, rash, itching, diarrhea, vomiting, increased appetite, tremor, numbness, uncontrolled eye movements, hearing impairment, sore throat, cough, speech difficulties, fatigue.

CAUTIONS
- Do not stop abruptly; gradually withdraw medication to minimize risk of increasing seizure frequency.
- Notify your doctor if you have liver impairment.
- Due to the confusion, sedation, and weakness side effects be cautious about performing tasks requiring alertness.
- Risk of serious rash including Stevens Johnson syndrome may occur.

DRUG INTERACTIONS
Valproate, primidone, phenobarbital, phenytoin, carbamazepine.

This drug is metabolized by a specific set of liver enzymes (cytochrome P450 enzymes 3A4). Several other drugs interfere with these liver enzymes, and thus may increase or decrease the clearance of tiagabine from the body, potentially increasing the risk of side effects or decreasing effectiveness. When these drugs are given in combination with tiagabine, dosage adjustments may be needed. As these are too numerous to list, you should always check with your doctor or pharmacist prior to starting a new medication, herbal, or nonprescription product.

FOOD INTERACTIONS
Alcohol

HERBAL INTERACTIONS
St. John's wort, valerian, kava kava, gotu kola

PREGNANCY AND BREAST-FEEDING CAUTIONS
FDA Pregnancy Risk Category C. Excreted in breast milk and is not recommended while breast-feeding.

SPECIAL INFORMATION
In 2005, the FDA published an advisory regarding new onset seizures when the drug is used for off-label indications in patients without epilepsy.

TICARCILLIN-CLAVULANTE
(tye-kar-SIL-in klav-yoo-LAN-ate)

NEWLY DISCOVERED USES (OFF-LABEL)
Diverticulitis

ORIGINAL USES (ON-LABEL)
Treatment of various infections, clavulanate expands activity of the penicillin

BRAND NAME
Timentin

DRUG CLASS
Antibiotic (penicillin)

DESCRIPTION
This drug inhibits bacterial cell wall synthesis.

POTENTIAL SIDE EFFECTS
Confusion, electrolyte imbalance, rash, Stevens-Johnson syndrome, severe diarrhea, leukopenia, liver toxicity, kidney toxicity, hypersensitivity reactions.

CAUTIONS
- Notify your doctor if you have congestive heart failure, a history of allergies to cephalosporins or penicillins, or kidney problems.
- Contains high sodium content.

DRUG INTERACTIONS
Probenecid, methotrexate, tetracyclines, aminoglycosides, neuromuscular blockers

FOOD INTERACTIONS
Unknown

HERBAL INTERACTIONS
Unknown

PREGNANCY AND BREAST-FEEDING CAUTIONS
FDA Pregnancy Risk Category B. Excreted in breast milk. Compatible with breast-feeding.

SPECIAL INFORMATION
Dosage adjustment required in kidney and liver dysfunction.

TICLOPIDINE
(tye-KLOE-pi-deen)

NEWLY DISCOVERED USES (OFF-LABEL)
Sickle cell anemia

ORIGINAL USES (ON-LABEL)
To reduce risk of stroke in patients who have had a stroke or stroke precursors and are intolerant or have failed aspirin, and to reduce incidence of subacute stent thrombosis in coronary stent implantation

BRAND NAME
Ticlid

DRUG CLASS
Antiplatelet, platelet aggregation inhibitor

DESCRIPTION
This drug prevents blood clots and increases bleeding time. It works by inhibiting platelet growth by interfering with the platelet

membrane function. The effect on platelet function is not reversible.

POTENTIAL SIDE EFFECTS

Diarrhea, nausea, upset stomach, rash, gastric pain, blood disorders (such as neutropenia, thrombocytopenia), increased cholesterol and triglycerides levels.

CAUTIONS

- Inform your doctor if you have active bleeding or a history of bleeding disorders, peptic or gastric ulcers, risks of bleeding, kidney or liver dysfunction. Notify your doctor if you are taking other drugs that affect bleeding.
- Notify your doctor two weeks prior to any scheduled surgery. Tell your doctor/dentist that you are taking this drug prior to any procedure or surgery.
- May cause life-threatening blood reactions (such as neutropenia—low white blood cells, thrombocytopenia—decreased platelets); requires blood monitoring before therapy is started and periodically thereafter.
- Notify your doctor if you develop any sign of infection (such as fever, chills, or sore throat), weakness, difficulty speaking, seizures, persistent diarrhea, yellowing of the skin or eyes, dark or bloody urine, or pinpoint red spots on the skin.

DRUG INTERACTIONS

Aspirin, anticoagulants, theophylline, NSAIDs, phenytoin, cimetidine, antacids, digoxin, cyclosporine.

This drug is metabolized by a specific set of liver enzymes (cytochrome P450 enzymes 3A4). Several other drugs interfere with these liver enzymes, and thus may increase or decrease the clearance of ticlopidine from the body, potentially increasing the risk of side effects or decreasing effectiveness. When these drugs are given in combination with ticlopidine, dosage adjustments may be needed. As these are too numerous to list, you should always check with your doctor or pharmacist prior to starting a new medication, herbal, or nonprescription product.

FOOD INTERACTIONS

Take with food to minimize stomach intolerance.

HERBAL INTERACTIONS

Avoid cat's claw, dong quai, evening primrose, feverfew, garlic, ginkgo, ginger, red clover, horse chestnut, green tea, ginseng (all have additional anti-platelet effects).

PREGNANCY AND BREAST-FEEDING CAUTIONS
FDA Pregnancy Risk Category B. Excretion in breast milk is unknown. Consult your doctor.

SPECIAL INFORMATION
This drug has a black box warning that describes the potential for developing life-threatening blood adverse reactions, (such as neutropenia/agranulocytosis, thrombotic thrombocytopenic purpura (TTP) and aplastic anemia). These may occur within a few days after the start of therapy and requires close blood monitoring throughout therapy.

TILUDRONATE
(tye-LOO-droe-nate)

NEWLY DISCOVERED USES (OFF-LABEL)
Bone loss reduction in spinal cord injury

ORIGINAL USES (ON-LABEL)
Treatment of Paget's disease in patients who have a serum alkaline phosphatase twice upper limit, are symptomatic, and are at risk for future complications

BRAND NAME
Skelid

DRUG CLASS
Biphosphonate derivative

DESCRIPTION
This drug reduces bone breakdown via inhibition of osteoclasts, which indirectly increases bone mineral density.

POTENTIAL SIDE EFFECTS
Pain, back pain, flu-like symptoms, headache, dizziness, numbness, diarrhea, nausea, upset stomach, vomiting, runny nose, sinusitis, upper respiratory tract infection.

CAUTIONS
- Notify your doctor if you have kidney impairment or gastric problems.
- Use with caution in patients with active upper GI problems.
- Maintain adequate vitamin D and calcium intake.

DRUG INTERACTIONS
Calcium salts, aluminum magnesium containing antacids, aspirin, indomethacin. (Should not be taken within two hours before or two hours after this drug.)

FOOD INTERACTIONS
Absorption is reduced 90% when given with food. Do not take within two hours of a meal.

HERBAL INTERACTIONS
Unknown

PREGNANCY AND BREAST-FEEDING CAUTIONS
FDA Pregnancy Risk Category C. Excretion in breast milk is unknown. Consult your doctor.

SPECIAL INFORMATION
Administer as a single oral dose with 6–8 ounces of plain water. Do not take within two hours of food or calcium and mineral supplements. Do not remove tablets from foil until you are ready to take them.

TIZANIDINE
(tye-ZAN-i-deen)

NEWLY DISCOVERED USES (OFF-LABEL)
Migraine prevention, tension headache treatment and prevention

ORIGINAL USES (ON-LABEL)
Treatment of muscle spasticity

BRAND NAME
Zanaflex

DRUG CLASS
Skeletal muscle relaxants (alpha-adrenergic agonist)

DESCRIPTION
This drug reduces spastic motions and relaxes muscles by inhibiting activity of spinal motor neurons.

POTENTIAL SIDE EFFECTS

Low blood pressure, fatigue, dizziness, drowsiness, constipation, dry mouth, sore throat, vomiting, urinary frequency, urinary tract infection, elevations in liver function tests, changes in vision.

CAUTIONS

- May cause liver toxicity, requiring periodic monitoring of liver function.
- May cause central nervous system effects, such as sedation, hallucinations, psychotic-like symptoms.
- Notify your doctor if you have decreased liver or kidney function as reduced doses may be needed or a decision to not use the drug.
- Notify your doctor if you have low blood pressure or heart disease.

DRUG INTERACTIONS

Diuretics, other alpha-adrenergic agonists, other antihypertensives, alcohol, baclofen, central nervous system depressants, oral contraceptives.

FOOD INTERACTIONS

May increase levels when taken with food.

HERBAL INTERACTIONS

Valerian, St. John's wort, kava kava, gotu kola (may increase central nervous system depression)

PREGNANCY AND BREAST-FEEDING CAUTIONS

FDA Pregnancy Risk Category C. Excretion into breast milk is unknown. Breast feeding not recommended during therapy.

SPECIAL INFORMATION

Avoid alcohol during therapy.

TOPIRAMATE
(TOE-pie-rah-mate)

NEWLY DISCOVERED USES (OFF-LABEL)

Alcoholism (cravings and dependence), binge eating disorder, cluster headache treatment and prevention, cocaine addiction, diabetic neuropathy, essential tremor, fibromyalgia, multiple sclerosis, migraine prevention in children, neuropathy, psoriasis, post-traumatic stress syndrome(PTSD), West syndrome

ORIGINAL USES (ON-LABEL)
Used in combination to treat partial onset seizures and generalized tonic-clonic seizures, treatment of seizures associated with Lennox-Gastaut syndrome, prevention of migraines

BRAND NAME
Topamax

DRUG CLASS
Anticonvulsant

DESCRIPTION
This drug decreases a patient's seizure frequency by blocking sodium channels in neurons and enhancing certain neurotransmitter activity.

POTENTIAL SIDE EFFECTS
Dizziness, muscle incoordination, drowsiness, insomnia, speech disorders, nervousness, uncontrolled movements of the eyes, numbness and tingling, memory impairment, tremor, confusion, difficulty concentrating, depression, language problems, agitation, aggressive reaction, emotional lability, abnormal gait, behavioral problems, rash, nausea, upset stomach, anorexia, abdominal pain, constipation, breast pain, weight loss, sinusitis, shortness of breath, blurred or double vision, fatigue, back pain, chest pain, flu-like syndrome, mood problems, increased sweating, loss of heat regulation resulting in increased body temperature.

CAUTIONS
- Report any sudden changes in vision to your doctor.
- Avoid abrupt withdrawal of topiramate and taper dose to minimize potential for increased seizure frequency.
- Notify doctor if you have liver or kidney impairment.
- Increase fluid intake to decrease risk of kidney stones.
- May cause numbness, sedation, psychomotor slowing, confusion, and mood disturbances.

DRUG INTERACTIONS
Other central nervous system depressants (such as alcohol, narcotics, etc.) may increase sedative effects, acetazolamide, phenytoin, antihistamines, cyclic antidepressants, antipsychotics, carbamazepine, digoxin, estradiol, valproic acid, oral contraceptives, digoxin.

This drug inhibits a specific set of liver enzymes (cytochrome P450 enzymes 2C19). Several other drugs are metabolized (cleared or activated) by these liver enzymes, and thus, coadministration with topiramate may potentially increase the risk of side effects or decrease effectiveness. When these drugs are given in combination, dosage adjustments may be needed. As these are too numerous to list, you should always check with your doctor or pharmacist prior to starting a new medication, herbal, or nonprescription product.

FOOD INTERACTIONS
Alcohol

HERBAL INTERACTIONS
Evening primrose

PREGNANCY AND BREAST-FEEDING CAUTIONS
FDA Pregnancy Risk Category C. Excreted in breast milk and is not recommended during breast-feeding.

SPECIAL INFORMATION
Contents of capsules may be sprinkled on a small amount of food (such as applesauce or custard). Swallow mixture immediately without chewing. Drink fluids immediately after ingesting to promote full swallowing. Do not save contents of capsule for future use.

TRAMADOL
(TRAM-a-dole)

NEWLY DISCOVERED USES (OFF-LABEL) ————
Fibromyalgia, diabetic neuropathy, neuropathy, restless legs syndrome

ORIGINAL USES (ON-LABEL)
Relief of moderate to moderately severe general and dental pain

BRAND NAME
Ultram

DRUG CLASS
Pain reliever

DESCRIPTION
This drug relieves pain by altering the body's perception and response to pain.

POTENTIAL SIDE EFFECTS

Dizziness, headache, sedation, constipation, nausea, agitation, anxiety, confusion, coordination impaired, itching, rash, menopausal symptoms, abdominal pain, anorexia, diarrhea, dry mouth, urinary frequency, urinary retention, spasticity, weakness, visual disturbances, sweating.

CAUTIONS

- Central nervous system (CNS) depression and respiratory depression may occur; risk increases with the coadministration of other CNS depressants. Consult with your doctor or pharmacist before starting new therapy with any prescription, nonprescription or herbal product.
- Increased risk of seizures may occur if taken with selective serotonin reuptake inhibitors (SSRIs—fluoxetine, sertraline, paroxetine, etc.), tricyclic antidepressants (such as amitriptyline, nortriptyline, etc.), neuroleptics, or monoamine oxidase inhibitors (MAOIs—phenelzine, etc.). See recommendation above regarding consultation with doctor or pharmacist.
- Inform your doctor if you currently experience seizures or have a history of seizures.
- Elderly patients with chronic respiratory disorders are at increased risk for adverse reactions.
- May impair alertness required for certain tasks (such as operation of machinery, driving, etc.).
- Caution in patients with increased intracranial pressure or head injury.
- Use caution and reduce dose in patients with liver disease, kidney, thyroid, or adrenal dysfunction.
- Tolerance or drug dependence may occur.
- Abrupt discontinuation should be avoided.

DRUG INTERACTIONS

Amphetamines, cimetidine, tricyclic antidepressants, SSRIs, linezolid, MAOIs, naloxone, neuroleptics, opioids, quinidine, carbamazepine, warfarin, digoxin. This drug is metabolized by a specific set of liver enzymes (cytochrome P450 enzymes 2D6). Several other drugs interfere with these liver enzymes, and thus may increase or decrease the clearance of tramadol from the body, potentially increasing the risk of side effects or decreasing effectiveness. When these drugs are given in combination with tramadol, dosage adjustments may be needed. As these are too numerous to list, you should always check with your doctor or pharmacist prior to starting a new medication, herbal, or nonprescription product.

FOOD INTERACTIONS
Alcohol

HERBAL INTERACTIONS
Valerian, St. John's wort, kava kava, gotu kola

PREGNANCY AND BREAST-FEEDING CAUTIONS
FDA Pregnancy Risk Category C. Excreted in breast milk. Consult your doctor.

SPECIAL INFORMATION
Withdrawal symptoms may occur if tramadol is discontinued abruptly. Do not take products which contain alcohol.

TRANEXAMIC ACID
(tran-eks-AM-ik AS-id)

NEWLY DISCOVERED USES (OFF-LABEL)
Menorrhagia

ORIGINAL USES (ON-LABEL)
Used for short-term in hemophilia patients during and following tooth extraction to reduce or prevent bleeding

BRAND NAME
Cyklokapron

DRUG CLASS
Antihemophilic, hemostatic

DESCRIPTION
This drug is used to reduce bleeding. It works by inhibiting elements in the body that promote bleeding.

POTENTIAL SIDE EFFECTS
Nausea, vomiting, diarrhea, low blood pressure, giddiness, blood clot events, visual abnormalities.

CAUTIONS
- Not for use if you have acquired defective color vision, a subarachnoid hemorrhage, or intravascular clotting.

- Eye exams are recommended in patients treated continually for longer than several days.
- Dose should be reduced if you have kidney impairment.
- Can cause ureteral obstruction due to clot formation in patients with upper urinary tract bleeding.
- Venous and arterial blood clots or thromboembolism have been reported. Patients with a previous history of thromboembolic disease may be at increased risk for venous or arterial blood clots.
- Requires close monitoring by doctor.

DRUG INTERACTIONS
Anti-inhibitor coagulant complexes, factor IX complex concentrates, trétinoin.

FOOD INTERACTIONS
Unknown

HERBAL INTERACTIONS
Unknown

PREGNANCY AND BREAST-FEEDING CAUTIONS
FDA Pregnancy Risk Category B. Excreted in breast milk. Consult your doctor.

TRAZODONE
(TRAZ-oh-done)

NEWLY DISCOVERED USES (OFF-LABEL)
Alzheimer's disease, chronic fatigue syndrome, insomnia, migraine prevention, post-traumatic stress disorder (PTSD)

ORIGINAL USES (ON-LABEL)
Treatment of depression

BRAND NAME
Desyrel

DRUG CLASS
Antidepressant

DESCRIPTION
This drug is used to control mood levels. It works by affecting the activity of serotonin, which promotes behavioral changes related to depression and mood disorders.

POTENTIAL SIDE EFFECTS

Blurred vision, constipation, dry mouth, changes in blood pressure, shortness of breath, fainting, anger, confusion, decreased concentration, disorientation, drowsiness, fatigue, headache, insomnia, nervousness, abdominal pain, diarrhea, nausea, musculoskeletal aches, tremors, weight gain or loss.

CAUTIONS

- Notify your doctor if you have heart disease or irregular heart rhythm.
- Has been associated with sedation. Caution in performing tasks that require alertness.
- This drug has been associated with the occurrence of priapism (prolonged, painful erection) and in some cases required surgery to reverse.
- Lowered blood pressure has occurred, particularly after standing from a sitting or lying down position. Do not stand too quickly.
- Therapeutic effects may take up to four weeks to occur. Therapy is normally maintained for several months after optimum response is reached to prevent recurrence of depression.

DRUG INTERACTIONS

Ritonavir, ketoconazole, indinavir, itraconazole, nefazodone, carbamazepine, digoxin, phenytoin, MAO inhibitors.

This drug is metabolized by a specific set of liver enzymes (cytochrome P450 enzymes 3A4). Several other drugs interfere with these liver enzymes, and thus may increase or decrease the clearance of trazodone from the body, potentially increasing the risk of side effects or decreasing effectiveness. When these drugs are given in combination with trazodone, dosage adjustments may be needed. As these are too numerous to list, you should always check with your doctor or pharmacist prior to starting a new medication, herbal, or nonprescription product.

FOOD INTERACTIONS

Take shortly after a meal or light snack. Risk of dizziness or lightheadedness may be increased when taken on an empty stomach.

HERBAL INTERACTIONS

Valerian, St. John's wort, SAMe, kava kava

PREGNANCY AND BREAST-FEEDING CAUTIONS

FDA Pregnancy Risk Category C. Excreted in breast milk. Do not breast-feed during therapy.

SPECIAL INFORMATION
This drug has a black box warning regarding the increased risk of suicidal thinking and behavior in children, adolescents, and adults with major depressive disorder. Discuss these risks with your doctor.

TRETINOIN
(TRET-i-noyn)

Topical

NEWLY DISCOVERED USES (OFF-LABEL)
Oral leukoplakia, keloids

ORIGINAL USES (ON-LABEL)
Acne, palliation of fine wrinkles (Renova) and mottled skin pigmentation

BRAND NAMES
Avita, Renova, Retin-A

DRUG CLASS
Topical acne drug, vitamin A derivative

DESCRIPTION
This drug is used primarily to fight acne. It works possibly by decreasing the cohesiveness of skin cells, which decreases acne formation.

POTENTIAL SIDE EFECTS
Local reactions, including peeling, dry skin, burning, stinging, redness, itching.

CAUTIONS
- Keep away from the eyes, mouth, and mucous membranes. For topical external use only.
- This drug is considered a skin irritant. The effects of the chronic use (greater than 48 weeks) of this drug is not known.
- May induce severe local redness, burning, stinging. May cause severe irritation to eczematous skin.
- Minimize exposure to sunlight and sunlamps. The use of this product causes heightened sun sensitivity.

DRUG INTERACTIONS
Topical sulfur, resorcinol, benzoyl peroxide, or salicylic acid. Other medicated or abrasive cleansers that may dry the skin (such as astringents, cosmetics, alcohol containing products, etc.). Consult your doctor or pharmacist prior to using other topical products. Other drugs that increase sensitivity to the sun (photosensitizers) such as thiazides, tetracyclines, fluoroquinolones, phenothiazines, sulfonamides.

FOOD INTERACTIONS
Unknown

HERBAL INTERACTIONS
Unknown

PREGNANCY AND BREAST-FEEDING CAUTIONS
FDA Pregnancy Risk Category C. Oral tretinoin is teratogenic. Not known if excreted in breast milk after topical use. Consult your doctor.

SPECIAL INFORMATION
Wash with mild soap and dry skin approximately 20 to 30 minutes prior to application. Ensure skin is entirely dry before application to minimize potential for irritation. Extreme weather conditions (wind, cold, heat) may be more irritating with the use of this drug.

TRIAMCINOLONE ACETONIDE
(try-am-SIN-oh-lone ah-SIT-oh-nide)

Injection

NEWLY DISCOVERED USES (OFF-LABEL)
Chalazia, cystoid macular edema, uveitis

ORIGINAL USES (ON-LABEL)
Treatment of various allergic and various inflammatory disorders, including those of the skin, endocrine system, gastrointestinal, lung, rheumatic, blood

BRAND NAMES
Kenalog 10, Tac 40, Tri-Kort, Trilog

DRUG CLASS
Corticosteroid, anti-inflammatory

DESCRIPTION
This drug decreases inflammation.

POTENTIAL SIDE EFFECTS
Insomnia, nervousness, increased appetite, indigestion, increased hair growth, diabetes mellitus, joint aches, cataracts, glaucoma, headache, impaired wound healing, thin fragile skin, loss of menstruation, sodium and fluid retention, loss of potassium or calcium, abdominal distention, nausea, vomiting.

CAUTIONS
- Therapy with this drug may mask the symptoms of infection and increase the susceptibility of infection via immunosuppression.
- Psychiatric symptoms may develop or be aggravated.
- Diabetics may require increased doses of insulin or oral drugs to treat diabetes.
- Notify your doctor if you have bacterial or viral infections, hyperthyroidism, cirrhosis, nonspecific ulcerative colitis, hypertension, osteoporosis, thromboembolic tendencies, congestive heart failure, convulsive disorders, myasthenia gravis, thrombophlebitis, peptic ulcer, diabetes.
- Acute adrenal insufficiency may occur with abrupt withdrawal after long-term therapy or with stress.

DRUG INTERACTIONS
Barbiturates, phenytoin, rifampin, vaccine and toxoid effects may be reduced

FOOD INTERACTIONS
Triamcinolone interferes with calcium absorption.

HERBAL INTERACTIONS
Cat's claw, echinacea

PREGNANCY AND BREAST-FEEDING CAUTIONS
FDA Pregnancy Risk Category C. Excretion in breast milk is unknown. Consult doctor.

TRIAMTERENE
(try-AM-ter-een)

NEWLY DISCOVERED USES (OFF-LABEL)
Primary hyperaldosteronism

ORIGINAL USES (ON-LABEL)
Edema either as monotherapy or in combination with another drug

BRAND NAME
Dyrenium

DRUG CLASS
Diuretic (potassium sparing)

DESCRIPTION
This drug interferes with sodium absorption in the kidneys and decreases potassium excretion from the body while promoting fluid excretion.

POTENTIAL SIDE EFFECTS
Headache, fatigue, dizziness, increased potassium levels, dehydration, reduced sodium levels, nausea, diarrhea, vomiting, constipation, abdominal and gas pain, appetite changes, impotence, muscle cramps, weakness, cough, shortness of breath, photosensitivity (skin reaction related to sun exposure), changes in electrolyte levels, increase in blood glucose.

CAUTIONS
- Not for use if you have severe liver or kidney dysfunction.
- Inform your doctor if you have a history of kidney stones or diabetes.
- Requires periodic monitoring of kidney function, electrolytes, and potassium levels. This drug may cause increased levels. Do not take concurrent potassium supplementation or potassium sparing drugs. Stop therapy if high levels of potassium occur.
- Not recommended if you have acute or chronic kidney insufficiency, or diabetic neuropathy disease.

DRUG INTERACTIONS
Potassium supplements, amantadine, ACE inhibitors (such as captopril, enalapril, lisinopril, etc.), cimetidine, indomethacin

FOOD INTERACTIONS
Take after meals to avoid gastric upset. Avoid eating large volumes of potassium-rich foods.

HERBAL INTERACTIONS
Unknown

PREGNANCY AND BREAST-FEEDING CAUTIONS
FDA Pregnancy Risk factor B. Not recommended during breast-feeding.

SPECIAL INFORMATION
If a single daily dose is prescribed, take early in the day to avoid frequent urination at night. Avoid prolonged exposure to sunlight.

TRICHLORMETHIAZIDE
(try-klor-met-THYE-a-zide)

NEWLY DISCOVERED USES (OFF-LABEL)
Hypercalciuria

ORIGINAL USES (ON-LABEL)
High blood pressure, swelling due to fluid retention (edema)

BRAND NAMES
Diurese, Metahydrin, Naqua

DRUG CLASS
Blood pressure medication (thiazide diuretic)

DESCRIPTION
This drug increases the excretion of sodium and chloride in urine, promoting fluid loss. It also promotes excretion of potassium and bicarbonate, but decreases excretion of calcium and uric acid.

POTENTIAL SIDE EFFECTS
Potassium loss, nausea, vomiting, loss of appetite, upset stomach, diarrhea, electrolyte imbalances, gout, changes in blood sugar or cholesterol levels, sudden drop in blood pressure upon standing from sitting or lying down position (orthostatic hypotension), dizziness, photosensitivity (skin reaction related to sun exposure).

CAUTIONS
- Notify your doctor if you have allergies to sulfonamide drugs; this drug is not for use in these patients. Inform your doctor if you have kidney disease, liver disease, diabetes, asthma, lupus, gout, or recently had surgery.
- Diabetics may require increased amounts of insulin or oral drugs commonly used to treat diabetes.
- Requires monitoring of electrolytes, and may require potassium supplementation during therapy.
- May cause dizziness and light-headedness when standing suddenly from a sitting or lying down position.

DRUG INTERACTIONS
ACE inhibitors (such as captopril, lisinopril, etc.), arsenic trioxide, calcitriol, calcium carbonate, cholestyramine, colestipol, digoxin, ketanserin, lithium, probenecid. Check with your pharmacist or doctor before starting new medications, herbal products, or nonprescription drugs.

FOOD INTERACTIONS
Avoid excessive ingestion of natural licorice.

HERBAL INTERACTIONS
Ginkgo, gossypol, ma huang, ephedra

PREGNANCY AND BREAST-FEEDING CAUTIONS
FDA Pregnancy Risk Category C according to manufacturer. May suppress lactation. Consult your doctor.

SPECIAL INFORMATION
This medication can cause dizziness or drowsiness.

TRIMETHOBENZAMIDE
(try-meth-oh-BEN-za-mide)

NEWLY DISCOVERED USES (OFF-LABEL)
Hyperemesis gravidarum

ORIGINAL USES (ON-LABEL)
To treat nausea and vomiting

BRAND NAME
Tigan

DRUG CLASS
Antiemetic, anticholinergic

DESCRIPTION
This drug reduces and suppresses vomiting by affecting nerve impulses to the part of the brain that controls the sensation of nausea and triggers vomiting.

POTENTIAL SIDE EFFECTS
Lowered blood pressure, blurred vision, disorientation, dizziness, diarrhea, drowsiness, depression.

CAUTIONS
- The suppository formulation contains benzocaine and should not be used by patients who have an allergy to this product or other similar type of anesthetics.
- Injection not for use in children; suppositories not for use in premature infants or neonates.
- May cause involuntary movements of muscles.

DRUG INTERACTIONS
Phenothiazines, barbiturates may cause additive effects on central nervous system

FOOD INTERACTIONS
Alcohol

HERBAL INTERACTIONS
Unknown

PREGNANCY AND BREAST-FEEDING CAUTIONS
FDA Pregnancy Risk Category D. Excretion into breast milk is unknown. Consult your doctor.

SPECIAL INFORMATION
May cause drowsiness; caution with using this drug if tasks require alertness. Report any restlessness or involuntary movement to your doctor.

TRIMETHOPRIM
(try-METH-oh-prim)

NEWLY DISCOVERED USES (OFF-LABEL)
Prevention and treatment of pneumocystis jiroveci pneumonia

ORIGINAL USES (ON-LABEL)
Treatment of initial uncomplicated urinary tract infections due to susceptible bacteria

BRAND NAMES
Primsol, Proloprim

DRUG CLASS
Antibiotic (folate antagonist)

DESCRIPTION
This drug fights bacterial growth by affecting bacterial metabolism of folinic acid; this interferes with the production of specific proteins in the bacteria.

POTENTIAL SIDE EFFECTS
Rash, itching, nausea, vomiting, stomach upset, various blood disorders (decreased red blood cells, decreased white blood cells, etc.), fever, changes in kidney or liver function.

CAUTIONS
- Rarely may cause blood disorders, especially if taken in high doses over chronic periods.
- Notify your doctor if you have decreased liver or kidney function.

DRUG INTERACTIONS
Phenytoin

FOOD INTERACTIONS
Unknown

HERBAL INTERACTIONS
Unknown

PREGNANCY AND BREAST-FEEDING CAUTIONS
FDA Pregnancy Risk Category C. Excretion into breast milk. Consult your doctor.

TRIMETHOPRIM-SULFAMETHOXAZOLE
(try-METH-oh-prim sul-fah-meth-OX-ahzole)

NEWLY DISCOVERED USES (OFF-LABEL)
Acne, atypical pneumonia (Legionnaire's), cholera, granuloma inguinale, nocardiosis, nonbacterial prostatitis, sinusitis

ORIGINAL USES (ON-LABEL)
Treatment of various infections due to susceptible bacteria

BRAND NAMES
Bactrim, Septra

DRUG CLASS
Antibiotic (folate antagonist, sulfonamide)

DESCRIPTION
This drug fights bacterial growth by affecting bacterial metabolism of folinic acid and dihydrofolic acid; this interferes with the production of specific proteins in the bacteria.

POTENTIAL SIDE EFFECTS
Rash, itching, nausea, vomiting, stomach upset, various blood disorders (decreased red blood cells, decreased white blood cells, etc.), fever, changes in kidney or liver function, local injection site reaction (injection), anorexia, severe skin reactions.

CAUTIONS
- Notify your doctor if you are allergic to sulfa drugs or sulfites, or have certain types of anemia (megaloblastic anemia due to folate deficiency).
- Not for use in infants less than two months of age, pregnant women at term, or women nursing infants less than two months of age.
- This drug may cause severe skin reactions, that although rare, may cause death. Discontinue this drug at the first sign of rash and notify your doctor immediately.
- Rash, sore throat, fever, joint pain, pallor, unusual bleeding or bruising, jaundice may be an early sign of serious reactions.
- Report any cough, shortness of breath may be indicative of a hypersensitivity reaction to the respiratory tract.
- Not for use in the treatment of group A beta-hemolytic streptococcal infections.
- Report chronic, persistent diarrhea that develops during or shortly after the completion of therapy.
- Notify your doctor if you have impaired kidney or liver function.

DRUG INTERACTIONS
Phenytoin, warfarin, cyclosporine, dapsone, diuretics, methotrexate, sulfonylureas, zidovudine

FOOD INTERACTIONS
Unknown

HERBAL INTERACTIONS
Unknown

PREGNANCY AND BREAST-FEEDING CAUTIONS
FDA Pregnancy Risk Category C. Excretion into breast milk. Consult your doctor.

SPECIAL INFORMATION
Maintain adequate fluid intake.

TRIMIPRAMINE
(try-MI-pra-meen)

NEWLY DISCOVERED USES (OFF-LABEL)
Panic disorder, post-traumatic stress disorder (PTSD)

ORIGINAL USES (ON-LABEL)
Depression

BRAND NAME
Surmontil

DRUG CLASS
Antidepressant (tricyclic)

DESCRIPTION
This drug increases the levels of chemicals in the body that affect mood by inhibiting uptake of these chemicals by neurons.

POTENTIAL SIDE EFFECTS
Dry mouth, sedation, dizziness, headache, nervousness, skin rash, tremors, hives, nausea, constipation, vision changes, sweating, lowered blood pressure, increased heart rate, decreased sodium levels, suicidal ideation, changes in heart rhythm and conduction, blurred vision, weight gain, sexual dysfunction.

CAUTIONS
- Do not use if you have been taking an MAO inhibitor (e.g., phenelzine, tranylcypromine, isocarboxazid) within the past 14 days. When used with MAO-Is fever, high blood pressure, increased heart rate, confusion, seizures, and deaths have been reported.
- Not for use immediately after a heart attack.
- Can cause sedation which may impair performance of tasks requiring alertness. Sedative effects may be additive with other drugs that cause similar effects (central nervous system depressants).
- May worsen psychosis or mania in patients with bipolar disease.
- Stop therapy with doctor permission and according to instructions (gradual taper) prior to elective surgery.

- Do not abruptly stop medication; taper gradually.
- Notify your doctor if you have low blood pressure, as this drug can cause low blood pressure episodes.
- Use with caution if you have urinary retention, a history of cardiac disease, seizure disorders, diabetes, benign prostatic hyperplasia, narrow angle glaucoma, dry mouth, visual problems, constipation, or a history of bowel obstruction.
- Possibility of suicide attempt may persist until remission occurs.
- Use with caution if you are hyperthyroid or if you receive thyroid supplementation.
- Use with caution in patients with liver or kidney dysfunction and in elderly.

DRUG INTERACTIONS
MAO inhibitors (such as phenelzine, tranylcypromine, isocarboxazid), ritonavir, bupropion, amphetamines, anticholinergics, sedatives, chlorpropamide, tolazamide, warfarin, fluoxetine, fluvoxamine, citalopram, escitalopram, paroxetine, sertraline, cimetidine, carbamazepine, haloperidol, smoking, methylphenidate, valproic acid, clonidine, venlafaxine, protease inhibitors, quinidine, diltiazem, verapamil, lithium, phenothiazines may affect the levels of trimipramine, drugs which prolong QT interval (see site: http://www.torsades.org/medical-pros/drug-lists/drug-lists.htm).

This drug is metabolized (inactivated) by a specific set of liver enzymes (cytochrome P450 enzymes). Several other drugs interfere with these liver enzymes, and thus may increase or decrease the clearance of trimipramine from the body, potentially increasing the risk of side effects or decreasing effectiveness. When these drugs are given in combination with trimipramine, dosage adjustments may be needed. As these are too numerous to list, you should always check with your doctor or pharmacist prior to starting a new medication.

FOOD INTERACTIONS
Alcohol, grapefruit juice

HERBAL INTERACTIONS
Valerian, St. John's wort, SAMe, kava kava

PREGNANCY AND BREAST-FEEDING CAUTIONS
FDA Pregnancy Risk Category C. Excreted in breast milk. Breast-feeding is not recommended during therapy with this drug.

SPECIAL INFORMATION

May take four to six weeks for the full therapeutic effects to be experienced. Avoid prolonged exposure to sunlight; wear sunscreen.

In 2005, the FDA announced new labeling for antidepressants regarding the need to closely monitor for worsening of depression and for the potential of increased suicidal thinking or suicidal behavior during therapy. Although this recommendation applies to all patients (adults, children, adolescents) treated with antidepressants for any indication, this is of particular importance in patients being treated for depression.

VALPROIC ACID
(val-PRO-ick acid)

NEWLY DISCOVERED USES (OFF-LABEL)

Migraine prevention in children, panic disorder, post-traumatic stress disorder (PTSD), schizoaffective disorder

ORIGINAL USES (ON-LABEL)

Used alone or in combination therapy for the treatment of complex partial seizures, simple and complex absence seizures, used in combination therapy for patients with multiple seizure types that include absence seizures and generalized seizures, for the treatment of mania associated with bipolar disorder, to prevent migraines

BRAND NAMES

Depacon, Depakene, Depakote Delayed Release, Depakote ER, Depakote Sprinkle

DRUG CLASS

Anticonvulsant, antimanic, antimigraine

DESCRIPTION

Valproic acid increases the availability of GABA, an inhibitory neurotransmitter, to the brain neurons.

POTENTIAL SIDE EFFECTS

Sleepiness, dizziness, insomnia, nervousness, hair loss, nausea, diarrhea, vomiting, abdominal pain, blood disorders, tremor, weakness, respiratory tract infection, shortness of breath, hypertension, sensation of changes in heart rhythm, peripheral edema, increased heart rate, amnesia, abnormal dreams, anxiety, confusion, bruising, dry skin, itching, loss of menstruation, painful menstruation, flatulence, increased appetite, urinary frequency, urinary incontinence, vaginitis, elevation in liver function tests, abnormal gait, joint pain, back pain, blurred vision, ringing in the ears, nosebleeds, double vision, weight gain, increased cough, pneumonia, sinusitis.

CAUTIONS

- Not recommended for use if you have liver dysfunction, urea cycle disorders, or if you are pregnant.
- May cause severe blood disorders, which increase the risk of bleeding.
- Use with other anticonvulsants requires monitoring for safety and efficacy.
- Tremors may be a sign of overdose.
- Cases of life-threatening pancreatitis have been reported with the use of this drug.
- Increased ammonia levels may occur and should be measured if you develop unexplained lethargy and vomiting, or changes in mental status.
- Do not discontinue abruptly because doing so may increase seizure frequency.
- Caution when performing tasks that require mental alertness. Sedative drugs or alcohol may increase these risks.
- The elderly may be at higher risk of sedation and require lower doses.
- Closely monitoring patients with psychiatric disorders for the development of suicidal ideation during initial drug therapy.

DRUG INTERACTIONS

Chlorpromazine, charcoal, cholestyramine, cimetidine, erythromycin, rifampin, aspirin and other salicylates, tricyclic antidepressants (such as amitriptyline, nortriptyline, etc.), carbamazepine, clonazepam, diazepam, ethosuximide, lamotrigine, phenobarbital, phenytoin, tolbutamide, warfarin, zidovudine

FOOD INTERACTIONS

Alcohol

HERBAL INTERACTIONS

Evening primrose

PREGNANCY AND BREAST-FEEDING CAUTIONS
FDA Pregnancy Risk Category D. Excreted in breast milk. Consult your doctor.

SPECIAL INFORMATION
This drug has a black box warning regarding the risks of liver toxicity during therapy. Increased risk for this toxic event is associated with use in small children (less than two years of age), those with congenital metabolic disorders, severe seizure disorders accompanied by mental retardation, and those with certain types of brain disease. This drug has also been reported to induce harmful effects during pregnancy (such as spina bifida). In addition, the use of this drug has caused life-threatening pancreatitis.

VALSARTAN
(val-SAR-tan)

NEWLY DISCOVERED USES (OFF-LABEL)
  Diabetic nephropathy

ORIGINAL USES (ON-LABEL)
For the treatment of high blood pressure and heart failure

BRAND NAME
Diovan

DRUG CLASS
Blood pressure medication (angiotensin II receptor antagonist [ARB])

DESCRIPTION
Valsartan works by blocking the substance that causes fluid retention and blood vessels to constrict.

POTENTIAL SIDE EFFECTS
Dizziness, fatigue, increased potassium levels, abdominal pain, dry cough, upper respiratory infection.

CAUTIONS
- Do not use if you have certain kidney problems (kidney artery stenosis, decreased kidney function).
- Do not use in pregnant patients who are in the second or third trimester.
- Avoid use if you are dehydrated.

DRUG INTERACTIONS
Lithium, amiloride, spironolactone and triamterene

FOOD INTERACTIONS
Unknown

HERBAL INTERACTIONS
Ma huang, yohimbine, limit intake of natural licorice

PREGNANCY AND BREAST-FEEDING CAUTIONS
FDA Pregnancy Risk Category C in first trimester, Category D in second and third trimesters. Do not use during second and third trimesters of pregnancy. Excreted in breast milk. Breast-feeding is not recommended.

SPECIAL INFORMATION
This drug has a black box warning regarding the fetal toxicities associated with the use of this drug class during the second and third trimesters of pregnancy. When pregnancy is detected, the drug should be discontinued as soon as possible.

VANCOMYCIN
(vank-coe-MY-sin)

NEWLY DISCOVERED USES (OFF-LABEL)
Hepatic encephalopathy, tonsillitis and peritonsillar abscess

ORIGINAL USES (ON-LABEL)
This drug is used for the treatment of serious bacterial infections

BRAND NAMES
Vancocin, Vancoled

DRUG CLASS
Antibiotic

DESCRIPTION
This drug inhibits the production of cell walls in susceptible bacteria.

POTENTIAL SIDE EFFECTS
Flushing, rash, hives, itching, dizziness, hearing loss.

CAUTIONS

- Inform your doctor of underlying hearing loss, kidney impairment.
- May cause vein or tissue irritation when administered intravenously.
- Requires monitoring of kidney function during therapy. Kidney damage is usually reversible.
- Requires blood monitoring of drug levels and ear examinations if treated for longer durations.
- Toxicity of the ears is proportional to dosage and duration of treatment.
- Red Man's syndrome may occur and includes a sudden decrease in blood pressure, rash, and flushing. It is usually related to too fast administration of the drug when given intravenously.

DRUG INTERACTIONS

Neuromuscular blocking drugs, other aminoglycosides, other kidney-toxic drugs (such as amphotericin, etc.) or nerve-toxic drugs

FOOD INTERACTIONS

Unknown

HERBAL INTERACTIONS

Unknown

PREGNANCY AND BREAST-FEEDING CAUTIONS

FDA Pregnancy Risk Category C, Category B for Oral pulvules. Excreted in breast milk. Consult with your doctor.

VARDENAFIL
(var-DEN-a-fil)

NEWLY DISCOVERED USES (OFF-LABEL)

Pulmonary hypertension

ORIGINAL USES (ON-LABEL)

Erectile dysfunction

BRAND NAME

Levitra

DRUG CLASS

Impotence drugs (5-phosphodiesterase inhibitors)

DESCRIPTION
This drug causes smooth muscle relaxation and flow of blood to the corpus cavernosum (erectile tissue of the penis).

POTENTIAL SIDE EFFECTS
Headache, stomach upset, diarrhea, nasal congestion, abnormal vision, flushing, dizziness, rash, urinary tract infection.

CAUTIONS
- Seek medical attention if prolonged erection (greater than four hours) occurs.
- There is a potential risk of a cardiac event associated with sexual activity in some patients. This drug is not for use in such patients. Discuss these risks with your doctor prior to initiation of therapy.
- May require lower doses in reduced liver function.
- Inform your doctor if you have an anatomical deformation of the penis or conditions that may put you at an increased risk for priapism (prolonged, painful erections greater than six hours), including but not limited to sickle cell anemia, multiple myeloma, and leukemia.
- Do not use nitrates in any form. See the following website for a list of such drugs (http://www.fda.gov/medwatch/safety/1998/viagra.htm). Check with your pharmacist or doctor before starting a new medication, herbal product or nonprescription drug while taking this drug.
- Use with other erectile dysfunction treatments is not recommended.

DRUG INTERACTIONS
Nitrates (see cautions), alpha-blockers (such as doxazosin, terazosin, etc.), heparin, phenytoin, carbamazepine, phenobarbital, rifampin, antihypertensives, nifedipine, ketoconazole, itraconazole, erythromycin, protease inhibitors.

This drug is metabolized by a specific set of liver enzymes (cytochrome P450 enzymes 3A4, 3A5). Several other drugs interfere with these liver enzymes, and thus may increase or decrease the clearance of vardenafil from the body, potentially increasing the risk of side effects or decreasing effectiveness. When these drugs are given in combination with vardenafil, dosage adjustments may be needed. As these are too numerous to list, you should always check with your doctor or pharmacist prior to starting a new medication, herbal, or nonprescription product.

FOOD INTERACTIONS
Grapefruit juice. May be taken with or without food. Avoid substantial alcohol intake.

HERBAL INTERACTIONS
St. John's wort

PREGNANCY AND BREAST-FEEDING CAUTIONS
FDA Pregnancy Risk Category B. Not for use in women; not recommended during breast-feeding.

SPECIAL INFORMATION
This medication is to be taken by mouth one hour prior to sexual activity. Do not take vardenafil with an alpha-blocker (may result in significant low blood pressure). This drug does not protect against sexually transmitted diseases. Do not take more than once daily.

In 2005, the FDA reported a safety alert that described changes in the product labeling for all drugs in this class. Specifically, the changes were based on a small number of post-marketing reports of sudden vision loss, attributed to NAION (non arteritis ischemic optic neuropathy), a condition where blood flow is blocked to the optic nerve. FDA advises patients to stop taking these medicines, and call a doctor or healthcare provider right away if they experience sudden or decreased vision loss in one or both eyes.

VASOPRESSIN
(veh-SO-prez-in)

NEWLY DISCOVERED USES (OFF-LABEL)
Acute upper gastrointestinal bleeding

ORIGINAL USES (ON-LABEL)
Diabetes insipidus, abdominal distention after surgery

BRAND NAME
Pitressin

DRUG CLASS
Pituitary hormone

DESCRIPTION
This drug increases reabsorption of water by the kidneys and causes contraction of smooth muscle in the gastrointestinal tract and blood vessels.

POTENTIAL SIDE EFFECTS
Tremor, vertigo, sweating, hives, abdominal cramps, change in heart rate, nausea, vomiting.

CAUTIONS
- Notify your doctor if you have vascular disease, since this drug may cause angina pain or the possibility of a heart attack with larger doses.
- May produce water intoxication by its effect to retain water. Notify your doctor if you develop drowsiness, headaches, or listlessness.
- May cause severe constriction of blood vessels, resulting in reduced circulation to the skin or changes in skin color. Notify your doctor if you notice skin blanching.
- Local allergy reactions may occur.
- Requires monitoring of fluid, electrolytes and cardiac function.

DRUG INTERACTIONS
Carbamazepine, chlorpropamide, clofibrate, urea, demecycline, lithium, heparin, ganglionic blocking drugs

FOOD INTERACTIONS
Unknown

HERBAL INTERACTIONS
Unknown

PREGNANCY AND BREAST-FEEDING CAUTIONS
FDA Pregnancy Risk Category C. Excretion in breast milk unknown. Consult your doctor.

SPECIAL INFORMATION
Abdominal cramping may be reduced if one to two glasses of water are taken with dose. It may be a transient effect.

VENLAFAXINE
(ven-la-FAX-een)

NEWLY DISCOVERED USES (OFF-LABEL)

Attention deficit/hyperactivity disorder (ADHD), chronic neuropathic pain, diabetic neuropathy, fibromyalgia, menopausal symptoms, migraine headache prevention, obsessive-compulsive disorder (OCD), panic disorder, premenstrual dysphoric disorder (PMDD), tension headache prevention

---

ORIGINAL USES (ON-LABEL)

Major depressive disorder, generalized anxiety disorder, social anxiety disorder, depression, social phobia

BRAND NAMES

Effexor, Effexor XR

DRUG CLASS

Antidepressant (serotonin/norepinephrine reuptake inhibitor [SNRI])

DESCRIPTION

This drug is used to treat mood disorders. It works by inhibiting serotonin and norepinephrine reuptake by brain neurons. This action is helpful in increasing levels of both these neurotransmitters.

POTENTIAL SIDE EFFECTS

Headache, dizziness, insomnia, nausea, dry mouth, constipation, anorexia, abnormal ejaculation/orgasm, weakness, sweating, changes in blood pressure, chest pain, anxiety, abnormal dreams, yawning, agitation, rash, itching, decreased libido, diarrhea, vomiting, stomach upset, flatulence, urinary frequency, impotence, impaired urination, orgasm disturbance, tremor, numbness, twitching, blurred vision, ringing in ears (tinnitus), infection, chills, trauma.

CAUTIONS

- Contraindicated in the use of MAO inhibitors (such as phenelzine, tranylcypromine, isocarboxazid) within 14 days and should not initiate a MAO inhibitor within seven days of discontinuing venlafaxine.

- Inform your doctor if you have current problems or a history of problems with kidney or liver failure, increased intraocular pressure, or glaucoma.
- Risk of suicide may be increased in patients with major depression.
- Abrupt discontinuation or dosage reduction after extended therapy may lead to agitation, mood changes, nervousness, anxiety, and other symptoms. Gradually taper dosage according to doctor's instructions.

DRUG INTERACTIONS

Buspirone, lithium, meperidine, nefazodone, selegiline, serotonin agonists, sibutramine, selective serotonin reuptake inhibitors (e.g., fluoxetine, sertraline, paroxetine, etc.), trazodone, tricyclic antidepressants, haloperidol, indinavir, phenobarbital, carbamazepine, phenytoin.

Concurrent use of MAO inhibitors or drugs with MAO inhibitor activity may result in serotonin syndrome; should not be used within two weeks of each other.

This drug is metabolized (activated) by a specific set of liver enzymes (cytochrome P450 enzymes 2D6, 3A4). Several other drugs interfere with these liver enzymes, and thus may increase or decrease the clearance of venlafaxine from the body, potentially increasing the risk of side effects or decreasing effectiveness. When these drugs are given in combination with venlafaxine, dosage adjustments may be needed. As these are too numerous to list, you should always check with your doctor or pharmacist prior to starting a new medication, herbal, or nonprescription product.

FOOD INTERACTIONS

Alcohol

HERBAL INTERACTIONS

Valerian, St. John's wort, SAMe, kava kava, tryptophan

PREGNANCY AND BREAST-FEEDING CAUTIONS

FDA Pregnancy Risk Category C. Excreted in breast milk. Do not use while breast-feeding.

SPECIAL INFORMATION

Neonates exposed to venlafaxine late in the third trimester of pregnancy have developed complications requiring prolonged hospitalization, respiratory support, and tube feeding. Such complications can arise immediately upon delivery.

This drug has a warning regarding that both adults and children with major depression, may experience worsening of their depression and/or the emergence of suicidal ideation and behavior (suicidality), whether or not they are taking antidepressant medications. The warning recommends patients being treated with antidepressants be observed closely for clinical worsening and suicidality, especially at the beginning of a course of drug therapy, or at the time of dose changes.

VERAPAMIL
(vur-AP-ah-mill)

NEWLY DISCOVERED USES (OFF-LABEL)
Cluster headache prevention, hypertrophic cardiomyopathy, migraine prevention, prevention of cyclosporine-induced nephrotoxicity, prevention of recurrence and sudden death in ventricular tachycardia, Raynaud's syndrome, ventricular tachycardia

ORIGINAL USES (ON-LABEL)
Angina, arrhythmias (irregular heart rhythm), high blood pressure

BRAND NAMES
Calan, Calan SR, Covera-HS, Isoptin SR, Verelan, Verelan PM

DRUG CLASS
Cardiac (calcium channel blocker)

DESCRIPTION
This drug relaxes coronary vascular smooth muscle and increases oxygen delivery to the heart. It works by blocking calcium ions from entering the "slow channels" or select voltage-sensitive areas of vascular smooth muscle and heart tissue.

POTENTIAL SIDE EFFECTS
Swelling of the gum tissue, constipation, low blood pressure, dizziness, headache, nausea, lowered heart rate, lightheadedness, constipation, wheezing.

CAUTIONS
- Notify your doctor if you have had an allergic reaction to a drug in this class.

- Inform your doctor if you have low blood pressure, severe left ventricular dysfunction or other types of heart problems, liver or kidney dysfunction.
- Abrupt withdrawal may cause increased duration and frequency of chest pain.
- The elderly may be at greater risk of experiencing low blood pressure and constipation associated with this therapy.

DRUG INTERACTIONS

Amiodarone, barbiturates, beta-blockers, calcium salts, cyclosporine, cimetidine, ranitidine, phenytoin, rifampin, disopyramide, flecainide, doxorubicin, antineoplastics, buspirone, carbamazepine, digoxin, dofetilide, statins (e.g., lovastatin, atorvastatin, etc.), imipramine, lithium, moricizine, certain muscle relaxants, prazosin, quinidine, sirolimus, tacrolimus, theophylline.

This drug is metabolized by and affects a specific set of liver enzymes (cytochrome P450 enzymes). Several other drugs interfere with these liver enzymes, and thus may increase or decrease the clearance of verapamil from the body, potentially increasing the risk of side effects or decreasing effectiveness. When these drugs are given in combination with verapamil, dosage adjustments may be needed. As these are too numerous to list, you should always check with your doctor or pharmacist prior to starting a new medication, herbal, or nonprescription product.

FOOD INTERACTIONS
Avoid grapefruit juice.

HERBAL INTERACTIONS
St. John's wort, dong quai, ephedra, yohimbe, ginseng, garlic

PREGNANCY AND BREAST-FEEDING CAUTIONS
FDA Pregnancy Risk Category C. Excreted in breast milk. Consult your doctor.

SPECIAL INFORMATION
Do not crush or chew the extended-release formulations. Do not be concerned if you see the outer shell of the Covera-HS tablets in the stools.

VINCRISTINE
(ven-CHRIS-teen)

NEWLY DISCOVERED USES (OFF-LABEL)
Therapy-resistant idiopathic thrombocytopenia purpura, therapy-resistant thrombotic thrombocytopenia purpura, thrombotic thrombocytopenic purpura

ORIGINAL USES (ON-LABEL)
Various cancers (acute leukemia, Hodgkin's disease, non-Hodgkin's malignant lymphoma)

BRAND NAME
Vincasar PFS

DRUG CLASS
Cancer chemotherapy (antineoplastic)

DESCRIPTION
This drug prevents cell growth and multiplication by interfering with DNA production.

POTENTIAL SIDE EFFECTS
Decreases in white blood cells (leukopenia), nerve pain, constipation, hair loss, sensory loss, numbness, difficulty walking, abnormal gait, loss of deep tendon reflexes, and muscle wasting.

CAUTIONS
- Only prescribed for intravenous administration.
- Acute shortness of breath and severe bronchospasm has occurred.
- Is known to cause nerve and neuromuscular toxicity, which requires periodic monitoring and testing.
- Has caused kidney damage related to uric acid production.
- Leukemia of the central nervous system has occurred in patients being treated with this drug.
- May be at increased risk of developing infection during therapy due to its immunosuppressive effects.

DRUG INTERACTIONS
Digoxin, L-asparaginase, mitomycin, phenytoin

FOOD INTERACTIONS
Unknown

HERBAL INTERACTIONS
Unknown

PREGNANCY AND BREAST-FEEDING CAUTIONS
FDA Pregnancy Risk Category D. Drug is excreted into the breast milk. Do not breast-feed while taking this drug.

SPECIAL INFORMATION
This drug has a black box warning regarding several blood adverse effects and adverse effects if infusion occurs outside of vein.

WARFARIN
(WAR-far-in)

NEWLY DISCOVERED USES (OFF-LABEL)
Peripheral artery disease, stroke risk reduction, thrombectomy in peripheral artery disease, transient ischemic attack

ORIGINAL USES (ON-LABEL)
Atrial fibrillation, prosthetic heart valve embolism prophylaxis, venous thromboembolism

BRAND NAMES
Coumadin, Jantoven

DRUG CLASS
Anticoagulant

DESCRIPTION
This drug interferes with production of coagulation factors that are essential in forming blood clots.

POTENTIAL SIDE EFFECTS
Bleeding, lethargy, malaise, asthenia, pain, headache, dizziness, rash, nausea, bruising.

CAUTIONS
- Do not switch brands once desired therapeutic response has been reached.
- Notify your doctor if you have active tuberculosis, diabetes, protein C and S deficiency, hemorrhagic tendencies, severe uncontrolled or malignant hypertension, severe liver disease, invasive procedures with potential for bleeding, risk of falls, pregnancy, warfarin-induced necrosis, ascorbic acid deficiency.

- Concurrent use with NSAIDs or aspirin may cause severe gastric irritation and increased risk of bleeding.
- Warfarin should be stopped three days prior to surgical procedures and blood monitoring checked prior to procedure.

DRUG INTERACTIONS

This drug is metabolized by a specific set of liver enzymes (cytochrome P450 enzymes). Several other drugs interfere with these liver enzymes, and thus may increase or decrease the clearance of warfarin from the body, potentially increasing the risk of side effects or decreasing effectiveness. When these drugs are given in combination with warfarin, dosage adjustments may be needed. As these are too numerous to list, you should always check with your doctor or pharmacist prior to starting a new medication, herbal, or nonprescription product.

FOOD INTERACTIONS

Avoid or decrease quantities ingested of foods rich in vitamin K, vitamin E, cranberry juice.

HERBAL INTERACTIONS

St. John's wort, alfalfa, coenzyme Q10, cat's claw, dong quai, bromelains, evening primrose, feverfew, red clover, horse chestnut, garlic, green tea, ginseng, ginkgo, avocado, boldo

PREGNANCY AND BREAST-FEEDING CAUTIONS

FDA Pregnancy Risk Category X. Do not take while pregnant. Consult your doctor regarding breast-feeding.

SPECIAL INFORMATION

It is important to not change dietary consumption of vitamin K once stabilized on warfarin therapy. Foods which contain vitamin K include, but are not limited to: beef liver, pork liver, green tea, leafy green vegetables.

ZAFIRLUKAST
(za-FIR-loo-kast)

NEWLY DISCOVERED USES (OFF-LABEL)
Seasonal allergic rhinitis

ORIGINAL USES (ON-LABEL)
Prevention and chronic treatment of asthma

BRAND NAME
Accolate

DRUG CLASS
Asthma (leukotriene receptor antagonist)

DESCRIPTION
This drug relaxes the bronchial system, reduces inflammatory response in the lungs, and decreases hyper-responsiveness.

POTENTIAL SIDE EFFECTS
Headache, dizziness, nausea, diarrhea, abdominal pain, vomiting, upset stomach, hives, rashes, infection.

CAUTIONS
- Not for use in the treatment of acute asthma attacks.
- Patients older than 55 years appear to be at increased risk of developing infections during therapy.
- Notify your doctor if you have liver impairment/disease.
- Report any signs of possible liver toxicity during therapy, including right upper quadrant abdominal pain, nausea, fatigue, lethargy, jaundice, etc.
- In rare instances, this drug has been associated with developing a blood disorder called eosinophilia.

DRUG INTERACTIONS
Aspirin, erythromycin, theophylline, warfarin

FOOD INTERACTIONS
Absorption decreased when taken with food. Take greater than one hour before or two hours after meals.

HERBAL INTERACTIONS
Unknown

PREGNANCY AND BREAST-FEEDING CAUTIONS
FDA Pregnancy Risk Category B. Excreted in breast milk. Do not breast-feed during therapy.

SPECIAL INFORMATION
Do not stop taking other anti-asthmatic drugs unless directed by physicians.

ZANAMIVIR
(zan-AH-meh-vir)

NEWLY DISCOVERED USES (OFF-LABEL)
Prevention of influenza

ORIGINAL USES (ON-LABEL)
Treatment of influenza

BRAND NAME
Relenza

DRUG CLASS
Antiviral

DESCRIPTION
This drug alters viral particle growth and release.

POTENTIAL SIDE EFFECTS
Diarrhea, nausea, vomiting, nasal signs and symptoms, bronchitis, cough, sinusitis, dizziness, headache, asthma, cough.

CAUTIONS
- Notify your doctor if you have underlying lung disease or disorders.
- No evidence to suggest that this is effective if started 48 hours after development of symptoms.

DRUG INTERACTIONS
No clinically significant drug interactions known at this time. Consult doctor or pharmacist prior to initiating therapy with any new prescription, herbal, or nonprescription product.

FOOD INTERACTIONS
None

HERBAL INTERACTIONS
Unknown

PREGNANCY AND BREAST-FEEDING CAUTIONS
FDA Pregnancy Risk Category C. Excreted in breast milk. Consult your doctor.

SPECIAL INFORMATION
Take complete course of therapy although you may feel better before therapy is finished. Therapy does not affect transmission of influenza to others.

ZIPRASIDONE
(ze-PRAZ-eh-don)

NEWLY DISCOVERED USES (OFF-LABEL)
Autism, Gilles de la Tourette syndrome, Huntington's disease

ORIGINAL USES (ON-LABEL)
Acute agitation in schizophrenia, manic episodes in bipolar disorders, schizophrenia

BRAND NAME
Geodon

DRUG CLASS
Antipsychotic

DESCRIPTION
This drug inhibits the reuptake of serotonin and norepinephrine, increasing the levels of these neurotransmitters in the brain.

POTENTIAL SIDE EFFECTS
Drowsiness, headache, nausea, decreased heart rate, high blood pressure, increased heart rate, decrease in blood pressure upon abrupt standing from sitting or lying down position, dizziness, uncontrolled involuntary muscle movements, rash, skin reactions, painful menstruation, upset stomach, diarrhea, dry mouth, vomiting, pain at injection site, weakness, numbness, abnormal vision, respiratory disorder, rhinitis, cough increased, accidental injury, sweating, changes in heart rate (QT prolongation), changes in blood glucose (increases).

CAUTIONS
- This drug may cause changes in heart rhythm (prolonged QT interval). Not for use if you have a history of certain heart problems including prolonged QT, recent heart attacks, history of irregular heart rate, uncompensated heart failure, concurrent use of other QT prolonging medications (see list of drugs at website: http://www.torsades.org/medical-pros/drug-lists/drug-lists.htm#).
- Immediately report symptoms of dizziness, sensations of increased heart rate, or fainting to your doctor.
- Use caution if you have Parkinson's disease due to the risk of extrapyramidal side effects (involuntary muscle movements).

- Notify your doctor if you have a history of seizures, are taking drugs which can lower seizure threshold. Inform your doctor if you are diabetic, have electrolyte imbalances, breast cancer, or other prolactin-dependent tumors.
- This drug may cause disturbances in temperature regulations and or neuroleptic malignant syndrome (NMS).

DRUG INTERACTIONS

This drug is metabolized by a specific set of liver enzymes (cytochrome P450 enzymes 3A4). Several other drugs interfere with these liver enzymes, and thus may increase or decrease the clearance of ziprasidone from the body, potentially increasing the risk of side effects or decreasing effectiveness. When these drugs are given in combination with ziprasidone, dosage adjustments may be needed. As these are too numerous to list, you should always check with your doctor or pharmacist prior to starting a new medication, herbal, or nonprescription product.

Concurrent use with other QT prolonging drugs may result in additive effects on cardiac conduction, potentially resulting in malignant or lethal changes in heart rate. See cautions.

FOOD INTERACTIONS

Avoid alcohol, grapefruit juice.

HERBAL INTERACTIONS

St. John's wort, kava kava, chamomile

PREGNANCY AND BREAST-FEEDING CAUTIONS

FDA Pregnancy Risk Category C. Excretion into breast milk is unknown. Refrain from breast-feeding while taking this drug.

SPECIAL INFORMATION

In 2005, the FDA published a safety alert that notified the public about an increased risk of death when atypical antipsychotics were used to treat behavioral disorders in elderly patients with dementia (unapproved use). The majority of deaths were attributed to cardiovascular events (such as heart failure or sudden death) or from infections (mostly pneumonia).

ZOLEDRONIC ACID
(ZOE-le-dron-ik AS-id)

NEWLY DISCOVERED USES (OFF-LABEL)
Postmenopausal osteoporosis

ORIGINAL USES (ON-LABEL)
Hypercalcemia (increased calcium) associated with cancers, multiple myeloma, and documented bone metastases from solid tumors

BRAND NAME
Zometa

DRUG CLASS
Bisphosphonate derivative

DESCRIPTION
This drug reduces bone breakdown via actions on osteoclasts, which indirectly increases bone mineral density and prevents release of calcium from the bone.

POTENTIAL SIDE EFFECTS
Low blood pressure, confusion, depression, dizziness, headache, insomnia, numbness, hair loss, skin reactions, abdominal pain, anorexia, decreased appetite, constipation, diarrhea, nausea, vomiting, decreased weight, anemia and other blood disorders, joint pain, back pain, bone pain, muscle aches, shortness of breath, sore throat, edema, fatigue, fever, dehydration, rigors. Urinary tract infection.

CAUTIONS
- Doses should not exceed 4 mg and duration of infusion should be no less than 15 minutes.
- This drug is associated with a risk of kidney toxicity; notify your doctor if you have any pre-existing kidney disease or risk factors.
- Requires monitoring of calcium, phosphate, and magnesium levels, blood factors, as well as for kidney function.
- Notify your doctor if you have aspirin sensitive asthma.
- Has caused osteonecrosis (breakdown of bone) in the jaw. Dental examinations and preventive dentistry procedures should be considered prior to starting therapy with this drug. Avoid dental procedures during therapy.

DRUG INTERACTIONS
Aminoglycosides, thalidomide

FOOD INTERACTIONS
None

HERBAL INTERACTIONS
Unknown

PREGNANCY AND BREAST-FEEDING CAUTIONS
FDA Pregnancy Risk Category D. Excretion into breast milk is unknown; do not breast-feed during therapy.

SPECIAL INFORMATION
In 2005, the manufacturer notified health professionals and patients regarding the possibility of osteonecrosis (bone breakdown) in the jaw, mainly in cancer patients who received intravenous bisphosphonates as part of their therapy. (See cautions.) Patients should receive a dental examination prior to the initiation of therapy and avoid invasive dental procedures during therapy.

ZOLMITRIPTAN
(zohl-mi-TRIP-tan)

NEWLY DISCOVERED USES (OFF-LABEL)
Migraine headaches in children

ORIGINAL USES (ON-LABEL)
To manage acute treatment of migraine with or without aura

BRAND NAMES
Zomig, Zomig ZMT

DRUG CLASS
Antimigraine

DESCRIPTION
Zolmitriptan works by causing constriction of certain blood vessels. It affects brain receptors for serotonin, a neurochemical in the body.

POTENTIAL SIDE EFFECTS
Chest pain, dizziness, drowsiness, pain, nausea, dry mouth, stomach upset, numbness, weakness, sweating, muscle aches

CAUTIONS

- Only for patients with clear diagnosis of migraine. Not for preventive treatment of migraine headaches.
- Do not take if you have certain cardiac problems with irregular heart rhythm, uncontrolled blood pressure.
- First dose may be given in healthcare setting.
- May make you drowsy and affect your judgment. Be careful when driving a car or operating machinery.
- You should be monitored for blood pressure changes.
- Zomig ZMT tablets contain phenylalanine.
- Alcohol may have added central nervous toxicity.
- Abdominal and bloody diarrhea have occurred.

DRUG INTERACTIONS

- Avoid concurrent use of SSRIs and sibutramine; may cause serotonin syndrome.
- Ergotamine containing drugs.
- Propranolol, cimetidine, oral contraceptives increase the levels of zolmitriptan and may increase toxicity.
- Do not use within 24 hours of ergotamines or another drug in this class.
- Do not use within two weeks of discontinuing MAO inhibitors (such as phenelzine, tranylcypromine, isocarboxazid).

FOOD INTERACTIONS

Limit use of alcohol.

HERBAL INTERACTIONS

Unknown

PREGNANCY AND BREAST-FEEDING CAUTIONS

FDA Pregnancy Risk Category C. Excretion in breast milk unknown. Consult physician regarding breast-feeding while taking this drug.

SPECIAL INFORMATION

Tell your doctor if you have high blood pressure, high cholesterol, or diabetes, or if you smoke. Oral disintegrating tablet must be taken whole; do not break, crush or chew. Place on tongue and allow to dissolve.

ZOLPIDEM
(zole-PE-dem)

NEWLY DISCOVERED USES (OFF-LABEL)
> Parkinson's disease

ORIGINAL USES (ON-LABEL)
Insomnia

BRAND NAME
Ambien

DRUG CLASS
Hypnotic, (non-benzodiazepine)

DESCRIPTION
This drug acts on the part of neurons that are responsible for inducing sedation.

POTENTIAL SIDE EFFECTS
Headache, drowsiness, dizziness, lethargy, drugged feeling, lightheadedness, nausea, upset stomach, diarrhea, abdominal pain, constipation, muscle ache, joint ache, upper respiratory infection, sinusitis, sore throat, allergy, back pain, dry mouth.

CAUTIONS
- Notify your doctor if you have impaired kidney or liver function, psychiatric disorders, taking other central nervous system depressants.
- Generally limit duration to seven to 10 days of use.
- May cause drowsiness; use caution when operating machinery, driving, or other tasks that require alertness.

DRUG INTERACTIONS
This drug is metabolized by a specific set of liver enzymes (cytochrome P450 enzymes 3A4). Several other drugs interfere with these liver enzymes, and thus may increase or decrease the clearance of zolpidem from the body, potentially increasing the risk of side effects or decreasing effectiveness. When these drugs are given in combination with zolpidem, dosage adjustments may be needed. As these are too numerous to list, you should always check with your doctor or pharmacist prior to starting a new medication, herbal, or nonprescription product.

FOOD INTERACTIONS
Grapefruit juice. May be taken with food if stomach upset occurs.

HERBAL INTERACTIONS
St. John's wort, valerian, kava kava, gotu kola

PREGNANCY AND BREAST-FEEDING CAUTIONS
FDA Pregnancy Risk Category B. Excreted into the breast milk.
Refrain from breast-feeding while taking this drug.

SPECIAL INFORMATION
May cause drowsiness; avoid driving or other tasks that require
being alert. Avoid alcohol.

ZONISAMIDE
(zoe-NIS-a-mide)

NEWLY DISCOVERED USES (OFF-LABEL)
> Obesity

ORIGINAL USES (ON-LABEL)
Epilepsy

BRAND NAME
Zonegran

DRUG CLASS
Anticonvulsant

DESCRIPTION
This drug may act on the sodium and calcium channels for neurons.

POTENTIAL SIDE EFFECTS
Somnolence, dizziness, anorexia, headache, agitation, fatigue,
tiredness, uncoordinated gait, confusion, depression, insomnia,
speech disorders, mental slowing, nervousness, rash, nausea, abdominal pain, diarrhea, double vision, anxiety, difficulty concentrating, memory impairment, uncontrolled eye movements,
numbness, speech abnormalities, flu syndrome.

CAUTIONS
- Notify your doctor if you are allergic to sulfonamide drugs, or if
  you have kidney or liver problems.
- Discontinue medication if rash or kidney problems develop.
- Decreased sweating and temperature irregulation (increased
  body temperatures) has been reported in children.

- Abrupt withdrawal may precipitate seizures; decrease dose gradually.

DRUG INTERACTIONS

Other drugs that cause sedation (central nervous system depressants), carbamazepine, phenobarbital, phenytoin, valproate, rifampin.

This drug is metabolized (cleared from the body) by a specific set of liver enzymes (cytochrome P450 enzymes 3A4). Several other drugs interfere with these liver enzymes, and thus may increase or decrease the clearance of zonisamide from the body, potentially increasing the risk of side effects or decreasing effectiveness. When these drugs are given in combination with zonisamide, dosage adjustments may be needed. As these are too numerous to list, you should always check with your doctor or pharmacist prior to starting a new medication, herbal, or nonprescription product.

FOOD INTERACTIONS

Alcohol

HERBAL INTERACTIONS

Unknown

PREGNANCY AND BREAST-FEEDING CAUTIONS

FDA Pregnancy Risk Category C. Discuss with your doctor if you are planning to become pregnant. Excretion in breast milk is unknown. Do not breast-feed while taking this medication.

SPECIAL CONSIDERATIONS

This medication can cause severe central nervous system depression (such as sedation, etc.), so use caution while performing certain tasks until effects upon performance can be determined. Contact your doctor if any of the following occur: skin rash, sudden back pain, abdominal pain, blood in the urine, fever, sore throat, oral ulcers, if seizures worsen, or easy bruising. Drink 6–8 glasses of water each day while using this medication.

PART III

DRUG
INFORMATION

Recently Approved FDA Drugs

INDICATION	GENERIC NAME	BRAND NAME
Alcohol dependence	Acamprosate calcium	Campral
Appendicitis, diagnosis equivocal	T99m TC	Fanolesomab, NeutroSpec
Bronchitis/sinusitis, acute, Community acquired pneumonia	Telithromycin	Ketek
Bronchospasm of chronic obstructive pulmonary disease, long-term therapy	Tiotropium bromide	Spiriva
Colon cancer, first line therapy for metastatic	Bevacizumab	Avastin
Colon cancer, refractory EGFR-expressing metastatic	Cetuximab	Erbitux
Complicated skin and skin structure Iinfections (cSSSI) and complicated intra-abdominal infections (cIAI)	Tigecycline	Tygacil
Depression, Diabetic neuropathy	Duloxetine	Cymbalta
Diabetes, Type 1 and 2, as an adjunct treatment in patients who use mealtime insulin therapy	Pramlintide acetate	Symlin

Diabetes, Type 2	Exenatide	Byetta
Diabetes, mellitus, Type 1 or Type 2	Insulin detemir	Levemir
Diabetes mellitus	Insulin glulisine	Apidra
Hepatitis B virus infection, chronic	Entecavir	Baraclude
HIV infection	Lamivudine/abacavir	Epzicom
HIV infection	Tenofovir/emtricitabine	Truvada
HIV, correction of lipoatrophy	Poly-L-Latctic acid	Sculptra
Antiretroviral HIV-1 infection	Tipranavir	Aptivus
Hypercholesterolemia	Ezetimibe/simvastatin	Vytorin
Increase absorption of injected drugs, improve resorption of radiopaque agents	Hyaluronidase (ovine)	Vitrase
Insomnia	Eszopiclone	Lunesta
Insomnia	Ramelteon	Rozerem
Leukemia, acute lymphoblastic (pediatrics)	Clofarabine	Clolar
Lung caner, metastatic nonsmall cell.	Erlotinib	Tarceva
Macular degeneration, age related	Pegaptanib	Macugen
Malignant pleural mesothelioma	Pemetrexed disodium	Alimta
MRI of central nervous system in adults	Gadobenate dimeglumine	Multihance

INDICATION	GENERIC NAME	BRAND NAME
Mucopolysaccharidosis	Naglazyme	Galsulfase
Multiple sclerosis	Natalizumab	Tysabri
Overactive bladder	Darifenacin	Enablex
Overactive bladder	Solifenacin succinate	VESIcare
Overactive bladder	Trospium chloride	Sanctura
Pain and inflammation associated with cataract surgery	Nevanac	Nepafenac
Parkinson's disease (hypomobility)	Apomorphine hydrochloride	Apokyn
Prophylaxis of *Candida* infections in patients undergoing hematopoietic stem cell transplantation	Micafungin sodium	Mycamine
Pulmonary hypertension	Iloprost	Ventavis
Refractory anemia, Chronic myelomonocytic leukemia	Azacitidine	Vidaza
Renal disease, end stage, serum phosphate reducer in	Lanthanum	Fosrenol
Secondary hyperparathyroidism in chronic kidney disease patients on dialysis	Cinacalcet hydrochloride	Sensipar

Seizure, neuropathy	Pregabalin	Lyrica
Severe chronic pain requiring intrathecal therapy	Ziconotide	Prialt
Short bowel syndrome	L-Glutamine	NutreStore
Short stature in children	Mecasermin	Increlex
Traveler's diarrhea (noninvasive E. Coli)	Rifaximin	Xifaxan
Trichomoniasis, Giardiasis, Amebiasis	Tinidazole	Tindamaz
Triglycerides, high levels	Omega-3 acid ethyl esters	Omacor

Sugar-Free Drugs

Listed below, by therapeutic category, is a selection of drugs that contain no sugar. Diabetic patients should keep in mind that many of these products may contain sorbitol, alcohol, or other sources of carbohydrates. This list should not be considered comprehen-sive. Generics and alternate brands of some products may be available. Check product labeling for a current listing of inactive ingredients.

Analgesics

Actamin Maximum Strength Liquid
Addaprin Tablet
Aminofen Tablet
Aminofen Max Tablet
Aspirtab Tablet
Back Pain-Off Tablet
Backprin Tablet
Buffasal Tablet
Dyspel Tablet
Febrol Liquid
I-Prin Tablet
Medi-Seltzer Effervescent Tablet
Ms. Aid Tablet
PMS Relief Tablet
Silapap Children's Elixir

Antacids/Antiflatulents

Almag Chewable Tablet
Alcalak Chewable Tablet
Aldroxicon I Suspension
Aldroxicon II Suspension
Baby Gasz Drops
Dimacid Chewable Tablet
Diotame Chewable Tablet
Diotame Suspension
Gas-Ban Chewable
Mallamint Chewable
Mylanta Gelcaplet

Neutralin Tablet
Tums E-X Chewable Tablet

Antiasthmatic/Respiratory Agents

Jay-Phyl Syrup

Antidiarrheals

Diarrest Tablet
Di-Gon II Tablet
Imogen Liquid

Blood Modifiers/Iron Preparations

I.L.X. B-12 Elixir
Irofel Liquid
Nephro-Fer Tablet

Corticosteroids

Pediapred Solution

Cough/Cold/Allergy Preparations

Accuhist DM Pediatric Drops
Accuhist DM Pediatric Liquid
Accuhist Pediatric Drops
Alacol DM Syrup
Amerifed DM Liquid
Amerifed Liquid
Amerituss AD Solution
Anaplex DM Syrup
Anaplex HD Syrup
Andehist DM Liquid
Andehist DM NR Liquid
Andehist DM NR Syrup
Andehist DM Syrup
Andehist Liquid
Andehist NR Liquid
Andehist NR Syrup
Andehist Syrup

Atuss EX Liquid
Atuss NX Solution
Baltussin Solution
Bellahist-D LA Tablet
Benadryl Allergy/Sinus Children's Solution
Biodec DM Drops
Biodec DM Syrup
Bromaxefed DM RF Syrup
Bromaxefed RF Syrup
Bromdec Solution
Bromdec DM Solution
Bromhist-DM Solution
Bromhist Pediatric Solution
Bromophed DX Syrup
Bromphenex DM Solution
Bromphenex HD Solution
Bromplex DM Solution
Bromplex HD Solution
Broncotron Liquid
Broncotron-D Suspension
Brovex HC Solution
B-Tuss Liquid
Carbaphen 12 Ped Suspension
Carbaphen 12 Suspension
Carbatuss-CL Solution
Carbetaplex Solution
Carbihist Solution
Carbinoxamine PSE Solution
Carbofed DM Syrup
Carbofed DM Drops
Carboxine Solution
Carboxine-PSE Solution
Cardec DM Syrup
Cetafen Cold Tablet
Cheratussin DAC Liquid
Chlordex GP Syrup
Codal-DM Syrup
ColdCough EXP Solution
ColdCough HC Solution
ColdCough PD Solution
ColdCough Solution
ColdCough XP Solution

Coldec DS Solution
ColdMist DM Syrup
Coldonyl Tablet
Colidrops Pediatric Liquid
Cordron-D Solution
Cordron-DM Solution
Cordron-HC Solution
Corfen DM Solution
Co-Tussin Liquid
Cotuss-V Syrup
Coughtuss Solution
Crantex HC Syrup
Crantex Syrup
Cypex-LA Tablet
Cytuss HC Syrup
Dacex-A Solution
Dacex-DM Solution
Dacex-PE Solution
Decahist-DM Solution
De-Chlor DM Solution
De-Chlor DR Solution
De-Chlor G Solution
De-Chlor HC Solution
De-Chlor HD Solution
De-Chlor MR Solution
De-Chlor NX Solution
Decorel Forte Tablet
Despec Liquid
Despec-SF Liquid
Dexcon-DM Solution
Diabetic Tussin Allergy Relief Liquid
Diabetic Tussin Allergy Relief Gelcaplet
Diabetic Tussin DM Liquid
Diabetic Tussin EX Liquid
Dimetapp Allergy Children's Elixir
Diphen Capsule
Double-Tussin DM Liquid
Drocon-CS Solution
Dynatuss Syrup
Dynatuss HC Solution
Dynatuss HCG Solution
Dytan-CS Tablet

Echotuss-HC Syrup
Emagrin Forte Tablet
Endacof DM Solution
Endacof HC Solution
Endacof XP Solution
Endacof-PD Solution
Endal HD Liquid
Endal HD Plus Liquid
Endotuss-HD Syrup
Enplus-HD Syrup
Entex Syrup
Entex HC Syrup
Exo-Tuss Syrup
Ganidin NR Liquid
Gani-Tuss NR Liquid
Gani-Tuss-DM NR Liquid
Genebronco-D Liquid
Genecof-HC Liquid
Genecof-XP Liquid
Genedel Syrup
Genedotuss-DM Liquid
Genelan Liquid
Genetuss-2 Liquid
Genexpect DM Liquid
Genexpect-PE Liquid
Genexpect-SF Liquid
Gilphex TR Tablet
Giltuss Liquid
Giltuss HC Syrup
Giltuss Pediatric Liquid
Giltuss TR Tablet
Guai-Co Liquid
Guaicon DMS Liquid
Guai-DEX Liquid
Guaitussin AC Solution
Guaitussin DAC Solution
Guapetex HC Solution
Guapetex Syrup
Guiatuss AC Syrup
Guiatuss DAC Syrup
Halotussin AC Liquid
Halotussin DAC Liquid

Hayfebrol Liquid
Histacol DM Pediatric Solution
Histex PD Liquid
Histex PD 12 Suspension
Histinex HC Syrup
Histinex PV Syrup
Histuss HC Solution
Histuss PD Solution
Hydex-PD Solution
Hydone Liquid
Hydro-DP Solution
Hydro GP Syrup
Hydro PC Syrup
Hydro PC II Plus Solution
Hydro Pro Solution
Hydrocof-HC Solution
Hydron CP Syrup
Hydron EX Syrup
Hydron KGS Liquid
Hydron PSC Liquid
Hydro-Tussin CBX Solution
Hydro-Tussin DM Elixir
Hydro-Tussin HC Syrup
Hydro-Tussin HD Liquid
Hydro-Tussin XP Syrup
Hytuss Tablet
Hytuss 2X Capsule
Iofen-C NF Liquid
Iofen-DM NF Liquid
Iofen-NF Liquid
Jaycof Expectorant Syrup
Jaycof-HC Liquid
Jaycof-XP Liquid
Kita LA Tos Liquid
Lemotussin-DM Liquid
Lodrane Liquid
Lortuss DM Solution
Lortuss HC Solution
Lusonal Solution
Marcof Expectorant Syrup
Maxi-tuss HCX Solution
M-Clear Syrup

Mintex PD Liquid
Mintuss NX Solution Syrup
Mytussin DAC Syrup
Nalex DH Liquid
Nalex-A Liquid
Nasop Suspension
Neotuss S/F Liquid
Nescon-PD Tablet
Norel DM Liquid
Norel SD Solution
Nycoff Tablet
Onset Forte Tablet
Orgadin Liquid
Orgadin-Tuss Liquid
Orgadin-Tuss DM Liquid
Organidin NR Liquid
Organidin NR Tablet
Palgic-DS Syrup
Pancof Syrup
Pancof EXP Syrup
Pancof HC Solution
Pancof XP Liquid
Pancof XP Solution
Panmist DM Syrup
Pediatex D
Pediatex DM Liquid
Pediatex HC Solution
Phanasin Syrup
Phanasin Diabetic Choice Syrup
Phanatuss Syrup
Phanatuss DM Diabetic Choice Syrup
Phanatuss-HC Diabetic Choice Solution
Phenabid DM Tablet
Phenydryl Solution
Pneumotussin 2.5 Syrup
Poly Hist PD Solution
Poly-Tussin Syrup
Poly-Tussin DM Syrup
Poly-Tussin HD Syrup
Poly-Tussin XP Syrup
Pro-Clear Solution
Pro-Cof Liquid

Pro-Cof D Liquid
Pro-Red Solution
Prolex DH Liquid
Prolex DM Liquid
Protex Solution
Protex D Solution
Protuss Liquid
Quintex Syrup
Quintex HC Syrup
Relacon-DM Liquid
Relacon-DM Solution
Relacon-HC Solution
Rhinacon A Solution
Rhinacon DH Solution
Rindal HD Liquid
Rindal HD Plus Solution
Rindal HPD Solution
Romilar AC Liquid
Romilar DM Liquid
Rondamine DM Liquid
Rondec Syrup
Rondec DM Syrup
Rondec DM Drops
Ru-Tuss A Syrup
Ru-Tuss DM Syrup
Scot-Tussin Allergy Relief Formula Liquid
Scot-Tussin DM Cough Chasers Lozenge
Scot-Tussin Original Liquid
Siladryl Allergy Liquid
Siladryl DAS Liquid
Sildec Syrup
Sildec Drops
Sildec-DM Syrup
Silexin Syrup
Silexin Tablet
Sil-Tex Liquid Liquid
Siltussin DM DAS Cough Formula Syrup
S-T Forte 2 Liquid
Statuss Green Liquid
Sudodrin Tablet
Sudafed Children's Cold & Cough Solution
Sudafed Children's Solution

Sudafed Children's Tablet
Sudanyl Tablet
Sudatuss-SF Liquid
Sudodrin Tablet
Supress DX Pediatric Drops
Suttar-SF Syrup
Triant-HC Solution
Tricodene Syrup
Trispec-PE Liquid
Trituss DM Solution
Trituss Solution
Tri-Vent DM Solution
Tusdec-DM Solution
Tusdec-HC Solution
Tusnel Solution
Tussafed Syrup
Tussafed-EX Pediatric Drops
Tussafed-HC Syrup
Tussall Solution
Tuss-DM Liquid
Tuss-ES Syrup
Tussi-Organidin DM NR Liquid
Tussi-Organidin DM-S NR Liquid
Tussi-Organidin NR Liquid
Tussi-Organidin-S NR Liquid
Tussi-Pres Liquid
Tussirex Liquid
Uni Cof EXP Solution
Uni Cof Solution
Uni-Lev 5.0 Solution
Vazol Solution
Vi-Q-Tuss Syrup
Vitussin Expectorant Syrup
Vortex Syrup
Welltuss EXP Solution
Welltuss HC Solution
Z-Cof HC Syrup
Ztuss Expectorant Solution
Zyrtec Syrup

Fluoride Preparations

Ethedent Chewable Tablet
Fluor-A-Day Tablet
Fluor-A-Day Lozenge
Flura-Loz Tablet
Lozi-Flur Lozenge
Sensodyne w/ Fluoride Gel
Sensodyne w/ Fluoride Tartar Control Toothpaste
Sensodyne w/ Fluoride Toothpaste

Laxatives

Citrucel Powder
Fiber Ease Liquid
Fibro-XL Capsule
Genfiber Powder
Konsyl Easy Mix Formula Powder
Konsyl-Orange Powder
Metamucil Smooth Texture Powder
Reguloid Powder

Miscellaneous

Acidoll Capsule
Alka-Gest Tablet
Bicitra Solution
Colidrops Pediatric Drops
Cytra-2 Solution
Cytra-K Solution
Cytra-K Crystals
Melatin Tablet
Methadose Solution
Neutra-Phos Powder
Neutra-Phos-K Powder
Polycitra-K Solution
Polycitra-LC Solution
Questran Light Powder

Mouth/Throat Preparations

Aquafresh Triple Protection Gum
Cepacol Maximum Strength Spray

Cepacol Sore Throat Lozenges
Cepacol Sore Throat Spray
Cylex Lozenges
Fisherman's Friend Lozenges
Fresh N Free Liquid
Isodettes Sore Throat Spray
Larynex Lozenges
Listerine Pocketpaks Film
Medikoff Drops
Oragesic Solution
Orasept Mouthwash/Gargle Liquid
Robitussin Lozenges
Sepasoothe Lozenges
Thorets Maximum Strength Lozenges
Throto-Ceptic Spray
Vademecum Mouthwash and Gargle Concentrate

Potassium Supplements

Cena K Liquid
Kaon Elixir
Kaon-CI 20% Liquid
Rum-K Liquid

Vitamins/Minerals/Supplements

Action-Tabs Made For Men
Adaptosode For Stress Liquid
Adaptosode R + R For Acute Stress Liquid
Alamag Tablet
Alcalak Tablet
Aldroxicon I Suspension
Aldroxicon II Suspension
Aminoplex Powder
Aminostasis Powder
Aminotate Powder
Apetigen Elixir
Apptrim Capsule
Apptrim-D Capsule
B-C-Bid Caplet
Bevitamel Tablet
Biosode Liquid

Biotect Plus Caplet
C & M Caps-375 Capsule
Calbon Tablet
Cal-Cee Tablet
Calcet Plus Tablet
Calcimin-300 Tablet
Cal-Mint Chewable Tablet
Cena K Solution
Cerefolin Tablet
Cevi-Bid Tablet
Choice DM Liquid
Cholestratin Tablet
Chromacaps Tablet
Chromium K6 Tablet
Citrimax 500 Plus Tablet
Combi-Cart Tablet
Daily Herbs Formulas
Delta D3 Tablet
Detoxosode Liquids
Dexfol Tablet
DHEA Capsule
Diabeze Tablet
Diatx Tablet
Diet System 6 Gum
Dimacid Tablet
Diucaps Capsule
Di-Phen-500 Capsule Electrotab Tablet
Endorphenyl Capsule
Ensure Nutra Shake Pudding
Enterex Diabetic Liquid
Essential Nutrients Plus Silica Tablet
Evening Primrose Oil Capsule
Evolve Softgel
Ex-L Tablet
Extress Tablet
Eyetamins Tablet
Fem-Cal Tablet
Fem-Cal Plus Tablet
Ferrocite F Tablet
Folacin-800 Tablet
Folbee Plus Tablet
Folplex 2.2 Tablet

Foltx Tablet
Gabadone Capsule
Gram-O-Leci Tablet
Hemovit Tablet
Herbal Slim Complex Capsule
Irofol Liquid
Lynae Calcium/Vitamin C Chewable Tablet
Lynae Chondroitin/Glucosamine Capsule
Lynae Ginse-Cool Chewable Tablet
Mag-Caps Capsule
Mag-Ox 400 Tablet
Mag-SR Tablet
Magimin Tablet
Magnacaps Capsule
Mangimin Capsule
Mangimin Tablet
Medi-Lyte Tablet
Multi-Delyn w/ Iron Liquid
Nephro-Fer Tablet
Neutra-Phos Powder
Neutra-Phos-K Powder
New Life Hair Tablet
Nutrisure OTC Tablet
O-Cal FA Tablet
Plenamins Plus Tablet
Powervites Tablet
Prostaplex Herbal Complex Capsule
Prostatonin Capsule
Protect Plus Liquid
Protect Plus NR Softgel
Pulmona Capsule
Quintabs-M Tablet
Re/Neph Liquid
Replace Capsule
Replace w/o Iron Capsule
Resource Arginaid Powder
Ribo-100 T.D. Capsule
Samolinic Softgel
Sea Omega 30 Softgel
Sea Omega 50 Softgel
Sentra AM Capsule
Sentra PM Capsule

Soy Care for Bone Health Tablet
Soy Care for Menopause Capsule
Span C Tablet
Strovite Forte Syrup
Sunnie Tablet
Sunvite Tablet
Super Dec B100 Tablet
Super Quints-50 Tablet
Supervite Liquid
Suplevit Liquid
Theramine Capsule
Triamin Tablet
Triamino Tablet
Ultramino Powder
Uro-Mag Capsule
Vinatal 600 Kit
Vitalize Liquid
Vitamin C/Rose Hips Tablet
Vitrum JR Chewable Tablet
Xtramins Tablet
Yohimbe Power Max 1500 For Women Tablet
Yohimbized 1000 Capsule
Ze-Plus Softgel

Alcohol-Free Drugs

The following is a selection of alcohol-free products grouped by therapeutic category. The list is not comprehensive. Generic and alternate brands may exist. Always check product labeling for definitive information on specific ingredients.

Analgesics

Acetaminophen Infants Drops
Actamin Maximum Strength Liquid
Addaprin Tablet
Aminofen Max Tablet
APAP Elixir
Aspirtab Tablet
Buffasal Tablet
Demerol Hydrochloride Syrup
Dolono Elixir
Dysepl Tablet
Genapap Children Elixir
Genapap Infants' Drops
Motrin Children's Suspension
Motrin Infants' Suspension
Silapap Children's Elixir
Silapap Infants' Drops
Tylenol Children's Suspension
Tylenol Extra Strength Solution
Tylenol Infants' Drops
Tylenol Infants' Suspension

Antiasthmatics

Dilor-G Liquid
Dy-G Liquid
Elixophyllin-GG Liquid

Anticonvulsants

Zarontin Syrup

Antivirals

Epivir Oral Solution

Cough/Cold/Allergy Preparations

Accuhist Pediatric Drops
Alacol DM Syrup
Allergy Relief Medicine Children's Elixir
Altarussin Syrup
Amerifed DM Liquid
Amerifed Liquid
Anaplex DM Syrup
Anaplex HD Syrup
Andehist DM Drops
Andehist HD Syrup
Andehist DM NR Liquid
Andehist DM NR Syrup
Andehist NR Syrup
Andehist Syrup
Aquatab DM Syrup
Atuss DR Syrup
Atuss EX Liquid
Atuss G Liquid
Atuss HC Syrup
Atuss MS Syrup
Baltussin Solution
Benadryl Allergy Solution
Benadryl Allergy/Sinus Children's Solution
Biodec DM Drops
Biodec DM Syrup
Bromaline Solution
Bromaline DM Elixir
Bromanate Elixir
Bromaxefed DM RF Syrup
Bromaxefed RF Syrup
Broncotron Liquid
Bromdec Solution
Bromdec DM Solution
Bromhist Pediatric Solution
Bromhist-DM Pediatric Syrup
Bromhist-DM Solution

Bromphenex HD Solution
Bromplex DM Solution
Bromplex HD Solution
Broncotron-D Suspension
Bron-Tuss Liquid
Brovex HC Solution
B-Tuss Liquid
Carbaphen 12 Ped Suspension
Carbaphen 12 Suspension
Carbafuss Liquid
Carbaxefed DM RF Liquid
Carbetaplex Solution
Carbihist Solution
Carbofed DM Drops
Carbofed DM Syrup
Carboxine Solution
Carboxine-PSE Solution
Cardec Syrup
Cardec DM Syrup
Cepacol Sore Throat Liquid
Chlordex GP Syrup
Chlor-Mes D Solution Chlor-Trimeton Allergy Syrup
Codal-DH Syrup
Codal-DM Syrup
Codofuss Liquid
Coldec DS Solution
Coldec-DM Syrup
Coldmist DM Solution
Coldmist DM Syrup
Coldmist S Syrup
Coldonyl Tablet
Coldfuss DR Syrup
Colidrops Pediatric Liquid
Complete Allergy Elixir
Cordron-D Solution
Cordron-DM Solution
Cordron-HC Solution
Corfen DM Solution
Co-Tussin Liquid
Cotuss-V Syrup
Crantex HC Syrup
Crantex Syrup

Creomulsion Complete Syrup
Creomulsion Cough Syrup
Creomulsion For Children Syrup
Cremulsion Pediatric Syrup
Cyfuss HC Syrup
Dacex-DM Solution
Decahist-DM Solution
De-Chlor DM Solution
De-Chlor DR Solution
Dehistine Syrup
Deituss Liquid
Deka Liquid
Deka Pediatric Drops Solution
Despec Liquid
Dex PC Syrup
Dexcon-DM Solution
Diabetic Tussin Allergy Relief Liquid
Diabetic Tussin C Expectorant Liquid
Diabetic Tussin Cold & Flu Tablet
Diabetic Tussin DM Liquid
Diabetic Tussin DM Maximum Strength Capsule
Diabetic Tussin DM Maximum Strength Liquid
Diabetic Tussin EX Liquid
Dimetapp Allergy Children's Elixir
Dimetapp Cold & Fever Children's Suspension
Dimetapp Decongestant Pediatric Drops
Double-Tussin DM Liquid
Drocon-CS Solution
Duradal HD Plus Syrup
Duratan DM Suspension
Dynatuss Syrup
Dynatuss EX Syrup
Dynatuss HC Solution
Dynatuss HCG Solution
Echotuss-HC Solution
Endacof DM Solution
Endacof HC Solution
Endacof XP Solution
Endagen-HD Syrup
Endal HD Solution
Endal HD Syrup
Endal HD Plus Syrup

Endotuss-HD Syrup
Enplus-HD Syrup
Entex Syrup
Entex HC Syrup
Exo-Tuss
Father John's Medicine Plus Drops
Friallergia DM Liquid
Friallergia Liquid
Ganidin NR Liquid
Gani-Tuss NR Liquid
Gani-Tuss-DM NR Liquid
Genahist Elixir
Genebronco-D Liquid
Genecof-HC Liquid
Genecof-XP Liquid
Genecof-XP Syrup
Genedel Syrup
Genedotuss-DM Liquid
Genepatuss Liquid
Genetuss-2 Liquid
Genexpect-DM Liquid
Genexpect-PE Liquid
Genexpect-SF Liquid
Giltuss HC Syrup
Giltuss Liquid
Giltuss Pediatric Liquid
Guai-Co Liquid
Guaicon DMS Liquid
Guai-Dex Liquid
Guaifed Syrup
Guaitussin AC Solution
Guaitussin DAC Solution
Guapetex HC Solution
Guapetex Syrup
Halotussin AC Liquid
Hayfebrol Liquid
H-C Tussive Syrup
Histacol DM Pediatric Solution
Histacol DM Pediatric Syrup
Histex HC Syrup
Histex Liquid
Histex PD Drops

Histex PD Liquid
Histinex HC Syrup
Histinex PV Syrup
Histuss HC Solution
Hi-Tuss Syrup
Hycomal DH Liquid
Hydex-PD Solution
Hydone Liquid
Hydramine Elixir
Hydro PC Syrup
Hydro PC II Plus Solution
Hydro Pro Solution
Hydrocof-HC Solution
Hydro-DP Solution
Hydron CP Syrup
Hydron EX Syrup
Hydron KGS Liquid
Hydron PSC Liquid
Hydro-Tussin DM Elixir
Hydro-Tussin HC Syrup
Hydro-Tussin HD Liquid
Hydro-Tussin XP Syrup
Hyphen-HD Syrup
Iofen-C NF Liquid
Iofen-DM NF Liquid
Iofen-NF Liquid
Jaycof Expectorant Syrup
Jaycof-HC Liquid
Jaycof-XP Liquid
Kita La Tos Liquid
Lemotussin-DM Liquid
Levall Liquid
Levall 5.0 Liquid
Lodrane Liquid
Lohist D Syrup
Lortuss DM Solution
Lortuss HC Solution
Marcof Expectorant Syrup
Maxi-Tuss HCX Solution
M-Clear Syrup
Medi-Brom Elixir
Mintex Liquid

Mintex PD Liquid
Mintuss DM Syrup
Mintuss EX Syrup
Mintuss G Syrup
Mintuss HD Syrup
Mintuss MR Syrup
Mintuss MS Syrup
Mintuss NX Solution
Motrin Cold Children's Suspension
Mytussin-PE Liquid
Nalex DH Liquid
Nalex-A Liquid
Nalspan Senior DX Liquid
Nasop Suspension
Neotuss S/F Liquid
Neotuss-D Liquid
Norel DM Liquid
Norel SD Solution
Nucofed Syrup
Nycoff Tablet
Orgadin-Tuss Liquid
Orgadin-Tuss DM Liquid
Organidin NR Liquid
Palgic-DS Syrup
Pancof Syrup
Pancof EXP Syrup
Pancof HC Liquid
Pancof XP Liquid
Panmist DM Syrup
Panmist-S Syrup
PediaCare Cold + Allergy Children's Liquid
PediaCare Cough + Cold Children's Liquid
PediaCare Decongestant Infants Drops
PediaCare Decongestant Plus Cough Drops
PediaCare Multi-Symptom Liquid
PediaCare Nightrest Liquid
Pediahist DM Syrup
Pedia-Relief Liquid
Pediatex Liquid
Pediatex-D Liquid
Pediox Liquid
Phanasin Syrup

Phanatuss Syrup
Phanatuss-HC Diabetic Choice Solution
Phena-S Liquid
Pneumotussin 2.5 Syrup
Poly Hist PD Solution
Poly-Tussin Syrup
Poly-Tussin DM Syrup
Poly-Tussin HD Syrup
Poly-Tussin XP Syrup
Primsol Solution
Pro-Clear Solution
Pro-Cof Liquid
Pro-Cof D Liquid
Prolex DH Liquid
Prolex DM Liquid
Pro-Red Solution
Protex Solution
Protex D Solution
Protuss Liquid
Protuss-D Liquid
Pyrroxate Extra Strength Tablet
Q-Tussin PE Liquid
Quintex Syrup
Quintex HC Syrup
Relacon-DM Solution
Relacon-HC Solution
Rescon-DM Liquid
Rescon-GG Liquid
Rhinacon A Solution
Rhinacon DH Solution
Rindal HD Liquid
Rindal HD Plus Solution
Rindal HPD Solution
Robitussin Cough & Congestion Liquid
Robitussin DM Syrup
Robitussin PE Syrup
Robitussin Pediatric Drops
Robitussin Pediatric Cough Syrup
Robitussin Pediatric Night Relief Liquid
Romilar AC Liquid
Romilar DM Liquid
Rondamine DM Liquid

Rondec Syrup
Rondec DM Drops
Rondec DM Syrup
Ru-Tuss A Syrup
Ru-Tuss DM Syrup
Scot-Tussin Allergy Relief Formula Liquid
Scot-Tussin DM Liquid
Scot-Tussin Expectorant Liquid
Scot-Tussin Original Syrup
Scot-Tussin Senior Liquid
Siladryl Allergy Liquid
Siladryl DAS Liquid
Sildec Liquid
Sildec Syrup
Sildec-DM Drops
Sildec-DM Syrup
Sil-Tex Liquid
Siltussin DAS Liquid
Siltussin DM Syrup
Siltussin DM DAS Cough Formula Syrup
Siltussin SA Syrup
Simply Cough Liquid
Simply Stuffy Liquid
S-T Forte 2 Liquid
Statuss DM Syrup
Sudafed Children's Cold & Cough Solution
Sudafed Children's Solution
Sudafed Children's Tablet
Sudal Liquid Solution
Sudanyl Tablet
Sudatuss DM Syrup
Sudatuss-2 Liquid
Sudatuss-SF Liquid
Triaminic Infant Decongestant Drops
Triant-HC Solution
Trispec-PE Liquid
Trituss DM Solution
Trituss Solution
Tri-Vent DM Solution
Tri-Vent DPC Syrup
Tusdec-DM Solution
Tusdec-HC Solution

Tusnel Pediatric Solution
Tusnel Solution
Tussafed Syrup
Tussafed-EX Syrup
Tussafed-EX Pediatric Liquid
Tussafed-HC Syrup
Tussall Solution
Tussbid Capsule
Tuss-DM Liquid
Tuss-ES Syrup
Tussex Syrup
Tussinate Syrup
Tussi-Organidin DM NR Liquid
Tussi-Organidin DM-S NR Liquid
Tussi-Organidin NR Liquid
Tuss-Organidin-S NR Liquid
Tussi-Pres Liquid
Tussirex Liquid
Tussirex Syrup
Tylenol Allergy-D Children's Liquid
Tylenol Cold Children's Liquid
Tylenol Cold Children's Suspension
Tylenol Cold Infants' Drops
Tylenol Cold Plus Cough Infants' Suspension
Tylenol Flu Children's Suspension
Tylenol Flu Nighttime Maximum Strength Liquid
Tylenol Sinus Children's Liquid
Uni-Lev 5.0 Solution
Vanex-HD Syrup
Vazol Solution
Vicks 44E Pediatric Liquid
Vicks 44M Pediatric Liquid
Vicks Dayquil Multi-Symptom Liquicap
Vicks Dayquil Multi-Symptom Liquid
Vicks 44 Liquid Capsules Cold, Flu, Cough
Vicks Nyquil Children's Liquid
Vicks Sinex 12 Hour Spray
Vicks Sinex Spray
Vi-Q-Tuss Syrup
V-Tann Suspension
Vitussin Expectorant Syrup
Vortex Syrup

Welltuss EXP Solution
Welltuss HC Solution
Z-Cof DM Syrup
Z-Cof HC Syrup
Ztuss Expectorant Solution

Ear/Nose/Throat Products

4-Way Saline Moisturizing Mist Spray
Ayr Baby Saline Spray
Bucalcide Solution
Bucalcide Spray
Bucalsep Solution
Bucalsep Spray
Cepacol Sore Throat Liquid
Cheracol Sore Throat Spray
Fresh N Free Liquid
Gly-Oxide Liquid
Isodettes Sore Throat Spray
Lacrosse Mouthwash Liquid
Larynex Lozenges
Listermint Liquid
Nasal Moist Gel
Orajel Baby Liquid
Orajel Baby Nighttime Gel
Oramagic Oral Wound Rinse Powder for Suspension
Orasept Mouthwash/Gargle Liquid
Tanac Liquid
Tech 2000 Dental Rinse Liquid
Throto-Ceptic Spray
Zilactin Baby Extra Strength Gel

Gastrointestinal Products

Axid
Baby Gasz Drops
Colidrops Pediatric Drops
Diarrest Tablet
Imogen Liquid
Kaodene NN Suspension
Liqui-Doss Liquid
Mylicon Infants' Suspension

Neoloid Liquid
Neutralin Tablet
Senokot Children's Syrup

Hematinics

Irofol Liquid

Miscellaneous

Cytra-2 Solution
Cytra-K Solution
Emetrol Solution
Fluorinse Solution
Rum-K Liquid

Psychotropics

Thorazine Syrup

Topical Products

Aloe Vesta 2-N-1 Antifungal Ointment
Blistex Complete Moisture Stick
Blistex Fruit Smoothies Stick
Blistex Herbal Answer Gel
Blistex Herbal Answer Stick
Dermatone Lips N Face Protector Ointment
Dermatone Moisturizing Sunblock Cream
Dermatone Outdoor Skin Protection Cream
Dermatone Skin Protector Cream
Eucapsulein Facial Lotion
Fleet Pain Relief Pads Fresh & Pure Douche Solution
Handclens Solution
Joint-Ritis Maximum Strength Ointment
Klenz Kloth Pads
Neutrogena Acne Wash Liquid
Neutrogena Antiseptic Liquid
Neutrogena Clear Pore Gel
Neutrogena T/Derm Liquid
Neutrogena Toner Liquid
Podiclens Spray

Propa pH Foaming Face Wash Liquid
Sea Breeze Foaming Face Wash Gel
Shade Uvaguard Lotion
Sportz Bloc Cream
Stri-Dex Pad
Stri-Dex Maximum Strength Pad
Stri-Dex Sensitive Skin Pad
Stri-Dex Super Scrub Pad
Therasoft Anti-Acne Cream
Therasoft Skin Protectant Cream
Tiger Balm Arthritis Rub Lotion

Vitamins/Minerals/Supplements

Adaptosode For Stress Liquid
Adaptosode R+R for Acute Stress Liquid
Apetigen Elixir
Biosode Liquid
Detoxosode Products Liquid
Folplex 2.2 Gel
Genesupp-500 Liquid
Genetect Plus Liquid
Multi-Delyn w/ Iron Liquid
Poly-Vi-Sol Drops
Poly-Vi-Sol w/ Iron Drops
Poly-Vi-Solution Liquid
Poly-Vi-Solution w/ Iron Liquid
Protect Plus Liquid
Soluvite-F Drops
Strovite Forte Syrup
Supervite Liquid
Suplevit Liquid
Tri-Vi-Sol Drops
Tri-Vi-Sol w/ Iron Drops
Vitafol Syrup
Vitalize Liquid
Vitamin C/Rose Hips Tablet Extended Release

Sulfite-Containing Drugs

The following is a selection of drugs that contain sulfites, a common allergic trigger. Please remember, however, that the list is not comprehensive. Always check product labeling for definitive information on specific ingredients.

Drug	Generic Name
Amikacin Sulfate Injection	Amikacin sulfate
Amikin Injectable	Amikacin sulfate
Apolyn	Apomorphine hydrochloride
Aramine Injection	Metaraminol
Betagan Liquifilm	Levobunolol
Campral (residual traces)	Acamprosate calcium
Claripel Cream	Hydroquinone
Coriopam Injection	Fenoldopam
Cortisporin Otic Solution	Hydrocortisone/ neomycin sulfate/ polymyxin B
Decadron Phosphate Ophthalmic Solution	Dexamethasone sodium phosphate
Decadron Phosphate Injection	Dexamethasone sodium phosphate
Dilaudid Oral Liquid; Dilaudid Tablets-8mg	Hydromorphone
Dobutrex Solution	Dobutamine
Duranest Injections	Etidocaine/epinephrine bitartrate
Epifrin	Epinephrine hydro-chloride
EpiPen Auto-Injector	Epinephrine
EpiPen Jr.	Epinephrine
Equin Micro	Hydroquinone
Equin Micro XD	Hydroquinone
Fungizone Oral	Amphotericin B
Garamycin Injectable	Gentamicin
Hydrocortone Phosphate Injection	Hydrocortisone sodium phosphate
Innohep Injection	Tinzaparin

Drug	Generic Name
Isuprel Hydrochloride Injection 1:5000 Inhalation Solution 1:200 & 1:100	Isoproterenol
Klaron Lotion 10%	Sodium sulfacetamide
Levophed Bitartrate Injection	Norepinephrine
Marcaine Hydrochloride/ Epinephrine 1:200,000	Bupivacaine/epinephrine bitartrate
Morphine Sulfate Injection	Morphine
Nebcin vials, Hyporets, Add-vantage	Tobramycin
Nizoral 2% Cream, Nizoral A-D	Ketoconazole
Norflex Injection, ER Tablets	Orphenadrine
Novocain Hydrochloride for Spinal Anesthesia	Procaine
Nubain ampules/Multiple Dose Vial	Nalbuphine
Numorphan Injection	Oxymorphone
Pamelor Capsules	Nortriptyline
Phenergan Injection	Promethazine hydrochloride
Pred Forte	Prednisolone acetate
Pred Mild	Prednisolone acetate
Propofol Injectable Emulsion	Propofol
ROWASA Suspension Enema	Mesalamine
Sensorcaine with Epinephrine Injection	Bupivacaine/epinephrine bitartrate
Sensorcaine-MPF with Epinephrine Injection	Bupivacaine/epinephrine bitartrate
Septra I.V. Infusion, ADD-Vantage Vials	Trimethoprim/ Sulfamethoxazole
Solaquin Forte 4% Cream; 4% Gel	Hydroquinone
Soma Compound with Codeine	Carisoprodol/ aspirin/codeine
Stelazine Concentrate	Trifluoperazine
Streptomycin Sulfate Injection	Streptomycin
Sulfamylon Cream	Mafenide acetate
Sumycin Suspension	Tetracycline hydrochloride
Talacen	Pentazocine hydrochloride/acetaminophen
Talwin Lactate Carpuject/ Multi-Dose Vials	Pentazocine lactate

Drug	Generic Name
Tensilon Injectable	Edrophonium
Terramycin Intramuscular Injection	Oxytetracycline
Thorazine Ampules/Multi-Dose Vials	Chlorpromazine
Torecan Injection	Triethylperazine maleate
Trilafon Injection/Tablets	Perphenazine
Tri-Luma	Fluocinolone acetonide/ hydroquinone/ tretinoin
Tylenol with Codeine Tablets	Acetaminophen/codeine
Tylox Capsules	Acetaminophen/ oxycodone
Vibramycin Calcium Syrup	Doxycycline calcium
Xylocaine with Epinephrine Injection	Lidocaine/epinephrine

Lactose- and Galactose-Free Drugs

Listed below is a selection of drugs that contain no lactose or galactose. This list should not be considered all-inclusive or comprehensive. Generics and alternate brands of some products may be available. Check product labeling for a current listing of inactive ingredients.

Brand Name (OTC)	Form
Advil	Tablets
Aleve	Caplets, Gelcaps, Tablets
Alimentum	Liquid
Alka-Mints	Tablets
Alka-Seltzer	Effervescent Tablets
Alka-Seltzer Plus Cold	Effervescent Tablets
Anti-Tuss DM	Syrup
Ascriptin	Tablets
Axid AR	Tablets
Benadryl	Liquid Tablets
Benadryl Allergy & Cold	Caplets
Benylin Expectorant	Liquid
Bufferin	Tablets
Caltrate 600 PLUS	Tablets
Casec	Powder
Cenafed	Syrup
Claritin-D	Tablets
Colace	Capsules
Doxidan Liqui-Gels	Capsules
Dramamine	Tablets
Elecare	Powder
Ensure	Liquid
Ensure High Calcium	Liquid
Ensure Plus	Liquid
Excedrin Extra-Strength	Tablets
Excedrin QuickTabs	Tablets
Ex-Lax Maximum Strength	Tablets
Fergon Iron	Tablets
Fibersource	Liquid
Fibersource HN	Liquid
Forta Drink	Powder

Brand Name (OTC)	Form
Gaviscon Regular Strength	Tablets
Hytinic	Capsules
Iberet	Tablets
Imodium A-D	Liquid, Tablets
Impact	Liquid
Impact with Fiber	Liquid
Isosource	Liquid
Isosource HN	Liquid
Jevity	Liquid
Kaopectate Children's	Liquid
Konsyl	Powder
Lactaid	Tablets
Lipisorb	Liquid
MCT Oil	Oil
Medi-Lyte	Tablets
Metamucil	Powder, Wafers
Modical	Powder
Motrin IB	Tablets
Mylanta Gas	Tablets
Mylicon Infants'	Drops
Naldecon Senior DX	Liquid
Naldecon Senior EX	Liquid
Nepro	Liquid
NoDoz Maxium Strength	Tablets
Nuprin	Tablets
Nu-Taste	Liquid
Ocuvite Vitamin and Mineral Supplement	Tablets
One-A-Day Active	Tablets
One-A-Day Garlic Softgels	Capsules
One-A-Day Maximum	Tablets
One-A-Day Men's	Tablets
One-A-Day Women's	Tablets
Orudis KT	Tablets
Osmolite	Liquid
Osmolite HN	Liquid
Pediasure	Liquid
Pepto-Bismol	Suspension, Tablets
Pepto-Bismol Max. Strength	Suspension
Percy Medicine	Liquid

Brand Name (OTC)	Form
Polycose	Liquid, powder
Poly-Vi-Sol	Drops
Poly-Vi-Sol with Iron	Drops
Portagen	Powder
Prilosec OTC	Tablets
Promote	Liquid
Pulmocare	Liquid
Purge	Oil
RCF	Liquid
Resource Plus	Liquid
Riopan	Suspension
Riopan Plus	Suspension
Similac with Iron	Concentrate, Powder
Simply Sleep	Caplets
St. Joseph Adult Low Strength Aspirin	Tablets
Sucrets Maximum Strength	Lozenges
Sudafed	Tablets
Sudafed Children's	Liquid
Sudafed Sinus	Tablets
Sunkist Vitamin C	Tablets
Surfak	Capsules
Titralac	Tablets
Titralac Plus	Tablets
Tri-Vi-Sol	Drops
Tri-Vi-Sol with Iron	Drops
Tums	Tablets
Tylenol	Drops, Liquid, Tablets
Unisom SleepTabs	Tablets
Vi-Daylin ADC Vitamins	Drops
Vi-Daylin ADC Vitamins Plus Iron	Drops
Vi-Daylin ADC Multi-Vitamin	Drops
Vi-Daylin ADC Multi-Vitamin Plus Iron	Drops
Zantac 75	Tablets

Brand Name (Rx)	Form
Accutane	Capsules
Actigall	Capsules
Advicor	Tablets

Brand Name (Rx)	Form
Aldactazide	Tablets
Aldactone	Tablets
Allegra	Tablets
Allegra-D	Tablets
Altace	Capsules
Amicar	Tablets
Antivert	Tablets
Aromasin	Tablets
Atrohist Pediatric	Capsules
Augmentin	Tablets
Augmentin XR	Tablets
Axid	Capsules
Bactrim	Tablets
Biaxin Filmtab	Tablets
Calan SR	Tablets
Carafate	Tablets
Cardene	Capsules
Cardizem CD	Capsules
Cardizem ST	Capsules
Ceclor	Capsules
Ceftin	Suspension, Tablets
Cefzil	Suspension, Tablets
Cipro	Tablets
Cipro XR	Tablets
Clinoril	Tablets
Combivir	Tablets
Comtan	Tablets
Covera-HS	Tablets
Creon	Capsules
Cytotec	Tablets
Darvon-N/Darvocet-N	Tablets
Daypro	Tablets
Deconsal II	Tablets
Demerol	Tablets
Depakene	Capsules
Depakote	Tablets
Depakote Sprinkle	Capsules
Desoxyn	Tablets
Detrol	Tablets
DiaBeta	Tablets

Brand Name (Rx)	Form
Diabinese	Tablets
Diovan	Capsules
Diovan HCT	Tablets
Dolobid	Tablets
Donnatal Extentabs	Tablets
Duricef	Capsules, Suspension, Tablets
E.E.S.	Suspension, Tablets
Entex LA	Tablets
Epivir	Tablets, Solution
Epivir-HBV	Tablets
Ery-Tab	Tablets
Esgic-Plus	Capsules, Tablets
Exelon	Capsules
Fero-Folic/Iberet Folic	Tablets
Fioricet	Tablets
Flomax	Capsules
Gleevec	Tablets
Glucotrol XL	Tablets
Glucovance	Tablets
Glyset	Tablets
GoLYTELY	Powder
Grifulvin V	Suspension, Tablets
Guaifed	Capsules
Hytrin	Capsules
Inderal LA	Capsules
Isoptin SR	Tablets
Kaletra	Capsules, Solution
K-Dur	Tablets
Keppra	Tablets
K-Lor	Powder
K-Phos Neutral	Tablets
K-Phos Original Formula	Tablets
K-Tab	Tablets
Lamisil	Tablets
Lanoxicaps	Capsules
Lescol	Capsules
Lescol XL	Tablets
Levaquin	Tablets
Levothroid	Tablets

Brand Name (Rx)	Form
Levoxyl	Tablets
Lexapro	Tablets
Librium	Capsules
Lomotil	Tablets
Lopid	Tablets
Malarone	Tablets
Malarone Pediatric	Tablets
Materna	Tablets
Maxzide	Tablets
Maxzide-25 mg	Tablets
Methylin ER	Tablets
Micardis	Tablets
Micro-K	Capsules
Micronase	Tablets
Minipress	Capsules
Minocin	Capsules
Motrin	Tablets
Mycostatin	Pastilles
Niaspan	Tablets
Nicomide	Tablets
Niferex-150	Capsules
Niferex-150-Forte	Capsules
Niferex-PN	Tablets
Nolvadex	Tablets
Norpramin	Tablets
Norvasc	Tablets
Omnicef	Capsules
Pamelor	Capsules
Pamine Forte	Tablets
Pancrease	Capsules
Pancrease MT	Capsules
Paxil	Tablets
Pepcid	Suspension, Tablets
Percocet	Tablets
Percodan	Tablets
PhosLo	Tablets
Plaquenil	Tablets
Pletal	Tablets
Prandin	Tablets
Precare	Tablets

Brand Name (Rx)	Form
Precose	Tablets
Prevacid	Capsules
Prinvil	Tablets
ProAmatine	Tablets
Procardia	Capsules
Procardia XL	Tablets
Prometrium	Capsules
Protonix	Tablets
Prozac	Capsules
Questran	Powder
Relafen	Tablets
Remeron SolTab	Tablets
Rifadin	Capsules
Robaxin	Tablets
Sarafem	Pulvules
Sectral	Capsules
Serzone	Tablets
Sinemet	Tablets
Sinemet CR	Tablets
Soma	Tablets
Stalevo	Tablets
StrongStart	Capsules
Symmetrel	Tablets
Tamiflu	Capsules
Tegretol/Tegretol-XR	Tablets
Tenoretic	Tablets
Tenormin	Tablets
Tequin	Tablets
Tessalon	Capsules
Tiazac	Capsules
Ticlid	Tablets
Tikosyn	Capsules
Tofranil-PM	Capsules
Toprol-XL	Tablets
Trental	Tablets
Trileptal	Tablets
Trilisate	Tablets
Trizivir	Tablets
Ultrase	Capsules
Uniphyl	Tablets

Brand Name (Rx)	Form
Valcyte	Tablets
Valium	Tablets
Valtrex	Caplets
Vibramycin Hyclate	Capsules
Vicodin	Tablets
Vicodin ES	Tablets
Vicodin HP	Tablets
Vicoprofen	Tablets
Videx	Tablets
Visicol	Tablets
Vistaril	Capsules
Welchol	Tablets
Wellbutrin	Tablets
Wellbutrin SR	Tablets
Xenical	Capsules
Yocon	Tablets
Zantac	Syrup, Tablets
Zarontin	Capsules
Zaroxolyn	Tablets
Zebeta	Tablets
Zestril	Tablets
Ziac	Tablets
Ziagen	Tablets
Zofran	Solution, Tablets (disintegrating)
Zoloft	Tablets
Zonegran	Capsules
Zyban	Tablets
Zyflo Filmtab	Tablets
Zymase	Capsules
Zyvox	Suspension, Tablets

Drugs That Should Not Be Crushed

Listed below is a selection of brand-name drugs that should not be crushed. This list should not be considered comprehensive. Generics and alternate brands of some products may be available. Check product labeling for a current listing of inactive ingredients.

Accuhist LA
Aciphex
Adalat CC
Adderall XR
Advicor
Aerohist
Aerohist Plus
Afeditab CR
Aggrenox
Aldex
Aleve Cold & Sinus
Aleve Sinus & Headache
Allegra-D
Allerx
Allerx-D
Allfen
Allfen-DM
Alophen
Altex-PSE
Altoprev
Ambifed-G
Ambifed-G DM
Amdry-C
Amdry-D
Amibid DM
Amibid LA
Amidal
Aminoxin
Ami-Tex PSE
Anextuss
Anti-Tussive
Aquabid-DM
Aquatab C

Aquatab D
Aquatab DM
Arthrotec
Asacol
Ascocid-1000
Ascocid-500-D
Ascription Enteric
ATP
Atrohist Pediatric
Augmentin XR
Avinza
Azulfidine Entabs
Bayer Aspirin Regimen
Bellahist-D LA
Biaxin XL
Bidex-DM
Bidhist
Biohist LA
Bisac-Evac
Biscolax
Blanex-A
Bontril Slow-Release
Bromfed
Bromfed-PD
Bromfenex
Bromfenex-PD
Bromfenex PE Pediatric
Budeprion SR
Buproban
Calan SR
Carbatrol
Cardene Sr
Cardizem CD
Cardizem LA
Carox Plus
Cartia XT
Catemine
Cemill 1000
Cemill 500
Certuss-D
Cevi-Bid
Chlorex-A

Chlor-Phen
Chlor-Trimeton Allergy
Chlor-Trimeton Allergy Decongestant
Cipro XR
Clorfed
Coldamine
Coldec D
Coldec TR
Coldex-A
Coldmist DM
Coldmist Jr
Coldmist La
Colfed-A
Concerta
Contac 12-Hour
Correctol
Cotazym-S
Covera-HS
Crantex ER
Crantex LA
Creon 10
Creon 20
Creon 5
Cymbalta
Cypex-LA
Dacex-PE
Dairycare
Dallergy
Dallergy-Jr
D-Amine-SR
Deconamine SR
Deconex
Decongest II
De-Congestine
Deconsal II
Depakote
Depakote ER
Depakote Sprinkles
Despec SR
Detrol LA
Dex GG TR
Dexaphen SA

Dexcon-PE
Dexedrine Spansules
D-Feda II
Diabetes Trio
Diamox Sequels
Dilacor XR
Dilantin Kapseals
Dilatrate-SR
Dilt-CD
Diltia XT
Dilt-XR
Dimetane Extentabs
Disophrol Chronotab
Ditropan XL
Donnatal Extentabs
Doryx
Drexophed SR
Drihist SR
Drituss G
Drituss GP
Drixomed
Drixoral
Drixoral Plus
Drixoral Sinus
Drize-R
Drysec
Dulcolax
Duradryl Jr
Durahist
Durahist PE
Duraphen DM
Duraphen II
Duratuss
Duratuss GP
Dynabac
Dynabac D5-Pak
Dynacirc CR
Dynahist-ER Pediatric
Dynex
Dytan-CS
Easprin
EC Naprosyn

Ecotrin
Ecotrin Adult Low Strength
Ecotrin Maximum Strength
Ecpirin
Ed A-Hist
Effexor-XR
Efidac 24 Chlorpheniramine
Efidac 24 Pseudoephedrine
Endal
Entab-DM
Entercote
Entex ER
Entex LA
Entex PSE
Entocort EC
Eryc
Ery-Tab
Eskalith-CR
Extendryl Jr
Extendryl SR
Extress-30
Extuss LA
Feen-A-Mint
Femilax
Fero-Folic 500
Fero-Grad 500
Ferro-Sequels
Ferro-Time
Ferrous Femarate DS
Fetrin
Flagyl ER
Fleet Bisacodyl
Folitab 500
Fortamet
Fumatinic
G/P 1200/75
Genacote
Gentlax
GFN 1000/DM 50
GFN 1200/DM 20/PE 40
GFN 1200/DM 60/PSE 60
GFN 1200/Phenylephrine 40

GFN 1200/PSE 50
GFN 500/DM 30
GFN 550/PSE 60
GFN 550/PSE 60/DM 30
GFN 595/PSE 48
GFN 595/PSE 48/DM 32
GFN 795/PSE 85
GFN 800/DM 30
GFN 800/PSE 25
GFN 800/PSE 60
Gilphex TR
Giltuss TR
Glucophage XR
Glucotrol XL
GP-1200
Guaifed
Guaifed-PD
Guaifenex DM
Guaifenex G
Guaifenex GP
Guaifenex LA
Guaifenex PSE 120
Guaifenex PSE 60
Guaifenex PSE 80
Guaifenex-Rx
Guaifenex-Rx DM
Guaimax-D
Gua-SR
Guia-D
Guiadex D
Guiadex PD
Guiadrine DM
Guiadrine G-1200
Guiadrine GP
Guiadrine PSE
H 9600 SR
Halfprin
Hematron-AF
Hemax
Histade
Histade Mx
Hista-Vent DA

Hista-Vent PSE
Histex CT
Histex I/E
Histex SR
Humavent LA
Humibid DM
Humibid LA
Hydro Pro DM SR
Hyoscyamine TR
Iberet-500
Iberet-Folic-500
Icar-C Plus SR
Imdur
Inderal LA
Indocin SR
Innopran XL
Iobid DM
Ionamin
Iosal II
Iotex PSE
Isochron
Isopro
Isoprotin SR
K-10
K-8
Kadian
Kaon-CL 10
K-Dur 10
K-Dur 20
Klor-Con 10
Klor-Con 8
Klor-Con M10
Klor-Con M15
Klor-Con M20
Klotrix
Kronofed-A
Kronofed-A-Jr
K-Tab
Lescol XL
Levall G
Levbid
Levsinex

Lexxel
Lipram 4500
Lipram-CR10
Lipram-CR20
Lipram-CR5
Lipram-PN10
Lipram-PN16
Lipram-PN20
Lipram-UL12
Lipram-UL18
Lipram-UL20
Liquibid-D
Liquibid-D 1200
Liquibid-PD
Lithobid
Lodine XL
Lodrane 12 Hour
Lodrane 12D
Lodrane LD
Lohist-12
Lohist-12D
Lusonex
Mag Delay
Mag64
Mag-SR
Mag-SR Plus Calcium
Mag-Tag SR
Maxifed
Maxifed DM
Maxifed DMX
Maxifed-G
Maxovite
Medent DM
Medent LD
Mega-C
Melfiat
Menopause Trio
Mescolor
Mestinon Timespan
Metadate CD
Metadate ER
Methylin ER

Micro-K
Micro-K 10
Mild-C
Mindal
Mindal DM
Mintab C
Mintab D
Mintab DM
Miraphen PSE
Modane
Ms Contin
MSP-BLU
Mucinex
Muco-Fen DM
Multi-Ferrous Folic
Multiret Folic-500
Myfortic
Nacon
Nalex-A
Naprelan
Nasatab LA
Nasex
Nd Clear
Nescon-PD
New Ami-Tex LA
Nexium
Niaspan
Nicomide
Nifediac CC
Nitrocot
Nitro-Time
Norflex
Norpace CR
Omnihist LA
Oramorph SR
Oruvail
Oxycontin
Palgic-D
Pancrease
Pancrease MT 10
Pancrease MT 16
Pancrease MT 20

Pancrecarb MS-4
Pancrecarb MS-8
Pangestyme CN-10
Pangestyme CN-20
Pangestyme EC
Pangestyme MT16
Pangestyme UL12
Pangestyme UL18
Pangestyme UL20
Panmist DM
Panmist Jr
Panmist LA
Pannaz
Papacon
Para-Time SR
Paser
Pavacot
Paxil CR
PCE Dispertab
PCM Allergy
PCM LA
Pendex
Pentasa
Pentopak
Pentoxil
Pharmadrine
Phenabid DM
Phenavent
Phenavent D
Phenavent LA
Phenavent Ped
Phendiet-105
Phenyleph 20/CPM 8/Methscop 2.5 LA
Phenytek
Plendil
Poly Hist Forte
Poly-Vent
Poly-Vent Jr
Prehist D
Prelu-2
Prevacid
Prilosec

Prilosec OTC
Procanbid
Procardia XL
Profen Forte
Profen Forte DM
Profen II DM
Prolex-PD
Prolix-D
Pronestyl-SR
Prosed EC
Proset-D
Protid
Protonix
Prozac Weekly
Pseubrom
Pseubrom-PD
Pseudo CM TR
Pseudo GG TR
Pseudocot-C
Pseudocot-G
Pseudovent
Pesudovent 400
Pseudovent DM
Pseudovent Ped
P-Tuss Dm
Q-Bid DM
Qdall
Quadra-Hist D
Quadra-Hist D Ped
Quibron-T/SR
Quindal
Reliable Gentle Laxative
Rescon-Jr.
Rescon-MX
Respa-1ST
Respa-A.R.
Respa-DM
Respahist
Respaire-120 SR
Respaire-60 SR
Respa-PE
Rhinabid PD

Rhinacon A
Ribo-2
Ritalin LA
Ritalin-SR
Rodex Forte
Rondec-TR
Ru-Tuss 800
Ru-Tuss 800 DM
Ru-Tuss Jr
Rythmol SR
Sam-E
Sinemet CR
Sinutuss DM
Sinuvent PE
Slo-Niacin
Slow Fe
Slow Fe With Folic Acid
Slow-Mag
Spacol T/S
St. Joseph Pain Reliever
Sta-D
Stahist
Stamoist E
Sudafed 12 Hour
Sudafed 24 Hour
Sudal 60/500
Sudal DM
Sudal SR
Sular
Sulfazine EC
Symax-SR
Tarka
Taztia XT
Tegretol-XR
Tenuate Dospan
Theo-24
Theocap
Theochron
Theo-Time
Thiamilate
Tiazac
Time-Hist

Toprol XL
Totalday
Touro Allergy
Touro CC
Touro CC-LD
Touro DM
Touro HC
Touro LA
Touro LA-LD
Tranxene-SD
Trental
Trikof-D
Trinalin Repetabs
Trituss-ER
Tussafed-LA
Tussall-Er
Tussbid
Tussi-Bid
Tussitab
Tylenol Arthritis
Ultrabrom
Ultrabrom PD
Ultrase
Ultrase MT12
Ultrase MT18
Ultrase MT20
Uniphyl
Uni-Tex
Urimax
Urocit-K 10
Urocit-K 5
Uroxatral
Utira
V-Dec-M
Veracolate
Verelan
Verelan PM
Versacaps
Videx EC
Vitamin C/Rose Hips
Vivotif Berna
Voltaren

Voltaren-XR
Vospire ER
WE Mist II LA
WE Mist LA
Wellbid-D
Wellbid-D 1200
Wellbutrin SR
Wellbutrin XL
Wobenzym N
Xanax XR
Xiral
Xpect-AT
Zaptec PSE
Z-Cof LA
Zephrex LA
Zorprin
Zyban
Zymase
Zyrtec-D

Drugs That May Cause Photosensitivity

Listed below is a selection of drugs that may cause photosensitivity. This list should not be considered comprehensive. Generics and alternate brands of some products may be available. Check product labeling for a current listing of inactive ingredients.

Generic	Brand
Acamprosate	Campral
Acetazolamide	Diamox
Acitrerin	Soriatane
Acyclovir	Zovirax
Alatrofloxacin	Trovan I.V.
Alendronate	Fosamax
Alitretinoin	Panretin
Almotriptan	Axert
Amiloride/hydrochlorothiazide	Moduretic
Aminolevulinic acid	Levulan Kerastick
Amiodarone	Cordarone, Pacerone
Amitriptyline	Elavil
Amitriptyline/chlordiazepoxide	Limbitrol
Amitriptyline/perphenazine	Triavil
Amlodipine/atorvastatin	Caduet
Anagrelide	Agrylin
Apripiprazole	Abilify
Atazanavir	Reyataz
Attenolol/chlorthalidone	Tenoretic
Atorvastatin	Lipitor
Atovaquone/proguanil	Malarone
Aurothioglucose	Solganal
Azatadine/pseudoephedrine	Rynatan, Trinalin
Azithromycin	Zithromax
Benazepril	Lotensin
Benazepril/hydrochlorothiazide	Lotensin HCT
Dendroflumethiazide/nadolol	Corzide
Bexarotene	Targretin
Bismuth/metronidazole/tetracycline	Helidac
Bisoprolol/hydrochlorothiazide	Ziac
Brompheniramine/dextromethorphan/ phenylephrine	Alacol DM

Generic	Brand
Brompheniramine/dextromethorphan/ pseudoephedrine	Bromfed-DM
Buffered aspirin/pravastatin	Pravigard PAC
Bupropion	Wellbutrin, Zyban
Candesartan/hydrochlorothiazide	Atacand HCT
Capecitabine	Xeloda
Captopril	Capoten
Captopril/hydrochlorothiazide	Capozide
Carbamazepine	Carbatrol, Tegretol, Tegretol-XR
Carbinoxamine/pseudoephedrine	Palgic-D, Palgic-DS, Pediatex-D
Carvedilol	Coreg
Celecoxib	Celebrex
Cetirizine	Zyrtec
Cetirizine/pseudoephedrine	Zyrtec-D
Cevimeline	Evoxac
Chlorhexidine gluconate	Hibistat
Chloroquine	Aralen
Chlorothiazide	Diuril
Chlorpheniramine/hydrocodone/ pseudoephedrine	Tussend
Chlorpheniramine/phenylephrine/ pyrilamine	Rynatan
Chloropromazine	Thorazine
Chlorpropamide	Diabinese
Chlorthalidone	Thalitone
Chlorthalidone/clonidine	Clorpres
Cidofovir	Vistide
Ciprofloxacin	Cipro
Citalopram	Celexa
Clemastine	Tavist
Clonidine/chlorthalidone	Clorpres
Clozapine	Clozaril, Fazaclo
Cromolyn sodium	Gastrocrom
Cyclobenzaprine	Flexeril
Cyproheptadine	Periactin
Dacarbazine	DTIC-Dome
Dantrolene	Dantrium
Demeclocycline	Declomycin

Generic	Brand
Desipramine	Norpramin
Diclofenac potassium	Cataflam
Diclofenac sodium	Voltaren
Diclofenac sodium/misoprostol	Arthrotec
Diflunisal	Dolobid
Dihydroergotamine	D.D.E. 45
Diltiazem	Cardizem, Tiazac
Diphenhydramine	Benadryl
Divalproex	Depakote
Doxepin	Sinequan
Doxycycline hyclate	Doryx, Periostat, Vibra-Tabs, Vibramycin
Doxycycline monohydrate	Monodox
Duloxetine	Cymbalta
Enalapril	Vasotec
Enalapril/felodipine	Lexxel
Enalapril/hydrochlorothiazide	Vaseretic
Enalaprilat	Vasotec I.V.
Epirubicin	Ellence
Eprosartan mesylate/ hydrochlorothiazide	Teveten HCT
Erythromycin/sulfisoxazole	Pediazole
Estazolam	ProSom
Estradiol	Gynodiol
Ethionamide	Trecator-SC
Etodolac	Lodine
Felbamate	Felbatol
Fenofibrate	Tricor, Lofibra
Floxuridine	Sterile FUDR
Flucytosine	Ancobon
Fluorouracil	Efudex
Fluoxetine	Prozac, Sarafem
Fluphenazine	Prolixin
Flutamide	Eulexin
Fluvastatin	Lescol
Fluvoxamine	Luvox
Fosinopril	Monopril
Fosphenytoin	Cerebyx
Furosemide	Lasix

Generic	Brand
Gabapentin	Neurontin
Gatifloxacin	Tequin
Gemfibrozil	Lopid
Gemifloxacin mesylate	Factive
Gentamicin	Garamycin
Glatiramer	Copaxone
Glimepiride	Amaryl
Glipizide	Glucotrol
Glyburide	DiaBeta, Glynase, Micronase
Glyburide/metformin HCl	Glucovance
Griseofulvin	Fulvicin P/G, Grifulvin, Gris-PEG
Haloperidol	Haldol
Hexachlorophene	pHisoHex
Hydralazine/hydrochlorothiazide	Apresazide
Hydrochlorothiazide	HydroDIURIL, Microzide, Oretic
Hydrochlorothiazide/fosinopril	Monopril HCT
Hydrochlorothiazide/irbesartan	Avalide
Hydrochlorothiazide/lisinopril	Prinzide, Zestoretic
Hydrochlorothiazide/ losartan potassium	Hyzaar
Hydrochlorothiazide/methyldopa	Aldoril
Hydrochlorothiazide/moexipril	Uniretic
Hydrochlorothiazide/propranolol	Inderide
Hydrochlorothiazide/quinapril	Accuretic
Hydrochlorothiazide/spironolactone	Aldactazide
Hydrochlorothiazide/telmisartan	Micardis HCT
Hydrochlorothiazide/timolol	Timolide
Hydrochlorothiazide/triamterene	Dyazide, Maxzide
Hydrochlorothiazide/valsartan	Diovan HCT
Hydroflumethiazide	Saluron
Hydroxychloroquine	Plaquenil
Hypericum	Kira, St. John's Wort
Hypericum/vitamin B1/vitamin C/ kava kava	One-A-Day Tension & Mood
Ibuprofen	Motrin
Imatinib mesylate	Gleevec

Generic	Brand
Imipramine	Tofranil
Imiquimod	Aldara
Indapamide	Lozol
Interferon alfa-2b, recombinant	Intron A
Interferon alfa-n3 (human leukocyte derived)	Alferon-N
Interferon beta-1a	Avonex
Interferon beta-1b	Betaseron
Irbesartan/hydrochlorothiazide	Avalide
Isoniazid/pyrazinamide/rifampin	Rifater
Isotretinoin	Accutane, Amnesteem
Itraconazole	Sporanox
Ketoprofen	Orudis, Oruvail
Lamotrigine	Lamictal
Leuprolide	Lupron
Levamisole	Ergamisol
Lisinopril	Prinivil, Zestril
Lisinopil/hydrochlorothiazide	Prinivil, Zestoretic
Lemefloxacin	Maxaquin
Loratadine	Claritin
Loratadine/pseudoephedrine	Claritin-D
Losartan	Cozaar
Losartan/hydrochlorothiazide	Hyzaar
Locastatin	Altoprev, Mevacor
Locastatin/niacin	Advicor
Maprotiline	Ludiomil
Mefenamic acid	Ponstel
Meloxicam	Mobic
Mesalamine	Pentasa
Methotrexate	Trexall
Methoxsalen	Uvadex, Oxsoralen, 8-MOP
Methyclothiazide	Enduron
Methyldopa/chlorothiazide	Aldoclor
Methyldopa/hydrochlorothiazide	Aldoril
Metolazone	Mykrox, Zaroxolyn
Minocycline	Dynacin, Minocin
Mirtazapine	Remeron
Moexipril	Univasc
Moexipril/hydrochlorothiazide	Uniretic

Generic	Brand
Moxifloxacin	Avelox
Nabumetone	Relafen
Nadolol/bendroflumethiazide	Corzide
Nalidixic acid	NegGram
Naproxen	Naprosyn, EC-Naprosyn
Naproxen sodium	Anaprox, Naprelan
Naratriptan	Amerge
Nefazodone	Serzone
Nifedipine	Adalat CC, Procardia
Nisoldipine	Sular
Norfloxacin	Noroxin
Nortriptyline	Pamelor
Ofloxacin	Floxin
Olansapine	Zyprexa
Olanzapine/fluoxetine	Symbyax
Olmesartan medoxomil/hydrochlorothiazide	Benicar HCT
Olsalazine	Dipentum
Oxaprozin	Daypro
Oxcarbazepine	Trileptal
Oxycodone	Roxicodone
Oxytetracycline	Terramycin
Pantoprazole	Protonix
Paroxetine	Paxil
Pastinaca sativa	Parsnip
Pentosan polysulfate	Elmiron
Pentostatin	Nipent
Perphenazine	Trilafon
Pilocarpine	Salagen
Piroxicam	Feldene
Polythiazide	Renese
Polythiazide/prazosin	Minizide
Porfimer sodium	Photofrin
Pravastatin	Pravachol
Prochlorperazine	Compazine, Compro
Promethazine	Phenergan
Protriptyline	Vivactil
Pyrazinamide	Pyrazinamide
Quetiapine	Seroquel

Generic	Brand
Quinapril	Accupril
Quinapril/hydrochlorothiazide	Accuretic
Quinidine gluconate	Quinidine
Quinidine sulfate	Quinidex
Rabeprazole sodium	Aciphex
Ramipril	Altace
Riluzole	Rilutek
Risperidone	Risperdal, Risperdal Consta
Ritonavir	Norvir
Rizatriptan	Maxalt
Ropinirole	Requip
Rosuvastatin	Crestor
Ruta graveolens	Rue
Saquinavir	Fortovase
Saquinavir mesylate	Invirase
Selegiline	Eldepryl
Sertraline	Zoloft
Sibutramine	Meridia
Sildenafil	Viagra
Simvastatin	Zocor
Simvastatin/ezetimibe	Vytorin
Somatropin	Serostim
Sotalol	Betapace, Betapace AF
Sulfamethoxazole/trimethoprim	Bactrim, Septra
Sulfasalazine	Azulfidine
Sulindac	Clinoril
Sumatriptan	Imitrex
Tacrolimus	Prograf, Protopic
Tazarotene	Tazorac
Telmisartan/hydrochlorothiazide	Micardis HCT
Tetracycline	Sumycin
Thalidomide	Thalomid
Thioridazine hydrochloride	Mellaril
Thiothixene	Navane
Tiagabine	Gabitril
Topiramate	Topamax
Tramcinolone	Azmacort
Triamterene	Dyrenium
Triamterene/hydrochlorothiazide	Dyazide, Maxzide

Generic	Brand
Trifluoperazine	Stelazine
Trimipramine	Surmontil
Trovafloxacin	Trovan
Valacyclovir	Valtrex
Valdecoxib	Bextra
Valproate	Depacon
Valproic acid	Depakene
Valsartan/hydrochlorothiazide	Diovan HCT
Vardenafil	Levitra
Venlafasxine	Effexor
Verteporfin	Visudyne
Voriconazole	Vfend
Zalcitabine	Hivid
Zalepion	Sonata
Ziprasidone	Geodon
Zolmitriptan	Zomig
Zolpidem	Ambien

Standard Medical Abbreviations

Abbreviation	Meaning
5-HIAA	5-hydroxyindoleacetic acid
5-HT	5-hydroxytryptamine (serotonin)
6-MP	6-mercaptopurine
17-OHCS	17-hydroxycorticosteroids
AA	Alcoholics Anonymous; amino acids
AACP	American Association of Clinical Pharmacy; American Association of Colleges of Pharmacy
AARP	American Association of Retired Persons
Ab	antibody
ABVD	Adriamycin (doxorubicin), bleomycin, vinblastine, (and) dacarbazine
ACCP	American College of Clinical Pharmacy
ACD	acid-citrate-dextrose
ACE	angiotensin-converting enzyme
ACEI	angiotensin-converting enzyme inhibitor
ACh	acetylcholine
ACLS	advanced cardiac life support
ACPE	American Council on Pharmaceutical Education
ACS	American Chemical Society
ACTH	adrenocorticotropic hormone
ADME	absorption, distribution, metabolism and elimination
ADP	adenosine diphosphate
ADR	adverse drug reaction
ADRRS	Adverse Drug Reaction Reporting System
Ag	antigen; silver (argentum)
AHA	American Hospital Association
AIDS	acquired immunodeficiency syndrome
AJHP	American Journal of Hospital Pharmacy
ALL	acute lymphocytic leukemia
ALT	alanine amniotransferase serum (previously SGPT)
AMA	American Medical Association
AML	acute myelogenous leukemia

Abbreviation	Meaning
AMP	adenosine monophosphate
ANA	antinuclear antibody(ies)
ANC	acid neutralizing capacity
APA	antipernicious anemia (factor)
APAP	acetaminophen
APhA	American Pharmaceutical Association
aPTT	activated partial thromboplastin time
ARC	AIDS-related complex
ARDS	adult respiratory distress syndrome
ARF	acute renal failure
ARV	AIDS-related virus
ASHD	arteriosclerotic heart disease
ASHP	American Society of Hospital Pharmacies
ATN	acute tubular necrosis
ATP	adenosine triphosphate
ATPase	adenosine triphosphatase
AV	atrioventricular
A-V	arteriovenous; atrioventricular (block, bundle, conduction, dissociation, extrasystole)
BAC	blood-alcohol concentration
BBB	blood brain barrier
BDZ	benzodiazepine
bm	bowel movement
BMR	basal metabolic rate
BP	blood pressure
BPH	benign prostatic hypertrophy
bpm	beats per minute
BSA	body surface area
BT	bleeding time
BUN	blood urea nitrogen
C	centigrade
°C	degrees Celsius
Ca	calcium
CA	cancer; carcinoma; cardiac arrest; chronologic age; croup-associated
CAD	coronary artery disease
cath	catheterize
CBC	complete blood count
CCBs	calcium channel blockers
CCU	coronary care unit; critical care unit

Abbreviation	Meaning
CD4	T-helper lymphocytes and macrophages
CDC	Centers for Disease Control and Prevention
CEA	cost effectiveness analysis
CF	cystic fibrosis
CFC	chlorofluorocarbon
CFU	colony-forming units
CHD	coronary heart disease
CHF	congestive heart failure
CMA	Certified Medical Assistant
CMI	cell-mediated immunity
CML	chronic myelocytic leukemia
CN	cranial nerve
CNM	Certified Nurse Midwife
CNS	central nervous system
CO	cardiac output
CO2	carbon dioxide
CoA	coenzyme A
COMT	catecholamine-o-methyl transferase
COPD	chronic obstructive pulmonary disease
CPAP	continuous positive airway pressure
CPR	cardiopulmonary resuscitation
Cr	creatinine; chromium
CRD	chronic respiratory disease
CRF	chronic renal failure
CRH	corticotropin-releasing hormone
CRNA	Certified Registered Nurse Anesthetist
CSA	Controlled Substances Act; cyclosporine A
CSF	cerebrospinal fluid; colony-stimulating factors
CSP	cellulose sodium phosphate
CV	cardiovascular
CVA	cerebrovascular accident
CVP	central venous pressure
CXR	chest x-ray
D&C	dilation and curettage; designation applied to dyes permitted for use in drugs and cosmetics
D&E	dilation and evacuation
DC	Doctor of Chiropractic
DDS	Doctor of Dental Surgery
DEA	Drug Enforcement Administration

Abbreviation	Meaning
DERM	dermatologic
DHHS	Department of Health and Human Services
DIC	disseminated intravascular coagulation
DIS	drug information source
DJD	degenerative joint disease
DKA	diabetic ketoacidosis
DMD	Doctor of Dental Medicine
DNA	deoxyribonucleic acid
DNR	do not resuscitate
DNS	Director of Nursing Service; Doctor of Nursing Services
DO	Doctor of Osteopathy
DOA	dead on arrival
DP	Doctor of Podiatry
DPH	Doctor of Public Health; Doctor of Public Hygiene
DPI	dry powder inhaler
DPM	Doctor of Physical Medicine; Doctor of Podiatric Medicine
DrPh	Doctor of Public Health; Doctor of Public Hygiene
DTP	diphtheria, tetanus toxoids & pertussis vaccine
DTRs	deep tendon reflexes
DUB	dysfunctional uterine bleeding
DVA	Department of Veterans Affairs
DVM	Doctor of Veterinary Medicine
DVT	deep venous thrombosis
E.	Enterococcus; Escherichia
EBV	Epstein-Barr virus
ECG	electrocardiogram
ECT	electroconvulsive therapy
ED	emergency department; effective dose
ED50	median-effective dose
EEG	electroencephalogram
EENT	eye, ear, nose, and throat
EF	ejection fraction
EKG	electrocardiogram
EMIT	enzyme-multiplied immunoassay test
ENL	erythema nodosum leprosum
ENT	ear, nose, and throat

Abbreviation	Meaning
EPA	Environmental Protection Agency
EPAP	expiratory positive airway pressure
EPO	erythropoietin
EPS	extrapyramidal syndrome (or symptoms)
ER	emergency room; estrogen receptor; extended release; endoplasmic reticulum
°F	degrees Fahrenheit
FAO	Food and Agriculture Organization
FAS	fetal alcohol syndrome
FBS	fasting blood sugar
FDA	Food and Drug Administration
FD&C	designation applied to dyes permitted for use in foods, drugs and cosmetics; Food, Drug and Cosmetic Act
Fe	iron (ferrum)
FEF	forced expiratory flow
FET	forced expiratory time
FEV₁	forced expiratory volume in 1 second
FSH	follicle-stimulating hormone
FTC	Federal Trade Commission
G-CSF	granulocyte colony-stimulating factor
GERD	gastroesophageal reflux disease
GGTP	gamma glutamyl transpeptidase
GH	growth hormone
GHRF	growth hormone-releasing factor
GHRH	growth hormone-releasing hormone
GI	gastrointestinal
H.	Haemophilus; Helicobacter
HCFA	Health Care Financing Administration
HCG	human chorionic gonadotropin
Hct	hematocrit
HDL	high-density lipoprotein
HEMA	hematologic
HEME	hematologic
HEPA	high efficiency particulate air
Hg	mercury (hydragyrum)
Hgb	hemoglobin
HGH	human pituitary growth hormone
Hib.	Haemophilus influenzae
His.	Haemophilus influenzae type b

Abbreviation	Meaning
HIV	human immunodeficiency virus
HMO	health maintenance organization
HPV	human papillomavirus
HR	heart rate
HSV-1	herpes simplex virus type 1
HSV-2	herpes simplex virus type 2
IBW	ideal body weight
IC	intracoronary
ICD	International Classification of Diseases of the World Health Organization
ICF	intracellular fluid
ICP	intracranial pressure
ICU	intensive care unit
ID	intradermal; infective dose
IDDM	insulin-dependent diabetes mellitus (type 1 diabetes)
IFN	interferon
Ig	immunoglobulin
IL	interleukin
IM	intramuscular
Inh	inhaled
INH	isoniazid
Inhal	inhalation
Inj	injection
INR	International Normalizing Ratio
IOP	intraocular pressure
IPA	International Pharmaceutical Abstracts
IPPB	intermittent positive pressure breathing
IPV	poliovirus vaccine inactivated
IQ	intelligence quotient
ISA	intrinsic sympathomimetic activity
ISF	interstitial fluid
ISI	Institute for Scientific Information
ISO	International Organization for Standardization
IT	intrathecal(ly)
IU	international unit(s)
IUD	intrauterine device
IV	intravenous
IVF	intravascular fluid

Abbreviation	Meaning
IVP	intravenous piggyback
JCAH	Joint Commission on Accreditation of Hospitals
JCAHO	Joint Commission on Accreditation of Healthcare Organizations
KVO	keep vein open
L.	*Legionella; Listeria*
LBW	low body weight
LD	lethal dose
LD-50	a dose lethal to 50% of the specified animals or microorganisms
LDL	low-density lipoprotein
LE	lupus erythematosus
LFT	liver function test
LH	luteinizing hormone
Lys	lysine
M.	*Moraxella; Mycobacterium; Mycloplasma*
MA	mental age
MADD	Mothers Against Drunk Driving
MAO	monoamine oxidase
MAOI	monoamine oxidase inhibitor
MAP	mean arterial pressure
max	maximum
MCV	mean corpuscular volume
MD	Doctor of Medicine (Medicina Doctor)
MDI	metered dose inhaler
MDR	minimum daily requirements
MEC	minimum effective concentration
MEDLARS	Medical Literature Analysis and Retrieval System
MEDLINE	National Library of Medicine medical database
MHC	major histocompatibility complex
MI	myocardial infarction
MIA	metabolite bacterial inhibition assay
MID	minimal infecting dose
MIP	maximum inspiratory pressure
MJ	mejajoule(s)
mmol	millimole
MMR	measles, mumps and rubella virus vaccine, live
MMWR	*Morbidity and Mortality Weekly Report*

Abbreviation	Meaning
MPH	Master of Public Health
MRI	magnetic resonance imaging
N.	*Neisseria*
NABP	National Association of Boards of Pharmacy
NAPA	N-acetyl procainamide
NCPA	National Association of Community Pharmacists
ND	Doctor of Naturopathic Medicine
NDA	new drug application
NF	National Formulary
NIDDM	non-insulin dependent diabetes mellitus (type 2 diabetes)
NIH	National Institutes of Health
NLM	National Library of Medicine
nm	nanometer(s)
NS	normal saline (as in solution)
NSAID	nonsteroidal anti-inflammatory drug
NTD	neural tube defect
OB/GYN	obstetrics and gynecology
OD	Doctor of Optometry; overdose
Ophth	ophthalmic
os	left eye (oculus sinister)
OSHA	Occupational Safety and Health Administration
OT	occupational therapy
otc	over-the-counter (nonprescription)
OPV	oral poliovirus vaccine, live
P&T	pharmacy and therapeutics (committee)
PA	Physician Assistant; Physician's Assistant
PABA	para-aminobenzoic acid
PAC	premature atrial contraction
PaCO2	arterial plasma partial pressure of carbon dioxide
PAW	pulmonary arterial wedge
PAWP	pulmonary artery wedge pressure
PCA	patient-controlled analgesia
PE	pulmonary embolism
PEEP	positive end expiratory pressure
PEG	polyethylene glycol

Abbreviation	Meaning
PERLA	pupils equal, react to light and accommodation
PET	positron emission tomography
PharmD	Doctor of Pharmacy
PhD	Doctor of Philosophy
Phe	phenylalanine
PhG	German Pharmacopeia
PHS	Public Health Service
PND	paroxysmal nocturnal dyspnea
PPI	patient package insert
PPO	preferred provider organization
Pr.	*Proteus*
Ps.	*Pseudomonas*
PSA	prostate-specific antigen
PSP	phenolsulfonphthalein
PSVT	paroxysmal supraventricular tachycardia
PT	prothrombin time; pharmacy and therapeutics; physical therapy
PTH	parathyroid hormone
PTT	partial thromboplastin time
PUD	peptic ulcer disease
PVC	premature ventricular contraction; polyvinyl chloride
PVD	peripheral vascular disease; premature ventricular depolarizations
R&D	research and development
RA	rheumatoid arthritis
RAI	radioactive iodine
RAS	renin-angiotension system; reticular-activating system
RAST	radioallergosorbent test
RBC	red blood (cell) count
RDA	Recommended Dietary (Daily) Allowance
RDS	respiratory distress syndrome
RDW	red-cell distribution width
RE	reticuloendothelial
rem	radio equivalent man
REM	rapid eye movement
RES	reticuloendothelial system
RF	releasing factor

Abbreviation	Meaning
Rh	Rhesus (RH blood group)
RIA	radioimmunoassay
RN	registered nurse
RNA	ribonucleic acid
ROM	range of motion
RPh	registered pharmacist
rpm	revolutions per minute
rps	revolutions per second
RR	respiratory rate
RT3U	total serum thyroxine concentration
RUL	right upper lobe (of lung)
RUQ	right upper quadrant (of abdomen)
Rx	prescription only; take; a recipe
S.	*Salmonella; Serratia*
S&S	signs and symptoms
S-A	sinoatrial
sat	saturated
SBE	self breast examination; subacute bacterial endocarditis
SC	subcutaneous(ly)
Scr	serum creatinine
SD	standard deviation; streptodornase
Se	selenium
sec	second
Ser	serine
sf	sugar free
SGGT	serum gamma-glutamyl transferase
Sh.	*Shigella*
SIADH	syndrome of inappropriate secretion of antidiuretic hormone
SIDS	sudden infant death syndrome
Sig.	Label; let it be printed
SI units	International System of Units
SK	streptokinase
SL	sublingual(ly)
SLE	systemic lupus erythematosus
SMA	sequential multiple analysis
Sn	tin
SNF	skilled nursing facility
sol	solution

Abbreviation	Meaning
soln	solution
solv	dissolve
sp	species
SPECT	single photon emission computerized tomography
sp gr	specific gravity
SPF	sun protection factor
SR	sedimentation rate; sustained-release
SSRI	selective serotonin reuptake inhibitors
Staph.	*Staphylococcus*
stat	immediately; at once
STD	sexually transmitted disease
STM	short-term memory
STP	standard temperature and pressure
Str.	*Streptococcus*
supp	suppository
suppl	supplement(s)
susp	suspension
SV	stroke volume
syr	syrup
t½	half-life
T3	triiodothyronine
T4	thyroxine
tab	tablet
tal	such
tal dos	such doses
TB	tuberculosis
TBG	thyroxine-binding globulin
TBP	thyroxine-binding proteins
TBPA	thyroxine-binding pre-albumin
TBW	total body weight
TCA	tricyclic antidepressant
TD50	median toxic dose
TEEC	transesophageal echocardiography
TEN	toxic epidermal necrolysis
TENS	transcutaneous electrical nerve stimulation
TG	total triglycerides
THC	tetrahydrocannabinol
Thr	threonine
TIA	transient ischemic attack

Abbreviation	Meaning
tid	three times daily
tbsp	tablespoon
tinct	tincture
TLC	total lung capacity; thin layer chromatography
Tmax	time to maximum concentration
TMJ	temporomandibular joint
TNF	tumor necrosis factor
TNM	tumor, node, metastasis
top	topical(ly)
TOPV	trivalent oral polio vaccine
tPA	tissue plasminogen activator
TPN	total parenteral nutrition
TPR	temperature, pulse, respirations
TQM	total quality management
tr	tincture
tRNA	transfer RNA
Trp	tryptophan
TSA	tumor-specific antigens
TSH	thyroid-stimulating hormone
tsp	teaspoon
TSS	toxic shock syndrome
TSTA	tumor-specific transplantation antigen
TT	thrombin time
TV	tidal volume
Tyr	tyrosine
U	unit
UD	unit-dose package
UK	United Kingdom
ung	ointment
URI	upper respiratory infection
USAN	United States Adopted Name(s)
USP	*United States Pharmacopeia*
USPHS	United States Public Health Service
UTI	urinary tract infection
UVA	ultraviolet A wave
V	volt
VA	Veterans Administration
vag	vaginal(ly)
Val	valine
var	variety

Abbreviation	Meaning
VHDL	very high density lipopotein
VLDL	very low density lipoprotein
VMA	vanillylmandelic acid
vol	volume
VS	vital signs
v/v	volume in volume
v/w	volume in weight
wa	while awake
WBC	white blood (cell) count
WBCT	whole blood clotting time
WDLL	well-differentiated lymphocytic lymphoma
WFI	water for injection
WHO	World Health Organization
wk	week
WNL	within normal limits
w/o	water in oil
wt	weight
w/v	weight in volume
w/w	weight in weight
yo	years old
yr	year
ZE	Zollinger-Ellison
Zn	zinc

Glossary

Aberrant: Irregular.

ACE Inhibitor: Angiotensin-converting enzyme. A drug that treats high blood pressure and heart failure.

Acidosis: High blood acidity.

ACTH: A hormone secreted from the pituitary gland.

Acuity: Sharpness.

Adenitis: Gland inflammation.

Adrenergic: Acting like adrenaline, a type of hormone.

Adrenolytic: Adrenaline-blocking drug.

Affinity: Attraction.

Agranulocytosis: Bone marrow poisoning.

Akinesia: Lack of movement.

Alkylate: Anti-cancer treatment.

Allergen: A foreign substance that causes an allergic reaction.

Allergy: A hypersensitivity reaction to a foreign substance such as drugs, food, and pollen.

Analgesic: A pain relieving drug.

Analogous: Similar.

Anaphylactic: Severe allergic response-related.

Androgenic: Masculine.

Anesthetic: Drug to deaden sensation.

Angiotensin II modifiers: A drug that lowers high blood pressure.

Anovulatory: A condition in which a woman's body does not produce an egg.

Antacid: A type of drug that neutralizes stomach acid.

Antagonist: Substance that nullifies the effects of another.

Antiarrhythmic: A drug used to treat abnormal heartbeats (arrhythmias).

Antibiotic: A type of drug that treats bacterial infections.

Anticholinergic: A drug that blocks the action of acetylcholine, a chemical that affects certain central nervous system activities.

Anticoagulant: A drug that prevents blood clotting.

Anticonvulsant: A drug that stops convulsions.

Antidepressant: A drug that treats mental depression.

Antidiabetic: A drug that helps control blood sugar levels.

Antiemetic: A drug that stops vomiting.

Antifibrinolytic: A drug that stops the breakdown of blood clots.

Antiflatulent: A drug that relieves excess gas in the stomach or intestines.

Antifungal: A drug that treats fungal infections.

Antigen: A foreign substance in the body.

Antihistamine: A drug that prevents or relieves allergy symptoms.

Antihypertensive: A drug that lowers high blood pressure.

Anti-inflammatory: A drug that reduces swelling.

Antineoplastic: A drug used to treat cancer.

Antipsychotic: A drug that treats serious mental disorders such as schizophrenia.

Antispasmodic: A drug that reduces smooth muscles spasms such as in the stomach, intestines, or urinary tract.

Antitubercular: A drug that treats tuberculosis (TB).

Anuria: A condition characterized by the non-production of urine.

Aortic stenosis: A narrowing of the aortic valve in the heart or one of the major blood vessels in the body (the aorta).

Aplasia: The non-development of an organ.

Arrhythmia: Irregular heartbeat.

Arteriosclerosis: A hardening of the arteries.

Arteriovenous: Artery and vein-related conditions.

Aspiration: The act of breathing in.

Asymptomatic: Without symptoms.

Ataxia: Lack of coordination.

Bactericide: A class of anti-bacteria drugs.

Barbiturate: A drug that produces drowsiness and/or a hypnotic state.

Benzodiazepines: A class of drug that treats nervousness, sleeping problems, muscle tension, and seizures.

Beta-blocker: A drug that blocks the action of the hormones epinephrine and norepinephrine on the heart.

Biphasic: Two-phase.

Bradycardia: Slow heartbeat.

Bradykinesia: Sluggishness.

Bronchodilator: A drug that improves airflow.

Bronchopulmonary: Chest-related conditions.

Buccal: Conditions relating to the cheek.

Calcification: Hardening.

Calcium channel blockers: A drug that lowers high blood pressure and controls heart rate by improving blood flow to the heart.

Cardiomyopathy: Chronic heart disease.

Cardiopathy: Heart disease.

Cardiopulmonary: Heart and lung-related conditions.

Cardiovascular: Heart and blood vessel-related conditions.

Cerebrovascular: Brain and blood vessel-related conditions.

Cholangitis: Bile duct inflammation.

Cholecystitis: Gall bladder inflammation.

Cholesteral-lowering drug: A drug that lowers cholesterol by either blocking the production of cholesterol or increasing cholesterol breakdown.

Claudication: Limping.

Coagulation: Clotting of blood.

Colonopathy: Colon disease.

Conjugated: Joined.

Contractility: Ability to contract.

Contraindication: Reason not to prescribe.

Corticosteroid: A type of hormone secreted by the adrenal gland; a drug that has anti-inflammatory properties and suppresses the immune system.

Cutaneous: Skin-related conditions.

Degenerative: Worsening.

Degradation: Break down.

Dermatitis: Skin problems.

Dermatological: Skin-related conditions.

Diastolic: Part of blood pressure when heart is in relaxation; the bottom number of a blood pressure measurement.

Distension: Enlarging.

Diuretic: A drug that increases urine output.

Dominance: Ability to influence.

Duodenum: Gut.

Dyskinesia: Jerky movements.

Dysplasia: Abnormality of development.

Dystrophy: Growth failure in tissue.

Dysuria: Painful urination.

Edema: Swelling in the body caused by the accumulation of fluid, most commonly in the feet and legs.

Effusion: Escape of fluid.

Electrocardiography: Heart monitor.

Electroencephalography: Brain scan.

Electrolytes: Chemicals such as sodium, potassium, calcium, magnesium, chloride, and bicarbonate that are present in the body tissues and fluids.

Embolism: Sudden blocking of an artery.

Emesis: Vomiting.

Emetic: Substance to cause vomiting.

Enzyme: A chemical that speeds up a chemical reaction.

Eosinophilia: Increase in white blood cells.

Epidermal: Skin-related conditions.

Epithelium: Covering of internal and external surfaces.

Erythropoiesis: Red cell production.

Exacerbation: Worsening.

Expectorant: A drug that thins mucus in the airway.

Extrapyramidal: Part of the central nervous system.

Febrile: Feverish.

Fibrosis: Fibrous tissue formation.

Fistula: Abnormal passage.

Fluoroquinolones: A family of antibiotics.

Gastroduodenal: Stomach and gut-related conditions.

Gonadotropic: A hormone that controls reproductive activity by affecting the ovaries and testes.

Gravidity: Pregnancy.

H2-blockers: Histamine-2 receptor antagonists. A class of drug that prevents the production of stomach acid.

Hemopoietic: Blood cell formation-related.

Hepatotoxic: Poisonous to liver cells.

Histamine: A chemical produced by the body in response to an allergen.

Homologous: Essentially similar.

Hormone: A substance usually produced in a gland that enters the bloodstream and helps organs and tissues to function.

Hyperemesis: Excessive vomiting.

Hyperkinesias: Hyperactivity.

Hyperreflexia: Exaggerated reflexes.

Hypersecretion: Excessive secretion.

Hypersensitivity: Over-sensitivity.

Hypertension: High blood pressure.

Hypotension: Low blood pressure.

Hypotrophy: Aging.

Hypoxemia: Blood oxygen deficiency.

Idiopathic: Of unknown cause.

Immunogenic: Producing immunity.

Immunosuppressant: A class of drug that stops the body's immune response.

Infusion: Transfusion not of blood.

Interstitial: In gaps between tissue.

Intramuscular: Within the muscle.

Intraocular: Within the eye.

Intravenous: Within a vein.

In vivo: In the body.

Ischemia: Inadequate blood flow.

Laxative: A drug that produces bowel movements.

Leukocytic: White blood cell-related conditions.

Leukotriene modifier: A type of asthma drug.

Lipoprotein: Any complex of fat and protein.

Liposome: Fatty or oily globule.

Malabsorption: Poor digestion.

Mastodynia: Breast pain.

Mediated: To act as an intermediate agent.

Monotherapy: One drug therapy.

Morbidity: Diseased state.

Mucolytic: A class of drug that breaks down mucus.

Narcotic: A class of morphine-like drug.

Nausea: Feeling sick.

Neonatal: New baby-related.

Nephritis: Kidney inflammation.

Nephropathy: Kidney disease.

Nephrotoxic: Destructive to the kidneys.

Neural: Nerve-related conditions.

Neurological: Nervous system-related conditions.

Neuromuscular: Muscle and nerve-related conditions.

Neuropathy: Nervous system disorder.

Neurotransmitter: A chemical released by nerve endings in the brain.

NSAID: Non-steroidal anti-inflammatory drugs. A drug that treats pain, fever, and swelling and does not contain corticosteroids.

Occlusion: Closing.

Occult: Concealed.

Oculogyric: Involving circular eye movements.

Oestrogen: Hormone produced by the ovaries that controls female sexual development.

Off-label: Indication, dosage form, dose regimen, population or other use parameter not mentioned in the FDA-approved product labeling.

On-label: Drug use according to FDA-approved product labeling.

Ossification: Bone formation.

Osteodystrophy: Defective bone formation.

Otitis: Ear inflammation.

Palliative: Giving relief but not cure.

Paroxysmal: In sudden attacks.

Pathogen: Disease-producing organism.

Peptic: Digestion-related conditions.

Percutaneous: Through the skin.

Photosensitivity: Over-sensitivity to light.

Polyneuritis: Inflammation of the nerves.

Preload: Heart muscle tension.

Presynaptic: Before a nerve/organ joint.

Progdrug: A drug that is administered as an inactive medication that becomes active once it is metabolized.

Progestogen: Female steroid hormone.

Psychomotor: Involving motor effects of mental activity.

Psychotropic: Mood-altering substances.

Reabsorption: Absorbing again.

Receptor agonist: A substance that binds to a receptor, a protein on the cell membrane, to trigger a response in a cell.

Recombinant: Produced from more than one source.

Refractory: Not responding to treatment.

Reuptake: Blocking the reuptake of the chemical by the nerves that release it, which allows more of the chemical to be available to be taken up by other nerves.

Sclerosis: Hardening.

Serotonin: A brain chemical responsible for feelings of well-being.

Spasmolytic: Anti-spasm drugs.

Spasticity: Muscle rigidity.

SSRI: Selective serotonin reuptake inhibitors, a class of drug that increases the amount of the neurotransimitter serotonin.

Statins: A family of cholesterol-lowering drugs.

Stenosis: Duct narrowing.

Subcutaneous: Below the skin.

Sublingual: Under the tongue.

Superinfection: Secondary infection.

Supraventricular: Above the heart chambers.

Systolic: Part of blood pressure when the heart is contracting, the top number of a blood pressure measurement.

Tachyarrhythmia: Irregular heartbeat.

Thromboembolism: Blood clotting.

Thrombolytic: A drug that dissolves blood clots.

Thrombus: Blood clot.

Transdermal: Through the skin.

Tricyclic anti-depressant (TCA): A drug that prevents that action of the neurotransmitters norepinephrine and serotonin.

Vasculitis: Blood vessel inflammation.

Vasoactive: Affecting blood vessels.

Vasodilatation: Widening of the blood vessels.

Vasomotor: Blood flow-related conditions.

Washout: A cleaning of various chemical substances from the body.

Index

Note to Readers

This book is intended only as a reference for use in an ongoing partnership between doctor and patient in the vigilant management of the patient's health. It is not a substitute for a doctor's professional judgment, and serves only as a reminder of concerns that may need discussion. It is sold with the understanding that the authors, editors and consultants, producer, and publisher are not engaged in rendering medical, health, or any other kind of personal professional services in the book. The reader should consult his or her medical, health, or other competent professional before drawing any inferences from this book or using any information contained in it.

While efforts have been made to ensure the accuracy of the drug information in this book, the book does not list every possible adverse reaction, interaction, precaution, and effect of a drug; and all information is presented without guarantees by the authors, consultants, producer, and publisher. The authors, editors and consultants, producer, and publisher specifically disclaim all responsibility for any liability, loss, or risk, personal or otherwise, which is incurred as a consequence, directly or indirectly, of the use and application of any of the contents of this book.

Brand names listed in this book are intended to represent only the more commonly used products. Inclusion of a brand name does not signify endorsement of the product; absence of a name does not imply a criticism or rejection of the product. The authors, editors and consultants, producer, and publisher do not advocate the use of any product described in this book, do not warrant or guarantee any of these products, and have not performed any independent analysis in connection with the product information contained herein.